PEDIATRIC CARDIAC ANESTHESIA

SECOND EDITION

PEDIATRIC CARDIAC ANESTHESIA

SECOND EDITION

Carol L. Lake, MD
Professor of Anesthesiology
Department of Anesthesiology
University of Virginia Health Sciences Center
Charlottesville, Virginia

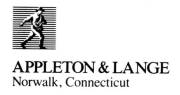

APPLETON & LANGE
Norwalk, Connecticut

Copyright © 1993 by Appleton & Lange
Simon & Schuster Business and Professional Group

93 94 95 96 97 / 10 9 8 7 6 5 4 3 2 1

Prentice Hall International (UK) Limited, *London*
Prentice Hall of Australia Pty. Limited, *Sydney*
Prentice Hall Canada, Inc., *Toronto*
Prentice Hall Hispanoamericana, S.A., *Mexico*
Prentice Hall of India Private Limited, *New Delhi*
Prentice Hall of Japan, Inc., *Tokyo*
Simon & Schuster Asia Pte. Ltd., *Singapore*
Editora Prentice Hall do Brasil Ltda., *Rio de Janeiro*
Prentice Hall, *Englewood Cliffs, New Jersey*

Library of Congress Cataloging-in-Publication Data
Pediatric cardiac anesthesia / [edited by] Carol L. Lake. — 2nd ed.
    p.   cm.
    Includes bibliographical references and index.
    ISBN 0-8385-7812-8
    1. Pediatric anesthesia.   2. Heart—Abnormalities—Surgery.
    3. Pediatric cardiology.   4. Therapeutics, Surgical.   I. Lake,
Carol L.
    [DNLM: 1. Anesthesia—in infancy & childhood.   2. Heart Defects,
Congenital—surgery.   3. Intraoperative Care—in infancy &
childhood.   WS 290 P37017 1993]
    RD139.P43   1993
    617.9′67412—dc20
    DNLM/DLC
    for Library of Congress   93-352
                                                               CIP

ISBN   0-8385-7812-8

90000

9 780838 578124

NB2I

Editor: Jane Licht
Production Supervisor: Karen Davis
Designer: Penny Kindzierski

PRINTED IN THE UNITED STATES OF AMERICA

Contents

Contributors

Desmond Bohn, MB, BCh, FRCPC
Assistant Director
Hospital for Sick Children
Associate Professor
University of Toronto
Toronto, Ontario
Canada

Frederick W. Campbell, MD
Vice Chairman, Department of Anesthesiology
Medical College Hospital
Professor of Anesthesiology
Medical College of Pennsylvania
Philadelphia, Pennsylvania

Martha A. Carpenter, MD
Department of Pediatrics
University of Virginia Medical Center
Charlottesville, Virginia

D. Ryan Cook, MD
Director of Anesthesiology
Children's Hospital of Pittsburgh
Professor of Anesthesiology
University of Pittsburgh School of Medicine
Pittsburgh, Pennsylvania

John R. Cooper, Jr, MD
Attending Anesthesiologist
Texas Heart Institute
Clinical Assistant Professor
University of Texas Health Science Center
Houston, Texas

Peter J. Davis, MD
Associate Director of Anesthesia
Children's Hospital of Pittsburgh
Associate Professor of Anesthesia, Critical Care
    Medicine, and Pediatrics
University of Pittsburgh School of Medicine
Pittsburgh, Pennsylvania

James A. DiNardo, MD
Clinical Associate Professor
Director, Cardiothoracic Anesthesia
Associate Head, Anesthesiology
University of Arizona Health Sciences Center
Tucson, Arizona

David M. Farrell, MA, CCP
Senior Clinical Cardiovascular Perfusionist
The Children's Hospital
Boston, Massachusetts

David D. Frankville, MD
Department of Anesthesiology
University of California at San Diego Medical Center
Assistant Clinical Professor of Anesthesiology
University of California at San Diego
San Diego, California

Willis G. Gieser, CCP
Chief Clinical Cardiovascular Perfusionist
The Children's Hospital
Boston, Massachusetts

William J. Greeley, MD
Associate Professor of Anesthesiology and Pediatrics
Duke University Medical Center
Durham, North Carolina

Howard P. Gutgesell, MD
Director, Pediatric Cardiology
University of Virginia Health Sciences Center
Children's Medical Center
Charlottesville, Virginia

David R. Jobes, MD
Senior Anesthesiologist
The Hospital of the University of Pennsylvania and
    The Children's Hospital of Philadelphia
Associate Professor
University of Pennsylvania School of Medicine
Philadelphia, Pennsylvania

Frank H. Kern, MD
Director of Pediatric Cardiac Anesthesia
Assistant Professor in Anesthesiology
Duke University Medical Center
Durham, North Carolina

C. Dean Kurth, MD
Department of Anesthesiology
The Children's Hospital of Philadelphia
Assistant Professor of Anesthesiology, Physiology, and
    Pediatrics
University of Pennsylvania School of Medicine
Philadelphia, Pennsylvania

Carol L. Lake, MD
Professor of Anesthesiology
Department of Anesthesiology
University of Virginia Health Sciences Center
Charlottesville, Virginia

William A. Lell, MD
Professor of Anesthesiology
Division of Cardiothoracic Anesthesia
The University of Alabama at Birmingham Medical
    Center
Birmingham, Alabama

David A. Lowe, MD, FCCM
Director, Anesthesia and Critical Care Medicine
St. Christopher's Hospital for Children
Associate Professor
Temple University School of Medicine
Philadelphia, Pennsylvania

Edward E. Lowe, MD
Clinical Professor of Anesthesia and Pediatrics
University of Cincinnati School of Medicine
Children's Hospital Medical Center
Cincinnati, Ohio

John J. McAuliffe III, MD, CM
Assistant Professor
Department of Anesthesia and Pediatrics
University of Cincinnati School of Medicine
Children's Hospital Medical Center
Cincinnati, Ohio

Roger A. Moore, MD
Chairman of Anesthesiology
Deborah Heart and Lung Center
Browns Mills, New Jersey
Associate Professor
University of Pennsylvania
Philadelphia, Pennsylvania

Susan Craig Nicolson, MD
Director, Cardiac Anesthesia
The Children's Hospital of Philadelphia
Associate Professor of Anesthesia
University of Pennsylvania School of Medicine
Philadelphia, Pennsylvania

Karen S. Rheuban, MD
Associate Professor of Pediatrics
Associate Dean
University of Virginia Health Sciences Center
Charlottesville, Virginia

David A. Rosen, MD
Director of Pediatric Cardiac Anesthesia
West Virginia University Children's Hospital
Associate Professor of Anesthesia and Pediatrics
West Virginia University School of Medicine
Morgantown, West Virginia

Kathleen R. Rosen, MD
Faculty, Pediatric Cardiac Anesthesia
West Virginia University Children's Hospital
Adjunct Associate Professor of Anesthesia and
    Pediatrics
West Virginia University School of Medicine
Morgantown, West Virginia

Paul N. Samuelson, MD
Director, Division of Cardiothoracic Anesthesia
Professor and Interim Chairman
Department of Anesthesiology
The University of Alabama at Birmingham Medical
    Center
Birmingham, Alabama

Alan Jay Schwartz, MD, MSEd
Professor and Chairman
Department of Anesthesiology
The Medical College of Pennsylvania
Philadelphia, Pennsylvania

Stephen A. Stayer, MD
Anesthesia and Critical Care Medicine
St. Christopher's Hospital for Children
Assistant Professor
Temple University School of Medicine
Philadelphia, Pennsylvania

James M. Steven, MD
Associate Anesthesiologist
The Children's Hospital of Philadelphia
Assistant Professor of Anesthesia and Pediatrics
University of Pennsylvania School of Medicine
Philadelphia, Pennsylvania

Douglas F. Willson, MD
Director, Pediatric Critical Care
Associate Professor, Department of Pediatrics and
    Anesthesiology
University of Virginia Health Sciences Center
Charlottesville, Virginia

Preface

This multiauthored book provides a comprehensive review of the anesthetic and perioperative management of patients with congenital cardiac abnormalities of all types. It begins with a historical perspective, the development of cardiac anesthesia as a subspecialty, as a result of special needs in children with congenital heart disease undergoing innovative palliative and definitive surgical treatment. The second chapter discusses the essential cardiac pathophysiology: shunting; outflow track obstruction; and altered pulmonary blood flow, produced by anatomic malformations. Then, as in the first edition, for each major cardiac pathology there are systematic descriptions including the diagnostic features, pathophysiology, natural history, anesthetic techniques, surgical therapy, and immediate and long-term postoperative care.

In the five years since the preparation of the first edition, research in pediatric cardiology, anesthesiology, and cardiac surgery has added greatly to the knowledge and skill with which patients with congenital cardiac lesions can be managed. Although much of the information in the chapters detailing specific cardiac lesions applies to both cardiac and noncardiac surgical patients, there is a new chapter describing the management of patients with congenital heart disease for noncardiac surgery or after repair of congenital lesions. Sections on circulatory assistance and cardiac transplantation have also been added. Current information on the physiology and pathophysiology of the neonatal myocardium is given in another new chapter. The increased use of epicardial and transesophageal echocardiography in pediatric cardiac anesthesia is reflected by the addition of a chapter on that subject. Other new monitors such as near infrared spectroscopy and transcranial Doppler are described in the chapter on monitoring. Because the subject of pediatric intensive care is beyond the scope of this text, the postoperative chapters have been rearranged to describe only anticipated cardiovascular changes; general respiratory management; and complications of the central nervous system and from hepatic, renal, and hemostatic origins in pediatric cardiac patients.

The second edition should be of interest to pediatric and cardiac anesthesiologists at either resident, fellow, or consultant levels; pediatric cardiac surgeons and their trainees; pediatric cardiologists; and specialists in pediatric intensive care, as well as medical students and nurses involved in the care of pediatric cardiac patients. The multiauthored format overcomes the inability of a single author to be expert in all subjects. Although many of the authors may have particular expertise with a specific cardiac lesion or technique, an attempt has been made to provide complete, authoritative information applicable to many situations.

ACKNOWLEDGMENTS

The editor wishes to thank especially the authors who contributed their time and experience in the writing of individual chapters on the preoperative evaluation and preparation of pediatric patients, various congenital cardiac lesions, and postoperative intensive care. Much of the artwork, graphic design, photography, and printing for the illustrations in the first edition that has been incorporated into the second edition was provided by Ms. Linda Hamme, Mr. Craig Harding, Ms. Cindy Hiter, and others in the Division of Biomedical Communications at the University of Virginia Health Sciences Center. Mrs. Barbara Lane of Lane Business Services, Charlottesville, provided skillful word-processing and formatting of the text. Numerous authors and publishers kindly permitted us to reprint figures and tables from their work. The staff of Appleton & Lange, particularly Ms. Jane Licht, were particularly helpful in the preparation of the manuscript and understanding about the inevitable and unavoidable delays. Finally, the editor is most grateful to residents and faculty at the University of Virginia and to pediatric cardiac anesthesiologists around the world who have provided numerous suggestions for the improvement of the second edition.

PEDIATRIC CARDIAC ANESTHESIA

SECOND EDITION

Chapter 1 | History of Pediatric Cardiac Anesthesia

Carol L. Lake

EARLY HISTORY

Congenital cardiac anomalies have existed for centuries. The early Babylonians, who were interested in omens and divinations, considered the birth of an infant with ectopia cordis to indicate forthcoming national calamities.[1] In the fourth century BC, Aristotle studied the embryology of the chick, noting the beating of the fetal heart. Later eighteenth century scientists confirmed these findings. Other notable historical events concerning congenital heart disease include the first description of dextrocardia by Benedetti in 1493, the discovery of the ductus arteriosus and foramen ovale in the sixteenth century, and the description of combined defects now known as the tetralogy of Fallot. Stensen in 1671,[2] Sandifort in 1777,[3] Farre in 1814, and Gintrac in 1824 described the classic combination of congenital cardiac anomalies in tetralogy, but Etienne-Louis Arthur Fallot did not present his comprehensive account until 1888 (Table 1–1).[4]

THE NINETEENTH CENTURY

Between 1836 and 1841, Bouillaud suggested that congenital anomalies resulted from inherent defects in development and diseases in the fetus. Pennock, in a discussion of J. Hope's *A Treatise on the Diseases of the Heart and Great Vessels*, noted that cardiac malformations were usually congenital imperfections in which there was a deficiency, a superabundance, or an anomalous configuration of the parts.[5] He catalogued the defects into 15 categories, including a single atrium and ventricle, two atria with one ventricle, patent foramen ovale, patent foramen ovale and ductus arteriosus, ventricular and atrial septal defects, transposition of the great vessels, aortic arch anomalies, ventricular outflow track anomalies, and tricuspid atresia, among others. Pennock recognized that right ventricular hypertrophy resulted

principally from obstruction of its outflow rather than introduction of excessive arterialized blood into the chamber.[5] He also noted that dilatation resulted from overdistention of a cardiac chamber.[5]

Peacock, who compiled in 1858 the most complete volume of his time of the congenital heart lesions, *On Malformations of the Human Heart*,[6] believed that cyanosis resulted from venous stasis rather than admixture of arterial and venous blood.[7] Peacock presented many of the congenital defects before the Pathological Society of London,[7] and his lectures to the medical students at St. Thomas' Hospital formed the basis of *On Malformations of the Human Heart* (see Table 1–1).[8] In his book, [6,8] Peacock described two cases of tetralogy of Fallot, 42 years before Fallot's report.[4] In addition to his lucid descriptions of the defects, Peacock surmised that the causes of death included cerebral disturbance from defective aeration of the brain, imperfect expansion and engorgement of the lungs, exhaustion of respiratory function, effusions from heart failure, and other diseases such as apoplexy from engorgement or extravasation of the blood in the brain. Peacock noted the association between cyanotic congenital heart disease and brain abscess, a process not fully recognized until the 1950s.[8] His second edition in 1866 revised and updated the first edition of *On Malformations of the Human Heart*, including the illustrations.[7]

During the late 1870s, Rokitansky described the origin and nature of congenital septal defects and Roger described the signs of interventricular septal defects.[9] In 1897, Eisenmenger described the complex that bears his name (see Table 1–1).[10]

THE TWENTIETH CENTURY

The clinical recognition and identification of congenital cardiovascular defects was enhanced by the extensive

TABLE 1–1. HISTORICAL MILESTONES IN PEDIATRIC CARDIAC SURGERY

16th century	Discovery of ductus arteriosus and foramen ovale
1858	Peacock's *On Malformations of the Human Heart* published
1879	Roger describes signs of interventricular septal defects
1888	Fallot describes tetralogy of ventricular septal defect, pulmonic stenosis, overriding aorta, and right ventricular hypertrophy
1897	Eisenmenger's complex described
1939	Closure of a patent ductus arteriosus performed by Gross
1945	Blalock and Taussig report the subclavian to pulmonary artery shunt to improve pulmonary blood flow
1945	Gross and Crafoord, working independently, report successful repair of coarctation of the aorta
1946	Potts performs the aorta to left pulmonary artery anastomosis to increase pulmonary blood flow
1949	Brock describes closed pulmonary valvulotomy
1952	Pulmonary artery banding to decrease pulmonary blood flow reported by Muller and Dammann
1953	Successful cardiopulmonary bypass using a pump oxygenator accomplished by Gibbon
1959	The Senning repair for transposition of the great vessels reported
1964	Mustard repair for transposition of the great vessels developed
1967	First pediatric heart transplant by Kantrowitz
1969	Rastelli describes use of a valve-bearing conduit between right ventricle and pulmonary artery to correct transposition of the great vessels and ventricular septal defect
1975	First successful arterial switch procedure by transposition of the great arteries by Jatene
1981	Norwood describes successful palliation of hypoplastic left heart syndrome
1985	First neonatal cardiac xenotransplantation by Bailey

study and knowledge of Maude Abbott in the early part of this century.[11] Despite recognition of the defects, however, little therapy was available and many of the lesions were fatal in early life or limited the patient to a life of invalidism. Medical therapy consisted of digitalis and rest.

In the 1930s and early 1940s, there were surgical attempts to correct congenital cardiac lesions. Historically, cardiac anesthesia began with the anesthetic management during surgical repair of these lesions.[12] Doyen attempted to relieve pulmonic stenosis using a closed valvulotomy procedure, but the patient died 4 hours postoperatively.[13] Sellors, in 1948, however, successfully opened a stenotic pulmonic valve using a hooked knife inserted through the valve.[14] Closure of the patent ductus arteriosus was accomplished in 1939 by Gross and Hubbard.[15] The landmark report in 1945 of the surgical creation of the subclavian to pulmonary artery shunt (Blalock-Taussig) to improve pulmonary blood flow in

infants with severe cyanosis using either cyclopropane or ether anesthesia was the dawn of pediatric cardiac anesthesia and surgery (see Table 1–1).[16] Both Gross and Crafoord repaired coarctation of the aorta within a short time of the initial Blalock-Taussig procedure.[17,18] In the late 1940s, Collett and Edwards reported a pathologic classification of truncus arteriosus by four types representing the various stages of arrested development.[19]

The improvement of systemic oxygenation during anesthesia was noted during some of these early Blalock-Taussig procedures. Other important findings from the use of the early Blalock-Taussig shunts were (1) patients could tolerate occlusion of either pulmonary artery for sufficient periods of time (30–90 minutes) for an anastomosis to be made, and (2) hypoxemia in cyanotic congenital heart disease resulted from reduced pulmonary blood flow, not that polycythemia interfered with alveolar-capillary gas exchange.[20]

Thus the feasibility of both definitive and palliative procedures for patients with congenital cardiac defects was rapidly demonstrated with a flurry of palliative procedures. The aorta to left pulmonary artery anastomosis was performed by Potts.[21] A superior vena cava to right pulmonary artery anastomosis was described by Glenn,[22] and Brock described the closed pulmonary valvulotomy.[23] However, it was not until 1955 that Kirklin at the Mayo Clinic and Lillihei at Minnesota reported successful intracardiac correction of tetralogy of Fallot.[24,25]

Because cardiopulmonary bypass was unavailable until 1953, various ingenious methods were developed to permit closure of atrial septal defects with the circulation intact. Among these methods were Bailey's atrioseptopexy,[26] Gross' atrial well,[27] and Glenn's operating diverticulum.[28] Operative maneuvers were guided by touch and facilitated by special intracardiac instruments. Sondegaard closed atrial septal defects by passing a heavy suture through the superior edge of the ventricular septum to pull the superior wall of the atrium down to close the defect.[29]

In addition to the previously described procedures to increase pulmonary blood flow, Muller and Dammann described the procedure of banding the pulmonary artery to prevent excessive pulmonary flow (see Table 1–1).[30] The operation to improve mixing of arterial and venous blood by open creation of an atrial septal defect in transposition of the great vessels also was described by Blalock in conjunction with Hanlon.[31] However, the anesthetic management of these patients was rarely or incompletely described.

Surgery for more complicated lesions was attempted as pump oxygenator technology evolved. An early attempt at arterial switching to correct transposition of the great arteries was reported by Mustard et al in 1954.[32] However, problems with coronary air embolism and generalized myocardial ischemia complicated these efforts.

Because of poor surgical outcome after the switching operation, attention was directed to correction of transposition at the atrial level (see Table 1–1).[33,34] The Mustard procedure, which creates an intra-atrial baffle of pericardium, diverts systemic venous blood across the mitral valve to the pulmonary artery while pulmonary venous blood crosses the tricuspid valve to the right ventricle and aorta. Because of the concern that the pericardium would not grow as the heart enlarged, Senning created an intra-atrial baffle using less prosthetic material by rearrangement of an atrial septal flap.[34] Anesthetic drugs and procedures are not described in most of these reports. However, the use of halothane anesthesia during closure of ventricular septal defects is noted by Kirklin.[35] It was also in this era that Waterston described the ascending aorta to right pulmonary artery anastomosis.[36] In 1969, Rastelli described the technique for repair of transposition of the great arteries and ventricular septal defect using a valve-bearing conduit from right ventricle to pulmonary artery[37] and reported three successful cases (see Table 1–1).[38]

Cardiac Catheterization

Cardiac catheterization was developed and refined as a diagnostic tool in the late 1940s. Angiocardiography facilitated accurate diagnosis and understanding of abnormal cardiac physiology. The anesthetic management of cardiac catheterization during this time included rectal thiobarbiturate, rectal avertin (tribromomethanol and amylene hydrate), intramuscular meperidine and barbiturates, or intravenous barbiturate.[39]

Pediatric Cardiac Anesthesia

An early description of pediatric cardiac anesthesia by Harmel and co-workers included numerous case reports and review of the literature for pulmonary valvulotomy for pulmonic stenosis performed by Blalock.[16,40] McQuiston advocated the use of cyclopropane for essentially all pediatric cardiac surgery because of its potency and rapid elimination.[41] However, Harmel et al were unable to demonstrate statistically significant differences in mortality between cyclopropane or ether anesthesia.[40] McQuiston discussed the anesthetic complications noted in 350 children undergoing cardiac procedures, including laryngeal edema in 15, cerebral anoxia in 5, atelectasis in 6, pneumonia in 2, as well as numerous other complications unrelated to anesthetic management.[42] Other early investigators[40,41] noted similar problems as well as postoperative hemorrhage, atrioventricular block, and hypothermia. Perioperative mortality often approached 25%.[40–42]

Subsequently, Patrick anesthetized a 5-year-old child with nitrous oxide and ether for closure of a ventricular septal defect using the Mayo-Gibbon oxygenator.[12] His review of the technical details of anesthetic management and supportive therapy appeared in 1955.[43]

Many important early contributions to pediatric cardiac anesthesia were made by Keats. Keats described the anesthetic problems in cardiopulmonary bypass,[44] heparin anticoagulation,[45] and its reversal with polybrene, the safety of endotracheal intubation in pediatric patients, the hemodynamic effects of anesthesia and controlled ventilation,[46,47] among many others. In a paper on anesthetic management for emergency cardiac surgery in 1963, Keats reviewed the perioperative management of 400 infants anesthetized between 1956 and 1963 as well as the specific problems associated with excessive airway pressure in patients with tetralogy or pulmonic stenosis.[48]

A very detailed review of the pathophysiology of congenital heart lesions and their impact upon anesthesia care was published by Smith in the journal *Anesthesiology* in 1952.[49] Except for the use of diethyl ether and other abandoned techniques, the principles of perioperative care for such lesions as tetralogy of Fallot and ligation of a patent ductus arteriosus remain remarkably similar more than 30 years later. The necessity for control of hypertension, bradycardia or other dysrhythmias, and blood volume were well described. In 1966, Strong et al reviewed the progress in anesthesias for cardiovascular surgery in infancy.[50] They noted that cardiac dysrhythmias, blood and fluid balance, respiratory insufficiency, and cerebral damage remained major problems. By this time, premedication with morphine and/or atropine and maintenance of anesthesia with halothane were common practices.[50]

Surface Cooling

McQuiston also described the use of surface cooling in the surgical treatment of severely hypoxic children to reduce the mortality from anoxia.[41,42] Techniques for profound hypothermia and circulatory arrest during surgical repair were further developed and perfected in the late 1960s by Dillard,[51] Barratt-Boyes,[52] and the group at Kyoto University.[53]

Extracorporeal Circulation

During the first unsuccessful attempt to use extracorporeal circulation in humans,[54] Van Bergen and Buckley administered cyclopropane anesthesia.[12] However, the anesthetic management of the first successful use of extracorporeal circulation for closure of an atrial septal defect is not detailed (see Table 1–1).[55] Another early report of the use of cardiopulmonary bypass for ventricular septal defect closure indicates the use of ether-oxygen anesthesia.[56] A ventricular septal defect was closed using cross-circulation in which the patient received cyclopropane anesthesia.[12] Mendelsohn and colleagues reviewed the intraoperative anesthetic management of patients undergoing extracorporeal circulation.[57] In the late 1960s, pediatric cardiac and heart-lung transplantation were first successfully performed. As in adults, however, post-transplantation survival was limited by the lack of effective immunosuppressive drugs.

1970 to 1980. The decade of the 1970s was one of perfection of the surgical and anesthetic techniques for children with congenital heart disease. New anesthetic drugs such as isoflurane and the neuromuscular blocking drug pancuronium were added to the pediatric cardiac anesthesiologist's armamentarium. Although Cooley and co-workers had used potassium cardioplegia during repair of ventricular septal defects in 1958, cardioplegia solutions were not widely used in pediatric myocardial preservation until the late 1970s.[58]

1980 to the Present. Although nearly all congenital cardiac lesions can be cured, or at least palliated, by surgical procedures, a few lesions, such as hypoplastic left heart, tricuspid atresia, endocardial fibroelastosis, and complex defects remain to challenge the imagination of the pediatric cardiologist, cardiac surgeon, and cardiac anesthesiologist. New anesthetic drugs, including sufentanil, alfentanil, vecuronium, atracurium, doxacurium, midazolam, propofol, and others, offer alternatives to potent volatile anesthetics for anesthesia during complex cardiac repair. Morbidity and mortality associated with pediatric cardiac procedures have decreased, with a 2% incidence of anesthetic complications and hospital mortality of 6% noted by Hickey and colleagues.[59]

The increased use of profound hypothermia and circulatory arrest during repair of complex congenital cardiac defects has increased research to determine the effects of these techniques on cerebral function.[60,61] Improved monitors of cerebral function, including direct measurement of cerebral blood flow, near-infrared spectroscopy, and transcranial Doppler ultrasonography, assess low-flow versus arrest or cerebral preservative drugs.

During the 1980s, many cardiac surgical teams recognized that methods of myocardial preservation that were successful in adults were not always similarly effective in neonates and children. Controversy continues over the resistance or sensitivity of the neonatal heart to hypoxia and ischemia.[62,63] Numerous animal studies attempt to define the optimum myocardial preservation technique and cardioplegia solution in immature hearts.

With the availability of cyclosporine and other effective immunosuppressive drugs, survival after pediatric cardiac transplantation approaches that in adults.[64] However, the limited supply of donor organs precludes widespread applicability of this therapeutic modality. Alternative animal sources have been explored as indicated by the successful baboon-to-human transplant performed by Bailey in an infant with hypoplastic left heart syndrome.[65] Intra-aortic balloon counterpulsation and extracorporeal membrane oxygenation offer cardiovascular support as a bridge to transplantation in children.

REFERENCES

1. Ballantyne JW: *Teratologia* (London and Edinburgh) **1**:127–143, 1894
2. Willius FA: Cardiac clinics. Unusually early description of socalled tetralogy of Fallot. *Mayo Clin Proc* **23**: 316–320, 1948
3. Bennett LR: Sandifort's "observations," Chapter 1, Concerning a very rare disease of the heart. I. Tetralogy of Fallot or Sandifort? *Bull Hist Med* **20**: 539–570, 1964
4. Fallot E-L: Contribution a l'anatomie pathologique de la maladie bleue (cyanose cardiaque). *Marseille-Med* **25**: 77–93, 138–158, 207–223, 270–286, 341–354, 403–420, 1888
5. Pennock CW: *Hope on the Heart (A Treatise on the Diseases of the Heart and Great Vessels* by J. Hope). Philadelphia: Lea and Blanchard, 1842
6. Peacock TB. *On Malformations of the Human Heart.* London: J. Churchill, 1858
7. Flaxman N: Peacock and congenital heart disease. *Bull Inst Hist Med* **7**:1061–1103, 1939
8. Porter IH: The nineteenth century physician and cardiologist Thomas Bevill Peacock (1812–1882). *Med Hist* **6**:240–254, 1962
9. Roger HL: Recherches cliniques sur la communication congenitale des deux coeurs par inocclusion du septum interventriculaire. *Bull Acad Med Paris* **8**:1074–1094, 1879
10. Eisenmenger V: Ursprung der Aorta aus beiden Ventrikeln beim Defekt des Septum Ventriculorum. *Wien Klin Wochenschr* **11**:25, 1898
11. Abbott M: *Atlas of Congenital Cardiac Disease.* New York: American Heart Association, 1936
12. Arens JF: Three decades of cardiac anesthesia. *Mt Sinai J Med* **52**:516–520, 1985
13. Doyen E: Chirurgie des malformations congenitales ou acquises du coeur. *Presse Med* **21**:860, 1913
14. Sellors TH: Surgery of pulmonary stenosis. *Lancet* **1**:988–989, 1948
15. Gross RE, Hubbard JP: Surgical ligation of a patent ductus arteriosus: Report of first successful case. *JAMA* **112**:729–731, 1939
16. Blalock A, Taussig HB: The surgical treatment of malformations of the heart in which there is pulmonary stenosis or pulmonary atresia. *JAMA* **128**:189–202, 1945
17. Gross RE, Hufnagel CA: Coarctation of the aorta: Experimental studies regarding its surgical correction. *N Engl J Med* **233**:287–293, 1945
18. Crafoord C, Nylin G: Congenital coarctation of the aorta and its surgical treatment. *J Thorac Surg* **14**:347–361, 1945
19. Collett RW, Edwards JE: Persistent truncus arteriosus: A classification. *Surg Clin North Am* **29**:1245–1270, 1949
20. McNamara DG: The Blalock-Taussig operation and subsequent progress in surgical treatment of cardiovascular diseases. *JAMA* **251**:2139–2141, 1984
21. Potts WJ, Smith S, Gibson S: Anastomosis of the aorta to a pulmonary artery: Certain types in congenital heart disease. *JAMA* **132**:627–631, 1946
22. Glenn WWL, Patino JF: Circulatory bypass of the right heart. I. Preliminary observations on the direct delivery of vena caval blood into the pulmonary arterial circulation—Azygous vein–pulmonary artery shunt. *Yale J Biol Med* **27**: 147–151, 1954

23. Brock RC: The surgery of pulmonary stenosis. *Br Med J* **2**:399–406, 1949

24. Lillehei CW, Cohen M, Warden HE, et al: Direct vision intracardiac surgical correction of the tetralogy of Fallot, pentalogy of Fallot, and pulmonary atresia defects: Report of the first ten cases. *Ann Surg* **142**:418–445, 1955

25. Kirklin JW, Karp RB: *The Tetralogy of Fallot from a Surgical Viewpoint*. Philadelphia: W.B. Saunders, 1970

26. Bailey CP, Bolton HE, Jamison WL, Neptune WB: Atrioseptopexy for interatrial septal defects. *J Thorac Surg* **26**:184–219, 1953

27. Gross RE, Watkins E, Pomeranz AA, Goldsmith EI: A method for surgical closure of interauricular septal defects. *Surg Gynecol Obstet* **96**:1–23, 1953

28. Glenn WWL, Jaeger C, Harned HS, et al: The diverticulum approach to the chambers of the heart and great vessels. *Surgery* **38**:872–885, 1955

29. Sondegaard T: Closure of atrial septal defects. *Acta Chir Scand* **107**:492–498, 1954

30. Muller WH, Dammann JF: The treatment of certain congenital malformations of the heart by the creation of pulmonic stenosis to reduce pulmonary hypertension and excessive pulmonary blood flow: A preliminary report. *Surg Gynecol Obstet* **95**:213–219, 1952

31. Blalock A, Hanlon CR: The surgical treatment of complete transposition of the aorta and pulmonary artery. *Surg Gynecol Obstet* **90**:1–15, 1950

32. Mustard WT, Chute AL, Keith JD, et al: A surgical approach to transposition of the great vessels with extracorporeal circuit. *Surgery* **36**:39–51, 1954

33. Mustard WT: Successful two-stage correction of transposition of the great vessels. *Surgery* **55**:469–472, 1964

34. Senning A: Surgical correction of transposition of the great vessels. *Surgery* **45**:966–980, 1959

35. Kirklin JW, DuShane JW: Repair of ventricular septal defect in infancy. *Pediatrics* **27**:961–966, 1961

36. Waterston DJ: Fallot's Tetralogy in children under one year of age. *Rozhl Chir* **41**:181–183, 1962

37. Rastelli GC: A new approach to "anatomic" repair of transposition of the great arteries. *Mayo Clin Proc* **44**:1–12, 1969

38. Rastelli GC, McGoon DC, Wallace RB: Anatomic correction of transposition of the great arteries with ventricular septal defect and subpulmonary stenosis. *J Thorac Cardiovasc Surg* **58**:545–552, 1969

39. Keown KK, Fisher SM, Downing DF, Hitchcock P: Anesthesia for cardiac catheterization in infants and children. *Anesthesiology* **18**:270–274, 1957

40. Harmel MH, Lamont A: Anesthesia in the surgical treatment of congenital pulmonic stenosis. *Anesthesiology* **7**:477–498, 1946

41. McQuiston WO: Anesthesia in cardiac surgery. Observations on 362 cases. *Arch Surg* **61**:892–902, 1950

42. McQuiston WO: Anesthetic problems in cardiac surgery in children. *Anesthesiology* **10**:590–600, 1949

43. Patrick RT, Ridley RW, Pender JW: Anesthesia and supportive therapy for patients undergoing cardiac surgery. *Surg Clin North Am* **August**:911–918, 1955

44. Keats AS, Kurosu Y, Telford J, Cooley DA: Anesthetic problems in cardiopulmonary bypass for open heart surgery. Experience with 200 patients. *Anesthesiology* **19**:501–504, 1958

45. Keats AS, Cooley DA, Telford J: Relative antiheparin potency of polybrene and protamine in patients undergoing extracorporeal circulation. *J Thorac Cardiovasc Surg* **38**:362–368, 1959

46. Keats AS: Mechanical ventilation for infants. *Anesthesiology* **29**:591–593, 1968

47. Keats AS: Carbon dioxide. *Anesthesiology* **17**:631–632, 1956

48. Keats AS: Anesthesia for emergency cardiovascular surgery. *Clin Anesth* **2**:47–70, 1963

49. Smith RM: Circulatory factors affecting anesthesia in surgery for congenital heart disease. *Anesthesiology* **13**:38–60, 1952

50. Strong MJ, Keats AS, Cooley DA: Anesthesia for cardiovascular surgery in infancy. *Anesthesiology* **27**:257–265, 1966

51. Dillard DH, Mohri H, Hessell EA: Correction of total anomalous pulmonary venous drainage in infants utilizing deep hypothermia and total circulatory arrest. *Circulation* **35**(suppl 1):1–105, 1967

52. Barratt-Boyes BG, Simpson M, Neutze JM: Intracardiac surgery in neonates and infants using deep hypothermia with surface cooling and limited cardiopulmonary bypass. *Circulation* **43**(suppl 1):1–25, 1971

53. Hikasa Y, Shirotani H, Satomura K, et al: Open heart surgery in infants with an aid of hypothermia anesthesia. *Arch Jpn Chir* **36**:495–508, 1967

54. Dennis C, Spreng DS, Nelson GE, et al: Development of a pump oxygenator to replace the heart and lungs: An apparatus applicable to human patients and application to one case. *Ann Surg* **134**:709–721, 1951

55. Gibbon JH: Application of a mechanical heart and lung apparatus to cardiac surgery. *Minn Med* **37**:171–180, 1954

56. Kirklin JW, DuShane JW, Patrick RT, et al: Intracardiac surgery with the aid of a mechanical pump-oxygenator system (Gibbon type): Report of eight cases. *Mayo Clin Proc* **30**:201–206, 1955

57. Mendelsohn D, MacKrell TN, MacLachlan MA, et al: Experiences using the pump-oxygenator for open cardiac surgery in man. *Anesthesiology* **18**:223–235, 1957

58. Cooley DA, Latson JR, Keats AS: Surgical considerations in repair of ventricular and atrial septal defects utilizing cardiopulmonary bypass. *Surgery* **43**:214–225, 1958

59. Hickey PR, Hansen DD, Norwood WI, Castaneda AR: Anesthetic complications in surgery for congenital heart disease. *Anesth Analg* **63**:657–664, 1984

60. Greeley WJ, Kern FH, Ungerleider RM, et al: The effect of hypothermic cardiopulmonary bypass and total circulatory arrest on cerebral metabolism in neonates, infants, and children. *J Thorac Cardiovasc Surg* **101**:783–794, 1991

61. Swain JA, McDonald TJ, Griffith PK, et al: Low-flow hypothermic cardiopulmonary bypass protects the brain. *J Thorac Cardiovasc Surg* **102**:76–84, 1991

62. Pridjian AK, Levitsky S, Krukenkamp I, et al: Developmental changes in reperfusion injury. *J Thorac Cardiovasc Surg* **93**:428–433, 1987

63. Magovern JA, Pae WE, Waldhausen JA: Protection of the immature myocardium. *J Thorac Cardiovasc Surg* **96**:408–413, 1988

64. Fricker FJ, Trento A, Griffith BP: Pediatric cardiac transplantation. *Cardiovasc Clin* **20**:223–235, 1990

65. Bailey LL, Nehlsen-Cannarella SL, Concepcion W, Jolley WB: Baboon-to-human cardiac xenotransplantaion in a neonate. *JAMA* **254**:3321–3329, 1985

Chapter 2 | Pathophysiologic Approach to Congenital Heart Disease

Alan Jay Schwartz and Frederick W. Campbell

The perioperative management of the child with congenital heart disease is a special challenge for the anesthesiologist. This is problematic because congenital heart disease consists of a vast array of anatomic variations that are infrequently encountered in daily clinical practice.[1] Each year in the United States, there are approximately 3.75 million live births. Slightly less than 1% of these children display some form of congenital heart disease (Table 2–1).[2–5] Some of these children will require palliative or corrective cardiac surgery early in their lives. Much of the cardiac surgery for congenital heart disease is performed in only a limited number of institutions. Many children with congenital heart disease will not require early cardiac surgical intervention, however, having relatively benign lesions that will go unrecognized or will be relatively asymptomatic or noncompromising. Most anesthesiologists, therefore, have very little clinical contact with the small number of children who have any one of the many presentations of congenital heart disease and are to undergo cardiac surgery. Anesthesiologists do encounter these children more frequently in the noncardiac surgical setting[6] (see Chapter 26). No matter what the exposure, it is crucial that anesthesiologists be familiar with the pathophysiologic alterations produced by the anatomic malformations of congenital heart disease.

CLASSIFICATION OF CONGENITAL HEART DISEASE

In order to make it possible to view the management of the child with congenital heart disease as a nonesoteric subject that is understandable to all, there needs to be a way to group the many anatomic varieties into a few common and understandable categories.[7–14] A pathophysiologic classification of congenital heart disease achieves this type of categorization. Assignment to the appropriate groups is based upon the answers to several basic questions:

1. Is there an abnormal *shunt* pathway for blood flow through an intracardiac, extracardiac, or combined defect?
2. Is there an *obstruction* to or reduction of blood flow due to a supravalvular, subvalvular, or primary valvular abnormality?
3. Is there an increase or decrease in pulmonary or systemic blood flow?

The pathophysiologic classification of congenital heart disease distills the numerous anatomic variations into three groups. In two of the groups, the primary problem is anatomic shunting of blood through abnormal circulatory pathways. The major alteration of these shunt lesions occurs with pulmonary blood flow. *Pulmonary blood flow* will either be *increased*, resulting in a volume or pressure overload to the pulmonary circulation (eg, ventricular or atrial septal defect, patent ductus arteriosus), or *decreased*, resulting in a relative inability to oxygenate blood (eg, tetralogy of Fallot). Also included in these groups are complex congenital heart lesions in which there is a functional shunt (eg, common ventricle, transposition of the great arteries, truncus arteriosus) that may or may not be associated with an anatomic obstruction to pulmonary or systemic blood flow. These more complex anatomic congenital heart malformations have the same effect of either increasing or decreasing the effective pulmonary blood flow. A functional decrease in pulmonary blood flow occurs, for example, when desaturated venous blood is shunted to the systemic circulation rather than to the pulmonary circulation because of the presence of a common mixing chamber such as a single ventricle.

There is no shunting of blood in the third group of congenital heart lesions (eg, aortic or pulmonic stenosis, coarctation of the aorta). The primary problem in this

TABLE 2–1. PERCENTAGE INCIDENCE OF CONGENITAL CARDIOVASCULAR MALFORMATIONS AMONG AFFECTED PERSONS IN THREE DIFFERENT AGE GROUPS (EXCLUDING NEONATES)

	Infants	Children	Older Children and Adults
Ventricular septal defect	28.3	24	15
Patent ductus arteriosus	12.5	15	15.5
Atrial septal defect	9.7	12	16
Coarctation	8.8	4.5	8
Transposition	8	4.5	2
Tetralogy of Fallot	7	11	15.5
Pulmonary stenosis	6	11	15
Aortic stenosis	3.5	6.5	5
Truncus	2.7	0.5	0
Tricuspid atresia	1	1.5	1
All others	12.5	9.5	7
Total	100.0	100.0	100.0

(Modified from Berman RE, Vaughan VC, Nelson WE: Nelson's Textbook of Pediatrics, 12th ed. Philadelphia: W.B. Saunders, 1983, with permission.)

TABLE 2–2. FLOW CHARACTERISTICS OF VARIOUS CONGENITAL CARDIAC LESIONS

Increased pulmonary blood flow lesions
Atrial septal defect
Ventricular septal defect
Patent ductus arteriosus
Endocardial cushion defect (atrioventricular canal abnormality)
Anomalous origin of coronary arteries
Transposition of the great arteries*
Anomalous pulmonary venous drainage*
Truncus arteriosus*
Single ventricle*

Decreased pulmonary blood flow lesions
Tetralogy of Fallot
Pulmonary atresia
Tricuspid atresia
Ebstein's anomaly
Truncus arteriosus*
Transposition of the great arteries*
Single ventricle*

Obstructive lesions
Aortic stenosis
Pulmonary stenosis
Coarctation of the aorta
Asymmetric septal hypertrophy

* Systemic hypoxemia occurs as a result of the mixing of systemic and pulmonary venous returns. Classification as an increased or decreased pulmonary blood flow lesion depends upon the absence or presence within the anatomic variation of obstruction to pulmonary blood flow.
(Modified from Schwartz AJ, Jobes DR: Congenital heart disease—Special anesthetic considerations. In Conahan TJ (ed): Cardiac Anesthesia. Menlo Park, CA: Addison-Wesley, 1982, with permission.)

group is *obstruction to blood flow*. The major consequences of obstruction to blood flow include the increased ventricular workload(s) necessary to overcome the obstruction(s) and the relatively reduced circulation distal to the obstruction(s). Common examples of the three groups of congenital heart lesions are listed in Table 2–2.

It is important to remember that the pathophysiologic classification being presented must be coupled with the clinical presentations seen in children with congenital heart disease. Cyanosis or congestive heart failure are the two major clinical states that result from the abnormal anatomy and pathophysiology of congenital heart lesions. Cyanosis occurs most commonly in lesions where (1) pulmonary blood flow is anatomically decreased or (2) pulmonary blood flow is functionally decreased as mixing of systemic and pulmonary venous blood occurs. Congestive heart failure occurs most commonly in (1) shunt lesions that excessively increase pulmonary blood flow or (2) obstructive lesions that stress the ventricle past its capacity to pump effectively.

Understanding the pathophysiology of shunting and obstruction to blood flow is essential to the comprehension of any individual anatomic presentation of congenital heart deformity. In addition, application of the same pathophysiologic concepts permits the design of rational perianesthetic management plans for children with congenital heart disease.[14]

PATHOPHYSIOLOGY OF CONGENITAL HEART DISEASE: THE "PLUMBING" PRINCIPLE

The pathophysiology of shunting of and obstruction to blood flow is explained by considering two fundamental principles of physics: Ohm's law and the Hagen-Poiseuille relationship.[15,16] Although neither of these are used quantitatively, in a qualitative sense they are very helpful in describing blood flow (Fig 2–1).

Ohm's law, as used in physics, relates the electromotive force producing an electric current to the actual flow of electricity and to its resistance.

$$\text{Ohm's Law}$$
$$I = \frac{E}{R}$$

where I = amperes (current flow), E = volts (electromotive force producing a current), R = ohms (resistance to current flow).

When applied to cardiovascular physiology, Ohm's law relates blood flow to the pressure generating it and the resistance impeding it.

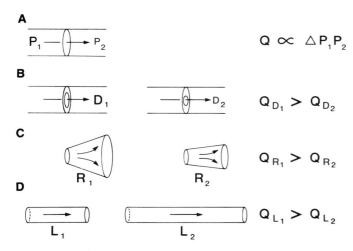

A

$$Q \propto \triangle P_1 P_2$$

B

$$Q_{D_1} > Q_{D_2}$$

C

$$Q_{R_1} > Q_{R_2}$$

D

$$Q_{L_1} > Q_{L_2}$$

Figure 2–1. Schematic representation of the individual factors that influence the flow of blood through vascular channels. The quantity of flow is determined by pressure gradients in vascular channels, the diameter of the vascular channel, the resistance offered by the circuit into which the vascular channels empties, and the length of the vascular channel. Abbreviations: Q, blood flow; Δ, difference between; P, pressure; D, diameter; R, resistance; L, length. (A) Q is proportional to the difference between P_1 and P_2. In the diagram, P_1 is $> P_2$, therefore, Q is in the direction of P_2. (B) Two vascular channels of different diameters are shown. Q through the channel with the larger diameter, D_1, is $>Q$ through the channel with the smaller diameter, D_2. (C) Two vascular channels of equal initial diameter (the opening of each on the left) are shown emptying into circuits offering different resistance. Q through the channel offering less resistance, R_1, is $>Q$ through the channel offering more resistance, R_2. (D) Two vascular channels of equal diameter and different length are shown. Q through the shorter channel, L_1, is $> Q$ through the longer channel, L_2.

Ohm's Law (Cardiovascular Equivalent)

$$Q = \frac{P}{R}$$

where Q = blood flow (cardiac output), P = blood pressure (generated within a ventricular chamber), R = vascular resistance (offered by the pulmonary or systemic vascular bed).

The Hagen-Poiseuille relationship describes the laminar flow of a homogeneous fluid through a rigid tube of constant caliber and length.[16] When applied to cardiovascular physiology, it is "assumed" that blood is a homogeneous fluid and the blood vessels are relatively constant-size conducting tubes. The factors that are related to flow in the Hagen-Poiseuille relationship as applied to cardiovascular physiology are expressed as:

Hagen-Poiseuille Relationship

$$Q = \frac{\Delta P \pi r^4}{8L\eta}$$

where Q = blood flow, ΔP = pressure drop in fluid as it flows through a vascular channel, r = radius of the vascular conduit, L = length of the vascular conduit, η = viscosity of fluid (assumed to remain constant). In this

relationship, $\pi r^4/L$ represents the cross-sectional area of the vascular conduit over its length. This is a more specifically defined resistance factor than that used in Ohm's law.

Combination and modification of Ohm's law and the Hagen-Poiseuille relationship yields a versatile learning tool that can be used to understand the pathophysiology of congenital heart disease. The reaggregation of these expressions results in a cardiovascular "plumbing" principle expressed as Equation 2–1.

$$Q \propto \frac{P \times D^4}{R} \qquad (2\text{–}1)$$

where Q = blood flow (cardiac output or shunt flow), P = pressure gradient (across valves, outflow tracts, or intracardiac or extracardiac communications), D = diameter (of valves or intracardiac or extracardiac communications), R = resistance to blood flow (ventricular outflow tracts, cross-sectional areas of vascular beds, or length of vascular channels).

Detailed examples of the application of this "plumbing" principle will demonstrate its utility in understanding the anatomic deformities and management of children with congenital heart disease. This same principle is utilized to understand the physiology of the fetal circulation and its transition to the adult pattern, which is discussed in Chapters 3 and 4.

APPLIED PATHOPHYSIOLOGY OF CONGENITAL HEART DISEASE

Ventricular septal defect (VSD) is an example of an increased pulmonary blood flow lesion (Fig 2–2).[8] Blood is shunted into the lungs because left ventricular pressure is higher than right ventricular pressure, and right ventricular outflow tract resistance (including that contributed by the pulmonary vasculature) offers less impedance to flow than that of the systemic circulation. The existence of *any* shunted blood and its total quantity is dependent upon the resistance to flow offered by the VSD itself. The larger the diameter of the VSD, the less resistance it offers, and the greater the flow across it from the higher pressure left ventricle to the lower pressure right ventricle and ultimately to the pulmonary circuit. This information would be expressed specifically by Equation 2–2. In a VSD:

$$Q\,(\text{pulmonary shunt}) \propto \frac{P(\text{LV} > \text{RV}) \times D^4(\text{VSD})}{R(\text{PVR} < \text{SVR})}$$

$$(2\text{–}2)$$

where LV = left ventricle, RV = right ventricle, PVR = pulmonary vascular resistance (cross-sectional area of the pulmonary vasculature), SVR = systemic vascular resistance (cross-sectional area of the systemic vasculature), D = diameter.

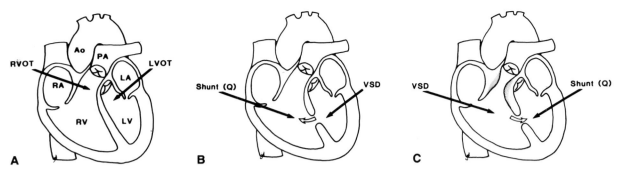

Figure 2–2. Diagrammatic representation of a normal heart and congenital heart lesions in which there is a pathophysiologic alteration in pulmonary blood flow (PBF). Abbreviations: Ao, aorta; LA, left atrium; LV, left ventricle; LVOT, left ventricular outflow tract; P, pressure; PA, pulmonary artery; Q, shunt blood flow; R, resistance to blood flow; RA, right atrium; RV, right ventricle; RVOT, right ventricular outflow tract; VSD, ventricular septal defect. (A) A normal heart showing the anatomic relationships between the cardiac chambers and the outflow tracts of the ventricles. (B) An increased PBF lesion is exemplified by a VSD. When (1) the VSD is large diameter offering low R and (2) RVOT and PA offer low R, then (3) $P_{LV} > P_{RV}$, and Q (indicated by the *open arrow*) is left-to-right increasing PBF. (C) A decreased PBF lesion is exemplified by tetralogy of Fallot. When (1) the VSD is large diameter offering low R, (2) RVOT is obstructed (subpulmonic muscular hypertrophy [indicated by the *shaded areas*]), (3) RVOT R>LVOT R, then (4) $P_{RV} \geq P_{LV'}$, and Q (indicated by the *open arrow*) is right-to-left decreasing PBF.

Tetralogy of Fallot (TOF) is an example of a decreased pulmonary blood flow lesion (Figs 2–2 and 2–3).[8] Blood is shunted away from the lungs because the muscular portion of the right ventricular outflow tract is obstructed (infundibular pulmonic stenosis) and offers

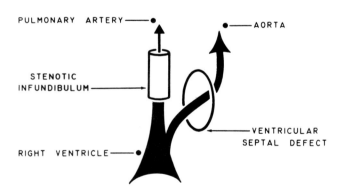

Figure 2–3. Schematic representation of the two pathophysiologically important components (stenotic infundibulum and ventricular septal defect) of tetralogy of Fallot. Blood flow is indicated by the arrows. There are two possible pathways for blood flow: (1) into the pulmonary artery (normal flow) and (2) across the ventricular septal defect (VSD) and subsequently into the aorta (shunt flow). In the classic form of the disease, more blood is shunted away from the pulmonary artery (*heavy solid arrow*) because the muscular portion of the right ventricular outflow tract is obstructed (stenotic infundibulum of the diagram), than is permitted to flow into the pulmonary circuit (*thin solid arrow*). The stenotic infundibulum offers more resistance to blood flow than the interventricular communication (ventricular septal defect of the diagram) that is present. The VSD actually serves as a "pop-off valve" that decompresses the right ventricle that cannot empty via the normal pathway owing to its obstructed outflow tract. (*From Fink BW: Congenital Heart Disease: A Deductive Approach to Its Diagnosis, 2nd ed. Chicago: Year Book Medical, 1985, p 91, with permission.*)

more resistance to blood flow than the interventricular communication, ie, the VSD, that is present. The VSD actually serves as a "pop-off valve" that decompresses the right ventricle that cannot empty normally owing to its obstructed outflow tract. The pressure in the right ventricle, which commonly equals or exceeds the pressure in the left ventricle, is elevated in response to the resistance of the normal pathway for right ventricular emptying. As long as the SVR is relatively low in comparison to the resistance offered by the obstructed right ventricular outflow tract, the left ventricle empties in a normal fashion and an additional quantity of blood will flow from the right ventricle through the VSD to the left ventricle and ultimately to the systemic circuit. This information would be expressed specifically by Equation 2–3. In tetralogy of Fallot:

$$Q \text{ (systemic shunt)} \propto \frac{P(RV > LV) \times D^4(VSD)}{R(RVOT > SVR)}$$

$$(2\text{–}3)$$

where RVOT = right ventricular outflow tract.

A limiting factor on the total amount of blood that will be shunted away from the right heart and pulmonary vasculature is the size of the VSD. If the anatomic deformity of the TOF includes a small-diameter VSD, shunt flow is limited. The significance of this is seen in the analysis of the so-called "pink Tet."[17] This is a child with TOF in whom the VSD may be of a small diameter and the right ventricular outflow tract obstruction of a mild enough degree that pulmonary blood flow is only minimally reduced. Under these conditions, there is usually sufficient blood flow into the pulmonary circuit under nonstressful conditions that clinically significant hypoxemia does not occur, nor do any of its manifestations such as cyanosis, clubbing, and polycythemia. Under these circumstances, this information would be expressed specifically in the relationship in Equation 2–4. In a "pink" TOF:

$$Q(\text{systemic shunt}) \propto \frac{P(\text{RV} = \text{or} < \text{LV}) \times D^4(\text{small VSD})}{R(\text{RVOT} = \text{or} < \text{SVR})}$$

(2–4)

Aortic stenosis (AS) is an example of a nonshunt obstructive lesion. The normal quantity of blood flows through the normal pathway. To satisfy the flow-pressure-resistance relationship, left ventricular pressure must be markedly increased in order to overcome the resistance offered by the reduced diameter of the aortic orifice. This is obvious as seen in Equation 2–5, which expresses these factors. In aortic stenosis:

$$Q(\text{systemic flow}) \propto \frac{P(\text{LV} > \text{Ao}) \times D^4(\text{aortic valve})}{R(\text{LVOT})}$$

(2–5)

where LVOT = left ventricular outflow tract.

Consideration of one of the more complex congenital heart malformations will demonstrate the utility of the pathophysiologic approach to classification. Transposition of the great vessels (TGV) is an ideal example for this because this lesion presents in at least one of three variations, each of which has a slightly different pathophysiologic consequence. The three types of TGV commonly encountered are (1) TGV with an intact ventricular septum; (2) TGV with a VSD; and (3) TGV with a VSD and subpulmonic stenosis (see Chapter 15).[8]

In the child with TGV with an intact ventricular septum, there are two circuits for blood flow that are parallel and independent of each other rather than connected in series fashion as they normally would be (Figs 2–4 and 2–5A). Viability under these circumstances depends upon some cross-mixing of the two separated circulations. The intermixing is permitted at the atrial level with the persistence of the foramen ovale and additionally by cross-communication of the circulations via a patent ductus arteriosus (PDA). Bidirectional flow across the patent foramen ovale depends upon its diameter and a pressure differential at the atrial level. The flow-pressure-resistance relationship explains the clinical course of a child with the circulation described. If the foramen ovale or PDA closes (their diameter becomes zero), then flow ceases and the child will die. If on the other hand, the foramen ovale remains open, as the child grows, the size (diameter) of the foramen will become relatively smaller and smaller and become less able to permit sufficient interatrial cross-mixing to sustain life. The diameter of the interatrial communication, therefore, is crucial for adequate blood flow.

Maintenance of an adequate-size interatrial connection is so important that there are two methods available to increase the diameter of this intracardiac communication. Surgically, a portion of the atrial septum may be excised (Blalock-Hanlon atrial septectomy).[18] The "medical" equivalent of this is the balloon atrial septostomy (Rashkind procedure).[19] Even when either of the options to increase atrial intermixing is exercised, there still comes a point at which the child's growth outstrips the diameter of the interatrial communication and blood flow into the pulmonary circuit becomes insufficient to adequately oxygenate blood. The flow-pressure-resistance relationship for TGV with an intact ventricular septum is expressed as Equation 2–6.

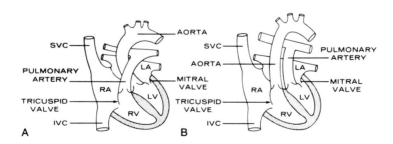

Figure 2–4. Diagrammatic representation of the anatomic malformations of transposition of the great vessels (TGV) (*B*) compared to the normal anatomy of the heart and great vessels (*A*). Abbreviations: IVC, inferior vena cava; LA, left atrium; LV, left ventricle; RA, right atrium; RV, right ventricle; SVC, superior vena cava. In the normal heart, the pulmonary circulation is connected in series with the systemic circulation via the pulmonary vascular bed. The great vessel of the pulmonary circuit, ie, the pulmonary artery, arises from the pulmonary (right) ventricle. The great vessel of the systemic circuit, ie, the aorta, arises from the systemic (left) ventricle. In TGV, the pulmonary and systemic circulations are parallel, not being connected. The great vessel of the pulmonary circuit arises from the systemic ventricle and the great vessel of the systemic circuit arises from the pulmonary ventricle. Viability under these abnormal circumstances depends upon some cross-mixing of the two separated circulations. Intermixing is permitted via an interatrial communication (see text for further description) and by a patent ductus arteriosus (neither are shown in the figure). (*From Fink BW: Congenital Heart Disease: A Deductive Approach to Its Diagnosis, 2nd ed. Chicago: Year Book Medical, 1985, p 112, with permission.*)

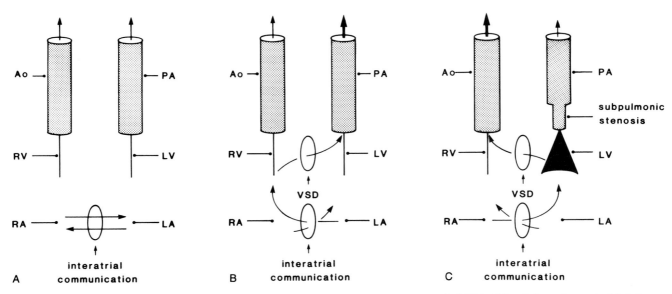

Figure 2–5. Schematic representation of three forms of transposition of the great vessels (TGV). Abbreviations: Ao, aorta; LA, left atrium; LV, left ventricle; PA, pulmonary artery; PBF, pulmonary blood flow; RA, right atrium; RV, right ventricle; VSD, ventricular septal defect. (*A*) In TGV with an intact ventricular septum, there are two circuits for blood flow that are parallel and independent of each other. Viability under these circumstances depends upon cross-mixing of the two separated circulations. Intermixing occurs through an interatrial communication that may be a patent foramen ovale, a surgically created atrial septal opening (Blalock-Hanlon atrial septectomy), or a "medically" created atrial septal opening (balloon atrial septostomy, ie, Rashkind procedure) (see text for further description). (*B*) In TGV with a VSD, there is shunting of blood at the ventricular level (*arrow through the VSD*) that tends to increase PBF (*larger arrow leaving the PA*). When pulmonary vascular resistance decreases during the neonatal period, blood is shunted across the VSD from the higher-pressure systemic (right) ventricle into the lower-pressure pulmonary (left) ventricle and ultimately into the PA. The shunt through the VSD increases PBF, which in turn increases pulmonary venous return to the LA. As a consequence of increasing left atrial return, cross-mixing at the interatrial communication is greater in the left-to-right direction (*longer arrow from LA to RA*) (see text for further description). (*C*) In TGV with a VSD and subpulmonic stenosis, there is shunting of blood at the ventricular level (*arrow through the VSD*) that tends to decrease PBF (*smaller arrow leaving the PA*). The subpulmonic stenosis offers resistance to emptying of the pulmonary (left) ventricle. This results in an increase in left ventricular pressure (*wide arrow base in the LV*). Blood is shunted across the VSD from the higher-pressure pulmonary (left) ventricle into the lower pressure systemic (right) ventricle and ultimately into the Ao. The shunt through the VSD decreases PBF, which in turn decreases pulmonary venous return to the LA. As a consequence of decreasing left atrial return, cross-mixing at the interatrial communication is greater in the right-to-left direction (*longer arrow from RA to LA*) (see text for further description). (*Modified from Fink BW: Congenital Heart Disease: A Deductive Approach to Its Diagnosis, 2nd ed. Chicago: Year Book Medical, 1985, pp 113, 118, 121, with permission.*)

Interatrial Q (bidirectional) $\propto$

$$\frac{P(\text{RA} >, =, < \text{LA}) \times D^4(\text{foramen ovale, Blalock-Hanlon atrial septectomy, or balloon atrial septostomy})}{R(\text{RV} >, =, < \text{LV})} \quad (2\text{–}6)$$

where RA = right atrium, LA = left atrium.

In this equation, the resistance factor, $R(\text{RV}>, =, <\text{LV})$, is intended to signify the fact that the outflow of each atrium across its respective atrioventricular valve depends upon the pressure differential from atrium to ventricle, which is a function of the ventricular volume and compliance, which in turn depends upon the vascular resistances against which the ventricles empty. Based upon these relationships, it will be the balance between the RA and its ability to empty into the RV and the LA and its ability to empty into the LV that will determine the direction of shunt at the interatrial communication.

TGV with a VSD represents a variation upon that described above for the simple form of TGV (Fig 2–5B). Initially, it is impossible to distinguish simple TGV from its counterpart with a VSD. This is because PVR is normally increased in the newborn. Maintenance of increased PVR limits shunt flow across the VSD, in this instance from the right (systemic) ventricle to the left (pulmonary) ventricle. During the 4- to 6-week normal neonatal maturation process, PVR decreases.[20] Even though the decrease in PVR in the child with TGV and a VSD may not be of the magnitude observed in the normal child, enough of a reduction occurs that shunt flow is permitted at the ventricle level. Although there may be a VSD of sufficient diameter to allow shunt blood flow, this will not happen until the resistance to flow offered by the pulmonary vessels is decreased. It is also important to recognize that the left ventricle in this situation is the pulmonary ventricle and, therefore, has a pressure lower than that in the right (systemic) ventricle, verifying the pressure gradient from right to left. An additional pathophysiologic consequence of the shunting of blood through the VSD increasing the pulmonary circulation is the increase in pulmonary venous return to the left atrium. Increasing pulmonary venous return increases (1) the size of the left atrium and ultimately the diameter of the interatrial communication; and (2) the left atrial pressure, both of which promote blood flow from the left (pulmonary) atrium to the right (systemic) atrium. In combination, the flow-pressure-resistance relationship explains how systemic venous desaturated blood is routed to the pulmonary circulation via the VSD and pulmonary venous oxygenated blood is routed to the systemic circulation via the interatrial communication in the child with TGV and VSD. These flow patterns are expressed in Equations 2–7A and 2–7B. In TGV with a VSD:

Q(pulmonary shunt) $\propto$

$$\frac{P[\text{RV(systemic ventricle)} > \text{(pulmonary ventricle)}] \times D^4(\text{VSD})}{R(\text{PVR} < \text{SVR})} \quad (2\text{–}7A)$$

In TGV with a VSD:

Interatrial Q(left to right) $\propto$

$$\frac{P(\text{LA} > \text{RA}) \times D^4(\text{foramen ovale, Blalock-Hanlon atrial septectomy, or balloon atrial septostomy})}{R(\text{RV} >, =, < \text{LV})} \quad (2\text{–}7B)$$

Like any other child with a shunt increasing pulmonary blood flow, the child with TGV and a VSD is at risk for the development of pulmonary vascular occlusive disease. Structural alteration of the pulmonary vasculature occurs as a result of both a volume and pressure load to its vessels.[21] The effect of pressure is greater in intensity and requires less time to occur. The early response of the pulmonary vessels is to constrict in an attempt to offset the volume and pressure load. In time, the medial muscular layer of the pulmonary arteries and arterioles hypertrophies. Up to this point, the pulmonary vascular changes are potentially reversible. If the volume and pressure stress on the pulmonary vessels is allowed to persist, however, irreversible vascular change develops. This is characterized as a nonspecific intimal fibrosis of the muscular arteries that progresses to an occlusive plexiform lesion of the intimal surfaces of both the small pulmonary arteries and the arterioles. These changes account for the increase in PVR and ultimately explain a reduction in pulmonary blood flow and reversal of the shunt through the VSD.

The third variation of TGV is that with a VSD and subpulmonic stenosis (Fig 2–5C). The pathophysiology

of this type of presentation of TGV is analogous to TOF. When the subpulmonic stenosis offers more impedance to left (pulmonary) ventricular emptying than that offered by the diameter of the VSD or outflow (SVR) of the right (systemic) ventricle, blood is shunted into the systemic circuit. Because the left (pulmonary) ventricular blood is being shunted to the systemic circuit, it might be expected that hypoxemia would be reduced. With clinically significant subpulmonic stenosis, however, pulmonary arterial blood flow is reduced and oxygenation limited. When pulmonary arterial blood flow is reduced, pulmonary venous blood flow is subsequently reduced. This results in a situation in which the left (pulmonary) atrium becomes small with a lower pressure than that in the right (systemic) atrium. This promotes interatrial mixing of more right (systemic) atrial desaturated venous blood with the left (pulmonary) atrial oxygenated blood. These flow patterns are expressed in Equations 2–8A and 2–8B. In TGV with a VSD and subpulmonic stenosis:

Q(systemic shunt) $\propto$

$$\frac{P[\text{LV(pulmonary ventricle)} > \text{RV(systemic ventricle)}] \times D^4(\text{VSD})}{R(\text{subpulmonic stenosis} > \text{SVR})} \quad (2\text{–}8A)$$

In TGV with a VSD and subpulmonic stenosis:

Interatrial Q (right to left) $\propto$

$$\frac{P(\text{RA} > \text{LA}) \times D^4(\text{foramen ovale, Blalock-Hanlon atrial septectomy, or balloon atrial septostomy})}{R(\text{RV} >, =, < \text{LV})} \quad (2\text{–}8B)$$

The net effect of decreased pulmonary arterial and venous blood flow is to reduce the quantity and the saturation of the blood entering the left ventricle, which thereby reduces the saturation of the blood shunted across the VSD into the right (systemic) ventricle. Systemic blood, therefore, is inadequately oxygenated in TGV with a VSD and subpulmonic stenosis.

In each of the three types of TGV that have been analyzed, it should be apparent that one of the major factors in determining the direction of blood flow into the systemic circulation and the quantity of that flow that is oxygenated is the diameter of the interatrial communication and the pressure differential across it. Even the more complicated congenital heart lesions can be simplified by analysis using the simple "plumbing" principle.

SURGICAL APPLICATION OF THE PATHOPHYSIOLOGIC PRINCIPLES OF CONGENITAL HEART DISEASE

Thinking about the pathophysiology of congenital heart disease not only makes the anatomic varieties understandable but in addition makes it possible to understand the thought process behind the development of the palliative and corrective surgical procedures for these lesions. This is quite relevant because many children with congenital heart disease present for cardiac anesthesia having had prior surgical palliation or correction. It is mandatory that the anesthesiologist understand the various types of surgical manipulations of the anatomy[22,23] in order to fully appreciate how this alters the pathophysiologic expression of the congenital heart lesion(s). Examples will make this obvious.

PA Banding

The pathophysiologic problem for the child with a VSD is an increase in the blood flow to the lungs. If the pulmonary blood flow is increased by a quantity of sufficient magnitude, the lungs will essentially be "drowned." Congestive heart failure or pulmonary edema results. If enough pulmonary interstitial water is present, there may even be an oxygen diffusion block with resultant cyanosis. Because the major problem is the increase in the pulmonary blood flow, surgical palliation or correction must be designed to reduce or eliminate this excess.

Pulmonary artery banding is the palliative procedure that offsets the increase in pulmonary blood flow of a VSD.[22,23] By placing a band (an artificial constriction) around the main pulmonary artery, the surgeon increases the resistance to blood flowing out of the right ventricle. In an effort to overcome this increased resistance to flow, the right ventricle attempts to generate a higher pressure. The pressure differential between the ventricles across their interconnection (the VSD) becomes less, resulting in less flow from the left ventricle to the right ventricle. The net result of the palliative pulmonary artery banding procedure is to reduce shunting of blood into the lungs. The amount of pulmonary artery constriction produced by the band must be balanced so that excessive pulmonary blood flow is reduced but sufficient pulmonary blood flow is permitted. Trading congestive heart failure for marked hypoxemia is unacceptable. Surgically manipulating the anatomy produces a different pathophysiologic outcome (Fig 2–6) expressed in Equation 2–9 for a banded VSD.

$$Q(\text{pulmonary shunt}) \propto \frac{P(\text{LV} > \text{or} = \text{RV}) \times D^4(\text{VSD})}{R(\text{pulmonary artery band} < \text{or} = \text{SVR})} \quad (2\text{–}9)$$

Septal Defect Closure

Total correction of a VSD eliminates the interventricular communication by direct suture closure or application of a patch to cover the defect. When the VSD is closed, its diameter becomes zero. Plugging this factor into the "plumbing" equation explains why shunt flow becomes zero, as shown in Equation 2–10. In a closed VSD:

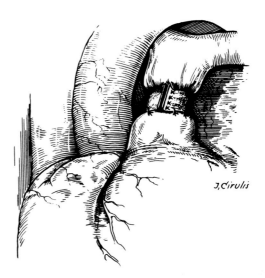

Figure 2–6. Diagrammatic representation of the placement of a band around the main pulmonary artery (PA) in order to surgically reduce the excessive pulmonary blood flow (PBF) associated with the presence of a ventricular septal defect (VSD). By placing a band, ie, an artificial constriction, around the main PA, the surgeon increases the resistance to blood flowing out of the right ventricle (RV) into the pulmonary circulation. This results in an increase in the pressure in the RV and a reduction in the pressure differential between the RV and left ventricle (LV) across the VSD. The net result of the palliative surgical PA banding procedure is to reduce the quantity of blood shunted from LV to RV and ultimately into the PA. (*From Bernhard WF, et al: Cardiac surgery in infants. In Norman JC (ed): Cardiac Surgery, 2nd ed. New York: Appleton-Century-Crofts 1972, p 254, with permission.*)

$$Q(\text{pulmonary shunt}) \propto \frac{P \times D^4(\text{VSD} = 0)}{R} \quad (2\text{–}10)$$

Shunt Reversal

Total correction of a VSD must be undertaken only after careful consideration of the pathophysiologic factors that control blood flow across the intracardiac communication. A VSD that is of large diameter and causes a large increase in pulmonary blood flow may eventually result in the development of sufficient irreversible pulmonary vascular occlusive disease that closure of the intracardiac communication will not be tolerated. In this situation (Eisenmenger complex),[24] were the VSD to be closed, the right ventricle would have to be able to generate sufficient pressure to produce pulmonary blood flow against an elevated PVR. Pathophysiologically, the Eisenmenger complex is expressed in Equation 2–11.

In the Eisenmenger complex VSD:

$$Q(\text{systemic shunt}) \propto \frac{P(\text{RV} > \text{LV}) \times D^4(\text{VSD})}{R(\text{PVR} > \text{SVR})} \quad (2\text{–}11)$$

If the increase in the PVR is of such magnitude, it may not be possible for the right ventricle to pump against this impedance to flow. Under these circumstances, the right ventricle would fail ("suicide" right ventricle) if the VSD were closed. The only appropriate pathophysiologic course of action in this situation is to allow the VSD to remain open to serve as a "pop off" for the right ventricle whose outflow is so severely and irreversibly obstructed. To prevent the development of the Eisenmenger complex in a child with a VSD, ongoing assessment of the flow-pressure-resistance factors would indicate when a reversal of its pathophysiology from the increase in pulmonary blood flow to the unusual and potentially lethal decrease in pulmonary blood flow might be likely and when surgical correction should be undertaken.

Systemic Arterial to Pulmonary Arterial Shunts

The pathophysiologic problem for the child with TOF is a decrease in the blood flow to the lungs. A variety of surgically created shunts are palliatively used to offset this type of problem by providing blood flow to the pulmonary circuit distal to its obstruction (Fig 2–7).[22,23]

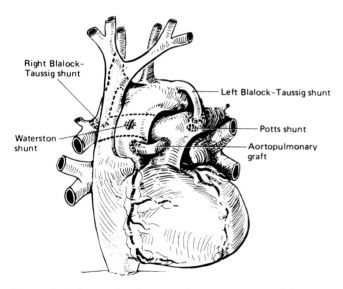

Right Blalock-Taussig shunt

Left Blalock-Taussig shunt

Potts shunt

Waterston shunt

Aortopulmonary graft

Figure 2–7. Composite diagrammatic representation of the commonly created surgical systemic arterial to pulmonary artery (PA) shunts that palliate congenital heart lesions associated with a reduction in pulmonary blood flow (PBF). In each instance, the systemic (higher-pressure) circulation is connected to the pulmonary (lower-pressure) circulation distal to an area of obstruction to normal PBF. The principle of operation of these shunts is analogous to the explanation of flow through a patent ductus arteriosus. The right or left Blalock-Taussig shunts connect the right or left subclavian artery to the right or left branch PA, respectively. The Potts shunt is a side-to-side anastomosis (aortopulmonary window) between the descending aorta and the left branch PA. The Waterston aortopulmonary window connects the ascending aorta to the right branch PA. The aortopulmonary graft signifies the fact that the systemic and pulmonary arterial circulations may be connected in any one of a variety of locations by the use of synthetic graft material. (*From Dillard DH, Miller DW: Surgery for Congenital Heart Disease: Atlas of Cardiac Surgery. New York: Macmillan, 1983, p 191, with permission.*)

The use of surgically created shunts in this fashion resulted from the recognition of the fact that some children with lesions that decreased pulmonary blood flow benefited from the presence of a PDA. The PDA is a systemic arterial to pulmonary arterial communication.[8] The direction and quantity of blood flow through a PDA depends upon the same factors listed in Equation 2–1 with the addition of the influence upon flow of the length of a vascular channel to which flow is inversely related. Shunt flow through an isolated PDA results in an increase in pulmonary blood flow specifically expressed as Equation 2–12.

PDA Q (pulmonary shunt) $\propto$

$$\frac{P(\text{Ao} > \text{PA}) \times D^4(\text{PDA})}{R(\text{SVR} > \text{PVR}) \times L(\text{PDA})} \quad (2\text{--}12)$$

where Ao = aorta, PA = pulmonary artery, L = length.

The Blalock-Taussig (BT) shunt is an example of a surgically created PDA-like systemic arterial to pulmonary arterial communication that takes advantage of the pathophysiologic factors controlling blood flow through such a vascular channel.[22,23,25] In this procedure, pulmonary blood flow is partially restored to the child with TOF when the subclavian artery is connected to the pulmonary artery distal to the obstruction of the pulmonary circulation as it exits the right ventricle. The subclavian artery thereby becomes an artificial PDA. Under these circumstances, blood flow is initially shunted away from the pulmonary vasculature as described by Equation 2–3, but subsequently shunted into the pulmonary vasculature as described in Equation 2–13, which expresses the surgically created equivalent of the PDA.

BT Q (pulmonary shunt) $\propto$

$$\frac{P(\text{SA} > \text{PA}) \times D^4(\text{SA})}{R(\text{SVR} > \text{PVR} \times L(\text{SA})} \quad (2\text{--}13)$$

where SA = subclavian artery.

Occasionally an artificial Blalock-Taussig anastomosis is created using synthetic graft material connected to both the aorta and the pulmonary artery. When this is done, the flow through this shunt will depend upon both the diameter and length selected by the surgeon. If the graft is too small in diameter and/or too long, pulmonary blood flow will be insufficiently increased and hypoxemia will persist. Conversely, if the graft is too large in diameter and/or short, pulmonary blood flow will be too great and congestive heart failure may result. This latter situation may be suspected if there is an excessive increase in arterial oxygenation upon initiating blood flow through the newly created anastomosis. An additional observation suggesting excessive pulmonary blood flow through an oversized shunt is a marked reduction in systemic diastolic blood pressure. This results from a large runoff through the shunt into the low-resistance pulmonary vasculature. The extremes of flow through the traditional Blalock-Taussig shunt do not seem to be a problem as the subclavian artery appears to be just the right diameter and length to increase pulmonary circulation a sufficient, but not excessive, quantity.

Other less commonly performed variations of systemic arterial to pulmonary arterial palliative shunts are the creation of aortopulmonary windows (side-to-side anastomosis).[22,23,26,27] In these procedures described by Potts and Waterston, the PDA-like shunt has no length and flow depends entirely upon the diameter of the window created by the surgeon and the pressure and resistance factors on both sides of this communication. The size of the aortopulmonary connection, therefore, becomes a critical pathophysiologic influence upon the adequacy of the increase in pulmonary blood flow.

Systemic Venous to Pulmonary Arterial Shunts

Another type of palliative procedure to improve pulmonary blood flow which is being used with increasing frequency is the systemic venous to pulmonary arterial shunt (Fig 2–8). Originally applied as the Glenn operation (superior vena cava to pulmonary artery anastomosis), this type of shunt is most commonly performed today as the Fontan operation (right atrial to pulmonary artery anastomosis).[28,29] The major controlling factor for blood flow from the right atrial venous circulation into the pulmonary artery is the pressure differential between these two circuits. Although all of the other factors influencing blood flow play a role, the pressure differential is most important because of the similarity in the actual pressures between these two circuits. Unless right atrial pressure is maintained in excess of the pulmonary runoff, adequate improvement of the pulmonary blood flow will not occur as a result of the creation of a Fontan anastomosis. This relationship is expressed as Equation 2–14.

$$\text{Fontan } Q \text{ (pulmonary shunt)} \propto$$
$$\frac{P(\text{RA} > \text{PA}) \times D^4(\text{Fontan})}{R(\text{PVR})} \quad (2\text{–}14)$$

Principles of Total Surgical Correction of Congenital Heart Lesions

Total correction of TOF or any of the other decreased pulmonary blood flow lesion is designed to reestablish a normal flow of blood in series fashion through the right heart into the pulmonary circuit and subsequently into the left heart and on to the systemic circuit. The ability to accomplish this depends upon the existence of four cardiac chambers and two great vessels or structures that can serve as their substitutes. Total surgical correction of hypoplastic left heart, on the other hand, cannot be ac-

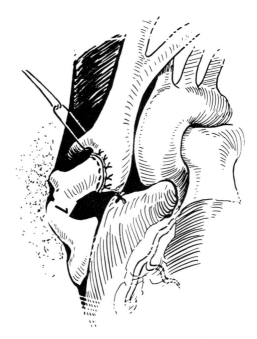

Figure 2–8. Diagramatic representation of the Glenn anastomosis. This palliative procedure improves pulmonary blood flow (PBF) for those congenital heart lesions associated with a reduction in PBF that cannot be improved by one of the more commonly performed systemic arterial to pulmonary artery (PA) palliative shunt procedures (see text and Fig 2–7 for further description). In the Glenn operation, or its modern-day counterpart, the Fontan operation (right atrial to PA anastomosis), the systemic venous blood is directed into the PA distal to an obstruction to normal PBF. The diagram displays a suture retracting the azygos vein as it joins the superior vena cava (SVC). The adjacent suture line indicates the connection created between the SVC and the right PA, which has been divided leaving the proximal end blind. The main PA can be seen as it exits from the right ventricle (midportion of the right border of the diagram) and the right branch PA can be seen passing behind the ascending aorta. The SVC has been divided from the right atrium (RA) to direct blood flow totally into the PA and not permit flow into the RA. The SVC must be disconnected from the RA in order for the Glenn shunt (systemic venous to PA) to function most efficiently. If the SVC were not divided from the RA at the time that it was anastomosed to the PA, then blood could flow from SVC to either the RA or PA depending upon which offered the least resistance to flow. (*From Dillard DH, Miller DW: Surgery for Congenital Heart Disease: Atlas of Cardiac Surgery. New York: Macmillan, 1983, p 193, with permission.*)

complished because of the presence in this lesion of only one functional ventricle and one great vessel. The one pumping chamber is needed for the production of systemic cardiac output. The one great vessel is used to create an aortic channel. Pulmonary blood flow is reestablished by the creation of an aortopulmonary PDA-like anastomosis during the first-stage repair and of a Fontan anastomosis at the later second-stage repair.[30]

There are many anatomic variations upon the two themes of shunt lesions presented, ie, congenital heart disease in which there is an intracardiac and extracardiac communication associated with either increased pulmonary blood flow or decreased pulmonary blood flow.

Many of the varieties may be viewed as falling upon a continuum of congenital heart disease. At one extreme of the continuum exist the congenital heart lesions in which blood flows across the communication toward the right ventricular outflow pathway because the flow-pressure-resistance relationship dictates this. At the other extreme of the continuum exist the congenital heart lesions that appear anatomically similar to those on the first end (possess an intracardiac or extracardiac communication) but in reality are much different. The pathophysiologic expression of these lesions is a reduction in pulmonary blood flow because of one common denominator; ie, at some point there is obstruction to right heart emptying. Whether the obstruction to right heart outflow occurs at the pulmonary valve, at the subvalvular muscular right ventricular outflow tract, in the supravalvular region with pulmonary atresia, or as far back as the tricuspid valve (ie, tricuspid atresia), blood cannot follow its normal course to the pulmonary vasculature. Its only way out of the obstructed right heart is via the intracardiac or extracardiac communication to the left heart.

Surgical correction of nonshunt obstructive lesions like AS involves increasing the diameter of the aortic orifice or totally replacing the aortic valve with a prosthesis that has sufficient diameter to allow unobstructed flow out of the left ventricle. Left ventricular outflow does not usually increase after repair of AS. Enlarging the diameter of the aortic valve and thus decreasing the resistance to flow through the left ventricular outflow tract therefore must result in a reduction of the pressure in the left ventricle (Equation 2–5).

ANESTHETIC APPLICATION OF THE PATHOPHYSIOLOGIC PRINCIPLES OF CONGENITAL HEART DISEASE

Anesthesia, like surgical manipulations, alters the pathophysiologic expression of congenital heart disease (Table 2–3). Anesthetic manipulations have the potential to affect several components of the flow-pressure-resistance relationship (eg, pressure and resistance).[6,14,31–44] Cardiac depressant effects of anesthesia may limit the ability of each ventricle to produce flow (cardiac output). If the ventricle's ability to generate pressure is affected, there may be a change in the pressure differential between chambers. Alteration in contractility may produce a desirable effect; ie, an induced muscular relaxation unobstructs a ventricular outflow pathway which had been offering resistance to blood flow. Vascular effects of anesthetic manipulations may alter pulmonary and/or systemic vascular resistance. These changes may have direct effects upon the blood flow in their respective circuits that results from the interplay of a balance between the PVR and SVR. Specific examples will clarify

TABLE 2–3. PERIANESTHETIC FACTORS INFLUENCING CARDIOVASCULAR FLOW AND RESISTANCE

Flow (cardiac output)	
Systemic and pulmonary circulations	
Increase:	Volume loading
	Chronotropic agents
	Inotropic agents
	Vasodilators (with adequate volume)
	Inhalation anesthetics*
	β-Adrenergic antagonists*
Decrease:	Inhalation anesthetics
	Hypovolemia
	Vasodilators (with inadequate volume)
	Dysrhythmias
	Ischemia
	Calcium slow channel blocking agents
	High mean airway pressure (with inadequate volume)
Resistance	
Systemic circulation	
Increase:	Sympathetic stimulation
	α-Adrenergic agonists
Decrease:	Anesthetics†
	Vasodilators
	α-Adrenergic antagonists
	β-Adrenergic agonists
	Calcium slow channel blocking agents
Pulmonary circulation	
Increase:	Hypoxia
	Hypercarbia
	Acidosis
	High mean airway pressure
	Sympathetic stimulation
	α-Adrenergic agonists
	Hypervolemia
	Anesthetics†
Decrease:	Oxygen
	Hypocarbia
	Alkalosis
	Prostaglandin E_1/prostacyclin
	α-Adrenergic antagonists
	Vasodilators
	Anesthetics†

* Indicated for congenital heart lesions in which there is hypertrophic cardiomyopathy producing ventricular outflow obstruction (right ventricle, eg, tetralogy of Fallot, or left ventricle, eg, idiopathic hypertrophic subaortic stenosis [asymmetric septal hypertrophy]) due to subvalvular muscular hypertrophy.
† Little definitive data exist that delineate the effects of anesthetics upon the pulmonary vasculature. The specific effects of anesthetics upon each individual patient's systemic or pulmonary vascular resistance are unpredictable and require physiologic assessment at the time of administration.

the effects of anesthesia upon blood flow in children with congenital heart disease.

In children with lesions that increase pulmonary blood flow, anesthetic manipulations are designed to reduce the shunt and increase systemic perfusion by increasing the ratio of right heart pressures to left heart pressures (Equation 2–2). Although it is not clinically feasible to independently regulate the right and left heart filling pressures (preload), chamber compliance, or inotropic state, right and left heart pressures may be altered by manipulation of the impedance to outflow of the respective ventricles. Less blood may be shunted into the lungs by increasing the ratio PVR/SVR (Equation 2–2). Increasing PVR promotes shunting of blood away from the lungs. Hypoxia, hypercarbia, acidosis, high mean airway pressure, sympathetic stimulation, and hypervolemia predispose to increased PVR. In the absence of clinically useful pulmonary vasoconstrictors, the avoidance of hypocarbia and the use of high mean airway pressures during ventilation (including positive end-expiratory pressure) are commonly used to maintain PVR. The use of vasodilators to reduce SVR, thereby increasing PVR/SVR, is of uncertain benefit. Vasodilators, including anesthetics, often exert similar actions on the pulmonary and systemic circulations resulting in no net change in PVR/SVR. Generalized vasoconstriction resulting from a high sympathetic tone due to light anesthesia or from vasopressor administration similarly may not alter the ratio of pulmonary blood flow to systemic blood flow.

In children with diminished pulmonary blood flow, anesthetic manipulations are designed to avoid further increases in right-to-left shunting leading to greater reductions in pulmonary blood flow. Pulmonary blood flow may be promoted and right-to-left shunting reduced by decreasing the ratio of right heart pressure to left heart pressure. This favorable alteration in the pressure gradient across the VSD may be accomplished by ameliorating the degree of right heart obstruction where possible and by maintaining of increasing SVR (Equation 2–3). Manipulation of SVR in the presence of an elevated and relatively fixed impedance to right heart outflow will produce observable alterations in shunt flow. Increasing SVR generally promotes shunting of blood into the lungs. Light levels of anesthesia and the administration of α-adrenergic agonists predisposes to maintenance or elevation of SVR. Infusion of phenylephrine into children with TOF reduces intracardiac shunting and increases systemic oxygen (O_2) tension.[45] In this instance, the vasopressor increases SVR and impedance to left heart outflow relative to right heart outflow (Equation 2–3). This results in a decrease in the right-to-left interventricular pressure gradient that reduces RV to LV shunting (Equation 2–3). Decreasing SVR, on the other hand, promotes shunting of blood away from the lungs and could intensify the shunt and create cyanosis. Vasodilators and deep levels of anesthesia can predispose to decreased SVR. If hypovolemia and systemic hypotension are superimposed on a congenital heart lesion with obstruction to pulmonary blood flow, both right-to-left shunt and cyanosis are intensified. This physiologic sequence leads to shock and cardiac arrest if unreversed. Reductions in PVR may also help in promoting pulmonary blood flow. These are accomplished by hyperventilation with a high inspired O_2 concentration and avoiding high mean airway pressure.

The flow-pressure-resistance relationship can also be applied to the non–shunt obstructive lesions. Reducing ventricular function limits the heart's ability to generate a pressure gradient and produce cardiac output in a setting in which obstruction to blood flow is present (Equation 2–5). The ability of the heart to eject stroke volume depends on the adequacy of ventricular filling and inotropic state. Excessive myocardial depression, hypovolemia, and loss of properly timed atrial systole are to be avoided. Adequate regulation of SVR is essential to provide important coronary perfusion pressure. Control of impedance to LV outflow is equally important, however, and excessive increases in this resistance to flow are to be avoided in nonshunt obstructive lesions (Equation 2–5).

Anesthetic depression of cardiac contractility is not always detrimental. In contrast to adults with valvular stenosis, AS and PS in children is often subvalvular (ie, infundibular) in location. Forward blood flow and myocardial O_2 balance may be altered by modifying the degree of infundibular obstruction in these lesions (Equation 2–3). In TOF, for example, the RV outflow tract is obstructed by a subvalvular muscular stenosis (subpulmonic muscular hypertrophy). Infundibular RV outflow tract obstruction can be exacerbated by tachycardia and hypovolemia, which reduce ventricular size, and by excessive contractility. This can increase the degree of muscular contraction and obstruction intensifying the abnormal shunt (Equation 2–3). Systemic vasodilation may also impair RV infundibular outflow by causing a reflex increase in heart rate and contractility. Avoidance of excessive sympathetic tone, provision of adequate venous return, and control of SVR are desirable in this setting (Equation 2–3). The negative chronotropic and inotropic actions of anesthetics and β-adrenergic agonists can be used to advantage to reduce muscular RV outflow tract obstruction.

Application of the flow-pressure-resistance principles in the selection of an anesthetic technique for children with congenital heart disease can be accomplished by use of a "cardiac grid" (Fig 2–9).[31] Once the desired hemodynamic parameters are decided, appropriate pharmacologic therapy can be selected to achieve them.

SUMMARY

The intent of this chapter is not to catalogue every congenital cardiac malformation, discuss its pathophysiology, and describe how it might be dealt with by either the surgeon or the anesthesiologist. Although these very things were done for many congenital heart lesions, these were selected only as examples. They serve as models for future reference in the analysis of unfamiliar anatomy

	Preload	Pulm. Vasc. Resistance	Syst. Vasc. Resistance	HR	Contractility
ASD	↑	↑	↓	N	N
VSD (R→L)	N	↓	↑	N	N
VSD (L→R)	↑	↑	↓	N	N
IHSS	↑	N	N-↑	*↓	*↓
PDA	↑	↑	↓	N	N
Coarct.	↑	N	↓	N	N
Valvular Pulm. Sten.	↑	↓	N	↓	↑
Infundibular Pulm. Sten.	↑	↓	N	↓	*↓
AS	↑	N	*↑	*↓	N-↑
MS	↑	N-↓	N	*↓	N-↑
AR	↑	N	↓	N-↑	N-↑
MR	↑	N-↓	↓	N-↑	N-↑

* — An overriding consideration.

Figure 2–9. Cardiac grid for common congenital heart diseases showing desired hemodynamic changes. A cardiac grid can be used for the selection of an anesthetic technique for a child with congenital heart disease. When the diagnosis is established, the desired control of hemodynamic parameters is identified. The utility of the grid is based upon the application of the relationship $Q \propto P/R$, where Q = flow; P = pressure gradient(s); and R = resistance(s) to blood flow. Abbreviations: ASD, atrial septal defect; VSD, ventricular septal defect; IHSS, idiopathic hypertrophic subaortic stenosis; PDA, patent ductus arteriosis; AS, aortic stenosis; MS, mitral stenosis; AR, aortic regurgitation; MR, mitral regurgitation. (*From Moore RA: Anesthesia for the pediatric congenital heart patient for noncardiac surgery. Anesthesiol Rev 8(12):23–29, 1981, with permission.*)

and its pathophysiologic expressions. It would be impossible to exhaust all considerations on this topic, for undoubtedly new and innovative surgical and medical (pharmacologic) therapies will be devised for congenital heart disease. When they are, it will be incumbent upon the anesthesiologists caring for these children to decipher the pathophysiologic consequences. This will be simple, however, if the flow-pressure-resistance "plumbing" relationship is applied in systematic fashion.

REFERENCES

1. Wegman ME: Annual summary of vital statistics—1985. *Pediatrics* **78**:983–994, 1986
2. Motoyama EK, Smith MS: *Anesthesia for Infants and Children*, 5th ed. St. Louis: C. V. Mosby, 1990
3. Keith JD: Prevalence, incidence and epidemiology. In Keith JD, Rowe RD, Vlad P (eds): *Heart Disease in Infancy and Childhood*, 3rd ed. New York: Macmillan, 1978, pp 3–11
4. Adams FH, Emmanouilides GC: *Moss' Heart Disease in Infants, Children, and Adolescents*, 4th ed. Baltimore: Williams & Wilkins, 1989
5. Morgan BC: Incidence, etiology, and classification of congenital heart disease. *Pediatr Clin North Am* **25**:721–723, 1978
6. Campbell FW, Schwartz AJ: Anesthesia for noncardiac surgery in the pediatric patient with congenital heart disease. *Refresher Courses Anesthesiol* **14**:75–98, 1986
7. Perloff JK: Introduction: Formulation of the problem. In

The Clinical Recognition of Congenital Heart Disease, 2nd ed. Philadelphia: W.B. Saunders, 1978, pp 1–7
8. Fink BW: *Congenital Heart Disease: A Deductive Approach to Its Diagnosis*, 2nd ed. Chicago: Year Book Medical, 1985
9. Stevenson JG: Acyanotic lesions with normal pulmonary blood flow. *Pediatr Clin North Am* **25**:725–742 1978
10. Stevenson JG: Acyanotic lesions with increased pulmonary blood flow. *Pediatr Clin North Am* **25**:743–758, 1978
11. Kawabori I: Cyanotic congenital heart defects with decreased pulmonary blood flow. *Pediatr Clin North Am* **25**:759–776, 1978
12. Kawabori I: Cyanotic congenital heart defects with increased pulmonary blood flow. *Pediatr Clin North Am* **25**:777–795, 1978
13. Young D: Pathophysiology of congenital heart disease. *Int Anesthesiol Clin* **18**:5–26, 1980
14. Schwartz AJ, Jobes DR: Congenital heart disease—Special anesthetic considerations. In Conahan TJ (ed): *Cardiac Anesthesia*. Menlo Park, CA: Addison-Wesley, 1982, pp 62–91
15. Ference M, Lemon HB, Stephenson RJ: *Analytical Experimental Physics*, 3rd ed. Chicago: University of Chicago Press, 1956, pp 278–310
16. MacIntosh R, Mushin WW, Epstein HG: *Physics for the Anaesthetist*, 3rd ed. Oxford, England: Blackwell Scientific, 1963, pp 156–167
17. Schlant RC: Altered cardiovascular function of congenital heart disease. In Hurst JW (ed): *The Heart*, 4th ed. New York: McGraw-Hill, 1978, pp 813–830
18. Blalock A, Hanlon CR: The surgical treatment of com-

plete transposition of the aorta and the pulmonary artery. *Surg Gynecol Obstet* **90**:1–15, 1950

19. Watson H, Rashkind WJ: Creation of atrial septal defects by balloon catheter in babies with transposition of the great arteries. *Lancet* **1**:403–405, 1967

20. Liebman J, Borkat G, Hirshfeld S: The heart. In Klaus MH, Fanaroff AA (eds): *Care of the High Risk Neonate*, 2nd ed. Philadelphia: W.B. Saunders, 1979, pp 294–323

21. Eliot RS, Edwards JE: Pathology of congenital heart disease. In Hurst JW (ed): *The Heart*, 4th ed. New York: McGraw-Hill, 1978, pp 782–783

22. Dillard DH, Miller DW: *Surgery for Congenital Heart Disease: Atlas of Cardiac Surgery*. New York: Macmillan, 1983, pp 165–255

23. Bernhard WF, Litwin SB, Jones JE: Cardiac surgery in infants. In Norman JC (ed): *Cardiac Surgery*, 2nd ed. New York: Appleton-Century-Crofts, 1972, pp 251–278

24. Wood P: The Eisenmenger syndrome or pulmonary hypertension with reversed central shunt. *Br Med J* **2**:701–709, 755–762, 1958

25. Blalock A, Taussig HB: The surgical treatment of malformations of the heart in which there is pulmonary stenosis or pulmonary atresia. *JAMA* **128**:189–202, 1945

26. Potts WJ, Smith S, Gibson S: Anastomosis of the aorta to a pulmonary artery. *JAMA* **132**:627–631, 1946

27. Kirklin JW, Pacifico AD: Tetralogy of Fallot. In Ravitch MM, Welch KJ, Berson CD, et al (eds): *Pediatric Surgery*, Vol 1, 3rd ed. Chicago: Year Book Medical, 1979, pp 706–714

28. Glenn WWL: Circulatory bypass of the right heart. *N Engl J Med* **259**:117–120, 1958

29. Fontan F, Baudet E: Surgical repair of tricuspid atresia. *Thorax* **26**:240–248, 1971

30. Norwood WI, Lang P, Hansen DD: Physiologic repair of aortic atresia-hypoplastic left heart syndrome. *N Engl J Med* **308**:23–26, 1983

31. Moore RA: Anesthesia for the pediatric congenital heart patient for noncardiac surgery. *Anesthesiol Rev* **8**(12):23–29, 1981

32. Aviado DM: The pharmacology of the pulmonary circulation. *Pharmacol Rev* **12**:159–239, 1960

33. Moffitt EA, McGoon DC, Ritter DG: The diagnosis and correction of congenital cardiac defects. *Anesthesiology* **33**:144–160, 1970

34. Laver MB, Bland JHL: Anesthetic management of the pediatric patient during open heart surgery. *Int Anesthesiol Clin* **13**:149–182, 1975

35. Hug CC: Pharmacology—Anesthetic drugs. In Kaplan JA (ed): *Cardiac Anesthesia*. New York: Grune & Stratton, 1979, pp 3–37

36. Reves JG, Kissin I: Pharmacology of anesthetic drugs: Intravenous anesthetics. In Kaplan JA (ed): *Cardiac Anesthesia*, Vol 2. New York: Grune & Stratton, 1983, pp 3–29

37. Moldenhauer CC: New narcotics. In Kaplan JA (ed): *Cardiac Anesthesia*, Vol 2. New York: Grune & Stratton, 1983, pp 31–78

38. Curling PE, Noback CR; Inhalational anesthetics: Isoflurane and nitrous oxide. In Kaplan JA (ed): *Cardiac Anesthesia*, Vol 2. New York: Grune & Stratton, 1983, pp 95–121

39. Strong MJ, Keats AS, Cooley DA: Arterial gas tensions under anaesthesia in tetralogy of Fallot. *Br J Anaesth* **39**:472–479, 1967

40. Landry LD, Emerson CW, Philbin DM, et al: The effect of nitrous oxide on pulmonary vascular resistance in children. *Anesth Analg* **59**:548–549, 1980

41. Schulte-Sasse M, Hess W, Tarnow V: Pulmonary vascular response to nitrous oxide in patients with normal and high pulmonary vascular resistance. *Anesthesiology* **57**:9–13, 1982

42. Hickey PR, Hansen DD: Fentanyl and sufentanil-oxygen-pancuronium anesthesia for cardiac surgery in infants. *Anesth Analg* **63**:117–124, 1984

43. Hickey PR, Hansen DD, Wessel DL, et al: Blunting of stress responses in the pulmonary circulation of infants by fentanyl. *Anesth Analg* **64**:1137–1142, 1985

44. Hickey PR, Hansen DD, Cramolini GM, et al: Pulmonary and systemic hemodynamic responses to ketamine in infants with normal and elevated pulmonary vascular resistance. *Anesthesiology* **62**:287–293, 1985

45. Nudel DB, Berman MA, Talner NS: Effects of acutely increasing systemic vascular resistance on oxygen tension in tetralogy of Fallot. *Pediatrics* **58**:248–251, 1976

Chapter 3 | Cardiovascular Embryology, Growth, and Development

Carol L. Lake

A knowledge of cardiac embryology is essential to the understanding of the congenital cardiac defects that are discussed in subsequent chapters. Cardiac anomalies occur in about 8 out of every 1000 births. Congenital heart disease is often associated with other major chromosomal abnormalities and appears to have little effect in utero.[1] Although older studies[2] suggested a prevalence of heart defects among stillborn infants, recent work suggests a similar spectrum in defects in both liveborn and stillborn infants.[1]

Screening for cardiac defects during prenatal life by echocardiography is now practical[3–5] (Fig 3–1). Indeed a recent study noted the occurrence of congenital cardiac anomalies in 1 of 52 fetuses with an affected sibling and in 1 of 10 fetuses with two siblings with cardiac disease.[6] No association of in utero cardiac anomalies and parental congenital cardiac defects was noted.[6] However, older studies suggested various familial and genetic factors as the etiology of cardiac malformations.[7]

EARLY CARDIAC DEVELOPMENT

Embryonic Development

Cardiac Tube Formation. The development of the embryonic heart occurs between 3 and 8 weeks of gestation. At about day 20, mesenchymal cells, known as angiogenic clusters, accumulate on the lateral sides of the embryo and spread cephalad. These cells subsequently arrange themselves into the cardiogenic area, the pericardial cavity, and the dorsal aortae. The tubes of angiogenic cells approach each other as the embryo lifts itself from the yolk sac. They also differentiate into three portions by means of two constrictions: the bulboventricular and atrioventricular sulci. The three major sections of the developing heart of the 1.5- to 2.0-mm embryo are (1) cephalic or bulbar, (2) middle ventricular, and (3) caudal atrial portions.[8] Fusion of these tubes ventral to the foregut occurs at 23 days of gestation (Fig 3–2). Between the tubes is an amorphous material termed the *cardiac jelly,* which is eventually invaded by mesenchymal cells. By this stage, the cardiac tube makes contact with the umbilicovitelline veins and the developing dorsal aortae. The atria join the extrapericardial venous channels to form the sinus venosus, which receives the umbilical and vitelline veins.

Cardiac Loop Formation. Subsequent development includes the formation of the atrioventriculobulbar loop in the 3.0- to 3.5-mm embryo (Fig 3–3). As the heart tube elongates, the cephalic portion bends ventrally, caudally, and rightward while the caudal portion bends leftward, dorsally, and cranially. With loop formation, the mesocardiac and bulboventricular regions are approximated. During loop formation, the atrioventricular junction remains narrow to form the atrioventricular canal.[9] The bulbus cordis is narrow except in the proximal third where the trabeculated portion of the right ventricle will form.[9] The junction of the bulbus cordis with the ventricle, which is indicated externally by the bulboventricular sulcus, remains narrow and is the primary interventricular foramen.[9] The primitive left ventricle and right ventricle are on either side of this foramen. Trabeculated areas developing proximally and distally to the interventricular foramen form the primitive left and right ventricles.

The right and left portions of the common atria emerge posteriorly (dorsal to the bulbus cordis and ventricle) from the loop as does the sinus venosus. Prior to this stage, the sinus venosus is connected to both atria, but deepening of the right and left atriovenous sulci occurs to remove the connection with the left atrium. The atrioventricular junction assumes a cranial position and becomes the atrioventricular canal. Right, left, and trans-

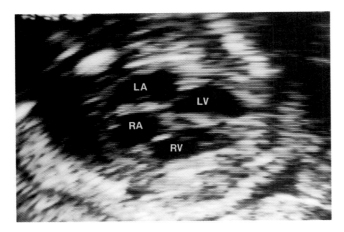

Figure 3–1. A normal four-chamber view of the fetal heart in utero. LA = left atrium; LV = left ventricle; RA = right atrium; RV = right ventricle. (*Photograph courtesy of Dr. Karen Rheuban.*)

verse horns are present in the sinus venosus.[8] The horns of the sinus venosus receive blood from (1) vitelline veins, (2) umbilical veins, and (3) common cardinal vein. In the 7.5-mm embryo at 4–5 weeks of gestation, blood flow shifts from the left umbilical vein to the right, which causes an enlargement of the right horn. This is further accentuated by the development of the anastomotic channel between right and left pericardial veins, which shifts blood to the right pericardial vein. The left horn loses importance when the left umbilical and left vitelline veins are obliterated. The right horn of the sinus venosus is absorbed into the developing right atrium, whereas the left horn becomes the coronary sinus and the oblique vein of the left atrium (oblique vein of Marshall).[8]

As the embryo increases in size from 4 to 17 mm, the atrial canal is reoriented to the bulbus portion, the bulbus portion is absorbed into the developing ventricle, septa develop in the atria and ventricle, and the common pulmonary vein is absorbed into the left atrium.

Resultant Anomalies

Initially the cardiogenic area is anterior to the neural crest and neural plate of the developing embryo. With rapid growth of the central nervous system, the developing cardiac structures are pulled forward and rotated to lie ventral to the neural structures. In a chick embryo model, removal of portions of the neural crest correlates with persistent truncus arteriosus, double outlet right ventricle, and ventricular septal defects.[10–12] Neural crest cells from the cranial region of the neural fold contribute to the cardiac outflow tract, and recent studies suggest an association between cardiac and noncardiac anomalies resulting from maldevelopment of the neural crest.[13] This region also contributes the cardiac ganglia.[11] The cardiac neural crest migrates through the branchial arches toward the outflow tract of the heart during the period when the heart is migrating craniocaudad.[10]

Cardiac Contraction and Circulation. During cardiac development, myogenic contraction occurs first in the ventriculobulbar portion, atrial portion, and last in the sinus venosus by the end of the fourth week of intrauterine life. The conducting system is formed somewhat later. Circulation is present in the 3- 4-mm embryo with blood flowing from the sinus venosus to right atrium, left atrium, the descending limb of the bulboventricular loop, the ascending limb of the bulboventricular loop, and out through the truncus.[14]

DEVELOPMENT OF THE ATRIAL AND VENTRICULAR SEPTA

The Interatrial Septum

The interatrial septum primum develops in the roof of the common atrium and grows toward the endocardial cushions in the atrioventricular canal. The space between the interatrial septum and the developing endocardial cushions is the ostium primum (Fig 3–4). When the interatrial septum is nearly completed by the growth of the endocardial cushions, perforations develop

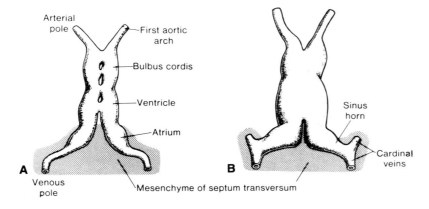

Figure 3–2. (*A*) Fusion of the paired cardiac tubes at 21 days' gestation; (*B*) the fused heart with the sinus horn. The three portions of the heart in its early development, the bulbus cordis, ventricle, and atrium, are demonstrated. (*From Sadler TW: Langman's Medical Embryology. Baltimore: Williams & Wilkins, 1990, p 182, with permission.*)

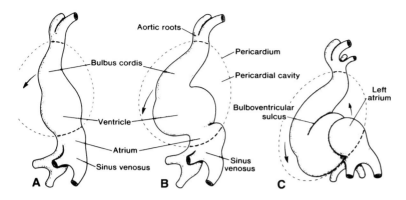

Figure 3–3. Formation of the cardiac loop. (*A*) The fused heart tube grows unequally on the right side and in its ventricular portion and must bend in response to cellular factors as well as limited space. (*B, C*) The cephalic portion bends ventrally and caudad, whereas the atrial portion shifts slightly to the left and cranially, so that mesocardial and bulboventricular portions are approximated. (*From Sadler TW: Langman's Medical Embryology. Baltimore: Williams & Wilkins, 1990, p 183, with permission.*)

in the septum primum that coalesce to form the ostium secundum. The septum secundum develops to close this defect by an infolding of the wall of the right atrium after the incorporation of the left sinus horn (Table 3–1). As the heart develops, the two septa approximate further leaving the foramen ovale, the remnant of the ostium secundum. The upper part of the septum primum becomes the valve of the foramen ovale. However, blood still flows from the higher-pressure right atrium into the left through an obliquely elongated passage until birth.

Resultant Congenital Defects. If the septum secundum is unable to approximate to the septum primum or the ostium secundum is unusually large, a secundum atrial septal defect is present. Persistence of the ostium primum usually results from faulty fusion of the anterior and posterior endocardial cushions and is associated with a cleft in the anterior leaflet of the mitral valve. The sinus venosus defect occurs when the sinus venosus is abnormally fused with the right atrium (see Chapter 13).

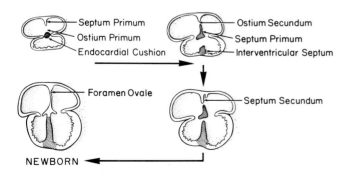

Figure 3–4. The embryologic development of the interatrial septum. The septum primum and ostium primum are the first stage. When the septum primum has grown to nearly close the ostium primum, a second opening, the ostium secundum, develops. To the right of the septum primum, the septum secundum develops to approximate with the septum primum to close the ostium secundum. (*From Lake CL: Cardiovascular Anesthesia. New York: Springer-Verlag, 1985, p 168, with permission. Drawn after description in Sadler TW: Langman's Medical Embryology. Baltimore: Williams & Wilkins, 1990.*)

The Interventricular Septum

Development of the interventricular septum occurs from the primordial septum of the original cardiac tube, the bulboventricular flange of the bulboventricular loop (bulbus cordis), and the endocardial cushions. This occurs in embryos of 5–6 mm. Initially the AV canal enters only the primitive left ventricle, but decreasing prominence of the bulboventricular flange and simultaneous growth of the right side of the AV canal allows blood to pass into both ventricles.[9] The medial walls of the growing ventricles become apposed and gradually fuse together to form the muscular portion of the interventricular sep-

TABLE 3–1. EVENTS IN HUMAN CARDIAC EMBRYOLOGY

Gestational Age (days)	Size of Embryo (mm)	Event
18	1.0–1.5	Earliest cardiac tissue appears
20	1.5–2.5	Sulci of cardiac tube appear, dividing it into bulbar, ventricular, and atrial portions
22	3.0–3.5	Cardiac loop formation; heart begins beating
26	3.5–5.0	Septum primum appears; AV canal defined
28	5–6	AV cushions present; conotruncal ridges form
32	6–7	AV cushions are approximating; truncus is dividing into aorta and pulmonary artery; sinus node present
33	7–9	AV bundle present; left and right AV canals defined
37	9–11	AV node present; semilunar cusps developing; ostium secundum formed
41	11–14	Ostium primum closed; papillary muscles present; pacemaker action potentials identified; coronary arteries developing
44	14–17	Interventricular septum closed; aortic and pulmonic valves formed; AV valves forming
47–57	17–31	General increase in cardiac size

(*Data from references 9, 16, 76, and 77.*)

tum. The membranous portion results from the merger of the lower portions of the conus arteriosus ridges with the endocardial cushions. Ventricular septation is usually completed between 35 and 42 days.

Resultant Congenital Defects. Failure of fusion of the endocardial cushions and other septa result in ventricular septal defects (VSDs). The location of the defect (membranous versus muscular) and the extent (single versus multiple) depend upon the specific portion that failed to approximate (see Chapter 13).

DEVELOPMENT OF THE ATRIOVENTRICULAR VALVES

Development of the atrioventricular valves occurs in the 6-mm embryo when the superior, inferior, and lateral atrioventricular endocardial cushions divide the atrioventricular canal. The lateral endocardial cushions develop on the right and left edges of the canal. These four cushions fuse to create right and left atrioventricular canals (see Table 3–1). There are three periods in valve development: (1) the leaflets are formed in the 11- to 23-mm embryo; (2) valves are attached to the ventricular wall by muscular cords, chordae tendineae; and (3) dense connective tissue replaces muscle in the cords, which are connected to the ventricular wall by trabeculations (papillary muscles). Both the aortic leaflet of the mitral valve and the anterior leaflet of the tricuspid valve are formed from fused anterior and posterior endocardial cushions. The lateral endocardial cushions form the inferior leaflets of the mitral and tricuspid valves.

Resultant Congenital Anomalies

Tricuspid atresia results when the atrioventricular canal migrates incompletely to the right. The tricuspid valve

forms normally from portions of the interventricular septum and endocardial cushions. Mitral stenosis may result from a hemodynamic origin, lack of blood flow on the left side of the heart, particularly when it is associated with generalized aortic hypoplasia. Because the endocardial cushions form portions of the interatrial and interventricular septa as well as the tricuspid and mitral valves, alterations in fusion result in a variable group of defects, including atrial septal defect, ventricular septal defect, cleft mitral or tricuspid leaflets, alone or in combination with one another. These defects are termed *endocardial cushion defects* and result in ostium primum defects, persistent common atrioventricular canal, or membranous ventricular septal defects (see Chapters 13 and 19).

DEVELOPMENT OF THE AORTA AND PULMONARY ARTERY

Aortic Arch and Valve

Aortic Arches. A total of six pairs of aortic arches develop from the distal truncus arteriosus or aortic sac. The arches disappear at various times during embryonic development but terminate in the two dorsal aortae (Fig 3–5). As the third arch forms in the 3- 5-mm embryo, the first two arches disappear with portions remaining as the maxillary, hyoid, and stapedial arteries. The third pair of arches form the origin of the carotid arteries and the dorsal aorta persists beyond the third arch as the carotid arteries themselves. External carotid arteries develop as separate vessels on the third arches. The dorsal aortae fuse at day 25, forming a single dorsal aorta. It atrophies between the third and fourth arches and between the common dorsal aorta and subclavian in the 14- to 16-mm embryo. The fourth arches, together with the third, draw

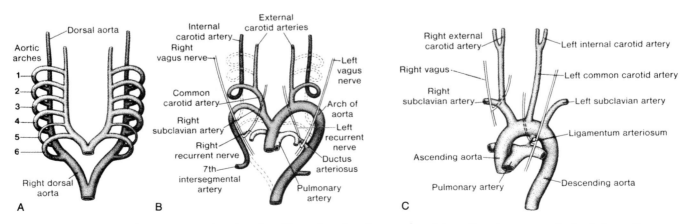

Figure 3–5. Normal development of aortic arches. The early embryo has a series of six aortic arches communicating between the dorsal and ventral aortas in (*A*). (*B*) The adult aorta and great vessels develop from the third, fourth, and sixth arches, whereas the first two arches largely disappear and the fifth arch forms only transiently. (*C*) The postnatal configuration of the great arteries is present. (*From Sadler TW: Langman's Medical Embryology. Baltimore: Williams & Wilkins, 1990, p 210, with permission.*)

out the aortic sac into right and left horns. Of these horns, the right becomes the brachiocephalic trunk, whereas the left (together with the left fourth arch) becomes the arch of the aorta. The aorta thus begins to assume its final configuration, having formed from the common dorsal aorta and the left fourth arch. The right fourth arch comprises the proximal subclavian artery. The fifth arch appears only transiently, if at all. The right portion of the sixth or pulmonary arch becomes the proximal right pulmonary artery. The left sixth arch persists as the ductus arteriosus. Thus, only the third, fourth, and sixth arches develop into permanent vessels.

Truncus Arteriosus Septation. Separation of the truncus arteriosus, or truncal artery, which is the main outlet from the developing heart into the aorta and pulmonary artery, occurs during the fourth week of gestation (Fig 3–6). The truncus arteriosus is joined to the ventricle by the conus arteriosus, a conical shaped portion of the heart at the level of the eventual aortic and pulmonic valves. The combination of the conus and truncus arteriosus is the conotruncal channel. In the lining of the conotruncal channel, two spiraled and opposed rows of swellings, the truncoconal cushions (formed from swellings in the truncus and the conus) form. Cells in the truncoconal cushions are of neural crest origin. The rotation of the spiral is clockwise. The truncoconal ridges spiral caudad to form a spiral septum dividing the conotruncal channel into two parts and also to join with the endocardial cushions and ventricular septum[15] (see Table 3–1). The truncoconal septum spirals through 180° so that the aortic channel, which is ventral at the level of the aortic arches (aortic sac), is dorsal of the bulbotruncal region at the site of aortic valve formation (see Fig 3–6).

The aortic valve develops from three tubercles within the aorta at the level of the truncus-conus junction at 6 to 9 weeks of gestation. Resorption of tissue from the aortic-tubercle junction results in the sinuses of Valsalva.

Resultant Congenital Defects. Aortic stenosis results from abnormal formation and fusion of the bulbar cushions but is also affected by hemodynamic alterations. If the division of the truncus is unequal, pulmonic infundibular stenosis results because the conotruncal septum was displaced anteriorly. Coarctation results from a lack of blood flow on the left side of the heart, an abnormality of the fourth arch (hypoplasia), or an abnormality in the media of the aorta with intimal proliferation. A right aortic arch occurs when the left fourth arch and left dorsal aorta are obliterated and replaced by the corresponding vessels on the right side. It may pass behind the esophagus and together with the ductus arteriosus form a vascular ring that constricts the trachea and esophagus. Double aortic arch results when the right fourth dorsal arch fails to regress. It may produce a vascular ring. In general, vascular rings around the trachea or esophagus (normally posterior to the great vessels) result from abnormal regression of structures that normally remain patent and failure of regression of structures that normally regress. Truncus arteriosus, resulting from failure of maturation of the truncoconal ridges, prevents the separation of the pulmonary and systemic circuits (see Chapter 20). Abnormal rotation during truncal separation produces transposition of the great vessels (see Chapter 15). Patent ductus arteriosus results when the distal portion of the sixth arch fails to involute after birth. A bicuspid aortic valve results from failure of formation of the truncoconal ridges.[15]

Coronary Arteries

Coronary arteries develop from thickenings in the aortic endothelium of the 10- to 12-mm embryo. The left coronary artery develops earlier than the right.[16] The coronaries pass to the side of the bulbus cordis. The circumflex artery is developed in the 14-mm embryo and all of the larger branches are present in the 20-mm embryo.[11] Cardiac veins appear before the coronary arteries.[16]

Anomalies of the Coronary Arteries. The most common situation is anomalous origin of the coronary arteries from the pulmonary artery. The left coronary may have a short common trunk or separate orifices for anterior descending and circumflex arteries. The right coronary artery may arise from the left coronary cusp of the aortic valve. The dominance (which coronary artery crosses the crux of the heart) of the coronary circulation may vary. Usually it is the right coronary that is dominant[17] (see Chapter 21).

Pulmonary Artery

The pulmonic valve and right ventricular infundibulum develop during 8–12 weeks of gestation. The valve forms from three tubercles within the pulmonary artery that initially enlarge and then thin out by resorption, whereas the infundibulum develops from the bulbus cordis. Simultaneously the division of the truncus arteriosus into aorta and pulmonary artery occurs. The sixth aortic arch develops into right, left, and distal pulmonary arteries.

Resultant Congenital Defects. Infundibular pulmonic stenosis results from abnormal incorporation of the bulbus into the right ventricle. Right ventricular outflow tract obstruction can also result from incomplete involution of the crista supraventricularis as right ventricular mass decreases during postnatal life.[18] The crista also may hypertrophy to obstruct right ventricular outflow.[18] Valvular stenosis results from faulty development of the bulbar cushions. Tetralogy of Fallot is a complex defect resulting from underdevelopment of the pulmonic infundibulum. It occurs when there is unequal division of the truncus arteriosus with an anterior displacement of the truncoconal septum (see Chapters 14, 15, 18, and 20).

Thoracic and Abdominal Aorta

The paired dorsal aortae fuse in the seventh week beginning at the level of the seventh cervical vertebra. Lateral, ventral, and dorsal arteries arising from the dorsal aortae supply each embryonic segment. From these segmental branches, the vertebral, intercostal, and lumbar arteries develop in the neck, thorax, and abdomen. Ventral segmental arteries, which become initially vitelline arteries, fuse to become the celiac, superior mesenteric, and inferior mesenteric arteries supplying the gut. Lateral segmental arteries supply the developing urogenital system.

Arteries to the upper and lower extremities develop from the aortic arches (subclavian) and the umbilical arteries (sciatic and external iliac arteries). The sciatic system eventually disappears and the ileofemoral system becomes the dominant supply. The subclavian arteries attach to the axillary, brachial, and anterior interosseus branches of the developing arm arteries.

Resultant Congenital Defects. Anomalies of peripheral arterial development are uncommon. They include persistent sciatic artery (0.05%), single umbilical artery (0.75–1.1%), and aberrant popliteal artery with entrapment by the gastrocnemius muscle.[19]

DEVELOPMENT OF THE VENOUS SYSTEM

Systemic Veins

There are three paired sets of veins in the 3-mm embryo. These are the cardinal veins draining the embryo, the vitelline veins draining the yolk sac, and the umbilical veins draining the chorion and carrying oxygenated blood to the fetus. Hepatic development affects the vitelline veins by converting them into hepatic sinusoids, portal vein, and hepatic veins. The umbilical veins pass through the hepatic sinusoids as the liver enlarges. Only a portion of the left umbilical vein remains as the right and proximal left umbilical vein disappear. Blood passes from the placenta through the left umbilical vein, which connects to the right hepatocardiac channel to form the ductus venosus for placental blood to bypass the liver sinusoids en route to the heart.

Inferior Vena Cava. The inferior vena cava forms between 6 and 10 weeks of gestation from the cardinal venous system consisting of posterior cardinal, supracardinal, sacrocardinal, and subcardinal veins (Fig 3–7). The posterior cardinal system that develops first at 6 weeks on the posterior aspect of the fetus atrophies in the 15-mm embryo when the supracardinal veins develop. During their existence, anterior and posterior cardinal veins join to form the duct of Cuvier, which opens into the sinus venosus.[20] The most distal portion of the cardinal system anastomoses to become the iliac bifurcation.[21] Subcardinal veins are the next to develop (at 7 weeks) to take over the function of the posterior cardinal veins and an anastomosis develops between them.[21] The left portion of this system regresses, whereas the right remains to form the suprarenal or prerenal inferior vena cava.[21] In the embryo of 11 mm, the hepatic portion of the inferior vena cava develops from the vitelline veins. Thus, the inferior vena cava develops from a fusion of the vitelline, subcardinal, and supracardinal veins.

Supracardinal veins develop at about 8 weeks of gestation. Subcardinal and supracardinal veins form extensive anastomoses at the level of the renal vein. The caudal portion of the supracardinals becomes the postrenal inferior vena cava, whereas anastomoses between supracardinal and subcardinal veins form the renal segment of the inferior vena cava. These channels unite to form a large vein, anterior and posterior to the kidney, that eventually joins the inferior vena cava.[21] Regression of the posterior vein occurs, whereas the anterior vein becomes the left renal vein.[21] In summary, the inferior vena cava from cephalad to caudad develops from the (1)

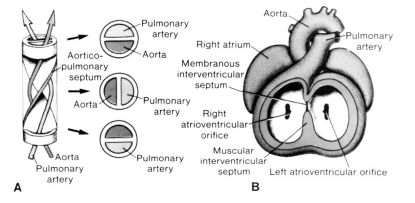

Figure 3–6. The division of the truncus arteriosus into the aorta and pulmonary artery. The truncoconal swellings grow toward each other in a spiral pattern (*A*). This produces not only division of the truncus into two great vessels but also the spiral orientation of the aorta and pulmonary artery to each other (*B*). (*From Sadler TW: Langman's Medical Embryology. Baltimore: Williams & Wilkins, 1990, p 197, with permission.*)

A

B

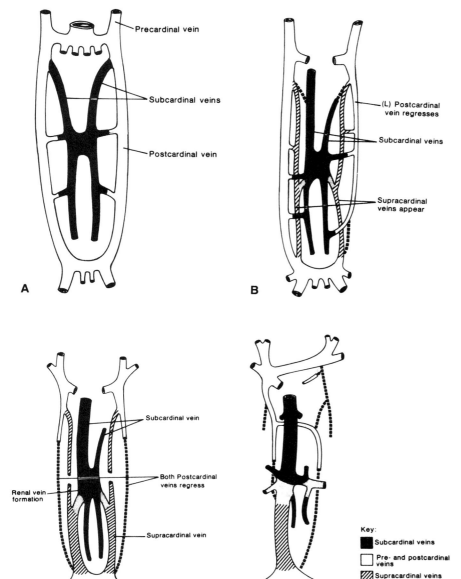

Figure 3–7. The development of the systemic veins. (*A*) The venous system at a gestational age of 6 weeks with the pre-, sub-, and postcardinal veins present. (*B*) The supracardinal veins appear at 7 weeks, whereas the left postcardinal vein regresses. (*C*) The formation of the suprarenal inferior vena cava from the subcardinal system at 8 weeks. (*D*) The fully developed or postnatal inferior vena cava, indicating its embryologic origins from the cardinal veins. Both subcardinal and supracardinal veins form the renal veins. (*From Giordano JM, Trout HH: Anomalies of the inferior vena cava. J Vasc Surg 3:924–928, 1986, with permission.*)

terminal right vitelline vein, (*2*) anastomosis of right vitelline and right cardinal veins, (*3*) right subcardinal vein, (*4*) caudal right supracardinal vein, and (*5*) posterior intercardinal anastomosis (see Fig 3–7).

Superior Vena Cava and Azygous System. The cranial portions of the right supracardinal vein plus a portion of the posterior cardinal vein becomes the azygous system.[21] The left supracardinal becomes the hemiazygous vein after a communication develops between the two supracardinal veins. The superior vena cava develops from the right anterior cardinal vein of the pericardial system and right common cardinal vein in the 20-mm embryo. The left superior vena cava is composed of the left superior intercostal vein, lower oblique vein, and a middle segment uniting the two. It normally atrophies when the left superior vena cava connects with the right via the brachiocephalic vein.[23] Left brachiocephalic and internal jugular veins form from the left pericardinal vein.

Resultant Venous Anomalies. Persistence of the left superior cava occurs when the communication between the left pericardinal and left common cardinal veins is retained. It is essentially a duplication of the superior vena cava.

Five anomalies result from abnormal embryogenesis of the inferior vena cava vasculature: (1) duplication or double inferior vena cava, (2) transposition or left-sided vena cava, (3) circumaortic left renal vein, (4) retroaortic left renal vein, and (5) azygous continuation or absent inferior vena cava.[20] Duplication occurs when the left renal supracardinal vein fails to regress. Retroaortic left renal vein occurs when the vein anterior to the aorta regresses and the vein posterior persists, exactly opposite to the normal situation. Circumaortic left renal vein results from failure of regression of the vein posterior to the aorta, so that the anterior and posterior veins form a collar around the aorta.[21] The left inferior vena cava results from failure of involution of the left cardinal system and regression of the right cardinal system.[24] Absence of the inferior vena cava occurs when the right supracardinal vein fails to join the hepatic vein and only the hepatic segment of the inferior vena cava is absent. Thus blood from the postrenal vena cava returns via the azygous or hemiazygous systems[20] (see Chapter 15).

Pulmonary Veins

The pulmonary vein originates from an outgrowth of endothelium-lined mesenchymal tissue from the lung buds that coalesces into a common pulmonary vein. The common pulmonary vein is absorbed into the left atrium at the same time the sinus venosus is absorbed into the right atrium. The absorption processes causes the four pulmonary veins to enter the left atrium separately.

Resultant Cardiac Anomalies. Anomalous pulmonary venous drainage results when the presplanchnic channels in the lung unite with the pericardinal veins (supracardiac anomalous pulmonary venous drainage), the right or transverse horns of the sinus venosus (cardiac connection), or the umbilicovitelline system (infracardiac connection). These connections may involve all or only some of the pulmonary veins (see Chapter 15).

DEVELOPMENT OF THE CONDUCTING SYSTEM

The embryologic origin of the cardiac conduction system remains controversial. It may develop from specialized rings of tissue, ie, the sinoatrial, atrioventricular, bulboventricular, and bulbotruncal rings.[25] The sinoatrial (SA) node develops from the sinoatrial ring or on the ventrolateral surface of the superior vena cava. The SA node is present by the sixth week of gestation and the SA artery by the tenth week.[26] The atrioventricular (AV) node and bundle of His develop separately from cells in the AV canal (AV ring) and sinus venosus in the 8- to 9-mm embryo[27,28] and are joined by the eighth week (see Table 3–1). Left and right bundle branches, present in 13-mm and 22- to 25-mm embryos, respectively, develop from the bulboventricular ring, whereas other small portions of the conducting system develop from the bul-

botruncal ring.[14] Action potentials typical of the AV node can be recorded as early as 12 weeks of gestation and by the sixteenth week of intrauterine life, the conducting system is fully mature.[26,29]

FETAL AND NEONATAL CIRCULATION

Fetal Circulation

In the fetus, umbilical venous blood, returning from the placenta, is relatively well oxygenated with a P_{O_2} of 33 mm Hg.[30] The abdominal portion of the umbilical vein enters the liver to join the portal vein. A trunk, the ductus venosus, unites the umbilical and portal veins. Only 40–60% of umbilical venous blood passes through the liver, with the remainder being shunted through the ductus venosus. A physiologic sphincter at the origin of the ductus venosus regulates the proportion of umbilical blood passing through the liver.[31] After mixing with the splanchnic circulation, the P_{O_2} of blood in the inferior vena cava is only 28–30 mm Hg. The ductus venosus connects to the inferior vena cava near the junction of the hepatic veins. As it enters the heart, about one third of the blood from the inferior vena cava is deflected across the foramen ovale by the crista dividens (lower end of the septum secundum) and eustachian valve[32] but some crosses the tricuspid valve to enter the right ventricle. Because the inferior vena cava receives the umbilical venous return, blood entering the left heart via the foramen ovale is better oxygenated than that entering the right ventricle. Superior vena cava blood, on the other hand, enters the right ventricle with only 2–3% crossing the foramen ovale.[33] The right ventricle pumps about two thirds and the left ventricle one third of the combined ventricular input in the fetal lamb.[33] Right ventricular blood is largely shunted to the systemic circulation via the ductus arteriosus, although 7–20% reaches the pulmonary circulation[33] (Fig 3–8). Interventricular septal motion, which tends to be flattened or paradoxic in the fetus, distorts the shape of the left ventricular cavity.[34] This probably results from relative volume overload of the right ventricle.[35] The left ventricle ejects its better oxygenated blood with a higher glucose content (about 15–20% to the brain)[35] into coronary circulation, cerebral circulation, upper extremity, and descending aorta.[31] The lower portion of the body receives blood with a lower oxygen content from the ductus arteriosus.

The P_{O_2} is higher (28–30 mm Hg) in the ascending aorta than in the descending aorta (20–22 mm Hg) because of preferential streaming at the atrial level.[33] From the dorsal aorta, the initially paired umbilical arteries carry blood to the placenta. In the fourth week of gestation, the umbilical arteries acquire a secondary connection to the common iliac artery and lose their initial origin. The umbilical artery blood, with a saturation of about 58%, returns to the placenta for oxygenation.

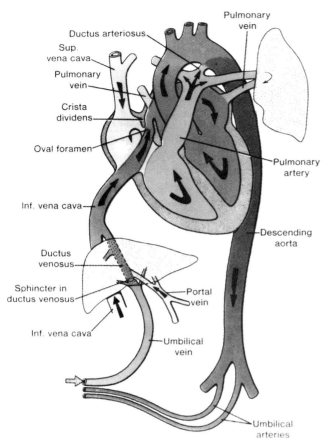

Pulmonary vein

Ductus arteriosus

Sup. vena cava

Pulmonary vein

Crista dividens

Oval foramen

Inf. vena cava

Ductus venosus

Sphincter in ductus venosus

Inf. vena cava

Pulmonary artery

Descending aorta

Portal vein

Umbilical vein

Umbilical arteries

Figure 3–8. The flow patterns of the fetal circulation. The inferior vena caval blood is largely diverted across the foramen ovale to the left atrium, whereas superior vena caval blood enters the right ventricle. Blood from the right ventricle is shunted away from the pulmonary circulation through the ductus arteriosus. (*From Sadler TW: Langman's Medical Embryology. Baltimore: Williams & Wilkins, 1990, p 210, with permission.*)

The fetal foramen ovale remains open as the result of kinetic energy from blood return from the inferior vena cava, not just the differences in pressure between the two atria.[36] Normally, the flap over the foramen ovale approximates to the atrial septum twice each cardiac cycle and reopens at the end of ventricular systole. Right atrial pressure in utero does not always exceed left atrial pressure, as it does in the neonate.[36]

Fetal echocardiography via the abdominal or transvaginal approaches demonstrates the apical four-chamber functional view of both atria, ventricles, the interventricular septum, and the mitral and tricuspid valves from the sixteenth week of gestation onward[4,5] (see Fig 3–1). Color flow mapping details blood flow direction across normal and abnormal communications and valvular regurgitation or stenosis.[37] Compared to conventional pulsed Doppler, color flow mapping increased the numbers of accurate observations, shortened observation time, and decreased intraobserver variation. Because

progressive deterioration of cardiac function is likely with continued gestation, serial echocardiographic examinations are helpful in predicting prognosis.[38] In a series of 170 prenatally diagnosed defects, 48% of the continued pregnancies resulted in stillbirth or early neonatal death.[39] In the surviving infants, extracardiac defects or aneuploidy (more or less than the normal diploid number of chromosomes) were present.[39] These findings substantiate older series.[40] A poor prognosis is suggested by the finding of an increased cardiothoracic ratio in early gestation.[38] Structural abnormalities of the tricuspid valve have been documented in 8% of prenatal cardiac malformations, a rate higher than noted postnatally. This finding probably results from greater intrauterine and immediate postbirth death rates.[38]

After the heart is completely partitioned, left ventricular, right ventricular, left atrial, pulmonic valve, aortic valve, and aortic size increase linearly[41,42] throughout gestation. Cardiac dimensions, such as that of the aortic root and the right and left ventricles, correlate with noncardiac dimensions, such as biparietal diameter, as growth occurs during gestation.[43,44] The pulmonic valve diameter is greater than the aortic throughout gestation. The diameter of the aortic isthmus is also larger than that of the ductus arteriosus, possibly due to increased flow to brain and other organs in late gestation.[42] The cardiothoracic ratio (linearly related to biparietal diameter)[45] remains constant throughout the second and third trimesters.[45] The mean ratio of septal to left ventricular wall thickness is about 1.14, which suggests that greater septal thickness indicates abnormalities of fetal or placental circulation.[46] The weights of right and left ventricular free walls and the ratio of chamber sizes remain similar throughout gestation, which questions the theory of right ventricular dominance in utero.[41,44,47] Nevertheless, Doppler echocardiography indicates that tricuspid flow velocities during early and late diastoles are greater than mitral flow, which suggests right ventricular dominance.[48] Tricuspid flow velocity also increases with gestational age.[48] During the last trimester, the diameters of both right and left ventricles increase as does left ventricular volume.[49] Cardiac output increases late in the third trimester, although ejection fraction remains constant.[50]

Contractility, measured by fractional shortening, is also constant throughout gestation.[47] The fetal ventricle is even less compliant than the neonatal ventricle. This finding is probably best explained by differences in the distribution of contractile and noncontractile elements in the fetal myocardium compared with the adult ventricle.[51] Although some investigators[52] suggest that contractility does not increase with volume loading in the fetus, Anderson and colleagues demonstrated that the Frank-Starling relationship operates in fetal lambs.[53,54] The left ventricle of the neonatal lamb, however, accomplishes greater work in response to volume infusion than the preterm lamb.[48]

Beat-to-beat variability of the fetal heart rate develops during the first trimester. Fetal heart rates are faster during the first trimester owing to parasympathetic immaturity. In a murine model, the response of the fetal heart to acetylcholine (bradycardia) increases with gestational age.[53] This finding probably results from an increase in cholinergic receptors during gestation.[55]

Fetal Dysrhythmias

Normal distribution of blood in the human fetus depends upon a rapid heart rate. The heart rate of the fetus, particularly during labor and delivery, has been monitored for more than 100 years.[56] The variability of the fetal heart rate depends upon not only a balance between the parasympathetic and sympathetic nervous systems but also upon resting cardioacceleratory drive of a non-neural type.[57] Many dysrhythmias are physiologic, occurring in response to cord compression, maternally administered drugs, thyrotoxicosis, or fever. Fetal breathing is associated with a small increase in beat-to-beat variation.[58] The heart rate accelerates with fetal movement.[58]

Correct diagnosis of fetal dysrhythmias is essential for appropriate therapy, recognition of associated congenital cardiac defects early enough for termination of pregnancy, and avoidance of unnecessary operative delivery.[59] The incidence of congenital heart disease is not increased if the arrhythmia is supraventricular extrasystoles, premature ventricular systoles, or other sinus node dysrhythmias in which the P-QRS complex, although distorted, is intact.[4] However, the incidence of structural cardiac disease is increased by the presence of supraventricular tachycardia (secondary to Wolff-Parkinson-White syndrome in 15% of cases),[55] atrial flutter or fibrillation, and heart block.[4,60,61] There is one reported case of coincidental maternal and fetal heart block causing bradycardia during labor, which prompted operative delivery of the infant.[62] Supraventricular tachycardia requires either therapy or delivery depending upon fetal condition and maturity.[4] Persistent supraventricular arrhythmias, particularly with heart rates over 200 beats/min increase end-diastolic dimensions and reduce fractional shortening.[63] The resulting cardiomyopathy is associated with heart failure and ascites. Sustained dysrhythmias, including complex arrhythmias, complete heart block, atrial flutter, or sinus bradycardia, are associated with a 36% incidence of fetal or early neonatal death.[64]

The diagnosis of the dysrhythmias can be made by M-mode echocardiography,[60] fetal electrocardiography, and ultrasonic flow measurements. Fetal electrocardiograms are often difficult to record because of interference from the maternal ECG, background noise, fetal movement and the low voltage of fetal ECG.[60] During labor, a fetal scalp electrode can be used to monitor the ECG. Specific criteria for differentiation of the various dysrhythmias are discussed in the review by Shenker.[26] Fetal M-mode echocardiography can demonstrate the atrial

and ventricular contractions independently, thus aiding in the diagnosis of the dysrhythmia. Ultrasonic measurements of aortic blood flow determine the significance of the dysrhythmia on cardiac function.[65,66]

In utero cardioversion of supraventricular tachycardia with digoxin,[67–70,71] procainamide,[72,73] verapamil,[74] or propranolol[75] (all of which cross the placenta) have been successful. Larger than usual doses of digoxin may be required to control the arrhythmia because of increased maternal intravascular volume, increased fetal digoxin metabolism, delayed gastric emptying, or increased glomerular filtration rate.[70,75] The need for large doses of procainamide has also been reported because its placental transfer may be limited.[73] Propranolol, however, which causes bradycardia, hypoglycemia, and decreased Apgar scores in the neonate, is best avoided. Insufficient data on verapamil therapy for pharmacologic cardioversion of fetal dysrhythmias are available.

REFERENCES

1. Ursell PC, Byrne JM, Strobino BA: Significance of cardiac defects in the developing fetus: A study of spontaneous abortuses. *Circulation* **72**:1232–1236, 1985
2. Hoffman JIE, Christianson R: Congenital heart disease in a cohort of 19,502 births with long-term follow-up. *Am J Cardiol* **42**:641–647, 1978
3. Allan LD, Crawford DC, Anderson RH, Tynan MJ: Echocardiographic and anatomical correlation in fetal congenital heart disease. *Br Heart J* **5**:542–548, 1984
4. McCallum WD: Fetal cardiac anatomy and vascular dynamics. *Clin Obstet Gynecol* **24**:837–849, 1981
5. Allan LD, Crawford DC, Chita SK, et al: Familial recurrence of congenital heart disease in a prospective series of mothers referred for fetal echocardiography. *Am J Cardiol* **58**:334–337, 1986
6. Allan LD, Tynan M, Campbell S, Anderson RH: Identification of congenital cardiac malformations by echocardiography in midtrimester fetus. *Br Heart J* **46**:358–362, 1981
7. Nora JJ, Nora AH, Wexler P: Hereditary and environmental aspects as they affect the fetus and newborn. *Clin Obstet Gynecol* **24**:851–861, 1981
8. Bharati S, Lev M: Direct entry of the right superior vena cava into the left atrium with aneurysmal dilatation and stenosis at its entry into the right atrium with stenosis of the pulmonary veins: A rare case. *Pediatr Cardiol* **5**:123–126, 1984
9. Sadler TW: *Langman's Medical Embryology.* Baltimore: Williams & Wilkins, 1990, pp 179–227
10. Besson WT, Kirby ML, Van Mierop LHS, Teabeaut JR: Effects of the size of lesions of the cardiac neural crest at various embryonic ages on incidence and type of cardiac defects. *Circulation* **73**:360–364, 1986
11. Kirby ML, Gale TF, Stewart DE: Neural crest cells contribute to normal aorticopulmonary septation. *Science* **220**:1059–1061, 1983
12. Kirby ML, Turnage KL, Hays BM: Characterization of conotruncal malformation following ablation of "cardiac" neural crest. *Anat Rec* **213**:87–93, 1985

13. Kappetein AP, Gittenberger-deGroot AC, Zwinderman AH, et al: The neural crest as a possible pathogenetic factor in coarctation of the aorta and bicuspid aortic valve. *J Thorac Cardiovasc Surg* **102**:830–836, 1991

14. Lev M, Bharati S: Embryology of the heart and great vessels. In Archiniegas E (ed): *Pediatric Cardiac Surgery.* Chicago: Year Book Medical, 1985, pp 1–12

15. Collett RW, Edwards JE: Persistent truncus arteriosus: A classification. *Surg Clin North Am* **29**:1245–1270, 1949

16. Hirakow R: Development of the cardiac blood vessels in staged human embryos. *Acta Anat* **115**:220–230, 1983

17. Schlesinger MJ: Relation of anatomic pattern to pathologic conditions of the coronary arteries. *Arch Pathol* **30**:403–415, 1941

18. James TN: Anatomy of the crista supraventricularis: Its importance for understanding right ventricular function, right ventricular infarction, and related conditions. *J Am Coll Cardiol* **6**:1083–1095, 1985

19. Giordano JM: Embryologic development of the vascular system. In Giordano JM, Trout HH, DePalma RG (eds): *The Basic Science of Vascular Surgery.* Mt Kisco, NY: Futura, 1988

20. Chuang VP, Mena CE, Hoskins PA: Congenital anomalies of the inferior vena cava. Review of embryogenesis and presentation of a simplified classification. *Br J Radiol* **47**:200–213, 1974

21. Giordano JM, Trout HH: Anomalies of the inferior vena cava. *J Vasc Surg* **3**:924–928, 1986

22. Mayo J, Gray R, St Louis E, et al: Anomalies of the inferior vena cava. *AJR* **140**:339–345, 1983

23. Huggins TJ, Lesar ML, Friedman AC, et al: CT appearance of persistent left superior vena cava. *J Comput Assist Tomogr* **6**:294–297, 1982

24. Siegfried MS, Rochester D, Bernstein JR, Miller JW: Diagnosis of inferior vena cava anomalies by computerized tomography. *Computerized Radiology* **7**:119–122, 1983

25. Anderson RH, Becker AE, Wenink AC, et al: The development of the cardiac specialized tissue. In Wellens HJ, Lie KI, Janse MJ (eds): *The Conduction System of the Heart: Structure, Function and Clinical Implications.* The Hague: Martinus Nijhoff, 1976, p 3–28

26. Shenker L: Fetal cardiac arrhythmias. *Obstet Gynecol Rev* **34**:561–572, 1979

27. Mall EP: On the development of the human heart. *Am J Anat* **13**:249–298, 1912

28. Field EJ: The development of the conductive system in the heart of sheep. *Br Heart J* **213**:129–147, 1951

29. Janse MJ, Anderson RH, Van Capelle FJL, et al: A combined electrophysiological and anatomical study of the human fetal heart. *Am Heart J* **91**:556–562, 1976

30. Rudolph AM: The changes in the circulation after birth. *Circulation* **41**:343–359, 1970

31. Rudolph AM: Hepatic and ductus venous blood flows during fetal life. *Hepatology* **3**:254–258, 1983

32. Allan LD, Joseph MC, Boyd EGCA, et al: M-mode echocardiography in the developing human fetus. *Br Heart J* **47**:573–583, 1982

33. Rudolph AM, Heymann MA: Fetal and neonatal circulation and respiration. *Ann Rev Physiol* **36**:187–209, 1974

34. Azancot A, Caudell TP, Allen HD, et al: Analysis of ventricular shape by echocardiography in normal fetuses, newborns, and infants. *Circulation* **68**:1201–1211, 1983

35. Kleinman CS, Donnerstein RL: Ultrasonic assessment of cardiac function in the intact human fetus. *J Am Coll Cardiol* **5**:84S–94S, 1985

36. Anderson DF, Faber JJ, Morton MJ, et al: Flow through the foramen ovale of the fetal and new-born lamb. *J Physiol (London)* **365**:29–39, 1985

37. Sharland GK, Chita SK, Allan LD: The use of colour Doppler in fetal echocardiography. *Int J Cardiol* **28**:229–236, 1990

38. Sharland GK, Chita SK, Allan LD: Tricuspid valve dysplasia or displacement in intrauterine life. *J Am Coll Cardiol* **17**:944–949, 1991

39. Smythe JF, Copel JAA, Kleinman CS: Outcome of prenatally detected cardiac malformations. *Am J Cardiol* **69**:1471–1474, 1992

40. Davis GK, Farquhar CM, Allan LD, et al: Structural cardiac abnormalities in the fetus: Reliability of prenatal diagnosis and outcome. *Br J Obstet Gynecol* **97**:27–31, 1990

41. St. John Sutton MG, Gewitz MH, Shah B, et al: Quantitative assessment of growth and function: A prospective longitudinal echocardiographic study. *Circulation* **69**:645–654, 1984

42. Ursell PC, Byrne JM, Fears TR, et al: Growth of the great vessels in the normal human fetus and in the fetus with cardiac defects. *Circulation* **84**:2028–2033, 1991

43. DeVore GR, Siassi B, Platt LD: Fetal echocardiography V. M-mode measurements of the aortic root and aortic valve in second- and third-trimester normal human fetuses. *Am J Obstet Gynecol* **152**:543–550, 1985

44. DeVore GR, Siassi B, Platt D: Fetal echocardiography IV. M-mode assessment of ventricular size and contractility during the second and third trimesters of pregnancy in the normal fetus. *Am J Obstet Gynecol* **150**:981–988, 1984

45. Filkins KA, Brown TF, Levine OR: Renal time ultrasonic evaluation of the fetal heart. *Int J Gynecol Obstet* **19**:35–39, 1981

46. Leslie J, Shen S, Thornton JC, Strauss L: The human fetal heart in the second trimester of gestation: A gross morphometric study of normal fetuses. *Am J Obstet Gynecol* **145**:312–316, 1983

47. St. John Sutton MG, Raichlen JS, Reicheck N, Huff DS: Quantitative assessment of right and left ventricular growth in the human fetal heart: A pathoanatomic study. *Circulation* **70**:935–941, 1984

48. Reed KL, Sahn DJ, Scagnelli S, et al: Doppler echocardiographic studies of diastolic function in the human fetal heart: Changes during gestation. *J Am Coll Cardiol* **8**:391–395, 1986

49. Wladimiroff JW, Vosters R, McGhie JS: Normal cardiac ventricular geometry and function during the last trimester of pregnancy and early neonatal period. *Br J Obstet Gynecol* **89**:938–944, 1982

50. Wladimiroff JW, McGhie J: Ultrasonic assessment of cardiovascular geometry and function in the human fetus. *Br J Obstet Gynecol* **88**:870–875, 1981

51. Romero T, Covell J, Friedman WF: A comparison of pressure-volume relations of the fetal, newborn, and adult heart. *Am J Physiol* **222**:1285–1290, 1972

52. Heymann MA, Rudolph AM: Effects of increasing preload on right ventricular output in fetal lambs in utero. *Circulation* **48**(suppl 4):37, 1973

53. Baylen BG, Ogata H, Ikegammi M, et al: Left ventricular performance and contractility before and after volume infusion: A comparative study of preterm and full-term newborn lambs. *Circulation* **73**:1042–1049, 1986

54. Anderson PAW, Manring A, Crenshaw C: Biophysics of the developing heart. II. The interaction of the force-interval relationship with inotropic state and muscle length (preload). *Am J Obstet Gynecol* **138**:44–54, 1980

55. Roeske WR, Wildenthal K: Responsiveness to drugs and hormones in the murine model of cardiac ontogenesis. *Pharmacol Ther* **14**:55–66, 1981

56. Solum T: Antenatal cardiotocography. *Acta Obstet Gynecol Scand* **96**(suppl):1–31, 1980

57. Dalton KJ, Dawes GS, Patrick JE: The autonomic nervous system and fetal heart rate variability. *Am J Obstet Gynecol* **146**:456–462, 1983

58. Dawes GS, Visser GHA, Goodman JDS, Levine DH: Numerical analysis of the human fetal heart rate: Modulation by breathing and movement. *Am J Obstet Gynecol* **140**:535–544, 1981

59. Shapiro I, Sharf M, Abinader EG: Prenatal diagnosis of fetal arrhythmias: A new echocardiographic technique. *J Clin Ultrasound* **12**:369–372, 1984

60. Bergmans MGM, Jonker GJ, Kock HCLV: Fetal supraventricular tachycardia. Review of the literature. *Obstet Gynecol Survey* **40**:61–68, 1985

61. Gochberg SH: Congenital heart block. *Am J Obstet Gynecol* **88**:238–241, 1964

62. Floyd HM, Dewan DM, James FM: Coincidental fetal and maternal heart block. *Anesth Analg* **69**:59–60, 1981

63. Koyanagi T, Hara K, Satoh S, et al: Relationship between heart rate and rhythm, and cardiac performance assessed in the human fetus in utero. *Int J Cardiol* **28**:163–171, 1990

64. Kleinman CS, Donnerstein RL, Jaffe CC, et al: Fetal echocardiography: A tool for evaluation of in utero cardiac arrhythmias and monitoring in utero therapy. Analysis of 71 patients. *Am J Cardiol* **51**:237–243, 1983

65. Lingman G, Dahlstrom J-A, Eik-Nes SH, et al: Haemo-dynamic assessment of fetal heart arrhythmias. *Br J Obstet Gynecol* **91**:647–652, 1984

66. Maulik D, Nanda NC, Moodley S, et al: Application of Doppler echocardiography in the assessment of fetal cardiac disease. *Am J Obstet Gynecol* **151**:951–957, 1985

67. Albers WH, Thompson RE: In utero diagnosis and management of fetal supraventricular tachycardia. *IMJ* **163**:269–271, 1983

68. Golichowski AM, Caldwell R, Hartsough A, Peleg D: Pharmacologic cardioversion of intrauterine supraventricular tachycardia. *J Reprod Med* **30**:139–144, 1985

69. Harrigan JT, Kangos JJ, Sikka A, et al: Successful treatment of fetal congestive heart failure secondary to tachycardia. *N Engl J Med* **304**:1527–1529, 1981

70. Heaton FC, Vaughan R: Intrauterine supraventricular tachycardia: Cardioversion with maternal digoxin. *Obstet Gynecol* **60**:749–751, 1982

71. Lingman G, Ohrlander S, Ohlin P: Intrauterine digoxin treatment of fetal paroxysmal tachycardia case report. *Br J Obstet Gynecol* **87**:340–342, 1980

72. Dumesic DA, Silverman NH, Tobias S, Golbus MS: Transplacental cardioversion of fetal supraventricular tachycardia with procainamide. *N Engl J Med* **307**:1128–1131, 1982

73. Given BD, Phillippe M, Sanders SP, Dzau VJ: Procainamide cardioversion of fetal supraventricular tachyarrhythmia. *Am J Cardiol* **53**:1460–1461, 1984

74. Wolff F, Brevker KH, Schlensker KH, Bolte A: Prenatal diagnosis and therapy of fetal heart rate anomalies with a contribution on the placental transfer of verapamil. *J Perinat Med* **8**:203–208, 1980

75. Rogers MC, Willerson JT, Goldblatt A, Smith TW: Serum digoxin concentration in the human fetus, neonate, and infant. *N Engl J Med* **287**:1010–1013, 1972

76. DeHaan RL, O'Rahilly R: Embryology of the heart. In Hurst JW (ed): *The Heart*, 4th ed. New York: McGraw-Hill, 1978

77. O'Rahilly R: The timing and sequence of events in human cardiogenesis. *Acta Anat* **79**:70–75, 1971

Chapter 4 | Neonatal Myocardial and Circulatory Function

Carol L. Lake

TRANSITIONAL CIRCULATION

At birth, there are several important changes in the heart and peripheral circulation. The circulation of the newborn is indeed in transition from the fetal to the adult pattern. It can shift back to the fetal pattern (but without the placenta) in the presence of congenital heart disease, prematurity, anesthesia, hypoxia, or other conditions for several days or longer[1] (Table 4-1). Shunting through the ductus arteriosus and across the foramen ovale is often referred to as persistence of the fetal circulation, although with the absence of the placenta and presence of pulmonary ventilation, it is not exactly fetal but rather transitional. Normally, it progresses rapidly toward the adult form.

An increase in systemic vascular resistance results from elimination of the low-resistance placental circulation.[2] Left ventricular output increases at birth owing to increases in stroke volume and percent fractional shortening.[3] Output is nearly maximal and remains constant or decreases slightly during the first 24 hours of life.[3,4] Fractional shortening of the ventricle is unchanged during the first 96 postnatal hours but stroke volume, heart rate, and ventricular end-diastolic dimensions decrease.[3]

Pulmonary vascular resistance decreases 75% and pulmonary flow increases 450% with the beginning of neonatal respiration.[5] From a prenatal pressure of 70/45, the pulmonary artery pressures decrease to 50/30 at 24 hours after birth and to 30/12 a few days later[5] (Fig 4-1). The reduction in pulmonary vascular resistance can be documented by the significant lengthening in the time to peak velocity in the pulmonary artery by 24 hours of age.[6] The size and number of pulmonary arteries increase rapidly during the first 2 months of life but subsequent increases occur at the same rate as the growth of alveoli. The media of the pulmonary artery decreases in thickness over the first 10 days of life and continues to

decrease for the first 3 months after birth.[7] These changes contribute to the continued progressive decrease in pulmonary vascular resistance over the first 3-6 weeks of life.[8] Vasoactive substances, including bradykinin, prostaglandins E_1, E_2, and I_2 and endothelium-derived relaxing factor also contribute to pulmonary vasodilation in the perinatal period.[8,9] Elaboration of these substances by lung or vascular endothelium is enhanced by oxygen, ventilation, and increased pulmonary blood flow. The increase in pulmonary blood flow secondarily increases left ventricular preload.

The ductus arteriosus begins to close within 10-15 hours of birth as a result of the increased arterial P_{O_2}, reflex neurogenic, or vasoactive factors.[10] Echocardiographic evidence of retrograde systolic aortic velocities and retrograde diastolic pulmonary artery velocities in 91% of infants in the first day of life indicates that flow continues to occur from the aorta into the ductus.[11] When the retrograde systolic velocity is still present in the aorta in the absence of retrograde diastolic velocity in the pulmonary artery, the ductus is beginning to close at the pulmonic end.[11] The ductus is usually physiologically closed by the second day of life in the majority of normal infants.[11] However, it can reopen in response to hypoxia or prostaglandin E_1.

Although the ductus arteriosus remains patent, pressures remain similar in both systemic and pulmonary circuits. However, there is preferential flow of blood to the lungs, a left-to-right shunt rather than the fetal right-to-left shunt. A decrease in flow or even reversal of flow ("diastolic steal") occurs in the renal, celiac, and superior mesenteric arteries as well as the descending thoracic aorta during diastole when the ductus remains patent.[12] Permanent anatomic closure of the ductus normally occurs within the first 3 weeks of life, forming the ligamentum arteriosum.[13]

Physiologic closure of the foramen ovale occurs

TABLE 4–1. CHARACTERISTICS OF THE TRANSITIONAL CIRCULATION

Patent ductus arteriosus (PDA), patent foramen ovale (PFO)
Increased pulmonary vascular resistance
Transient right-to-left shunting (possible at PFO and PDA)

shortly after birth, but some degree of left-to-right shunting may be present during the first day of life.[14] Right-to-left shunting may also occur because left ventricular relaxation occurs earlier than right ventricular relaxation, causing opening of the mitral valve before the tricuspid valve and bowing of the interatrial septum and valve of the foramen ovale toward the left atrium.[15] Anatomic closure may be delayed as long as 1 year.[16] Many healthy infants demonstrate tricuspid insufficiency in the first 24 hours of life.[11,15]

The umbilical arteries close within a few minutes after birth by contraction of musculature within their walls. Fibrous proliferation over the first 2–3 months produces complete obliteration. Eventually the medial umbilical ligaments form from the distal portions of the arteries, whereas the proximal umbilical arteries remain as the superior vesical arteries. Umbilical veins close shortly after the umbilical arteries, eventually becoming the ligamentum teres. The ductus venosus also closes to form the ligamentum venosum.

NEONATAL MYOCARDIAL FUNCTION

Myocardial Ultrastructure

Immediately after birth, the left ventricular end diastolic diameter and volume increase.[17] Because of the marked

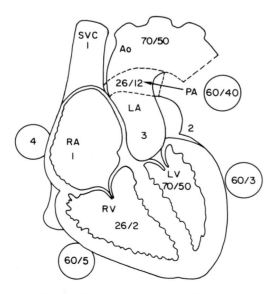

Figure 4–1. Intracardiac pressures in the fetal (circled numbers outside the chambers) and the neonatal heart (within the chambers) demonstrating the changes occurring with birth. Not shown is the ductus arteriosus between the pulmonary artery and aorta or the foramen ovale between the right and left atria.

increase in the pressure load on the left ventricle, the left ventricular myocardium grows more rapidly (more rapid increase in the myocyte population) than that of the right ventricle.[18] In addition to these gross anatomic changes, ultrastructural changes in size, number, and architecture of myocardial cells occur. Before a discussion of the ultrastructural changes that contribute to myocardial growth, the ultrastructure of the cardiac cell must be reviewed (Fig 4–2). Myocardium consists of myocytes interconnected by collagen fibers that form an interstitial network. There is considerable interaction between individual cells via intercalated discs that allow electric, chemical, and physical communication.

Contractile Apparatus. Each myocardial cell is surrounded by its sarcolemma or plasma membrane. The T system of tubules develops from invaginations of the sarcolemma. Within the sarcolemma are the myofibrils consisting of thin F actin and thick myosin myofilaments running parallel to the long axis of the cell in repeating units called sarcomeres. The sarcomeres are interconnected via the Z bands or lines, from which the thin filaments project. Where thin filaments overlap with thick filaments, an A band is present, whereas the I band results when there is no overlap. Changes in myofibril length depend upon the extent of overlap of actin and myosin and the actions of the regulatory proteins tropomyosin and troponin. Troponin has three subunits: troponin I (inhibitory), troponin T (tropomyosin-binding), and troponin C (calcium-binding). Cross-linking between actin and myosin is inhibited by troponin I and tropomyosin that bind to actin.

Tropomyosin exists as two isoforms: α and β, with the α form predominating in the fetus and newborn. Because tropomyosin in the α isoform binds more efficiently to troponin T, the presence of more α-tropomyosin may be due to the need for rapid relaxation at faster heart rates. As maturation proceeds and heart rate decreases, less α-tropomyosin is present until the β form predominates in adults.[19] A greater proportion of the tropomyosin is phosphorylated in the fetus, which may affect the relationship between tropomyosin and troponin T as well as the sensitivity of the myofilaments to calcium.[19] Tropomyosin increases about 50%, but its phosphorylation decreases during the transition from fetus to adult.[20] The decreased phosphorylation with maturation results from a decreased need for rapid relaxation at slower adult heart rates.

Myosin, the major protein in the thick filaments of the contractile apparatus, consists of a globular head composed of light chains and a tail section with heavy chains. It exists as three isoenzymes in the ventricular myocardium, V_1, V_2, and V_3, and as two isoenzymes in the atria, A_1 and A_2. These isoenzymes consist of two heavy chains, α and β. Myosin isoenzyme V_1, consisting of two α chains, has the highest adenosine triphosphatase

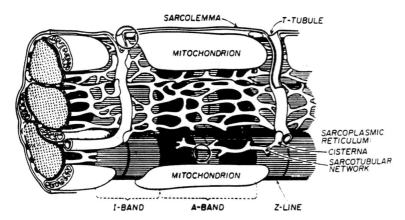

Figure 4–2. The ultrastructure of a myocardial cell. The extensive intracellular network of sarcoplasmic reticulum, T tubule system, and Z bands of the sarcomeres enhances physical, chemical, and electric interactions between cardiac myocytes. (*From Katz AM: Congestive heart failure. Role of altered myocardial cellular control. N Engl J Med 293:1184–1191, 1975, with permission.*)

(ATPase) activity and, therefore, the fastest shortening velocity. Isoenzyme V_2, with an α and a β chain, has intermediate activity, and V_3 with two β chains has the lowest ATPase activity. Although myosin isoenzymes vary with stage of development in other species,[21] in humans, V_3 is predominant in all ages from newborns to the elderly. However, a nonphosphorylatable myosin light chain, similar to adult atrial myosin, is present in the fetus.[19] Adult atrial myosin is composed of α chains and has high ATPase activity.

Cytoskeleton. The decreased contractility of the immature ventricle results in part from lack of organization in the cytoskeleton of the myocytes. During development, the myocardial cell changes from a short, round form to a long, rodlike form and its myofibrils become oriented to the long axis of the cell. The transverse tubular (T system) develops within the cell during this maturational process. Structural changes in the cardiac myocyte cytoskeleton occur, with maturation progressing from chaotically arranged myofibrils, through myofibrils located together in a thin subsarcolemmal cell with the cell nucleus and mitochondria in the center, to the mature, longitudinally oriented myofibrillar pattern with mitochondria surrounding each myofilament. Changes in the cytoskeleton proteins desmin, spectrin, ankyrin, and vinculin also occur. Desmin is diffusely distributed in newborn rats, but it localizes to the Z band by 4 weeks of age.[22] Receptor sites for spectrin also change in isoforms.[23]

Sarcoplasmic Reticulum. In the rat and other species, the number of cardiac myocytes increases rapidly immediately after birth.[18] The myocyte diameter also increases because of an increase in the myofibrillar volume of the myocyte and extensive changes in the sarcoplasmic reticulum (SR), a closed intracellular membranous network that surrounds the myofibrils.[18,19,24] Sarcoplasmic reticulum can be divided into several regions: the terminal cisternae, the release site of calcium, junctional SR, and longitudinal SR. Terminal cisternae are connected to the T tubules at the Z band by foot proteins. Portions of the terminal cisternae in the heart do not connect to the T tubules and are called the corbular SR. Longitudinal SR connects the two terminal cisternae at the ends of the sarcomere. Junctional SR has foot processes that extend toward the sarcolemma, allowing transmission of cell membrane depolarization to the SR.

The neonatal SR is structurally immature and undergoes substantial changes in organization during maturation. Principal differences in immature SR include the absence of a fixed repetitive relationship of the corbular SR to the sarcomere, obscured demarcations between the corbular SR and the longitudinal SR, and peripheral coupling between the junctional SR and the sarcolemma.[19] During maturation, the SR becomes functionally differentiated and demarcated, whereas internal couplings of sarcolemma and SR are acquired with the formation of the transverse tubular system.[19] The mitochondrial/sarcoplasmic area increases in parallel with increased mitochondrial enzymatic activity.

The SR and cytosolic calcium concentrations are reduced, making the immature heart more dependent upon trans-sarcolemmal fluxes of calcium for regulation of contractility and excitation-contraction coupling. Variation in cytosolic calcium alters the loaded shortening and force development during individual myocardial contractions. When cytosolic calcium is increased, there are more cross bridges between actin, myosin, and the thin filament regulatory proteins (tropomyosin, troponin I, troponin C, and troponin T that are present even in embryos). The neonate's reduced sarcoplasmic reticular calcium may decrease susceptibility to free radical injury during reperfusion.

Biochemical and Metabolic Differences in Neonatal Myocardium

Although fetal myocardial oxygen consumption is similar to that of the adult, right ventricular oxygen consumption is greater than the left. Marked changes in myocardial metabolism occur within hours of birth, among which is the increased oxygen consumption of the left ventricle. Myocardial glycogen content decreases throughout gestation and continues to decrease in early postnatal life and the heart shifts from primarily anaerobic to aerobic metabolism. Enzymatic activity increases in the mitochondria to increase lipolysis, gluconeogenesis, and regulation of cytosolic calcium concentration (excitation-contraction coupling).[25] The activities of enzymes involved in the citric acid cycle and respiratory chain increase markedly after birth, particularly by 15–20 days of age.[26] Although the immature heart uses lactate as its primary substrate and glucose only under hypoxic conditions, the myocardium completely converts to fatty acid oxidation by 1–2 years of age. The increased oxidation of fatty acids by the myocardium with maturation is primarily due to increased mitochondrial number and size, which enhances enzyme activity.[26] However, in neonates, a small amount of glucose is necessary even when myocardial fatty acid metabolism is present.[27]

However, hypoxia impairs fatty acid oxidation, and glucose metabolism produces more energy without the decreased contractility and arrhythmias caused by unmetabolized lipids.[25] Children with cyanotic heart disease do not demonstrate myocardial acidosis.[28] Whether the neonatal heart is more resistant to hypoxia or ischemia is a subject with important implications for intraoperative myocardial preservation discussed in Chapter 11. It is more resistant to calcium paradox.[29]

Newborn hearts develop contracture more quickly during ischemia. However, newborn hearts recover systolic and diastolic function after normothermic ischemia faster than do adult hearts.[30] Myocardial adenosine triphosphate content is better preserved during ischemia and normalizes more quickly during reperfusion, probably because of higher glycogen stores and greater glycolytic flux.

Electrophysiology in the Neonatal Myocardium

Electric activation of the myocardium produces an action potential resulting from the rapid influx of sodium into the cardiac cell. The action potential is similar to that in the adult, starting from a resting potential of -80 mVs, proceeding through a rapid upstroke to $+20$ mVs, and finally arriving at a plateau lasting 200–300 ms. Depolarization spreads throughout the cell via the transverse tubular system and the sarcolemma. Calcium moves intracellularly through the voltage-sensitive slow calcium channels. The increased entry of calcium into the cell causes additional calcium to be released from the sarcoplasmic reticulum.

Excitation Contraction Coupling. Increased intracellular free calcium combines with troponin C on the actin myofilaments causing a conformational change in tropo-

myosin and exposure of the actin and myosin binding sites. This excitation-contraction coupling results from the increased intracellular calcium. Energy from ATP obtained from an actomyosin ATPase is necessary for the binding of actin and myosin via cross bridges to produce contraction.

Depolarization initiates tension development in the newborn myocardium. Tension development in immature myocardium is dependent upon the influx of calcium across the sarcolemma.[31] As the myocardium matures, tension development becomes more dependent upon intracellular calcium storage sites such as the sarcoplasmic reticulum.[32] Peak tension is reached during the plateau of the action potential and tension declines during repolarization.[32]

Relaxation occurs when the excess calcium is extruded by the sodium-calcium exchanger and pumped from the cytoplasm by the sarcolemmal calcium ATPase pump. Although normally one calcium ion (Out) is exchanged for three sodium ions (In), the reverse reaction is possible. Calcium release from the mitochondria is also regulated by the sodium-calcium exchanger but the process is too slow to affect either cardiac muscle contraction or relaxation. The troponin-tropomyosin complex inhibits the actin-myosin interaction when intracellular calcium decreases. An age-related decrease in the myocardial relaxation time constant has been reported between the last week of gestation and the first week of life.[33] This finding may result from increases in calcium ATPase activity and phospholamban content.[34] Phospholamban phosphorylation by protein kinase C, calcium-calmodulin–dependent protein kinase, or cyclic AMP–dependent protein kinase affects the affinity of calcium ATPase for calcium.

β-Adrenergic Receptor Function. β-Adrenergic receptors appear in the fetal myocardium prior to the development of the adrenergic nervous system. Stimulation of the β-adrenergic receptors, probably by circulating catecholamines in the absence of the sympathetic nervous system, increases adenylate cyclase and cyclic adenosine monophosphate. Parasympathetic innervation occurs during the period of cardiac growth and muscarinic receptor numbers decrease.

The fetal myocardial stores of norepinephrine are substantially less than those of neonates, which, in turn, are less than adults'[24] (Fig 4–3). This finding suggests that sympathetic innervation may be incomplete or binding and uptake of catecholamines in the heart is in an immature state in the newborn.[24] Myocardial uptake of norepinephrine increases throughout human gestation.[35] Sympathetic innervation of the heart is incomplete at birth. Development continues during the first 6 weeks of life. As norepinephrine concentrations increase toward normal adult levels in mice, the number of adrenergic receptors, increased in the fetus, de-

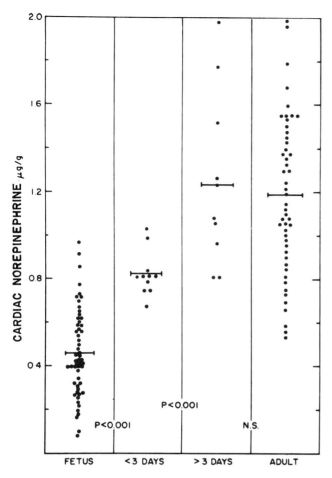

Figure 4–3. Cardiac norepinephrine content probably reflects the incomplete sympathetic innervation that increases from the fetal to the adult state. The lower norepinephrine content and sympathetic activity in neonates explains their limited response to either endogenous or exogenous catecholamines. (*From Friedman WF: The intrinsic properties of the developing heart. Prog Cardiovasc Dis 15: 87–111, 1972, with permission.*)

TABLE 4–2. DIFFERENCES BETWEEN THE IMMATURE AND ADULT HEART

	Neonate	Adult
Cardiac output	Rate dependent	Increased by stroke volume/ heart rate
Contractility	Reduced	Normal
Starling Response	Limited	Normal
Catecholamine Response	Reduced	Normal
Compliance	Reduced	Normal
Afterload Mismatch	Susceptible	Resistant
Ventricular Interdependence	Increased	Normal

volume elasticity resulting from sarcolemmal rupture, mitochondrial swelling, and deposition of calcium in mitochondria.[41] Such myocardial changes, which include intracellular calcium overload, altered sodium-calcium exchange in sarcolemma and sarcoplasmic reticulum, depressed myocardial oxidation of fatty acids, and decreased phosphorylase activity, are considered irreversible.[41] Although the epinephrine doses are somewhat higher than used clinically, these doses might be necessary for hemodynamic support before or after cardiac surgery.

Neonatal Myocardial Physiology

The major differences between the immature and adult heart are summarized in Table 4–2. Myocytes in immature hearts shorten less rapidly than those of adult hearts.

Myocardial Contractility. Cardiac index and stroke volume increase progressively during the first 6 weeks of extrauterine life[43] (Fig 4–4). Cardiac output in infants

creases.[36,37] A similar finding has been noted in fetal lambs.[38] Downregulation of the β-adrenergic receptor/ adenylate cyclase system in left ventricular myocardium has been demonstrated in newborn lambs with chronic hypoxemia secondary to right-to-left shunt.[39] The cause of the downregulation is chronic sympathetic stimulation, a compensatory mechanism to maintain oxygen delivery. β receptor density is also decreased by hypoxemia.

These findings suggest a diminished response of the neonatal heart to exogenous catecholamines given for left ventricular failure.[40] In neonatal pigs, epinephrine infusions increased cardiac output by an increase in heart rate rather than contractility.[41] However, catecholamine concentrations increase at birth in humans.[42]

Neonatal pigs also are more susceptible to cardiotoxicity from circulating epinephrine (2-hour infusion at 2 μg/kg/min) as indicated by an increase in left ventricular

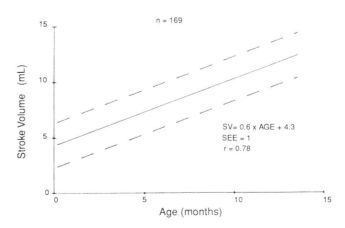

Figure 4–4. Stroke volume versus age. Cardiac output increases during the first year of life. (*From Sholler GF, et al: Am J Cardiol 60:1112, 1987, with permission.*)

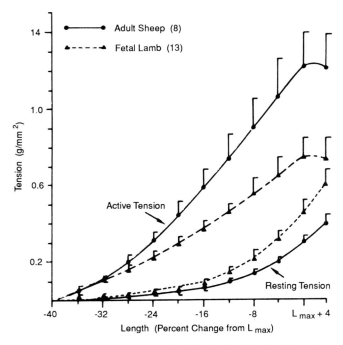

Figure 4–5. Length-tension relationships in fetal lambs (triangles) and adult sheep (circles) demonstrating the lower resting tension and greater active tension development in adult sheep. Fetal myocardium has a higher resting tension but less active tension development, which may explain why neonatal myocardium is less compliant than adult. (*From Friedman WF: The intrinsic properties of the developing heart. Prog Cardiovasc Dis 15:87–111, 1972, with permission.*)

less than 12 months of age correlates well with height, weight, or body surface area, but the best correlation for predicting normal cardiac output is with height.[43] The correlation of stroke volume with age is slightly higher than that with cardiac output. Ventricular dP/dt max increases at birth as demonstrated in chronically instrumented fetal and neonatal lambs.[44] These changes probably result from increased pulmonary venous return, heart rate, and inotropy in addition to changes in diastolic and systolic ventricular interactions.[44]

Left ventricular mechanics are abnormal in the neonate. At end diastole, the left ventricular cavity is circular, but significant ventricular distortion occurs with systole due to septal flattening associated with right ventricular hypertension. Ventricular septal and free wall systolic motion are increased during the first 3 days of life but become normal by day 4.[45]

In animal studies, postextrasystolic potentiation (PESP) increases during the last part of gestation or the first neonatal weeks.[44] However, experimental studies demonstrate that the neonatal increase in inotropy is associated with decreased postextrasystolic potentiation.[44] Within the first few weeks of life, both dP/dt max and PESP return toward fetal levels but PESP remains above

fetal levels. These changes reflect the alterations in cytosolic calcium associated with maturation.

In normal children aged 1 week to 19 years, Colan and co-workers noted that systolic function decreased with age as a substantial increase in wall stress occurred (most rapidly in the first 2 years of life).[46] However, velocity of shortening decreased more than expected from increased afterload alone.

In children aged 2 to 12 years, Franklin and co-workers noted that shortening and ejection fractions, velocity of circumferential fiber shortening, and wall stress were unchanged with growth. However, left ventricular end-systolic and end-diastolic length, diameter, wall thickness, volume, and mass increased linearly with body surface area.[47] Whether these normal developments in myocardial mechanics exist in the presence of cardiac pathology is unknown.

Myocardial Compliance. The neonatal myocardium is significantly less compliant than the adult myocardium[48] (Fig 4–5). Left ventricular compliance is greater than that of the right ventricle.[15] Thus, increases in preload do not improve stroke volume to the same extent as in adults.[24,48] Because of the reduced compliance, the neonatal heart is also more sensitive to increased afterload[49] (Fig 4–6).

Frank-Starling Relationship. Although both the fetal and neonatal heart follow the Frank-Starling relationship, the response of the neonatal heart to volume overload is distinctly limited compared with the adult.[50] The ascending limb of the Starling curve is short and steep

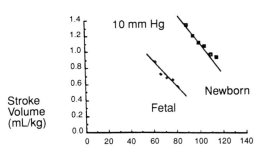

Figure 4–6. At a constant preload (left atrial pressure = 10 mm Hg), both fetal and newborn lamb hearts are sensitive to increased mean arterial pressure. In response to increased afterload, stroke volume decreases to a similar extent in both fetus and newborn (same slope). However, the newborn heart operates at greater mean pressures and stroke volumes than does the fetal heart. The differences in the position of the curves may result from changes in wall stress, intrathoracic pressure, or intrinsic contractility associated with birth. (*From Van Hare GF, et al: The effects of increasing mean arterial pressure on left ventricular output in newborn lambs. Circ Res 67: 78–83, 1990, with permission.*)

and plateaus at much lower filling pressures (5–7 mm Hg) than in the adult[51] (Fig 4–7). In younger infants, the plateau occurs at lower filling pressures than in older infants. Experimental evidence in newborn lambs indicates that the plateau in the Starling curve results from increases in mean arterial pressure. If mean arterial pressure remains constant, stroke volume continues to increase as left atrial pressure increases to 10 mm Hg when volume is infused.[49] The neonatal heart increases cardiac output by increasing rate rather than stroke volume. However, as in adults, excessive heart rates reduce biventricular stroke volume and output.[52]

Neonatal Circulatory Physiology

Although there are conflicting reports, cerebral blood flow appears to be lower in neonates than in adults, particularly in premature infants. In animal studies, cerebral blood flow increases during the first few weeks of life.[53,54] The qualitative response to changes in P_{CO_2} is similar in all age groups, but quantitative responses to hypocapnia are reduced in neonates.[55] As in adults, cerebral blood flow increases during hypoxia and decreases during hyperoxia. Autoregulatory mechanisms are easily impaired in neonates, causing cerebral blood flow to passively follow changes in mean arterial pressure.

The human neonatal kidney receives a slightly lower proportion of the cardiac output than the adult. Less of the renal blood flow is distributed to the superficial cortical nephrons in neonates.[56] Outer cortical flow increases during maturation. Renal blood flow increases with age owing to increased cardiac output and decreased renal vascular resistance. The development of renal autoregulation and adrenergic innervation with maturation also enhances compensatory mechanisms.

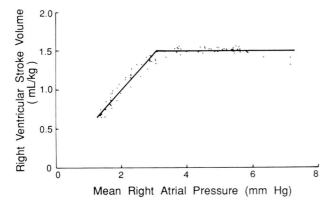

Figure 4–7. The neonatal heart obeys Starling's law, but the ascending limb of the Starling curve is short and steep with a plateau at 5–7 mm Hg. (*From Thornburg KL: Filling and arterial pressures as determinants of RV stroke volume in the sheep fetus. Am J Physiol 144:H656–H663, 1983, with permission.*)

In animals, gastrointestinal and hepatic blood flow increases during the first few days of life in response to increased organ weight. Weight-adjusted flows are greater than in adults.[57,58] An additional increase in gastrointestinal blood flow, oxygen consumption, and oxygen extraction is associated with feeding.[58]

PATHOPHYSIOLOGIC CONDITIONS

Hypoxia

In neonates, acute moderate hypoxia increases cardiac output if metabolic acidosis is absent. However, in the presence of acidosis, cardiac output decreases. Although heart rate increases with hypoxia, acute severe hypoxia causes bradycardia. Other changes associated with hypoxia are decreased myocardial contractility, increased central blood volume, increased pulmonary vascular resistance, increased cerebral blood flow, and reopening of the ductus arteriosus with right to left shunting.[59]

Chronic intrauterine fetal lamb hypoxia is characterized by initially unchanged right ventricular function, subsequently reduced output and stroke volume, and recovery of function within 2 weeks.[60] Thus, adaptive mechanisms, such as increased oxygen-carrying capacity, maintain normal fetal myocardial function during chronic hypoxia.

Ischemia

Neonatal hearts respond to ischemia by a rapid, proportional reduction in mechanical function to preserve critical energy stores and prevent irreversible myocardial injury. This property of myocardial hibernation is similar to that in adults and is characterized by increased oxygen extraction, decreased myocardial oxygen consumption, decreased glucose oxidation, lactate production and release, and preservation of ATP at 76% of control.[61] Glycolytic capacity and glycogen content is greater in neonates than in adult hearts. Lactate dehydrogenase in neonatal myocardium accelerates conversion of pyruvate to lactate, generating nicotinamide adenine dinucleotide for the glycolytic pathway.

Acidosis

Acidosis depresses myocardial function in adults. Recent evidence suggests that both respiratory and metabolic acidosis in newborns (rabbits) cause less depression of contractility.[62] The greater resistance of the newborn myocardium results from a smaller change in intracellular pH with acidosis as intracellular calcium increases to a similar extent in newborn and adult myocardium during acidosis[62] (Fig 4–8). Intracellular buffer capacity is greater in immature myocardium. The sensitivity of the contractile proteins and myofibrillar ATPase activity to acidosis in less in newborn than in adult animals.

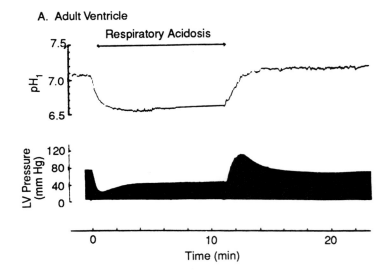

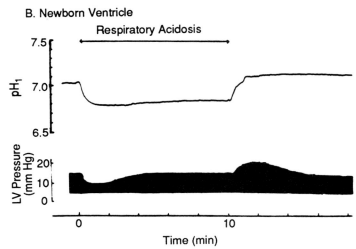

Figure 4–8. Respiratory acidosis produces less depression of intracellular pH and myocardial contractility in newborn (*B*) than in adult (*A*) rabbit ventricle. Similar effects occur with metabolic acidosis. (*From Nakanishi T, et al: Effect of acidosis on intracellular pH and calcium concentration in the newborn and adult rabbit myocardium. Circ Res 67:111–123, 1990, with permission.*)

REFERENCES

1. Hickey PR, Hansen DD: Anesthesia and cardiac shunting in the neonate: Ductus arteriosus, transitional circulation, and congenital heart disease. *Semin Anesth* **3:**106–116, 1984

2. Pang LM, Mellins RB: Neonatal cardiorespiratory physiology. *Anesthesiology* **43:**171–196, 1975

3. Agata Y, Hiraishi S, Oguchi K, et al: Changes in left ventricular output from fetal to early neonatal life. *J Pediatr* **119:**441–445, 1991

4. Takenaka K, Waffern F, Dabestani A, et al: A pulsed Doppler echocardiographic study of the postnatal changes in pulmonary artery and ascending aortic flow in normal term newborn infants. *Am Heart J* **113:**759–766, 1987

5. Farooki ZQ, Green EW: Physiology of the circulation. In Arciniegas E (ed): *Pediatric Cardiac Surgery*. Chicago: Year Book Medical, 1985, pp 13–18

6. Wilson N, Reed K, Allen HD, et al: Doppler echocardiographic observations of pulmonary and transvalvular velocity changes after birth and during the early neonatal period. *Am Heart J* **113:**750–758, 1987

7. Haworth SG, Hislop AA: Pulmonary vascular development: Normal values of peripheral vascular structure. *Am J Cardiol* **52:**578–583, 1983

8. Heymann MA: Regulation of the pulmonary circulation in the perinatal period and in children. *Intensive Care Med* **15:**S9–S12, 1989

9. Abman SH, Chatfield BA, Hall SL, McMurtry IF: Role of endothelium-derived relaxing factor during transition of pulmonary circulation at birth. *Am J Physiol* **259:**H1921–H1927, 1990

10. Rudolph AM, Heymann MA: Fetal and neonatal circulation and respiration. *Ann Rev Physiol* **36:**187–209, 1974

11. Mahoney LT, Coryell KG, Lauer RM: The newborn transitional circulation: A two-dimensional Doppler echocardiographic study. *J Am Coll Cardiol* **6:**623–629, 1985

12. Wong S-N, Lo RN, Hui P-W: Abnormal renal and splanchnic arterial Doppler pattern in premature babies with symptomatic patent ductus arteriosus. *J Ultrasound Med* **9:**125–130, 1990

13. Heymann MA, Rudolph AM: Control of the ductus arteriosus. *Physiol Rev* **55:**62–78, 1975

14. Rudolph AM, Scarpelli EM, Golinko RJ: Hemodynamic basis for clinical manifestations for patent ductus arteriosus. *Am Heart J* **68:**447–458, 1964

15. Steinfeld L, Almeida OD, Rothfeld EL: Asynchronous atrioventricular valve opening as it related to right to left interatrial shunting in the normal newborn. *J Am Coll Cardiol* **12:**712–718, 1988

16. Lev M, Bharati S: Embryology of the heart and great vessels. In Arciniegas E (ed): *Pediatric Cardiac Surgery.* Chicago: Year Book Medical, 1985, pp 1–12

17. Wladimiroff JW, Vosters R, McGhie JS: Normal cardiac ventricular geometry and function during the last trimester of pregnancy and early neonatal period. *Br J Obstet Gynecol* **89:**938–944, 1982

18. Anversa P, Ricci R, Olivetti G: Quantitative structural analysis of the myocardium during physiologic growth and induced cardiac hypertrophy: A Review. *J Am Coll Cardiol* **7:**1140–1149, 1986

19. Anderson PAW: Maturation and cardiac contractility. *Cardiol Clin* **7:**209–225, 1989

20. Humphreys JE, Cummins P: Regulatory protein of the myocardium. Atrial and ventricular tropomyosin and troponin in the developing and adult bovine and human heart. *J Mol Cell Cardiol* **16:**643–657, 1984

21. Sweeney LJ, Nag AC, Eisenberg B, et al: Developmental aspects of cardiac contractile proteins. *Basic Res Cardiol* **80**(suppl 2):123–127, 1985

22. Carlsson E, Kjorell U, Thornell LE, et al: Differentiation of the myofibrils and the intermediate filament system during postnatal development of the rat heart. *Eur J Cell Biol* **27:**62–73, 1982

23. Nelson WJ, Lazarides E: Expression of the beta subunit of spectrin in nonerythroid cells. *Proc Natl Acad Sci USA* **80:** 363–367, 1983

24. Friedman WF: The intrinsic physiologic properties of the developing heart. *Prog Cardiovasc Dis* **15:**87–111, 1972

25. Tripp ME: Developmental cardiac metabolism in health and disease. *Pediatr Cardiol* **10:**150–158, 1989

26. Veerkamp JH, Glatz JFC, Wagenmakers AJM: Metabolic changes during cardiac maturation. *Basic Res Cardiol* **80**(suppl 2):111–114, 1985

27. Werner JC, Whitman V, Vary TC, et al: Fatty acid and glucose utilization in isolated, working newborn pig hearts. *Am J Physiol* **244:**E19–E23, 1983

28. White RD, Moffitt EA, Feldt RH, Ritter DG: Myocardial metabolism in children with heart disease. *Anesth Analg* **51:**6–10, 1972

29. Chizzonite RA, Zak R: Calcium-induced cell death: Susceptibility of cardiac myocytes is age-dependent. *Science* **213:**1508–1511, 1981

30. Nakamura H, del Nido PJ, Jimenez E, et al: Age-related differences in cardiac susceptibility to ischemia/reperfusion injury. *J Thorac Cardiovasc Surg* **104:**165–172, 1992

31. Chin TK, Friedman WF, Klitzner TS: Developmental changes in cardiac myocyte calcium regulation. *Circ Res* **67:**574–579, 1990

32. Klitzner TS: Maturational changes in excitation-contraction coupling in mammalian myocardium. *J Am Coll Cardiol* **17:**218–225, 1991

33. Hoerter J, Mazet F, Vassort G: Perinatal growth of the rabbit cardiac cell: Possible implications for the mechanism of relaxation. *J Mol Cell Cardiol* **13:**725–740, 1981

34. Mahony L, Jones LR: Developmental changes in cardiac sarcoplasmic reticulum in sheep. *J Biol Chem* **261:**15257–15265, 1986

35. Saarikoski S: Functional development of adrenergic uptake mechanisms in the human fetal heart. *Biol Neonate* **43:**158–163, 1983

36. Roeske WR, Wildenthal K: Responsiveness to drugs and hormones in the murine model of cardiac ontogenesis. *Pharmacol Ther* **14:**55–66, 1981

37. Yamada S, Yamamura HI, Roseke WR: Ontogeny of mammalian cardiac alpha$_1$ adrenergic receptors. *Eur J Pharmacol* **68:**217–221, 1980

38. Cheng JB, Cornett LE, Goldfien A, Roberts JM: Decreased concentration of myocardial alpha-adrenoceptors with increasing age in fetal lambs. *Br J Pharmacol* **70:**515–517, 1980

39. Bernstein D, Voss E, Huang S, et al: Differential regulation of right and left ventricular beta-adrenergic receptors in newborn lambs with experimental cyanotic heart disease. *J Clin Invest* **85:**68–74, 1990

40. Driscoll DJ, Park I-S, Baron P, Michael L: Developmental changes in response of dog isolated ventricular myocardium to norepinephrine. *Texas Heart Inst J* **10:**397–403, 1983

41. Caspi J, Coles JG, Benson LN, et al: Age-related response to epinephrine-induced myocardial stress. *Circulation* **84**(suppl III):III394–III399, 1991

42. Eliot RJ, Lam R, Leake RD, et al: Plasma catecholamine concentrations in infants at birth and during the first 48 hours of life. *J Pediatr* **96:**311–315, 1980

43. Sholler GF, Celermajer JM, Whight CM, Baumann AE: Echo Doppler assessment of cardiac output and its relation to growth in normal infants. *Am J Cardiol* **60:**1112–1116, 1987

44. Anderson PAW, Manring A, Glick KL, et al: Biophysics of the developing heart. III. A comparison of the left ventricular dynamics of the fetal and neonatal lamb heart. *Am J Obstet Gynecol* **143:**195–203, 1982

45. Rein AJJT, Sanders SP, Colan SD, et al: Left ventricular mechanics in the normal newborn. *Circulation* **76:**1029–1036, 1987

46. Colan SD, Parness IA, Spevak PJ, Sanders SP: Developmental modulation of myocardial mechanics: Age and growth-related alterations in afterload and contractility. *J Am Coll Cardiol* **19:**619–629, 1992

47. Franklin RCG, Wyse RKH, Graham TP, et al: Normal values for noninvasive estimation of left ventricular contractile state and afterload in children. *Am J Cardiol* **65:** 505–510, 1990

48. Romero T, Covell J, Friedman WF: A comparison of pressure-volume relations of the fetal, newborn, and adult heart. *Am J Physiol* **222:**1285–1290, 1972

49. Van Hare GF, Hawkins JA, Schmidt KG, Rudolph AM: The effects of increasing mean arterial pressure on left ventricular output in newborn lambs. *Circ Res* **67:**78–83, 1990

50. Rudolph AM: Developmental considerations in neonatal failure. *Hosp Pract* **20:**53–57, and 61–67, 1985

51. Thornburg KL, Morton MJ: Filling and arterial pressures as determinants of RV stroke volume in the sheep fetus. *Am J Physiol* **144:**H656–H663, 1983

52. Anderson PA, Glick KL, Killiam AP: The effect of heart rate on in utero left ventricular output in the fetal sheep. *J Physiol (Lond)* **372:**557–573, 1986

53. Kennedy C, Grave GD, Jehle JW, et al: Blood flow to white matter during maturation of the brain. *Neurology* **20:**613–621, 1970

54. Kennedy C, Grave GD, Jehle JW, et al: Changes in blood flow in the component structures of the dog brain during postnatal maturation. *Neurochemistry* **19:**137–140, 1972

55. Shapiro HM, Greenberg JH, Naughton KV, et al: Heterogeneity of local cerebral blood flow-PaCo2 sensitivity in neonatal dogs. *J Appl Physiol* **49:**113–118, 1980

56. Olbing H, Blaufox MD, Aschinberg LC, et al: Postnatal changes in renal glomerular blood flow distribution in puppies. *J Clin Invest* **52:**2885–2895, 1973

57. Edelstone DI, Holzman IR: Oxygen consumption by the gastrointestinal tract and liver in conscious newborn lambs. *Am J Physiol* **240:**G297–G304, 1981

58. Touloukian RJ, Spencer RP, Stinson KK: Alimentary circulation in the pup during the postnatal period. *Arch Surg* **102:**516–520, 1981

59. Einzig S, Zhang S-L: Neonatal systemic vasculature. In Moller JH, Neal WA (eds): *Fetal, Neonatal, and Infant Cardiac Disease.* East Norwalk, CT: Appleton & Lange, 1990, pp 133–157

60. Alonso JG, Oaki T, Longo LD, Gilbert RD: Cardiac function during long-term hypoxemia in fetal sheep. *Am J Physiol* **257:**H581–589, 1989

61. Downing SE, Chen V: Myocardial hibernation in the ischemic neonatal heart. *Circ Res* **66:**763–772, 1990

62. Nakanishi T, Seguchi M, Tsuchiya T, et al: Effect of acidosis on intracellular pH and calcium concentration in the newborn and adult rabbit myocardium. *Circ Res* **67:**111–123, 1990

Chapter 5 | Preoperative Evaluation of the Pediatric Cardiac Patient

Karen S. Rheuban

The evaluation of the child with congenital heart disease requires a multidisciplinary approach. The techniques of a carefully recorded history and physical examination combined with radiographic and electrocardiographic studies serve as an introduction to the cardiovascular anatomy and physiology of the child with congenital heart defects.

Echocardiographic tools (two-dimensional, M-mode, Doppler, and color flow Doppler) provide precise noninvasive anatomic diagnoses along with measurements of cardiac flow patterns, velocities, and assessments of ventricular function. When further hemodynamic and/or angiographic data are necessary, cardiac catheterization and angiography offer confirmation of noninvasive diagnoses as well as documentation of intracardiac pressures, shunts, cardiac output, and systemic and pulmonary vascular resistances.

HISTORY AND PHYSICAL EXAMINATION

History

The initial assessment of the child with cardiac disease should include a review of historical parameters referable to the cardiovascular system, obtained in a somewhat chronologic fashion beginning with the prenatal period.

1. *Family history:* Is there a family history of congenital heart disease (the recurrence risk is approximately 3% when one sibling has congenital heart disease), sudden death (hypertrophic cardiomyopathy, long QT syndrome, congenital coronary artery anomalies), premature cardiovascular death (hypertension, atherosclerotic coronary artery disease)?
2. *Prenatal period:* Maternal health should be ascertained with attention to possible viral infections (such as rubella), drug and alcohol exposure, first trimester bleeding, and maternal glucose homeostasis.
3. *Neonatal period:* Attention should be paid to birth weight, gestational age, Apgar scores, the presence or absence of respiratory distress, cyanosis or oxygen requirement. Was a cardiac murmur noted in the nursery? Did the infant require cardiac catheterization or surgery?
4. *Infancy:* Did the patient feed well, gain weight normally, and meet developmental milestones? Were there episodes of central or peripheral cyanosis, dyspnea, pallor, or extremes of diaphoresis?
5. *Preschool and school age:* Does the child keep up with his or her peers? Does the child tire more readily, squat with activity, complain of chest pain, palpitations, or syncope? Is there any history of arthritis, rash, fever, chorea, streptococcal disease, subcutaneous nodules, blood transfusion, or drug abuse?

Physical Examination

The physical examination of the child with heart disease is best performed in the least threatening environment, often most satisfactorily in the arms of a parent. One can usually readily ascertain if the patient is in good health or acutely or chronically ill. The detection of cyanosis is of critical importance. Cyanosis is clinically apparent in the presence of 5 g of unsaturated hemoglobin. Thus, an anemic child with significant arterial desaturation may not appear cyanotic. Conversely, an infant with extreme polycythemia may appear severely cyanotic even in the face of mild systemic desaturation. Cyanosis may be exacerbated with crying or with activity in older patients. Respiratory distress, as manifested by tachypnea, intercostal or subcostal retractions, alar flaring, and grunting, is often plainly seen upon inspection of the patient.

Measurement of vital signs should include height, weight, pulse rate, respiratory rate, and temperature, and measurement of the blood pressure in the right arm and a lower extremity. Normal blood pressure measurements are indicated in Fig 5–1.[1]

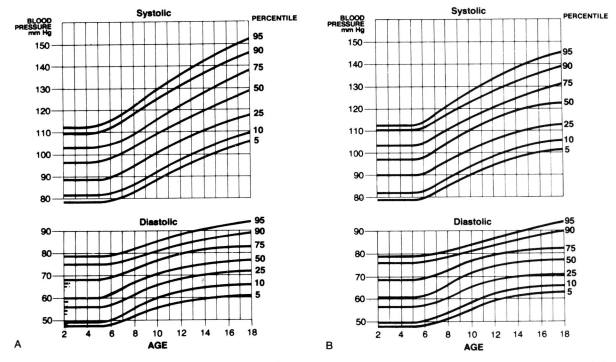

Figure 5–1. Summary of normal blood pressures in children. (*A*) Males. (*B*) Females. (*From Blumenthal S, et al: Standards for Children's Blood Pressure. Pediatrics 59:803, 1977, with permission.*)

Cardiac Examination. The external examination of the heart includes an assessment of the precordial activity. Is the precordium quiet or is there increased precordial activity? Is it there a precordial bulge or a pectus excavatum? Palpation of the precordial impulse will locate the point of maximal intensity and indicate the presence or absence of thrills.

Auscultation of the heart should be performed in a quiet setting with maximum patient cooperation. The heart sounds are evaluated in various body positions (lying, sitting, decubitus, standing). S_1 is normally split only at the lower left sternal border. The presence of splitting of the first heart sound at other locations should raise the suspicion of the presence of an ejection click. S_2, consisting of the aortic and pulmonic closure sounds, is best evaluated at the upper left sternal border. In inspiration, the pulmonic closure sound may normally be delayed by 0.04–0.06 seconds. The two components of the second sound should merge during expiration. Wide splitting of the second heart sound may be heard in association with atrial septal defect, pulmonic stenosis, or right bundle branch block, all of which are conditions that delay right ventricular emptying. Reverse splitting may be heard in association with aortic stenosis, with delayed closure of the aortic valve.

Clicks and Murmurs. Systolic ejection clicks are generally heard in early systole in patients with pulmonic

and aortic valve abnormalities and in mid-systole in patients with mitral valve prolapse. Diastolic sounds are heard in association with atrioventricular valve abnormalities (such as the diastolic rumble and opening snap associated with mitral stenosis). A third heart sound is normal in children, but a fourth heart sound or summation gallop always indicates diminished myocardial compliance.

Cardiac murmurs may occur in systole, diastole, or may be classified as continuous, beginning in systole and extending into diastole (Table 5–1). Systolic murmurs may be innocent (such as a Still's murmur) or may occur secondary to true stenosis of a semilunar valve, outflow tract or an artery (such as in aortic stenosis, subaortic stenosis, or coarctation of the aorta), increased flow through a normal valve (as in the pulmonary flow murmur in atrial septal defect), secondary to insufficiency of an atrioventricular valve (as in mitral or tricuspid regurgitation), or secondary to a ventricular septal defect. Diastolic murmurs may reflect insufficiency of a semilunar valve (as in aortic insufficiency), stenosis of an atrioventricular valve (mitral, tricuspid stenosis), or "relative stenosis" of an atrioventricular valve (increased volume of flow across a normal atrioventricular valve, as in the mitral flow rumble associated with a large ventricular septal defect). Continuous murmurs may occur in the presence of a patent ductus arteriosus, a surgical shunt (such as the Blalock-Taussig shunt), an aorticopulmo-

TABLE 5–1. CLASSIFICATION OF CARDIAC MURMURS

Systolic
    Aortic stenosis
    Pulmonic stenosis
    Atrial septal defect
    Tricuspid regurgitation
    Mitral regurgitation
    Ventricular septal defect
    Coarctation
    Still's murmur

Diastolic
    Pulmonic insufficiency
    Aortic insufficiency
    Tricuspid stenosis
    Mitral stenosis
    Mitral flow rumble
    Tricuspid flow rumble

Continuous
    Patent ductus arteriosus
    Venous hum
    Surgical shunt
    Aorticopulmonary window
    Arteriovenous fistula
    Bronchial collaterals
    Severe peripheral pulmonic stenosis

nary septal defect, an arteriovenous malformation, or a coronary artery fistula. Generally, these continuous murmurs are accentuated in systole. A continuous murmur with diastolic accentuation heard at the upper right sternal border in the upright position is usually a benign venous hum.

Heart sounds and murmurs may be greatly influenced by changes in posture and respiration. A simple maneuver, such as changing from the supine to the sitting position, decreases venous return and exacerbates the murmurs of hypertrophic cardiomyopathy and mitral valve prolapse. Auscultation in the supine position increases venous return to the heart and thus increases the intensity of an innocent murmur as well as the murmurs of aortic and pulmonic stenosis. By augmenting venous return to the right heart, inspiration increases the murmur of pulmonic stenosis and tricuspid regurgitation. By increasing systemic vascular resistance, squatting decreases the murmur of hypertrophic cardiomyopathy and mitral prolapse but increases the murmur of ventricular septal defect.

Pulmonary Examination. A careful lung examination will help to identify the patient with abnormal pulmonary compliance secondary to large left-to-right shunts, pulmonary edema, or the presence of a pulmonary infection. Wheezing may occur in patients with pulmonary infection and air trapping (as in infants with bronchiolitis) but may also be heard in patients with a vascular ring or bronchomalacia secondary to bronchial compression,

as in the absent pulmonary valve syndrome. The presence of rales may indicate pulmonary edema but more commonly reflects underlying pneumonitis.

Chest Radiograph. Although extremely helpful in the evaluation of the child with congenital heart disease, the chest radiograph frequently appears normal during the early neonatal period despite the presence of complex congenital heart disease. In evauating the chest radiograph of a child with possible heart disease, the following parameters should be carefully evaluated: (1) the position of the heart, (2) the cardiac size, (3) the cardiac shape, (4) the pulmonary artery, (5) the pulmonary vascularity, and (6) the aortic contour.

Cardiac malposition may be secondary to congenital abnormalities of the lungs, skeleton, or diaphragm or may be due to atelectasis or pneumothorax. True cardiac malpositions may be associated with the syndromes of asplenia, polysplenia, and situs inversus. In assessing the child with cardiac malposition, it is of the utmost importance to identify visceral situs by assessing the location of the gastric bubble and liver.

In ascertaining heart size, one needs to consider the method by which the chest radiograph was obtained. If it was obtained in the supine rather than the upright position, the cardiothoracic ratio may be slightly >50% (Fig 5–2). The presence of a prominent thymic shadow may further complicate the assessment of heart size. During the first year of life, the thymic shadow generally regresses and the cardiothoracic ratio should diminish to ≤50% in an upright position.[2]

Various configurations of cardiac shape have been described that suggest a specific cardiac diagnosis. The "egg on its side" has been used to describe D-transposition of the great arteries; the "coeur en sabot," or

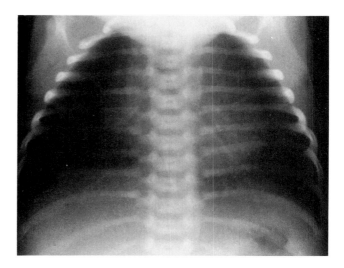

Figure 5–2. A normal chest radiograph of a 2-week-old child. Note the cardiothoracic ratio is approximately 50%.

boot-shaped heart, for tetralogy of Fallot (Fig 5–3); the "snowman" or "figure-of-eight" for total anomalous pulmonary venous return to the vertical vein (Fig 5–4); and the "water bottle" heart for pericardial effusion.[3]

An evaluation of the pulmonary vascular pattern is essential in attempting to diagnose congenital heart disease using radiologic tools. The vascular pattern may be increased, decreased, or normal. Enlarged pulmonary arteries and veins occur secondary to left-to-right shunt lesions. When a pulmonary artery is seen and is larger than its companion bronchus on end, increased pulmonary vascularity is suggested. In general, engorgement of the pulmonary vascular bed occurs when the pulmonary to systemic flow ratio is >2:1 (Fig 5–5).[4] A pulmonary edema pattern secondary to extravasation of fluid into the pulmonary interstitium may be seen in patients with large left-to-right shunts or with left heart obstruction.

Dilatation of the main pulmonary artery may be seen in left-to-right shunt lesions, the syndrome of idiopathic dilatation of the main pulmonary artery, and in valvular pulmonic stenosis, where frequently the left pulmonary artery is dilated as well. Aneurysmal dilatation of the pulmonary arteries may be seen in patients with tetralogy of Fallot with an absent pulmonary valve.

Decreased pulmonary vascularity associated with right-to-left shunt lesions is manifested radiographically by a small main pulmonary artery and pulmonary vessels that extend only to the middle third to one half of the

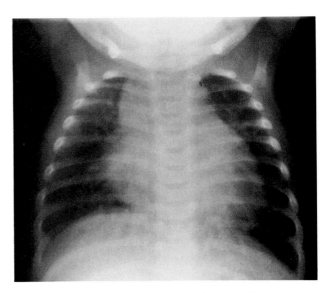

Figure 5–4. The classic "snow-man" or "figure of eight" is seen on the chest radiograph of an infant with total anomalous pulmonary venous connection to the vertical vein.

lung fields. An absent pulmonary artery segment may be seen in association with tetralogy of Fallot and truncus arteriosus.

The aortic contour and location of the aortic arch are helpful in the diagnosis of specific cardiac lesions. Dilatation of the ascending aorta suggests valvular aortic stenosis, whereas a notch in the descending aorta (the so-called "3 sign") is seen with coarctation of the aorta. A right aortic arch is seen in 30% of patients with truncus arteriosus and 25% of patients with tetralogy of Fallot.

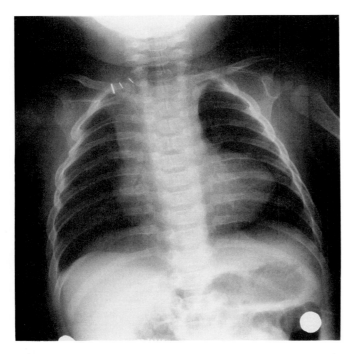

Figure 5–3. The classic chest radiograph of a child with tetralogy of Fallot is seen. Note the boot-shaped heart secondary to an absent main pulmonary artery segment and a tipped up apex.

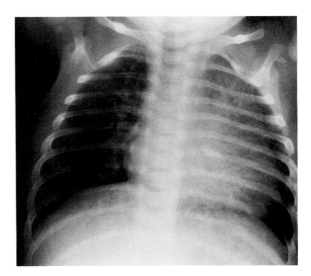

Figure 5–5. Chest radiograph of an infant with large ventricular septal defect showing cardiomegaly, increased vascularity, and a prominent thymic shadow.

TABLE 5-2. SUMMARY OF NORMAL ELECTROCARDIOGRAPHIC VALUES IN CHILDREN

Age Group	*Heart Rate (BPM)	Frontal Plane QRS Vector (degrees)	PR Interval (s)	†Q III (mm)§	†Q V6 (mm)	RV1 (mm)	SV1 (mm)	R/S V1	RV6 (mm)	SV6 (mm)	R/S V6	†SV1 + RV6 (mm)	†R + S V4 (mm)
< 1 d	93–154 (123)	+59 to −163 (137)	0.08–0.16 (0.11)	4.5	2	5–26 (14)	0–23 (8)	0.1–U (2.2)	0–11 (4)	0–9.5 (3)	0.1–U (2.0)	28	52.5
1–2 d	91–159 (123)	+64 to −161 (134)	0.08–0.14 (0.11)	6.5	2.5	5–27 (14)	0–21 (9)	0.1–U (2.0)	0–12 (4.5)	0–9.5 (3)	0.1–U (2.5)	29	52
3–6 d	91–166 (129)	+77 to −163 (132)	0.07–0.14 (0.10)	5.5	3	3–24 (13)	0–17 (7)	0.2–U (2.7)	0.5–12 (5)	0–10 (3.5)	0.1–U (2.2)	24.5	49
1–3 wk	107–182 (148)	+65 to +161 (110)	0.07–0.14 (0.10)	6	3	3–21 (11)	0–11 (4)	1.0–U (2.9)	2.5–16.5 (7.5)	0–10 (3.5)	0.1–U (3.3)	21	49
1–2 mo	121–179 (149)	+31 to +113 (74)	0.07–0.13 (0.10)	7.5	3	3–18 (10)	0–12 (5)	0.3–U (2.3)	5–21.5 (11.5)	0–6.5 (3)	0.2–U (4.8)	29	53.5
3–5 mo	106–186 (141)	+7 to +104 (60)	0.07–0.15 (0.11)	6.5	3	3–20 (10)	0–17 (6)	0.1–U (2.3)	6.5–22.5 (13)	0–10 (3)	0.2–U (6.2)	32	61.5
6–11 mo	109–169 (134)	+6 to +99 (56)	0.07–0.16 (0.11)	8.5	3	1.5–20 (9.5)	0.5–18 (4)	0.1–3.9 (1.6)	6–22.5 (12.5)	0–7 (2)	0.2–U (7.6)	32	53
1–2 yr	89–151 (119)	+7 to +101 (55)	0.08–0.15 (0.11)	6	3	2.5–17 (9)	0.5–21 (8)	0.05–4.3 (1.4)	6–22.5 (13)	0–6.5 (2)	0.3–U (9.3)	39	49.5
3–4 yr	73–137 (108)	+6 to +104 (55)	0.09–0.16 (0.12)	5	3.5	1–18 (8)	0.2–21 (10)	0.03–2.8 (0.9)	8–24.5 (15)	0–5 (1.5)	0.6–U (10.8)	42	53.5
5–7 yr	65–133 (100)	+11 to +143 (65)	0.09–0.16 (0.12)	4	4.5	0.5–14 (7)	0.3–24 (12)	0.02–2.0 (0.7)	8.5–26.5 (16)	0–4 (1)	0.9–U (11.5)	47	54
8–11 yr	62–130 (91)	+9 to +114 (61)	0.09–0.17 (0.13)	3	3	0–12 (5.5)	0.3–25 (12)	0–1.8 (0.5)	9–25.5 (16)	0–4 (1)	1.5–U (14.3)	45.5	53
12–15 yr	60–119 (85)	+11 to +130 (59)	0.09–0.18 (0.14)	3	3	0–10 (4)	0.3–21 (11)	0–1.7 (0.5)	6.5–23 (14)	0–4 (1)	1.4–U (14.7)	41	50

* 2.98% (mean).
† Ninety-eighth percentile.
§ Millimeters at normal standardization.
U, undefined.
Note: Numbers in parentheses are means. U = unknown.
(From Garson A, et al: The Science and Practice of Pediatric Cardiology. Philadelphia: Lea & Febiger, 1990, p 714, with permission.)

Electrocardiography. The pediatric electrocardiogram differs greatly from that of the adult in that the electrocardiogram of the child reflects the evolution from fetal anatomy and physiology to more adult patterns after the first few years of life. In the neonatal period, profound changes in pulmonary and systemic vascular resistance occur causing gradual reductions in ventricular muscle mass. Thus, in infancy, the electrocardiogram reflects this increased right ventricular mass as "normal" right ventricular hypertrophy.[5]

As regression of the right ventricular hypertrophy occurs, the normal adult pattern develops. Heart rate, mean frontal plane QRS axis, PR interval, and QRS duration are all variables that change with age.[5,6] For this reason, the criteria for ventricular hypertrophy vary with the age of the patient (Table 5–2).[6]

Echocardiography. Echocardiography is an important noninvasive diagnostic tool that has revolutionized pediatric cardiology practices. A variety of imaging and flow analysis techniques including M-mode, two-dimensional, Doppler, contrast, color flow, and esophageal echocardiography have become routine diagnostic tools that are invaluable to the pediatric cardiologist. An extensive review of echocardiographic techniques is in Chapter 6.

REFERENCES

1. Blumenthal S, Epps R, Heavenrich, R: Report of the task force on blood pressure control in children. *Pediatrics* **59:** 797–798, 1977
2. Burnard E, James L: Radiographic heart size in apparently healthy newborn infants. *Pediatrics* **27:**726–739, 1961
3. Elliot LP, Scheibler G: *X-ray Diagnosis of Congenital Heart Disease.* Springfield, IL: Charles C Thomas, 1968
4. Moes CAF: Noninvasive investigations: The chest roentgenogram in congenital heart disease. In Keith JD, Rowe RD, Vlad P (eds): *Heart Disease in Infants, Children and Adolescents.* New York: Macmillan, 1978, pp 45–50
5. Davignon A, Rautaharju P: Normal ECG standards for infants and children. *Pediatr Cardiol* **1:**123–152, 1979
6. Garson A: *The Electrocardiogram in Infants and Children: A Systematic Approach.* Philadelphia: Lea & Febiger, 1983, p 404

Chapter 6 | Pediatric Echocardiography

William J. Greeley

The complexity of congenital heart defects, the diversity of surgical repairs, and the critical alterations in blood flow patterns and ventricular function are challenges to the anesthesiologist and surgeon during operative management of patients with congenital heart disease. Echocardiography with Doppler color flow imaging improves the intraoperative assessment of quality of surgical repair of congenital heart defects.

PRINCIPLES OF ECHOCARDIOGRAPHY

Sound is propagated as a series of mechanical waves of compression through the medium traversed. Sound transmission through a medium sets up a series of compressions and refractions causing pressure waves that oscillate regularly. The distance between successive pressure wave cycles determines the wavelength. The nature, impedance, density, and homogeneity of the medium determine the speed of transmission and wave propagation.[1] Sound waves can be further characterized by their velocity and frequency, which are interrelated. Frequency is a fundamental characteristic of any wave phenomenon, including sound, and is defined as the number of waves that pass a given point in 1 second. It is usually described in units of cycles per second or hertz (Hz). Emitted frequencies of sound inaudible to the human ear are referred to as ultrasound.

Echocardiography uses the principles of ultrasound wave transmission to produce images and assess blood flow.[1,2] The echocardiographic transducer (pulse generator) emits ultrasound beams and receives reflected waves. Ultrasound transducers possess piezoelectric crystals that are capable of producing a burst of ultrasound at a specific frequency in a selected direction. As ultrasound waves travel through a homogeneous media, part of the energy will be absorbed and the remainder transmitted. When ultrasound waves are propagated through an inhomogeneous medium, some of the energy is absorbed, some of the energy is reflected back (reflected wave), and the remainder passes through the medium (refracted wave) into the next medium or is scattered. Because all human tissues are inhomogeneous, ultrasound waves passed through the chest wall or esophagus have this pattern of partial absorption, partial reflection, partial refraction, and partial scattering. The degree of reflection versus refraction depends on two properties: (1) the difference between density and impedance of the two media through which the ultrasound wave travels and (2) the angle of incidence of the ultrasound beam.[1,2] Large differences in homogeneity of the media, eg, the endocardial surface of the heart and adjacent blood-filled ventricular cavity, produce strong reflections of ultrasound waves. Likewise, surfaces perpendicular to the line of beam propagation, eg, tricuspid and mitral valve motion in a four-chamber view of the heart, have very prominent reflected waves and an intense signal. Owing to the fact that the intensity of ultrasound waves is attenuated with increasing transmission distance, reflectance is diminished and the resultant analysis of the beam decreases in quality. Therefore, for a given transducer with a set frequency, image quality is poorer when the area of interest is farther from the transducer.[3] Because frequency and speed of transmission are known, the distance of wave propagation to a specific point can be easily determined by the time required for the echo wave to be reflected back to the transducer. Because each ultrasound wave encounters many surfaces of inhomogeneity, the reflected echo waves return at times corresponding to the depth of reflection. Consequently, each pulsed-wave transmission generates information and corresponds to the structures encountered along the line of ultrasound beam transmission. From this information, an image is processed and constructed.

M-Mode Echocardiography
M-mode echocardiography takes advantage of these principles of wave transmission along a single line.[3] With M-mode or motion-mode display, structural information is plotted as distance from the transducer on the vertical

axis and time on the horizontal axis. The combination of depth information and time provides a visual display of cardiac structures in motion in real time. With the M-mode technique, all ultrasonic waves are propagated along the same axis in different parts of the heart and studied by changing the direction of the beam manually. The M-mode echocardiogram depicts structural change during the cardiac cycle. This method does not provide information about the spatial relationships of different parts of the heart to each other. Because only a restricted view of cardiac structures is displayed with M-mode, its use is selective and limited. However, M-mode provides an excellent method for precise quantitation of the timing of cardiac events.

Two-Dimensional Echocardiography

Using multiple individual lines of wave transmission, ie, multiple lines of M-mode echocardiographic transmission, a two-dimensional image of the heart can be obtained.[3] Two-dimensional echocardiographic systems emit high-frequency bursts of sound (ultrasound) into tissues. A given pulse of ultrasound is transmitted into the body and then reflected back from the various tissues. The best ultrasound images are made when the target is perpendicular to the sound waves. Because the speed of ultrasound wave propagation in tissue is known, two-dimensional echocardiography waits for a given time for the transmitted pulse to travel to the target and then back, where information is received, processed, and recorded. Using repetitive scanning along a sector arch of approximately 90°, two-dimensional cardiac images are obtained and constructed in real time. With conventional two-dimensional imaging systems, this alternating process is repeated in a variety of directions hundreds of times each second. A series of matrixes of electronic memory cells allow digitizing of the image. The resultant sector image is formatted using a digital scan converter. Images from the scan converter can be transferred directly onto a videotape for storage or immediate playback.

Doppler Echocardiography

Doppler echocardiography is a method for detecting the direction and velocity of moving blood in the heart.[4,5] The Doppler methods extend the use of cardiac ultrasound into the evaluation of normal and abnormal flow states and provide quantitative data that are essential to the clinical decision-making process about patients with heart disease. Understanding Doppler echocardiography begins with knowledge of the Doppler principle. This principle was first described by Johan Doppler in 1892 when he postulated that certain properties of light emitted from the stars depended on the relative motion of the observer and the wave source. The Doppler principle states that the frequency of transmitted sound is changed when the source of the emitted waves is moving. The original frequency of the moving sound emitter does not change; however, the received frequency of the signal changes as the emitter is moving toward or away from the receiver. The Doppler principle applies to all types of wave propagation where the source and receiver are moving relative to one another.

When applied to echocardiography, the Doppler principle states that the frequency of ultrasound waves reflected from moving red blood cells and other cardiac tissues are different from the original frequency emitted from the transducer.[4,5] Doppler systems depend entirely on the changes in the frequency of transmitted ultrasound, resulting from the encounter of the wave front with moving red blood cells. Doppler systems analyze the transmitted waveform and the received waveform for a change in frequency. These changes, called phase shifts, are automatically determined within the Doppler instrument. The Doppler instrument is a complex analyzer detecting red blood cell motion and measuring its velocity.

The change in frequency from the original and received ultrasound waves is related to the velocity and direction of blood flow as well as to other factors such as the angle between the ultrasound beam and the blood flow. The resultant Doppler frequency change (Doppler shift) is of the magnitude that produces an audible signal. Analysis of the spectrum of frequencies can be transformed into frequency display and corresponding amplitude. Depending on the relative changes of the returning frequencies, Doppler echocardiographic systems measure direction, velocity, and turbulence of disturbed flow. This feature allows differentiation between normal and abnormal flow patterns and quantifies those characteristics that are helpful in determining the severity of abnormal flow states.[4,5]

Thus, Doppler echocardiography produces graphic displays of frequency, signal change, or velocity versus time and distinguishes directions of Doppler flow signals. Currently, Doppler technology is used in echocardiography to measure blood flow velocity and direction: (1) continuous-wave Doppler, (2) pulsed-wave Doppler, and (3) Doppler color flow imaging (echo-Doppler).

Continuous-Wave Doppler. As the name implies, continuous-wave Doppler involves continuous generation of ultrasound beams coupled with continuous reception.[4,5] This dual function is accomplished by a two-crystal transducer with one crystal devoted to each function. Discrete pulses of ultrasound wave are not used. The main advantage of continuous-wave Doppler is the ability to measure accurately high blood flow velocities. Maximum flow velocity can be measured precisely and very accurately compared with techniques utilizing discrete pulses of ultrasound wave such as with pulsed-wave Doppler or color flow mapping. Continuous-wave Doppler can accurately record the highest velocities produced by valvular or congenital heart disease (Fig 6–1). This methodology is particularly useful

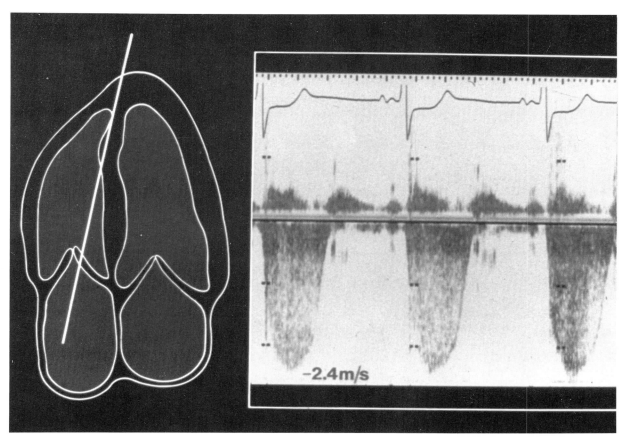

Figure 6–1. Continuous-wave spectral recording of tricuspid regurgitation. The peak flow velocity of the regurgitant jet measures 2.4 m/s.

for the evaluation of blood flow across stenotic lesions or septal defects. It can also be used to derive hemodynamic data in the assessment of pressure gradients or regurgitation.

The main disadvantage of continuous-wave Doppler is its lack of selectivity or depth discrimination. The output from a continuous-wave examination contains Doppler shift data from every red blood cell reflecting ultrasound back to the transducer along the course of the ultrasound beam (see Fig 6–1). Because continuous-wave Doppler is constantly transmitting and receiving from two different transducer heads, there is no provision for range gating to selectively place a given Doppler sample volume in space. Owing to the lack of depth resolution, blood flow velocities cannot be precisely localized in a selected area of the heart or great vessel.

Pulsed-Wave Doppler. With pulsed-wave Doppler, blood velocities can be determined at precise locations within the heart. Pulsed-wave Doppler systems use a transducer that alternates transmission and reception of ultrasound beams in a way similar to an M-mode transducer.[4,5] This method involves repetitive, short bursts of

ultrasound transmission at a specific rate called the pulse repetition frequency (PRF). An ultrasound pulse is transmitted into tissue, traveling for a given time until it is reflected back by a moving red blood cell. The reflected wave returns to the transducer over the same time but at a shifted frequency. The resultant Doppler shifts can be analyzed referable to a specific time resulting in the ability to determine the depth of the targeted tissue. This range gating is therefore dependent on a timing mechanism that only samples returning Doppler shift data from a given region. Depth of sampling is varied by changing the time delay between emission of the signal and the sampling of the reflected wave. In practice, the sample volume is placed along the Doppler beam as displayed on the monitoring screen and moved to the desired intracardiac target by a cursor.

The main advantage of pulsed-wave Doppler is its ability to provide Doppler shift data selectively from a small area along the ultrasound beam referred to as the "sample volume." Blood flow velocity and direction can be sampled in a specific area and at the certain depth. The desired target of the sample volume is operator controlled. Another advantage of pulsed-wave Doppler is that concurrent two-dimensional imaging may be carried on simultaneously with the Doppler data analysis. The cursor can be steered through a two-dimensional field that can be viewed in real-time on the monitor. In practice, the cursor is directed to the specific area of interest, such as an area of stenosis or disturbed flow, where additional assessments of flow velocity and direction can be obtained.

The main disadvantage of the pulsed-wave Doppler is its inability to measure accurately high blood flow velocities, such as those encountered with certain types of congenital heart disease and valvular lesions. In attempting to assess localized targets, the limits of this technology as they relate to the PRF are exceeded at maximum frequencies. The Nyquist limit describes the relationship between transmission frequency and beam distance. At certain distances or at high frequencies, artifacts are created that give discrepant information regarding blood flow velocities. This limitation is technically known as "aliasing" and results in an inability of the pulsed-wave Doppler instrument to record true blood flow velocities. To a degree, it is possible to overcome and control aliasing by using a lower-frequency transducer as well as by adjusting the "baseline shift" of the instrument.

Doppler Color Flow (Echo-Doppler). Blood flow through the heart in great vessels has certain characteristics and, as discussed above, can be measured using Doppler instrumentation.[4,6] In general, laminar flow exists in the great vessels and in the heart, where red blood cells are moving approximately at the same speed. In contrast, turbulent or disturbed flow is present when there is some obstruction or defect that results in disruption of the normal laminar pattern. This causes the orderly movement of red blood cells to become disorganized and produces blood flow of different velocities and directions within cardiac chambers and great vessels. The turbulent flow is characterized by disordered direction of flow in combination with many given red blood cell velocities. Abnormal flows are therefore generally characterized by turbulence and an increase in velocity.

Doppler color flow mapping is a very useful method for noninvasively imaging normal and abnormal blood flow through the heart by displaying flow data on a two-dimensional echocardiographic image (echo-Doppler). In understanding echo-Doppler, it is important to realize that the characteristics of blood flow (direction, velocity, and size) are displayed onto the two-dimensional echocardiographic image by means of color encoding of the Doppler-generated flow signal.[5] This flow information is obtained in the same manner as with the pulsed-wave Doppler technique, with multiple sample volumes interrogated sequentially. With echo-Doppler, the colors red and blue represent direction of a given jet; the various hues from dull to bright represent varying velocities. By convention, red is generally represented as flow toward the transducer, whereas blue is represented as flow away from the transducer. This pattern results in a color map of a given jet with ready identification of size and direction. Consequently, the Doppler information is given a spatial orientation that makes flow information more readily understood when compared to conventional approaches.

In addition to simple direction, velocity information also is displayed. Intensity of the color reflects the magnitude of the mean velocity of flow.[6,7] Progressively increasing velocities are coded in varying hues of either red or blue. The more dull the hue, the slower the velocity; the brighter the hue, the faster the relative velocity. Color also is used to display turbulent flow and allows a discrimination between normal and abnormal flow states. Varying velocities of red blood cells moving through a ventricular septal defect will appear as a mosaic pattern of colors representing turbulent flow.

Because echo-Doppler allows for the simultaneous display of cardiac structural data accompanied by blood flow information, this display of echocardiographic information is considered to be an essential part of patient evaluation. This technique is ideal for imaging blood flow abnormalities through cardiac chambers and large blood vessels as well as imaging intracardiac defects such as ventricular septal defects.[6,7] Since its introduction, echo-Doppler has dramatically changed the preoperative cardiac evaluation as well as intraoperative evaluation of patients with congenital heart disease. For example, a limited or no cardiac catheterization for the evaluation of some routine cardiac defects is a direct consequence of this technique.

There are limitations to the color flow technique. Owing to the high PRF required by echo-Doppler and the need to satisfy temporal resolution of this gated signal, it is not possible to assess mean blood flow velocities accurately. Therefore, the Nyquist limitations apply particularly for Doppler color flow imaging and aliasing of blood flow jets may be seen. In addition, the velocities displayed are mean velocities rather than peak velocities.

EQUIPMENT

Transmission, reception, and analysis of ultrasound waves and their conversion into visual images is a complex process that involves several electronic, mechanical, and digital conversions. Detailed discussion of echocardiographic equipment and instrumentation are beyond the scope of this chapter.[3,5] It is sufficient to say that current conventional echocardiographic systems have the full capability of providing two-dimensional image processing and complete Doppler ultrasound technology, including continuous-wave and pulsed-wave Doppler and color flow mapping. Each echocardiographic technique provides information complementary to the other techniques. Familiarity with equipment controls, including power, gain, log compression, baseline shifting, dampening, and dynamic range manipulations, are essential to the appropriate operation of these systems.

Transducers

In general, the transducer requirements for imaging and Doppler studies differ according to the needs of the specific examination (eg, continuous-wave Doppler versus echo-Doppler) and the study examination condition (transthoracic for preoperative evaluation or transesophageal or epicardial for intraoperative evaluation). The objective in echocardiographic imaging is to aim the transducer beam in the area of interest, which is accomplished with the various techniques by changing transducers. Echocardiographic transducers have size and frequency variations.[3] The larger and flatter the transducer head, the better the resolution in the far field and the greater the depth of the focal zone. Larger transducers will not yield good images in the near field. In epicardial echo-Doppler, where near-field imaging is of primary importance, special short-focused transducers are available. A second consideration in selecting the appropriate transducer is choice of frequency. The higher the frequency of the transducer, the better the resolution of the image. However, higher frequencies have limited tissue penetration. Therefore, consideration should be given to using the highest frequency that allows adequate penetration to the depth required. For most pediatric studies, transducers with a frequency range of 2.5–5.0 MHz are adequate.

Conventional transducers use a linear array of crystals that emit synchronized ultrasound waves resulting in a flat beam that moves in a direction perpendicular to the array. These transducer systems minimize beam divergence and enhance resolution of images. The targeted tissue is scanned in a sector with either a mechanical or a phased-array two-dimensional sector scanner.

With a mechanical sector transducer, an oscillating transducer head scans the tissues.[3] The mechanical transducers use a crystal that is mechanically aimed for each scan line. Three crystals are mounted in the transducer head and rotated continuously in one direction sending and receiving sequentially pulsed waves. As each crystal passes over the heart, it transmits and receives ultrasound waves. The result is a tomographic image of the heart showing moving cardiac structures in the selected plane. Because of the moving transducer head within the mechanical scanner, Doppler ultrasound with color flow imaging is not possible because it requires multiple pulses along the same line. Newer systems of mechanical scanning have now included an annular phased-array transducer that allows for more uniform imaging and at the same time provides simultaneous Doppler flow mapping.

Phased-array transducers consist of many independent elements consisting of piezoelectric crystals in a linear arrangement, each of which can be pulsed independently.[3] Current systems include up to 128 elements in a transducer head. In these systems, the individual elements are essentially small transducers that are pulsed in a very rapid, precisely controlled sequence. Individual waves are combined to make one compound wave that travels in a single wave front in an angle perpendicular to the axis of the transducer and subtends the wave propagation along the entire sector arc, maintaining a planar, flat wave front across the 90° arc. The ultrasound beam is aimed not by the moving parts within the transducer head, such as with the mechanical scanner, but by electronic steering of the beam through appropriate timing of the pulses from each element. The ultrasound beam is steered electrically without moving the transducer. Consequently, this scanner allows simultaneous acquisition of imaging and Doppler data, with sample volumes shown on two-dimensional display for guidance.

ECHOCARDIOGRAPHIC VIEWS

An echo-Doppler examination usually scans along three basic planes: a *long-axis plane*, which is parallel to the major axis of the left ventricle; a *short-axis plane*, which is perpendicular to the major axis of the left ventricle; and a *four-chamber plane*, which is a coronal view through the cardiac apex.[3,4–7] Within each plane, a series of additional views are obtained by aiming the transducer with varying degrees of tilt along each axis. Using the transthoracic approach, all three planes can be obtained by imaging from four areas on the chest: (1) along the parasternum, (2) the suprasternal notch, (3) the cardiac apex, and (4) the subcostal area. During epicardial intraoperative echo-Doppler, the same planes can usually be imaged; however, the four-chamber view is foreshortened owing to the inability to put the probe at the apex of the heart.[8,9] The imaging planes are confined to the short-axis and the four-chamber views with a transesophageal approach.

Long-Axis Plane

The long-axis view in a normal patient provides simultaneous imaging of the left ventricular inflow and outflow tracts (Fig 6–2). The long-axis plane transects the heart from the aortic root to the left ventricular apex and includes the aortic and mitral valves.[10,11] In a long-axis view, the outflow portion of the right ventricle is at the top and the plane cuts across the anterior portion of the intraventricular septum below. The aortic root is seen below the septum, where the right coronary and noncoronary cups of the aortic valve are visualized. Below the aortic root, the left atrium is viewed as well as the apex and body of the left ventricle. Separating the left atrium from the left ventricle is the mitral valve. This view shows the motion of the aortic and mitral valve and per-

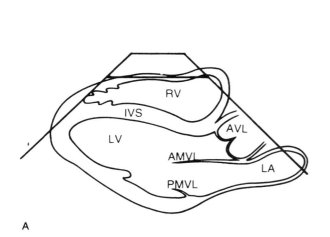

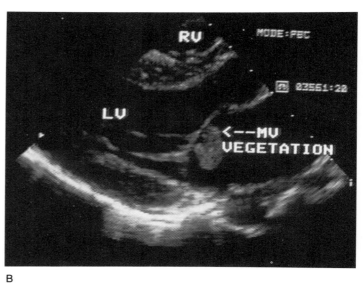

A

B

Figure 6–2. Diagram of the long-axis plane (*A*). Epicardial two-dimensional echocardiogram in the long-axis plane (*B*). Note the vegetation attached directly to the mitral valve. Abbreviations: RV, right ventricle; IVS, intraventricular septum; LV, left ventricle; AVL, aortic valve leaflet; AMVL, anterior mitral valve leaflet; PMVL, posterior mitral leaflet; LA, left atrium.

mits measurement of left atrial, aortic root, and left ventricular cavity dimensions. Stenotic and regurgitant lesions of the aortic and mitral valve are especially well visualized in this imaging plane. It also allows visualization of the intraventricular septum for septal defects and posterior ventricular wall. Different types of left ventricular outflow obstruction can be evaluated.

Short-Axis Plane

The short-axis view is obtained when the transducer is rotated clockwise through 90° from the long-axis plane (Fig 6–3). This view can be obtained from the transthoracic, epicardial, or transesophageal approaches.[10,11] In this tomographic view, the left ventricle, within the left ventricular cavity, the two leaflets, and supporting apparatus of the mitral valve are seen. The motion of the mitral valve leaflets and the dynamic function of the left ventricular outflow track is assessed. A family of short-axis planes is generated by tilting the transducer from the base of the heart superiorly to the apex. If the transducer head is tilted toward the apex of the heart, a cross section of the left ventricle and the right ventricle can be obtained. The left ventricle is sectioned across the middle of its two papillary muscles. This section also cuts

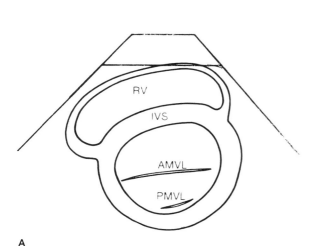

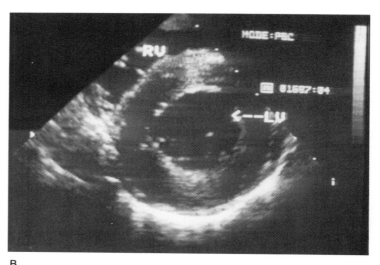

A

B

Figure 6–3. Diagram of the short-axis plane at the level of the mitral valve (*A*). Epicardial two-dimensional echocardiogram in the short-axis plane (*B*). Abbreviations: RV, right ventricle; IVS, intraventricular septum; AMVL, anterior mitral valve leaflet; PMVL, posterior mitral valve leaflet.

across the right ventricle, usually visualized anteriorly. This plane is particularly good for obtaining information about left and right ventricular function as well as segmental analysis of wall motion.

By tilting the transducer toward the base of the heart, the great vessels are imaged. In this view, a cross section of the aorta is usually seen in the middle of the image, where the right ventricular outflow track courses around the aorta, and the tricuspid valve and pulmonary valve are visualized. The right ventricular inlet and outflow tract are also visualized (Fig 6–4). This view is especially useful to analyze the tricuspid valve, the intraventricular septum, and the right ventricular outflow track, including the bifurcation of the main pulmonary artery. Tricuspid valve regurgitation, ventricular septal defect, right ventricular outflow obstruction (valvular or subvalvular), and patent ductus arteriosus can be seen. With even more angulation of the probe, the intra-atrial septum is seen and atrial septal defects identified.

Four-Chamber Plane

The third basic imaging plane is the four-chamber view (Fig 6–5). Four-chamber imaging is performed transthoracically by placing the transducer at the cardiac apex or subcostally; transesophageally, by increasing angulation of the transducer head; or epicardially, by approximating a position near the cardiac apex, rendering a foreshortened view.[10,11] The four-chamber plane runs from the apex to the base of the heart and is approximately perpendicular to both the intraventricular and intra-atrial septa. As its name implies, the four-chamber view includes an image of each of the four cardiac chambers. This view usually shows the intraventricular and intra-atrial septa in the center as well as the balance between

right ventricular and left ventricular musculature. With anterior angulation of the transducer, a view of the aortic root as it originates from the left ventricle is visualized. The origins of the right and left coronary arteries can be identified. This view is a satisfactory way to visualize the right and left atrium, mitral or tricuspid valve, and defects in the cardiac septa.

IMAGING APPROACHES

Transthoracic Echo-Doppler

The transthoracic approach to echocardiographic imaging is utilized diagnostically in the preoperative evaluation of congenital heart disease in children.[6] In addition, postoperative evaluation and long-term follow-up is done by this approach. Because most of the heart is covered anteriorly by the sternum, ribs, or lungs, which are relatively impenetrable to ultrasound, the transthoracic approach for echo-Doppler must be performed through certain "windows" on the chest surface. The left parasternal area provides the best access because the left lung does not completely cover the heart in most individuals. Additional access can be obtained from the cardiac apex and by a subcostal approach near the xiphisternum. In small infants and particularly in neonates, the transducer can be placed almost anywhere on the chest for imaging.

Transesophageal Echo-Doppler

The transesophageal approach to echocardiographic imaging is generally utilized intraoperatively where continuous imaging can be obtained.[12,16] In selective circumstances preoperatively, the diagnostic evaluation of

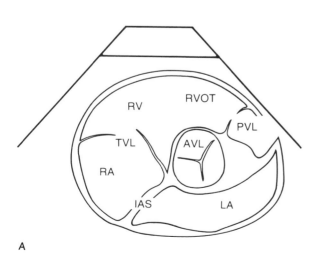

A

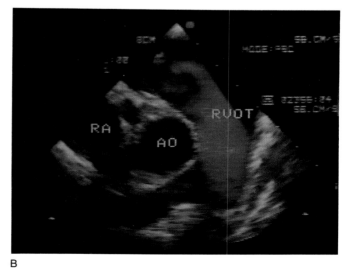

B

Figure 6–4. Diagram of the short-axis plane at the level of the great vessels (*A*). Epicardial two-dimensional echocardiogram with color flow imaging in the short-axis plane (*B*). Abbreviations: RA, right atrium; RV, right ventricle; RVOT, right ventricular outflow tract; TVL, tricuspid valve leaflet; IAS, intra-atrial septum; AVL, aortic valve leaflet; PVL, pulmonary valve leaflet; LA, left atrium; Ao, aorta.

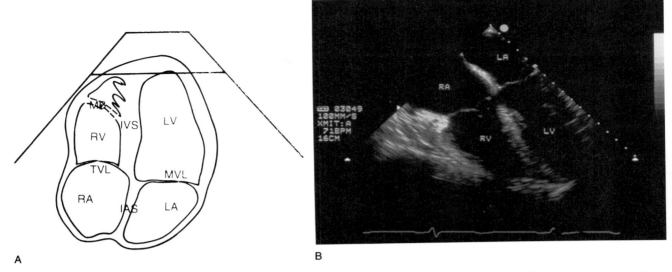

A   B

Figure 6–5. Diagram of the four-chamber plane with the probe at the cardiac apex (*A*). Transesophageal two-dimensional echocardiogram in the four-chamber plane (*B*). Abbreviations: RA, right atrium; RV, right ventricle; LA, left atrium; LV, left ventricle; TVL, tricuspid valve leaflet; IAS, intra-atrial septum; IVS, intraventricular septum; MB, moderator band.

patients with mitral and aortic valve disease is aided with this approach. The incorporation of the echo-Doppler transducer on a flexible gastroscope allows the ultrasound beam to be directed at the heart. The standard transesophageal transducer consists of a 15-mm width transducer head containing 64 elements. The transducer head can be rotated within the esophagus to obtain the imaging planes discussed above. The proximity of the probe to cardiac structures provides an unobstructed view of the heart compared with standard transthoracic techniques that must penetrate intrathoracic structures such as the lung. Because of its location behind the heart, this technique is superior to the epicardial and transthoracic approaches in visualization of left atrial, mitral, and aor-

tic valve anatomy (Fig 6–6). In patients with previous operations where ventricular septal prosthetic patches or valves are present, preventing beam transmission from the epicardial or transthoracic approach, the transesophageal approach permits adequate views to assess valvular insufficiency.[17] The other obvious advantage to transesophageal echocardiography is its use as a continuous intraoperative monitor during surgery without operator interruption of the procedure.[16] The surgeon does not need to interrupt the repair to obtain an echocardiographic study. Another advantage is the probe does not threaten the sterility of the operative field. This technique is particularly helpful for monitoring ventricular function, where sequential evaluation of segmental wall

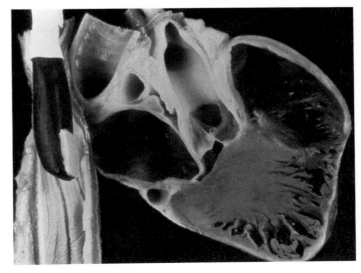

Figure 6–6. Anatomic section demonstrating a transesophageal probe within the esophagus and the adjacent cardiac structures. Note the proximity of the probe to the left atrium and mitral valve apparatus.

motion in the short-axis view at a fixed position is possible.[14,15,18] When required, the transducer can be left in place for postoperative monitoring.

There are certain limitations of the transesophageal echo-Doppler. First, because of the limited probe manipulations, the imaging planes are restricted. Transesophageal probes are less maneuverable, especially in small patients and, therefore, less capable of imaging certain aspects of the anatomy.[8] It is difficult to obtain a long-axis plane using the transesophageal approach, thereby limiting an evaluation of the left ventricular outflow tract and intraventricular septum. Also, the transesophageal approach does not allow as accurate a description of the right ventricular outflow tract, descending aorta, and atrial septum as the epicardial approach. For example, visualization of a sinus venosus atrial septal defect is easily seen in the epicardial view but can be readily missed with the transesophageal approach. To a certain degree this problem is solved by the use of bi-plane transducers. Bi-plane devices permit sector arc scanning from two pulsed-wave transducers in perpendicular directions. Each individual transducer mounted on the gastroscope has 32 elements, operates at a frequency of 5 MHz, and is approximately 15–17 mm at its widest point. With the bi-plane transducer, new tomographic cardiac images are obtained, including views of blood flow patterns in orthogonal planes.

Another limitation is the actual size of the transducer. The small size of many patients undergoing congenital heart surgery limits the application of transesophageal techniques using adult transesophageal transducers.[8] Because of the probe size of the transducer head, the adult gastroscope can only be used in large children and adolescents. In our experience, children weighing >12 kg are suitable candidates for transesophageal echo-Doppler using the adult probe. When utilizing the adult transducer in these patients, the operator must be aware of the possibility of airway obstruction with the probe as well as the possibility of descending aortic compression. As a consequence, peak airway pressure and femoral arterial pressure should be monitored for obstruction.

The problem of transducer size may be alleviated by the development of a pediatric-size transducer attached to a gastroscope. Technologic advances are now providing echo-Doppler capabilities with smaller esophageal probes. Several groups have recently used the smaller pediatric transducers in neonatal patients without any complications.[19-21] The current pediatric systems available for use have 24 elements in the transducer head. This system is not ideal, however, because of the poor resolution. Because the pediatric probe incorporates fewer elements (24 as opposed to 64 in the conventional adult transducer), resolution of the two-dimensional image is considerably inferior. For example, difficulties are encountered in visualizing the endocardial/epicardial surfaces for the determination of ventricular wall motion. When compared with epicardial or transesophageal echo-Doppler using the adult transducer, both of which have more piezoelectric crystals, the resolution is inferior with the pediatric transducer.

Quantitative image analysis is available through intraoperative transesophageal echo-Doppler.[16-22] On-line analysis is available with current echocardiographic systems and consists of flow velocities and timing intervals. Off-line analysis is also available and can be performed by digitizing information from replay of the videotape. The latter function largely consists of sophisticated operations, such as wall motion or wall thickness analysis, to obtain functional data regarding ventricular function. With future improvements in the existing transesophageal technology, this approach to intraoperative assessment of the pediatric patient with congenital heart disease will become more routine.

Epicardial Echo-Doppler

The epicardial approach is useful in patients of all ages and sizes who undergo repair of congenital heart defects through a median sternotomy.[23] The complex nature of these lesions favors the more versatile epicardial approach that views the anatomy from a variety of orientations and demonstrates each defect in exquisite detail. Using this approach, all major cardiac structures, including all valves, chambers, septal structure, and great vessels, are reviewed.[8,9,23-27] Not only does epicardial imaging require participation (and, therefore, concentration on the images) by the surgeon and the anesthesiologist, the variety of views enables superior interrogation of the numerous components of complex congenital defects and assessment of ventricular function or loading conditions. This approach is applied at any time before, during, or after bypass.

Epicardial transducer selection varies with patient size and disease entity. Although the 5.0-MHz short-focus transducer is used in the vast majority of patients, in certain cases a 2.5-MHz or 3.5-MHz transducer will be necessary.[25] When deemed necessary, epicardial scans can be performed with a nonimaging 1.9-MHz continuous-wave Doppler probe. Prior to imaging, the transducer and cable are cleaned with a commercially available glutaraldehyde solution and left wrapped in a glutaraldehyde-soaked towel for at least 10 minutes. It is not necessary to gas sterilize the transducers that are to be used for epicardial images. Particular care should be taken to keep the liquid from entering the electric contacts on the transducer assembly. The transducer is then wiped with sterile saline and taken to the patient's head, where it is introduced into a sterile sheath containing 20 mL of sterile ultrasound gel. The sheath is then secured to the surgical side of the anesthesia screen, where it is available for use at any time during the operation. This method is not associated with an increased risk of infec-

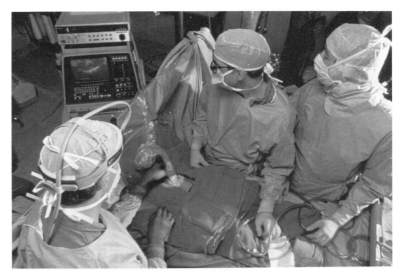

Figure 6–7. Intraoperative photograph showing how the epicardial transducer is readily available for use by the surgeon after insertion into a sterile sheath over the top of the anesthesia drapes. The echo-Doppler monitor is easily positioned in a location where the surgeon and anesthesiologist can view the images in an on-line, real-time fashion as epicardial echo is performed. (*From Ungerleider RM, et al: The use of intraoperative echocardiography with Doppler color flow imaging in the repair of congenital heart defects. Echocardiography 7:289–304, 1990, with permission.*)

tion or prolonged arrhythmias.[23] The operator places the transducer on the heart and manipulates it to obtain the views discussed previously (Fig 6–7). Angulation of the probe in a to-and-fro motion will obtain the family of tomographic views required in each plane.

The epicardial technique of intraoperative echocardiography (Fig 6–8) has several limitations. First, the technique requires placement of transducer on the heart, which may expose the patient to increased risk of infection or produce life-threatening arrhythmias. To date, concerns about infection or sustained arrhythmias have not been substantiated despite extensive use.[23,25] Second, the four-chamber view is difficult to obtain from an epicardial approach. Because the transducer probe cannot be placed exactly at the apex of the heart, a foreshortened view of the four chambers as well as the mitral valve is often seen. The third limitation is its

restricted use due to interruption of surgical repair. However, surgical groups that view epicardial echocardiography as an essential part of the procedure both before and after repair do not consider echocardiography an interruption or inconvenience. The actual amount of time in assessing intracardiac anatomy averages 3–4 minutes and is usually performed before or after cardiopulmonary bypass.[8,23–25]

PREOPERATIVE DIAGNOSTIC ECHOCARDIOGRAPHY

Preoperative echocardiographic evaluation details abnormal cardiac anatomic structure and function even more accurately than cardiac catheterization. Two-dimensional echocardiography with Doppler color flow imaging

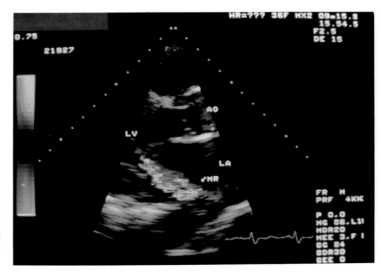

Figure 6–8. Epicardial two-dimensional echocardiogram with Doppler color flow imaging demonstrating mitral regurgitation (MR), depicted as the mosaic pattern of various color hues representing varying mean velocities. Abbreviations: AO, aorta; LV, left ventricle; LA, left atrium.

has made a major impact on the ability to diagnose even the most complex congenital heart defects.[6] Current cardiology practice uses this approach as a complementary technique in the overall evaluation of the child with congenital heart disease.[28]

It is necessary to use a logical and systematic approach in evaluation of cardiovascular disease by echo-Doppler in children,[6] including sequential cardiac chamber analysis of the atria and ventricles, description of the atrioventricular (AV) and ventriculoarterial (VA) connections, and an analysis of the great artery connections and any supravalvular abnormalities. The three basic planes, as discussed previously, obtain a family of views and an adequate analysis of chambers, valves, and great vessels. Coupling the echocardiographic information with angiography ensures adequate identification of the specific congenital heart defect, its functional effect, and resultant blood flow patterns. Such evaluations ensure the most precise anatomic and functional repair during congenital cardiac surgery.

INTRAOPERATIVE ECHOCARDIOGRAPHY

The broad spectrum of cardiac defects and complexity of operations confound the intraoperative anesthetic and surgical management of patients undergoing repair of congenital heart disease. Many elements during the repair influence overall outcome. The most critical element is performance of a technically accurate and efficient surgical correction. In order to obtain good technical results, a clear description of the anatomy and the ways these anatomic variations affect physiology is necessary. This information enables formulation of the most appropriate surgical procedure. Furthermore, after completion of the reconstruction, the quality of repair is evaluated to ensure that these patients have the most optimal result possible. Because intracardiac repair radically alters blood flow patterns and cardiac structure, the effect of the surgery on cardiac function and physiology is also determined.

Current methods of intraoperative assessment during and after surgery for congenital heart disease are restricted to visual inspection of the heart and isolated pressure measurements, usually central venous pressure with occasional use of transthoracic catheters for measurement of pulmonary artery and left atrial pressures. By utilizing a combination of pressure measurements, oxygen saturation data, and dye-dilution cardiac output curves, an indirect and relatively insensitive appraisal of the adequacy of a repair is obtained. None of these methods enables the surgical team to judge visually the degree of anatomic and functional normalcy achieved by the repair. Improved quantitative and qualitative methods for functional assessment of the heart and adequacy of surgical repair are needed.

Stimulated by the increasing preoperative usefulness of echo-Doppler and the development of the transesophageal transducer, cardiac surgeons and anesthesiologists became aware of the value of intraoperative echocardiography,[6,16,29,30] especially in adult cardiac patients.[12,16] However, the transesophageal approach is not as useful in neonates, infants, and small children undergoing cardiac surgery owing to the large size of the probe and the restricted views from within the esophagus that do not clearly assess the spectrum of cardiac anomalies in congenital heart disease. Nonetheless, the utility of echo-Doppler in providing new information on cardiac function, structure, and blood flow patterns in congenital heart disease has encouraged its continued intraoperative use in children. Several recent studies demonstrated that intraoperative epicardial and transesophageal echo-Doppler can be quickly and efficiently performed during operations for the repair of congenital heart defects even in small infants and neonates.[8,9,19,23–27] Because intraoperative echocardiography visualizes cardiac chamber and valve anatomy, ventricular function, and blood flow patterns, its use in the operating room has dramatically increased. The same echo-Doppler techniques used for preoperative diagnostic evaluation, when employed in the operating room prior to surgical repair using the epicardial or transesophageal approach, often better identify cardiac abnormalities of structure, blood flow, or function. After repair, they provide instant feedback about the quality of repair as well as ventricular function.

Johnson first reported the use of intraoperative epicardial echocardiography for the evaluation of results of mitral commissurotomy in 1972 using M-mode techniques.[31] Since then, there have been multiple reports of the use of epicardial echocardiography for a variety of specialized purposes using the two-dimensional technique.[32–34] Intraoperative transesophageal echocardiography is an effective technique to assess cardiac function and anatomic defects in adult patients with valvular and ischemic heart diseases.[12,13,15,17]

Takamoto and co-workers[35] first reported the use of intraoperative echo-Doppler with color flow mapping for a wide variety of cardiac diseases, including repair of congenital heart defects. Recently, the usefulness of intraoperative echocardiography during the repair of congenital heart lesions has been reported by several groups. Gussenhoven and colleagues[26] reported the use of two-dimensional echocardiography in combination with contrast methods for intraoperative epicardial assessment in 195 patients with congenital heart disease. In addition, Hagler and co-workers reported a preliminary series of 30 patients in whom echo-Doppler was used in the operating room to assess repair of congenital heart lesions.[27] Recent reports suggest the potential advantages of echo-Doppler when used to evaluate repair of certain congenital cardiac defects.[8,19,24,25]

Utility of Intraoperative Echocardiography

Before the institution of cardiopulmonary bypass and surgical repair, echo-Doppler accurately determines the integrity of the intra-atrial or ventricular septa and the function of the aortic, mitral, tricuspid, and pulmonary valves. Intraoperative echo-Doppler is superior to transthoracic echocardiography in assessing valve function, with particular reference to the mitral and aortic valves.[7,34,36,38] The degree of valvular or subvalvular stenosis can be quantitated and regurgitation qualitatively assessed.[8,24–25] Echo-Doppler determines the precise anatomy of the mitral valve leaflets, identifying leaflet redundancy and prolapse or perivalvular leaks, as well as chordal and papillary muscle integrity. This information indicates when valve repair or replacement is more suitable than valvoplasty.[17]

After bypass, echo-Doppler evaluates and quantitates residual defects, assesses ventricular function,[8,17,19,23–25,39–41] and indicates ventricular volume in the patient.[14,15,18] From this qualitative assessment, the surgeon and anesthesiologist can determine preload and contractility. Two-dimensional echocardiography is a very sensitive and accurate indicator of regional and global ventricular function.[14,15,18,22] It is superior to the 7-lead ECG or pulmonary artery catheter in detecting wall motion abnormalities associated with ischemia. Although qualitative visualization of wall motion abnormalities lacks sensitivity and precision, it reliably detects ischemia-related abnormalities. Computerized analysis of regional wall motion abnormalities is superior to qualitative visual assessment in detecting ischemia-related changes in ventricular function.[22] However, off-line analysis of wall motion is often difficult and cumbersome. Analysis in real-time is now possible.

Efficacy of Intraoperative Echocardiography

The value of intraoperative echo-Doppler has been prospectively evaluated by several groups during congenital cardiac surgery.[8,17,21,23–27] In these studies, intraoperative assessment using echo-Doppler was performed systematically from epicardial or transesophageal approaches before the initiation of cardiopulmonary bypass (CPB) and again at the conclusion of the procedure, usually after the patient had been weaned from CPB. The echo-Doppler examination included all cardiac chambers and valves, including venous inflows and great vessel outflows. During this examination, all images were analyzed on-line in real-time and decisions were made in each case on the basis of echo-Doppler as well as any other relevant clinical observations available. Using the combination of epicardial and transesophageal echocardiography, Ungerleider and colleagues[23] demonstrated the feasibility of performing echo-Doppler for any simple or complex cardiac defect, in any size patient (smallest, 1.8 kg), and at any age (youngest, 1 day). Although contact of the transducer with the epicardial

surface necessary to obtain good images occasionally induced a few ectopic beats, the vast majority of the patients had no significant arrhythmias. Further, there was no increased risk of mediastinal infections with the epicardial approach. With the epicardial approach, routine intraoperative echo-Doppler added an average of less than 10 minutes to each case, most of this as non-CPB time.

The transesophageal approach avoids the concerns regarding infections and arrhythmias and does not disrupt the operative procedure.[19] However, the quality of the images in children, excepting those of the mitral valve and, possibly, the four-chamber view, are inferior to the epicardial images.[8] Although the adult and pediatric transesophageal probes are purported to be equally feasible for intraoperative echo-Doppler for congenital heart surgery, the restricted views permitted by transducer manipulation within the esophagus, the poor resolution of the pediatric transducer, and the size limitation of the adult transducer (patients must weigh >12–15 kg) render the transesophageal approach less useful. This is especially true for neonates and small infants, who constitute the majority of complex pediatric cardiovascular surgical patients.

Pre-CPB Evaluation. Prior to CPB and operative repair, a complete echo-Doppler examination demonstrates the structural features and some functional features and loading conditions at a time when the surgeon is planning the operative repair (Table 6–1).[8,23,25] Not infrequently, previously unappreciated details of anatomy are observed. Analysis of prebypass echo-Doppler data has identified several factors influencing the operative procedure. In one series, the pre-CPB echo-Doppler examination assisted anesthetic and surgical management 233 times in 175 patients. The most common effects on surgical management were changes in the intraoperative surgical plan or the intraoperative surgical approach.

TABLE 6–1. IMPACT OF PREOPERATIVE ECHO-DOPPLER ON PATIENT MANAGEMENT

Influence Operative Plan Prior to CPB (N = 92)	
Change diagnosis	4
Change operation	20
Repair unsuspected lesion	20
Influence approach to lesion	32
Altered CPB plan	16
Guide the Intraoperative Approach (N = 121)	
Clarify valve and/or chordal commitments	28
Indicate best manner for valve repair	19
Identify precise location of defect	18
Specify how to repair	56
Alter Anesthesia Conduct Before CPB (N = 20)	

(*Data from Duke Medical Center Congenital Heart Databank.*)

The changes in anesthetic management initiated by pre-CPB echo-Doppler occurred in a minority of patients and were usually of minor significance. Examples of echo-Doppler impact on anesthetic management include increasing anesthetic depth to reduce left ventricular outflow obstruction in a patient with unsuspected subaortic stenosis physiology, the identification and treatment of pulmonary hypertension in neonates to reduce right ventricular distention, and the diagnosis and treatment of tetralogy of Fallot spells (Fig 6–9).[42]

Post-CPB Evaluation. The post-CPB echo-Doppler examination assesses the quality of surgical repair and changes in ventricular function (Fig 6–10). There is good evidence that echo-Doppler is an invaluable tool for assessing the quality of surgical repair in the immediate post-CPB period.[8,19,23–27,42,43] Echo-Doppler is much more accurate in judging the adequacy of repair than the surgeon's opinion of the repair. In 15% of the cases where the surgeon was "satisfied" with the reconstruction, echo-Doppler disclosed a residual problem of some concern (Fig 6–11).[8,39] In addition, when the surgeon was dissatisfied with the reconstruction, echo-Doppler demonstrated acceptable repair in 32% of cases. Most large series estimate that 7–12% of patients have immediate successful revision of their procedure in the same operative setting based entirely on the information displayed by echo-Doppler after the initial repair.[8] Patients without suspicious clinical problems would have left the operating room with a suboptimal repair without routine echo-Doppler evaluation.

Epicardial and transesophageal echo-Doppler are also extremely sensitive methods for examining intraoperative ventricular function.[8,14,15,18,19,22] This particular assessment is performed simply by obtaining a short-axis view of the ventricles before and after repair. Contractility and chamber dimension of each ventricle is compared to the preoperative state. Qualitatively, ventricular

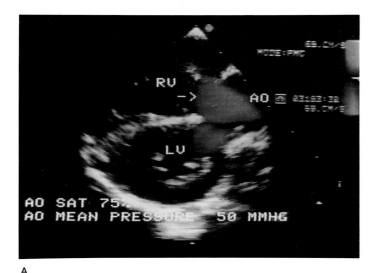

A

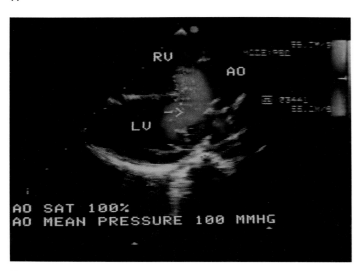

B

Figure 6–9. Right-to-left shunting (*arrow*) across the ventricular septal defect in a patient with tetralogy of Fallot. ("tet spell") is treated by increasing the mean arterial pressure using phenylephrine (*A*). After institution of therapy, the shunt is reversed and systemic arterial saturation increased from 75 to 100% (*B*). Abbreviations: AO, aorta; LV, left ventricle; RV, right ventricle. (*From Greeley WJ, et al: Intraoperative hypoxic spells in tetralogy of Fallot: An echocardiographic analysis of diagnosis and treatment. Anesth Analg 68:815–819, 1989, with permission.*)

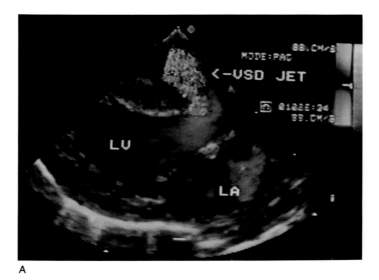

A

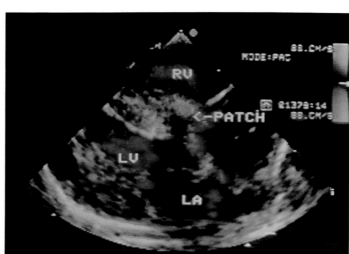

B

Figure 6–10. A left-to-right shunt across a perimembranous VSD is easily imaged in this 1800-g infant (*A*). After the repair, the patch can be seen to obliterate completely any residual shunt flow (*B*). Abbreviations: VSD, ventricular septal defect; LV, left ventricle; LA, left atrium. (*From Ungerleider RM, et al: Routine use of intraoperative epicardial echocardiography and Doppler color flow imaging to guide and evaluate repair of congenital heart defects. A prospective study. J Thorac Cardiovasc 100:297–309, 1990, with permission.*)

dysfunction is defined as a change in wall motion (akinesis or dyskinesis) or absence of systolic thickening on the post-CPB echo-Doppler examination when compared with the baseline, pre-CPB examination. Although it is the goal of an efficient procedure to produce an accurate reconstruction without damaging cardiac function, 15–25% of the patients in some series have some alteration of ventricular function (by echo) immediately post-CPB.[8] This is not always clinically significant and does not always require treatment. The finding of decreased contractility is not necessarily an indication for inotropic therapy but should be considered within the context of the physiology of the cardiac lesion and the patient's course. For example, increased right ventricular chamber size and decreased right ventricular contractility as visualized by echo-Doppler caused by pulmonary hypertension is best treated with hyperventilation. Left ventricular dysfunction from intramyocardial air is best treated by transient elevation of the blood pressure with

phenylephrine rather than with the use of inotropes (Fig 6–12).[42] For evaluating ventricular function after repair of congenital heart defects, echocardiography is a sensitive method to identify dysfunction and assess subsequent therapeutic interventions.

Outcome Studies Using Intraoperative Echocardiography

Little prospective information about identification of operative risk factors predictive of patient outcome for congenital heart surgery is available. Echo-Doppler may be useful in this regard. The post-CPB echo-Doppler examination evaluates the surgical repair for residual problems and associations between residual defects and outcome have been demonstrated. In patients with no residual structural problems after repair identified by echo-Doppler, reoperation and mortality rates are very low (Table 6–2).[8,23–25] However, in patients with residual structural defects leaving the operating room, the

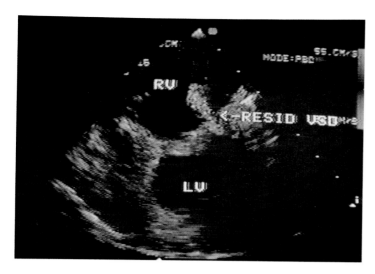

Figure 6–11. This postrepair image is obtained from an infant after attempted correction of a ventricular septal defect. There is a large residual VSD shunt in the subaortic position. Despite the size of the shunt depicted by epicardial color flow imaging, the patient was clinically well and had been weaned from cardiopulmonary bypass without difficulty. The infant was replaced on cardiopulmonary bypass and additional sutures were placed to close the defect. Abbreviations: LV, left ventricle; RV, right ventricle. (*From Ungerleider RM, et al: Routine use of intraoperative epicardial echocardiography and Doppler color flow imaging to guide and evaluate repair of congenital heart defects. A prospective study. J Thorac Cardiovasc 100:297–309, 1990, with permission.*)

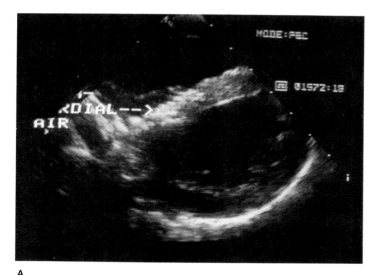

A

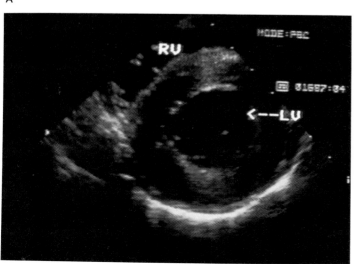

B

Figure 6–12. After CPB, the short-axis view in this patient revealed a regional wall motion abnormality of the right ventricle, flattening of the intraventricular septum, and evidence of intramyocardial air in the distribution of the right coronary artery (*A*). Obscured label in (*A*) should read myocardial air. After reperfusion on bypass and treatment with phenylephrine, repeat echo-Doppler demonstrated normal wall motion, normal position of the intraventricular septum, and evacuation of intramyocardial air (*B*). Abbreviations: LV, left ventricle; RV, right ventricle. (*From Greeley WJ, et al: Intramyocardial air causes right ventricular dysfunction after repair of a congenital heart defect. Anesthesiology 73: 1042–1046, 1990, with permission.*)

TABLE 6–2. PATIENT OUTCOME AND POSTOPERATIVE ECHO-DOPPLER RESULTS

Residual Defect (Echo)	N	Accept-able Out-come	Reoper-ated	Surgical Death	Later Death
No residual defect	295 (71%)*	273 (93%)	8(3%)	9(3%)	4(2%)
Residual defect	119 (28%)*	54 (45%)†	15 (13%)†	45 (38%)†	5 (4%)
Cannot evaluate	4 (1%)*	2 (50%)	0	2 (50%)	0

* Of entire series.
† P <.006 by chi square (compared to "no residual defect").
(*Data from Duke Medical Center Congenital Heart Databank.*)

chance of reoperation at a later date and mortality rates were greatly increased: 13 and 38%, respectively (see Fig 6–11). In other words, after completion of surgery if post-CPB echo-Doppler demonstrates good anatomic repair, the prognosis for a good outcome is better than 93%. However, if there is any concern regarding the postrepair study, the likelihood of a good outcome is substantially decreased to about 55%.

Likewise, concerns about ventricular dysfunction identified by echo-Doppler after repair are also predictive of outcome (see Table 6–2).[8,23–25] The identification of a new right ventricular contraction abnormality as determined by a change in wall motion carries a mortality rate estimated to be 33%, left ventricular wall motion abnormality of 25%, and biventricular dysfunction of 69%. When no left or right ventricular changes are observed by echo-Doppler, the operative mortality rate is 4%. It is not known whether the early identification of ventricular dysfunction will improve outcome.

All data that led to the generation of these rates regarding structural defects and cardiac function were provided prospectively in the operating room at the time of surgery.[8,23–25] This means that the surgeon and anesthesiologist who become familiar with the interpretation of echo-Doppler have the ability to quickly generate predictive information about the quality of the operative repair before the patient leaves the operating room. Furthermore, the nature of this information guides the direct and efficient modification of the procedure where appropriate to repair residual defects, to revise technical problems, or to initiate early therapeutic interventions for ventricular dysfunction.

During the repair of complex congenital heart defects, the anesthesiologist and surgeon are occasionally confronted with a patient who is difficult to wean from CPB. Under these circumstances, identification of the problem, ie, residual structural defect requiring re-repair versus a functional abnormality requiring pharmacologic support, is difficult to assess. Neonates, infants, and children with minimal cardiac reserve may not tolerate he-

modynamic instability for long periods of time under these conditions. Interventions must be made quickly and be rationally based on available clinical information. The subjective experiences of the surgeon and the anesthesiologist often become the primary determinants for altering support or assessing the adequacy of repair. Echo-Doppler provides an additional method for rapidly diagnosing functional and structural abnormalities and assisting the anesthesiologist and surgeon in selecting the appropriate medical or surgical therapy. For the anesthesiologist, echo-Doppler identification of intramyocardial air or a new wall motion abnormality may direct specific pharmacologic interventions and provide a means of assessing the results of these interventions.[42] For the surgeon, identification of residual anatomic defects may lead to immediate reinstitution of cardiopulmonary bypass, correction of the defect, and subsequent weaning from bypass.

Although the nature of the data is subjective, experience indicates that a surgical team can learn to interpret their intraoperative echo-Doppler data with respect to repair of congenital cardiac defects.[8,23–27] The information provided by echo-Doppler shortens the learning curve by teaching the surgical team where problems occurred and giving immediate positive reinforcement to techniques that avoided these problems in subsequent patients.

TRAINING REQUIREMENT

Echocardiographic techniques are becoming more widely used in the operating room to define normal and abnormal cardiac anatomy, evaluate cardiac chamber sizes and dynamics, and assess valvular disease both before and after repair. Surgeons and anesthesiologists must be trained in the conduct and interpretation of echo-Doppler examinations to assure high-quality data. A long, intensive cooperative effort between experienced cardiologists with surgeons and anesthesiologists less experienced in ultrasound methods is required.

A knowledge of cardiac anatomy, transducer manipulation, and echocardiographic features is essential for successful performance from the epicardial, transthoracic, or transesophageal approaches. When performing two-dimensional echocardiography with Doppler color flow imaging, complex maneuvers are sometimes necessary in order to align the scan plane with the desired anatomic axis of the heart. Tilting the transducer displaces the scan to form a series of radial planes. These maneuvers take some experience. Isolated, nonsystematic use confined to problem cases will probably not produce sufficient experience for the operative team to use intraoperative echo-Doppler effectively and efficiently.

Intraoperative echocardiographic evaluation of the patient with congenital heart disease involves the use of several related ultrasonic techniques that require a requisite understanding of the underlying principles, instrumentation, and application advantages and limitations. What constitutes optimal physician training in echocardiography in order to attain the technical expertise in these diagnostic techniques has not been firmly established. Proper development of these skills requires training under the guidance of an experienced echocardiographer. The American Society of Echocardiography's Committee for Physician Training in Echocardiography has identified three levels of training (introductory, intermediate, and advanced) in echocardiography and recommend that physicians obtain the equivalent levels of expertise appropriate to their needs.[44] Specialized expertise (intermediate level) is needed for the physician (cardiologist, surgeon, and anesthesiologist) who uses intraoperative echocardiography during the repair of complex congenital heart disease. In general, two levels of training are required. Identification of ventricular wall motion abnormalities and function in the short-axis view using either an epicardial or transesophageal approach requires approximately 3 months of consistent training and includes the application of 100–200 examinations intraoperatively. Identification of wall motion abnormalities has been shown to be easily learned. The second level, ie, the ability to generate diagnostic information and render an interpretation requires significantly more experience and expertise. It is difficult to specify the length of training necessary for a physician to achieve this level of competence. It appears that the ability to evaluate complex congenital heart defects requires approximately 1 year of continuous training and at least 250 patient studies in the operating room before sufficient expertise is developed to make independent diagnostic judgments and to use results to determine patient management. Because the decision to reoperate and place the patient back on bypass is of critical magnitude, application of echocardiographic techniques in this regard becomes very important.

These guidelines represent only a general framework. Ideally, the best approach to intraoperative echocardiographic analysis is a cooperative team of competent physicians including an experienced echocardiographer, surgeon, and cardiac anesthesiologist well practiced in the discipline. Echocardiographic information must be viewed in the context of overall patient status, including surgical assessment and interpretation of hemodynamic data.

REFERENCES

1. Wells PNT: *Biomedical Ultransonics.* London: Academic Press, 1977
2. Hatle L, Angelsons B: *Doppler Ultrasound in Cardiology: Physical Principles and Clinical Applications,* 2nd ed. Philadelphia: Lea & Febiger, 1985
3. Feigenbaum HS: *Echocardiography.* Philadelphia: Lea & Febiger, 1986
4. Pearlman AS, Stevenson JG, Baker DW: Doppler echocardiography: Theory, instrumentation, technique and application. *Mayo Clin Proc* **60:**321–343, 1980
5. Kisslo J, Belkins AD, Belkins RN: *Doppler Color Flow Imaging.* New York: Churchill Livingstone, 1988
6. Sahn D: Real-time two dimensional Doppler echocardiographic flow mapping. *Circulation* **71:**849–853, 1985
7. Sutherland GR, Fraser AG: Colour flow mapping in cardiology: Indications and limitations. *Br Med Bull* **45:** 1076–1091, 1989
8. Ungerleider RM, Greeley WJ, Kisslo J: Intraoperative echocardiography in congenital heart disease surgery: Preliminary report on a current study. *Am J Cardiol* **63**(suppl 1): 3F–8F, 1989
9. Sutherland GR, Balaji S, Monro JL: Potential value of intraoperative Doppler colour flow mapping in operations for complex intracardiac shunting. *Br Heart J* **62:**467–469, 1989
10. Omoto RS: *Color Atlas of Real-Time Two Dimensional Doppler Echocardiography.* Tokyo: Shindan-To-Chinyo Co, 1984
11. Waller BJ, Taliercio CP, Slack JD, et al: Tomographic views of normal and abnormal hearts: The anatomic basis for various cardiac imaging techniques. Part I. *Clin Cardiol* **13:**804–812, 1990
12. de Bruijn NE, Clements F, Kisslo J: Intraoperative transesophageal color flow mapping: Initial experience. *Anesth Analg* **66:**386–390, 1987
13. Cahalan M, Litt L, Botvinick E, Schiller N: Advances in noninvasive cardiovascular imaging: Implications for the anesthesiologist. *Anesthesiology* **66:**356–372, 1987
14. Matsumoto M, Oka Y, Strom J, et al: Application of transesophageal echocardiography to continuous intraoperative monitoring of left ventricular performance. *Am J Cardiol* **46:**95–105, 1980
15. Smith J, Cahalan M, Benefiel D, et al: Intraoperative detection of myocardial ischemia by echocardiography. *Circulation* **72:**1015–1021, 1985
16. Thys DM, Hillel Z, Konstadt SN, Goldman ME: Intraoperative Echocardiography. In Kaplan JA (ed): *Cardiac Anesthesia,* 2nd ed. Orlando, FL: Grune & Stratton, 1987, pp 255–318
17. Sheikh KH, de Bruijn NP, Rankin JS, et al: The utility of transesophageal echocardiography and Doppler color flow imaging in patients undergoing cardiac valve surgery. *J Am Coll Cardiol* **15:**363–372, 1990
18. Konstadt S, Thys D, Mindich B, et al: Validation of quantitative intraoperative transesophageal echocardiography. *Anesthesiology* **65:**418–421, 1986
19. Muhiudeen IA, Roberson DA, Silverman NH, et al: Intraoperative echocardiography in infants and children with congenital cardiac shunt lesions; transesophageal versus epicardial echocardiography. *J Am Coll Cardiol* **16:**1687–1695, 1990
20. Ritter SB, Thys DM: Pediatric transesophageal color flow imaging: Smaller probes for smaller hearts. *Echocardiography* **6:**431–436, 1989
21. Dan M, Bonato R, Mazzucco A, et al: Value of transesophageal echocardiography during repair of congenital heart defects. *Ann Thorac Surg* **50:**637–643, 1990
22. Skorton DJ, Collins SM: Quantitation in echocardiography. *Cardiovasc Intervent Radiol* **10:**316–331, 1987

23. Ungerleider RM, Greeley WJ, Sheikh KH, et al: Routine use of intraoperative epicardial echocardiography and Doppler color flow imaging to guide and evaluate repair of congenital heart lesions. A prospective study. *J Thorac Cardiovasc Surg* **100**:297–309, 1990

24. Ungerleider RM: Decision making in pediatric cardiac surgery using intraoperative echo. *Int J Card Imaging* **4**:33–35, 1989

25. Ungerleider RM, Kisslo JA, Greeley WJ, et al: Intraoperative prebypass and postbypass epicardial color flow imaging in the repair of atrioventricular septal defects (see comments). *J Thorac Cardiovasc Surg* **98**:90–99, 1989

26. Gussenhoven EJ, vanHerwerden LA, Roelandt J, et al: Intraoperative two-dimensional echocardiography in congenital heart disease. *J Am Coll Cardiol* **9**:565–572, 1987

27. Hagler DJ, Tajik AJ, Seward JB, et al: Intraoperative two-dimensional Doppler echocardiography. A preliminary study for congenital heart disease. *J Thorac Cardiovasc Surg* **95**:516–522, 1988

28. Currie PJ, Seward JB, Hagler DJ, Tajik AJ: Two dimensional/Doppler echocardiography and its relationship to cardiac catheterization for diagnosis and management of congenital heart disease. *Cardiovasc Clin* **17**:301–322, 1986

29. Goldman, ME, Mindich BP: Intraoperative two-dimensional echocardiography: New application of an old technique. *J Am Coll Cardiol* **7**:374–382, 1986

30. Lazar HL, Plehn J: Intraoperative echocardiography. *Ann Thorac Surg* **50**:1010–1018, 1990

31. Johnson M, Holmes J, Spangler R, Patton B: Usefulness of echocardiography in patients undergoing mitral valve surgery. *J Thorac Cardiovasc Surg* **64**:922–934, 1972

32. Spotnitz HM, Malm JR: Two-dimensional ultrasound and cardiac operations. *J Thorac Cardiovasc Surg* **83**:43–51, 1982

33. Maurer G, Czer LSC, Chaux A: Intraoperative Doppler color flow mapping for assessment of valve repair for mitral regurgitation. *Am J Cardiol* **60**:333–337, 1987

34. Mindich BP, Guarino T, Goldman ME: Aortic valvuloplasty for acquired aortic stenosis. *Circulation* **74**:I130–I135, 1986

35. Takamoto S, Kyo S, Adachi H, et al: Intraoperative color flow mapping by real-time two-dimensional Doppler echocardiography for evaluation of valvular and congenital heart disease and vascular disease. *J Thorac Cardiovasc Surg* **90**:802–812, 1985

36. Goldman ME, Mora F, Guarino T, et al: Mitral valvuloplasty is superior to valve replacement for preservation of left ventricular function: An intraoperative two-dimensional echocardiographic study. *J Am Coll Cardiol* **10**:568–575, 1987

37. Goldman ME, Fuster V, Guarino T, Mindich BP: Intraoperative echocardiography for the evaluation of valvular regurgitation: Experience in 263 patients. *Circulation* **74**: I143–I149, 1986

38. Goldman ME, Guarino T, Mindich BP: Localization of aortic dissection intimal flap by intraoperative two-dimensional echocardiography. *J Am Coll Cardiol* **6**:1155–1159, 1985

39. VanHerwerden LA, Gussenhoven WJ, Roelandt J, et al: Intraoperative epicardial two-dimensional echocardiography. *Eur Heart J* **7**:386–395, 1986

40. Canter CE, Sekarski DC, Martin TC, et al: Intraoperative evaluation of atrioventricular septal defect repair by color flow mapping echocardiography. *Ann Thorac Surg* **48**:544–550, 1989

41. Canter CE, Gutierrez FR, Molina P, et al: Noninvasive diagnosis of right-sided extracardiac conduit obstruction by combined magnetic resonance imaging and continuous-wave Doppler echocardiography. *J Thorac Cardiovasc Surg* **101**:724–731, 1991

42. Greeley WT, Stanley T, Ungerleider R, Kisslo J: Intraoperative hypoxemic spells in tetralogy of Fallot: An echocardiographic analysis of diagnosis and treatment. *Anesth Analg* **68**:815–819, 1989

43. Greeley WJ, Kern FH, Ungerleider RM, Kisslo JA: Intramyocardial air causes right ventricular dysfunction after repair of a congenital heart defect. *Anesthesiology* **73**:1042–1046, 1990

44. Pearlman AS, Gardin JM, Martin RP: Guidelines for optimal physician training in echocardiography: Recommendations of American Society of Echocardiography Committee for Physician Training in Echocardiography. *Am J Cardiol* **60**:158–163, 1987

Chapter 7 | Diagnostic Cardiac Catheterization, Angiography, and Interventional Catheterization

Karen S. Rheuban and Martha A. Carpenter

DIAGNOSTIC CARDIAC CATHETERIZATION

The use of cardiac catheterization and angiography as a diagnostic tool for patients with congenital heart disease was first described in 1947 by Bing and co-workers, who described the hemodynamic data of 48 patients with cyanotic congenital heart disease.[1] Over the past four decades, refinements in techniques, catheter technology, and imaging equipment have vastly improved the safety and efficacy of pediatric cardiac catheterization.

As stated by the Committee on Cardiac Catheterization and Angiography of the American Heart Association, cardiac catheterization should be used to "identify specific congenital or acquired lesions, to establish their functional significance, to trace their physiological course and finally to evaluate the results of surgical procedures."[2] The development of superb noninvasive imaging and Doppler techniques has significantly reduced the number of cardiac catheterizations performed to those cases in which the acquisition of hemodynamic data is mandatory. Indeed, many patients with uncomplicated patent ductus arteriosus, atrial septal defect, hypoplastic left heart syndrome, and other lesions routinely undergo surgical correction based on data obtained by echocardiographic techniques.

Techniques

Sedation and Anesthesia. Following a minimum fast of 4 hours in infants and 6 hours in children, patients receive premedication prior to transfer to the cardiac catheterization laboratory. The method of anesthesia varies among centers from light sedation to general anesthesia, although most cardiologists prefer light sedation for routine procedures. General anesthesia is generally reserved for those cases requiring complicated interventions (such as clam-shell occlusion of ventricular septal defects) or for extremely uncooperative patients.

Sedation and Local Anesthesia. Neonates are often sedated with chloral hydrate (50–75 mg/kg) prior to transfer to the cardiac catheterization laboratory, although some cardiologists prefer not to premedicate hemodynamically unstable newborns and administer agents such as midazolam (0.05–0.08 mg/kg IV) during the procedure. Older infants and young children may be premedicated with meperidine (2 mg/kg IM, maximum dose 50 mg), promethazine (0.5 mg/kg IM, maximum dose 12.5 mg), and chlorpromazine (0.5 mg/kg IM, maximum dose 12.5 mg). The dosage is reduced by 50% for cyanotic infants. Other methods of sedation in older infants and young children include chloral hydrate 75–100 mg/kg PO with or without diphenhydramine 1 mg/kg PO. Additional sedation with diazepam or midazolam may be added during the procedure. Other agents reported to provide effective sedation during cardiac catheterization include fentanyl and droperidol or morphine and secobarbital.[3] Ketamine (1 mg/kg IV) may be administered during the procedure when patient cooperation is limited.

It has been documented that premedicants adversely affect hemodynamic parameters by causing alveolar hypoventilation, increased pulmonary vascular resistance, depression of cardiac output, and changes in systemic vascular resistance.[3] Although one must be cautious to prevent respiratory and cardiovascular depression from sedative agents, hemodynamic data obtained from an agitated child is equally misleading.

Patients are positioned on the fluoroscopy table, and small infants are placed on a heating pad to prevent acidosis from thermal losses. Following sterile preparation of both groin areas, the inguinal region is infiltrated with 1% lidocaine for local anesthesia (dosage: 1–2 mL in neonates, 3–4 mL in infants, and 2–8 mL in older children and adults). These doses are well below those producing either cardiac or neurotoxicity.

General Anesthesia. General anesthesia, using a variety of agents, can be performed in the cardiac disease laboratory.[4] The choice of anesthetic drugs must carefully consider their cardiovascular effects as detailed in Chapter 9. The anesthesiologist should aim to avoid major changes in pulmonary or systemic resistance, cardiac contractility, heart rate, or venous return that may alter the hemodynamic measurements being made. In addition, the necessity for an anesthesia machine, ventilator, waste gas scavenging apparatus, and expired gas monitoring equipment near the patient, but not impairing the mobility of radiology equipment, makes general anesthesia quite cumbersome. Although some catheterizations may be accomplished with heavy sedation (i.e., monitored anesthesia care) and supplemental oxygen by mask or cannula, most general anesthetic techniques will require airway control by endotracheal intubation. Invasive hemodynamic monitoring may be necessary in some patients. Postanesthesia recovery areas should be available in reasonable proximity to the catheterization laboratory. Finally, the anesthesiologist may need to provide inotropic, vasodilator, or fluid support to the patient experiencing heart failure or other cardiac complications during catheterization.

Vascular Access. Most pediatric cardiac catheterizations are performed via the Seldinger (percutaneous) technique. The femoral vessels are punctured with a thin-walled needle and an appropriate sized guidewire (Table 7–1) is advanced with fluoroscopic guidance.[5]

TABLE 7–1. SUMMARY OF COMMONLY USED GUIDEWIRE, SHEATH, AND DILATOR SETS

Dilator/ Sheath/Catheter Size (French)	Puncture Needle (Gauge)	Guidewire Diameter (in)
4	21	0.018
5	21	0.018
	19	0.021, 0.025
6	19	0.021, 0.025
7	18	0.035
8	18	0.035

When placement into the inferior vena cava and descending aorta are confirmed via fluoroscopy, a small stab wound is made over the wire. An appropriate sized dilator and sheath are advanced into the vessel, and the dilator is removed and the fully flushed catheter is inserted into the sheath. When retrograde catheterization is not required, a small femoral artery catheter can be placed for monitoring arterial pressure. The umbilical artery is commonly used for this purpose in neonates, and in some cases, the umbilical vein is used for venous access. When groin access is impossible, the basilic, jugular, or subclavian venous system can be used.

Opinion varies as to the necessity for anticoagulation during cardiac catheterization. Most pediatric cardiologists administer heparin, 50–100 U/kg, intravenously when an arterial sheath is inserted to prevent the complications of femoral artery thrombosis and embolization. Others administer heparin, 50 U/kg, to all patients regardless of the site of catheter entry and repeat the dose every 90 minutes.

Equipment. A diverse variety of cardiac catheters have been designed to provide maximum safety and accuracy and tailored specifically to the study desired. Hemodynamic assessments are best performed with an end-hole catheter (such as a Lehman catheter) or with a flow-directed balloon-tipped catheter (balloon wedge catheter). Thermodilution catheters are designed in all sizes (4, 5, 6, and 7 French) to measure cardiac output and are useful in the absence of shunts.

Angiographic catheters deliver contrast material through side holes, so as to prevent myocardial staining during the injection. A number of catheters have been devised for this purpose, including the NIH catheter, the pig-tail catheter, the multipurpose catheter (with both end and side holes), and the Berman angiographic catheter with side holes and a latex balloon to facilitate catheter manipulations.

Hemodynamic Data

The objective of cardiac catheterization is the attainment of meaningful hemodynamic data in addition to angiographic confirmation of diagnoses previously made by noninvasive techniques. Most children undergoing cardiac catheterization have shunt lesions and/or stenotic valves. Therapeutic decisions are made based on the hemodynamic data obtained at cardiac catheterization. Hemodynamic data are obtained in a systematic fashion using an end-hole catheter. In each chamber or vessel entered, pressure measurements and oxygen saturations are obtained.

Cardiac Output Determination. Cardiac output may be calculated by several different methods, including the Fick method, thermodilution, and indicator dilution techniques.[5,6] Because most patients with congenital heart disease have either left-to-right or right-to-left shunts, the Fick principle used to calculate blood flows is the common method.

Oxygen Measurements. When blood is exposed to oxygen, the oxygen is both bound to hemoglobin and dissolved in plasma. When calculating oxygen content, one must consider both these factors, although at a Pa_{O_2} of under 100, the amount of dissolved oxygen is negligible.

Oxygen Capacity. Oxygen capacity refers to the maximal amount of oxygen that can be bound by hemoglobin. This is obtained by multiplying the patient's hemoglobin by 1.34 and is expressed as milliliters per 100 mL.[7] Oxygen content indicates the amount of oxygen present in any particular sample of blood, and it is obtained by multiplying the oxygen capacity times the percent saturation and adding the amount of oxygen dissolved in plasma.[8–10]

Oxygen capacity = hemoglobin × 1.34
Oxygen content = oxygen capacity × percent saturation plus dissolved oxygen
Dissolved oxygen = Pa_{O_2} × 0.003 mL/100 mL

Thus when the Pa_{O_2} is increased in the presence of oxygen administration, the amount of oxygen dissolved in plasma will increase significantly and should not be neglected in oxygen content measurements.

Oxygen Saturation. In evaluating oxygen saturations obtained at cardiac catheterization, it is important to obtain samples as close in time as possible. It is usually desirable to obtain more than one sample from each site. Vena caval saturations are quite variable, although superior vena caval samples are subject to less fluctuation than those obtained from the inferior vena cava. Right atrial saturations are best obtained at the midlateral right atrial wall, where the best mixing of caval blood occurs. A slight step down in saturation normally occurs in the right ventricle secondary to the addition of desaturated coronary venous blood. Pulmonary artery blood should be considered to be mixed venous blood when shunts are absent. Left heart saturations should be obtained whenever possible, and an attempt to enter the left atrium and pulmonary veins to obtain a sample of fully saturated blood should be made. Low pulmonary venous saturations are generally secondary to alveolar hypoventilation, whereas low left atrial, ventricular, or arterial oxygen saturations may be due to intracardiac right-to-left shunting or pulmonary disease.

Oxygen Consumption. Oxygen consumption measurements should be performed in order to calculate cardiac output precisely. This is generally achieved with a Douglas bag, collecting and measuring oxygen and carbon dioxide in expired gas, and comparing these values to those of ambient air. In infants and younger children, oxygen consumption may be measured with a hood analyzer, but it may be difficult to obtain because of a lack of patient cooperation.[11] Although oxygen consumption varies under different circumstances, oxygen consumption may be estimated using heart rate and age as variables[12] (Table 7–2).

Shunts. Measurements of oxygen consumption are utilized to calculate blood flows by the Fick method. The Fick method of determining cardiac output utilizes the principle that if a known amount of a given indicator (oxygen) is added to a volume of fluid (blood), and one knows the amount of indicator utilized (oxygen consumption), the flow may be calculated.

$$Q = \frac{\text{Oxygen consumption}}{Ca_{O_2} - Cv_{O_2}} \quad \text{(per m}^2)$$

where Q = cardiac index (L/min/m²), Ca_{O_2} = arterial O_2 content (mL/L), Cv_{O_2} = mixed venous O_2 content (mL/L).

In the presence of cardiac shunts, the Fick method may be used to calculate the pulmonary blood flow (Qp), the systemic blood flow (Qs), and left-to-right or right-to-left shunts.

$$Qp = \frac{\text{Oxygen consumption}}{Cpv_{O_2} - Cpa_{O_2}} \quad \text{(per m}^2)$$

where Cpv_{O_2} = pulmonary venous oxygen content, Cpa_{O_2} = pulmonary arterial oxygen content.

$$Qs = \frac{\text{Oxygen consumption}}{Ca_{O_2} - Cmv_{O_2}} \quad \text{(per m}^2)$$

where Ca_{O_2} = systemic arterial oxygen content, Cmv_{O_2} = mixed venous oxygen content (obtained from the proximal to the shunt).

When bidirectional shunting occurs, the effective pulmonary blood flow (Qep) is calculated. This represents the quantity of mixed venous blood that ultimately reaches the lungs.

TABLE 7–2. OXYGEN CONSUMPTION TABLES.

Age (y)	\multicolumn{13}{c}{Heart rate (bpm)}												
	50	60	70	80	90	100	110	120	130	140	150	160	170
Men													
3				155	159	163	167	171	175	178	182	186	190
4			149	152	156	160	163	168	171	175	179	182	186
6		141	144	148	151	155	159	162	167	171	174	178	181
8		136	141	145	148	152	156	159	163	167	171	175	178
10	130	134	139	142	146	149	153	157	160	165	169	172	176
12	128	132	136	140	144	147	151	155	158	162	167	170	174
14	127	130	134	137	142	146	149	153	157	160	165	169	172
16	125	129	132	136	141	144	148	152	155	159	162	167	
18	124	127	131	135	139	143	147	150	154	157	161	166	
20	123	126	130	134	137	142	145	149	153	156	160	165	
25	120	124	127	131	135	139	143	147	150	154	157		
30	118	122	125	129	133	136	141	145	148	152	155		
35	116	120	124	127	131	135	139	143	147	150			
40	115	119	122	126	130	133	137	141	145	149			
Women													
3				150	153	157	161	165	169	172	176	180	183
4			141	145	149	152	156	159	163	168	171	175	179
6		130	134	137	142	146	149	153	156	160	165	168	172
8		125	129	133	136	141	144	148	152	155	159	163	167
10	118	122	125	129	133	136	141	144	148	152	155	159	163
12	115	119	122	126	130	133	137	141	145	149	152	156	160
14	112	116	120	123	127	131	134	133	143	146	150	153	157
16	109	114	118	121	125	128	132	136	140	144	148	151	
18	107	111	116	119	123	127	130	134	137	142	146	149	
20	106	109	114	118	121	125	128	132	136	140	144	148	
25	102	106	109	114	118	121	125	128	132	136	140		
30	99	103	106	110	115	118	122	125	129	133	136		
35	97	100	104	107	111	116	119	123	127	130			
50	94	98	102	105	109	112	117	121	124	128			

(Modified from La Farge C, Miettinen O: Cardiovasc Res 4:23, 1970, with permission.)

$$Qep = \frac{\text{Oxygen consumption}}{Cpvo_2 - Cmvo_2} \quad \text{(per m}^2\text{)}$$

The left-to-right shunt may be calculated by subtracting Qep from Qp. The right-to-left shunt may be calculated by subtracting Qep from Qs.

In patients with congenital heart disease, the relationship between pulmonary and systemic blood flows (Qp:Qs) is often important. A ratio of 1:1 indicates no shunt or a bidirectional shunt of equal magnitude. A ratio of 2:1 indicates pulmonary flow that is twice the volume of systemic blood flow, and a ratio of 0.5:1 indicates a right-to-left shunt, with a pulmonary flow that is one half systemic. Shunts may also be detected by indicator dilution techniques or by the use of a hydrogen catheter.

Pressure Measurements. Pressures in the heart and great vessels are measured with a fluid-filled catheter and transducer system. One should exercise great caution to ascertain that the transducers are at the cardiac level and electronically balanced and that no air bubbles or clots are present in the system that may cause distortion of the

desired waveform. Phasic and mean pressures are recorded in all venous, atrial, and arterial positions; phasic pressures are recorded in the ventricles. End-diastolic pressures in the ventricles are amplified so as to facilitate precise recordings.

The normal intracardiac and great artery pressures are shown in Table 7–3.[13,14] Atrial tracings are analyzed and the a, c, and v wave amplitudes are measured. The a wave is due to atrial systole, the c wave is associated

TABLE 7–3. NORMAL INTRACARDIAC PRESSURES (mm Hg)

Location	Newborn	Child
Right atrium (mean)	0–4	2–6
Right ventricle	65–80/0–6	15–25/3–7
Pulmonary artery	65–80/35–50	15–25/10–16
Pulmonary wedge (mean)	6–9	8–11
Left atrium (mean)	3–6	5–10
Left ventricle	65–80/0–6	90–110/7–9
Aorta	65–80/45–60	90–110/65–75

with ventricular systole, and the v wave represents atrial filling. The right ventricular and pulmonary artery systolic pressures should be equal and the right ventricular end-diastolic pressure should equal the right atrial a wave. The pulmonary capillary wedge pressure, obtained by either passing an end-hole catheter distally into a branch pulmonary artery or by inflating a latex balloon in a branch pulmonary artery, approximates the left atrial and pulmonary venous pressure although it may actually be 2–3 mm Hg higher. The left ventricular systolic pressure and the central aortic systolic pressure normally are equal. The left ventricular end-diastolic pressure normally correlates, in the absence of mitral stenosis, with the left atrial a wave. The pressure in the ascending aorta differs from that of the peripheral arteries in that peripheral pressure waveforms are characterized by a higher systolic and lower diastolic pressure. This phenomenon is related to the flow characteristics in smaller arteries with higher vascular resistance.[15]

Gradients. Pressure pullbacks are obtained so as to assess accurately any gradient across the cardiac valves or central vessels. In the presence of large left-to-right shunts, however, "flow gradients" may be measured in the absence of any structural valvular lesions. Gradients of 30 mm Hg have been measured across the pulmonic valve in patients with large shunts in the absence of true pulmonic stenosis, presumably secondary to a "relative" stenosis caused by excess flow across a normal valve.[16]

Resistances. The concept of vascular resistance has been used to provide an assessment of the response of various vascular beds to physiologic and pharmacologic interventions. Vascular resistance is based on the Pouseille formula relating flow, pressures, and the cross-sectional area of the vessel.

The pulmonary vascular resistance has been extensively used to assess the effects of various cardiac lesions on the pulmonary vascular bed and to determine the presence or absence of pulmonary vascular obstructive disease. The degree to which the pulmonary vascular resistance is elevated and the actual ratio of pulmonary to systemic vascular resistance has been utilized to determine the potential risk of corrective surgery, and/or the suitability of patients for cardiac transplantation. Pulmonary arteriolar resistance is calculated from the following equation:

$$PVR = \frac{MPAP - MPCWP \text{ (or MLAP)}}{Qp}$$

where PVR = pulmonary arteriolar resistance, MPAP = mean pulmonary artery pressure, MLAP = mean left atrial pressure, MPCWP = mean pulmonary capillary wedge pressure, Qp = pulmonary blood flow (per m²).

The normal pulmonary vascular resistance is ≤2 Wood units in older children and adults and in neonates is considerably higher.[17,18]

An increased pulmonary vascular resistance may be secondary to reversible pulmonary vasoconstriction or to fixed pulmonary vascular obstructive disease. The administration of 100% oxygen or a pulmonary vasodilator such as tolazoline (1 mg/kg IV) may decrease pulmonary resistance with an increase in pulmonary blood flow.[19]

Systemic vascular resistance is calculated from the following formula:

$$SVR = \frac{MAP - RAP}{Qs}$$

where SVR = systemic vascular resistance, MAP = mean arterial pressure, RAP = mean right atrial pressure, Qs = systemic blood flow

The systemic vascular resistance rises from a range of 10–15 U per m² in the neonatal period to 20 U per m², where it generally remains after infancy.[9] The systemic vascular resistance varies in response to sympathetic tone and may be considerably elevated in patients with congestive heart failure.

Valve Areas. The calculation of valve area, in addition to the measurement of a transvalvar gradient, has been extensively used to assess the degree of severity of mitral and aortic valve stenosis. The formula for valve area considers the gradient as well as the cardiac output through that valve:

$$A = \frac{Q \text{ (m}^2)}{K\sqrt{\Delta P}}$$

where A = valve area per square meter, Q = cardiac output through that valve per square meter, K = a devised constant for each specific valve, P = mean pressure gradient.

For the aortic valve, the flow in systole is calculated, and the K is 44.5. For the mitral valve, transvalvar flow is measured in diastole, and the K is 37.5.

A normal valve area, indexed per m², is 2.5 cm²/m². Critical valvar stenoses have been associated with a valve area of less than 0.75 cm²/m².[20,21]

ANGIOGRAPHY

Angiography has been available since 1937 when the right heart was first imaged, followed in 1938 by imaging of the left heart.[22,23] Selective angiography, performed at the site of the cardiac defect, has evolved over the past 40 years as a result of advances in the technology of cardiac catheters, imaging equipment, contrast material, and the development of biplane cineangiography.

Contrast Media

Modern contrast materials are radiopaque water-soluble organic iodide preparations. Conventional ionic agents are highly concentrated, hyperosmolar, and often cause discomfort when injected. New nonionic contrast agents have lower osmolarity than the ionic agents and are subject to fewer side effects, although these agents are more viscous and can cause hyperaggregability of red blood cells. No more than 5 mL/kg of ionic contrast material should be administered as a total dose, although higher doses can be used with the nonionic (and much more expensive) agents. Contrast materials should be injected into as short and large a catheter as possible so as to optimize the quality of the angiogram.

Fifteen minutes should elapse between angiograms to allow for return of the preangiogram hemodynamic state. Anaphylactic reactions are rare but should be treated with epinephrine, fluid administration, steroids, and diphenhydramine.

Views

Selective biplane angiography now may be performed with an "C-arm" in which the sedated patient need not be moved to obtain angiograms in different projections. The anterior posterior (AP) and lateral projections demonstrate many anatomic details, and complex oblique views provide superb images of ventricular septal defects, the right ventricular outflow tract, and the great arteries (Figs 7–1 to 7–3).[24]

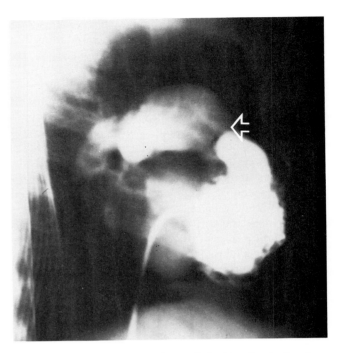

Figure 7–2. Right ventricular angiogram in the lateral projection demonstrating a domed thickened pulmonic valve (*arrow*), with the post-stenotic dilation.

COMPLICATIONS OF CARDIAC CATHETERIZATION

The morbidity and mortality rates associated with cardiac catheterization are related to the age, diagnosis, and condition of the patient. The highest mortality rates are seen in patients with complex congenital heart disease undergoing cardiac catheterization in the first week of life (9.6% of 685 infants at the Hospital for Sick Children in Toronto).[25] These data were obtained in the era prior to the use of prostaglandin E_1 manipulation of the ductus arteriosus.[26,27] Current data suggest a significant reduction in catheterization-related morbidity and mortality since the introduction of prostaglandin therapy in the late 1970s.

Major catheterization-related complications include dysrhythmias, cardiac perforation, air embolization, hemorrhage with either inguinal or retroperitoneal hematoma, arterial or venous thrombosis, seizures, respiratory depression, catheter knotting, and anaphylaxis. Advances in medical therapy, percutaneous techniques, and improved equipment have significantly reduced the incidence of these complications.

Blood loss during catheterization is not uncommon, particularly during a lengthy interventional catheterization or during the catheterization of a neonate. In general, blood losses in excess of 5 mL/kg require treatment with volume expansion. Packed red blood cells should be administered if the hemoglobin is <10 g/100 mL;

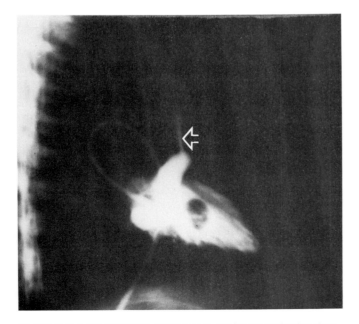

Figure 7–1. Left ventricular angiogram in the lateral projection demonstrating critical aortic stenosis with a jet of contrast through the dysplastic valve.

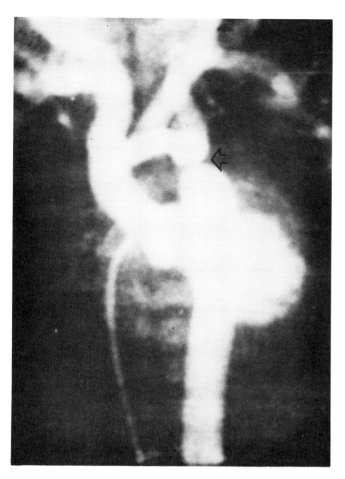

Figure 7–3. Left ventricular angiogram in the AP projection showing a discrete coarctation of the aorta (*arrow*) distal to the left subclavian artery.

volume expanders such as lactated Ringer's solution or 5% albumin are used at the discretion of the cardiologist if the hemoglobin is higher.

INTERVENTIONAL CARDIAC CATHETERIZATION

Recent modifications in techniques of interventional cardiac catheterization, initially designed for the palliation of certain life-threatening cyanotic congenital cardiovascular lesions, now enable pediatric cardiologists to treat a number of congenital cardiovascular malformations nonsurgically. The development of the double-lumen balloon-tipped atrioseptostomy catheter by Rashkind and Miller in 1966 was the first innovation in nonsurgical therapy of congenital heart disease.[18] Blade atrial septostomy followed in 1973, and further advances in therapeutic techniques such as embolization, umbrella and clam-shell occlusion, balloon dilation valvuloplasty, and

angioplasty have revolutionized pediatric catheterization.[29–32,33]

Balloon Atrial Septostomy

Balloon atrial septostomy, introduced by Rashkind and Miller in 1966, was the first nonsurgical therapeutic procedure in pediatric cardiac catheterization.[28] Although initially designed for palliation of transposition of the great arteries, this technique has proven effective in the palliation of a number of other congenital cardiovascular defects, where the presence of a nonrestrictive atrial septal defect may significantly improve hemodynamics, including tricuspid atresia, pulmonary atresia with an intact ventricular septum, mitral atresia, total anomalous pulmonary venous return, double-outlet right ventricle with a restrictive ventricular septal defect, some cases of mitral stenosis, and the hypoplastic left heart syndrome.[33]

The success of balloon atrial septostomy is generally limited to the neonatal period, when the lower margin of the foramen ovale is very thin and can be torn by forcibly withdrawing a balloon filled with dilute contrast material from the left to right atrium (Fig 7–4). Complications include avulsion of the inferior vena cava, tricuspid valve damage (when the catheter is improperly positioned in the right ventricle), cardiac perforation, dysrhythmias, low cardiac output, and balloon rupture.

Successful balloon atrial septostomy causes (1) an improvement in oxygen saturation, (2) a reduction in atrial pressure gradient, and (3) a reduction in the left atrial pressure. Successful septostomy can be readily confirmed by echocardiographic techniques (Fig 7–5).

The results of balloon atrial septostomy have been extremely rewarding. Of Rashkind's initial 60 patients reported in 1971, 85% were successfully discharged from hospital.[33] Nine patients died in the hospital despite the presence of an adequate atrial communication; they died from acidosis or during further palliative surgery.[33] These data, obtained prior to the use of prostaglandin therapy, demonstrates a remarkable clinical response in a group of patients previously doomed to high mortality rates.

Blade Atrial Septostomy

In some patients, the foramen ovale has closed or the atrial septum is too thick to perform successful balloon atrial septostomy. These patients are generally older than 1 month of age, may have premature closure of the foramen ovale, may have had an inadequate balloon septostomy, or may have an inadequate natural atrial communication. In 1973, Park devised a catheter equipped with a built-in retractable blade that may be used to incise the lower portion of the fossa ovalis (Fig 7–6). This procedure is then followed by a balloon atrial septostomy.[29]

Criteria for a successful blade septostomy have been established depending on the lesion in need of pallia-

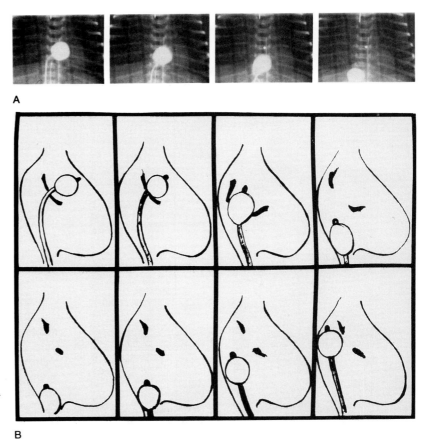

A

B

Figure 7–4. (*A*) Angiogram of the technique of balloon atrial septostomy, forcibly withdrawing a contrast filled balloon from left atrium to right atrium. (*B*) Diagram of balloon atrial septostomy. (*From Rashkind WJ: Atrioseptostomy by balloon catheter in congenital heart disease. Radiol Clin North Am 9:196, 1971, with permission.*)

tion. Most important is a reduction in the pressure gradient between the two atria, combined with echocardiographic confirmation of enlargement of the atrial septal defect.

A collaborative study to review the overall results of blade septostomy reported clinical improvement in 70–100% of patients treated via this technique.[34] Complications, including cardiac perforation and seizures, were reported in 10% of patients.

Embolization Techniques

In some patients with extreme forms of tetralogy of Fallot or other complex cyanosis-producing lesions, abundant bronchial collateral vessels may supply the pulmonary vascular bed. These collateral vessels may in fact cause excessive pulmonary blood flow either before or after surgical correction. Surgical ligation is often impossible because the collateral vessels are technically difficult to reach. Balloon and coil embolization techniques have been developed to occlude these collateral arteries successfully (Fig 7–7A,B).[30,35–39]

Indications for embolization include (1) the elimination of right-to-left shunts through pulmonary arteriovenous malformations; (2) the reduction of left ventricular volume overload from bronchial collaterals; (3) protection of the pulmonary vascular bed from ex-

cessive flow; (4) reduction in the flow from collaterals that may prevent either a successful Fontan procedure or Glenn shunt; and (5) closure of previously placed systemic-pulmonary shunt. Complications of embolization techniques include inadvertent embolization of normal vascular structures and failure of embolization secondary to improper coil or balloon positioning.

Umbrella Occlusion Techniques

Rashkind, in 1983, reported the use of a device for the nonoperative closure of a patent ductus arteriosus.[40] This technique, implemented by insertion of a double-umbrella prosthesis retrograde through the ductus arteriosus has been reported to occlude the ductus successfully in 83% of patients.[39] Because surgical closure of patent ductus offers excellent results with low morbidity and mortality rates, transcatheter ductal closure still remains limited to 12 centers enrolled in a collaborative study.

Occlusion techniques have been applied to transcatheter closure of atrial septal defects, initially utilizing a spring-loaded single-umbrella device advanced prograde across the atrial septum, which is withdrawn and hooked into the left side of the atrial septum. Technical difficulties limited the use of this device to atrial defects of 1.5–2.0 cm in diameter and to patients greater than 20

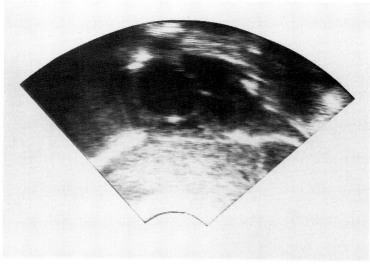

A

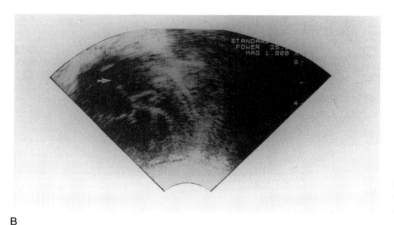

B

Figure 7–5. Echocardiographic demonstration of interatrial septum before (*A*) and after (*B*) balloon atrial septostomy. (*Arrow*) Atrial septal defect.

kg in weight. The device cannot be retrieved through a catheter system should it be improperly implanted or if it embolizes. Thus, transcatheter techniques for closure of atrial septal defects remain both controversial and experimental.[39]

The Lock clamshell occluder (a double-umbrella device) has been successfully used to close both atrial and ventricular septal defects, but these techniques also remain experimental at this time.[41]

Balloon Dilation Angioplasty

Although the first attempts to relieve congenital cardiovascular disease with catheters were described in 1954 by Rubio and co-workers, interest in this field lay dormant until suitable catheter systems and imaging techniques were developed.[42] In 1964, Dotter and Judkins introduced the technique of transluminal angioplasty for the treatment of atherosclerotic obstructions of the femoral artery.[43] Gruntzig, in 1979, reported the development of a new double-lumen catheter with an elastic balloon for the percutaneous treatment of coronary and renal artery

stenoses.[44] Interest in balloon angioplasty for congenital heart disease was stimulated by a report of a successful postmortem balloon dilation of a coarctation of the aorta in an infant with the hypoplastic left heart syndrome.[45] Since that report, balloon dilation angioplasty has been successfully used as therapy for recurrent coarctation of the aorta. Successful balloon dilation angioplasty of coarctation of the aorta has been defined as >50% reduction in gradient across the coarcted segment plus a 30% or greater increase in the aortic diameter at the site of the angioplasty. Gradient reductions of 70% have been reported by many investigators.[46] (See Fig 7–8.)

The issue of balloon dilation of native coarctation of the aorta is more controversial.[47] The development of aneurysmal changes in the aorta 6–12 months following angioplasty in as many as 10% of patients has led most cardiologists to reserve this intervention for recurrent coarctation of the aorta.

Balloon angioplasty for coarctation of the aorta is achieved through a femoral artery approach. A large femoral artery sheath is inserted via the percutaneous tech-

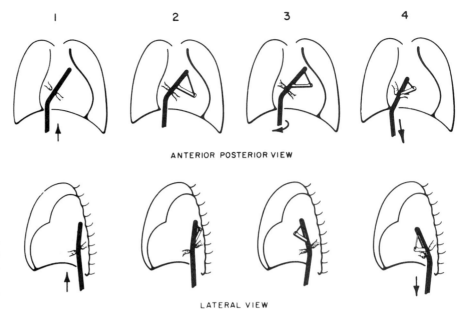

Figure 7-6. Technique of blade atrial septostomy. (*From Park SC, Neches WH, Mullins CE, et al: Blade atrial septostomy: A collaborative study. Circulation 66:258-266, 1982, with permission from the American Heart Association.*)

nique, the patient is anticoagulated, and a guidewire is advanced into the root of the aorta following a baseline cardiac catheterization. A polyethylene dilating balloon is selected with an inflation diameter that measures the size of the normal aorta proximal to the coarctation and is advanced through the coarctation and inflated several times to ensure satisfactory dilation of the coarctation. Immediate complications of balloon angioplasty of coarctation include femoral artery compromise, aortic tears,

and systemic hypotension from vagal reactions. Patients should receive intravenous fluids for 12 hours following the angioplasty to maintain intravascular volume and brisk flow through the angioplasty site.

Other vascular lesions amenable to balloon dilation angioplasty include peripheral pulmonic stenosis, a lesion typically poorly amenable to surgical therapy, but that may be effectively treated by angioplasty techniques in as many as 50% of patients.[48] Additionally, stenotic

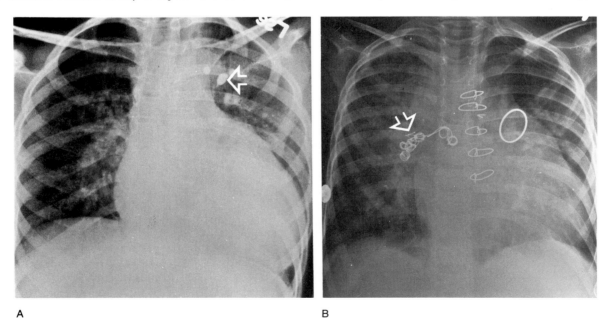

A   B

Figure 7-7. (*A*) Silicon balloons (arrow) in bronchial arteries in a patient postrepair of tetralogy of Fallot with pulmonary atresia. (*B*) Coils (arrow) in bronchial collaterals of another patient with tetralogy of Fallot.

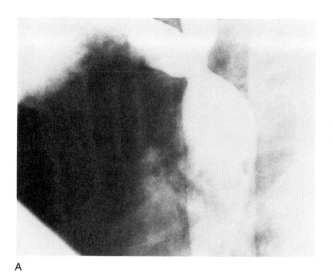 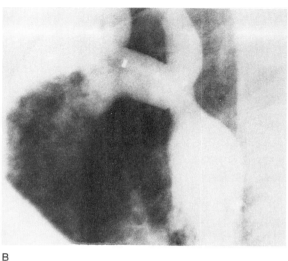

A B

Figure 7–8. Balloon dilatation angioplasty of a patient with a recoarctation at the site of a previous end-to-end anastomosis. (*A*) Angiogram before balloon angioplasty; (*B*) angiogram demonstrating relief of obstruction.

systemic-to-pulmonary shunts may be successfully dilated (Fig 7–9), as may be obstructed baffles (Fig 7–10) following the Mustard operation.

Balloon Valvuloplasty

In 1982, Kan reported the first successful balloon dilation valvuloplasty of a stenotic pulmonic valve.[32] Since that time, this procedure has become the accepted procedure of choice for treatment of valvular pulmonic stenosis in both children and adults, although some cases with an extremely dysplastic pulmonary valve or hypoplastic annulus may not be amenable to valvuloplasty. The results of valvuloplasty have been rewarding, with gradient reductions of 70% reported in most series.[49,50]

The technique of pulmonary valvuloplasty has been well described. After baseline hemodynamic catheterization and angiography, a "J" wire is advanced across the pulmonic valve into the left lower lobe pulmonary artery.

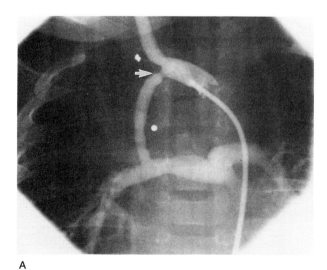 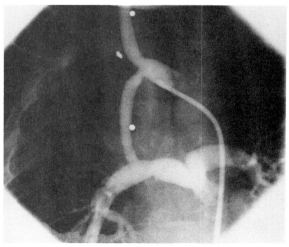

A B

Figure 7–9. (*A, B*) Balloon dilatation angioplasty of a stenotic Blalock-Taussig shunt. Note the disappearance of the "waist" (*arrow*) upon inflation of the balloon.

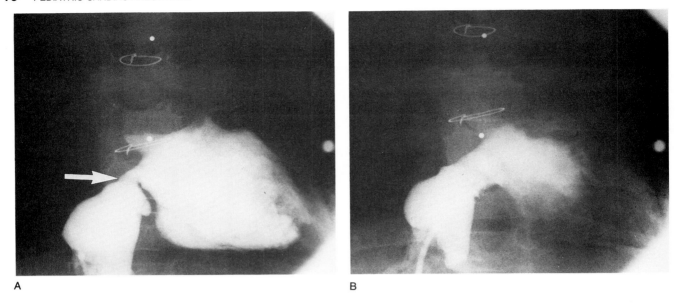

Figure 7–10. Balloon dilatation of the obstructed lower limb of a Mustard operation predilatation (*A*) and postdilatation (*B*).

A single balloon with an inflation diameter 1.2–1.4 times the diameter of the pulmonary annulus (measured angiographically) or a double balloon measuring 1.5–1.6 times the annulus is advanced over the wire and inflated several times (Fig 7–11). Continuous monitoring of the systemic blood pressure is mandatory, and the patient should be adequately hydrated prior to the procedure. A satisfactory result is confirmed by a reduction in right ventricular pressure and a gradient reduction to less than 20 mm Hg. (See Figs 7–12 and 7–13.) All patients are

placed in an intensive care setting for 6–12 hours postvalvuloplasty, and intravenous fluids are administered during this period. Feedings are reinstituted when the patient is awake with stable vital signs. The patient is discharged the morning after valvuloplasty.

Balloon valvuloplasty of the aortic valve has become an accepted therapeutic technique in the treatment of valvular aortic stenosis in older infants and children and in some centers in neonates.[51,52] This technique requires the retrograde passage of a guidewire across the aortic

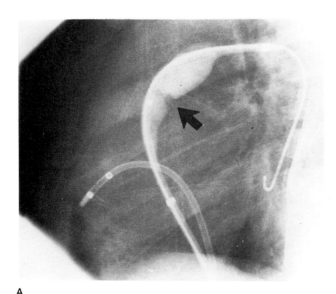
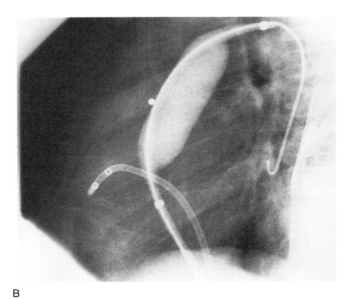

Figure 7–11. Technique of balloon dilatation angioplasty of a stenotic pulmonic valve. It shows the constriction at the *arrow* (*A*) prior to dilatation and unobstructed pulmonic outflow (*B*) after dilatation.

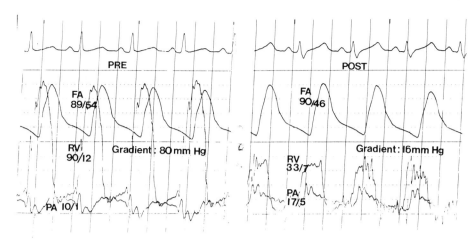

Figure 7–12. Balloon dilatation angioplasty of a patient with severe valvular pulmonic stenosis. Note that the pulmonic gradient (RV systolic–PA systolic) after angioplasty has decreased from 80 to 16 mm Hg.

valve, followed by a valvuloplasty catheter, the size of the aortic annulus measured angiographically at the cardiac catheterization. Patients are anticoagulated with heparin during the procedure to minimize the embolic complications of a left heart intervention and to prevent vascular insufficiency following placement of a large femoral artery catheter. Patients with significant aortic insufficiency (>2+) are not treated by valvuloplasty techniques for fear of worsening the valvar leak and obviating valve replacement. Success rates, as reported by Sholler et al, in 1988, are high, with gradient reductions in 55%.[53] However, the incidence of significant aortic regurgitation postvalvuloplasty approached 26%.[53] Nearly one third of the patients experienced a pulse loss (60% under age 2, 10% over age 2), and three infants died (4%)

of complications related to the procedure. Another investigator reported a reduction in left ventricular outflow tract gradient of 70% with only mild residual aortic insufficiency.[53] Balloon dilation valvuloplasty is now also performed in adults as treatment for calcific aortic stenosis, and it has also been attempted as treatment for both congenital and acquired mitral valve stenosis.

POSTCATHETERIZATION CARE

Most patients undergo diagnostic cardiac catheterization on an outpatient basis, with the exception of neonates and infants with extreme cyanosis and/or severe congestive heart failure, and those patients who undergo inter-

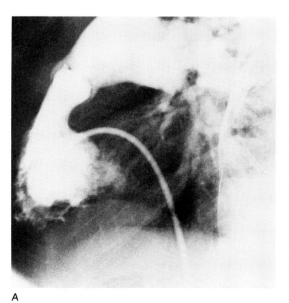

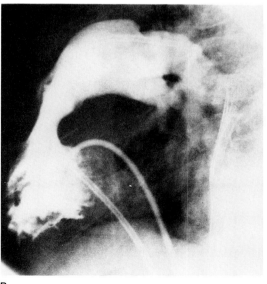

A   B

Figure 7–13. The angiograms demonstrate doming of the pulmonic valve in systole preangioplasty (*A*) with marked improvement postangioplasty (*B*).

ventional catheterization. All patients are observed in a recovery room postcatheterization. Vital signs are obtained every 15 minutes for 1 hour, every 30 minutes for 2 hours, and then on an hourly basis. Attention is given to the catheterization site, which is usually dressed with an elastic bandage dressing, and occasionally with a sandbag to prevent further bleeding from the arterial catheter site. Distal pulses and perfusion of the extremity through which the catheter was inserted are evaluated as well. An absent pulse reflects either arterial spasm or thrombosis and requires treatment if capillary refill is delayed, the extremity is cool, and the pulse remains absent for 2 hours after conclusion of the catheterization. Treatment with intravenous heparin for 24–48 hours generally is sufficient to restore the pulse; however, thrombolytic agents such as streptokinase or urokinase are occasionally necessary when anticoagulation fails. Acetaminophen is administered for fever and/or pain, and fluids are administered orally when the patient is fully awake. Should oral intake or the patient's state of hydration be inadequate, intravenous fluids may be administered. Patients may be discharged home 4–6 hours postcardiac catheterization when they are awake, taking food/fluids, and have palpable peripheral pulses and stable vital signs.

REFERENCES

1. Bing RJ, Vandam L, Gray F: Physiological studies in congenital heart disease. *Bull Johns Hopkins Hosp* **80**:107–120, 1947
2. Cournand A, Bing R, Dexter L, et al: Report of the Committee on Cardiac Catheterization and Angiography of the American Heart Association. *Circulation* **7**:769–773, 1953
3. Goldberg S, Linde L, Gaal P, Sachs D: The pulmonary and systemic hemodynamic effects produced by meperidine and hydroxyzine. *J Pharmacol Exp Ther* **159**:306–313, 1968
4. Topkins MJ: Anesthetic management of cardiac catheterization. *Int Anesth Clin* **18**:59–69, 1980
5. Seldinger S: Catheter replacement of the needle in percutaneous arteriography. *Acta Radiol* **39**:368–376, 1953
6. Alpert J, Dexter L: Blood flow measurement: The cardiac output. In Grossman W (ed): *Cardiac Catheterization and Angiography*. Philadelphia: Lea & Febiger, 1976, pp 61–72
7. Swan HJC: Indicator dilution methods in the diagnosis of congenital heart disease. *Prog Cardiovasc Dis* **2**:143–165, 1959
8. Jarmakani JM: Cardiac catheterization and angiography. In Adams FH, Emmanouilides GC (eds): *Heart Disease in Infants, Children and Adolescents*. Baltimore: Williams & Wilkins, 1983, pp 83–100
9. Rudolph AM: Cardiac catheterization and angiography. In Rudolph AM (ed): *Congenital Diseases of the Heart*. Chicago: Year Book Medical, 1974, pp 49–167
10. Yang SS: *Cardiac Catheterization Data to Hemodynamic Parameters*. Philadelphia: FA Davis, 1972
11. Wessel HU, Rorem D, Muster AJ, et al: Continuous determination of oxygen uptake in sedated infants and chil-

dren during cardiac catheterization. *Am J Cardiol* **24**:376–385, 1969
12. LaFarge C, Miettinen OS: The estimation of oxygen consumption. *Cardiovasc Res* **4**:23–30, 1970
13. Krovetz LJ, McLoughlin TG, Mitchell MB, Schiebler GL: Hemodynamic findings in normal children. *Pediatr Res* **1**:122–130, 1967
14. Krovetz LJ, Goldbloom S: Normal standards for cardiovascular data. *Johns Hopkins Med J* **130**:187–195, 1972
15. O'Rourke MF, Blazek JV, Morreels CL, Krovetz LJ: Pressure wave transmission along the human aorta: Changes with age and in arterial degenerative disease. *Circulation Res* **23**:567–579, 1968
16. Rudolph A, Nadas A, Goodale W: Intracardiac left-to-right shunt with pulmonic stenosis. *Am Heart J* **48**:808–816, 1954
17. Emmanouilides GC, Moss AJ, Duffie ER, Adams FH: Pulmonary arteriolar changes in human newborn infants from birth to three days of age. *J Pediatr* **65**:327–333, 1964
18. Rudolph A, Nadas A: The pulmonary circulation and congenital heart disease. *N Engl J Med* **267**:968–974, 1962
19. Rao BNS, Moller JH, Edwards JE: Primary pulmonary hypertension in a child: Response to pharmacologic agents. *Circulation* **40**:583–587, 1969
20. Gorlin R, Gorlin S: Hydraulic formula for calculation of the stenotic mitral valve, other cardiac valves and central shunts. *Am Heart J* **41**:1–19, 1951
21. Dexter L: Profiles in valvular heart disease. In Grossman W (ed): *Cardiac Catheterization and Angiography*. Philadelphia: Lea & Febiger, 1976, pp 253–268
22. Castellanos A, Pereiras R, Garcia A: La angiocardiographica radio opaca. *Arch Soc Estud Clin Habana* **31**:523, 1937
23. Robb G, Steinberg I: Visualization of the chambers of the heart, pulmonary circulation and great blood vessels in man; practical method. *Am J Roentgenol* **41**:1–17, 1939
24. Freedom R, Culham J, Moes C: *Angiocardiography of Congenital Heart Disease*. New York: Macmillan, 1984
25. Rowe RD: Cardiac catheterization. In Keith JD, Rowe RD, Vlad P (eds): *Heart Disease in Infants, and Children, and Adolescents*. New York: Macmillan, 1978, pp 81–115
26. Heyman M, Rudolph A: Ductus arteriosus dilatation by prostaglandin E1 in infants with pulmonary atresia. *Pediatrics* **59**:325–329, 1977
27. Heyman MA, Berman W, Rudolph AM, Whitman V: Dilatation of the ductus arteriosus by Prostaglandin E1 in aortic arch abnormalities. *Circulation* **59**:169–173, 1979
28. Rashkind SJ, Miller WW: Creation of an atrial septal defect without thoracotomy. *JAMA* **196**:991–992, 1966
29. Park SC, Zuberbuhler JR, Neches WH, et al: A new atrial septostomy technique. *Cathet Cardiovasc Diagn* **1**:195–201, 1975
30. Fellows KE, Khaw KT, Schuster S, Schwachman H: Bronchial artery embolization in cystic fibrosis: Technique and long term results. *J Pediatr* **95**:959–963, 1979
31. Porstmann W, Wierny L, Warnke H, et al: Catheter closure of patent ductus arteriosus. *Radiol Clin North Am* **9**:203–218, 1971
32. Kan JS, White RI, Mitchell SE, Gardner TJ: Percutaneous balloon valvuloplasty: A new method for treating congenital pulmonary valve stenosis, *N Engl J Med* **307**:540–542, 1982

33. Rashkind WJ: Atrioseptostomy by balloon catheter in congenital heart disease. *Radiol Clin North Am* **9**:193–202, 1971

34. Park SC, Neches WH, Mullins CE, et al: Blade atrial septostomy: A collaborative study. *Circulation* **66**:258–266, 1982

35. Fuhrman B, Bass JL, Castaneda-Zuniga W, et al: Coil embolization of congenital thoracic vascular anomalies in infants and children. *Circulation* **70**:285–289, 1984

36. Terry PB, White RI, Barth KH, et al: Pulmonary arteriovenous malformations: Physiologic observations and results of therapeutic balloon embolization. *N Engl J Med* **308**:1197–1200, 1983

37. Kaufman SL, Gorandberg JD, Barth KJ, et al: Therapeutic embolization with detachable silicone balloons; long term effects in swine. *Invest Radiol* **14**:156–161, 1979

38. Perry S, Radtke W, Fellows K, et al: Coil embolization to occlude aorticopulmonary collateral vessels. *J Am Coll Cardiol* **13**:100–108, 1989

39. Mullins CC: Therapeutic cardiac catheterization. In Garson A, Bricker JT, McNamara DG (eds): *Science and Practice of Pediatric Cardiology*. Philadelphia: Lea & Febiger, 1990, pp 2183–2209

40. Rashkind WJ: Transcatheter treatment of congenital heart disease. *Circulation* **67**:711–716, 1983

41. Lock J, Black P, McKay R, et al: Transcatheter closure of ventricular septal defects. *Circulation* **78**:361–368, 1988

42. Rubio V, Limon-Larson R: *Treatment of Pulmonary Valvar Stenosis and of Tricuspid Stenosis Using a Modified Catheter.* Second World Congress of Cardiology, Washington, DC, 1954

43. Dotter CT, Judkins, MP: Transluminal treatment of arteriosclerotic obstruction. *Circulation* **30**:654–670, 1964

44. Gruntzig AR, Senning A, Siegenthaler WE: Nonoperative dilatation of coronary artery stenosis. *N Engl J Med* **301**:61–68, 1979

45. Sos T, Sniderman KW, Retek-Sos B, et al: Percutaneous transluminal dilatation of coarctation of the thoracic aorta post mortem. *Lancet* **2**:970–971, 1979

46. Lock JE, Bass JL, Amplatz K, et al: Balloon dilatation angioplasty of aortic coarctations in infants and children. *Circulation* **68**:109–116, 1983

47. Marvin WJ, Mahoney LT: Balloon angioplasty of unoperated coarctation in young children. *J Am Coll Cardiol* **5**:405, 1985 (abstr)

48. Lock JE, Castaneda-Zuniga WR, Furman BP, Bass JL: Balloon dilatation angioplasty of hypoplastic and stenotic pulmonary arteries. *Circulation* **67**:962–967, 1983

49. Kan JS, White RI, Mitchell SE, et al: Percutaneous transluminal balloon valvuloplasty for pulmonary valve stenosis. *Circulation* **69**:554–560, 1984

50. Rocchini AP, Kveselis DA, Crosley D, et al: Percutaneous balloon valvuloplasty for treatment of congenital pulmonary valvar stenosis in children. *J Am Coll Cardiol* **3**:1005–1012, 1984

51. Lock JE, Keane JF, Fellows KE: The use of catheter intervention procedures for congenital heart disease. *J Am Coll Cardiol* **7**:1420–1423, 1986

52. Lababidi Z, Wu JR, Walls JT: Percutaneous balloon aortic valvuloplasty results in 23 patients. *Am J Cardiol* **53**:194–197, 1984

53. Sholler G, Keane J, Perry S, et al: Balloon dilatation of congenital aortic valve stenosis. *Circulation* **78**:351–360, 1988

Chapter 8 | Monitoring of the Pediatric Cardiac Patient

Carol L. Lake

Monitoring is an essential part of anesthesia for pediatric cardiac surgery. Basic monitoring of the electrocardiogram (ECG), blood pressure, and cardiorespiratory sounds can usually be established prior to induction of anesthesia. However, if a child is upset or crying, even these monitors can be delayed until the induction is started. In older children, even some invasive monitoring such as intra-arterial catheters can be inserted before anesthetic induction. This chapter discusses primarily intraoperative monitors, although many of the same monitors are used in both the operating room and intensive care unit.

ELECTROCARDIOGRAPHIC MONITORING

Basic ECG

The details of ECG monitoring in operating rooms and intensive care units are presented in the American Heart Association's Task Force 1989 report.[1] ECG electrodes are usually placed on the upper arms and iliac crests for cardiovascular surgical procedures. Disposable silver-silver chloride electrodes are commonly used. These must be applied correctly, assuring that the electrode gel is present and moist. The skin should be lightly abraded with an alcohol swab to minimize skin resistance. The differences between the neonatal, child, and adult ECG have been previously described in Chapter 5. Changes in the axis of the T wave and right ventricular dominance are the prevailing features in the neonatal ECG.

An ECG lead measures the potential difference between two electrodes. The difference between the right and left arms is lead I. Lead II is the difference between right arm and left leg, whereas the difference between left arm and left leg is lead III. Unipolar limb leads are also used. The inactive central terminal is the right and left arm, with the left leg the active electrode in lead

aVF. Lead aVR has the active electrode on the right arm, whereas lead aVL has the left arm as active electrode, with the inactive central terminal provided by the left leg and the opposite arm. The precordial leads are unipolar leads with the four limb leads forming a central indifferent lead. V_1 is placed in the fourth right intercostal space and V_2 in the left fourth intercostal space. Lead V_5 is in the left fifth intercostal space in the midaxillary line. Leads V_3 and V_4 are intermediate between V_2 and V_5. Lead V_6 is in the left sixth intercostal space in the midaxillary line.

Oscilloscope artifacts can be the major problem leading to misdiagnosis of ECG abnormalities. Many monitors have two filter systems. One is the diagnostic setting that filters frequencies below 0.14 Hz. This results in an ECG that is reasonably close to that of a standard ECG machine. However, it is sensitive to baseline drift, patient motion, respiration, and electrode movement. The monitor mode filters all frequencies below 4 Hz and removes interference from patient movement, but it also distorts P and T waves and especially the ST segment, although the baseline is more stable.

The principal use of ECG is the detection of dysrhythmias. In children, tachycardia often makes diagnosis of dysrhythmias difficult. Greeley et al[2] noted that only 20% of surface ECG waveforms permitted accurate diagnosis, whereas Bushman[3] reported esophageal ECG leads were required for diagnosis in 38% of pediatric cardiac surgical patients. Factors associated with dysrhythmias requiring esophageal ECG diagnosis include younger age, prolonged cardiopulmonary bypass, prolonged aortic occlusion, and longer time with more interventions to achieve normal rhythm on cardiac reperfusion.[2]

Specialized Electrocardiography

Lead V_5 is often monitored during cardiac surgery by covering the electrode with an adhesive drape to protect it from surgical scrub solutions.[4] A right atrial ECG can be obtained by converting the central venous pressure catheter using the Arrow Johans (Arrow International, Inc., Reading, PA) adapter. Either a right atrial electrogram or an esophageal ECG lead will demonstrate P waves in atrial dysrhythmias that are not apparent on other leads.[2]

ST Segment Monitoring

Although myocardial ischemia is relatively uncommon in pediatric patients, some children with congenital heart disease develop significant myocardial ischemia during cardiac surgery as reported by Bell et al[5] (Fig 8–1). Newer ECG monitors provide automated analysis of the ST segment. The ST segment trend analysis compares the change in the ST segment (measured 60–80 ms after the J point to the isoelectric point 40 ms before the QRS complex). Three leads, usually I, II, and V are evaluated, compared with the learned complex, and displayed (Fig 8–2A). The learned ST template or morphology is displayed as a low-intensity waveform with the current ST segment as a brighter waveform indicating changes. The point for ST measurement can be adjusted to avoid erroneous measurement, as timing depends upon heart rate and T wave configuration. A magnified complex facilitates these adjustments (Fig 8–2B). With tachycardia, it may be necessary to measure at 40 ms after the J point to avoid blending of the J point into the T wave.

The representative QRS complex, or median complex, is determined by the automatic evaluation of a certain minimum number of complexes (in the Marquette Electronics system, 16 beats). Signals that are abnormal, ie, with long QRS duration (PVC), are rejected. After the dominant normal QRS shape has been determined on beats 1 through 17, that waveform becomes the template for the second phase of analysis of 16 more beats. A process called incremental averaging, rather than determination of the mean or median of the incoming beat waveforms, is used to determine positive or negative changes on subsequent complexes. The algorithm tracks these changes and alters the template at selected points from the prior shape. However, the degree of allowable change, before the incrementally averaged template becomes the learned template to which subsequent ST changes are compared, varies among manufacturers.

Both short- and long-term trending are possible. At the end of the three monitored leads, the Marquette system provides a 28-minute trend summation of the three leads in which deviations from the baseline up or down are displayed (Fig 8–2C). Cautery artifacts result in spikes in the trended waveform. The presence of the designation x.x with a lead indicates that ST segment measurements cannot be made in that lead. Longer-duration trend analysis from any of the three leads can be displayed over 1-, 2-, 4-, or 8-hour periods (Fig 8–2D).

Recent comparisons between the Marquette system and the Hewlett Packard 78534C automated ST segment analysis in adults indicated greater sensitivity but lower specificity for the Marquette system as compared with a standard ECG.[6] However, compared to transesophageal echocardiographic detection of wall-thickening abnormalities, the Marquette system was nearly twice as sensitive as the Hewlett Packard system.[6] Because transesophageal echocardiography is generally not used prior to endotracheal intubation in perioperative settings and may not be feasible in the smallest infants, automated ST segment analysis is a valuable monitor for perioperative ischemia.

MONITORING OF THE ARTERIAL BLOOD PRESSURE

Arterial blood pressure in infants and children can be measured by palpation, auscultation, observation of skin flush on cuff deflation, return of flow on Doppler after cuff deflation, oscillometry, or an invasive catheter. It provides an index of peripheral perfusion, cardiac output, and vascular volume. Auscultatory pressures are difficult to obtain in small children. Palpation and skin flush methods are usually impossible during anesthesia. Thus, return to flow, indicated by Doppler sounds, oscillometric methods, and direct intra-arterial catheters are the usual techniques for measurement of blood pressure in pediatric patients.

Indirect Methods

An indirect method of monitoring the arterial pressure should always be available in addition to an indwelling arterial catheter during most pediatric cardiac surgery.

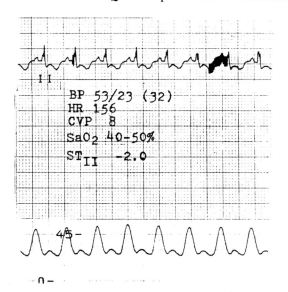

Figure 8–1. Depression of the ST segments as detected by the Marquette ECG ST segment analysis system in an infant undergoing creation of the systemic-to-pulmonary shunt. Although systemic arterial pressure is maintained, severe desaturation and myocardial ischemia accompany partial occlusion of the pulmonary artery.

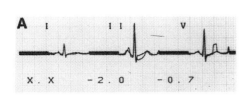

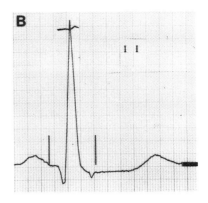

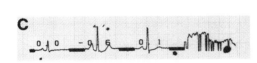

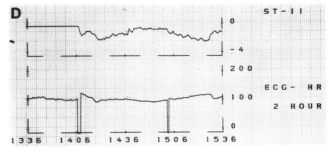

Figure 8–2. (*A*) Three electrocardiogram leads, usually I, II, and V_5 are compared to a learned waveform to detect ST segment changes. The designation x.x indicates that the ST segments cannot be measured in that waveform. (*B*) A magnified waveform facilitates adjustment of the measurement points (isoelectric point 40 ms before the QRS complex and 60–80 ms after the J point). (*C*) Short-term ST segment trend summation of the positive or negative ST segment changes in the three monitored leads. The spikes in the waveform are electrocautery artifacts. (*D*) Long-term trend analyses of ST segment changes from 0 to ± 4 mm can be performed for 1, 2, 4, or 8 hs.

Korotkoff Method. In the auscultatory method, the Korotkoff sounds are detected when an occlusive cuff, which is 20% wider than the diameter of the limb, is deflated over a decreasing pressure range. The sounds are produced with resumption of blood flow through a previously collapsed artery. This method is useless during cardiopulmonary bypass with nonpulsatile flow. It is also difficult to use when the peripheral circulation is constricted or hypotension is present. Too small a cuff results in artificially high systolic and diastolic pressures.[7]

Doppler Method. Blood pressure can also be measured using a 10-Hz Doppler probe placed over the brachial, radial, dorsalis pedis, or posterior tibial artery with a cuff on arm or leg. As in the auscultatory method, cuff size is important because too large a cuff falsely decreases measurements. The Doppler is a radio frequency oscillator driving a crystal in a transducer assembly with a receiver that detects the difference in frequency between the transmitted and reflected sound. The pitch of its output is proportional to the velocity of the reflective surface, whereas the volume is proportional to the area. Movement of the arterial wall as blood flow returns allows detection of a Doppler shift signal, the systolic blood pressure. Diastole is a soft, sloshing sound that is only detected with difficulty with a Doppler. Doppler sounds, unlike Korotkoff sounds, are generated when there is any movement of the blood. Doppler measurements yield higher pressure than either flush or palpation methods.[8] Doppler pressures are slightly lower than direct intra-aortic pressures.[9]

Oscillometric Method. Automated noninvasive blood pressure measurement devices such as the Dinamapp (Critikon, Tampa, FL) use the oscillometric technique. The systolic pressure occurs at the point of the rapid increase in oscillation, the mean at the maximum point of oscillation, and the diastolic at the fade of oscillations. The Dinamapp cuff is both actuator and transducer, one tube to the cuff producing cuff inflation and the other transmitting the sensed pressure to the transducer of the instrument. With the oscillometric method, there are two pressure indicators, one for the cuff pressure and one for the amplitude of pulsation. Generally the Dinamapp initially inflates to above the systolic pressure and then deflates in 3-mm Hg increments. Under low noise conditions, two cardiac cycles are compared at each increment. With patient or cuff movement, the inflation is held until successive comparative beats occur, making the measurement time dependent.

The accuracy of the Dinamapp oscillometric technique has been documented with pressures similar to those of the central aorta.[10,11] Other investigators, however, have noted good correlation between peripheral and central pressure only with systolic pressure. Diastolic pressure showed an 8- to 13-mm Hg variation between direct arterial and Dinamapp measurements.[12] The clinical accuracy of the Dinamapp in premature and term infants as compared with direct arterial or Doppler measurements has also been documented.[13,14] However, it is less accurate with arterial pressures below 40 mm Hg.[15] To ensure accurate pressures, a cuff of appropriate size, 50% of the circumference or 120% of the diameter of the limb, must be used with automated oscillometry.[14]

The advantages of the automated oscillometric technique are independence from Korotkoff sounds and greater accuracy than auscultatory measurements.[11] Such devices cannot replace direct arterial cannulation when there is large beat-to-beat variability of the arterial pressure. Severe upper extremity venostasis was reported by Showman and Betts in an infant after 90 minutes of automated oscillometric pressure measurements.[16] Repeated or continuous inflation of the device during unsuccessful attempts to measure blood pressure has been reported to result in radial nerve palsy.[17]

Direct Arterial Blood Pressure Measurement

The use of an indwelling arterial cannula is essential when continuous pressure recordings are necessary or serial arterial blood samples without additional trauma to the artery must be obtained. Direct intra-arterial cannulas continue to function even during deterioration of the peripheral circulation. Thus, it is indicated for all open-heart procedures using cardiopulmonary bypass and in many pediatric closed-heart procedures, particularly those performed in neonates. The contour of the arterial pressure tracing itself provides a qualitative approximation of circulatory alterations, although it is affected by stroke volume, myocardial performance, and peripheral vascular resistance. Indwelling arterial cannulas are connected to automatic flushing devices and electronic pressure transducers.

Transducers. Intravascular pressures are monitored using strain gauge transducers operating on the principle of the Wheatstone bridge. Careful assembly of transducers, tubings, and stopcocks is essential to prevent contamination, entrainment of air, or inadequate sealing to the nondisposable portion. The drip chamber is the major source of air bubbles in the system owing to the high-velocity jet when fluid flows.[18] These bubbles not only affect the dynamic response of the system but may cause air emboli in the patient. Only the dead space of the transducer-tubing system must be cleared for accurate determination of blood gases or coagulation tests.[19]

The transducer should first be placed with its reference point at heart level. The transducer is then calibrated to zero by opening it to the atmosphere. If the patient is moved, the transducer must also be moved so that it remains at the level of the patient's heart (midchest level). Transducer, tubing, and catheter dynamics have been discussed in detail elsewhere.[20,21] However, the use of resonance eliminators improves the in vivo performance of vascular monitoring systems.[22] Nonadjustable resonance eliminators provide the most accurate systolic pressure measurements.[22]

Flushing Devices. Transducers should also have a continuous flushing device located near the transducer to avoid a static column of fluid.[23,24] The continuous flush systems (CFS) administer 2–4 mL/h of fluids slowly through the catheter with rapid flushes of 1–2 mL/s.[24] In infants, infusion pumps[25] or gravity-driven weighted syringes[26] are often used to administer small volumes of fluid to prevent volume overload.[27] The resistor on the CFS eliminates any pulsatile artifacts from the infusion pump.[25] Saline, not dextrose, should be used for the flushing solution as bacterial growth is less likely in saline.

Sites and Techniques of Cannulation

Radial Artery Cannulation. Although the brachial, dorsalis pedis, femoral, peroneal, temporal, and axillary arteries may be cannulated, the radial artery is most often used. Both radial arteries should be palpated to assess equality of pulsation. Allen's test[28] is performed to assure adequacy of the collateral circulation. Allen's test is performed in the following way in children: First, the examiner compresses the radial artery and ulnar artery while an assistant compresses the patient's hand ten times. If the palmar arterial arch is patent, the hand blanches during compression, but on release of ulnar compression and partial relaxation of the hand, the normal color returns within 5–7 seconds. Delayed return of color greater than 7 seconds indicates inadequate flow. With ulnar artery occlusion, pallor of the hand occurs and is maintained as long as the radial artery is compressed. When compression of the radial artery is released, reactive hyperemia occurs, causing the hand to become red. Repetition of the test with compression of the ulnar artery demonstrates the presence or absence of a lesion of the radial artery.[29] Excessive extension of the hand occludes the transpalmar arch resulting in artifactually inadequate flow.[30–32] Slogoff and co-workers question the need to perform Allen's test, reporting cannulation of the radial artery in 16 patients with abnormal Allen's test (>15-second refill) without ischemic damage.[33] A report of a large series of patients from the Great Ormond Street Hospital for Sick Children also noted the absence of complications after radial artery cannulation in children without performance of Allen's test except in previously cannulated arteries.[34]

Technique of Radial Cannulation. After satisfactory collateral circulation has been demonstrated, the wrist should be hyperextended over a small support. The course of the artery is traced on the skin and is very superficial in children. After povidone-iodine skin preparation, local anesthesia is infiltrated into the area over the artery if the child is unanesthetized. A small nick in the skin is made with a needle through which a 20-gauge Teflon catheter in children over age 5 years or weighing 25 kg (a 22-gauge catheter in infants and small children and a 24-gauge for infants weighing <3 kg) is introduced through the skin nick and along the line of the radial artery at an angle of 20–30 degrees to the skin[35] (Fig 8–3). Any catheter that gives a grating sensation on passage through tissue or artery should be discarded because it may have a damaged tip and therefore may injure the arterial intima and predispose to thrombus formation.[36] The cannula is advanced until arterial pulsation is transmitted to the needle. The arterial wall is then pierced and freely spurting blood flow obtained. The angle be-

tween the artery and the cannula is then quickly reduced to about 10 degrees, and the catheter is gently advanced from the needle into the artery. If the artery appears to have been missed completely, remove the needle and withdraw the cannula slowly to assess possible arterial entry. If no freely spurting flow is obtained, put the catheter-needle unit together, check the patency of the needle, reestablish the palpable course of the artery, and try again. Because the radial artery easily develops spasm with attempted cannulation, multiple attempts may be difficult unless the arterial course is located with a Doppler.[37–39,40] If the posterior wall is inadvertently pierced when attempting to advance the catheter-needle unit, remove the needle and slowly withdraw the plastic cannula until briskly spurting blood flow is obtained. Then attempt to advance the cannula longitudinally into the artery. An assistant wearing sterile gloves should be immediately available to introduce a J wire into the catheter if brisk, spurting blood flow is obtained but the operator is unable to advance the cannula into the artery. In obese patients, placement of a pulse oximeter distal to the cannulation site and repeated palpation over the likely arterial site while observing for cessation of the

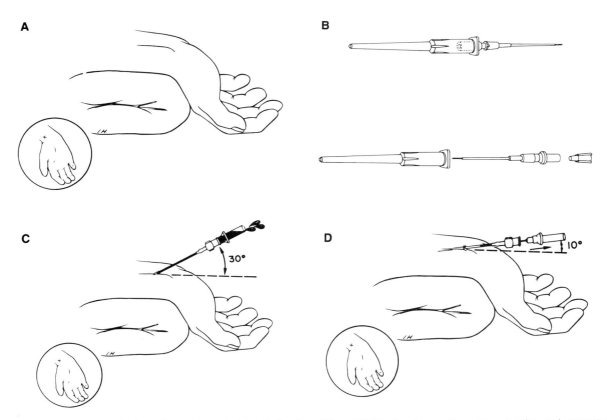

Figure 8–3. Technique for insertion of intra-arterial catheters in children. (*A*) The hand is positioned in extension and supported by a small pad. (*B*) Attachment of the catheter cover over the end of the catheter allows visualization of blood return without contamination of patient and operator. (*C*) The catheter is inserted at a 30-degree or smaller angle to the course of the artery. (*D*) When brisk, spurting flow is obtained, the angle of the catheter is further reduced to 10 degrees or less and the catheter is advanced into the artery. (*From Lake CL: Cardiovascular Anesthesia. New York: Springer-Verlag, 1985, with permission.*)

distal pulse can facilitate location of an optimal site to attempt arterial puncture.[41]

After cannulation, the catheter is connected to a transducer and taped using the Venigard (Conmed, Utica, NY) system after application of povidone-iodine ointment to the area around the cannula. The support used to dorsiflex the wrist is removed to prevent damage to the median nerve from prolonged extension.

The tip of the cannula should be carefully positioned by observing the response to a bolus injection of 3–4 mL of heparinized saline through the cannula.[42] The preferred response is a large area of slight pallor rather than a localized area of a few square centimeters of intense blanching. This response suggests that there is less interference with local cutaneous circulation by the flushing fluid.

PROBLEMS AND COMPLICATIONS OF RADIAL ARTERY CATHETERS

Studies indicate that radial arterial pressures are often inaccurate during the immediate postbypass period in both adults and children.[43–45] Pressure in the radial artery is considerably lower than that in the central aorta or femoral artery. Although previous studies suggested that this problem resulted from peripheral vasoconstriction[44] or a decrease in forearm vascular resistance on rewarming from hypothermic cardiopulmonary bypass,[43] recent investigations in adults demonstrated no effect of either vasoconstrictor or vasodilator drugs on the gradient that developed on initiation of bypass.[45] The gradient often persists for 1 hour or more after discontinuation of bypass.[43] When this condition occurs, measurement of blood pressure indirectly using a cuff or directly in the central aorta can be performed until the peripheral circulation returns to normal.[43]

Intra-arterial cannulas can be left in place up to 3 days or longer, but then should be removed immediately if evidence of vascular insufficiency, hematomata, or infection occur. After prolonged catheterization, catheters may become nonfunctional owing to thrombotic occlusion of the artery. Passage of a wire through the cannula and replacement with a new cannula can be performed. Aspiration of the cannula and proximal and distal arterial occlusion as it is removed permits removal of thrombotic material.[46] Compression over the site should be applied for 10 minutes or longer.

An infrequent but potentially lethal complication of arterial cannulation is hemorrhage in the event of accidental disconnection of the catheter and tubing. Other complications include radial artery thrombosis,[35,46–49] decreased peripheral circulation with ischemic changes in the skin of the forearm,[42,49] vasospasm,[50] central and peripheral embolization,[51] hematoma,[48] median and radial nerve injuries, aneurysm and pseudoaneurysm,[52,53]

and infection.[54,55] The differential diagnosis of hand ischemia in the presence of a radial arterial catheter can be difficult.[56] Proximal pulses should be completely examined and, if absent, an arteriogram should be considered to rule out embolization.[56] However, the incidence of transient ischemia is about 4% and permanent ischemia is rare when adequate collateral circulation is present in radial arterial cannulation in newborns.[57]

The incidence of positive arterial catheter tip cultures in children undergoing heart surgery has been reported at 5–13% depending upon age.[58] Lower rates of 0–5% have been reported in adults.[55,59] Positive cultures and bacteremia have been reported when arterial catheters remain for more than 4 days.[54] However, Leroy and co-workers were unable to document either catheter-related or infusate-related bacteremia in patients having arterial cannulation for as long as 9 days provided strict sterile insertion and maintenance were practiced.[59]

Alternative Arterial Cannulation Sites

Dorsalis Pedis Arterial Cannulation. Although the dorsalis pedis artery is absent in about 3–12% of humans,[60] it is often easy to cannulate in children. Systolic and pulse pressures are higher in dorsalis pedis[61,62] than brachial or radial pressures, particularly in children.[63] In adults, mean arterial and diastolic pressures are higher in the radial or brachial artery than in the dorsalis pedis.[61,62] Careful interpretation of pedal pressures in children must be made to avoid overtreatment of hypertension or undertreatment of shock.

Collateral flow for the dorsalis pedis artery is verified by occluding it with external pressure and compressing the great toenail. Release of the nail and observation of flushing as the blood returns indicates adequate lateral plantar flow from the posterior tibial artery. Youngberg and Miller[62] suggest compression of both the dorsalis pedis and posterior tibial arteries while the great and second toes are blanched. A Doppler probe is placed over the dorsalis pedis artery as well. When pressure over the posterior tibial artery is released, flow is checked both by Doppler and by observation of flushing in the toes. The test is repeated by releasing the occlusion of the dorsalis pedis to check its flow. Cannulation is not recommended unless the toes flush in less than 10 seconds.[64]

Johnstone and Greenhow describe the technique for insertion of a dorsalis pedis cannula.[65] The artery, which is the continuation of the anterior tibial artery, lies subcutaneously on the dorsum of the foot, parallel and lateral to the extensor hallucis longus tendon. A 20- or 22-gauge cannula is recommended.

The incidence of thrombosis is 6.7[62]–25%.[62,66] Although recannulization occurs, the artery does not return to its previous condition.[66] Indications for removal of a dorsalis pedis cannula are the same as for a radial cannula.

Femoral Arterial Cannulation. Because of its large size, the femoral artery may be cannulated directly in children with an 18- or 20-gauge (approximately No. 3 French) 6- to 8-cm catheter. Alternatively, the Seldinger technique with a guidewire is performed. The rate of successful cannulation is 95%, with 60% of the insertions on the first attempt in Graves' series in which 50% of the children weighed less than 10 kg and were less than 1 year of age.[67] Disadvantages of the femoral approach are the need for postoperative immobilization of the leg and its position in the surgical field with the need for removal in the event of femoral cannulation for cardiopulmonary bypass or insertion of an intra-aortic balloon.

Like other arterial cannulation sites, potential complications include transient vascular insufficiency (11%), infection (1–4% incidence), or ischemia (1–4%).[67,68] Transient vascular insufficiency, characterized by decreased distal pulses, pallor, and prolonged capillary refill, may be due to vascular spasm, direct mechanical obstruction, or transient thrombosis.[67] Although vascular complications are infrequent and usually not limb threatening, Taylor and colleagues noted that about 35% of femoral arteries demonstrate chronic occlusion after diagnostic femoral catheterization.[69]

Umbilical Arterial Cannulation. A cutdown technique is usually performed by pediatricians shortly after birth of the infant to cannulate the umbilical vessels with a No. 3.5 or 5.0 French (depending upon infant size) umbilical artery catheter.[70] However, a percutaneous method in which a 15-gauge intravenous catheter is placed peripherally in the umbilical cord and a 3.5 French umbilical artery catheter is then guided through it into the aorta has been described.[71] The umbilical arterial catheter should lie just above the aortic bifurcation but below the inferior mesenteric artery or above the diaphragm in the middorsal aorta.[72] Once the catheter is correctly placed, the remainder of the umbilical cord is carefully dissected away.[71] Complications include lower extremity ischemia secondary to iliac spasm, abdominal organ ischemia if the catheter is deflected into specific intra-abdominal vessels, thrombosis,[73] or embolism.[72]

Brachial or Axillary Arterial Cannulation. Although brachial cannulation has been used in adults for many years,[74,75] it is infrequently used in children. Chronic vascular occlusion may occur after brachial cannulation, resulting in arterial insufficiency. Axillary catheters also are infrequently used, but they may be required in children who have had multiple catheterizations or surgical procedures.[76] The position of the patient and the point of needle insertion is the same as that for an axillary brachial plexus block. The Seldinger technique, using 20- to 24-gauge, 9- to 12-cm catheters, is recommended.[77] In Cantwell's series of 11 patients, vascular insufficiency occurred

in only one patient.[78] Other potential complications include brachial plexus injuries and infection.

CENTRAL VENOUS PRESSURE MONITORING

Central venous cannulation is often required in children for rapid administration of drugs, fluids, or blood in the absence of adequate peripheral veins, measurement of the central venous pressure, insertion of pulmonary artery or pacing catheters, or postoperative hyperalimentation. Sites used for placement of central venous catheters are the internal or external jugular, antecubital (basilic), axillary, femoral, and subclavian veins. All of these sites have disadvantages, including the inconstancy of external jugular venous anatomy,[79] risk of thrombosis in the femoral vein, and venospasm and small size in the brachiocephalic system. However, the interval without complications is about 23 days in children having jugular, subclavian, femoral, or antecubital catheters, with infection being the most common complication.[80] Nevertheless, cannulation of the internal jugular vein eliminates many of the disadvantages or hazards of the other sites in both children and adults.

Sites and Techniques of Insertion

Internal Jugular Venous Cannulation

Anatomy. The internal jugular vein is essentially a straight line from the right internal jugular vein to the right atrium.[81–83] Its anatomic position is relatively constant, and during its course through the neck, the internal jugular becomes lateral and then anterolateral to the carotid artery. The left internal jugular vein should generally be avoided in pediatric cardiac patients because it may connect to a persistent left superior vena cava which may be ligated during surgery, the left innominate may be sacrificed during the difficult surgical dissection or a reoperation, and the thoracic duct is located on the left.[82,83] Careful cannulation of the right internal jugular vein in children with transposition of the great vessels or a right aortic arch should be performed because accidental cannulation of the ascending aorta has been reported.[84]

Insertion Technique. The central technique of percutaneous internal jugular vein cannulation is as follows[82,83,85]: The patient is placed in an at least 15-degree Trendelenburg position to distend the vein[86] and reduce the hazard of air embolism. A shoulder roll is placed to hyperextend the child's neck.[83] The triangular gap between the sternal and clavicular heads of the sternocleidomastoid muscle with its base on the medial end of the clavicle is identified with the patient's head turned slightly toward the opposite side (Fig 8–4). Pulsation

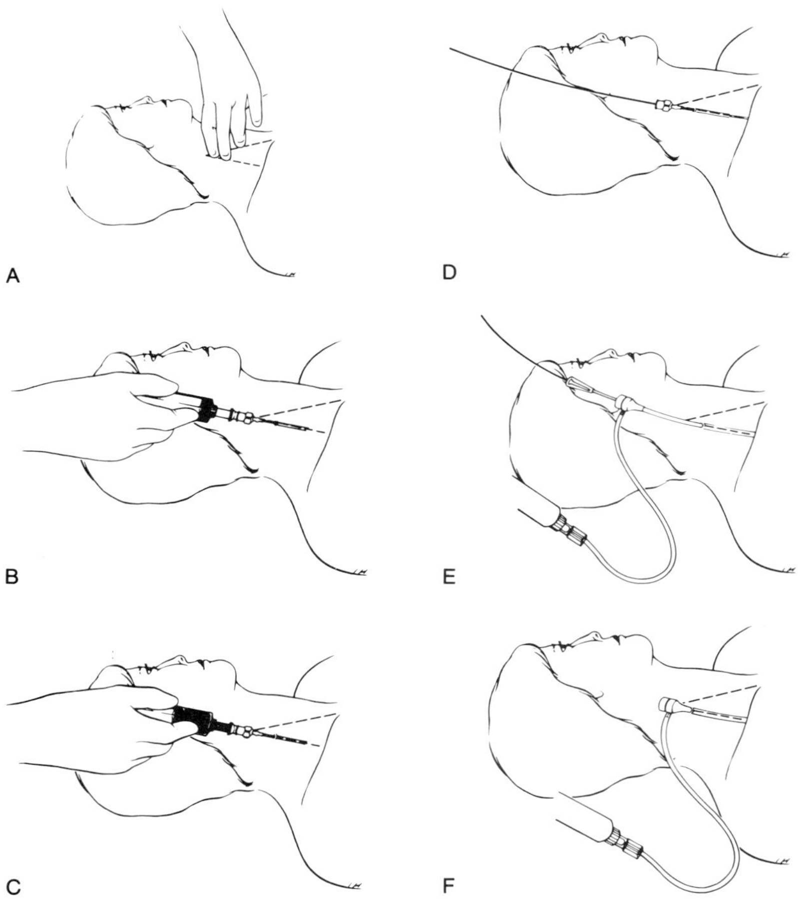

A

D

B

E

C

F

Figure 8–4. The Seldinger technique for insertion of vascular catheters. (*A*) Position of the neck for insertion of an internal jugular catheter. (*B*) A 21-gauge needle with attached syringe is directed laterally at a 30-degree angle to the plane of the neck at the point where the sternal and clavicular heads of the sternocleidomastoid muscle converge. (*C*) The small-gauge needle in the vein is replaced by a larger (usually 18-gauge) needle or catheter-needle. (*D*) After the pressure and waveform verify the venous position, a wire is passed into the vein through the needle or catheter. (*E*) The catheter or needle is removed and a dilator or introducer-dilator passed over the wire. (*F*) The wire and dilator are removed leaving the introducer for passage of a pulmonary artery catheter. Alternatively, a central venous catheter can be passed directly over the guidewire. (*From Lake CL: Cardiovascular Anesthesia. New York: Springer-Verlag, 1985, with permission.*)

from the carotid artery must be felt against the tips of two fingers after rotation of the head has aided in the separation of the common carotid artery and the bulk of the stenocleidomastoid. Care should be taken to avoid extreme rotation of the head or continuous palpation of the carotid pulse as both maneuvers tend to decrease internal jugular size.[86,87] If the patient is unanesthetized, the skin near the apex of this triangle is infiltrated with local anesthetic. The Seldinger technique is recommended.[88] Ultrasound devices may be used to facilitate vein location. Use of Doppler devices to locate the internal jugular vein was suggested by Ullman and Stoelting in 1978.[89] Standard echocardiographic transducers have also been used in adults but may be cumbersome in infants or children.[90] Recently developed Doppler devices such as the Smart (Peripheral Systems Group, Mountainview, CA) needle makes location of the vein by flow characteristics a practical technique, especially in children. A 21-gauge needle with attached 6-mL syringe is then inserted through the infiltrated area near the apex of the triangle at an angle of 45 degrees to the skin surface and advanced caudally and laterally.[91] In children, Rao and co-workers have recommended a lower approach just above the palpable notch on the superior

aspect of the clavicle just lateral to the sternoclavicular junction.[92] The needle is aimed caudad and parallel to the sagittal plane at an angle of 30–45 degrees to the skin. A distinct "give" is felt as the vein is entered, and this is confirmed by aspiration of venous blood. If the internal jugular is not entered on the first attempt, the needle point is directed 5–10 degrees laterally and readvanced. Occasionally, if venous pressure is likely to be very low, an infusion of crystalloid will be helpful.[93] Gentle compression of the right upper quadrant of the abdomen increases venous pressure in children in heart failure. In adults, use of ultrasound-guided venous cannulation increased first-time success from 54 to 73% and decreased cannulation time and the incidence of carotid puncture.[94]

After successful venous puncture is confirmed with the 21-gauge needle, an 18-gauge long needle or catheter with 10-mL syringe attached is introduced into the vein. A straight or J wire is inserted through the catheter on needle. A soft polyurethane or silastic central venous catheter is then advanced over the wire, and then the wire is removed and connected to a transducer. A device that permits passage of a J wire through the plunger into an 18-gauge needle appears particularly useful for pediatric patients with small, difficult-to-locate veins.[95]

Double- and triple-lumen central venous pressure catheters are available in various sizes and lengths (Fig 8–5). These catheters increase the usefulness of a single intravascular site by permitting simultaneous monitoring and drug infusion.

Coté et al compared the standard and lower approach techniques in children.[96] Success rates of 74–97% have been demonstrated by Coté, Nicolson, Hayashi, and their co-workers in children.[96–98] However, greater morbidity (2% incidence of pneumothorax and nearly 4% incidence of hematoma) was associated with the lower approach.[96] The success rate and time to completed venous catheterization were unaffected by operator experience as demonstrated by Hayashi and co-workers.[98] Body weight less than 4 kg significantly reduced the success rate to 78%.[98] However, Garrick and colleagues reported a 95% success rate during cardiac catheterization of children, but the success rate was not detailed by body weight.[99] Failure to locate and successfully cannulate the internal jugular vein occurs in 8–9% of patients in the perioperative period.[82,83,100]

Alternative Approaches. Other approaches used in internal jugular cannulation are the posterior route,[101] in which the needle is introduced under the sternocleidomastoid just above the point where the distended exter-

nal jugular vein crosses this border and is aimed ventrally and caudally toward the suprasternal notch or the anterior route[101] in which the carotid is retracted medially at a point 5 cm above the clavicle and 5 cm below the angle of the mandible. The needle is introduced at this point at a 30- to 45-angle with the skin and directed caudally in the sagittal plane toward the ipsilateral nipple and the junction of the middle and inner third of the clavicle.

Complications. One of the most frequent complications of internal jugular cannulation is a 2–4% incidence[102,103,104] of carotid artery puncture,[82,83,85,103] which can be recognized by rapid reflux of blood into the catheter, the increased pressure, the color of the blood, or the use of a pressure transducer to display the waveform.[103] In patients with cyanotic congenital heart disease, the color of the blood is an unreliable guide to rule out carotid puncture. If the carotid artery is accidentally punctured with a 16-gauge or smaller catheter or needle, the needle should immediately be removed and firm compression applied for 15 minutes. Life-threatening hemorrhage secondary to 16-gauge arterial puncture can occur.[105] In the unanesthetized patient, the level of consciousness or any neurologic symptoms can be assessed. Cannulation of the carotid artery with a larger-gauge cannula, such as a No. 8 French sheath introducer, should

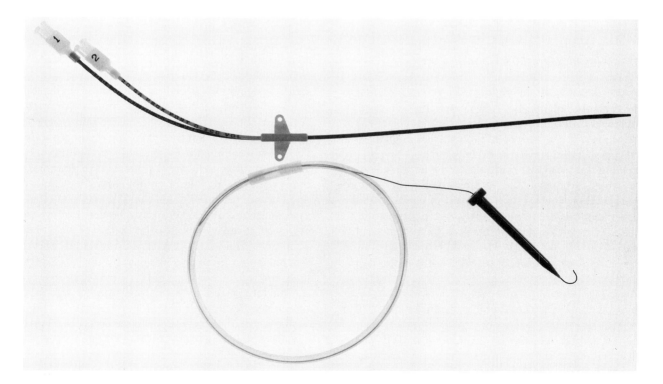

Figure 8–5. A double-lumen central venous pressure catheter of No. 4 French size, suitable for insertion in children of 8–10 kg body weight. Smaller catheters of No. 3.5 French size are used in neonates, whereas larger catheters of Nos. 5–7 French are used in larger children or teenagers. A double- or triple-lumen catheter allows monitoring of central venous pressure and infusion of fluids or drugs through the same venipuncture in the central veins.

be managed in a similar fashion, although direct surgical exploration may be required and elective surgery, particularly that requiring anticoagulation, should be postponed.[103] Failure to remove a catheter unintentionally placed in the carotid artery of an infant during attempted jugular cannulation resulted in massive extravasation of blood during cardiopulmonary bypass and subsequent demise.[106]

Other complications of internal jugular cannulation include arterial[107] and venous[79,101] air embolism, which is not always prevented by the Trendelenburg position, particularly with a No. 8 French introducer[107] in patients with a right-to-left shunt or a malfunctioning self-sealing valve[108]; neurologic complications such as phrenic[109,110,111] or sympathetic pupillodilator pathway damage[112]; catheter malposition[83,113]; thoracic duct injury (when left vein is used); puncture of endotracheal tube cuff[114]; thrombophlebitis[79], pneumothorax,[102,115] mediastinal widening; left pleural effusion, hydrothorax[116] and hydromediastinum[117]; hematomas, and 10–30%[118-120] incidence of venous thrombosis, chylothorax, and infection. Internal jugular venous thrombosis can be documented by sonographic evidence of an intraluminal mass.[121] The incidence of positive catheter tip cultures from central venous catheters inserted in children undergoing cardiac surgery has been reported at 6%.[104] Risk factors for infection in pediatric cardiac patients were younger age, longer duration of cannulation, and need for inotropic support.[104] However, the overall complication rate has been lower than with the subclavian approach.[82]

External Jugular Venous Cannulation

Insertion Technique. In children or other patients in whom the internal jugular vein cannot be successfully cannulated, the external jugular vein may be used. There are two sets of valves in the external jugular vein, one about 4 cm superior to the clavicle and one at the entrance to the subclavian vein that must be traversed by intravascular catheters. The Seldinger technique is used for most external jugular vein cannulations using a J wire to ensure central placement.[122] A J wire is preferable to a straight wire with a flexible tip because the success of passage is 100% with a J versus 44% with a straight wire.[123] Although it is uncertain whether it is the radius of curvature or the lesser external diameter, a 3-mm J wire accomplishes external jugular cannulation in 90% of cases as opposed to 70% success with a 6-mm J wire.[124] If a No. 8 French sheath introducer is placed in the external jugular vein, it should not be introduced its full length because tearing of the vein at its junction with the subclavian may occur. Among the reasons for failure to cannulate the central circulation via the external jugular vein are an inability to cannulate the vein initially and an inability to thread the wire or catheter into the chest veins.[125] Successful cannulation occurred in 65% of ex-

ternal jugular veins in Nicolson's pediatric series.[97] However, a 77% successful placement of pulmonary artery catheters via the external jugular vein has been reported in adults.[125]

Complications. The complications of infection, malposition, thrombosis, and perforation seen with internal jugular vein cannulation also occur with external jugular cannulation. Either a catheter whose tip reaches the right atrium or a short catheter should be used from an external jugular insertion site so that the catheters do not lie transversely at the innominate-subclavian junction where perforation may occur.[126] Eichold and Berryman report a case of contralateral hydrothorax after external jugular venous cannulation.[127] The incidence of silent external jugular thrombosis has been reported at 27% in children.[119]

Subclavian Venous Cannulation

Technique of Insertion. Because the subclavian vein is large and constant in position, it can easily be cannulated in children.[128,129] Although the left subclavian vein is often preferred because it makes a more gradual curve into the right atrium, damage to the thoracic duct may occur on the left, so the right is generally used. However, either vein can be cannulated. The patient is placed in slight Trendelenburg position with the head turned toward the opposite side, as head position has not been demonstrated to affect the incidence of misplacement in the internal jugular vein.[130] A needle or needle-catheter combination, usually of 18-gauge size is inserted at the junction of the medial and middle thirds of the clavicle, aiming posteriorly, medially, and slightly cephalad.[131] Aspiration should be maintained while the needle is advanced, so that venous entrance is immediately apparent. The needle or catheter-needle assembly is advanced slightly so that freely flowing blood is obtained. A J or straight wire is then threaded through the needle or catheter into the vein. Over the wire, the definitive catheter or introducer-dilator combination is passed. Introduction of the needle too far laterally may result in pneumothorax. Pleural entry can be detected when air is aspirated through the needle. The needle should be withdrawn and an upright chest radiograph performed. Arterial puncture is also avoided by not attempting the puncture too far laterally.[131] If arterial puncture occurs, it can be recognized by color, pressure, or arterial waveform. Needles should always be completely withdrawn before redirection to prevent laceration of the vein. Successful cannulation occurs in 70–80% of children, but the rate is lower in infants and children under age 6.[132]

Complications. The most common complications of subclavian cannulation are pneumothorax (2–10% incidence), arterial puncture (8% incidence), and infection (5–40% incidence).[132,133] Acute airway obstruction after accidental subclavian arterial puncture has also been reported.[134] Other complications are lymph leakage secondary to thoracic duct injury, brachial plexus damage, misplacement into the internal jugular veins (5% incidence in Sanchez' series),[130] thrombosis, and hemothorax. Subclavian venous thrombosis is suspected in the presence of painful swelling of the arm and distended subcutaneous veins. It may be confirmed by ultrasound.[135] The incidence of complications increases in younger and smaller children.[132]

Antecubital or Axillary Vein Cannulation. Basilic or cephalic venous cannulation at the antecubital fossa is occasionally a practical route to the central circulation of infants or children. Ragasa and co-workers reported 54% successful cannulations of the central veins in adults.[136] Success rate is increased by turning the patient's head toward the ipsilateral side and applying pressure to the supraclavicular fossa.[136,137] These maneuvers obviated the inability to pass the subclavian-internal jugular vein junction.[136] Catheter kinking or fracture, guidewire retention,[138] infection, and problems common to other cannulation sites may occur with antecubital venous cannulations.

Cannulation of the axillary vein medially and superficially to the axillary artery has been reported in infants by Oriot and co-workers.[139] In the recent series of Metz and colleagues, the success rate was 79%, which was improved in older infants.[140] There was a 3.7% incidence of complications, including pneumothorax, hematoma, venous stasis or thrombosis, infiltration, and catheter-related sepsis.[140]

Umbilical Venous Cannulation. The umbilical vein is usually cannulated by a pediatrician in the newborn nursery using a cutdown technique similar to that described previously for the umbilical artery.[70] Under ideal conditions, the umbilical venous catheter should be threaded into the intrathoracic inferior vena cava or right atrium. It should not be located within the liver (intrahepatic portal vein) where portal vein thrombosis or hepatic necrosis may result from injection of hypertonic solutions.

Direct Right Atrial Catheterization. Central venous catheters may also be placed directly into the right atrium during cardiac surgery. Complications from this technique include hemorrhage on discontinuation and pericardial tamponade if the catheter becomes displaced from the right atrium and fluids continue to be infused.

PULMONARY ARTERY PRESSURE MONITORING

In many types of congenital heart disease, left and right heart function are quite different, unlike the parallel function in normal humans. The central venous pressure reflects right heart filling pressure and blood volume status.[141] The Swan-Ganz catheter, introduced in 1970,[142] provides continuous monitoring of pulmonary pressures. The pulmonary wedge pressure monitors left heart-filling pressure (left ventricular end-diastolic pressure) indirectly by means of the pulmonary artery wedge pressure (PAW) or pulmonary artery occlusion pressure (PAo). Generally, left ventricular end-diastolic pressure (LVEDP) equals left atrial pressure (LAP) equals pulmonary artery wedge pressure (PAo) equals pulmonary artery diastolic pressure (PAD) in the absence of tachycardia, mitral valve disease, pulmonary hypertension, or severe pulmonary disease.[143] However, PAD is normally equal to or only 1–3 mm Hg higher than PAW when pulmonary vascular resistance is normal. Thus PAD can be used as an index of left ventricular filling when the PAW is unobtainable.[144] The magnitude of the A wave magnitude in PAW reading indicates a closer agreement for end-diastolic ventricular pressure. Pulmonary artery diastolic pressure is usually only slightly greater than LAP, although inconsistencies between LAP and PAW have been noted by several investigators.[145,146]

However, PAW does not reflect LVED volume owing to variations in ventricular compliance.[147,148] PAW is a poor indicator of myocardial ischemia as indicated by the work of van Daele, Haggmark, and their colleagues in adult patients.[149,150] Unlike wall-thickening abnormalities detected on echocardiography or ST segment changes on electrocardiogram, PAW is an insensitive and unreliable monitor for ischemia.

Indications
Monitoring of the pulmonary artery pressure is indicated in patients with congestive heart failure, poor left ventricular function, pulmonary hypertension, and aortic and mitral valve disease.[151] The risks of placement outweigh their benefit in patients with normal ventricular function.

Types of Catheters
Although a pulmonary artery catheter of No. 7 French size with four lumens, one for measuring pressure at the tip, another for inflating a latex balloon located approximately 1.0 mm from the tip with 1.5 mL of air, one at 20–30 cm for monitoring right atrial pressure, and the fourth containing a thermistor, is used in older children and adults, Nos. 4 and 5 French pulmonary artery catheters are available for smaller children usually less than 8 years of age (Fig 8–6). There are separate No. 3.5 French injectate catheters with No. 2.5 French thermodilution probes as well as No. 4 French thermodilution probes with lumens (Fig 8–7). The injectate catheter is placed during surgery via pursestring sutures

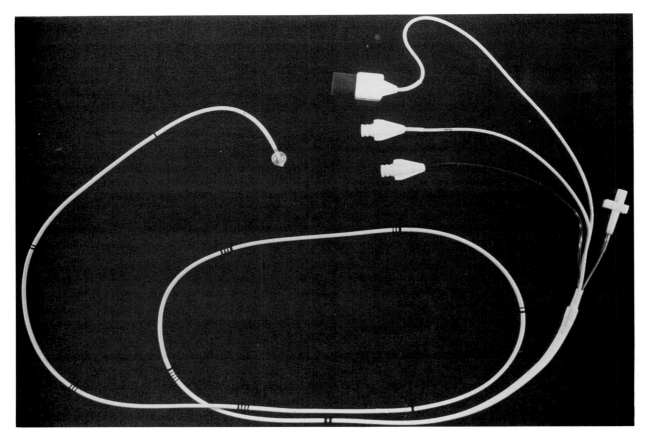

Figure 8–6. A quadruple-lumen, No. 7 French thermodilution pulmonary artery catheter for use in older children and adults. The 1.5-mL volume balloon is at the left. On the right are (*top*), the thermistor for thermodilution cardiac output determinations; (*middle*), the distal lumen at the tip of the catheter; (*bottom*), the proximal lumen at 30 cm. At the far right is the balloon lumen. (*From Lake CL: Cardiovascular Anesthesia. New York: Springer-Verlag, 1985, p 62, with permission.*)

in the right atrium and the thermistor in the pulmonary artery[152] (Fig 8–8). Careful positioning is essential because these catheters have been reported to migrate through a patent ductus arteriosus into the aorta.[153] The lumens of all catheters should be tested for patency, the balloon for inflation, and the thermistor for electrical continuity prior to insertion.

Catheters with pacing electrodes at atrial and ventricular levels or ports for passage of pacing wires are available. However, because of the difficulty in positioning such catheters in hearts of different sizes, they are of little use in pediatric patients. If such a catheter is needed in an older child or teenager, it is inserted in the same fashion as a regular catheter, but the pacing capability should be checked before final securing of the catheter. In adult patients,[154] acceptable pacing thresholds and atrial, ventricular, and sequential pacing were achieved in more than 80% of patients. Potential complications of these catheters are electrode dislodgement[155] or ventricular fibrillation if an uncovered ventricular electrode contacts an improperly grounded electrical circuit.

Insertion Technique

After the vein has been cannulated by the Seldinger technique,[88] a No. 6, 7, or 8 French introducer is placed over the wire (see Fig 8–4). The wire and dilator are removed, leaving the sheath in the vein. The pulmonary artery catheter is attached to pressure transducers and inserted to the 10- to 15-cm mark. Slight withdrawal of the introducer from the external jugular may be necessary for the pulmonary catheter to negotiate the external jugular-subclavian junction. Generally about 5–10 cm of additional catheter from the external jugular insertion site must be added to the distances indicated for internal jugular insertion site. Advancement to the 20-cm mark results in a right atrial waveform from the internal jugular insertion site. The balloon is then inflated. Further advancement results in a right ventricular tracing at about 30 cm. Contact with the ventricular wall usually results in ventricular extrasystoles and the catheter should be quickly withdrawn with the balloon deflated when this occurs. Readvancement should proceed only after the cardiac rhythm is stable. Prophylactic administration of lidocaine is unnecessary during catheter passage[156] be-

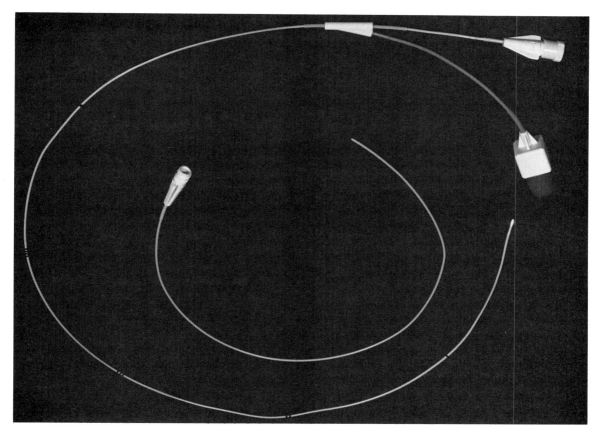

Figure 8–7. Separate central venous catheter and pulmonary artery thermistor for direct insertion into the pulmonary artery during cardiac surgery. These catheters are particularly useful in children in whom a standard pulmonary artery catheter would be too large or when its placement prior to surgery would interfere with the surgical procedure.

cause careful insertion and the balloon covering the tip of the catheter are sufficient to prevent ventricular extrasystoles. A PAW should be present at 40–50 cm; therefore, insertion to 50 cm without obtaining a pulmonary artery tracing indicates coiling in the right atrium or ventricle. The catheter should be withdrawn to the 15- to 20-cm distance and readvanced (Fig 8–9). Placement in the pulmonary artery is indicated by a sudden change in configuration of the tracing with a higher diastolic reading. Advancement is continued until the catheter is wedged and a waveform similar to the atrial waveform and a pressure of 10–12 mm Hg or less are present. Deflation of the balloon returns the pulmonary artery waveform.

Criteria for Pulmonary Wedge Pressure. The PAW is recognized by (1) pressure and waveform lower than pulmonary artery pressure and (2) presence of A and V waves in sinus rhythm.[143,157] Either mixed venous blood (balloon deflated) or arterialized blood[158] (balloon inflated) can be aspirated from the pulmonary artery lumen depending upon balloon inflation.[159,160] The principle of the measurement of wedge pressure is that the balloon isolates the catheter tip from the pulmonary arterial pres-

sure. Flow between the catheter tip and the point where the veins served by the occluded artery join the other veins, which have blood flow, ceases. The pressure in the catheter equilibrates with the pressure at this junction.

Ideally, the tip of the catheter should be in a large-size pulmonary artery where the catheter can advance to "wedge" on inflation and withdraw itself on deflation. Pulmonary artery catheters should never remain continuously wedged because infarction of a lung segment will occur. Continuous wedging is recognized by the absence of pulmonary artery waveform and the presence of the pulmonary artery waveform only during deep inspiration or a Valsalva maneuver. The balloon should be slightly withdrawn until the pulmonary artery waveform is seen consistently. If significantly less air than the maximum balloon volume is needed, the catheter should be withdrawn 1–2 cm. Inflation in a small vessel may result in eccentric inflation, forcing the tip of the catheter against the vessel wall, resulting in loss of the waveform, a rise in pressure due to "overwedging," and possible rupture of the pulmonary artery.[161] The relationship between PAD, PAW, and LAP should be noted so that the other

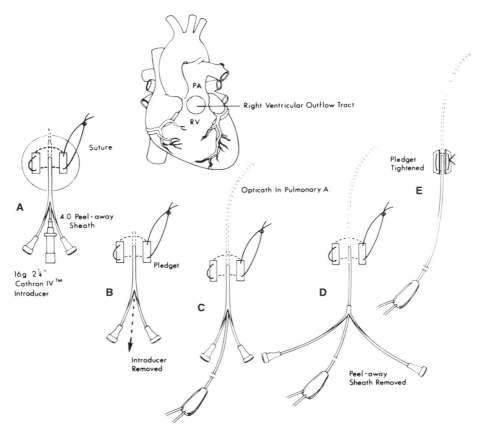

Figure 8–8. The technique of direct surgical insertion of catheters through the right ventricular outflow tract into the pulmonary artery. (*From Rah KH, et al: A method for continuous postoperative measurement of mixed venous oxygen saturation in infants and children after open heart procedures. Anesth Analg 63:873–881, 1984, with permission of the International Research Society.*)

pressure measurements can be used without need for additional balloon inflations or catheter repositioning if catheter failure or failure to wedge occurs. Although the position of the catheter may be confirmed by chest radiograph, fluoroscopy is unnecessary for catheter placement.

Problems with Catheter Positioning. Difficulties in passing the catheters to the wedge position occur in patients with enlarged hearts, poor myocardial contractil-

ity, pulmonary hypertension, or atrial fibrillation. In patients with mitral regurgitation, it may be difficult to differentiate the "wedge" position due to the large V waves from the pulmonary artery waveform. If the catheter becomes soft after prolonged contact with the body, flushing with room temperature saline may produce stiffening. Repositioning of the catheter after changes in cardiac function or cardiac surgery may be necessary. This is facilitated by the use of a plastic sheath over the catheter.[162,163] Although there is always a possibility of

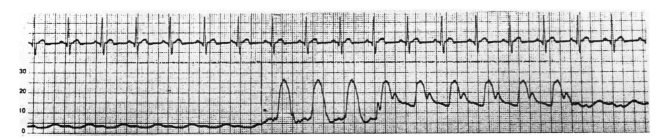

Figure 8–9. Typical pressure waveforms seen during passage of a pulmonary artery catheter from the right atrium to the wedge position. (*From American Edwards Laboratories, Santa Ana, CA, with permission.*)

contamination of such shields,[164] their safety has been demonstrated over years of use.[165]

Measurement of Pulmonary Pressures. Pressure measurements should be made at end expiration because inspiratory effort lowers mean intrathoracic pressure and decreases the pulmonary vascular pressure during spontaneous ventilation.[166] Many hemodynamic monitor systems incorporate airway pressure[167] or temperature measurements[166] to determine the optimum time for pressure recording[167] and improve their accuracy.[168] During controlled ventilation, less variability occurs because there is less change in pleural pressure with mechanical ventilation to cause changes in wedge pressure.[168] During positive-pressure ventilation, inspiration elevates pressure readings.

Benumof and co-workers[169] reported that most catheter tips go to the right lung and caudal, although 6.9% have a high cephalad, extreme lateral placement. The latter catheters may be in a zone I region of the lung where measurements will be erroneously low because alveolar pressure exceeds pulmonary artery pressure in such a region. A catheter wedged in zone 1 or 2 is relatively free of cardiac pulsation but exhibits marked respiratory variation[159] in its pressures. PAW reflects pulmonary venous pressure only when the pulmonary venous pressure is greater than alveolar pressure as in West's zone 3; otherwise the PAW will reflect alveolar pressure. Zone 3 is a physiologic zone, not an anatomic one, and may decrease in size as a result of shock, hypovolemia, or PEEP.[159] A non–zone 3 position should be suspected if PAW is greater than PAD[159] or if PAW increases by more than half of the increment of added positive end-expiratory pressure (PEEP) during expiration.[159] However, positioning of the catheter tip in a specific lung segment can be facilitated by patient position during insertion. Upward flotation of the air-filled balloon predominates over pulmonary artery flow allowing preferential placement.[170]

Abnormal pressure measurements occur with valvular heart disease, altered myocardial contractility, PEEP, cardiac tamponade, and pulmonary embolism. LAP is greater than LVEDP in mitral stenosis and acutely in mitral regurgitation. As PEEP is applied, the incremental increase in PWP should be noted because it is impractical to measure intrapleural pressure in order to subtract it from the PWP reading or to remove the patient from PEEP during measurements. Aortic regurgitation may cause LVEDP to be greater than LAP because the mitral valve closes early. When ventricular distensibility (compliance) is decreased, the LAP after the A wave may be lower than LVEDP owing to the "atrial kick."[159] The development of pulmonary edema at any specific PAW depends on vascular endothelial integrity, blood oncotic pressure, and interstitial fluid oncotic pressure. In pericardial tamponade, right atrial, right

ventricular end-diastolic, pulmonary artery diastolic, and pulmonary wedge pressures are equal and elevated.

Complications
Major complications of catheter insertion occur in 3% of catheterizations with a mortality of 0.016-to 0.3%.[171,172]

Rupture of the Pulmonary Artery. Rupture of the pulmonary artery[173–179] with massive hemoptysis is associated with advanced age (over age 60),[180] pulmonary hypertension,[181] anticoagulation, distal balloon placement, eccentric inflation of the balloon pushing the catheter tip through the artery, and hyperinflation of the balloon.[180,182] However, rupture has been reported in a patient without pulmonary hypertension.[183] Retrograde dissection of the pulmonary artery with rupture has been reported in a patient with pulmonary hypertension.[181] Pulmonary hemorrhage without demonstrable pulmonary artery injury has occurred.[184]

Diagnosis and Management. An early indication of catheter-induced pulmonary artery rupture is the presence of a small amount of hemoptysis.[185] However, Yellin and co-workers noted only minimal hemoptysis in a patient with rupture of a pseudoaneurysm induced by a pulmonary artery catheter.[186] The management of pulmonary artery rupture includes reversal of anticoagulation (if present and feasible),[187] endobronchial intubation facilitated by continuation of cardiopulmonary bypass during placement,[188] withdrawal of the catheter into the main or proximal pulmonary artery, and institution of PEEP.[189,190] Possible mechanisms for successful treatment with PEEP: (1) increased intrathoracic pressure might mechanically compress the ruptured arterial segment; (2) PEEP may decrease the pressure gradient between the damaged vessels and surrounding lung parenchyma; and (3) endobronchial pressure should increase with PEEP, leading to decreased pressure gradient from the pulmonary artery to the bronchus, and resulting in cessation of blood flow.[190] Lateral positioning of the patient with the affected side up should decrease the pulmonary artery pressure in the area of laceration.[190] Pulmonary angiography or a contrast-enhanced computed tomographic scan should be performed as soon as the patient is hemodynamically stable. Insertion of a chest tube, direct ligation of ruptured pulmonary vessel, or pulmonary resection may also be required.[191]

Successful treatment of catheter-induced pulmonary artery rupture may result in the development of a false aneurysm of the artery.[191,192] Therapy for false aneurysms, which may spontaneously rupture, includes transcatheter embolization or pulmonary resection.

Thrombocytopenia and Thromboembolism. Significant thrombocytopenia with decreased platelet survival is associated with the use of pulmonary artery catheters in dogs[194] and humans.[194] Thromboembolic complications are occasionally reported.[120,161,195–198] Heparin bonding of the catheters reduces their thrombogenicity.[197] Blood drawn through nonbonded catheters demonstrates increased platelet factor 4, thromboxane B_2, β-thromboglobulin, and fibrinopeptide A, which are absent in blood from heparin-bonded catheters.[199] Thrombosis occurs even when only the pulmonary artery catheter, not the introducer and catheter, remains in the vein. However, Perkins and co-workers[200] did not find thrombi in the internal jugular either before or after pulmonary artery catheter removal, probably as a result of continuous infusion through the side port of the introducer sheath.

Other Complications. Dysrhythmias are among the most common complications, occurring in 72% in one series of patients during catheter passage through the right heart.[171] They include persistent atrial arrhythmias,[160] ventricular arrhythmias,[172,202] and complete heart block.[202,203] Heart block may also result from contact of a guidewire with the bundle of His or its branches.[204] Dysrhythmias such as ventricular tachycardia are minimized by patient positioning in a right lateral decubitus and head-up position.[205] Other complications include pulmonary ischemia, infarction,[206,207] and valvular damage[207,208]; right-sided endocarditis[207,209]; air embolism[210]; fracture of the catheter[211]; ruptured tricuspid valve chordae[212]; entrapment by sutures in the right atrium during cardiac surgery[161,213,214]; hydromediastinum[215]; intracardiac knot formation[216]; and infections.[217]

LEFT ATRIAL PRESSURE MONITORING

Because of the inability to place pulmonary artery catheters in pediatric patients, direct measurements of the left atrial pressure is often performed. A left atrial pressure catheter is usually inserted by the surgeon during cardiac surgery via the superior pulmonary vein. The disadvantages are the need for thoracotomy for placement, danger of systemic embolization of clots and foreign material, and the risk of hemorrhage or tamponade with removal.[218]

CARDIAC OUTPUT DETERMINATION

Cardiac output may be determined by several methods, including the Fick principle, indicator dilution technique, the echo-Doppler method, or thermodilution technique. Advantages and disadvantages of the various methods in the child with congenital cardiac disease is detailed by Talner and Lister[219] (Table 8–1). The overall error of most clinical methods of cardiac output determination is 15–20%.

Techniques

Fick Method. The Fick principle states that the size of the stream may be readily calculated if the amount of substance entering or leaving the stream and the concentration difference resulting from the entry or removal are known. The measurement of oxygen uptake across the lungs and the arteriovenous difference of oxygen across the lungs are measured to determine pulmonary blood flow, which is essentially the same as the cardiac output. The Fick method is cardiac output (mL/min) = $\dot{V}o_2/(Cao_2 - C\bar{v}o_2) \times 100$, where $\dot{V}o_2$ is the uptake of oxygen per minute (mL/min) and $Cao_2 - C\bar{v}o_2$ is the arterial minus the venous oxygen content difference (mL/100 mL) $\cdot CO_2 = \alpha Po_2 + 1.34 Hb \times So_2$ where α = solubility of O_2 in whole blood (0.0031 mL 100 mL^{-1} mm Hg^{-1}), So_2 = % oxyhemoglobin saturation, and Hb = hemoglobin in grams per 100 mL^{-1}.

To measure oxygen uptake a steady state of 3–4 minutes, an accurate spirometer, and oximeter are necessary. The Fick equation assumes that pulmonary oxygen consumption is negligible compared with oxygen consumption of the body as a whole and that the rate of oxygen removal by blood equals the rate of oxygen uptake at the mouth. Either a closed- or open-circuit method is used to measure oxygen uptake, as described by Fagard and Conway.[220]

TABLE 8–1. CARDIAC OUTPUT METHODS

Method	Equipment	Advantages	Disadvantages
Fick Principle	Arterial oxygen contents in right atrium, systemic, pulmonary arteries	Shunt detection Small blood samples	Oxygen consumption measurement cumbersome
Dye Dilution	Arterial, central venous catheters	Shunt detection	Cumbersome calibration, large blood samples
Thermodilution	Central venous, pulmonary artery catheters	No blood samples Frequent repetition possible	Inaccurate with right-to-left shunts
Doppler	Tracheal, esophageal, pulmonary artery transducer	Semi-invasive	Inaccurate

The Fick technique has several limitations. The need for sampling of arterial blood precludes repeated measurements on multiple occasions. Expired air must be collected over at least 3 minutes to ensure accurate measurement of oxygen uptake. However, Morton described a three-breath technique for determination of the oxygenated mixed venous P_{CO_2} that, when combined with the end-tidal carbon dioxide and carbon dioxide production, allows noninvasive determination of cardiac output in children after cardiopulmonary bypass.[221] Phasic changes in the composition of arterial blood and blood flow with respiration cause errors of up to 4% in calculated output at rest and greater errors during exercise. The method assumes steady-state conditions. Finally, the contribution of the bronchial circulation to pulmonary blood flow produces a small error.[220]

Indicator-Dilution Method. This technique is derived from the Fick principle and the concentration gradient of an indicator, such as indocyanine green, is measured. Indocyanine green is (1) nontoxic, (2) rapidly mixed with blood, (3) nondiffusible into the lungs, (4) rapidly metabolized in the liver, and (5) easily and accurately measured with a photodensitometer owing to its maximal absorption of light at 805 μm, with the measurement not being influenced by hemoglobin concentration.[222] Indocyanine green is injected into the peripheral or central venous system. At a convenient arterial site, blood is continuously withdrawn into a photodensitometer, the concentration of indicator measured, and the curve relating the concentration of dye to time elapsed plotted. The total concentration of dye during the entire time interval represented by the curve is determined. Ordinarily, this quantity could be derived by measuring the total area under the curve. However, because of the early recirculation of the dye, some of the dye would be measured twice. Instead, the downslope of the curve is extrapolated to near zero to eliminate this redundancy. Other details of the method are described by Lund-Johansen.[223]

The general formula for indicator-dilution technique is:

$$\text{Cardiac output (L/min)} = \frac{60 \times \text{Indicator dose (mg)}}{\text{Average concentration} \times \text{Time (s)}}$$

In the absence of shunt, the indicator-dilution curve shows an uninterrupted build-up slope, a sharp concentration, a steep disappearance slope (short disappearance time), and a prominent recirculation peak. Central shunting distorts the curve as follows: (1) right-to-left shunting causes an abnormal early-appearing hump or reflection on the build-up slope and (2) left-to-right shunting causes decreased peak concentration of dye, prolonged disappearance time, and absence of the recirculation peak (Fig 8–10).

Dye dilution cardiac outputs have been used in the past in children and were noted to predict outcome, assess hemodynamic status, and monitor therapeutic interventions.[224] However, at present, they are infrequently used in either children or adults because of the need to withdraw blood and to assure a steady state during measurement of 20–30 seconds, precluding measurement of beat-to-beat changes. In addition, the simplicity and accuracy of the thermodilution method have encouraged its preferential use.[223] Under ideal conditions, dye dilution cardiac outputs have an error rate of less than 5% and are considered the standard for comparison of other techniques.[223] However, calculation of the curve may be erroneous during low flow states such as shock because recirculation ocurs so early that its recognition may be impossible. The calculated cardiac output is correspondingly reduced because the area under the curve after elimination of recirculation is increased. Mitral or aortic regurgitation also causes recirculation-induced distortion of the curve.

Thermodilution Technique. The thermodilution method, which is a modification of the indicator-dilution technique in which cooled dextrose is injected into the central venous system and a thermistor is used to measure the change of temperature in the pulmonary artery, is particularly useful in pediatric patients. Thermodilution has many advantages over the Fick or dye dilution

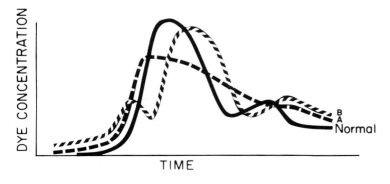

Figure 8–10. Examples of cardiac output curves obtained by the dye dilution method. The normal curve shows a rapid peak, sharp disappearance slope and prominent recirculation. Curve A is seen in the presence of a left-to-right intracardiac shunting and demonstrates the decreased peak concentration of dye, prolonged disappearance time, and absence of the recirculation peak characteristic of a left-to-right shunt. Curve B occurs with right-to-left shunting, which produces an abnormal early-appearing hump on the build-up slope. (*From Lake CL: Cardiovascular Anesthesia. New York: Springer-Verlag, 1985, with permission.*)

methods. The advantages are (1) rapid dissipation of heat eliminates recirculation problems and permits rapidly repeatable determination, (2) withdrawal of blood is not necessary, (3) the indicator is completely safe, and (4) rapid mixing occurs.[222] Unlike dye dilution, which is inaccurate in low cardiac output or left-heart regurgitant lesions, thermodilution cardiac output determinations are accurate in most clinical situations.[225]

Determination of Cardiac Output. The theory of this method is that if a known quantity of (negative) heat is introduced into the circulation, the resulting cooling curve recorded at a position sufficiently downstream to permit even distribution of the injected (negative) heat in the flowing blood allows computation of cardiac output. Adequate mixing of blood with the cold injectate has been found to occur during passage of the mixture through two valves and one cardiac chamber. The equation for this determination is:

$$\text{Cardiac output} = V_I \frac{(T_B - T_I) \times 60 \times 1.08}{A(\text{L/min})}$$

where 1.08 = correction factor for the specific heat and specific gravity of indicator and blood; V_I = volume of injectate in liters; T_B = initial blood temperature in °C; T_I = injectate temperature; A = the area under the curve multiplied by time for curve inscription.[226] The temperature change with time is measured by the computer as a resistance change. Both the injectate temperature and patient temperature are entered prior to the cardiac output determination, either directly or automatically. The computer then determines the difference between injectate and patient temperature. The temperature-time curve is integrated automatically by the computer and a correction factor for cutting off the curve at 30% of baseline is applied. The operator's manual for the specific system should be consulted to determine exactly how the curve is calculated. A critical analysis of the technique is provided by Conway and Lund-Johansen.[226]

Injection Technique. Either room-temperature or cooled injectate in 3-, 5-, or 10-mL volumes may be used. The injectate is delivered into a separate central venous catheter or the proximal port of a triple- or quadruple-lumen pulmonary artery catheter. Cooled injectate can be prepared in separate prefilled syringes or using a closed injectate system in which a coil of intravenous tubing is placed in an ice bath and connected to a reservoir of fluid. The connecting tubing must also be cooled; otherwise inaccuracies in output will occur.[227] Atrial fibrillation,[228] bradycardia,[229] or transient arrhythmias[222] may occur with injection of iced injectate. Even room-temperature injectate has been reported to cause ventricular fibrillation in one patient.[230]

Injections are preferably performed during apnea at end expiration because there is least fluctuation in the pulmonary artery temperature at that time.[231] Injections at peak inspiration are also reproducible.[230] Pulmonary artery temperature varies about 0.05 degrees with respiration as a result not only of cooling of the surface of the right ventricle and great veins by the overlying lung[232] but also to changes in superior and inferior venae cavae flows related to respiration. However, fluctuations of up to 0.11°C have been reported.[233] Variation in cardiac output due to respiration occurs in both mechanically ventilated and spontaneously ventilating patients. For this reason, automated systems with pneumatically driven pumps controlled by a microcomputer connected to a capnometer synchronize injections with the respiratory cycle. Use of the automated technique results in increased cardiac output as compared with manual injections at end expiration.[234] Significant temperature changes affecting the baseline temperature measurement occur during deep spontaneous respiration, panting, shivering, attempted breathing against a closed glottis, and diaphragmatic respiratory efforts.[233] Cardiac output is also increased in either the right or left lateral position as compared with the supine position.[235]

Thermodilution cardiac output measurements should not be made during or immediately (within 30 seconds) after rapid volume infusion.[236] When the output is recorded immediately after rapid volume infusion, the recorded output is low, whereas volume infusion during the injection of indicator results in falsely high output.[236] The inaccuracies occur because of variation in the baseline blood temperature as volume is administered via a peripheral vein. The curve is essentially a combination of the infused volume and the injectate. Although there is less error if the infusion is warmed than if it is at room temperature, an inaccuracy of 80% is created.[236]

Significant changes in pulmonary artery temperature are also seen immediately after discontinuation of extracorporeal circulation.[237] The changing baseline temperature may substantially underestimate thermodilution cardiac output during the first 10 minutes after bypass.[237]

Cardiac Output Curves. Cardiac output curves should always be recorded to check for baseline drift that can introduce a 50% error in measurement. The recorded curve can also be used to calculate the output by planimetry as a check of computer accuracy. The normal curve is smooth and characterized by a rapid peak and slow return to baseline (Fig 8–11). There may be underlying baseline fluctuations due to either respiratory or cardiac cycling. Low-amplitude curves result from an inadequate temperature difference between the blood and injectate (usally less than 10°C), too small an injectate volume, or the thermistor being positioned either too far distally in the pulmonary artery or slipping back in the right ventricle.[233] An anomalous slowly rising curve results when

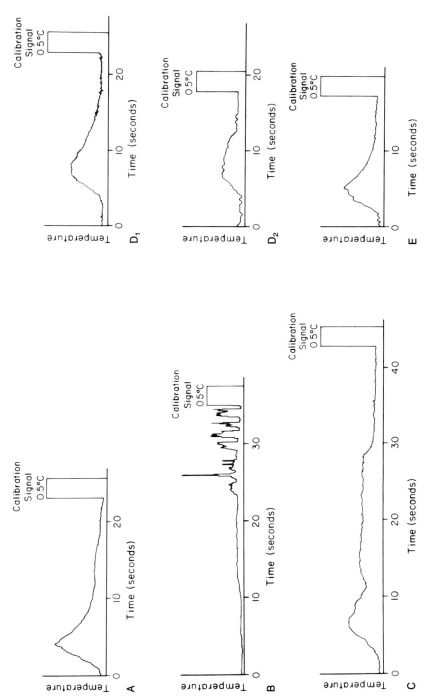

Figure 8–11. Normal and abnormal thermodilution cardiac output curves. (*A*) Normal curve. (*B*) The curve is delayed and of low amplitude when the injectate is administered slowly over 15 s. (*C*) The curve is an irregular, low-amplitude curve that results from the thermistor being against the vessel wall in a wedge position. (*D₁*) A curve resulting from injection of 10 mL of injectate. (*D₂*) An erroneously increased output resulting from injection of only 5 mL of injectate. (*E*) Patient motion during injection produces a curve with an unsteady baseline. (*From Lake CL: Clinical Monitoring. Philadelphia: WB Saunders, 1990, p 263, with permission.*)

the thermistor is positioned too peripherally in the pulmonary artery.[233] Irregular curves are caused by inadequate mixing, contact between the vessel wall and thermistor, or rapid changes in heart rate, respiration, or blood pressure.

In tricuspid insufficiency, significant recirculation occurs in the right heart affecting the downslope and preventing accurate measurement of the cardiac output. Recirculation also occurs with central shunting.[233,238] The recorded thermodilution curve can be used to determine the magnitude of the left-to-right cardiac shunt.[239] At the point just before recirculation, the curve is extrapolated to baseline and its area (A) measured by planimetry. The entire area, including recirculation ($A + B$), is also measured. Shunt size is calculated as the ratio of the total area to the area before recirculation ($[A + B]/A$). This correlates well with shunt ratio determined by the Fick method.[239]

Errors in Determination of Cardiac Output. The factors that cause inaccuracies in thermodilution measurements of cardiac output are type of injectate, volume of injectate, patient and injectate temperatures, mixing, injection technique, rewarming of injectate, and thermistor factors. Normally, curves should be reproducible to within 0.5 L/min at outputs of 5 L.[226]

TYPE AND VOLUME OF INJECTATE. Although 5% dextrose in water is the recommended injectate, the product of specific gravity and specific heat of either dextrose or saline is so similar that either fluid can be used.[233] Differences in the types of syringes will induce small errors in the volume of injectate. If the volume in the syringe is less than that entered in the computer, the area under the curve is smaller than it should be, resulting in overestimation of the cardiac output.[240]

INJECTATE AND PATIENT TEMPERATURES. If an adequate injectate volume is used (i.e., 10 mL), room-temperature injectates are as accurate and reproducible as iced injectate.[241,242] If the temperature of the injectate is not entered accurately into the computer, a 1°C error in injectate temperature would introduce an error of 2.7% using iced injectate and 77% using room-temperature injectate in a patient at 37°C.[233] Because the signal reflecting the temperature change is two to three times smaller when the solution is at room temperature than when it is at 0–5°C, the use of room-temperature injectates is not recommended in patients with significant respiratory fluctuations in pulmonary artery temperatures. Cold is also preferable in patients with very high cardiac outputs. Iced injectate is essential for accurate cardiac output determinations using 3-mL volumes, unlike the use of 10-mL injectate volumes.[241] Accurate thermodilution outputs can be performed in hypothermic patients as well.[243,244]

RECIRCULATION, MIXING, AND THERMISTOR FACTORS. The cold charge radiating off the catheter following injection arrives 5–35 seconds following injection and is eliminated as recirculation. The cold charge lost to the walls of a vessel is regained as warmed blood following the cooled is in turn cooled by the vessel wall. This accounts for the diminution in the peak of the thermodilution curve and its longer tail as compared with dye curves. Mixing of the injectate with the bloodstream is adequate at distances longer than 20 cm. Wessel and co-workers[245] observed a thermal gradient between the blood flowing centrally and that near the wall of a vessel. The intravascular position of the thermistor must be central (at least 2 mm from the vessel wall) for agreement of 2% between determinations. If the thermistor is placed so that an undamped pulmonary artery waveform is seen, good reproducibility is found. An unusual cause of inaccurate measurements is an intracatheter septal defect in which the injectate is flushed through both proximal and distal channels.[246] Mechanical injectors are advisable to control consistency of injections, particularly with large volumes.[247] At least 90 seconds should elapse between determinations to allow resumption of a steady blood temperature.[232]

Echo-Doppler Method. In critically ill infants, noninvasive methods such as the echo-Doppler may be useful to guide pharmacologic manipulations. A Doppler probe placed either externally at the sternal notch, in the esophagus or trachea, directly on the ascending aorta, or on a pulmonary artery catheter quantitates aortic blood flow, whereas the cross-sectional aortic area is determined by echocardiograph.[248–251] Ascending aortic flow is measured from transducers on endotracheal tubes and descending aortic flow from transducers on esophageal stethoscopes. The stroke volume is estimated as mean aortic root flow velocity times aortic cross-sectional area times R-R interval divided by the cosine θ, where θ is the angle between the ultrasound beam and direction of blood flow.[249]

In children, ultrasound cardiac output measurements correlate well with Fick-, electromagnetic flowmeter-, and thermodilution-measured cardiac output.[251–253] Some investigators also report good correlations with thermodilution measurements during rest and exercise in adult patients with correlation coefficients of 0.84–0.85.[253] Because the ultrasound method is less invasive when esophageal or external transducers are used, it would appear advantageous in children when thermodilution pulmonary artery catheters are not feasible. However, ultrasound measurements underestimate cardiac output and are inaccurate with patent ductus arteriosus, stenosis, insufficiency, or replacement of the aortic valve, mitral regurgitation, and very low stroke volumes. Among the causes of inaccuracy are the exclusion of coronary blood flow,[254] changes in aortic diameter and cross-sectional area, and technical difficulties related to the fixed angle of insonation.[250] Recent reviews have failed to confirm the accuracy of the ultrasound measurements reported in the early studies[252,255–257] and detail both the theoretic and practical inadequacies of the technique.[258–261] Among the problems reported are prolonged time to position the ultrasound transducer, operator dependency of measurements, need for frequent repositioning of transducer with surgical manipulation or patient movement, and pulmonary aspiration when the Doppler device is attached to endotracheal tube and requires cuff deflation for repositioning. Directly applied aortic ultrasound probes have not achieved widespread use in children owing to potential complications associated with removal, difficulties in maintaining useful ultrasound signals, and availability of less invasive ultrasound transducers.

Impedance Cardiography. Beat-to-beat stroke volume can be measured using impedance cardiography. The change in impedance to a 2.5-mA current passed through the chest (as a result of changes in the volume of blood in the chest during the cardiac cycle) is measured. The measurement is based upon the theoretic formula described by Kubicek and co-workers[262] and modified by Sramek, Bernstein and co-workers:

$$SV = \frac{\rho L^2 - T}{Z_o^2} \, dZ/dt_{max}$$

where SV is stroke volume in milliliters, ρ is blood resistivity in ohms per centimeter, L is the mean midline distance between dorsal and ventral recording electrodes in centimeters (thoracic length constant), Z_o is mean thoracic impedance in ohms, T is ejection time, dZ/dt_{max} is the maximum rate of change of impedance during ventricular ejection in ohms per second. Electrodes are placed on the neck and thorax with the outer two electrodes connected to a current source and the inner two recording the ECG, thoracic impedance (Z_o), and the change in impedance that occurs during the cardiac cycle plus its first derivative. Careful skin preparation and electrode placement are essential to accurate measurements.

Early studies suggested that bioimpedance cardiography would be useful in children with intra- and extracardiac shunts.[263] However, when recently compared with dye dilution, bioimpedance measurements of cardiac output differed by 0.28–0.29 L/min, with a standard deviation of 0.47 L/min.[264] Attempts to improve the accuracy of the bioimpedance technique include the use of a thoracic length constant determined from thermodilution measurements of cardiac output[265] or by actual measurement of anatomic thoracic length and circumference.[266]

Further critical analysis of the method has been performed by White and co-workers.[267] Blood resistivity changes with fluctuations in hematocrit. Intrathoracic blood flow distribution is not always homogeneous but depends upon cardiovascular function. These and similar assumptions inherent in the bioimpedance method cause inaccuracies that preclude its use in critically ill pediatric cardiac patients. However, bioimpedance technology has been recently reported to estimate total body water in children after cardiac surgery noninvasively.[268]

Calculation of Hemodynamic Parameters. Pulmonary and systemic vascular resistance, stroke volume, cardiac index, right and left ventricular stroke work are calculated from the measurements of systemic and pulmonary pressure, heart rate, and cardiac output. The formulas and normal values are in Table 8–2. Cardiac outputs, systemic and pulmonary vascular resistances, right and left ventricular stroke work are usually converted to indices by relating them to body surface area (BSA) to permit comparison between patients of different sizes. The BSA is usually determined from a table of normal values. Systemic and pulmonary resistance are expressed as absolute resistance units or hybrid (Wood)

TABLE 8–2. CALCULATION OF HEMODYNAMIC VARIABLES

Systemic vascular resistance (dynes-s-cm^{-5}) = $\dfrac{\text{MAP (mm Hg)} - \text{CVP (mm Hg)} \times 79.9}{\text{Cardiac output (L/min)}}$		Normal values: 1200–1500 dynes-s-cm^{-5}
Pulmonary vascular resistance (dynes-s-cm^{-5}) = $\dfrac{\text{Mean PAP} - \text{Mean PWP} \times 79.9}{\text{Cardiac output (L/min)}}$		Normal values: 100–300 dynes-s-cm^{-5}
Cardiac index (L/min/m^2) = $\dfrac{\text{Cardiac output (L/min)}}{\text{Body surface area (m}^2)}$		Normal values: 2.8–4.2 L/min/m^2
Stroke volume (mL/beat) = $\dfrac{\text{Cardiac output (mL/min)}}{\text{Heart rate (beats/min)}}$		Normal values: 60–90 mL/beat
Stroke index (mL/beat/m^2) = $\dfrac{\text{Stroke volume (mL/beat)}}{\text{Body surface area}}$		Normal values: 30–65 mL/beat/m^2
Left ventricular stroke work (g-m/beat/m^2) = 0.0136 (MAP − Mean PWP) × Stroke index		Normal values: 45–60 g-m/beat/m^2
Right ventricular stroke work (g-m/beat/m^2) = 0.0136 (Mean PAP − Mean CVP) × Stroke index		Normal values: 5–10 g-m/beat/m^2

Abbreviations: CVP, central venous pressure; PWP, pulmonary wedge pressure; MAP, mean arterial pressure; and PAP, pulmonary artery pressure.

units. The absolute resistance units are given as dynes-s-cm^{-5}. Division of the absolute resistance units by 80 converts them to Wood units in mm Hg/L/min. Because the calculated pulmonary vascular resistance is influenced by flow (cardiac output, pulmonary vascular tone, left heart filling pressure), the effects of drugs and interventions on pulmonary resistance are often best expressed by the pulmonary diastolic–pulmonary wedge pressure gradient rather than pulmonary resistance or direct pulmonary flow.[269]

MONITORING OF THE CENTRAL NERVOUS SYSTEM

Electroencephalography (EEG)

Although monitoring of the EEG, particularly during cardiopulmonary bypass, has been attempted since the early years of cardiac surgery,[270] the equipment was so cumbersome and the results were so difficult to interpret and uncertain in significance that EEG was infrequently monitored. However, despite the inability of EEG to detect all critical events,[271] many critical events can be recognized,[272] and no better or more practical method to continuously evaluate the function of the central nervous system has been developed.[273] The multilead EEG is a sensitive indicator of cerebral cortical function but not of brain stem function. Its use is facilitated by a constant depth of anesthesia and by filter-processor systems providing density spectral array and compressed spectral analysis.

Multilead EEG. Although the continuous multichannel EEG can be correlated with cerebral blood flow,[274] the EEG does not show changes until cerebral metabolism is profoundly altered. EEG activity commonly shifts from the occipital to the frontal areas during anesthesia because occipital alpha activity is lost and frontal beta activity increases in amplitude. A standard EEG can document cerebral dysfunction secondary to low blood flow, low perfusion pressure, or malpositioned bypass cannulas.[275]

Density and Compressed Spectral Array. A density spectral array (DSA) is a two-dimensional display of EEG frequency versus time with amplitude represented by the intensity of shading or dot size. The record has the appearance of multiple utility poles. The spectral edge is the frequency below which 95% of the power of the EEG is located. Anesthetic induction or hypothermia during cardiopulmonary bypass changes the power from the high-frequency alpha activity to lower frequencies, but the activity is symmetrically reduced over both cerebral hemispheres. Global cerebral hypoperfusion or hypoxia also reduce frequency or eliminate all cerebral activity (Fig 8–12). Compressed spectral array (CSA) is

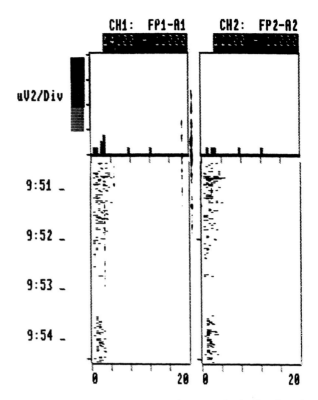

Figure 8–12. Density spectral array of an anesthetized patient during hypothermic cardiopulmonary bypass. Channel 1 (CH1: FP1-A1) results from left frontotemporal leads, whereas channel 2 (CH2: FP2-A2) is from patient's right side. The frequency of activity is in the 4-Hz range (0–20 horizontal, scale) but at time 9:52 (vertical scale), a decrease in oxygen supply to the oxygenator results in severe systemic hypoxia and loss of cerebral activity at 9:53. Restoration of the oxygenator oxygen supply produces rapid return of cerebral activity at 9:54.

a three-dimensional display of the EEG power spectrum with amplitude and time compressed on the vertical axis. A CSA record appears to have mountains and valleys. The augmented delta quotient, the ratio of the mean amplitude of the delta waves of the raw EEG to the mean amplitude of the entire EEG signal, correlates well with changes in CSA in children with congenital heart disease undergoing cardiopulmonary bypass.[276]

Cerebral Spectroscopy

Devices capable of measuring the oxygen saturation of brain hemoglobin using near infrared light have recently become available. Brain oximetry measures regional oxygen saturation in the cerebral microvasculature, which is composed of 20% arterial, 5% capillary, and 75% venous blood. Pulsation is not essential to the measurements. The sensor that is placed just lateral to the midline of the forehead emits near infrared light at wavelengths between 650 and 1100 nanometers, which penetrates the scalp, skull, and brain tissue where it is reflected and refracted before being returned to the surface. Samplers of the returning light are located either near the source (for shallow portions) or several centimeters away (for deep portions of the brain). The light is attenuated by passage through the brain because of light-absorbing iron-porphyrin in oxyhemoglobin or deoxyhemoglobin and copper in cytochrome c oxidase.[277] Data are normalized to a reference wavelength of 803 nm, the isosbestic point of reduced and oxyhemoglobin.

Normal cerebral oxygen saturation is about 70% owing to the large contribution of venous blood. Hampson and co-workers demonstrated decreased oxyhemoglobin and oxidized cytochrome and increased deoxyhemoglobin during induced hypoxia at normo- or hypocarbia.[278] Cerebral oxyhemoglobin also decreases rapidly during endotracheal suctioning of premature infants.[279] Reasonably good correlations of cerebral oximeter saturations with directly measured jugular venous bulb saturations have been reported.

Jugular Venous Oximetry

Oximeter catheters transmitting three wavelengths of light are inserted into the cerebral venous circulation to measure cerebral venous oxygen saturation directly and continuously. Commercially available devices are modifications of catheter oximeters originally developed for the pulmonary circulation. External preinsertion calibration of the catheter and documentation of catheter position in the jugular bulb are required for accurate measurements. In vivo calibrations against co-oximeter samples can also be performed. Reflected light signals are averaged, filtered, and displayed. Conditions affecting the accuracy of these measurements include catheter kinking, blood flow around the catheter, changes in hematocrit, fibrin deposition on the catheter, and changes in temperature.

Transcranial Doppler Flow Velocity

Transcranial Doppler permits noninvasive measurement of blood flow velocity in the cerebral arteries. A 1- to 2-MHZ pulsed ultrasound transducer emits and receives energy. Low frequencies of sound are used to minimize artifacts from skull-reflected sound. The Doppler-shifted signal is subjected to fast Fourier transform to create a directional display over time (horizontal axis). On the vertical axis, flow away from the transducer is displayed below the zero line while flow toward the transducer is above the zero line. Normal middle cerebral artery flow in a healthy human is 60 cm/s. The other measured variable is the pulsatility index, determined as peak systolic–peak diastolic/time mean velocities, which indicates the pulsatile dynamics of the cerebral circulation. Normal values are 0.71 ± 0.10.[280]

If the assumption that the diameter of the cerebral arteries remains constant during various conditions, the flow velocity is considered proportional to cerebral blood flow. Points of measurement are principally transtemporal (determination of middle cerebral artery flow) or transorbital (determination of ophthalmic artery flow) although other "windows" into the skull may be used, including the foramen magnum. The absence of an appropriate window precludes measurements in about 10% of patients. Present technology precludes accurate detection of flow less than 3–4 cm/s.

However, the measurement is affected by age (lower flows at younger ages), viscosity (changes in hematocrit during cardiac surgery), intracranial pressure, and with turbulent flow. Electrocautery use also interferes with the signal. Pilato and co-workers demonstrated that cerebral blood flow velocity decreased with hypocarbia and increased logarithmically with end-tidal carbon dioxide in anesthetized children.[281] The pulsatility index also decreased as end-tidal carbon dioxide increased.[281] Low concentrations of halothane (0.8% inspired), isoflurane (1.2% inspired), or enflurane (1.7% inspired) had little effect on middle cerebral artery systolic, diastolic, or mean flow velocities in adults.[282] However, hyperventilation decreased blood flow velocities, whereas halothane (1.6% inspired) increased flow velocity. At higher anesthetic concentrations, a constant diameter of the middle cerebral arteries cannot be assumed and cerebral flow velocity may not be proportional to cerebral blood flow.[282]

Transcranial Doppler was used by van der Linden and co-workers to demonstrate the decrease in cerebral flow velocity and oxygen consumption associated with profound hypothermia in children undergoing cardiac surgery.[283] They noted that flow velocity was unaffected by perfusion pressures between 20 and 42 mm Hg but was related to pump flow rates. Because the diameter of the middle cerebral artery remained constant during cardiac surgery in the children studied, van der Linden and co-workers considered that cerebral flow velocity could be used as a estimate of cerebral blood flow.[283] Combined with measurements of arterial and jugular venous oxygen content, cerebral oxygen consumption was also determined.

MONITORS OF OXYGENATION

Noninvasive methods to monitor arterial oxygenation include oximetry, transcutaneous oxygen electrodes (TCo_2), and optode sensors. The newest technique is the optode, which uses the oxygen-sensitive fluorescence-quenching phenomenon to measure Po_2. The optode, a fiberoptic, heparin-bonded probe containing the fluorescent dye hydroxypyrene trisulfonic acid can be placed within an intravascular catheter.[284,285] Carbon dioxide and pH sensors are also incorporated into these probes. Clinically acceptable performance of optode technology has been demonstrated in animal experiments, normal volunteers, and anesthetized patients.[284]

Pulse Oximeters

Pulse oximeters are a combination of an oximeter with a pulse plethysmograph. Relevant physics and physiology are extensively reviewed by Tremper and Barker,[286] whereas their uses, accuracy, and limitations have been critically evaluated by Severinghaus and Kelleher.[287] The oximeter functions by positioning any pulsating arterial vascular bed between a two-wavelength light source and detector.[288] Unlike the co-oximeter, which measures the fractional saturation of hemoglobin and includes the contributions of carboxy- and methemoglobin, the functional oxygen saturation of hemoglobin is approximated by most pulse oximeters according to the relationship:

$$\frac{Oxyhemoglobin}{Hemoglobin\ +\ Oxyhemoglobin}$$

Two wavelengths of light (660 and 940 nm) are passed through the tissue being measured to a photodetector. The pulsatile and nonpulsatile components of both wavelengths are compared to yield a value that varies nonlinearly with hemoglobin saturation. The intensity of the color reaching the photodetector depends upon the color, the thickness of the skin, the brightness of the light, and the absorption of arterial and venous blood in the tissues. Pulsation creates a change in the light path length that modifies the amount of light detected. The amplitude of varying detected light depends upon the size of the arterial pulse change, the wavelength of light used, and the oxygen saturation. Several types of sensors are available in various sizes for use on the nose, fingers, or ear lobes.

The reliability of a pulse oximeter will be affected by hypotension, hypothermia, vasoconstriction, abnormal hemoglobins (carboxy- or methemoglobin), low signal to noise ratios (patient motion, increased venous pressure, electrocautery), or exposure to room light (avoided by providing an opaque cover).[288,289] However, fetal hemoglobin has no effect.[290] Dyes such as methylene blue and indocyanine green cause falsely low readings. Placement of the pulse oximeter on the dependent arm of a patient in the lateral decubitus position may cause false readings due to increased venous pulsation in that extremity. A close correlation (0.96) between pulse oximeter readings, ear lobe oximeter, and in vitro measurements of arterial saturation has been noted[289,291] (Fig 8–13).

Although pulse oximeters are generally used during all types of surgical procedures,[287] they are especially useful in pediatric cardiovascular procedures in which an intra-arterial catheter cannot be placed or in addition to the intra-arterial catheter to provide immediate information about oxygenation. During pulmonary artery banding, desaturation detected by the pulse oximeter indicates that the band is too tightly applied even before vital signs deteriorate[292,293] (Fig 8–14). However, oximeters are relatively insensitive to blood flow. Accurate pulse oximeter readings are present at only 8.6% of control flow.[294]

Oximeter Catheters

Mixed venous oxygen saturation, which reflects tissue oxygenation, quantitates the extent to which the organism is relying on compensatory mechanisms to match oxygen consumption with demand.[295] A mixed venous oxygen saturation of less than 40% indicates the limits of compensation are being reached.[295]

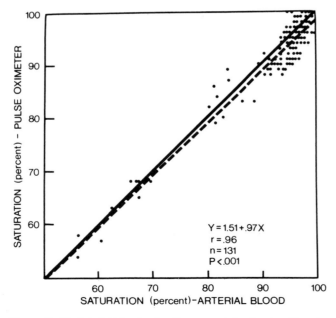

Figure 8–13. Arterial blood saturations correlate closely with saturation measured by a pulse oximeter. (*From Mihm FG: Noninvasive detection of profound arterial desaturations using a pulse oximetry device. Anesthesiology 62:85, 1985, with permission.*)

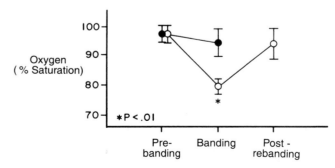

Figure 8–14. During banding of the pulmonary artery, an unacceptable decrease in arterial oxygen saturation is detected by pulse oximetry (*open circles*). Reapplication of the band less tightly restores oxygen saturation to acceptable values. The *closed circles* indicate an acceptable decrease in pulmonary blood flow producing mild desaturation. (*Data from Casthely PA, et al: Pulse oximetry during pulmonary artery banding. J Cardiothorac Anesth 1:297–299, 1987, with permission.*)

The pulmonary artery contains mixed venous blood and is an ideal site to monitor venous oxygen saturation (Svo_2) continuously. Mixed venous blood is defined as (1) blood that has traversed capillary beds capable of extracting oxygen but not those incapable of oxygen extraction[295] and (2) thoroughly mixed blood with a single oxygen saturation throughout. The reflection spectrophotometry employed consists of light-emitting diodes generating alternating pulses of two or three different wavelengths at 244 times per second.[296,297] Light is transmitted through the catheter using a fiberoptic channel. The light is absorbed, refracted, and reflected by the passing erythrocytes. Another fiberoptic channel conducts the reflected light to a photodetector that determines the saturation of hemoglobin from the relative intensities corresponding to the three different wavelengths and a computer averages these values over the preceding 5 seconds.[296] The accuracy of the catheter oximeter compared with laboratory oximeters has been well documented.[291,296,298,299]

Although oximeter catheters of No. 7.5 French size are made for adults (see Fig 8–8), smaller sizes suitable for direct placement in the pulmonary artery during surgery are also available. These latter catheters are particularly useful to monitor children during and after repair of congenital cardiac defects and were originally designed to be inserted into the umbilical artery for continuous monitoring of arterial oxygen saturation in neonates.

Oximeter catheters can be calibrated either prior to induction or in vivo. Their readings are inaccurate if the tip of the catheter is lodged against the vessel wall or covered with fibrin deposits.

Postoperatively, mixed venous oxygen saturation serves as an early warning of deteriorating cardiac function in children.[291,296,298,301,302] Venous oxygen saturation decreases acutely with endotracheal suction, bucking, or coughing against the endotracheal tube or mucous plugging of the endotracheal tube. Svo_2 measurements can be used during application of PEEP to determine the "best PEEP" without the need for repeated blood gases.[299] However, the measurements are erroneous with patient motion or shivering. In sepsis, the mixed venous oxygen saturation may reach 60% even in the presence of lactic acidosis due to an inability of the tissue to extract oxygen from blood, contamination of mixed venous blood with arterial blood in peripheral shunts, and abnormalities in the distribution of blood flow.[301]

RESPIRATORY GAS ANALYSIS

Carbon Dioxide

The concentration of carbon dioxide in the expired gases is usually measured by an infrared detector, a mass spectrometer, or a Raman scattering device. Either mainstream (directly at the airway) or sidestream (aspiration of a gas sample via a small tube at a rate of 50–250 cc/min) analysis of carbon dioxide is performed. Mainstream analyzers are rapid and avoid the problems of blocked tubing, need for water traps, or sampling errors. However, their size, weight, placement at the endotracheal tube, and cost are disadvantages. Mainstream analyzers are available only for carbon dioxide and not for other respiratory gases or anesthetic vapors.

The infrared capnograph passes infrared light through a sample of gas where carbon dioxide molecules absorb part of the infrared light. Unabsorbed light passes through the end of the chamber and impinges on heat detectors. Differential heating of the sampling and a reference detector is transduced to a meter calibrated directly in percent carbon dioxide. Because infrared absorption also detects nitrous oxide, the instrument must be calibrated against a known gas mixture or a correction factor applied to the reading. Infrared detectors are unable to measure asymmetric molecules such as nitrogen and oxygen.

Raman scattering analyzers are sidestream devices in which laser light interacts with gas molecules in the sample to produce spectra that identify components of the gas mixture. All molecules, including oxygen, nitrogen, and volatile anesthetics, can be identified. Atoms, such as helium, cannot be identified with Raman scattering because the scattering relates to bond energies in the gas molecules.

Mass spectrometers separate the ions in a gas sample according to their mass/charge ratios using a magnetic field. The separated beams leaving the magnetic field are directed to detectors of the ion currents for oxygen, carbon dioxide, nitrogen, nitrous oxide, enflurane, halothane, isoflurane, and others. Compounds with similar mass:charge ratios are fragmented to produce different breakdown products to enhance their detection. Unlike infrared or Raman scattering devices, mass spectrometers are usually shared or multiplexed among many sampling sites.

The normal capnogram, the waveform of exhaled carbon dioxide over time, is nearly a square wave (Fig 8–15). The carbon dioxide concentration in its first portion (phase I) is usually 0, the last gas entering and the first gas exiting the lung, ie, anatomic and equipment dead space. Phase II begins with the increase in carbon dioxide concentration due to exhalation of alveolar gas and continues as a plateau (phase III). During phase III, the exhaled gas is a mixture of alveolar dead space gas and alveolar gas from well-perfused alveoli with a nearly arterial Pco_2.

End-tidal carbon dioxide increases with malignant hyperthermia, providing an earlier warning sign than the increase in temperature.[303] Decreases in pulmonary blood flow during pulmonary artery banding or creation

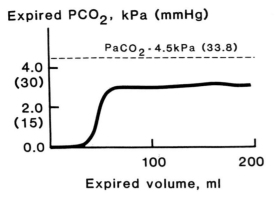

Figure 8–15. This single-breath expired carbon dioxide waveform demonstrates the increase in alveolar dead space (the area between the line representing arterial carbon dioxide and the expired carbon dioxide waveform) in a child with congenital heart disease and right-to-left shunt. (*From Fletcher RL: The relationship between the arterial to end-tidal PCO_2 difference and hemoglobin saturation in patients with congenital heart disease. Anesthesiology 75:210–216, 1991, with permission.*)

of systemic-to-pulmonary shunts are detected by decreased end-tidal carbon dioxide[304] (Fig 8–16). In Fig 8–15, the difference between the carbon dioxide concentration of the alveolar plateau of phase III and arterial P_{CO_2} is equivalent to alveolar dead space. Fletcher demonstrated a curvilinear negative correlation between the

arterial and end-tidal carbon dioxide gradient in children with congenital heart disease.[305] He also noted that the slope of the regression of arterial to end-tidal carbon dioxide correlated positively with hemoglobin concentration and respiratory quotient[305] (Fig 8–17). End-tidal carbon dioxide also decreases with venous air embolism because there is a progressive reduction in lung perfusion relative to ventilation causing an increase in physiologic dead space. Other causes of absence of the capnogram are cardiac arrest, ventilator disconnection, tracheal tube obstruction, and esophageal intubation.

MISCELLANEOUS MONITORS

Monitors such as heart sounds, temperature, blood gases, electrolytes, hematocrit, and urine output are routinely used in all pediatric cardiac surgical procedures. Generally, a precordial stethoscope is used initially and subsequently replaced by a multipurpose esophageal stethoscope. Such stethoscopes contain thermistors for temperature monitoring and electrodes for esophageal ECG leads.[306]

Stethoscopy

The precordial stethoscope is a simple, inexpensive, easily applied device providing a direct, continuous link between the anesthesiologist and the pediatric patient for assessment of cardiorespiratory sounds.[290] However, the amount of information derived from the

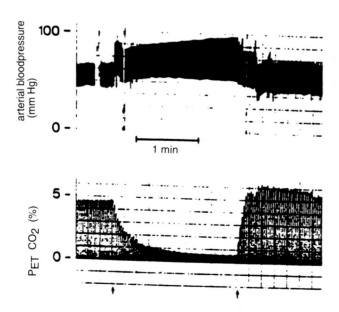

Figure 8–16. During banding of the pulmonary artery, occlusion of the pulmonary artery decreases end-tidal P_{CO_2} (*lower panel*) while increasing systemic arterial blood pressure (*upper panel*). (*From Schuller JL, et al: Severe reduction in end-tidal PCO_2 following unilateral pulmonary artery occlusion in a child with pulmonary hypertension. Anesth Analg 68:792–794, 1989, with permission.*)

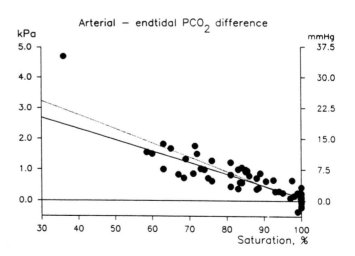

Figure 8–17. In children with congenital heart disease, there is a curvilinear negative correlation between the arterial to end-tidal carbon dioxide gradient and arterial oxygen saturation and a positive correlation with hemoglobin concentration and respiratory quotient. (*From Fletcher R: The relationship between the arterial to end-tidal PCO_2 difference and hemoglobin saturation in patients with congenital heart disease. Anesthesiology 75:210–216, 1991, with permission.*)

precordial stethoscope is limited; in the case of heart sounds, the information includes increases/decreases in rate and the subtle "muffling" of heart sounds associated with decreasing cardiac output.[290] Information on respiration, limited by the ability to monitor only a small portion of one lung, requires attention to each breath.[307]

Esophageal stethoscopes are also simple and inexpensive but require endotracheal intubation prior to their use. Thermistors, Doppler ultrasound transducers, and electrocardiographic leads are commonly incorporated into esophageal stethoscopes (Fig 8–18). In general, stethoscopes should be used during patient transportation between operating room and intensive care or as adjuncts to more sophisticated electronic devices for intraoperative monitoring of the cardiorespiratory system.

Blood Gases

Arterial blood gases, including pH, P_{CO_2}, P_{O_2}, are frequently sampled at intervals determined by the stage of the operative procedure, such as opening of the chest and initiation of cardiopulmonary bypass as well as at hemodynamic changes. Although arterial blood gases were corrected for temperature during cardiopulmonary bypass for many years, temperature-correction or pH-stat versus uncorrected or alpha-stat strategy has been a subject of controversy in recent years.[239,240]

Murkin and co-workers noted an uncoupling of cerebral oxygen consumption from cerebral blood flow during hypothermic cardiopulmonary bypass in humans when the pH-stat method was used.[310] In experimental animals, Hindman and co-workers noted that the increase in cerebral blood flow associated with pH-stat management occurred only at perfusion flow rates of 100 mL/kg/min. Except in neonates, such flow rates are substantially greater than flows used clinically.[311] However, Bashein and colleagues were unable to demonstrate any differences on neuropsychologic testing of adult patients managed by either pH or alpha-stat strategy.[312] More recently, however, Stephan and co-workers suggested that neurologic dysfunction occurred more frequently in pH-stat–managed adult patients.[313] Watanabe and co-workers suggested that brain oxygenation recovered more rapidly and acidosis was less severe with alpha-stat management in experimental animals.[314] Baraka and colleagues recently reported that whole-body oxygen consumption and oxyhemoglobin dissociation was not significantly affected by blood gas management in humans.[315] Likewise, Badner and co-workers noted no

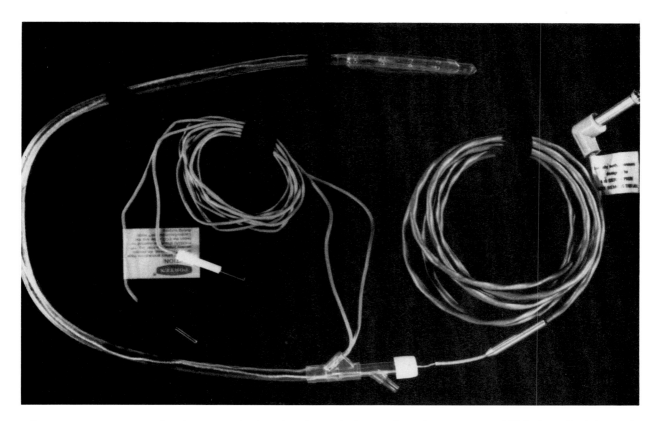

Figure 8–18. An esophageal stethoscope with a thermistor for monitoring esophageal temperature and ECG electrodes (wires and black bands on stethoscope) for recording an esophageal ECG lead.

differences in perioperative renal function with blood gas strategy.[316]

Temperature

Body temperature should be monitored during every pediatric cardiac surgical procedure to detect malignant hyperthermia or accidental hypothermia and to monitor induced hypothermia. Sites commonly used include the esophagus, nasopharynx, rectum, tympanic membrane, and bladder. During noncardiac surgery, all sites give similar values, but during cardiac surgery central (core) temperature should be monitored from the distal esophagus, pulmonary artery, tympanic membrane, or nasopharynx.[317] Although temperature-sensitive liquid crystal skin-surface thermometers may be used during induction or recovery, skin temperature poorly reflects core temperature and thermocouples in other sites are preferable.

Nasal thermistors are useful because their values reflect brain (hypothalamic) temperature because they are close to the high blood flow of the turbinates. However, they must be carefully positioned just behind the soft palate. In children, nasopharyngeal temperature may be affected by the temperature of inhaled gases because of leakage around uncuffed endotracheal tubes.[318] Tympanic probes are useful indicators of brain temperature because a branch of the internal carotid artery supplies the tympanic membrane. The esophageal temperature closely approximates cardiac temperature, particularly when the temperature probe is located in the distal esophagus at the tip of a well-positioned esophageal stethoscope and good heart sounds are heard. However, esophageal temperature measurements are also affected by the temperature of respiratory gases in children.[319]

Foley catheters with thermistors can be used in older children[320] but are too large for infants. Bladder temperatures tend to lag behind nasopharyngeal and esophageal temperatures during cardiopulmonary bypass in adult patients.[320] However, bladder temperatures are quite similar to pulmonary artery temperatures in the ICU.[320,321] Bladder temperatures correlate well with esophageal and rectal temperatures, particularly at temperatures greater than 34° C. Although rectal temperatures are often measured in children, they are inaccurate unless the rectum is empty. The use of upper extremity skin or muscle temperature probes may be helpful in cardiac surgery to assure complete rewarming during cardiopulmonary bypass.[322] Particularly in patients with large muscle masses, the nasopharyngeal temperature does not adequately indicate the completeness of rewarming.[322]

Urine Output

Urine flow rate, sodium concentration, and osmolarity reflect renal perfusion. Urinary output is measured at 30-minute intervals during most cardiovascular surgery.

The placement of an indwelling Foley catheter is dictated not only by the type of procedure but also its length and potential for hemodynamic change. For short procedures, an external drainage system can be placed instead of a Foley catheter. Urine output in the perioperative period is affected by blood glucose, administration of diuretics such as mannitol or furosemide, and hemodilution. Diuretics increase both urine volume and urinary sodium excretion. Determination of urine sodium, osmolarity, specific gravity, protein, glucose, and sediment usually reveals a specific cause for oliguria.

REFERENCES

1. Mirvis DM, Berson AS, Goldberger AL, et al: Instrumentation and practice standards for electrocardiographic monitoring in special care units. *Circulation* **79**:464–471, 1989
2. Greeley WJ, Kates RA, Bushman GA, et al: Intraoperative esophageal electrocardiography for dysrhythmia analysis and therapy in pediatric cardiac surgical patients. *Anesthesiology* **65**:669–672, 1986
3. Bushman GA: Clinical correlates of dysrhythmias requiring an esophageal ECG for accurate diagnosis in patients with congenital heart disease. *J Cardiothorac Anesth* **3**:290–294, 1989
4. Kaplan JA, King SB: The precordial electrocardiographic lead (V[5]) in patients who have coronary artery disease. *Anesthesiology* **45**:570–574, 1976
5. Bell C, Rimar S, Barash P: Intraoperative ST segment changes with myocardial ischemia in the neonate: Report of three cases. *Anesthesiology* **7**:601–604, 1989
6. Ellis JE, Shah MN, Briller JE, et al: A comparison of methods for the detection of myocardial ischemia during noncardiac surgery: Automated ST-segment analysis systems, electrocardiography, and transesophageal echocardiography. *Anesth Analg* **75**:764–772, 1992
7. Manning DM, Kuchirka C, Kamienski J: Miscuffing: Inappropriate blood pressure cuff application. *Circulation* **68**:763–766, 1983
8. Kirkland RT, Kirkland JL: Systolic blood pressure measurement in the newborn infant with the transcutaneous Doppler method. *J Pediatr* **80**:52–55, 1972
9. Hernandez A, Goldring D, Hartmann AF: Measurement of blood pressure in infants and children by the Doppler ultrasound technique. *Pediatrics* **48**:788–794, 1971
10. Yelderman M, Ream AK: Indirect measurement of mean blood pressure in the anesthetized patient. *Anesthesiology* **50**:253–256, 1979
11. Borow KN, Newburger JW: Noninvasive estimation of central aortic pressure using the oscillometric method for analyzing systemic artery pulsatile blood flow: Comparative study of indirect systolic, diastolic, and mean brachial artery pressure with simultaneous direct ascending aortic pressure measurements. *Am Heart J* **103**:879–886, 1982
12. Nystrom E, Reid KH, Bennett R, et al: A comparison of two automated indirect arterial blood pressure meters: With recordings from a radial arterial catheter in anesthetized surgical patients. *Anesthesiology* **62**:526–530, 1985

13. Friesen RH, Lichtor JL: Indirect measurement of blood pressure in neonates and infants utilizing an automatic non-invasive oscillometric monitor. *Anesth Analg* **60**:742–745, 1981

14. Kimble KJ, Darnall RA, Yelderman M, et al: An automated oscillometric technique for estimating mean arterial pressure in critically ill newborns. *Anesthesiology* **54**:423–425, 1981

15. Diprose GK, Evens DH, Archer LN: Dinamapp fails to detect hypotension in very low birthweight infants. *Arch Dis Child* **61**:771–773, 1986

16. Showman A, Betts EK: Hazard of automatic noninvasive blood pressure monitoring. *Anesthesiology* **55**:717–718, 1981

17. Bickler PE, Schapera A, Bainton CR: Acute radial nerve injury from use of an automated blood pressure monitor. *Anesthesiology* **73**:186–188, 1990

18. Gardner RM, Bond EL, Clark JS: Safety and efficacy of continuous flush systems for arterial and pulmonary artery catheters. *Ann Thorac Surg* **23**:534–538, 1977

19. Palermo LM, Andrews RW, Ellison N: Avoidance of heparin contamination in coagulation studies drawn from indwelling lines. *Anesth Analg* **59**:222–224, 1980

20. Lake CL (ed): *Clinical Monitoring.* Philadelphia: WB Saunders, 1990, p. 85–113

21. Gardner RM: Direct blood pressure measurements—Dynamic response requirements. *Anesthesiology* **54**:227–236, 1981

22. Hipkins SF, Rutten AJ, Runciman WB: Experimental analysis of catheter-manometer systems in vitro and in vivo. *Anesthesiology* **71**:893–906, 1989

23. Shinozaki T, Deane R, Mazuzan JE, et al: Bacterial contamination of arterial lines: A prospective study. *JAMA* **249**:223–225, 1983

24. Gibbs N, Hart G, Cameron PD, et al: A comparison of continuous flush devices. *Anesth Intens Care* **13**:184–187, 1985

25. Gardner RM, Parker J, Feinauer R: System for umbilical artery monitoring. *Crit Care Med* **10**:456–458, 1982

26. Haselby KA, Dierdorf SF: A gravity-driven continuous flush system for vascular catheters. *Anesth Analg* **61**:871–872, 1982

27. Morray J, Todd S: A hazard of continuous flush systems for vascular pressure monitoring in infants. *Anesthesiology* **58**:187–189, 1983

28. Allen EV: Thromboangiitis obliterans: Methods of diagnosis of chronic occlusive arterial lesion distal to the wrist with illustrative cases. *Am J Med Sci* **178**:237–244, 1929

29. Meyer RM, Katele GV: The case for a complete Allen's test. *Anesth Analg* **62**:947–948, 1983

30. Greenhow DE: Incorrect performance of Allen's test: Ulnar artery flow erroneously presumed inadequate. *Anesthesiology* **37**:356–357, 1972

31. Kamienski RW, Barnes RW: Critique of Allen test for continuity of palmar arch assessed by Doppler ultrasound. *Surg Gynecol Obstet* **142**:861–864, 1976

32. Hirai M, Kawai S: False positive and negative results in Allen test. *J Cardiovasc Surg* **21**:353–360, 1980

33. Slogoff S, Keats AS, Arlund C: On the safety of radial artery cannulation. *Anesthesiology* **59**:42–47, 1983

34. Marshall AG, Erwin DC, Wyses RKH, Hatch DJ: Percu-taneous arterial cannulation in children. *Anaesthesia* **39**:27–31, 1984

35. Bedford RF: Percutaneous radial-artery cannulation. Increased safety using Teflon catheters. *Anesthesiology* **42**:219–222, 1975

36. Talmadge EA: Shearing hazard of intra-arterial teflon catheters. *Anesth Analg* **55**:597–598, 1976

37. Morray JP, Brandford HG, Barnes LF, Furman EB: Doppler-assisted radial artery cannulation in infants and children. *Anesth Analg* **63**:346–348, 1984

38. Brodsky JB, Wong AL, Meyer JA: Percutaneous cannulation of weakly palpable arteries. *Anesth Analg* **56**:448, 1977

39. Buakham C, Kim JM: Cannulation of a nonpalpable artery with the aid of a Doppler monitor. *Anesth Analg* **56**:125–126, 1977

40. Chinyanga HM, Smith JM: A modified Doppler flow detector probe—An aid to percutaneous radial arterial cannulation in infants and small children. *Anesthesiology* **50**:256–258, 1979

41. Introna RPS, Silverstein PI: A new use for the pulse oximeter. *Anesthesiology* **65**:342, 1986

42. Johnson RW: Complication of radial artery cannulation. *Anesthesiology* **40**:598–600, 1974

43. Stern DH, Gerson JI, Allen FB, et al: Can we trust the direct radial artery pressure immediately following cardiopulmonary bypass? *Anesthesiology* **62**:557–561, 1985

44. Gallagher JD, Moore RA, McNicholas KW, Jose AB: Comparison of radial and femoral arterial blood pressures in children after cardiopulmonary bypass. *J Clin Monit* **1**:168–171, 1985

45. Rich GF, Lubanski RE, McLoughlin TM: Differences between aortic and radial artery pressure associated with cardiopulmonary bypass. *Anesthesiology* **77**:63–66, 1992

46. Bedford RF: Removal of radial-artery thrombi following percutaneous cannulation for monitoring. *Anesthesiology* **46**:430–432, 1977

47. Bedford RF: Radial artery function following percutaneous cannulation with 18 and 20 gauge catheters. *Anesthesiology* **47**:37–39, 1977

48. Bedford RF, Wollman H: Complications of percutaneous radial-artery cannulation: An objective prospective study in man. *Anesthesiology* **38**:228–236, 1973

49. Miyasaka K, Edmonds JF, Conn AW: Complications of radial artery lines in the pediatric patient. *Can Anaesth Soc J* **23**:9–14, 1976

50. Dalton B, Laver MB: Vasospasm with an indwelling radial artery cannula. *Anesthesiology* **34**:194–197, 1973

51. Lowenstein E, Little JW, Lo HH: Prevention of cerebral embolization from flushing radial artery cannulas. *N Engl J Med* **285**:1414–1415, 1971

52. Wolf S, Mangano DT: Pseudoaneurysm, a late complication of radial-artery catheterization. *Anesthesiology* **52**:80–81, 1980

53. Mathieu A, Dalton B, Fischer JE, Kumar A: Expanding aneurysm of radial artery after frequent puncture. *Anesthesiology* **38**:401–403, 1973

54. Freeman R, King B: Analysis of results of catheter tip culture in open-heart surgery patients. *Thorax* **30**:26–30, 1975

55. Band JD, Maki DG: Infections caused by arterial catheters

used for hemodynamic monitoring. *Am J Med* **67**:735–741, 1982

56. Vender JS, Watts DR: Differential diagnosis of hand ischemia in the presence of an arterial cannula. *Anesth Analg* **61**:465–468, 1982

57. Hack WWM, Vos A, Okken A: Incidence of forearm and hand ischaemia related to radial artery cannulation in newborn infants. *Intensive Care Med* **16**:50–53, 1990

58. Damen J, Van der Tweel I: Positive tip cultures and related risk factors associated with intravascular catheterization in pediatric cardiac patients. *Crit Care Med* **16**:221–228, 1988

59. Leroy O, Billiau V, Beuscart C, et al: Nosocomial infections associated with long-term radial artery cannulation. *Intensive Care Med* **15**:241–246, 1989

60. Huber JF: The arterial network supplying the dorsum of the foot. *Anat Rec* **80**:373–391, 1941

61. Spoerel WE, Deimling P, Aitken R: Direct arterial pressure monitoring from the dorsalis pedis artery. *Can Anaesth Soc J* **22**:91–99, 1975

62. Youngberg JA, Miller ED: Evaluation of percutaneous cannulations of the dorsalis pedis artery. *Anesthesiology* **44**:80–83, 1976

63. Park MK, Robotham JL, German VF: Systolic pressure amplification in pedal arteries in children. *Crit Care Med* **11**:286–289, 1983

64. Palm T, Husum B: Blood pressure in the great toe with simulated occlusion of the dorsalis pedis artery. *Anesth Analg* **57**:453–456, 1978

65. Johnstone RE, Greenhow DE: Catheterization of the dorsalis pedis artery. *Anesthesiology* **39**:654–655, 1973

66. Husum B, Palm T, Eriksen J: Percutaneous cannulation of the dorsalis pedis artery. *Br J Anaesth* **53**:635, 1981

67. Graves PW, Davis AL, Maggi JC, et al: Femoral artery cannulation for monitoring in critically ill children: Prospective study. *Crit Care Med* **18**:1363–1366, 1990

68. Glenski JA, Beynen FM, Brady J: A prospective evaluation of femoral artery monitoring in pediatric patients. *Anesthesiology* **66**:227–229, 1987

69. Taylor LM, Troutman R, Feliciano P, et al: Late complications after femoral artery catheterization in children less than five years of age. *J Vasc Surg* **11**:297–306, 1990

70. Vidyasagar D, Downes JJ, Boggs TR: Respiratory distress syndrome of newborn infants: II. Technic of catheterization of umbilical artery and clinical results of treatment. *Clin Pediatr* **9**:332–336, 1970

71. Cole AFD, Rolbin SH: A technique for rapid catheterization of the umbilical artery. *Anesthesiology* **53**:254–255, 1980

72. Paster SB, Middleton P: Roentgenographic evaluation of umbilical artery and vein catheters. *JAMA* **231**:742–746, 1975

73. McFadden PM, Ochsner JL: Neonatal aortic thrombosis: Complication of umbilical artery cannulation. *J Cardiovasc Surg* **24**:1–4, 1983

74. Barnes RW, Foster EJ, Janssen GA, Boutros AR: Safety of brachial arterial catheters as monitors in intensive care unit: Prospective evaluation with Doppler ultrasonic velocity detector. *Anesthesiology* **44**:260–264, 1976

75. Gordon LH, Brown M, Brown OW, Brown EM: Alternative sites for continuous arterial monitoring. *South Med J* **77**:1498–1500, 1984

76. Lawless S, Orr R: Axillary arterial monitoring of pediatric patients. *Pediatrics* **84**:273–275, 1989

77. Adler DC, Bryan-Brown CW: Use of the axillary artery for intravascular monitoring. *Crit Care Med* **1**:148–150, 1973

78. Cantwell GP, Holzman BH, Caceres MJ: Percutaneous catheterization in the pediatric patient. *Crit Care Med* **18**:880–881, 1990

79. Jernigan WR, Gardner WC, Mahr MM, Milburn JL: Use of the internal jugular vein for placement of central venous catheter. *Surg Gynecol Obstet* **130**:520–524, 1969

80. Stenzel JP, Green TP, Fuhrman BP, et al: Percutaneous central venous catheterization in pediatric intensive care unit: A survival analysis of complications. *Crit Care Med* **17**:984–988, 1989

81. Civetta JM, Gabel JC, Gemer M: Internal-jugular-vein puncture with a margin of safety. *Anesthesiology* **36**:622–623, 1972

82. Daily PO, Griepp RB, Shumway NE: Percutaneous internal jugular vein cannulation. *Arch Surg* **101**:534–536, 1970

83. English IC, Frew RM, Pigott JF, Zaki M: Percutaneous catheterization of the internal jugular vein. *Anaesthesia* **24**:521–531, 1969

84. Schwartz AJ: Percutaneous aortic catheterization—A hazard of supraclavicular internal-jugular-vein catheterization. *Anesthesiology* **46**:77, 1977

85. Mostert JP, Kenny GM, Murphy GP: Safe placement of central venous catheter into internal jugular veins. *Arch Surg* **101**:431–432, 1970

86. Mallory DL, Shawker T, Evans RG, et al: Effects of clinical maneuvers on sonographically determined internal jugular vein size during venous cannulation. *Crit Care Med* **18**:1269–1273, 1990

87. Bazaral MG, Harlan S: Ultrasonographic anatomy of the internal jugular vein relevant to percutaneous cannulation. *Crit Care Med* **9**:307–310, 1981

88. Seldinger SI: Catheter replacement of the needle in percutaneous arteriography. *Acta Radiol* **39**:368–376, 1953

89. Ullman JI, Stoelting RK: Internal jugular vein location with the ultrasound Doppler blood flow detector. *Anesth Analg* **57**:118, 1978

90. Troianos CA, Savino JS: Internal jugular vein cannulation guided by echocardiography. *Anesthesiology* **74**:787–789, 1991

91. Prince SR, Sullivan RL, Hackel A: Percutaneous catheterization of the internal jugular vein in infants and children. *Anesthesiology* **44**:170–174, 1976

92. Rao TLK, Wong AY, Salem MR: A new approach to percutaneous catheterization of the internal jugular vein. *Anesthesiology* **46**:362–364, 1977

93. English JB, Hodges MR, Sentker C, et al: Comparison of aortic pulse wave contour analysis and thermodilution methods of measuring cardiac output during anesthesia in the dog. *Anesthesiology* **52**:56–61, 1980

94. Troianos CA, Jobes DR, Ellison N: Ultrasound-guided cannulation of the internal jugular vein, a prospective, randomized study. *Anesth Analg* **72**:823–826, 1991

95. Ellermeyer WP, Keifer P: Central venous cannulation: A new and efficient device. *Anesthesiology* **65**:341–342, 1986

96. Coté CJ, Jobes DR, Schwartz AJ, Ellison N: Two approaches to cannulation of the child's internal jugular vein. *Anesthesiology* **50**:371–373, 1979

97. Nicolson SG, Sweeney MF, Moore RA, et al: Comparison of internal and external jugular cannulation of the central circulation in the pediatric patient. *Crit Care Med* **13:**747–749, 1985

98. Hayashi Y, Uchida O, Takaki O, et al: Internal jugular vein catheterization in infants undergoing cardiovascular surgery: An analysis of the factors influencing successful catheterization. *Anesth Analg* **74:**688–693, 1992

99. Garrick ML, Neches WH, Fricker FJ, et al: Usefulness of the internal jugular venous route for cardiac catheterization in children. *Am J Cardiol* **65:**1276–1278, 1990

100. Belani KG, Buckley JJ, Gordon JR, Castenada W: Percutaneous cervical central venous line placement: A comparison of the internal and external jugular vein routes. *Anesth Analg* **59:**40–44, 1980

101. Defalque RJ: Percutaneous catheterization of the internal jugular vein. *Anesth Analg* **53:**116–121, 1974

102. Escarpa A, Gomez-Arnau J: Internal jugular vein catheterization: Time required with several techniques under different clinical situations. *Anesth Analg* **62:**97–99, 1983

103. Jobes DR, Schwartz AJ, Greenhow DE, et al: Safer jugular vein cannulation: Recognition of arterial puncture and preferential use of the external jugular route. *Anesthesiology* **59:**353–355, 1983

104. Damen J, Bolton D: A prospective analysis of 1400 pulmonary artery catheterizations in patients undergoing cardiac surgery. *Acta Anaesthesiol Scand* **30:**386–392, 1986

105. McEnany MT, Austen WG: Life-threatening hemorrhage from inadvertent cervical arteriotomy. *Ann Thorac Surg* **24:**233–236, 1977

106. Milo S, Sawaed S, Adler Z, et al: Misplaced arterial catheter in an infant causes intraoperative death. *J Cardiothorac Vasc Anesth* **6:**101–104, 1992

107. Horrow JC, Laucks SO: Coronary air embolism during venous cannulation. *Anesthesiology* **56:**212–214, 1982

108. Cohen MB, Mark JB, Morris RW, Frank E: Introducer sheath malfunction producing insidious air embolism. *Anesthesiology* **67:**573–575, 1987.

109. Stock MC, Downs JB: Transient phrenic nerve blockade during internal jugular vein cannulation using the anterolateral approach. *Anesthesiology* **57:**230–233, 1982

110. Vest JV, Pereira MB, Senior RM: Phrenic nerve injury associated with venipuncture of the internal jugular vein. *Chest* **78:**777–779, 1980

111. Depierraz B, Essinger A, Morin D, et al: Isolated phrenic nerve injury after apparently atraumatic puncture of the internal jugular vein. *Intensive Care Med* **15:**132–134, 1989

112. Forestner JE: Ipsilateral mydriasis following carotid-artery puncture during attempted cannulation of the internal jugular vein. *Anesthesiology* **52:**438–439, 1980

113. Quigley RC, Petty C, Tobin G: Unusual placement of a central venous catheter via the internal jugular vein. *Anesth Analg* **53:**478, 1974

114. Blitt CD, Wright WA: An unusual complication of percutaneous internal jugular vein cannulation, puncture of an endotracheal tube cuff. *Anesthesiology* **40:**306–307, 1974

115. Cook TL, Dueker CW: Tension pneumothorax following internal jugular cannulation and general anesthesia. *Anesthesiology* **45:**554–555, 1976

116. Galvis A, Nakagawa T: Hydrothorax as a late complication of central venous catheterization in children: Diagnosis and management. *Anaesth Intensive Care* **20:**75–98, 1992

117. Mason MS, Wheeler JR, Jaffe AT, Gregory RT: Massive bilateral hydrothorax and hydromediastinum: An unusual complication of percutaneous internal jugular vein cannulation. *Heart Lung* **9:**883–886, 1980

118. DeBruijn NP, Stadt HH: Bilateral thrombosis of internal jugular veins after multiple percutaneous cannulation. *Anesth Analg* **60:**448–449, 1981

119. Moore RA, McNicholas KW, Naidech H, et al: Clinical silent venous thrombosis following internal and external jugular central venous cannulation in pediatric cardiac patients. *Anesthesiology* **62:**640–643, 1985

120. Ducatman BS, McMichan JC, Edwards WD: Catheter-induced lesions of the right side of the heart. *JAMA* **253:**791–795, 1985

121. Gaitini D, Kaftori JK, Pery M, Engel A: High-resolution real-time ultrasonography. *J Ultrasound Med* **7:**621–627, 1988

122. Blitt CD, Wright WA: Central venous catheterization via the external jugular vein. A technique employing the J-wire. *JAMA* **229:**817–818, 1974

123. Blitt CD, Carlson GL, Wright WA, Otto CW: J-wire versus straight wire for central venous system cannulations via the external jugular vein. *Anesth Analg* **61:**536–537, 1982

124. Nordstrom L, Fletcher R: Comparison of two different J-wires for central venous cannulation via the external jugular vein. *Anesth Analg* **62:**365, 1983

125. Schwartz AJ, Jobes DR, Levy WJ, et al: Intrathoracic vascular catheterization via the external jugular vein. *Anesthesiology* **56:**400–402, 1982

126. Ghani GA, Berry AJ: Right hydrothorax after left external jugular vein catheterization. *Anesthesiology* **58:**93–94, 1983

127. Eichold BH, Berryman CR: Contralateral hydrothorax: An unusual complication of central venous catheter placement. *Anesthesiology* **62:**673–674, 1985

128. Kron IL, Rheuban K, Miller ED, et al: Subclavian vein catheterization for central line placement in children under two years of age. *Am Surg* **51:**272–273, 1985

129. Pybus DA, Poole JL, Crawford MC: Subclavian venous catheterization in small children using the Seldinger technique. *Anaesthesia* **37:**451–453, 1982

130. Sanchez R, Halck S, Walther-Larsen S, Heslet L: Misplacement of subclavian venous catheters: Importance of head position and choice of puncture site. *Br J Anaesth* **64:**632–633, 1990

131. Borja AR, Hinshaw JR: A safe way to perform infraclavicular subclavian vein catheterization. *Surg Gynecol Obstet* **130:**673–676, 1970

132. Bonventre EV, Lally KP, Chwals WJ, et al: Percutaneous insertion of subclavian venous catheters in infants and children. *Surg Gynecol Obstet* **169:**203–205, 1989

133. Hoyt DB: A surgeon's view: The subclavian vein. *J Clin Monit* **1:**61–63, 1985

134. O'Leary AM: Acute upper airway obstruction due to arterial puncture during percutaneous central venous cannulation of the subclavian vein. *Anesthesiology* **73:**780–782, 1990

135. Hubsch PJS, Stiglbauer RL, Schwaighofer BWAM, et al:

Internal jugular and subclavian vein thrombosis caused by central venous catheters. *J Ultrasound Med* 7:629–636, 1988

136. Ragasa J, Shah N, Watson RC: Where antecubital catheters go: A study under fluoroscopic control. *Anesthesiology* 71:378–380, 1989

137. Sparks CJ, McSkimming I, George L: Shoulder manipulation to facilitate central vein catheterization from the external jugular vein. *Anaesth Intens Care* 19:567–568, 1991

138. Cucchiara RF, Muzzi DA: Guide-wire retention after right atrial catheter insertion. *Anesth Analg* 74:303–304, 1992

139. Oriot D, Defawe G: Percutaneous catheterization of the axillary vein in neonates. *Crit Care Med* 16:285–286, 1988

140. Metz RI, Lucking SE, Chaten FC, et al: Percutaneous catheterization of the axillary vein in infants and children. *Pediatrics* 85:531–533, 1990

141. Toussaint GPM, Burgess JH, Hampson LG: CVP and PWP in critical surgical illness. *Arch Surg* 109:265–269, 1974

142. Swan HJC: Cardiac surgery and hemodynamic monitoring. *Can Anaesth Soc J* 29:336–340, 1982

143. Lappas DG, Lell WA, Gabel JC, et al: Indirect measurement of left atrial pressure in surgical patients— Pulmonary capillary wedge and pulmonary-artery diastolic pressures compared with left atrial pressures. *Anesthesiology* 38:394–397, 1973

144. Buchbinder N, Ganz W: Hemodynamic monitoring: Invasive techniques. *Anesthesiology* 45:146–155, 1976

145. Mammana RB, Hiro S, Levitsky S, et al: Inaccuracy of pulmonary capillary wedge pressure when compared to left atrial pressure in the early postsurgical period. *J Thorac Cardiovasc Surg* 84:420–425, 1982

146. Humphrey CB, Oury JH, Virgilio RW, et al: An analysis of direct and indirect measurements of left atrial filling pressure. *J Thorac Cardiovasc Surg* 71:643–647, 1976

147. Ellis RJ, Mangano DT, Van Dyke DC: Relationship of wedge pressure to end diastolic volume in patients undergoing myocardial revascularization. *J Thorac Cardiovasc Surg* 78:605–613, 1979

148. Hansen RM, Viquerat CE, Matthay MA, et al: Poor correlation between pulmonary artery wedge pressure and left ventricular end-diastolic volume after coronary artery bypass graft surgery. *Anesthesiology* 64:764–770, 1986

149. van Daele MERM, Sutherland GR, Mitchell MM, et al: Do changes in pulmonary capillary wedge pressure adequately reflect myocardial ischemia during anesthesia. *Circulation* 81:865–871, 1990

150. Haggmark S, Hohner P, Ostman M, et al: Comparison of hemodynamic, electrocardiographic, mechanical and metabolic indicators of intraoperative myocardial ischemia in vascular surgical patients with coronary artery disease. *Anesthesiology* 70:19–25, 1989

151. Swan HJC: Cardiac surgery and haemodynamic monitoring. *Can Anaesth Soc J* 29:336–340, 1982

152. Romano A, Niguidula FN: Technique of intraoperative placement of thermodilution catheter for cardiac output measurement in children. *J Cardiovasc Surg* 21:267–270, 1980

153. Moore RA, McNicholas K, Gallagher JD, et al: Migration of pediatric pulmonary artery catheters. *Anesthesiology* 58:102–104, 1982

154. Zaidan JR, Freniere S: Use of pacing pulmonary artery catheter during cardiac surgery. *Ann Thorac Surg* 35:633–636, 1983

155. Lawson D, Kushins LG: A complication of multipurpose pacing pulmonary artery catheterization via the external jugular vein approach. *Anesthesiology* 62:3776–3778, 1985

156. Salmenpera M, Pelotola K, Rosenberg P: Does prophylactic lidocaine control cardiac arrhythmias associated with pulmonary artery catheterization? *Anesthesiology* 56:210–212, 1982

157. Pace NL: A critique of flow-directed pulmonary arterial catheterization. *Anesthesiology* 47:455–465, 1977

158. Lappas D, Lell WA, Gabel JC, et al: Indirect measurement of left atrial pressure in surgical patients— Pulmonary-capillary wedge and pulmonary artery diastolic pressures compared with left atrial pressures. *Anesthesiology* 38:394–397, 1973

159. O'Quin R, Marini JJ: Pulmonary artery occlusion pressure: Clinical physiology, measurement and interpretation. *Am Rev Respir Dis* 128:319–326, 1983

160. Suter PM, Lindauer JM, Fairley HB, Schlobohm RM: Errors in data derived from pulmonary artery blood gas values. *Crit Care Med* 3:175–181, 1975

161. Shin B, Ayella R, McAslan TC: Problems with measurement using the Swan-Ganz catheter. *Anesthesiology* 43:474–476, 1975

162. Bessette MC, Quinton L, Whalley DG, et al: Swan Ganz contamination: A protective sleeve for repositioning. *Can Anaesth Soc J* 28:86–87, 1981

163. Kopman EA, Sandza JG: Manipulation of the pulmonary arterial catheter after placement: Maintenance of sterility. *Anesthesiology* 48:373–374, 1978

164. Groeger J, Carlon GC, Howland WS: Contamination of shields for pulmonary artery catheters. *Crit Care Med* 11:320, 1983

165. Johnston WE, Prough DS, Royster RL, et al: Short-term sterility of the pulmonary artery catheter inserted through an external plastic shield. *Anesthesiology* 61:461–464, 1984

166. Oden R, Mitchell MM, Benumof JL: Detection of end-exhalation period by airway thermistor: An approach to automated pulmonary artery pressure measurement. *Anesthesiology* 58:467–471, 1983

167. Berryhill RE, Benumof JL, Rauscher LA: Pulmonary vascular pressure reading at the end of exhalation. *Anesthesiology* 49:365–368, 1978

168. Cengiz M, Crapo RO, Gardner RM: The effect of ventilation on the accuracy of pulmonary artery and wedge pressure measurements. *Crit Care Med* 11:502–507, 1983

169. Benumof JL, Saidman LJ, Arkin DB, Diamant M: Where the pulmonary artery catheters go: Intrathoracic distribution. *Anesthesiology* 46:336–338, 1977

170. Parlow JL, Milne B, Cervenko FW: Balloon flotation is more important than flow direction in determining the position of flow-directed pulmonary artery catheters. *J Cardiothorac Vasc Anesth* 6:20–23, 1992

171. Shah KB, Rao TLK, Laughlin S, El Etr AA: A review of pulmonary artery catheterization in 6245 patients. *Anesthesiology* 61:271–275, 1984

172. Sise MJ, Hollingsworth P, Bumm JE, et al: Complica-

tions of the flow-directed pulmonary artery catheter. *Crit Care Med* **9**:315–318, 1981

173. Cuasay RS, Lemole GM: Rupture of pulmonary artery by Swan Ganz catheter: A cause of postoperative bleeding after open heart operation. *Ann Thorac Surg* **32**:415–419, 1981

174. Golden MS, Pinder T, Anderson WT, Cheitlin MD: Fatal pulmonary hemorrhage complicating use of flow directed balloon-tipped catheter in a patient receiving anticoagulant therapy. *Am J Cardiol* **32**:865–867, 1973

175. Krantz EM, Viljoen JF: Hemoptysis following insertion of a Swan Ganz catheter. *Br J Anaesth* **51**:457–459, 1979

176. Lemen R, Jones JG, Cowan G: Mechanism of pulmonary artery perforation by Swan Ganz catheters. *N Engl J Med* **292**:211, 1975

177. McDaniel DD, Stone JG, Faltas AN, et al: Catheter-induced pulmonary artery hemorrhage. *J Thorac Cardiovasc Surg* **82**:1–4, 1981

178. Pape LA, Haffajee CI, Markis JE, et al: Fatal pulmonary hemorrhage after use of the flow-directed balloon tipped catheter. *Ann Intern Med* **90**:344–347, 1979

179. Paulson DM, Scott SM, Sethe GK: Pulmonary hemorrhage associated with balloon flotation catheters. *J Thorac Cardiovasc Surg* **80**:453–458, 1980

180. Hardy J-F, Morisette M, Taillefer J, Vauclair R: Pathophysiology of rupture of the pulmonary artery by pulmonary artery balloon catheters. *Anesth Analg* **62**:925–930, 1983

181. Gomez-Arnau J, Montero CG, Luengo C, et al: Retrograde dissection and rupture of pulmonary artery catheter after catheter use in pulmonary hypertension. *Crit Care Med* **10**:694–695, 1982

182. Barbieri LT, Kaplan JA: Artifactual hypotension secondary to intraoperative transducer failure. *Anesth Analg* **62**:112–114, 1983

183. Kopman EA: Hemoptysis associated with the use of flow-directed catheter. *Anesth Analg* **58**:153–154, 1979

184. Connors JP, Sandza JG, Shaw RC, et al: Lobar pulmonary hemorrhage. *Arch Surg* **115**:883–885, 1980

185. Rosenbaum L, Rosenbaum SH, Askanazi J, et al: Small amounts of hemoptysis as an early warning sign of pulmonary artery rupture by a pulmonary artery catheter. *Crit Care Med* **9**:319–320, 1981

186. Yellin LB, Filler JJ, Barnette RE: Nominal hemoptysis heralds pseudoaneurysm induced by a pulmonary artery catheter. *Anesthesiology* **74**:370–373, 1991

187. Cervenko FW, Shelley SE, Spence DG, et al: Massive endobronchial hemorrhage during cardiopulmonary bypass: Treatable complication of balloon tipped catheter damage to the pulmonary artery. *Ann Thorac Surg* **35**:326–328, 1983

188. Stein JM, Lisbon A: Pulmonary hemorrhage from pulmonary artery catheterization treated with endobronchial intubation. *Anesthesiology* **55**:698–699, 1981

189. Rice PL, Pifarré R, El Etr AA, et al: Management of endobronchial hemorrhage during cardiopulmonary bypass. *J Thorac Cardiovasc Surg* **81**:800–801, 1981

190. Scuderi PE, Prough DS, Price JD, Comer PB: Cessation of pulmonary artery catheter-induced endobronchial hemorrhage associated with the use of PEEP. *Anesth Analg* **62**:236–238, 1983

191. Kron IL, Piepgrass W, Carabello B, et al: False aneurysm of the pulmonary artery: A complication of pulmonary artery catheterization. *Ann Thorac Surg* **33**:629–630, 1982

192. Feng WC, Singh AK, Drew T, Donat W: Swan-Ganz catheter-induced massive hemoptysis and pulmonary artery false aneurysm. *Ann Thorac Surg* **50**:644–646, 1990

193. Richman KA, Kim YL, Marshall BE: Thrombocytopenia and altered platelet kinetics associated with prolonged pulmonary-artery catheterization in the dog. *Anesthesiology* **53**:101–105, 1980

194. Kim JM, Arakawa K, Bliss J: Arterial cannulation: Factors in the development of occlusion. *Anesth Analg* **54**:836–841, 1975

195. Devitt JH, Noble WH, Byrick RJ: A Swan Ganz related complication in a patient with Eisenmenger's syndrome. *Anesthesiology* **57**:335–337, 1982

196. Goodman DJ, Rider AK, Billingham ME, Schroeder JS: Thromboembolic complications with the indwelling balloon tipped pulmonary artery catheter. *N Engl J Med* **291**:777, 1974

197. Hoar PF, Stone JG, Wicks AE, et al: Thrombogenesis associated with Swan Ganz catheters. *Anesthesiology* **48**:445–447, 1978

198. Chastre J, Ciornud F, Bouchama A, et al: Thrombosis as a complication of pulmonary artery catheterization via the internal jugular vein. *N Engl J Med* **306**:278–281, 1982

199. Nichols AB, Owen J, Grossman BA, et al: Effect of heparin bonding on catheter-induced fibrin formation and platelet activation. *Circulation* **70**:843–850, 1984

200. Perkins NAK, Bedford RF, Buschi AJ, Cail WS: Internal jugular vein function after Swan Ganz catheterization. *Anesthesiology* **61**:456–459, 1984

201. Geha DG, Davis NJ, Lappas DG: Persistent atrial arrhythmias associated with placement of a Swan Ganz catheter. *Anesthesiology* **39**:651–653, 1973

202. Abernathy WS: Complete heart block caused by Swan Ganz catheter. *Chest* **65**:349, 1976

203. Thomson IR, Dalton BC, Lappas DG, Lowenstein E: Right bundle branch block caused by the Swan Ganz catheter. *Anesthesiology* **51**:359–362, 1979

204. Eissa NT, Kvetan V: Guide wire as a cause of complete heart block in patients with preexisting left bundle branch block. *Anesthesiology* **73**:772–774, 1990

205. Keusch DJ, Winters S, Thys DM: The patient's position influences the incidence of dysrhythmias during pulmonary artery catheterization. *Anesthesiology* **70**:582–584, 1989

206. Foote GA, Schabel SI, Hodges M: Pulmonary complication of the flow-directed balloon-tipped catheter. *N Engl J Med* **290**:927–931, 1974

207. Lange HW, Galliani CA, Edwards JE: Local complications associated with indwelling Swan-Ganz catheters. Autopsy study of 36 cases. *Am J Cardiol* **52**:1108–1111, 1983

208. O'Toole JD, Wurtzbacher JJ, Wearner NE, Jain AC: Pulmonary-valve injury and insufficiency during pulmonary-artery catheterization. *N Engl J Med* **301**:1167–1168, 1979

209. Green JF, Fitzwater JE, Clemmer TP: Septic endocardi-

tis and indwelling pulmonary artery catheters. *JAMA* **233:** 891–892, 1975

210. Conahan TJ: Air embolism during percutaneous Swan-Ganz catheter placement. *Anesthesiology* **50:**360–361, 1979

211. Parulkar DS, Grundy EM, Bennett EJ: Fracture of a float catheter. *Br J Anaesth* **50:**201–203, 1978

212. Smith WR, Glauser FL, Jemison P: Ruptured chordae of tricuspid valve: Consequence of flow-directed Swan Ganz catheterization. *Chest* **70:**790–792, 1976

213. Block PC: Snaring of the Swan-Ganz catheter. *J Thorac Cardiovasc Surg* **71:**918–919, 1976

214. Culpeper JA, Setter M, Rinaldo JE: Massive hemoptysis and tension pneumothorax following pulmonary artery catheterization. *Chest* **82:**380–382, 1982

215. Gordon EP, Quan SF, Schlobohm RM: Hydromediastinum after placement of a thermodilution pulmonary arterial catheter. *Anesth Analg* **59:**159–160, 1980

216. Daum S, Shapira M: Intracardiac knot formation in a Swan Ganz catheter. *Anesth Analg* **52:**862–863, 1973

217. Michel L, Marsh HM, McMichan JC, et al: Infection of pulmonary artery catheters. *JAMA* **245:**1032–1036, 1981

218. Bricker DL, Dalton ML: Cardiac tamponade following dislodgement of a left atrial catheter after coronary artery bypass. *J Thorac Cardiovasc Surg* **66:**636–638, 1973

219. Talner NS, Lister G: Perioperative care of the infant with congenital heart disease. *Cardiol Clin* **7:**419–437, 1989

220. Fagard R, Conway J: Measurement of cardiac output: Fick principle using catheterization. *Eur Heart J* **11**(suppl I):1–5, 1990

221. Morton WD: The non-invasive determination of cardiac output in children: A three-breath technique. *Anesthesiology* **69:**223–226, 1988

222. Weisel RD, Berger RL, Hechtman HB: Measurement of cardiac output by thermodilution. *N Engl J Med* **292:**682–684, 1975

223. Lund-Johansen P: The dye dilution method for measurement of cardiac output. *Eur Heart J* **11**(suppl I):6–12, 1990

224. Truccone NJ, Spotnitz HM, Gersony WM, et al: Cardiac output in infants and children after open heart surgery. *J Thorac Cardiovasc Surg* **71:**410–411, 1976

225. Hillis LD, Firth BG, Winniford MD: Comparison of thermodilution and indocyanine green dye in low cardiac output or left-sided regurgitation. *Am J Cardiol* **57:**1201–1202, 1986

226. Conway J, Lund-Johansen P: Thermodilution method for measuring cardiac output. *Eur Heart J* **11**(suppl I):17–20, 1990

227. Platchetka JR, Larson DF, Salomon NW, Copeland JG: Comparison of two closed systems for thermodilution cardiac outputs. *Crit Care Med* **9:**487–489, 1981

228. Todd MM: Atrial fibrillation induced by the right atrial injection of cold fluids during thermodilution cardiac output determination. A case report. *Anesthesiology* **59:**253–255, 1983

229. Nishikawa T, Dohi S: Slowing of heart rate during cardiac output measurement by thermodilution. *Anesthesiology* **57:**538–539, 1982

230. Katz RI, Teller ED, Poppers PJ: Ventricular fibrillation during thermodilution cardiac output determination. *Anesthesiology* **62:**376–377, 1985

231. Stevens JH, Raffin TA, Mihm FG, et al: Thermodilution cardiac output measurement. *JAMA* **253:**2240–2242, 1985

232. Fegler G: Measurement of cardiac output in anesthetized animals by a thermodilution method. *Q J Exp Physiol* **39:** 153–164, 1954

233. Levett JM, Replogle RL: Thermodilution cardiac output: A critical analysis and review of the literature. *J Surg Res* **27:**392–404, 1979

234. Thrush DN, Varlotta D: Thermodilution cardiac output: Comparison between automated and manual injection of indicator. *J Cardiothorac Vasc Anesth* **6:**17–19, 1992

235. Nakao S, Come PC, Miller MJ, et al: Effects of supine and lateral positions on cardiac output and intracardiac pressures: An experimental study. *Circulation* **73:**579–585, 1986

236. Wetzel RC, Latson TW: Major errors in thermodilution cardiac output measurement during rapid volume infusion. *Anesthesiology* **62:**684–687, 1985

237. Bazaral MG, Petre J, Novoa R: Errors in thermodilution cardiac output measurements caused by rapid pulmonary artery temperature decreases after cardiopulmonary bypass. *Anesthesiology* **77:**31–37, 1992

238. Fischer AP, Benis AM, Jurado RA, et al: Analysis of errors in measurement of cardiac output by simultaneous dye and thermal dilution in cardiothoracic surgical patients. *Cardiovasc Res* **112:**190–199, 1978

239. Morady F, Brundage BH, Gelberg HJ: Rapid method for determination of shunt ratio using a thermodilution technique. *Am Heart J* **106:**369–373, 1983

240. Reininger EJ, Troy BL: Error in thermodilution cardiac output measurement caused by variation in syringe volume. *Cathet Cardiovasc Diagn* **2:**415–417, 1976

241. Pearl RG, Rosenthal MH, Nielson L, et al: Effect of injectate volume and temperature on thermodilution cardiac output determination. *Anesthesiology* **64:**798–801, 1986

242. Vennix CV, Nelson DH, Pierpoint GL: Thermodilution cardiac output in critically ill patients: Comparison of room-temperature and ice injectate. *Heart Lung* **13:**574–578, 1984

243. Merrick SH, Hessel EA, Dillard DH: Determination of cardiac output by thermodilution during hypothermia. *Am J Cardiol* **46:**419–422, 1980

244. Shellock FG, Reidinger MS, Bateman TM, Gray RJ: Thermodilution cardiac output determination in hypothermic postcardiac surgery patients: Room versus ice injectate. *Crit Care Med* **11:**668–670, 1983

245. Wessel HU, Paul MH, James GW, Grahn AR: Limitations of thermal dilution curves for cardiac output determination. *J Appl Physiol* **30:**643–652, 1971

246. Kiggins CM, Lake CL, Ross WT: The shunting Swan Ganz catheter. *J Cardiothorac Anesth* **3:**229–234, 1989

247. Nelson LD, Houtchens BA: Automatic versus manual injection for thermodilution cardiac output determinations. *Crit Care Med* **10:**190–192, 1982

248. Abrams JH, Weber RE, Holman KD: Continuous cardiac output determination using transtracheal Doppler: Initial results in humans. *Anesthesiology* **71:**11–15, 1989

249. Alverson DC, Eldridge N, Dillon T, et al: Noninvasive pulsed Doppler determination of cardiac output in neonates and children. *J Pediatr* **101:**46–50, 1982

250. Lees MH: Cardiac output determination in the neonate. *J Pediatr* **102:**709–711, 1983

251. Keagy BA, Wilcox BR, Lucas CL, et al: Constant postoperative monitoring of cardiac output after correction of congenital heart defects. *J Thorac Cardiovasc Surg* **93**: 658–664, 1987

252. Morrow WR, Murphy DJ, Fisher DJ, et al: Continuous wave Doppler cardiac output: Use in pediatric patients receiving inotropic support. *Pediatr Cardiol* **9**:131–136, 1988

253. Rose JS, Nanna M, Rahimtoola S, et al: Accuracy of determination of changes in cardiac output by transcutaneous continuous-wave Doppler computer. *Am J Cardiol* **54**: 1099–1101, 1984

254. Berman W, Alverson DC: Assessment of hemodynamic function with pulsed Doppler ultrasound. *J Am Coll Surg* **5**:104S–112S, 1985

255. Siegel LC, Fitzgerald DC, Engstrom RH: Simultaneous intraoperative measurement of cardiac output by thermodilution and transtracheal Doppler. *Anesthesiology* **74**: 664–669, 1991

256. Kumar A, Minagoe S, Thangathurai D, et al: Noninvasive measurement of cardiac output during surgery using a new continuous-wave Doppler esophageal probe. *Am J Cardiol* **64**:793–798, 1989

257. Siegel LC, Pearl RG: Noninvasive cardiac output measurement: Troubled technologies and troubled studies. *Anesth Analg* **74**:790–792, 1992

258. Maedra M, Yokota M, Iwase M, et al: Accuracy of cardiac output measured by continuous wave Doppler echocardiography during dynamic exercise testing in the supine position in patients with coronary artery disease. *J Am Coll Surg* **13**:76–83, 1989

259. Wong DH, Watson T, Gordon I, et al: Comparison of changes in transit time ultrasound, esophageal Doppler, and thermodilution cardiac output after changes in preload, afterload, and contractility in pigs. *Anesth Analg* **72**: 584–588, 1991

260. Wong DH, Mahutte CK: Two-beam pulsed Doppler cardiac output measurement: Reproducibility and agreement with thermodilution. *Crit Care Med* **18**:433–437, 1990

261. Hausen B, Schafers H-J, Rohde R, Haverich A: Clinical evaluation of transtracheal Doppler for continuous cardiac output estimation. *Anesth Analg* **74**:800–804, 1992

262. Kubicek WG, Karnegis JN, Patterson RP, et al: Development and evaluation of an impedance cardiac output system. *Aerospace Med* **37**:1208–1212, 1966

263. Miles DS, Gotshall RW, Golden JC, et al: Accuracy of electrical impedance cardiography for measuring cardiac output in children with congenital heart defects. *Am J Cardiol* **61**:612–616, 1988

264. Tibballs J, Hochmann M, Osborne A, Carter B: Accuracy of the BoMED NCCOM3 bioimpedance cardiac output monitor during induced hypotension: An experimental study in dogs. *Anaesth Intensive Care* **20**:326–331, 1992

265. Introna RPS, Pruett JK, Crumrine RC, Cuadrado AR: Use of transthoracic bioimpedance to determine cardiac output in pediatric patients. *Crit Care Med* **16**:1101–1105, 1988

266. O'Connell AJ, Tibballs J, Coulthard M: Improving agreement between thoracic bioimpedance and dye dilution cardiac output estimation in children. *Anaesth Intensive Care* **19**:434–440, 1991

267. White SW, Quail AW, DeLeeuw PW, et al: Impedance cardiography for cardiac output measurement: An evaluation of accuracy and limitations. *Eur Heart J* **11**(suppl I):79–92, 1990

268. Novak I, Elliott MJ: Noninvasive estimation of total body water in critically ill children after cardiac operations. *J Thorac Cardiovasc Surg* **104**:585–589, 1992

269. Hilgenberg JC: Pulmonary vascular impedance: Resistance versus pulmonary artery diastolic-pulmonary artery occluded pressure gradient. *Anesthesiology* **58**:484–485, 1983

270. Davenport HT, Arfel G, Sanchez FR: The electroencephalogram in patients undergoing open heart surgery with heart-lung bypass. *Anesthesiology* **20**:674–684, 1959

271. Bashein G, Nessly ML, Bledsoe SW, et al: Electroencephalography during surgery with cardiopulmonary bypass and hypothermia. *Anesthesiology* **76**:878–891, 1992

272. El-Fiki M, Fish KJ: Is the EEG a useful monitor during cardiac surgery? A case report. *Anesthesiology* **67**:575–578, 1987

273. Levy WJ: Intraoperative EEG patterns: Implications for EEG monitoring. *Anesthesiology* **60**:430–434, 1984

274. Sharbrough FW, Messick JM, Sundt TM: Correlation of continuous electroencephalogram with cerebral blood flow measurements during carotid endarterectomy. *Stroke* **4**:676–683, 1973

275. Salerno TA, Lince DP, White DN, et al: Monitoring of the electroencephalogram during open heart surgery. *J Thorac Cardiovasc Surg* **76**:97–100, 1978

276. Burrows FA, Volgyesi GA, James PD: Clinical evaluation of the augmented delta quotient monitor for intraoperative electroencephalographic monitoring of children during surgery and cardiopulmonary bypass for repair of congenital cardiac defects. *Br J Anaesth* **63**:565–573, 1989

277. McCormick PW, Stewart M, Goetting MG, et al: Noninvasive cerebral optical spectroscopy for monitoring cerebral oxygen delivery and hemodynamics. *Crit Care Med* **19**:89–97, 1991

278. Hampson NB, Camporesi EM, Stolp BW, et al: Cerebral oxygen availability by NIR spectroscopy during transient hypoxia in humans. *J Apply Physiol* **69**:907–913, 1990

279. Shah AR, Kurth CD, Gwiazdowski SG, et al: Fluctuations in cerebral oxygenation and blood volume during endotracheal suctioning in premature infants. *J Pediatr* **120**:769–774, 1992

280. Lindegaard KF, Bakke SJ, Grolimund P, et al: Assessment of intracranial hemodynamics in carotid artery disease by transcranial Doppler ultrasound. *J Neurosurg* **63**: 890–898, 1985

281. Pilato MA, Bissonnette B, Lerman J: Transcranial Doppler: Response of cerebral blood-flow velocity to carbon dioxide in anaesthetized children. *Can J Anaesth* **38**: 37–42, 1991

282. Thiel A, Zickmann B, Zimmermann R, Hempelmann G: Transcranial Doppler sonography: Effects of halothane, enflurane and isoflurane on blood flow velocity in the middle cerebral artery. *Br J Anaesth* **68**:388–393, 1992

283. Van der Linden J, Priddy R, Ekroth R, et al: Cerebral perfusion and metabolism during profound hypothermia in children. *J Thorac Cardiovasc Surg* **102**:103–114, 1991

284. Barker SJ, Hyatt J: Continuous measurement of intraarterial pHa, $PaCO_2$, and PaO_2 in the operating room. *Anesth Analg* **73**:43–48, 1991

285. Greenblott GB, Tremper KK, Barker SJ, et al: Continuous blood gas monitoring with an intra-arterial optode during one-lung anesthesia. *J Cardiothorac Vasc Anesth* **5:**365–367, 1991

286. Tremper KK, Barker SJ: Pulse oximetry. *Anesthesiology* **70:**98–108, 1989

287. Severinghaus JW, Kelleher JF: Recent developments in pulse oximetry. *Anesthesiology* **76:**1018–1038, 1992

288. Yelderman M, New W: Evaluation of pulse oximetry. *Anesthesiology* **59:**349–352, 1983

289. Mihm FG, Halperin BD: Noninvasive detection of profound arterial desaturations using a pulse oximetry device. *Anesthesiology* **62:**85–87, 1985

290. Yemen TA: Noninvasive monitoring in the pediatric patient. *Int Anesth Clin* **30:**77–90, 1992

291. Mackenzie N: Comparison of a pulse oximeter with an ear oximeter and an in vitro oximeter. *J Clin Monit* **1:**156–160, 1985

292. Casthely PA, Redko V, Dluzneski J, et al: Pulse oximetry during pulmonary artery banding. *J Cardiothorac Anesth* **1:**297–299, 1987

293. Friesen RH: Pulse oximetry during pulmonary artery surgery. *Anesth Analg* **64:**376, 1985

294. Lawson D, Norley I, Korbon G, et al: Blood flow limits and pulse oximeter signal detection. *Anesthesiology* **67:**599–603, 1987

295. Kandel G, Aberman A: Mixed venous oxygen saturation. *Arch Intern Med* **143:**1400–1402, 1983

296. Baele PL, McMichan JC, Marsh HM, et al: Continuous monitoring of mixed venous oxygen saturation in critically ill patients. *Anesth Analg* **61:**513–517, 1982

297. McMichan JC: Continuous monitoring of mixed venous oxygen saturation in clinical practice. *Mt Sinai J Med* **51:**569–572, 1984

298. Waller JL, Kaplan JA, Bauman DI, Craver JM: Clinical evaluation of a new fiberoptic catheter oximeter during cardiac surgery. *Anesth Analg* **61:**676–679, 1982

299. Fahey PJ, Harris K, Vanderwarf C: Clinical experience with continuous monitoring of mixed venous oxygen saturation in respiratory failure. *Chest* **86:**748–752, 1984

300. Rah KH, Dunwiddie WC, Lower RR: A method for continuous postoperative measurement of mixed venous oxygen saturation in infants and children after open heart operations. *Anesth Analg* **63:**873–881, 1984

301. Jamieson WRE, Turnbull KW, Larrieu AJ, et al: Continuous monitoring of mixed venous oxygen saturation in cardiac surgery. *Can J Surg* **25:**538–543, 1982

302. Schranz D, Schmitt S, Oelert H, et al: Continuous monitoring of mixed venous oxygen saturation in infants after cardiac surgery. *Intensive Care Med* **15:**228–232, 1989

303. Baudendistel L, Goudsouzian N, Cote C, et al: End-tidal CO_2 monitoring. *Anaesthesia* **39:**1000–1003, 1984

304. Schuller JL, Bovill JG: Severe reduction in end-tidal PCO_2 following unilateral pulmonary artery occlusion in a child with pulmonary hypertension. *Anesth Analg* **68:**792–794, 1989

305. Fletcher R: The relationship between the arterial to end-tidal PCO_2 differences and hemoglobin saturation in patients with congenital heart disease. *Anesthesiology* **75:**210–216, 1991

306. Baker AB, McLeod C: Oesophageal multipurpose monitoring probe. *Anaesthesia* **38:**892–897, 1983

307. Cooper JO, Cullen BF: Observer reliability in detecting surreptitious random occlusions of the monaural esophageal stethoscope. *J Clin Monit* **6:**271–275, 1991

308. Andritsch RF, Muravchick S, Gold MI: Temperature correction of arterial blood-gas parameters. *Anesthesiology* **55:**311–316, 1981

309. Ream AK, Reitz BA, Silverberg G: Temperature correction of pCO_2 and pH in estimating acid-base status. *Anesthesiology* **56:**41–44, 1982

310. Murkin JM, Farrar JK, Tweed A, et al: Cerebral autoregulation and flow/metabolism coupling during cardiopulmonary bypass: The influence of $PaCO_2$. *Anesth Analg* **66:**825–832, 1987

311. Hindman BJ, Funatsu N, Harrington J, et al: Differences in cerebral blood flow between alpha-stat and pH-stat management are eliminated during periods of decreased systemic flow and pressure. *Anesthesiology* **74:**1096–1102, 1991

312. Basheín G, Townes BD, Nessly MC, et al: A randomized study of carbon dioxide management during hypothermic cardiopulmonary bypass. *Anesthesiology* **72:**7–15, 1990

313. Stephan H, Weyland A, Kazmaier S, et al: Acid-base management during hypothermic cardiopulmonary bypass does not affect cerebral metabolism but does affect blood flow and neurological outcome. *Br J Anaesth* **69:**51–57, 1992

314. Watanabe T, Miura M, Inui K, et al: Blood and brain tissue gaseous strategy for profoundly hypothermic total circulatory arrest. *J Thorac Cardiovasc Surg* **102:**497–504, 1991

315. Baraka AS, Baroody MA, Haroun ST, et al: Effect of alpha-stat versus pH-stat strategy on oxyhemoglobin dissociation and whole-body oxygen consumption during hypothermic cardiopulmonary bypass. *Anesth Analg* **74:**32–37, 1992

316. Badner NH, Murkin JM, Lok P: Differences in pH management and pulsatile/nonpulsatile perfusion during cardiopulmonary bypass do not influence renal function. *Anesth Analg* **75:**696–701, 1992

317. Cork RC, Vaughan RW, Humphrey LS: Precision and accuracy of intraoperative temperature monitoring. *Anesth Analg* **62:**211–214, 1983

318. Bissonnette B: Temperature monitoring in pediatric anesthesia. *Intensive Anesth Clin* **30:**63–76, 1992

319. Bissonnette B, Sessler DI, LaFlamme P: Temperature monitoring sites in infants and children and the effect of inspired gas warming on esophageal temperature. *Anesth Analg* **69:**192–196, 1989

320. Moorthy SS, Winn BA, Jallard MS, Smith ND: Monitoring urinary bladder temperature. *Heart Lung* **14:**90–93, 1985

321. Lilly JK, Boland JP, Zekan S: Urinary bladder temperature monitoring: A new index of body core temperature. *Crit Care Med* **8:**742–744, 1980

322. Muravchick S, Conrad DP, Vargas A: Peripheral temperature monitoring during cardiopulmonary bypass operation. *Ann Thorac Surg* **29:**36–41, 1980

Chapter 9 | Pediatric Anesthesia Pharmacology

D. Ryan Cook and Peter J. Davis

During the first several months of life, there is rapid physical growth and maturation that causes a rapid change in the factors involved in the uptake, distribution, redistribution, metabolism, and excretion of drugs.[1-6] Important differences in these processes between the infant and adult explain the young infant's altered quantitative responses to many anesthetic drugs and adjuncts. Variations in drug penetration of the blood-brain barrier and in the sensitivity of the neuromuscular junction have been observed in infants for some anesthetics and neuromuscular blocking agents. Although physical growth and physiologic maturation gradually take place over childhood, pharmacologic maturation takes place in the first six months of life. The purposes of this chapter are to discuss the factors that influence the infant's handling of drugs in general; to site specific pharmacologic differences in the responses to certain anesthetic drugs and adjuncts in children and adults; and to review the pharmacology of newer induction agents commonly used for cardiac anesthesia. Few age-related comparative studies of the cardiovascular effects of these drugs have been performed for many of the anesthetic agents and adjuncts.

DEVELOPMENTAL PHARMACOLOGY

Drug Absorption

Most anesthetic drugs (other than inhalation anesthetics) are given parenterally. The intravenous route is the most direct, bypassing the absorption barriers. Drugs in aqueous solution injected intramuscularly are often absorbed fairly rapidly; subcutaneously injected drugs are usually more slowly absorbed. Absorption from intramuscular and subcutaneous sites depends mainly on tissue perfusion, and if perfusion is adequate, this absorption is similar in children and adults. The vasomotor instability in

the newborn period theoretically might delay absorption from peripheral sites, although in practice the therapeutic effectiveness of drugs given via these routes suggests that this is not an important factor.[7]

On rare occasions, anesthesiologists give either oral or rectal medication (sedative-hypnotics) to infants, usually for diagnostic procedures. Such drugs are given in solution, not as tablets or capsules, so that disintegration and dissolution are irrelevant. They are absorbed across the gut by passive diffusion that depends upon the physicochemical properties of the drug and the surface area of the gut available for diffusion.[8-9] Because most drugs are weak acids or weak bases, the un-ionized fraction that is available for diffusion will vary with the pH of the fluid in the gut (eg, the pH of gastric fluid varies between 1.5 and 6.0, whereas the intestinal fluid is considerably more alkaline).

In adults, the total absorptional area of the small intestine is probably 200 m^2 compared with 1 m^2 for the stomach. Because of this larger surface area, acidic drugs are absorbed more rapidly from the alkaline small intestine than from the acidic stomach in spite of their being highly un-ionized in the intestine. In large part, therefore, the rate of gastric emptying is a controlling factor in drug absorption from the gut (ie, slower gastric emptying delays a drug's access to the small intestine and vice versa). Gastric emptying may be slowed by food, drugs, or surgical conditions. Once a drug is in the small intestine, up to 4-10 hours are available for absorption; however, most drugs reach peak concentrations by 30-40 minutes. Thus, changes in intestinal transit time have little effect on drug absorption. Likewise, very few drugs are absorbed rapidly enough for blood flow to be a rate-limiting factor. There are no functional differences among the older infant, child, and adult that should affect gastrointestinal absorption. The rate, but not extent, of absorption of many drugs may be increased by using liquid preparations. In the newborn period and after the first day of life, gastric contents are less acidic and the gastric emptying time and intestinal transit time are considerably slower than at any other age.[10] Consequently, drugs such as penicillin G and ampicillin, which are partially inactivated by a low pH, have greater overall absorption when swallowed. The slow gastric emptying time reduces the absorption of some drugs, whereas other drugs may achieve greater absorption because of prolonged contact with the bowel wall during the longer transit period through the intestine.

Drug Distribution

The distribution process regulates the amount of drug reaching specific body compartments or tissues and hence the concentration of the drug at the receptor site. Distribution is influenced mainly by protein binding, red blood cell binding, tissue volumes, tissue solubility coefficients, and blood flow to various tissues. Extracellular inert binding to plasma proteins depends on the amount of binding protein available (albumin or other serum proteins) and the drug affinity constant for proteins; these factors are directly or indirectly modified by pathophysiologic conditions and by other drugs and compounds.[11–18]

The degree of binding to proteins is usually measured as the percentage of total nondialyzable drug in the blood, ie, that bound to large molecules. Binding to nonreceptor proteins also takes place outside the vascular compartment and may account for a significant fraction of the total drug in the body. The volume of distribution of a drug is directly proportional to the fraction of free drug in the plasma. Drug molecules bound to inert binding sites are not available for diffusion or interaction with receptors but are, however, in equilibrium with free drug. Thus alterations in the concentration of free drug will result in changes in the amount (but not the percentage) bound. Nonreceptor protein binding sites are not very specific, ie, many weak acids with different pharmacologic effects bind to the same or closely related plasma protein sites. Therefore, different drugs may compete for the same binding sites. This can have important consequences when a high percentage of a potent drug (A) is bound; the binding sites must be loaded to achieve a therapeutic concentration of free drug in the plasma. Addition of a second drug (B) that competes for the same inert binding site (but not the receptor site) may result in a marked increase in the concentration of free drug A and thereby precipitate toxicity. A quantitative and qualitative reduction in plasma protein binding occurs in the newborn period.[19–21] Infants, particularly preterm infants, have lower plasma albumin concentrations than at other ages (30–40 g/L); the albumin is qualitatively different and has a low affinity for drugs. Further modification of plasma protein binding is likely to occur at this age as a result of the

higher free fatty acid and bilirubin concentrations and the lower blood pH. Concentrations of α-acid glycoproteins that bind many alkaline drugs are lower in the newborn than in the adult. Decreased protein binding may, therefore, contribute to the larger apparent volume of distribution for many drugs (eg, ketamine).[22]

In the neonate, differences in the size of the body fluid compartments, relatively smaller muscle mass and fat stores, and presumably greater blood flow per unit of organ weight influence the distribution of drugs to their active site and secondary redistribution. Age-related differences in tissue solubility coefficients also exist. Metabolism and excretion may take place during redistribution. Total body water, extracellular fluid, and blood volume of the neonate are larger on a weight basis than those of an adult.[23–24] The initial larger volume for distribution of a parenterally administered drug may explain, in part, why neonates appear to require larger amounts of some drugs on a weight basis to produce a given effect. Table 9–1 gives developmental estimates of tissue volumes and tissue blood flow derived from physiologic studies and from autopsy of normal tissue at the Children's Hospital in Pittsburgh.[24–27] A high proportion of the cardiac output is distributed to the vessel-rich organs, particularly to the brain. Smaller muscle mass and fat stores provide less uptake to inactive sites and tend to keep plasma concentration higher. The smaller amount of fat tissue in neonates provides a relatively small reservoir for fat-soluble drugs.

Blood-Brain Barrier. The blood-brain barrier, a lipid membrane interface between the endothelial cells of the brain vasculature and the extracellular fluid of the brain,

TABLE 9–1. TISSUE VOLUME AND BLOOD FLOW IN INFANTS AND ADULTS

	Infants	Adults
Brain volume (mL/kg)	90	21
Brain blood flow (% CO)	34 %	14.3%
Heart volume (mL/kg)	4.5	4
Coronary blood flow (% CO)	3	4.3
Splanchnic organ volume (mL/kg)	70	57
Splanchnic flow (% CO)	25	28.6
Kidney volume (mL/kg)	10	6
Renal blood flow (% CO)	18	25.7
Muscle volume (mL/kg)	180	425
Muscle blood flow (% CO)	10	11.4
Volume of poorly perfused tissues (mL/kg)	270	270
Flow to poorly perfused tissue (% CO)	5	10
Fat volume (mL/kg)	100	150
Fat blood flow (% CO)	5	10

Abbreviation: CO, cardiac output.
(Data compiled from references 24–27.)

may be "immature" at birth.[28–35] The intercellular clefts of brain are closed, the so-called tight junctions. Transport of drugs into and out of brain depends on principles identical to those determining the movement of substances across other biologic membranes. The rate of penetration of un-ionized drugs into brain increases with the degree of lipid solubility. Active transport mechanisms or specific carrier systems allow rapid changes of certain biologically active compounds and of certain inorganic and organic anions either into or from the brain. Some polar metabolites are cleared from the brain by diffusion into cerebral spinal fluid (ie, sink action).

Oldendorf[36–38] has measured the blood-brain barrier permeability during a single capillary pass for a number of drugs relative to a highly diffusible tracer like water or butanol. The uptake of the drug is expressed as a percentage of the uptake of the highly diffusable tracer, the brain uptake index (BUI). Drugs with an oil-water partition coefficient less than 0.01 hardly penetrate the cerebral capillaries during a single pass, whereas those with a partition coefficient greater than 0.1 are likely to have 50% or more penetration. Drugs having a partition coefficient greater than about 0.03 will undergo substantially complete clearance during a single brain passage. If the lipid solubility of a compound is very high, rapid diffusion across the barrier leads to rapid equilibration between blood and brain. The rate of entry is then determined by blood flow. Because in the infant the brain receives a large proportion of cardiac output, it is not surprising that the brain concentration of many drugs is higher in the infant than in the adult. Regional differences in brain perfusion will also affect the uptake of compounds into brain.

Neuromuscular System. Throughout infancy the neuromuscular junction matures physically and biochemically, the contractile properties of skeletal muscle change, the amount of muscle in proportion to body weight increases, and the neuromuscular junction is variably sensitive to neuromuscular blocking drugs.[39] The structural and functional development of the neuromuscular system is incomplete at birth.[40–44] The conduction velocity of motor nerves increases throughout gestation as nerve fibers myelinate. The myotubules connect to mature muscle fibers in the latter part of intrauterine life and in the first several weeks after birth. Some slow-contracting muscles (intrinsic muscles of the hand) are progressively converted to fast-contracting muscles, with a concomitant change in the force-velocity relationship. Both the diaphragm and intercostal muscles in infants increase the percentage of slow muscle fibers in the first months of life. Synaptic transmission is relatively slow at birth, but more important, the rate at which acetylcholine is released during repetitive nerve stimulation is limited in the infant. This margin of safety for neurotransmission is reduced in infants compared with adults.

Unanesthetized newborn infants appear to have less neuromuscular reserve during tetanic stimulation than do adults. In neonates, there is no fade of twitch height with repetitive stimulation at rates of 1–2 Hz; at 20 Hz, however, there is significant fade. Premature infants may show post-tetanic exhaustion for 15–20 minutes.[45] Goudsouzian[46] noted slower contraction times of the thumb following slow and rapid rates of stimulation in term infants (1–10 days of age, anesthetized with halothane) than in older children. The percent of fading at 20, 50, or 100 Hz did not differ between the infants and the older children; however, the tetanic stimulus was applied for only 5 seconds. The train-of-four ratio (the ratio of the amplitude of the fourth evoked response to the amplitude of the first response in the same train), the degree of post-tetanic facilitation, and the tetanus twitch ratio increase with age. Crumrine and Yodlowski[47] noted a decrease in the amplitude of the frequency sweep electromyogram (FS-EMG) at frequencies of 50–100 Hz in infants less than 12 weeks of age (Fig 9–1). The FS-EMG is a recording of the action potential from an electrical stimulus rate that increases expotentially from 1 pulse per second to 100 Hz over a stimulation period of 10 seconds. The exponential increase in frequency allows assessment of neuromuscular transmission of tetanic rates without inducing fatigue. In older infants and children, Crumrine and Yodlowski[47] found that there was little or no decrement in the FS-EMG at the higher frequencies of stimulation. Similarly, the FS-EMG response of full-term infants less than 12 weeks old was depressed after administration of 70% nitrous oxide, whereas that of the older patients did not change.

Biotransformation and Excretion

Renal Excretion. Renal excretion plays a pivotal role in terminating the biologic activity of a few drugs that have small molecular sizes or have polar characteristics at physiologic pH. Most drugs do not possess such physiochemical properties. Pharmacologically active organic molecules tend to be highly lipophilic and remain un-ionized or only partially ionized at physiologic pH. They are often strongly bound to plasma proteins. Such substances are not readily filtered at the glomerulus. The lipophilic nature of renal tubular membranes also facilitates the reabsorption of hydrophobic compounds following their glomerular filtration. Consequently, most drugs would have a prolonged duration of action if their termination depended solely on renal excretion.

Nevertheless, the ultimate route of elimination of most drugs or their metabolites is by way of the kidney. Because many drugs are simply filtered by the kidney, glomerular filtration rate influences drug excretion and action. Inulin and thiosulfate clearances, which reflect the glomerular filtration rate (GFR), are lower in newborns and young children then in adults. Volume clear-

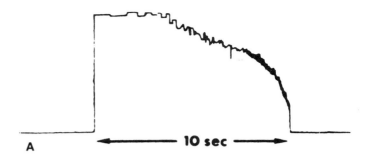

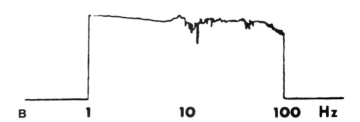

Figure 9–1. (*A*) Frequency sweep electromyogram of a 1-day-old infant. Note the decrease in amplitude of twitch in the newborn infant compared to (*B*) from a 4-month-old infant. (*From Crumrine RS, et al: Assessment of neuromuscular function in infants. Anesthesiology 54:29–32, 1981, with permission.*)

ance, when related to surface area, approaches adult values at about 3 months. If, on the other hand, clearance is related to weight, adult values are reached in about 10 days to 2 weeks. The time-clearance method resolves the question of which basis to select. The elimination half-life for thiosulfate is about three times slower in newborns than in older children or adults; by 3 weeks of age, these differences disappear. The maturation of glomerular function may be related to changes in the permeability of the glomerular membrane or to conversion of nonfunctional glomeruli to functional participants in the process of filtration. Proximal tubular secretion assumes adult values in the first 4–5 months of age.[48] The glucuronide and sulfate metabolites of drugs may be secreted through the proximal tubules by an acid pump mechanism.

Metabolism. An alternative process that may lead to the termination of alteration of biologic activity is metabolism. In general, lipophilic drugs are transformed to more polar and hence more readily excretable products. Most metabolic biotransformations occur at some point between absorption of the drug into the general circulation and its renal elimination. A few transformations occur in the intestinal lumen or intestinal wall. In general, all of these reactions can be assigned to two major categories called phase I and phase II reactions. Phase I reactions usually convert the parent drug to a more polar metabolite by introducing or unmasking a functional group (-OH, -NH$_2$, -SH). Often these metabolites are inactive, although in some instances activity is only modified. Metabolic products are often less active than the

parent drug and may even be inactive. However, some biotransformation products have enhanced activity or toxic properties, including mutagenicity, teratogenicity, and carcinogenicity. Some phase I metabolites are readily excreted, whereas others undergo conjugation or phase II metabolism.

Although at all ages every tissue has some ability to metabolize drugs, the liver is the principal organ of drug metabolism. The overall rate of metabolism probably depends on both the size of the liver and the metabolizing ability of the appropriate microsomal enzyme system. Liver volume relative to body weight decreases from birth to adulthood, with the relative volume in the first year of life being twice that at 14 years (see Table 9–1). Other sites of considerable metabolic activity include gastrointestinal tract, lungs, skin, and kidney. After oral administration many drugs (eg, isoproterenol, meperidine, and morphine) are absorbed intact from the small intestine and transported first via the portal system to the liver, where they undergo extensive metabolism. This process is called the first-pass effect. Some orally administered drugs are more extensively metabolized in the intestine than in the liver. Thus, intestinal metabolism may contribute to the overall first-pass effect. First-pass effects may so greatly limit the bioavailability of orally administered drugs that alternative routes of administration must be used to achieve therapeutically effective blood levels.

Enzyme Induction. Although drug biotransformation in vivo can occur by spontaneous, noncatalyzed chemical reactions, the vast majority are catalyzed by specific cellular enzymes. Many drug-metabolizing enzymes are located in the lipophilic membranes of the endoplasmic reticulum of the liver and other tissues. When these lamellar membranes are isolated by homogenization and fractionation of the cell, they re-form into vesicles called microsomes. Microsomes retain most of the morphologic and functional characteristics of the intact membranes, including the rough and smooth surface features of the rough (ribosome-studded) and smooth (no ribosomes) endoplasmic reticulum. Whereas the rough microsomes tend to be dedicated to protein synthesis, the smooth microsomes are relatively rich in enzymes responsible for oxidative drug metabolism. In particular, they contain the important class of enzymes known as the mixed-function oxidases.

Microsomal drug oxidations require cytochrome P-450, cytochrome P-450 reductase, nicotine adenine diphosphate hydrogenase (NADPH), and molecular oxygen. The relative abundance of cytochrome P-450, as compared with that of the reductase in the liver, contributes to making cytochrome P–450 reduction of heme the rate-limiting step in hepatic drug oxidations. The potent oxidizing properties of this activated oxygen permit oxidation of a large number of substrates. Substrate specificity is very low for this enzyme complex. High solubility in lipids is the only common feature of the wide variety of structurally unrelated drugs and chemicals that serve as substrates in this system.

A variety of dissimilar drugs on repeated administration can "induce" the cytochrome P-450 systems by enhancing the rate of their synthesis or reducing their rate of degradation. In infants, the enzyme activity of the cytochrome P-450 systems can be increased by benzopyrene or phenobarbital. Thus, the low enzyme activity for various substrates reflects lack of stimulation rather than inability of the enzyme system to be stimulated.[49] The age from birth is important for maturation of these enzyme systems, not the duration of gestation. Premature infants and mature-born infants develop the ability to metabolize drugs to the same degree at the same time period after birth. Of the phase I reactions, drug oxidation is most deficient in neonates, substrate reduction less so, and hydrolyzation nearly as effective as in adults. Oxidative and reduction enzymes increase to adult levels within the first few days of life. Other drug substrates may inhibit cytochrome P-450 enzyme activity.[50–51]

Phase II Reactions. Phase II reactions involve the coupling or conjugation reactions of either parent drug or phase I metabolite with an endogenous substance to yield drug conjugates. In general, conjugates are polar molecules that are readily excreted and often inactive. Certain conjugation reactions (*O*-sulfation of *N*-hydroxy-acetylaminofluorene and *N*-acetylation of isoniazid) may lead to the formation of reactive species responsible for the hepatotoxicity of the drug. Conjugate formation involves high-energy intermediates and specific transfer enzymes. Such enzymes (transferases) may be located in microsomes or in the cytosol. They catalyze the coupling of an activated endogenous substance (such as the uridine 5′-diphosphate [UDP] derivative of glucuronic acid) with a drug or of an activated drug with an endogenous substrate. Because the endogenous substrates originate in the diet, nutrition plays a critical role in the regulation of drug conjugations.

The hepatic enzyme systems responsible for the metabolism of drugs are incompletely developed or absent in the neonate. Phase II processes, conjugation with sulfate, acetate, glucuronic acid, or amino acids are severely limited at birth.[48,52] Neonatal hepatic tissues, for example, are unable to synthesize glucuronides because of low tissue levels of UDP, glucuronic acid, and UDP-transferase, the latter of which catalyses transfer of glucuronic acid to foreign molecules.[53] Conjugation reactions with acetate occur by 1 month of age, with glucuronide by 2 months, and with amino acids by 3 months. Some of these metabolized drugs are recirculated and excreted in the urine; other metabolites or unmetabolized drugs are excreted in the bile.

Biotransformation of Inhalation Anesthetics. Significant biotransformation of inhalation anesthetics occur in the liver. The metabolites may be toxic to tissue. Carbon tetrachloride and chloroform are hepatotoxic in adult animals; however, they are not hepatotoxins in animals less than 1–2 weeks of age. In the newborn rat, the metabolism of halothane takes several weeks to reach adult levels.[54] Free fluoride concentration, a nephrotoxic metabolite of methoxyflurane, is lower in infants and children.[55] Nephrotoxicity from free fluoride, reported after enflurane anesthesia in obsese patients, is unlikely in infants because of their limited fat deposits. Likewise, biotransformation of isoflurane is unlikely. Differences in the relative rates of metabolism of inhalation anesthetics in infants and adults have not been compared nor has any determination been made of differences in intermediate metabolites.

INHALATION ANESTHETICS

Uptake and Distribution

The uptake of nitrous oxide and halothane is more rapid in infants and small children than in adults.[56–60] Salanitre and Rackow compared the uptake of nitrous oxide among infants 0–6 months of age, 15-year-old children, and two groups of adults.[57] An end-tidal concentration/inspired concentration (FE/FI) ratio of 1 occurred in infants in about 25 minutes, in children in about 30 minutes, and in adults at about 60 minutes. Steward and Creighton[58] likewise noted more rapid washout of nitrous oxide in infants than in adults. These age-related differences in anesthetic uptake are more striking with halothane, which has a fivefold higher blood solubility than nitrous oxide. Salanitre and Rackow showed that the uptake of halothane was more rapid in children 15 years of age than in adults.[57] However, the uptake of halothane was determined concurrently with that of nitrous oxide. The rapid uptake of nitrous oxide may have influenced the early uptake of halothane because of the so-called "second gas effect." More recently, Brandom et al noted that the uptake of halothane is, indeed, more rapid in infants than in adults[60] (Fig 9–2).

Major differences between adults and infants in blood gas solubility coefficients, body composition, alveolar ventilation, and the distribution of cardiac output explain the concomitant differences in their rates of uptake of anesthetic. Tidal volume on a weight basis (7 mL/kg) is relatively constant throughout life. However, the infant has a relatively high alveolar ventilation, particularly in relation to its functional residual capacity (FRC). The alveolar ventilation to FRC ratio is about 5:1 in infants contrasted with 1.4:1 in adults. The lung time constant is estimated to be 0.19 minutes in infants and 0.73 minutes in adults for a gas with limited blood solubility (helium

and nitrous oxide). Thus, lung washin or lung washout of inhalation anesthetics is relatively more rapid in infants than in adults. In infants, controlled ventilation that increased alveolar ventilation would further increase this ratio; in adults, it would appear difficult to utilize tidal breaths approaching FRC in magnitude.

The blood gas solubility coefficients for halothane have been shown to vary with age.[60–61] Halothane is less soluable in blood taken from the fetal circulation of the placenta than it is in blood taken from adults. The influence of hematocrit, hemoglobin type, and plasma protein fractions on anesthetic solubility has not been well defined. The blood gas solubility coefficient of nitrous oxide varied about 3% as hematocrit increased from 30 to 52%. If all other things were equal, the high cardiac output of the infant (on a weight basis about twice that of the adult) would retard the uptake of inhalation anesthetics. However, this effect is minimized by other factors. More important, a larger percentage of the infant's cardiac output is distributed to the vessel-rich tissue group. Compared with the adult, the infant has increased brain mass and limited muscle mass and fat; significant differences in tissue blood flow correspond to these differences in tissue compartments.

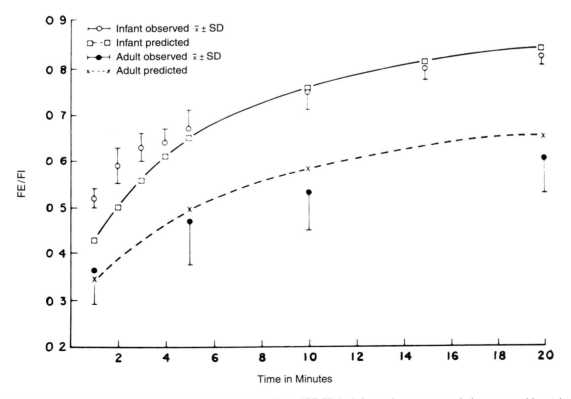

Figure 9–2. The observed ratio of expired to inspired halothane (FE/FI) in infants demonstrates their more rapid uptake of halothane compared with adults. (*Observed data for adults are from Sechzer PM, et al: Uptake of halothane by the human body. Anesthesiology 24:779–783, 1963, and Eger EI II, et al: The effect of age on the rate of increase of alveolar anesthetic concentration. Anesthesiology 35:365–372, 1971. Predicted curves were generated from a computer model from Brandom BW, et al: Uptake and distribution of halothane in infants: In vivo measurements and computer simulations. Anesth Analg 62:404–410, 1983, reprinted with permission from the International Anesthesia Society.*)

The concentration of halothane in tissues (eg, the brain and heart) will increase more rapidly in infants than in adults given the same inspired concentration of halothane[60,63] (Fig 9–3). The reduced muscle mass of the infant compared with the adult, and the concurrent reduction of the proportion of cardiac output perfusing muscle, tends to concentrate the cardiac output in infants toward the more highly perfused vessel-rich organs such as the brain and heart. Early in an anesthetic induction, the infant has a higher tissue concentration of anesthetic than the adult; at some relatively infinite time, both will have the same tissue concentrations if one assumes the partition coefficients to be the same in infants and adults. Another way to state this difference is in terms of tissue time constants, Vi/Q (blood-tissue solubility coefficient times volume divided by tissue blood flow). Given the same concentration of anesthetic in arterial blood, the anesthetic concentration will increase more rapidly in a tissue with a shorter time constant. Time constants of infant tissues are less than the corresponding time constants in the adult.

Effects of Shunting on Uptake.

Intracardiac shunts can alter the uptake of inhalation anesthetics.[64–65] Their influence is more pronounced with relatively insoluble agents. A right-to-left shunt slows the uptake of anesthetic as the anesthetic tension or concentration in the arterial blood increases more slowly.[65] Induction of anesthesia is prolonged. Using overpressure to achieve a more rapid induction in infants with significant right-to-left shunts from congenital heart disease can be hazardous. If significant cardiovascular depression occurs from a relative anesthetic overdose, it is equally difficult to decrease the anesthetic concentration. The influence of a left-to-right shunt on anesthetic uptake depends on the size of the shunt and on whether a right-to-left shunt exists.[66] A large (>80%) left-to-right shunt increases the rate of anesthetic transfer from the lungs to the arterial blood; smaller shunts (<50%) have a neglible effect on uptake. A left-to-right shunt may speed induction when it coexists with a large right-to-left shunt. Increases in pulmonary vascular resistance or decreases in systemic vascular resistance occasionally can reverse left-to-right shunts.

Anesthetic Requirements

The anesthetic requirements for various inhalation anesthetics (halothane and enflurane) generally are related inversely to age.[66–70] Anesthetic requirements are usually quantitated by MAC, the maximum alveolar concentration of anesthetic at which 50% of the patients move (or do not move) in response to a surgical stimulus. Alternatively, one can estimate MAC for an individual patient as an intermediate concentration between a concentration associated with movement and a concentration associated with no movement. The MAC (or ED_{50}, median effective dose) for halothane in infants and children has been determined by several groups of investigators.

In the first months of life, the relation between age and MAC is somewhat complex. During the first week of

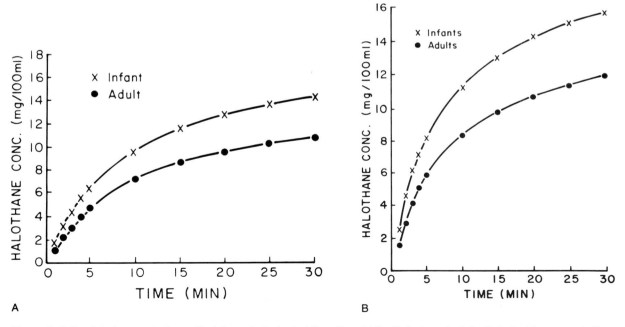

Figure 9–3. Predicted concentrations of halothane in the brain (*A*) and heart (*B*) of infants and adults. Note that the concentrations of halothane in both organs increases more rapidly in the infant. (*From Brandom BW, et al: Uptake and distribution of halothane in infants: In vivo measurements and computer simulations. Anesth Analg 62:404–410, 1983, reprinted with permission from the International Anesthesia Research Society.*)

life, the response of the newborn to pain is attenuated even in the awake state. During the first few months of life, both the sensitivity to pain and the behavioral response to pain rapidly mature. Gregory and co-workers[70] noted that the MAC for halothane is lower in the fetal lamb than in the newborn lamb; in addition, the MAC for halothane increased over the first 12 hours of life in the newborn lambs. The increase in MAC in the newborn lambs was associated with a decrease in serum progesterone (Fig 9–4). At pharmacologic doses, progesterone is an anesthetic in the rat. No causal relationship exists.[71] Increased metabolic rate and oxygen consumption after birth may also contribute to the increase in anesthetic requirements. Increased plasma peptide concentrations have been documented in newborns during the immediate postnatal period; in the first month of life, these concentrations decrease to adult concentrations.[72] In adults, peptides do not cross the blood-brain barrier. In neonates, one could postulate increased permeability of the blood-brain barrier to these peptides, although cerebrospinal fluid (CSF) concentrations have not been documented. However, Gregory and colleagues could not reverse the early "analgesia" in newborn lambs with naloxone.[70]

Equally as perplexing as the progressive increase in MAC through the first month or so of life is the gradual and progressive decrease after 6 months. Is this related to changes in oxygen consumption, is it related to differences in anesthetic solubilities, or is it a conundrum of definition? MAC is an indirect measurement of the anesthetic partial pressure at the anesthetic sites of action. At equilibrium the partial pressure of anesthetic is equal in all tissue compartments of the body. However, the tissue concentration (mg/100 g tissue) of anesthetic will vary with the solubility of the anesthetic in that tissue. Miller and co-workers[73] have suggested that a certain anesthetic molar concentration at the sites of action is necessary to produce anesthesia. The molar concentration of anesthesia at the site of action is the product of the anesthetic partial pressure and the anesthetic solubility at the site. Measurement of anesthetic concentration in the brain allows one to estimate the molar concentration required in the brain to produce anesthesia. Cook and colleagues[63] noted that the ED_{50} for halothane was higher in 15-day-old rats than in 30- or 60-day-old rats. In contrast, the concentration of halothane in the brain under anesthesia was lower in the 15-day-old rats than in the older rats. This difference in brain concentration for halothane as a function of age is most likely due to the difference in water content in the younger rats. When corrected for differences in water content, the estimated halothane concentrations in brain dry weight appear comparable in the three age groups of rats. This suggests that nearly equal concentrations of halothane in the nonaqueous phase of the brain are achieved at the endpoint of anesthesia in different aged animals. A higher partial pressure of anesthetic (ED_{50} or MAC) may be necessary in the younger animal to compensate for the high water content of the developing brain.

Age-related differences in blood gas solubility coefficients may also influence the brain anesthetic concentration and hence contribute to age-related differences in MAC. One can alter the blood gas solubility coefficient of halothane while holding all other physiologic variables constant to assess the effect of this change on brain anesthetic concentrations (B.W. Brandom, unpublished data). With a blood gas solubility coefficient of 2.3, the FE/FI ratio was 0.813 after 45 minutes of exposure to 0.5% halothane; the corresponding estimate of brain halothane concentration was 15.6 mg/100 mL. With a solubility coefficient of 1.9, that measured in neonatal cord blood, the FE/FI ratio was 0.843 after 45 minutes; the corresponding brain halothane concentration was

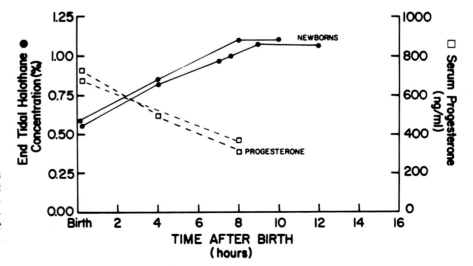

Figure 9–4. The increase in MAC after birth is demonstrated in two lambs. Although not causally related, progesterone decreases during the first few hours after birth. (*From Gregory GA, et al: Fetal anesthetic requirement (MAC) for halothane. Anesth Analg 62:9–14, 1983, with permission.*)

13.2 mg/100 mL. The decrease in blood gas solubility coefficient caused a more rapid increase in FE/FI and a slower increase in tissue anesthetic concentration. FE/FI was 3% higher with the less soluable anesthetic but the associated brain concentration was 17% lower. These data suggest that changes in blood gas solubility may contribute to age-dependent differences in the movement of anesthetic through the body to the brain and hence to age-dependent differences in anesthetic requirements.

Cardiovascular Effects of Inhalation Anesthetics

The incidence of bradycardia, hypotension, and cardiac arrest during induction of anesthesia is higher in infants and small children than in adults.[68,74-76] This has been attributed to an increased sensitivity of the cardiovascular system to potent agents. Rao and colleagues[77] noted that halothane, isoflurane, and enflurane depress the force of contraction in isolated neonatal rat atria significantly more than in the adult atria (Fig 9–5). This may be related to the decreased contractile element in the neonatal myocardium. However, the greater incidence of untoward effects can be attributed partly to differences in uptake and to the use of higher than necessary inspired concentrations of potent agents. The myocardial and brain concentration of anesthetic at equal inspired concentrations may be higher early in anesthetic induction in the infant than in the adult. These higher tissue concentrations may produce what appears to be augmented cardiovascular effect. To define clearly the issue of age-related cardiovascular sensitivity, it is necessary to measure simultaneously the determinants of cardiac output in anesthetized patients (or animals) at known end-tidal concentrations of anesthetic and at known MAC multiples. In addition, it is necessary to define the sensitivity of cardiovascular "protective" reflexes (baroreceptor reflex) at MAC multiples of the anesthetic. Direct measurement of cardiac output, contractility, preload, and afterload involves invasive techniques. Few patient studies have been done, but the results of several key animal studies are available.

The hemodynamic effects of halothane have been determined in the developing piglet.[78] MAC for halothane in piglets (111 days) was 0.87% (range 0.73–0.099%).[78] Cardiac index (CI), mean arterial pressure (MAP), heart rate (HR), and all contractility indexes (LV [left ventricular] peak dp/dt, shortening fraction, and mean rate of LV circumferential fiber shortening) decreased relative to concentration after 0.5 and 1.0% halothane. When heart rate was kept constant with atrial pacing, dp/dt/DP_{40}, CI, and MAP remained severely depressed at the two concentrations of halothane. Estimates of preload, stroke volume index, and total peripheral vascular index did not change significantly. Thus, the major adverse hemodynamic effect of

halothane was its negative inotropic action, not negative chronotropic or loading activity. This effect occurred at a concentration less than MAC. These cardiovascular changes were not age related. In piglets studied by Bailie and co-workers,[79] profound bradycardia and hypotension were associated with an unexplained increase in peripheral resistance. The change in cardiovascular response to halothane with age in the piglet is similar to that in newborn infants and children. In the study of Boudreaux and co-workers,[78] the degree of change of each variable with the administration of 1% halothane did not correlate with age over the first 2.5 weeks of life. However, the pattern of cardiovascular response to halothane in pigs appears to change with increasing age beyond this period. At equal end-tidal halothane concentrations supplemented by 60–70% nitrous oxide, 3-month-old pigs (21–28 kg) studied by Merin and colleagues[80] had a depression of CI comparable to that observed in younger animals. However, MAP was considerably lower in the older animal study than it was in Boudreaux and co-workers' study[78] and was accompanied by peripheral vasodilation and marked reduction in the first derivative of developed pressure over time (dp/dt). In Boudreaux and colleagues' study,[78] newborn piglets had less profound reductions in CI, MAP, and dp/dt and no important change in peripheral resistance (SVR, systemic vascular resistance). Of note, bradycardia occurred regularly only in the newborn piglets (Table 9–2). These differences in HR among pigs of different ages under halothane anesthesia were probably due to the more highly developed baroreceptor responses of the older animals.[81] Lerman and co-workers[69] found that at equipotent concentrations of halothane, the incidence of hypotension and bradycardia was equal in neonates and infants. These data agree with our findings that the maximal degrees of change in MAP and HR did not correlate significantly with age.

In a similar study of Schieber and co-workers, the MAC for isoflurane in piglets was determined to be 1.20% ± 0.4%.[82] At 0.5 MAC, isoflurane caused a large, significant reduction in MAP, SVR index, and dp/dt at a developed pressure of 40 mm Hg (dp/dt/DP_{40}). At 1 MAC, MAP and dp/dt/DP_{40} decreased further and SVR index shortening fraction remained depressed. At 1.3 MAC, these four variables remained low. Preload (LVEDP, left ventricular end-diastolic pressure) and stroke volume index (SVI) did not change significantly during the study period. CI and HR were significantly less than baseline only at 1.3 MAC, although bradycardia did not occur in all animals. Atrial pacing at baseline HR was used in five piglets that developed bradycardia at 1.3 MAC to determine the influence of HR on the other variables. CI then remained within 2% of baseline, whereas MAP and SVR index each decreased 49% and dp/dt/DP_{40} decreased 45% from baseline values. The large decrease in MAP at 1 MAC isoflurane was offset by

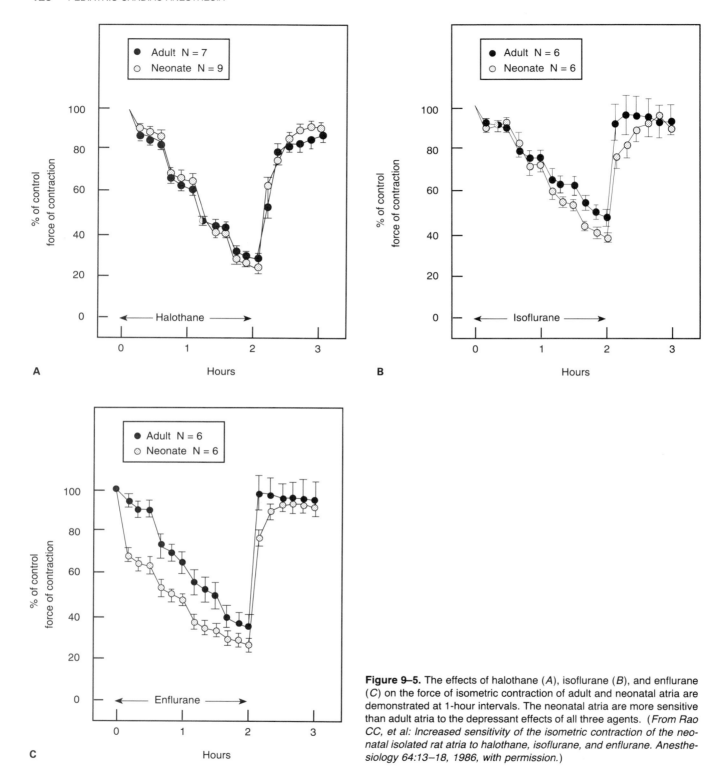

Figure 9–5. The effects of halothane (*A*), isoflurane (*B*), and enflurane (*C*) on the force of isometric contraction of adult and neonatal atria are demonstrated at 1-hour intervals. The neonatal atria are more sensitive than adult atria to the depressant effects of all three agents. (*From Rao CC, et al: Increased sensitivity of the isometric contraction of the neonatal isolated rat atria to halothane, isoflurane, and enflurane. Anesthesiology 64:13–18, 1986, with permission.*)

a similar decrease in afterload, leaving CI unchanged. During pacing dp/dt/DP$_{40}$ is a particularly reliable indicator of LV contractility because it is independent of changes in HR, preload, and afterload. The large reduction in afterload may have also partly offset the effect of reduced contractility on CI. However, the reduced MAP should have caused tachycardia via the baroreceptor response. The lack of tachycardia signifies either an immature baroreflex or a drug-induced attenuation of baroreceptor responsiveness.

TABLE 9–2. CARDIOVASCULAR RESPONSES TO HALOTHANE IN NEWBORN AND OLDER SWINE EXPRESSED AS PERCENT OF CONTROL

Cardiovascular Response	0.05% Halothane		1% Halothane	
	Older (%)	Newborn (%)	Older (%)	Newborn (%)
HR	110	86	111	73
MAP	67	84	45	66
LVEDP	118	120	132	161
dp/dt	42	68	25	43
CO	90	82	68	71
SV	82	81	61	89
SVR	71	98	57	89

(Data for older swine (3 months) from Merin RG, et al: Dose dependent depression of cardiac function and metabolism in swine (Sus scrofa). Anesthesiology 46:417–423, 1977. Data for newborn swine from Boudreaux JP, et al: Hemodynamic effects of halothane in the newborn piglet. Anesth Analg 63:731–737, 1984.)

Isoflurane had fewer adverse cardiovascular effects than 1.3 MAC halothane in the same animal model. Although the drugs reduced dp/dt and HR at 1.3 MAC, isoflurane reduced SVR index three times as much and MAP one and a half times as much as did halothane; the resulting reduction in CI with isoflurane was thus only half that with halothane. At 0.5 MAC, isoflurane increased CI, whereas halothane reduced it. During anesthesia in the newborn, isoflurane may permit greater hemodynamic stability than halothane. The alarming reduction in MAP caused by isoflurane may reflect only a decrease in peripheral resistance in the face of normal cardiac output.

Effects of Anesthetics on Baroreceptor Reflexes

Baroreceptor reflexes modulate changes in blood pressure by altering heart rate, myocardial contractility, and systemic vascular resistance. In the unanesthetized infant, particularly the premature infant, these protective reflexes may be limited. Anesthetic agents may further blunt these reflexes. To evaluate baroresponses, Gregory[83] examined the relationship among changes in heart rate and blood pressure in premature infants anesthetized with halothane having ligation of a patent ductus arteriosus (PDA). After the ductus was ligated and systemic blood flow increased, the arterial pressure had increased 38% (to about control values) without a change in heart rate. These data suggest that potent anesthetics abolish baroreceptor activity in premature infants.

In subsequent studies, the effect of halothane and nitrous oxide on the baroresponse in adult and baby rabbits was evaluated.[84–85] In these studies, the baroreceptor response was tested by increasing the systolic pressure 20–30% with phenylephrine. When the baroreflexes are intact, this increase in systolic pressure decreases heart rate. The slope of the heart rate versus systolic pressure curve, a reflection of baroreflex sensitivity, was decreased in adults and babies with

halothane in a concentration (dose)–dependent manner. More important, the sensitivity of the reflex was lower in the awake baby rabbits than in the awake adults; at equal MAC multiples of halothane, the reflex was attenuated more in the baby rabbits than in the adult rabbits. Halothane (1 MAC) effectively abolished the baroresponse in baby rabbits (Fig 9–6). In the newborn rabbit, nitrous oxide also diminishes baroreceptor activity in a concentration-dependent manner to the same degree as does halothane (at equal MAC multiples).

The reasons why anesthesia depresses the baroreceptor reflexes more in baby rabbits are unknown. Most likely, they are related to developmental differences in the autonomic nervous system (see Chapter 3). Baroresponses may be mediated in part by acute changes in plasma catecholamines. Young animals have significant amounts of norepinephrine in their adrenergic terminals, but the nerves fail to arborize and incompletely penetrate the myocardium. In addition, the vascular response to vasopressors is also less in the neonate than in the adult. The baroresponse included a reduction in sympathetic outflow. Because the neonate's sympathetic nervous system is inadequately developed, an increase in systolic pressure may not permit the heart rate to decrease as much. The parasympathetic nervous system is very active in the newborn.

The lack of responsiveness of the baroreflexes places the infant at considerable disadvantage during anesthesia with potent inhalation anesthetics. For reasons previously discussed, the incidence of hypotension and bradycardia is high in this age group.

Margin of Safety

The separation between MAC and the lethal concentration of a potent inhalation anesthetic defines the safety margin or therapeutic ratio. Wolfson and colleagues[86,87] determined the therapeutic ratio (TR) of the potent anesthetic in adult rats:

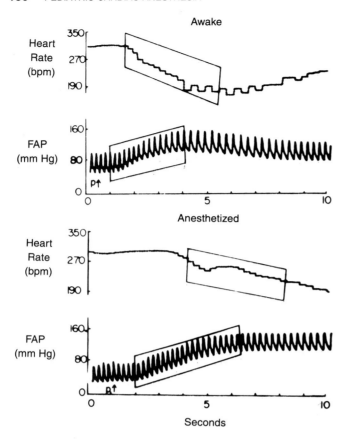

Figure 9–6. The abolition of the baroreceptor response during halothane anesthesia in a baby rabbit is demonstrated. P is the point of injection of phenylephrine. In the awake state, heart rate decreases within three beats of the pressure increase, whereas in the anesthetized state, there is no response until nine beats. (*From Wear R, et al: The effect of halothane on the baroresponse of adult and baby rabbits. Anesthesiology 56:188–191, 1982, with permission.*)

$$TR = \frac{\text{Mean anesthetic heart concentration at cardiovascular failure}}{\text{Mean anesthetic heart concentration at anesthesia}}$$

In Wolfson et al's study,[86,87] isoflurane had a higher therapeutic ratio than did halothane. Kissen and co-workers[88] confirmed these findings and in addition noted that the standard safety margin, the percentage by which the ED_{95} (effective dose in 95% of test subjects) has to be increased before the LD_{50} (median lethal dose) is reached, is also higher with isoflurane than with halothane.

Cook and colleagues[63] noted that the therapeutic ratio for halothane was decreased about 50% in young rats compared with older rats. Their study suggests that at higher anesthetic concentrations myocardial contractility and protective cardiovascular reflexes are not preserved in the infant. Isoflurane and halothane were found

to have similar therapeutic ratios in the newborn piglet (2.5:1.0).[82]

New Anesthetic Agents

A new potent inhalational anesthetic, desflurane has recently been released. Another new agent sevoflurane is currently undergoing clinical trials. Because of their low blood gas solubilities, these agents should demonstrate rapid uptake and elimination.

Desflurane. This is a potent inhalational anesthetic with a blood gas solubility of 0.46 and an oil gas coefficient of 18.7. The boiling point of the gas is room temperature. Consequently, it requires a pressurized, heated vaporizer for delivery of anesthetic gases. In healthy adults, the minimal alveolar concentration is between 6 and 7. In children, Lerman has noted age-related changes in MAC that are similar to the other potent inhalational agents. On exposure to soda lime, desflurane is markedly stable and undergoes negligible metabolism or degradation.[89]

Little information is available on the cardiovascular effects of desflurane in humans. In swine, the cardiovascular effects of desflurane appear similar to the effects of isoflurane.[90] In humans, desflurane appears to decrease mean arterial blood pressure and vascular resistance more than isoflurane. At concentrations less than 1.5 MAC, desflurane maintained cardiac output by increasing HR.[91]

In chronically instrumented dogs with multivessel coronary artery obstruction, desflurane does not appear to redistribute coronary blood flow away from collateral-dependent myocardium.[92] Studies in pediatric patients are limited. Although hemodynamic stability appears maintained with desflurane, coughing and laryngospasm upon induction of anesthesia are major problems. Clinical experience suggests that these side effects will significantly delay the onset of anesthesia regardless of the low solubility of the gas.

Sevoflurane. This is a potent halogenated inhalation anesthetic undergoing investigational trials. Its low blood gas solubility provides a rapid induction of anesthesia. It has a blood gas solubility of 0.6 and an oil gas partition coefficient of 47.2.[93] In healthy adults the MAC required for sevoflurane was 1.71% ± 0.07% and the ED_{95} was 2.07%. The addition of N_2O can reduce the MAC of sevoflurane by 61%.[94] Sevoflurane has been reported to be unstable on exposure to soda lime, with the degradation amounting to a few percent during a 3-hour exposure.[95] More recently, Eger has reported that the rate of anesthetic degradation increases with temperature and that compared with desflurane, isoflurane, and halothane, sevoflurane undergoes the greatest amount of degradation.[89] In dogs, sevoflurane is metabolized to inorganic fluoride and hexafluoroisopropanol.[96] Studies by Strum of rats pretreated with phenobarbital and placed in a hypoxic environment demonstrated that sevoflurane passed through soda lime was no more toxic than isoflurane and less toxic than halothane.[93]

Little information is available on the cardiovascular effects of sevoflurane in humans. In the animal model, Bernard et al noted that at 1.2 and 2.0 MAC, except for the changes in HR, the effects of sevoflurane on blood pressure, coronary blood flow, left ventricular dp/dt, stroke volume, and cardiac output were similar to equipotent concentrations of isoflurane.[97] In neonatal piglets, Lerman has shown that 1.5 MAC sevoflurane decreased HR and MAP but had little effect on the CI.[98]

INTRAVENOUS DRUGS

Sedative-Hypnotics

A variety of sedative-hypnotic drugs appear to have increased toxic effects in the neonate.[99] The mechanism of this increased sensitivity has been elucidated for some of the barbiturates and benzodiazepines.

Barbiturates. On a milligram per kilogram basis, barbiturates are more lethal to newborns than to more mature animals.[100–102] The sleeping times of newborn animals are markedly prolonged at sublethal doses given on an equal milligram per kilogram basis.[102] Greater penetration of the blood-brain barrier by barbiturates has been found in neonates as opposed to older animals.[103] The BUI of pentobarbital at 15 seconds has been determined in developing rats (Cook DR, unpublished observations). The BUI was higher in the younger rats and exceeded 100% (Table 9–3). These data suggest that capillary transit time is less than 15 seconds in younger rats. High brain blood flow rather than differential permeability probably explains these observations for pentobarbital, which is highly lipid soluble. In addition, the brain levels of hexobarbital on arousal or following death from respiratory failure are lower in neonates than in adults. This suggests that the barbiturates are more potent in the neonatal brain.

Neonates have a decreased ability to metabolize barbiturates.[104] The longer-acting barbiturates, which are in part excreted unmetabolized in the urine, would be expected to have prolonged or elevated blood levels.[105–106] Glucuronic acid conjugation of barbiturates develops rapidly and increases 30-fold during the first 3 weeks of life.[52] For the ultra–short-acting barbiturates, redistribution is as important as metabolism in the liver in lowering the brain concentration.[107] Blood concentrations of thiopentone decrease about as rapidly in newborns as in their mothers.[108] The use of these ultra–short-acting barbiturates for induction of anesthesia is, therefore, not a pharmacologic problem, although the lack of a suitable intravenous route is often a practical deterrent.

Benzodiazepines

Diazepam. This is a widely used sedative-hypnotic and anticonvulsant. Infants born of mothers who have had diazepam for sedation during labor have shown lethargy and impaired thermoregulation for several days. The probable reasons for this prolongation of effect are several. Brain levels of diazepam and *N*-demethyldiazepam, a metabolite, have been noted to be higher in newborn rats and guinea pigs for up to 180 minutes after subcutaneous administration. This higher brain concentration probably explains why diazepam also gives greater protection against metrazol convulsions in newborn rats and guinea pigs than in adult animals.[109]

The plasma half-life of diazepam varies with maturity. The ability of the liver to metabolize diazepam is reduced in newborns as compared with adults. A demethylated derivative of diazepam, *N*-demethyldiazepam, could not be measured in plasma in premature infants until 4 hours after injection, although its plasma concentration was still rising at 48 hours. In contrast, *N*-demethyldiazepam was measured in the plasma of older children by 1 hour and had peaked by 24 hours. In adults, 71% of diazepam or its metabolites was excreted in the urine and about 10% in the feces. Urinary excretion of diazepam has not been quantitated in infants and children. Older children were shown to excrete a considerable amount of hydroxylated metabolites in urine, term infants a limited amount, and premature infants none. All three groups had trace amounts of diazepam and *N*-demethyldiazepam in the urine.[110]

Midazolam. Midazolam is a new water-soluble short-acting benzodiazepine. Its chemical configuration confers a pH-dependent ring phenomenon. At a pH of 4, the diazepine ring opens and a highly stable water-soluble compound results. At physiologic pH ranges the ring closes and thereby increases the drug's lipophilic activity.[110] Cardiovascular stability, transient mild respiratory depression, minimal venous irritation, antegrade amnesia, and short duration of action are all useful anesthetic properties of midazolam. Midazolam is metabolized in the liver; less than 1% is excreted unchanged in the urine. The terminal elimination phase ranges from 1

TABLE 9–3. BRAIN UPTAKE INDEX (%) OF MORPHINE AND PENTOBARBITAL IN RATS AT VARIOUS AGES

Age (ds)	Pentobarbital	Morphine
7	213.3 ± 20.6	36.2 ± 3.5
15	78.0 ± 1.5	17.2 ± 3.2
30	61.2 ± 5.0	7.4 ± 0.8
60	44.0 ± 3.0	5.6 ± 1.3

to 4 hours.[111] Protein binding is extensive with a free fraction of 3–6%. Following oral administration, midazolam has an intermediate rate of absorption (0.5–1.5 hours) and a bioavailability of 30–50%.

Anesthesia induction times following midazolam are comparable with those of diazepam.[103] Numerous studies of midazolam as an induction agent have documented its ability to maintain cardiovascular stability, its wide margin of safety, and its effective sedative hypnotic action. Massout and co-workers[112–117] evaluated the hemodynamic effects of 0.2 mg/kg of midazolam in anesthetized patients with coronary artery disease.[118] In patients already anesthetized with nitrous oxide, oxygen, etomidate, and fentanyl, midazolam decreased mean arterial and pulmonary capillary wedge pressures, HR, systemic vascular resistance and CI, whereas stroke volume increased. The overall result was an increase in the endocardial viability ratio; ie, an increase in the myocardial oxygen supply to demand ratio. Reves and colleagues observed that 0.2 mg/kg midazolam as an induction agent in patients with ischemic heart disease produced modest changes in the hemodynamic parameters.[119] They concluded it was a safe drug for induction of anesthesia in patients with compromised myocardial function. In healthy patients,[120] there is no significant difference in hemodynamic effects between induction doses of 0.25 mg/kg midazolam or 4 mg/kg of thiopental. Midazolam can cause transient respiratory depression and apnea in some individuals.[117] It can also inhibit the ventilatory response to carbon dioxide.

In children, midazolam has been used as an effective preanesthetic medication. In a double-blind study, Rita has shown that intramuscular midazolam (0.8 mg/kg) was a better drug for preanesthetic sedation than morphone (0.15 mg/kg).[121] More recently, Feld demonstrated in a randomized, double-blind, placebo-controlled study that orally administered midazolam (0.5–0.75 mg/kg) is an effective preanesthetic medication.[122] Transmucosal administration is another means of administering midazolam.

Following rectal administration, Saint-Maurice reported that 0.35 mg/kg of midazolam produced a noticeable effect by 10 minutes but required 20–30 minutes for more reliable sedation.[123] Wilton has shown 0.2 mg/kg of intranasal midazolam can provide anxiolysis and sedation in pre–school-aged children.[124]

Plasma concentrations following 0.1 mg/kg intravenous and intranasal administration of midazolam have been reported by Walbergh.[125] Intranasal midazolam achieved peak concentrations of 72.2 ng/mL ± 27.3 (means ±SD) 10 minutes following administration. These peak plasma concentrations were 57% of that observed in the intravenous group after 10 minutes. In pediatric patients of similar age and weight undergoing closed or open cardiac surgical procedures, the pharmacokinetic profile of midazolam was determined following

a single intravenous dose (in the group undergoing open-heart procedures, midazolam was administered after cardiopulmonary bypass). There was no significant difference between these two groups with respect to half-life (2.8 ± 0.89 h vs 3.3 ± 0.53), clearance (719 ± 400 mL · kg^{-1} · h^{-1} vs 512 ± 108), or volume of distribution at steady state (1.89 ± 0.243 L/kg vs 1.85 ± 0.283).[126] However, the half-life observed in the children with cardiac disease was longer than the values reported in healthy children (1.42 ± 0.49 h) undergoing elective surgery with a variable anesthetic background.[127]

Flunitrazepam. Flunitrazepam (RO5-4200) is a benzodiazepine 10 times more potent than diazepam. Its hypnotic and amnesic effects predominate over its sedative, anxiolytic, muscle-relaxing, and anticonvulsant effects. Like other benzodiazepines, it has a selective effect on the γ aminobutyric acid (GABA)–mediated receptor synapses in the brain. The drug is insoluble in water and is characterized as having a slow onset, a slow recovery time, and marked individual variability.[128–129] Flunitrazepam is 80% protein bound. It is metabolized in the liver by the mixed oxidase system; some of the metabolites are pharmacologically active; excretion of the metabolites is via the urine. In patients with renal insufficiency, metabolic cumulation occurs. In objective psychomotor studies, patients show residual impairment on testing up to 16 hours following injection.[130] Its major advantage lies in its reliably amnesic properties. Flunitrazepam has a volume of distribution at steady state of 4.63 L/kg, a terminal half-life of 23 hours, and a clearance of 2.7 mL/min/kg.

The variability of response to flunitrazepam appears to be related to pharmacodynamic alterations of receptor levels. Its cardiovascular, amnesic, and sedative hypnotic effects are similar to diazepam.[131–133] The cardiovascular effects have been studied in healthy patients as well as patients with myocardial compromise. Rolley and co-workers noted in healthy patients given 0.03 mg/kg of intravenous flunitrazepam as an induction dose, a decrease in cardiac output and stroke volume.[134] However, these reductions were less than those seen with induction doses of thiopental. List and colleagues[135] using systolic time intervals noted a negative inotropic effect of flunitrazepam. However, this attenuation in inotropy was less than that of thiopental. Coleman and co-workers[136] observed that flunitrazepam decreased peripheral vascular resistance and central venous pressure. These changes were associated with clinical evidence of vasodilation. Hennert and colleagues[137] investigated the cardiovascular properties of flunitrazepam in adult cardiac surgical patients anesthetized with fentanyl, etomidate, and pancuronium. Flunitrazepam slightly decreased systemic arterial pressure and cardiac output but did not change systemic vascular resistance. Clarke and Lyons[132] noted significant decreases in blood pressure with flunitrazepam in cardiac surgical patients. However, fluni-trazepam did not suppress the tachycardia and hypertension associated with laryngoscopy and intubation. In addition to its cardiovascular effects, flunitrazepam appears to be a respiratory depressant.[132] The depressant effects are affected by route and rate of administration. Studies in children have been limited to its use as a premedication. It appears that flunitrazepam is an effective premedicant in both adults and children.[138–140]

Etomidate. This is a potent, short-acting, nonbarbiturate sedative-hypnotic agent that lacks analgesic properties. It produces its central depressant effects by its GABA mimetic effects. Administered intravenously, etomidate has been used for induction and maintenance of anesthesia as well as for prolonged sedation in critically ill patients. The drug can be administered by single injections or by continuous infusions. It is a drug with rapid onset of action and rapid recovery.[141] Cardiovascular stability is maintained[142–144] and histamine release is not induced.[145] Little or no information is available about etomidate in infants and small children.

Etomidate is a safe drug ($LD_{50}:ED_{50}$ of 26).[146] It is metabolized in the liver; only 2% of the drug appears unchanged in the urine. Etomidate has an apparent volume of distribution of 4.5 times the body weight.[147] Because 75% of the drug is protein bound to albumin,[148] this actually may be an underestimate of the drug's apparent volume of distribution. Van Hamme and co-workers[147] also noted that the distribution phases t ½ alpha and t ½ gamma were 2.6 and 28.7 minutes, respectively.

Etomidate produces little change in cardiovascular function in both healthy and cardiovascularly compromised patients.[143–144] Intravenous infusions increased HR and CI by 9 and 14%, respectively. LVEDP and MAP remained unchanged. Coronary blood flow increased by approximately 20%, whereas myocardial oxygen extraction decreased by 10%. In addition to minimal cardiovascular effects, etomidate exhibits minimal respiratory depression. Etomidate produces a slight decrease in respiratory rate and minute volume. These decreases are less than those changes seen with thiopental.

Myoclonic movements not associated with epileptiform EEG activity[149] occur in 30–75% of patients following etomidate induction. The incidence of side effects is uneffected by prior fentanyl administration.[150] Gancher and co-workers[151] noted enhanced epileptogenic activity in two patients with complex partial seizures given etomidate.

The major concern about etomidate is the increased mortality seen in patients receiving prolonged infusions.[135] Numerous investigators[152–154] indicate that the mortality associated with etomidate is secondary to suppression of the adrenal cortex. Etomidate blocks adrenal steroid synthesis by inhibition of two mitochondrial cytochrome P-450–dependent enzymes, cholesterol side chain cleavage enzyme and 11-β-hydroxylase.[155] This inhibition of steroid synthesis occurs not only with prolonged continuous infusions but also with single induction doses.[154] This inhibition of the adrenal cortex by etomidate has created controversy regarding its use as an anesthetic agent.[156]

Propofol (Disoprofol). This is a rapidly acting hypnotic agent with no analgesic properties. Its rapid redistribution and metabolism make for a short duration of action and allow for repeat injections or continuous infusions without any cumulation of drug.[157] Induction time is dependent on dose and speed of injection.[158] Initial studies involving disoprofol were done with the drug's dissolution in 16% Cremophor El. As a result of anaphylactoid hypersensitivity reactions[159] associated with Cremophor El, disoprofol is now being reconstituted in 10% Intralipid. The pharmacokinetics of disoprofol have been evaluated by Adam and co-workers.[160]

Propofol compares favorably with althesin in smoothness of induction and lack of excitatory side effects.[161] Because of its short duration of action and noncumulative properties, continuous infusion regimens both with and without the use of nitrous oxide have been developed.[162–164] Following 2 mg/kg induction doses, Al-Khudhairi and colleagues[165] noted a 19% increase in heart rate, 23% decrease in mean arterial pressure, 19% decrease in systemic vascular resistance, and a 26% decrease in stroke volume, with no change in the cardiac output. Propofol causes minimal respiratory depression following induction doses.

Little information on disoprofol is available in children. Hannallah et all noted in children that the ED_{50} and ED_{95} for loss of eyelash reflex were 1.3 and 2.0 mg/kg, and the ED_{50} and ED_{95} for acceptance of a face mask were 1.5 and 2.3 mg/kg.[166] In this study, blood pressure decreased by 20% in 48% of the children who received 1–3% halothane following the disoprofol infusion. In a study comparing bolus and continuous infusion disoprofol to thiopental bolus followed by halothane maintenance, Borgeat noted that children receiving disoprofol had significantly shorter times to extubation, shorter times to discharge, and fewer side effects (nausea, vomiting, and agitation were less than the thiopental/halothane–anesthetized children).[167] Following the bolus of disoprofol, arterial pressure decreased 14%, similar to the decline following thiopental. Similar hemodynamic results have been demonstrated by Valtonen et al.[168]

The pharmacokinetics of disoprofol in children have been characterized by Valtonen.[168] In children anesthetized with nitrous, oxygen, and fentanyl, the disoprofol pharmacokinetic profile fits a three-compartment model. Their results suggested that the final elimination phase, the volumes of distribution, and the clearance volumes were similar to values obtained in adults. However, fentanyl is thought to decrease the clearance of disprofol. Thus, these values may underestimate the kinetic parameters in children. As with adult studies, the clearance values of disoprofol observed in children surpasses hepatic blood flow. Therefore, extrahepatic sites of metabolism probably are involved with disoprofol metabolism and elimination.

Ketamine. This is a nonbarbiturate cyclohexamine derivative that produces dissociation of the cortex from the limbic system; it may also act on the brain stem. There is frequently electroencephalographic seizure activity, particularly in the limbic system and cortex without clinical manifestations. This may be the mechanism of its action. On a microgram per kilogram basis, the amount of ketamine required to prevent gross movements is four times greater in infants under 6 months than in 6 year olds.[169] Acute studies show little metabolism of ketamine by the newborn.[170]

Waterman and Livingstone[171] noted that after ketamine, the sleeping times of rats decreased with increasing age; the onset time of sleep was significantly shorter in younger rats than in older ones. The demethylated metabolite of ketamine was present at recovery from anesthesia in 1-week-old rats; the oxidated metabolite was not present until 2–4 weeks of age. A dramatic decrease in sleeping time after ketamine was associated with the appearance of the oxidated metabolite. Recently, the pharmacokinetics of ketamine in patients of different ages were determined (Table 9–4). In infants less than 3 months of age, the volume of distribution was similar to that in older infants but the elimination half-life was prolonged. Hence, clearance was reduced in the younger infants. Reduced metabolism and renal excretion in the young infant are the likely causes.

In the "anesthetic" state associated with ketamine, respiration and blood pressure are usually well maintained. However, the use of ketamine in infants, particularly at the high doses required for lack of movement, has been associated with respiratory depression and apnea.[172] Generalized extensor spasm with opisthotonus

also has been seen in infants.[173] Intracranial pressure may increase in infants with hydrocephalus.[174] In addition, acute increases in pulmonary artery pressure have occasionally occurred in infants with congenital heart disease during ketamine anesthesia for cardiac catheterization.[175] Recent studies suggest that pulmonary vascular resistance is not changed by ketamine in infants with either normal or elevated pulmonary vascular resistance as long as the airway and ventilation are maintained.[176–177]

Narcotics

Morphine and Meperidine. Meperidine (0.5–1.0 mg/kg) and morphine (0.05–0.1 mg/kg) are used to reinforce nitrous oxide–oxygen anesthesia in the neonate. Such low doses attentuate the cardiovascular responses to surgical stress. In the past, high-dose meperidine and morphine anesthesia was given with oxygen-air to critically ill infants, particularly those requiring palliative heart surgery. The cardiovascular effects of these narcotics seemed minimal.

Narcotics are more toxic to newborn animals than to older animals.[99] In neonates, morphine depresses respiration more than meperidine does in a ratio of 1:10; in adults 10 mg of morphine produces respiratory depression equal to that from 100 mg meperidine.[178] The blood-brain barrier is more permeable to morphine and dihydromorphinone in newborn animals than in older animals. Brain concentration of morphine several hours after injection was two to four times greater in brains of younger rats despite equal blood concentration. This finding may be related to greater perfusion, to greater permeability, or both in the newborn. When the BUI for morphine was determined (Cook DR, unpublished data) in developing rats, it was higher in the younger than in older rats (see Table 9–3). Such developmentally increased permeability is not seen with meperidine.[179] This is not surprising because the lipid solubility of meperidine is quite high.

Morphine is inactivated by *N*-demethylation and glucuronide conjugation; the inactive forms are largely excreted in the urine. In spite of the inefficient metabolism of morphine, there is little difference in the plasma half-life of morphine beween newborn and older animals.[180] The pharmacokinetics of morphine in early infancy have been reported by Lynn and Slattery.[181] Compared with older infants, infants 2–4 days of age demonstrated longer elimination half-lives and similar volumes of distribution at steady-state compared with older infants 17–65 days of age. Meperidine in inactive forms is also largely excreted. De-esterification and *N*-demethylation occur mainly in the liver. In adults, the rate of transformation ranges from 10 to 20% per hour.[53] In newborn animals, the plasma half-life of meperidine is about twice that of the adult. Neonates excrete 25–

TABLE 9–4. PHARMACOKINETICS OF KETAMINE: EFFECT OF AGE

Age	$t_{1/2}\,\beta$ (min)	Vdss (L/kg)	Clearance (mL/min/kg)
<3 months	184.7	3.46	12.9
4–12 months	65.1	3.03	35.0
4 yrs	31.6	1.18	25.1
Adult	107.3	0.75	20.0

Abbreviations: $t_{1/2}\,\beta$, elimination half-life; Vdss, volume of distribution at steady state.

40% of a dose of meperidine in about 48 hours, almost exclusively in the demethylated form.[180]

Fentanyl. This (3–5 μg/kg) is used to reinforce nitrous oxide–oxygen anesthesia in the neonate; high-dose fentanyl (25–50 μg/kg) is popular as the primary anesthetic in infants undergoing cardiac anesthesia. Bradycardia and chest wall rigidity are potential features of high-dose fentanyl anesthesia. For these reasons, it is common to administer neuromuscular blocking drugs with wanted cardiovascular side effects (ie, pancuronium or gallamine) to ameliorate the effects of fentanyl. The cardiovascular effects of fentanyl at doses of 30–75 μg/kg fentanyl (with pancuronium) are minimal.[182] Modest decreases in mean arterial pressure and systemic vascular resistance index were noted by Hickey and co-workers.[182] Other indexes of cardiac function were unchanged. Schieber and colleagues[183] documented that the cardiovascular effects of fentanyl (without neuromuscular blocking drugs) are concentration dependent; a similar relationship between decreases in systolic blood pressure and concentration was noted by Koren.[184] Respiratory depression is also concentration related.

The dose of fentanyl for satisfactory anesthesia for infants is unknown but depends on the type and duration of surgery. In neonates, Yaster noted that fentanyl at initial doses of 10.0–12.5 μg/kg provided adequate anesthesia (as defined by changes in HR and blood pressure) for 75 minutes.[185] Ellis and Steward reported that infants receiving more than 50 μg/kg of fentanyl before hypothermic cardiopulmonary bypass and limited exogenous dextrose infusions had a reduced stress response as indicated by blood glucose concentrations less than 200 mg/dL.[186] Decreased stress responses and improved postoperative outcome were similarly noted by Anand and Hickey with sufentanil as compared with morphine-halothane anesthesia.[187] Age-related differences in the kinetics and sensitivity to fentanyl and changes in kinetics associated with profound pathophysiologic conditions make generalizations difficult.[188–191] In neonates, the volume of distribution is larger, the elimination half-life longer, and the clearance comparable or faster compared with adults. In premature infants undergoing patent ductus arteriosus (PDA) ligation, Collins noted prolongation of the elimination half-life of fentanyl, ranging from 6 to 32 hours.[192] In addition to age-related pharmacokinetic changes, the disease process may influence fentanyl pharmacology. Koehntop, in a study of newborns undergoing various types of surgery, noted that fentanyl half-life was markedly prolonged[188] in neonates with increased intra-abdominal pressure. In a study of children undergoing repair of congenital heart disease, changes in fentanyl volume of distribution depended on the severity of the hemodynamic disturbance, whereas changes in drug clearance were a function of patient age.[193]

In addition to intravenous routes of administration,

fentanyl can be administered transmucosally. In healthy pediatric patients, oral transmucosal fentanyl citrate (OTFC) in doses of 15–20 μg/kg is a safe and efficacious preanesthetic medication.[122,194–195] However, in patients with congenital heart disease, Goldstein-Dresner et al noted that when compared with a standard oral premedication of atropine, demerol, and diazepam, higher doses of OTFC (20–25 μg/kg) resulted in similar emotional status scores at the time of parental separation and anesthetic induction, but OTFC was associated with significantly more side effects, namely, preoperative emesis and pruritus.[196]

Sufentanil. This N–4 substituted derivative of fentanyl is a new potent synthetic opioid. It is a highly lipophilic compound that is distributed rapidly and extensively to all tissues. Sufentanil is approximately 5–10 times more potent than fentanyl and has an extremely high margin of safety. The median lethal to median effective dose ($LD_{50}:ED_{50}$) is about 10:1.[197] Dogs have survived intravenous doses of 5 mg/kg without respiratory assistance. Infusions of 40 μg/kg in mechanically ventilated animals given atropine produced little hemodynamic change.[198] Little is known about the effects of sufentanil on human cerebral metabolism, cerebral blood flow, and intracranial pressure. The major pathways for sufentanil metabolism involve *O*-demethylation and *N*-dealkylation; minimal amounts are excreted unchanged in urine.

Pharmacokinetic and pharmocodynamic studies of sufentanil have been conducted in infants, children, and adults. In adults, compared with fentanyl, sufentanil's smaller volume of distribution (2.48 L/kg) and high clearance rate (11.3 mL/kg/min) contribute to its short terminal elimination half-life (149 minutes). Meuldermans and co-workers[199] demonstrated that sufentanil is more protein bound (92%) than fentanyl (84%) and that pH affects protein binding. Decreasing pH from 7.4 to 7.0 increased protein binding by 28%; conversely, increasing pH from 7.4 to 7.8 decreased protein binding by 28%. The shorter elimination half-life of sufentanil should allow for a shorter duration of action. Clinical studies by deLange, Howie, and colleagues[200–201] using recovery times or time to extubation have not demonstrated significant clinical differences between sufentanil and fentanyl, whereas studies by Smith and co-workers[202] support shorter periods of postoperative ventilation in patients treated with sufentanil.

Clinical studies assessing the hemodynamic and endocrine stress response of sufentanil have been conducted in patients undergoing cardiopulmonary bypass. In patients maintained on high-dose β-adrenergic blocking agents and with good left ventricular function, sufentanil produced no significant hemodynamic changes.[200,203–204] In a study comparing comparable doses of fentanyl and sufentanil, Bovill and colleagues[205] found the incidence of hypertension necessitating vasodilator therapy was less in the patients anesthetized with sufentanil. If hypertension did occur, supplemental doses of sufentanil were more effective in blood pressure control than equipotent doses of fentanyl.[200] However, in a double-blind study, Rosow[206] found the drugs to be comparable with regard to hemodynamic stability. The neuroendocrine response in patients undergoing cardiothoracic surgery has been evaluated following sufentanil infusions[204,207] and is variable. Sufentanil appears to block some of the stress responses to cardiac surgery. Stress-induced increases in antidiuretic hormone (ADH) and growth hormone (GH) appear to be blocked before, during, and after cardiopulmonary bypass, whereas the catecholamines (norepinephrine, epinephrine, and dopamine) show a large surge during the bypass and postbypass periods.

The pharmacodynamic and pharmacokinetic effects of sufentanil in children are relatively unknown. Hickey and Hansen[208] compared the hemodynamic response of 5 and 10 μg/kg of sufentanil to 50–75 μg/kg of fentanyl in patients with complex congenital heart disease. Although HR and blood pressure changed slightly, they noted marked improvement in the patient's oxygenation with both fentanyl and sufentanil. The authors concluded that both sufentanil and fentanyl were safe anesthetics in high doses, and that both agents favorably decreased pulmonary vascular resistance and thereby increased pulmonary blood flow and systemic oxygenation in patients with cyanotic heart disease.[208] Davis and colleagues[209] examined both the pharmacodynamics and pharmacokinetics of high-dose sufentanil (15 μg/kg^{-1}) and oxygen in infants and children undergoing cardiac surgery. Sufentanil provided marked hemodynamic stability after an infusion and during the stress periods of incision and sternotomy. The hemodynamic responses to sufentanil were similar to those noted by Hickey and Hanson.[208] The pharmacokinetic data best fit a two-compartment model. In infants younger than 10 months and children older than 10 months who were not surface cooled, elimination half-lives were similar as were clearance values. However, the volume of distribution were significantly smaller in the infants compared with the older children. In infants younger than 10 months who were surface cooled, elimination half-life was longer and the volume of distribution larger but clearance rate was similar compared with age- and weight-matched infants.

As with fentanyl, transmucosal administration of sufentanil has also been reported. Henderson and others have reported that in doses of 1.5–3.0 μg/kg, nasal sufentanil is an effective preanesthetic medication. However, in doses greater than 3.0 μg/kg, truncal rigidity with decreased ventilatory compliance occur, thereby decreasing the usefulness of the drug.[209] Helmers et al have studied the pharmacodynamics and plasma decay curves of intravenous and nasal sufentanil.[210] In this study, onset of sedation was rapid in both groups but more so with the intravenous group. After 20 minutes, the degree of sedation was similar in both groups. After 30 minutes, the plasma concentrations were identical regardless of the route of administration.

Alfentanil. This new potent ultra–short-acting analogue of fentanyl is rapidly distributed to brain and central organs and then rapidly redistributed to more remote sites. It is about one fourth as potent as fentanyl and has one third the duration of action. It is a safe drug; the $LD_{50}:ED_{50}$ ratio is 1080:1.[211] Alfentanil's ultrashort duration of action, relative hemodynamic stability, and lack of cardiac-depressant effect provide great flexibility in anesthetic management. The drug's decreased volume of distribution results in a significantly shorter elimination half-life. Its low lipid solubility allows less penetration of the blood-brain barrier. Thus, brain tissue concentration is markedly less than that of the plasma. The duration of narcotic effect appears to be governed by distribution and elimination. These two mechanisms are influenced by dosage and method of infusion (bolus injection or constant infusion). The redistribution principle operates in small single-dose infusions, whereas elimination determines the effect of a large single bolus, multiple small bolus infusions, or continuous infusions. Alfentanil is metabolized in the liver by oxidative *N*-dealkylation and *O*-demethylation. The pharmacologically inactive metabolites are excreted in the urine.[212]

Protein binding has a significant influence on the pharmacokinetics of alfentanil. Protein binding is independent of alfentanil concentrations and is independent of changes in blood pH. Alfentanil is 88–95% protein bound in the plasma. The plasma protein most responsible for binding of alfentanil is α_1-acid glycoprotein. Changes in the binding and in the pharmacokinetics of alfentanil occur during and after cardiopulmonary bypass.[213] These changes have been associated with altered concentrations of α_1-acid glycoprotein. The pharmacokinetics of alfentanil have been studied in both pediatric and adult patients. In children, renal failure and cholestatic liver disease do not appear to affect alfentanil's pharmacokinetics.[214] Large interpatient variability with respect to alfentanil pharmacokinetics occurs in both children and adults. Little information is available on the developmental pharmacology of alfentanil. In children, the half-life of alfentanil appears shorter than in adults. In the study by Meistelman comparing children with adults, the shorter half-life in children was influenced by the smaller volume of distribution,[215] whereas in the study by Roure et al, volumes of distribution were similar but children had smaller clearance values than did adult patients.[216]

In studies of alfentanil in premature infants, Davis et al demonstrated that newly born, premature infants in the first 3 days of life had larger volumes of distribution, longer elimination half-lives, and smaller clearance rates compared with older children.[217] Killian et al noted that there was no correlation of gestational age to the pharmacokinetic parameters of alfentanil.[218]

The pharmacodynamics of alfentanil have been extensively investigated in adults but not in infants and children.[219–221] McDonnell and co-workers[219] have shown the ED_{50} and ED_{90} of unconsciousness to be 111 and 164 μg/kg, respectively, in the unpremedicated healthy patient. Nauta and colleagues found that the ED_{50} and ED_{90} could be reduced to 40 and 50 μg/kg in patient premedicated with atropine and lorazepam.[220] Premedication also affects the drug's onset time. In patients premedicated with lorazepam, alfentanil has an onset time of 75 seconds, whereas in unpremedicated patients, the onset time is 135 seconds.[220] In addition to a rapid onset time, recovery time from alfentanil infusions is rapid. Rapid recovery from alfentanil is felt to be a function of the drug's redistribution and elimination mechanics as well as the drug's ability to dissociate from its opioid receptors in the central nervous system.[222]

As with other narcotics, alfentanil produces a shift to the right in the ventilatory response curve. Although this shift is dose dependent, the ventilatory depressant effects are dissipated by 30–50 minutes following the dose.[223–224]

The cardiovascular effects of alfentanil have been assessed during both low- and high-dose infusions. In low-dose infusions (1.6 and 6.4 μg/kg) administered at slow rates to healthy volunteers no hemodynamic changes occurred.[223] In patients undergoing minor surgical procedures, Kay and Stephenson[224] demonstrated hemodynamic stability of low-dose alfentanil. At higher doses 150 μg/kg, HR, MAP, and SVR were noted to decrease. Pulmonary capillary wedge pressure, pulmonary vascular resistance, right atrial pressure, and pulmonary artery pressure increased slightly.[225] In other studies following induction with high-dose alfentanil, small transient decreases in MAP and systolic pressure occurred. These changes were not associated with changes in cardiac output or venous pressures. However, with the surgical stimulus of sternotomy, both arterial and central venous pressures increased.

The neuroendocrine stress response has been studied by Stanley[226] and deLange and co-workers.[227] The ability of high-dose alfentanil to blunt the stress response is incomplete. In Stanley's study, high-dose alfentanil was found to blunt the stress response of GH, ADH, and cortisol before, during, and after bypass. In deLange's study,[227] catecholamines (epinephrine and norepinephrine) were measured following high-dose alfentanil infusion. They noted plasma norepinephrine and epinephrine concentrations were unaltered until the bypass period. With the onset of bypass, there was a marked elevation in their concentrations.

Local Anesthetics. The rates of plasma decay for lidocaine and mepivacaine are similar in adults and newborns. However, the plasma levels of lidocaine and me-pivacaine in the neonate that produce cardiovascular and respiratory depression are about one-half those in adults.[180] The convulsive dose for infants on a milligram per kilogram basis of either ester-type (benzocaine) or amide-type (lidocaine) local anesthetics is not known. The rate of metabolism of the ester-type local anesthetics is decreased in the infant because pseudocholinesterase levels are low.[228] The newborn metabolizes lidocaine[229]; the rates of metabolism of the remaining amide-type local anesthetics in the neonate are not known.[230–231] The kinetics of intravenous lidocaine are similar in older infants, children, and adults.[232] However, lidocaine has a longer elimination half-life and larger volume of distribution in children than in adults following either intratracheal or caudal lidocaine.[233–234] Bokesch and co-workers[235] demonstrated higher plasma lidocaine levels in the systemic circulation in animals with right-to-left shunts. Because 60–80% of lidocaine is absorbed in the lung, it is speculated that in children with right-to-left shunts reduced amounts of lidocaine should be given to avoid possible systemic toxicity.

Atropine. Strong cholinergic stimulation, such as from cyclopropane, halothane, methoxyflurane, and succinylcholine, can produce profound bradycardia and reduce cardiac output in infants. The primary purpose of atropine in pediatric anesthesia is to protect against cholinergic challenge; its secondary purpose is to inhibit the production of secretions.

If atropine is given intravenous in incremental doses, more atropine is needed in children less than 2 years of age on a weight basis to accelerate the heart rate; however, acceleration uniformly occurs with 14.3 μg/kg.[236] A dose of 30 μg/kg appears to be vagolytic in infants, children, and adults. This dose provides adequate protection against a cholinergic challenge. In all age groups, 5–10 μg/kg atropine will minimally decrease salivation.[237] Children with the Down syndrome have an increased sensitivity to atropine. In such children, dilation of the pupils occurs in response to atropine and there are large increases in HR following repeated doses of atropine.[238–240]

NEUROMUSCULAR BLOCKING AGENTS

Depolarizing Neuromuscular Blocking Drugs

Succinylcholine. On a weight basis, more succinylcholine is needed in infants than in older children or adults to produce apnea, to depress respiration, or to depress neuromuscular transmission. Cook and Fischer[241] noted that in infants succinylcholine (1 mg/kg) produced neuroblockade about equal to that produced by 0.5 mg/kg in children (6–8 years). At these equipotent doses, there is no statistically significant difference between the times to recover to 50% (T_{50}) and 90% (T_{90}) neuromuscular transmission in the two groups. Complete neuromuscular blockade develops in children given 1 mg/kg of succinylcholine. The ED_{95} of succinylcholine (the estimated dose of relaxant required to give 95% neuromuscular blockade) in infants is 2.2 mg/kg.[241–242]

Goudsouzian and Liu[243] needed threefold higher infusion rates of succinylcholine (mg/kg/h) to maintain 90% twitch depression in young infants than in older infants or children. Phase II block occured after a slightly larger dose of succinylcholine in infants than in the other age groups. Differences in cholinesterase activity, receptor sensitivity, or volume of distribution may explain these age-related differences in succinylcholine requirements.

The infant has about one half the pseudocholinesterase activity of the older child or adult. Thus, it is unlikely that augmented cholinesterase activity is responsible for the infant's resistance to succinylcholine. When succinylcholine was given in equal doses on a surface area basis (40 mg/m²), Walts and Dillon[244] found no difference between infants and adults in the times to recover to 10, 50, or 90% neuromuscular transmission; this dose of succinylcholine produced complete neuromuscular blockade in all patients. Cook and Fischer[241] noted a linear relationship between the log dose on a milligram per square meter basis and the maximum intensity of neuromuscular blockade for infants, children, and adults (Fig 9–7). They also saw a linear relationship between the logarithm of the dose on a milligram per square meter basis and to either 50 or 90% recovery time for infants and children as a combined group. Because of its relatively small molecular size, succinylcholine is rapidly distributed throughout the extracellular fluid (ECF). The blood volume and ECF volume of the infant are significantly greater than that of the child or adult on a weight basis. Therefore, on a weight basis (mg/kg), twice as much succinylcholine is needed in the infant as in adults to produce 50% neuromuscular blockade. Because ECF and surface area bear a nearly constant relationship throughout life (6–8 L/m²), it is not surprising that there is a good correlation between succinylcholine dose (in mg/m²) and response throughout life. The data of Goudsouzian and Liu[243] suggest that relative resistance to succinylcholine persists in some infants even when the dose is transformed to milligrams per square meter per minute. These data suggest that the acetylcholine receptor matures with age.

Nondepolarizing Neuromuscular Blocking Drugs

Long-acting Neuromuscular Blocking Agents

Curares. On the basis of clinical criteria, it has been suggested that the newborn is sensitive to d-tubocurarine (dTC). However, electromyographic (EMG) studies

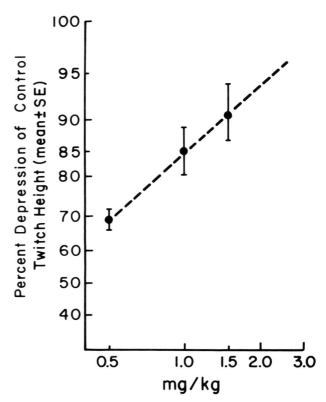

Figure 9–7. Log probit dose response curves for succinylcholine in infants. (*Data calculated from Cook DR, Fischer CG: Neuromuscular blocking effects of succinylcholine in infants and children. Anesthesiology 42:662–665, 1975, and Cook DR, Fischer CG: Characteristics of succinylcholine in infants and children. Anesth Analg 57:63–66, 1978.*)

demonstrate no increased sensitivity of hand muscles to dTC in infants compared with adults. In infants, respiratory depression parallels the neuromuscular blockade noted in the hands; in adults, neuromuscular blockade of the hand occurs before respiratory depression.[245] This important observation suggests that either the respiratory muscles of the infant may be more sensitive to dTC than those of the adult or that the infant has less respiratory reserve than the adult.

In adults, Donlon and colleagues[246] have determined cumulative dose-response curves and noted recovery times for dTC, gallamine, pancuronium, and metocurine during nitrous oxide–oxygen–narcotic anesthesia. At equipotent doses of these relaxants, the recovery time from 95–50% block averaged 45 minutes. Similar studies have been performed in children during halothane and balanced anesthesia by other investigators[247–251] (Table 9–5). The ED_{95} for these relaxants during balanced anesthesia in children tended to be higher than that in adults and the recovery times tended to be shorter. The dose requirements (ED_{95}) for pancuronium, metocurine, dTC, and gallamine are reduced by halothane anesthesia in children as they are in

TABLE 9–5. COMPARISON OF AGE-RELATED DOSE REQUIREMENTS OF NONDEPOLARIZING RELAXANTS AND RECOVERY TIMES

Relaxant	Age	ED$_{95}$ (mg/kg)	Recovery Time (min)
d-Tubocurarine			T$_5$–T$_{25}$
	1–7 yr	0.32	28.3
	2–12 mo	0.29	17.8
	11–60 d	0.34	22.4
	1–10 d	0.34	32.7
Metocurine			
	1–7 yr	0.18	49.7
	10 d–1 yr	0.22	36.7
	0–9 d	0.19	25.7
Pancuronium			
	5 wk–7 hr	0.05	23.6
	2–10 yr	0.06	–
Gallamine	2–10 yr	1.90	–

Abbreviations: ED$_{95}$, estimated dose of relaxant to produce 95% neuromuscular blockade; T$_5$–T$_{25}$, time for neuromuscular transmission to recovery from 5% to 25%.
(*Data compiled from references 238–245 and the authors' unpublished work.*)

adults. During halothane–nitrous oxide anesthesia, there is little difference in the ED$_{95}$ on a weight basis for the longer-acting muscle relaxants in infants and children. However, it has been noted that the ED$_{95}$ of pancuronium is less for infants from 3 through 6 months of age than for older children (Blinn A, et al, unpublished data).

Cook[252] estimated the dose of dTC on a surface area basis that would be needed to produce 95% twitch depression in infants, in children, and in adults during halothane anesthesia. In this estimate, compensation is needed for the wide variation in extracellular fluid volume that exists in infants, children, and adults. The extracellular fluid volume mirrors the volume of distribution for the nondepolarizing muscle relaxants. Also, the comparison is between like anesthetics—halothane with halothane. The adult and child require about 7–8 mg/m^2 of dTC; and the 6- to 9-month-old infants require 5–6 mg/m^2 but the neonate requires only about 4 mg/m^2. This suggests that the neonate, and to a lesser degree the infant, is quite sensitive to dTC if compensation is made for the wide variation in volumes of distribution.

Fisher and colleagues[253] documented the sensitivity to dTC of infants as compared with older patients during equipotent nitrous oxide–halothane anesthesia. Because the MAC of halothane is higher in infants than in adults, infants received higher end-tidal concentrations of halothane. The volume of distribution for dTC is quite high in the newborn infant compared with the older child or adult, but plasma clearance of dTC does not differ with age. However, the volume of distribution for dTC appears relatively constant on a liter per square meter basis. More important, the plasma concentration associated with 50% neuromuscular block (Cpss$_{50}$) was age related; Cpss$_{50}$ in neonates was about one third that

noted for adults. The largest variability in elimination half-life and volumes of distribution was seen in the data for the neonates. Likewise, Goudsouzian and co-workers[250] noted wide variations in the ED$_{95}$ for dTC in neonates during halothane anesthesia. Some infants were paralyzed with 0.18 mg/kg and others required 0.6 mg/kg; the mean ED$_{95}$ was similar to that in older children. This suggests that the neonate's response to nondepolarizing relaxants is quite unpredictable and that the clinician should titrate the dose of relaxant to produce the desired effect. The recovery times from all relaxants is dose related: if the infant were overdosed by a factor of 2, recovery time would be quite prolonged.

Pipecuronium and doxacurium, new long-acting relaxants without cardiovascular effects, have recently been introduced into clinical practice. Both have a duration of action in adults and children similar to that of pancuronium, but unlike pancuronium, they appear to be devoid of cardiovascular effects.[254–256] Renal failure can prolong the effect of these relaxants.[257–258] Children require higher doses of each relaxant than adults to achieve the same degree of neuromuscular blockade during equivalent anesthetic backgrounds. At equipotent doses of pipecuronium and doxacurium, the time to recovery of neuromuscular transmission to T$_{25}$ are shorter in children than adults. Infants appear to be more sensitive to the neuromuscular blocking effects of pipecuronium. However, the clinical duration of action (T$_{25}$) of pipecuronium following cumulative dosing is about 20 minutes in infants and 30 minutes in children. Spontaneous recovery indexes are not prolonged in the younger patients.

Intermediate-acting Relaxants

Atracurium. This is a muscle relaxant of intermediate duration that is metabolized by nonspecific esters and spontaneously decomposes by Hofmann degradation. Both processes are sensitive to pH and temperature. Under physiologic conditions, the breakdown of atracurium is mainly by ester hydrolysis; Hofmann elimination plays a minor role. Deficient or abnormal pseudocholinesterases have little or no effect on atracurium degradation.[259–260]

Cook and others have studied the effects of both age and potent inhalation agents on dose-response relationships of atracurium in infants, children, and adolescents.[261–265] On a weight basis (μg/kg), the ED$_{95}$ for atracurium was similar in infants (1–6 months of age) and adolescents, whereas children had a higher dose requirement. On a surface area basis (μg/m^2) the ED$_{95}$ for atracurium was similar in children and adolescents; the ED$_{95}$ (μgm^2) for atracurium in infants was much lower (Table 9–6; Fig 9–8).

At equipotent doses (1 × ED$_{95}$) the duration of effect (time from injection to 95% recovery) was 23 minutes in infants and 29 minutes in children and adoles-

TABLE 9–6. MEAN ED$_{50}$ AND ED$_{95}$ VALUES FOR ATRACURIUM IN ANESTHETIZED CHILDREN

Anesthetic	ED$_{50}$ (μg/kg)	ED$_{95}$ (μg/kg)	ED$_{50}$ (μg/m^2)	ED$_{95}$ (μg/m^2)
Thiopental-Fentanyl	170	350	3900	8200
Halothane	130	260	3300	6600
Isoflurane	120	280	3000	8600

cents compared with 44 minutes in adults. The time from injection to T$_{25}$ (25% neuromuscular transmission) was 10 minutes in infants, 15 minutes in children and adolescents, and 16 minutes in adults. At T$_{25}$, supplemental doses are needed to maintain relaxation for surgery. At higher multiples of the ED$_{95}$, the duration of effect (i.e., the time to T$_5$) will be longer but the times from T$_5$ to T$_{25}$ will be the same. The shorter duration of effect in the infant may represent a difference in pharmacokinetics.

The pharmacokinetics of atracurium differ among infants, children, and adults.[266] The volume of distribution is larger and the elimination half-life is shorter in infants than in children or adults. For both reasons, clearance in infants is more rapid. Although there is little

difference in the kinetics of atracurium among children aged 2–10 years, there are age-related differences in the volume of distribution, elimination half-life, and clearance. The volume of distribution is higher in the younger patients and the elimination half-life is shorter; clearance is little different (Table 9–7).

In children, "light" isoflurane anesthesia (1% end-tidal) reduces the atracurium required by about 30% from that needed with thiopental-narcotic anesthesia. There was no statistically significant difference in the isoflurane or halothane dose response curve. For clinical purposes, both potent agents should be viewed as potentiating atracurium to the same degree[263] (Fig 9–9).

A continuous infusion of dilute atracurium (200 μg/mL) following a bolus has been used to maintain neuromuscular blockade at 95 ± 5%.[263] To maintain this degree of steady-state block, an infusion rate of 4–5 μg/kg/min was required during halothane or isoflurane anesthesia and 8–10 μg/kg/min was required with thiopental-narcotic anesthesia following an initial bolus. No cumulation was seen with prolonged infusion; recovery of neuromuscular transmission was prompt. An infusion rate of 226/μg/m^2/min was needed. The recovery of neuromuscular transmission from the same degree of blockade was similar with all three anesthetics.

From these infusion data, one can estimate the removal of atracurium. At steady state, the infusion rate (Iss) equals the removal rate (Rss) of atracurium. Removal is directly related to the clearance and steady-state plasma concentration associated with 95% neuromuscular blockade (CPss$_{95}$). Hence Iss = Rss = clearance × CPss$_{95}$. From this relationship, one can estimate CPss$_{95}$ from clearance and the steady-state infusion rate. In children, during the potent anesthetics, CPss$_{95}$ is about 1 μg/mL; during balanced anesthesia, it is about 2 μg/mL. Atracurium infusion requirements in children during nitrous oxide–narcotic anesthesia can be compared to those noted in several age groups of adults during similar anesthesia. D'Hollander and co-workers[267] noted that in patients 16–85 years of age, the steady-state atracurium infusion rate averaged 14.4 mg/m^2/h; this corresponds to 240 μg/m^2/min.

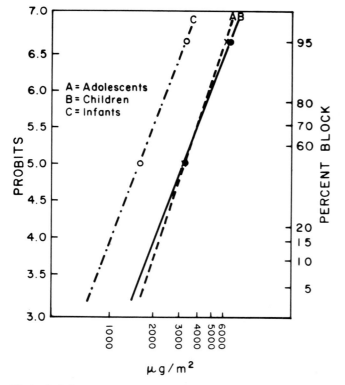

Figure 9–8. Dose-response curves for atracurium in infants, children, and adults. Note that the ED$_{95}$ for infants is much lower than that of children and adults when calculated on the basis of surface area.

A = Adolescents
B = Children
C = Infants

TABLE 9–7. AGE-RELATED PHARMACOKINETICS OF ATRACURIUM

Parameter	Children	Infants
$t_{1/2}\alpha$	2.1 ± 0.56	1.04 ± 0.34*
$t_{1/2}\beta$	19.1 ± 4.5	13.6 ± 1.4*
Vd (mL/kg)	139.0 ± 23.48	176.6 ± 22.2*
Clearance (mL/kg/min)	5.1 ± 0.56	9.0 ± 1.65*

Abbreviations: $t_{1/2}\alpha$, distribution half-life; $t_{1/2}\beta$, elimination half-life; Vd, volume of distribution.
* $P < 0.05$.

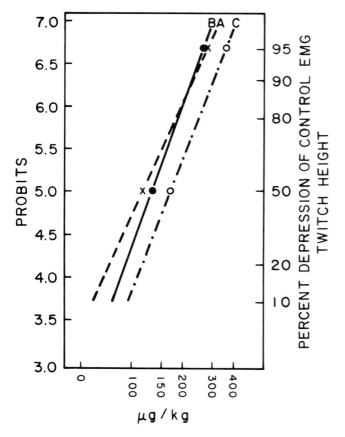

Figure 9–9. Dose-response curves for atracurium during halothane (*A*), isoflurane (*B*), or nitrous oxide-narcotic (*C*) anesthesia. Both halothane and isoflurane potentiate atracurium, so the atracurium requirement is reduced by 30%.

Vecuronium. A steroidal relaxant related to pancuronium, vecuronium is taken up largely by the liver and then excreted unchanged via the hepatobiliary system (40–50%) or alternatively excreted through the kidneys (4–14%). Limited biotransformation of vecuronium to the 3-hydroxy, 17 hydroxy, and 3,17-dihydroxy metabolites occurs. Only 3-hydroxyvecuronium has neuromuscular blocking effects.[268] These routes of elimination

may be affected by physiologic changes at the extremes of life.[269–270]

The ED_{95} for vecuronium is somewhat higher in children than in infants and adults.[269–271] At equipotent doses (two times ED_{95}) of vecuronium, the duration of effect (time from injection to 90% recovery) was longest for infants (73 minutes) compared with that for children (35 minutes) and adults (53 minutes). Thus, vecuronium does not have intermediate duration in infants. Vecuronium is potentiated by potent inhalation anesthetics but not in a dose-dependent manner[272–273] (Table 9–8).

Fisher et al have recently determined the pharmacodynamics and pharmacokinetics of vecuronium in infants and children[274] (Table 9–9). The volume of distribution and mean residence time were greater in infants than in children. Clearance was similar in the two groups; the $CPss_{50}$ was lower in infants than in children. The combination of a large volume of distribution in infants and fixed clearance results in a longer mean residence time. After a single dose of relaxant, recovery of neuromuscular transmission depends on both distribution and elimination. The combination of a longer mean residence time and a lower sensitivity for vecuronium explain the prolongation of neuromuscular blockade in infants.

Rocuronium (ORG–9426). An intermediate steroidal derivative of vecuronium, ORG–9426 is less potent than vecuronium but has a shorter onset time of neuromuscular blockade and a similar duration of action. It has minimal cardiovascular effects. The ED_{95} of ORG–9426 in adults receiving balanced anesthesia is 300 µg/kg.[275] At 2 × ED_{95}, the onset time of complete neuromuscular blockade is about 1.5 minutes. At these doses, the clinical duration (ie, time to T_{25}) was 40 minutes, which is comparable to that of vecuronium at equal multiples of the ED_{95}. Cardiovascular changes were minimal. The ED_{50} and ED_{95} of ORG–9426 has been determined in children during halothane anesthesia to be 179 µg · kg^{-1} and 303 µg · kg^{-1}, respectively (Woelfel SK et al, unpublished data). The initial recovery index (T_{10}–T_{25}) after an ED_{95} dose (given in incremental doses) was 3.2 minutes. Thus, the duration of neuromuscular blockade is somewhat shorter in children than in adults.

Short-acting Relaxants

Mivacurium. This is a short acting relaxant that is metabolized by plasma cholinesterase. When administered in doses less than two times the ED_{95} in adults, mivacurium appears to be devoid of cardiovascular effects; larger doses may be associated with a transient decrease in blood pressure from histamine release. Compared with adults, children require significantly more mivacurium (µg/kg) during comparable anesthetics. When refer-

TABLE 9–8. POTENCY AND TIME COURSE FOR VECURONIUM EFFECT IN RELATION TO AGE

	Potency			Time Course (70 µg/kg)	
	ED_{50} (µg/kg)	ED_{95} (µg/kg)	ED_{95} Multiple	Onset Time (min)	Duration (min)
Infants	16.5	27.7	2.5	1.5 ± 0.6	73 ± 27
Children	19.0	45.5	1.5	2.4 ± 1.4	35 ± 6
Adults	15.0	33.8	2	2.9 ± 0.2	53 ± 21

TABLE 9–9. PHARMACOKINETICS AND PHARMACODYNAMICS OF VECURONIUM

	$t_{1/2}\beta$ (min)	Clearance (mL/kg/min)	Vdss (mL/kg)	$CPss_{50}$ (ng/mL)
Infants	64.7	5.6	357	57.3
	±30.2	±1	±70	±17.7
Children	41.0	5.9	204	109.8
	±15.1	±24	±116	±28.1
Adult	70.7	5.2	269	93.7
	±20.4	±0.7	±42	±33.5

Abbreviations: $t_{1/2}\beta$, elimination, half-life; Vdss, volume of distribution at steady state; $CPss_{50}$, plasma concentration associated with 50% neuromuscular blockade.

enced to body surface area ($\mu g/m^2$), however, the dosage requirements are not significantly different. This suggests that age-related dosage requirements for mivacurium may be associated with age-related differences in volume of distribution. At equal potent doses, the onset time of mivacurium is faster in children than in adults; the clinical duration is likewise shorter in children. We observed cutaneous flushing in three children given high doses of mivacurium and a transient 32% decrease in mean arterial pressure in one of these patients. Flushing was not always associated with hypotension. Pseudocholinesterase activity influences the clearance and hence infusion roles in children. Mivacurium can be administered by infusion for several hours with no evidence of cumulation and with rapid spontaneous or pharmacologically induced return of neuromuscular function after termination of the infusion. The mivacurium infusion rates are higher in children than in adults.[276]

Cardiovascular Effects of Relaxants

Succinylcholine exerts variable and seemingly paradoxical effects on the cardiovascular system. Typically, intravenous succinylcholine produces initial bradycardia and hypotension followed after 15–30 seconds by tachycardia and hypertension. In the infant and small child, profound sustained sinus bradycardia (rates of 50–60 per minute) is commonly observed[277–278]; asystole rarely occurs. Nodal rhythm and ventricular ectopic beats are seen in about 80% of children given a single intravenous injection of succinylcholine; such dysrhythmias are rarely seen following intramuscular succinylcholine.

As in adults, the incidence of bradycardia and other dysrhythmias is higher in children following a second dose of succinylcholine. Atropine (0.1 mg) appears to offer adequate protection against these bradyarrhythmias in all age groups. In infants, vagolytic doses of atropine (0:03 mg/kg) are required for protection; in older children, adequate protection is provided by doses of 0.005 mg/kg.

Cook and colleagues reported several young infants who developed fulminant pulmonary edema following intramuscular succinylcholine (4 mg/kg).[279] The pulmonary edema occurred with minutes of the intramuscular injection and responded to continuous positive pressure ventilation (CPAP). They noted additional cases of pulmonary edema and pulmonary hemorrhage following intravenous succinylcholine as well. In each instance, the patient was lightly anesthetized. This pulmonary edema may result from an acute elevation of systemic vascular resistance and an acute decrease in pulmonary vascular resistance. In addition, "leaky" capillaries appear to be involved. Whether these cardiovascular changes are mediated by succinylcholine itself or some other vasoactive substance (ie, histamine) is not known.

The cardiovascular effects of the nondepolarizing relaxants are related to the magnitude of histamine release, ganglionic blockade, and vagolysis. In addition, the cardiovascular effects seem age related.

In infants and children, minimal cardiovascular effects are seen following atracurium, metocurine, and vecuronium at several multiples of the ED_{95}. In adults, atracurium at three times the ED_{95} causes slightly less histamine release than two times the ED_{95} of metocurine and less than half as much histamine release as one times the ED_{95} of dTC. Vecuronium (at any multiple of ED_{95}) is not associated with histamine release. Infants and children appear less susceptible to histamine release following relaxants than adults. In a small series of infants, five times the ED_{95} of atracurium did not elicit flushing or alteration of heart rate or blood pewssure. However, when atracurium is injected directly intravenously in infants and children, local signs of histamine release have been described. Rarely, flushing with or without mild hypotension is seen at high multiples of the ED_{95}. At high doses, dTC may cause hypotension and histamine release in children.

Keon and Downes (unpublished data) compared changes in heart rate, changes in blood pressure, and differences in intubating conditions in infants (average age 5.6 months) "anesthetized" with nitrous oxide–oxygen following either dTC (0.6 mg/kg) or pancuronium (0.1 mg/kg). None had received premedication. In both groups, there were modest increases in pulse rate; transient episodes of bradycardia occurred in some infants in both groups during intubation. No infant given pancuronium developed significant hypotension or hypertension (>10% change from control levels). In contrast, 25% of the infants given dTC experienced decreases in blood pressure greater than 10% from control (range 11–26%).

In children anesthetized with halothane and nitrous oxide, one times the ED_{95} of gallamine increases the HR by 42 beats per minute and one times the ED_{95} of pancuronium increases the HR by 19 beats per minute. Both drugs increase MAP under these conditions by about 10 mm Hg. At two times the ED_{95}, further increases in the

HR were seen with pancuronium but not with gallamine. In contrast, minimal effects of gallamine or pancuronium were noted on the HR in infants. Unless the HR has slowed from halothane, neither gallamine or pancuronium exhibited any vagolytic effects. In an occasional infant, however, gallamine or pancuronium significantly increases the HR. Because the infant responds to a variety of stimuli with bradycardia (eg, potent inhalation agents, hypoxia, intubation), the potential vagolytic effects of pancuronium and gallamine may be wanted side effects. For example, in adults, pancuronium is usually administered with high-dose fentanyl anesthesia to minimize the bradycardia seen with fentanyl; substitution of atracurium or vecuronium for pancuronium has resulted in profound bradycardia from the fentanyl—a totally predictable side effect. Whether profound bradycardia will be seen in infants anesthetized with deep halothane given atracurium, vecuronium, doxacurium, or pipecuronium remains to be seen. No significant change in the HR and only a minimal (7 mm Hg) decrease in blood pressure were noted in infants anesthetized with halothane 1% end-tidal and nitrous oxide and given 0.3 mg/kg of atracurium.[261] No changes in the HR or blood occurred after 70 μg/kg of vecuronium in pediatric patients also anesthetized with halothane and nitrous oxide.[269]

ANTAGONISM OF NEUROMUSCULAR BLOCKADE

Fisher and co-workers have recently examined the dose of neostigmine and edrophonium required in infants, children, and adults to reverse a 90% block from a continuous dTC infusion.[280–281] In infants and children, 15 μg/kg of neostigmine produced a 50% antagonism of the dTC block; in adults, 23 μg/kg was required. It was claimed that the duration of antagonism was equal in all three groups, although the elimination half-life was clearly shorter for infants. A larger dose than that seemingly recommended would give a higher sustained blood concentration. Whether this is of pharmacologic benefit in the absence of a continuous infusion of relaxant is doubtful. The dissociation between the elimination half-life and the duration of antagonism may result from the carbamylation of cholinesterase by neostigmine. In infants, 145 μg/kg of edrophonium produced a 50% antagonism of the dTC tubocurarine block, in children, 233 μg/kg was required, and in adults 128 μg/kg was required. The volume of distribution of edrophonium was similar in all age groups. The elimination half-life of edrophonium was shorter in infants than in children or adults; hence, clearance was more rapid in infants. Because the molecular interaction between edrophonium and cholinesterase is readily reversible, Fisher et al suggest that the shorter elimination half-life for edropho-

nium might limit the value of edrophonium in pediatric patients. This is doubtful.

Meakin and colleagues[232] compared the rate of recovery from pancuronium-induced neuromuscular blockade with several doses of neostigmine (0.036 or 0.07 mg/kg) or edrophonium (0.7 or 1.43 mg/kg) in infants and children. In the first 5 minutes, recovery of neuromuscular transmission was more rapid after edrophonium than neostigmine in all age groups; the speed of recovery was faster in infants and children than in adults. By 10 minutes, there was no difference in neuromuscular transmission achieved in infants and children with either reversal agent (at either dose); adults had lower neuromuscular transmission at the lower dose (0.036 mg/kg) of neostigmine. Thus, if speed of initial recovery is a critical issue, then edrophonium is better than neostigmine and a high dose of neostigmine is better than a low dose. At 30 minutes after injection of either reversal agent (at any dose) there was no differences between neuromuscular transmission between age groups.

REFERENCES

1. Sereni F: Developmental pharmacology. *Annu Rev Pharm* **8**:453–470, 1968
2. Jusko WJ: Pharmacokinetic principles in pediatric pharmacology. *Pediatr Clin North Am* **19**:1:81–100, 1972
3. Brown TCK: Pediatric pharmacology. *Anaesth Intensive Care* **1**:473–479, 1973
4. Cook DR: Neonatal anesthetic pharmacology: A review. *Anesth Analg* **53**:544–548, 1974
5. Yaffe SJ, Juchau MR: Perinatal pharmacology. *Ann Rev of Pharm* **14**:219–238, 1974
6. Cook DR: Pediatric anesthesia: Pharmacological considerations. *Drugs* **12**:212–221, 1976
7. Rylance G: Clinical pharmacology: Drugs in children. *Br Med J* **282**:50–51, 1981
8. Orme M: Drug absorption in the gut. *Br J Anaesth* **56**:59–67, 1984
9. DeBoer AG, DeLeede LGJ, Breimer DD: Drug absorption by sublingual and rectal routes. *Br J Anaesth* **56**:69–82, 1984
10. Huang NN, High RH: Comparison of serum levels following the administration of oral and parenteral preparations of penicillin in infants and children of various age groups. *J Pediatr* **42**:567–568, 1958
11. Borga G, Piafsky KM, Nilsen OG: Plasma protein binding of basic drugs I. Selective displacement from alpha-1 acid glycoprotein by tris-butoxyethyl phosphate. *Clin Pharmacol Ther* **22**:539–544, 1977
12. Brem RF, Giardina EGV, Bigger JT: Time course of alpha-1 acid glycoprotein and its relationship to imipramine plasma binding. *Clin Pharmacol Ther* **31**:206, 1982
13. Edwards DJ, Lalka D, Cerra G, Slaughter RL: Alpha-1 acid glycoprotein concentration and protein binding in trauma. *Clin Pharmacol Ther* **31**:62–67, 1982
14. Grossman SH, Davis D, Kitchell BB, et al: Diazepam and

lidocaine plasma protein binding in renal disease. *Clin Pharmacol Ther* **31**:350–357, 1982

15. Kornguth ML, Hutchins LG, Eichelman BS: Binding of psychotropic drugs to isolated alpha–1 acid glycoprotein. *Biochem Pharmacol* **30**:2435–2441, 1981

16. Piafsky KM: Disease-induced changes in the plasma binding of basic drugs. *Clin Pharmacokinet* **5**:246–262, 1980

17. Piafsky KM, Borga O, Odar-Cederlog I, et al: Increased plasma protein binding of propranolol and chlorpromazine mediated by disease-induced elevations of plasma acid glycoprotein. *N Engl J Med* **299**:1435–1439, 1978

18. Pike E, Skuterud B, Kierugg P, et al: Binding and displacement of basic, acidic and neutral drugs in normal and orosomucoid-deficient plasma. *Clin Pharmacokinet* **6**:367–374, 1981

19. Nation RL: Meperidine binding in maternal and fetal plasma. *Clin Pharmacol Ther* **29**:472–479, 1981

20. Pruitt AW, Dayton PG: A comparison of the binding of drugs to adult and cord plasma. *Eur J Clin Pharmacol* **4**:59–62, 1971

21. Wood J, Wood AJJ: Changes in plasma drug binding and alpha-1 acid glycoprotein in mother and newborn infant. *Clin Pharmacol Ther* **29**:522–526, 1981

22. Dayton PG, Stiller RL, Cook DR, Perel JM: The binding of ketamine to plasma proteins: Emphasis on human plasma. *Eur J Clin Pharmacol* **24**:825–831, 1983

23. Friss-Hansen B: Body composition during growth. *Pediatrics* **47**:264–274, 1971

24. Widdowson EM: Changes in body proportions and composite during growth. In Davis JA, Dobbing J (eds): *Scientific Foundations of Pediatrics*. Philadelphia: WB Saunders, 1974, pp 153–163

25. Smith CA, Nelson NM: *The Physiology of the Newborn Infant*, 4th ed. Springfield, IL: Charles C Thomas, 1976

26. Guignard JP, Torrado A, Cunha OD, Gautier E: Glomerular filtration rate in the first three weeks of life. *J Pediatr* **87**:268–272, 1975

27. Altman PL, Dittmer DS: *Respiration and Circulation Handbook* (rev ed). Bethesda, MD: Federation of American Societies of Experimental Biology, 1971, pp 426–427

28. Oldendorf WH: The blood-brain barrier. In Bito LZ, Davson H, Fenstermacher JD (eds): *The Ocular and Cerebrospinal Fluids*. New York: Academic Press, 1977, pp 177–190

29. Behnsen G: Farbstoffversuche mit Trypanblan an der Schranke zwischen Blut und Zentralnervensystem der wachsenden Maus. *Munch Med Wochr* **73**:1143–1147, 1926

30. Behnsen G: Uber die Farbstoffspeicherung im Zentralnervensystem der weissen Maus in verschiedenen Alterszugstanden. *Z Zellforsch* **4**:515–572, 1927

31. Barlow CF, Domek NS, Goldberg MA, Roth LJ: Extracellular brain space measured by ^{35}S-sulphate. *Arch Neurol* **5**:102–110, 1961

32. Davson H: *Physiology of the Cerebral Spinal Fluid*. London, Churchill, 1967

33. Ferguson RK, Woodbury DM: Penetration of ^{14}C-inulin and ^{14}C-sucrose into brain, cerebrospinal fluid, and skeletal muscle in developing rats. *Exp Brain Res* **7**:181–194, 1969

34. Evans CAN, Reynolds JM, Reynolds ML, et al: The development of a blood-brain barrier mechanism in foetal sheep. *J Physiol (Lond)* **238**:371–386, 1974

35. Evans CAN, Reynolds JM, Reynolds ML, Saunders NR: The effect of hypercapnia on a blood-brain barrier mechanism in foetal and newborn sheep. *J Physiol (Lond)* **255**:701–714, 1976

36. Oldendorf WH: Measurement of brain uptake of radio-labelled substances using a tritiated water internal standard. *Brain Res* **24**:372–376, 1970

37. Oldendorf WH, Braun LD: [^{3}H]-Tryptamine and ^{3}H water as diffusible internal standard for measuring brain extraction of radio-labelled substances following carotid injection. *Brain Res* **113**:219–224

38. Oldendorf WH, Hyman S, Braun L, Oldendorf SZ: Blood-brain barrier: Penetration of morphine, codeine, heroin and methadone after carotid injection. *Science* **178**:984–986, 1972

39. Cook DR: Clinical use of muscle relaxants in infants and children. *Anesth Analg* **60**:335–343, 1981

40. Anggard L, Ottoson D: Observations on the functional development of the neuromuscular apparatus in fetal sheep. *Exp Neurol* **7**:294–304, 1963

41. Close R: Dynamic properties of fast and slow skeletal muscles of the rat during development. *J Physiol (Lond)* **173**:74–95, 1964

42. Close R: Force-velocity properties of mouse muscles. *Nature* **206**:718–719, 1965

43. Close R: Effects of cross-union of motor nerves to fast and slow skeletal muscles. *Nature* **206**:831–832, 1965

44. Buller AJ: Developmental physiology of the neuromuscular system. *Br Med Bull* **22**:45–48, 1966

45. Koenigsberger MR, Patten B, Lovelace RE: Studies of neuromuscular function in the newborn—A comparison of myoneural function in the full term and premature infant. *Neuropadiatrie* **4**:350–361, 1973

46. Goudsouzian NG: Maturation of neuromuscular transmission in the infant. *Br J Anaesth* **52**:205–213, 1980

47. Crumrine RS, Yodlowski EH: Assessment of neuromuscular function in infants. *Anesthesiology* **54**:29–32, 1981

48. Gladtke E, Heimann G: The rate of development of elimination functions in kidney and liver of young infants. In Morselli PC, Garattini S, Sereni F (eds): *Basic and Therapeutic Aspects of Perinatal Pharmacology*. New York: Raven Press, 1975, pp 377–392

49. Yaffe SJ: Neonatal pharmacology. *Pediatr Clin North Am* **13**:527–532, 1966

50. Somogyi A, Gugler R: Drug interactions with cimetidine. *Clin Pharmacokinet* **7**:23–41, 1982

51. Katzung GB: *Basic and Clinical Pharmacology*. Los Altos, CA: Lange, 1984

52. Brown AK, Zwelzin WW, Burnett HH: Studies on the neonatal development of the glucuronide conjugating system. *J Clin Invest* **37**:332–337, 1958

53. Greene NM: The metabolism of drugs employed in anesthesia. *Anesthesiology* **29**:127–137, 1968

54. Uehleke H, Werner T: Postnatal development of halothane and other halothane metabolism and covalent binding in rat liver microsomes. In Morselli PL, Garattini S, Sereni F (eds): *Basic and Therapeutic Aspects of Perinatal Pharmacology*. New York: Raven Press, 1975, pp 277–287

55. Stoelting RK, Peterson C: Methoxyflurane anesthesia in pediatric patients: Evaluation of anesthetic metabolism and renal function. *Anesthesiology* **42**:26–29, 1975

56. Eger EI II: *Anesthesia Uptake and Action*. Baltimore: William & Wilkins, 1974
57. Salanitre E, Rackow H: The pulmonary exchange of nitrous oxide and halothane in infants and children. *Anesthesiology* **30**:388–394, 1969
58. Steward DJ, Creighton RE: The uptake and excretion of nitrous oxide in the newborn. *Can Anaesth Soc J* **25**:215–217, 1978
59. Eger EI II, Bahlman SH, Munson ES: The effect of age on the rate of increase of alveolar anesthetic concentration. *Anesthesiology* **35**:365–372, 1971
60. Brandom BW, Brandom RB, Cook DR: Uptake and distribution of halothane in infants: In vivo measurements and computer simulations. *Anesth Analg* **62**:404–410, 1983
61. Gibbs CP, Munson ES, Tham MK: Anesthetic solubility coefficients for maternal and fetal blood. *Anesthesiology* **43**:100–103, 1975
62. Lerman J, Gregory GA, Willis MM, Eger EI II: Age and solubility of volatile anesthetics in blood. *Anesthesiology* **61**:139–143, 1984
63. Cook DR, Brandom BW, Shiu G, Wolfson BW: The inspired median effective dose, brain concentration at anesthesia, and cardiovascular index for halothane in young rats. *Anesth Analg* **60**:182–185, 1981
64. Stoelting RK, Longnecker DE: Effect of right-to-left shunt on rate of increase in arterial anesthetic concentration. *Anesthesiology* **36**:352–356, 1972
65. Tanner GE, Angers DG, Barash PG, et al: Effect of left-to-right, mixed left-to-right, and right-to-left shunts on inhalational anesthetic induction in children: A computer model. *Anesth Analg* **64**:101–107, 1985
66. Deming MV: Agents and techniques for induction of anesthesia in infants and young children. *Anesth Analg* **31**:113–117, 1952
67. Gregory GA, Eger EI II, Munson ES: The relationship between age and halothane requirements in man. *Anesthesiology* **30**:488–491, 1969
68. Nicodemus HF, Nassiri-Rahimi C, Bachman L: Median effective dose (ED_{50}) of halothane in adults and children. *Anesthesiology* **31**:344–348, 1969
69. Lerman J, Robinson S, Willis MM, Gregory G: Anesthetic requirements for halothane in young children 0–1 month and 1–6 months of age. *Anesthesiology* **59**:421–424, 1983
70. Gregory GA, Wade JG, Beihl DR, et al: Fetal anesthetic requirement (MAC) for halothane. *Anesth Analg* **62**:9–14, 1983
71. Moss IR, Conner H, Yee WFH, et al: Human B-endorphin in the neonatal period. *J Pediatr* **101**:443–446, 1982
72. Bayon A, Shoemaker WJ, Bloom FE, et al: Perinatal development of the endorphin- and enkephalin-containing systems in rat brain. *Brain Res* **179**:93, 1979
73. Miller KM, Paton WDM, Smith EB, Smith RA: Physiochemical approaches to the mode of action of general anesthetics. *Anesthesiology* **36**:339–351, 1972
74. Rackow H, Salanitre E, Green LT: Frequency of cardiac arrest associated with anesthesia in infants and children. *Pediatrics* **28**:697–704, 1961
75. Friesen RH, Lichtor JL: Cardiovascular depression during halothane anesthesia in infants: A study of three induction techniques. *Anesth Analg* **61**:42–45, 1982
76. Friesen RH, Lichtor JL: Cardiovascular effects of inhalation induction with isoflurane in infants. *Anesth Analg* **62**:411–414, 1983
77. Rao CC, Bayer M, Krishna G, Paradise RR: Increased sensitivity of the isometric contraction of the neonatal isolated rat atria to halothane, isoflurane, and enflurane. *Anesthesiology* **64**:13–18, 1986
78. Boudreaux JP, Schieber RA, Cook DR: Hemodynamic effects of halothane in the newborn piglet. *Anesth Analg* **63**:731–737, 1984
79. Bailie MD, Alward CT, Sawyer DC, Hook JB: Effect of anesthesia on cardiovascular and renal function in the newborn piglet. *J Pharmacol Exp Ther* **208**:298–302, 1979
80. Merin RG, Verdouw PD, deJong JW: Dose-dependent depression of cardiac function and metabolism by halothane in swine (Sus scrofa). *Anesthesiology* **46**:417–423, 1977
81. Gootman PM, Gootman N, Buckley BJ: Maturation of central autonomic control of the circulation. *Fed Proc* **42**:1648–1655, 1983
82. Schieber RA, Namnoum A, Sugden A, et al: Hemodynamic effects of isoflurane in the newborn piglet: Comparison with halothane. *Anesth Analg* **65**:633–638, 1986
83. Gregory GA: The baroresponses of preterm infants during halothane anesthesia. *Can Anaesth Soc J* **29**:105–107, 1982
84. Duncan P, Gregory GA, Wade JA: The effects of nitrous oxide on the baroreceptor response of newborn and adult rabbits. *Can Anesth Soc J* **18**:339–341, 1981
85. Wear R, Robinson S, Gregory GA: The effect of halothane on the baroresponse of adult and baby rabbits. *Anesthesiology* **56**:188–191, 1982
86. Wolfson B, Kielar CM, Lake C, et al: Anesthetic index—A new approach. *Anesthesiology* **38**:583–586, 1973
87. Wolfson B, Hetrick WD, Lake C, Siker ES: Anesthetic indices—Further data. *Anesthesiology* **48**:187–190, 1978
88. Kissin I, Morgan PL, Smith LR: Comparison of isoflurane and halothane safety margins in rats. *Anesthesiology* **58**:556–561, 1983
89. Eger EI: Stability of I-653 in soda lime. *Anesth Analg* **66**:983–985, 1987
90. Weiskopf RB, Holmes MA, Eger EI II, et al: Cardiovascular effects of I653 in swine. *Anesthesiology* **69**:303–309, 1988
91. Weiskopf RB, Cahalan MK, Yasuda N, et al: Cardiovascular actions of desflurane (I-653) in humans. *Anesth Analg* **70**:S426, 1990 (abstr)
92. Hartman JC, Pagel PS, Kampine JP, et al: Influence of desflurane on regional distribution of coronary blood flow in chronically instrumented canine model of multivessel coronary artery obstruction. *Anesth Analg* **72**:289–299, 1991
93. Strum DP, Eger EI, Johnson BH, et al: Toxicity of sevoflurane in rats. *Anesth Analg* **66**:769–773, 1987
94. Katoh T, Ikeda K: The minimum alveolar concentration (MAC) of sevoflurane in humans. *Anesthesiology* **66**:301–303, 1987
95. Wallin RF, Napoli MD: Sevoflurane, a new inhalational anesthetic agent. *Anesth Analg* **54**:758–765, 1975
96. Martis L, Lynch S, Napoli MD, Woods EF: Biotransformation of sevoflurane in dogs and rats. *Anesth Analg* **60**:186–191, 1981
97. Bernard JM, Wouters PF, Doursout MF, et al: Effects of sevoflurane and isoflurane on cardiac and coronary dy-

namics in chronically instrumental dogs. *Anesthesiology* **72**: 659–662, 1990

98. Lerman J, Oyston JP, Gallagher TM, et al: The minimum alveolar concentration (MAC) and hemodynamic effects of halothane, isoflurane, and sevoflurane in newborn swine. *Anesthesiology* **72**:717–721, 1990

99. Goldenthal EI: A compilation of LD$_{50}$ values in newborn and adult animals. *Toxicol Appl Pharmacol* **18**:185–207, 1971

100. Carmichael EB: The median lethal dose (LD$_{50}$) of pentothal sodium for both young and old guinea pigs and rats. *Anesthesiology* **8**:589–593, 1947

101. Carmichael EB: The median lethal dose of nembutal (pentobarbital sodium) for young and old rats. *J Pharmacol Exp Ther* **62**:284–286, 1938

102. Weatherall JA: Anaesthesia in newborn animals. *Br J Pharmacol* **15**:454–459, 1960

103. Domek NS, Barlow CF, Roth LJ: An octogenetic study of phenobarbital C-14 in cat brain. *J Pharmacol Exp Ther* **130**:285–290, 1960

104. Mirkin BL: Perinatal pharmacology. *Anesthesiology* **43**: 156–169, 1975

105. Boreus LO, Jalling B, Kallberg N: Clinical pharmacology of phenobarbital in the neonatal period. In Morselli PL, Garattini S, Sereni F (eds): *Basic and Therapeutic Aspects of Perinatal Pharmacology.* New York: Raven Press, 1975, pp 331–340

106. Knauer B, Draffen GA, Williams FM: Elimination kinetics of amobarbital in mothers and their newborn infants. *Clin Pharmacol Ther* **14**:442–447, 1973

107. Sorbo S, Hudson RJ, Loomis JC: The pharmacokinetics of thiopental in pediatric surgical patients. *Anesthesiology* **61**:666–670, 1984

108. Kosaka Y, Takahashi T, Mark LC: Intravenous thiobarbituate anesthesia for cesarean section. *Anesthesiology* **31**: 489–506, 1969

109. Marcucci F, Mussini E, Airoldi L, et al: Diazepam metabolism and anticonvulsant activity in newborn animals. *Biochem Pharmacol* **22**:3051–3059, 1973

110. Morselli PL, Mandelli M, Tognoni G, et al: Drug interactions in the human fetus and in the newborn infant. In Morselli PL, Cohen SN (eds): *Drug Interactions.* New York: Raven Press, 1974, pp 320–333

111. Greenblatt D, Arendt R, Abernethy D, et al: In vitro quantitation of benzodiazepine lipophilicity, relation to in vivo distribution. *Br J Anesth* **55**:985–989, 1983

112. Smith M, Eadie M, Brophy T: The pharmacokinetics of midazolam in man. *Eur J Clin Pharmacol* **19**:271–278, 1981

113. Fragen R, Gahl F, Caldwell N: A water soluble benzodiazepine, RO21–3981, for induction of anesthesia. *Anesthesiology* **49**:41–43, 1978

114. Nilsson A, Lee P, Revenas B: Midazolam as induction agent prior to inhalation anesthesia: A comparison with thiopentone. *Acta Anaesth Scand* **28**:249–251, 1984

115. Gamble J, Kawar P, Dundee J, et al: Evaluation of midazolam as an intravenous induction agent. *Anaesthesia* **36**:868–873, 1981

116. Berggren L, Eriksson I: Midazolam for induction of anesthesia in outpatients: A comparison with thiopentone. *Acta Anaesth Scand* **25**:492–496, 1981

117. Brown C, Sarnquist F, Canup C, Pedley T: Clinical electroencephalographic and pharmacokinetic studies of a water soluble benzodiazepine midazolam maleate. *Anesthesiology* **50**:467–470, 1979

118. Massaut J, D'Hollander A, Barvais L, Dubois-Primo J: Haemodynamic effects of midazolam in the anaesthetized patients with coronary artery disease. *Acta Anaesth Scand* **27**:299–302, 1983

119. Reeves J, Samuelson P, Lewis S: Midazolam maleate induction in patients with ischemic heart disease: Haemodynamic observation. *Can Anaesth Soc J* **26**:402–407, 1979

120. Lebowitz P, Coté E, Daniels A, et al: Comparative cardiovascular effects of midazolam and thiopental in healthy patients. *Anesth Analg* **61**:771–775, 1982

121. Rita L, Seleny FL, Goodarzi M: Intramuscular midazolam for pediatric preanesthetic sedation: A double-blind controlled study with morphine. *Anesthesiology* **63**:528–531, 1985

122. Feld LH, Champeau MW, van Steennis CA, Scott JC: Preanesthetic medication in children: A comparison of oral transmucosal fentanyl citrate versus placebo. *Anesthesiology* **71**:374–377, 1989

123. Saint-Maurice C, Meistelman C, Rey E, et al: The pharmacokinetics of rectal midazolam for premedication in children. *Anesthesiology* **65**:536–538, 1986

124. Wilton NCT, Leigh J, Rosen DR, Pandit UA: Preanesthetic sedation of preschool children using intranasal midazolam. *Anesthesiology* **69**:972–975, 1988

125. Walbergh EJ, Wills RJ, Eckhert J: Plasma concentrations of midazolam in children following intranasal administration. *Anesthesiology* **74**:233–235, 1991

126. Mathews HML, Carson IW, Lyons SM, et al: A pharmacokinetic study of midazolam in paediatric patients undergoing cardiac surgery. *Br J Anaesth* **61**:302–307, 1988

127. Salonen M, Kanto J, Iisalo E, Himberg JJ: Midazolam as an induction agent in children: A pharmacokinetic and clinical study. *Anesth Analg* **66**:625–628, 1987

128. Mattila M, Saila K, Kokko T, Karkkainen T: Comparison of diazepam and flunitrazepam as adjuncts to general anaesthesia in preventing arousal following surgical stimuli. *Br J Anaesth* **51**:229–331, 1979

129. Hovi-Viander M, Aaltonen L, Kangas L, Kanto J: Flunitrazepam as an induction agent in the elderly, poor risk patients. *Acta Anaesth Scand* **26**:507–510, 1982

130. Kortilla K, Linnoila M: Skills related to driving after intravenous diazepam, flunitrazepam or droperidol. *Br J Anaesth* **46**:961–969, 1974

131. Vega D: Induction of anaesthetic sleep by means of a new benzodiazepine derivative. *Rev Drug Anesthesiol* **5**:41–44, 1971

132. Clarke R, Lyons S: Diazepam and flunitrazepam as induction agents for cardiac surgical operations. *Acta Anaesth Scand* **21**:282–292, 1977

133. George K, Dundee J: Relative amnestic actions of diazepam, flunitrazepam and lorazepam in man. *Br J Clin Pharmacol* **4**:45–50, 1977

134. Rolly G, Lamote D, Cosgert D: Hemodynamic studies of flunitrazepam or RO5-4200 injection in man. *Acta Anesth Belg* **25**:359–370, 1974

135. List W: Monitoring of myocardial function with systolic time intervals. *Acta Anaesth Belg* 29:271–285, 1978

136. Coleman A, Downing J, Mayes D, O'Brien A: Acute cardiovascular effects of RO5-4200: A new anesthetic induction agent. *S Afr Med J* 47:382–384, 1973

137. Hennart D, D'Hollander D, Primo-Dubois J: The haemodynamic effects of flunitrazepam in anesthetized patients with valvular or coronary artery lesions. *Acta Anaesth Scand* 26:183–188, 1982

138. Kanto J, Kangas L, Mansrikka M: Flunitrazepam versus placebo premedication for minor surgery. *Acta Anaesth Scand* 23:561–566, 1979

139. Richardson F, Manfold M: Comparison of flunitrazepam and diazepam for oral premedication in older children. *Br J Anaesth* 51:313–314, 1979

140. Lindgren L, Saarnivarra L, Himberg J: Comparison of i.m. pethidine, diazepam and flunitrazepam as premedicants in children undergoing otolaryngological surgery. *Br J Anaesth* 51:321–327, 1979

141. Kay B: A dose-response relationship for etomidate, with some observation on cumulation. *Br J Anaesth* 48:213–216, 1976

142. Criado A, Maseda J, Navarro E, et al: Induction of anaesthesia with etomidate: Haemodynamic study of 36 patients. *Br J Anaesth* 52:803–805, 1980

143. Gooding J, Corssen G: Effects of etomidate on the cardiovascular system. *Anesth Analg* 56:717–719, 1977

144. Gooding J, Weng J, Smith R, et al: Cardiovascular and pulmonary responses following etomidate induction of anesthesia in patients with demonstrated cardiac disease. *Anesth Analg* 58:40–41, 1979

145. Doenicke A, Lorenz W, Beigl R, et al: Histamine release after intravenous application of short-acting hypnotics. *Br J Anaesth* 45:1097–1104, 1973

146. Kissen I, Motoyama S, Aultman DF, Reves JG: Inotropic and anesthetic potencies of etomidate and thiopental in man. *Anesth Analg* 62:961–965, 1983

147. Van Hamme M, Ghoneim M, Ambre J: Pharmacokinetics of etomidate, a new intravenous anesthetic. *Anesthesiology* 49:274–277, 1978

148. Meuldermans W, Heykants J: The plasma protein binding and distribution of etomidate in dog, rat and human blood. *Arch Int Pharmacodyn Ther* 221:150–162, 1976

149. Ghonheim M, Yamanda T: Etomidate: A clinical and electroencephalographic comparison with thiopental. *Anesth Analg* 56:479–485, 1977

150. Horrigan R, Moyers J, Johnson B, et al: Etomidate vs. thiopental with and without fentanyl—A comparative study of awakening in man. *Anesthesiology* 52:362–364, 1980

151. Gancher S, Laxer K, Krieger W: Activation of epileptogenic activity by etomidate. *Anesthesiology* 61:616–618, 1984

152. Ledingham I, Watt I: Influence of sedation on mortality in critically ill multiple trauma patients. *Lancet* 1:1270, 1983

153. Fragen R, Shanks C, Molteni A, Avram M: Effects of etomidate on hormonal response to surgical stress. *Anesthesiology* 61:652–656, 1984

154. Wagner R, White P: Etomidate inhibits adrenocortical function in surgical patients. *Anesthesiology* 61:647–651, 1984

155. Wagner R, White P, Kan P, et al: Inhibition of adrenal steroidogenesis by the anesthetic etomidate. *N Engl J Med* 310:1415–1421, 1984

156. Longnecker DE: Stress free: To be or not to be? *Anesthesiology* 61:643–644, 1984

157. Kay B, Rolly G: ICI 35868 a new intravenous induction agent. *Acta Anaesth Belg* 28:303–316, 1977

158. Kay B, Stephenson D: Alfentanil (R39209) initial clinical experience with a new narcotic analgesic. *Anaesthesia* 35:1197–1201, 1980

159. Briggs L, Clarke R, Watkins J: An adverse reaction to the administration of disoprofol (Diprivam). *Anaesthesia* 37:1099–1101, 1982

160. Adam H, Briggs L, Bahar M, et al: The pharmacokinetic evaluation of ICI 35868 in man. Single induction dose with different rates of infusion. *Br J Anaesth* 55:97–103, 1983

161. Rogers K, Dewar K, McCubbin T, Spence A: Preliminary experience with ICI 35,868 as an I.V. induction agent: Comparison with althesin. *Br J Anesth* 35:807–810, 1980

162. Fragen R, Hanssen H, Denissen P, et al: Disoprofol (ICI 35868) for total intravenous anaesthesia. *Acta Anaesth Scand* 27:113–116, 1983

163. Prys-Roberts C, Davies J, Calverley R, Goodman N: Haemodynamic effects of infusions of di-isopropyl phenol (ICI 35,868) during nitrous oxide anaesthesia in man. *Br J Anaesth* 55:105–111, 1983

164. O'Callaghan A, Normandale J, Grundy E, et al: Continuous intravenous infusion of disoprofol (ICI 35,868, Diprivan) comparison with althesin to cover surgery under local analgesia. *Anaesthesia* 37:295–300, 1982

165. Al-Khudhairi D, Gordon G, Morgan M, Whitman J: Acute cardiovascular changes following disoprofol. *Anaesthesia* 37:1007–1010, 1982

166. Hannallah RS, Baker SB, Casey W, et al: Propofol: Effective dose and induction characteristics in unpremedicated children. *Anesthesiology* 74:217–219, 1991

167. Borgeat A, Popovic V, Meier D, Schwander D: Comparison of propofol and thiopental/halothane for short-duration ENT surgical procedures in children. *Anesth Analg* 71:511–515, 1990

168. Valtonen M, Iisalo E, Kanto J, Rosenberg P: Propofol as an induction agent in children: Pain on injection and pharmacokinetics. *Acta Anaesth Scand* 33:152–155, 1989

169. Lockhart CH, Nelson WL: The relationship of ketamine requirements to age in pediatric patients. *Anesthesiology* 40:507–508, 1974

170. Chang T, Glazko T: Biotransformation and distribution of ketamine. *Int Anesth Clin* 12:157–177, 1974

171. Waterman AE, Livingston A: Effects of age and sex on ketamine anesthesia in the rat. *Br J Anaesth* 50:885–889, 1978

172. Eng M, Bonica JJ, Akamatsu TJ, et al: Respiratory depression in newborn monkeys at cesarean section following ketamine administration. *Br J Anaesth* 47:917–920, 1975

173. Radney PA, Badola RP: Generalized extensor spasm in infants following ketamine anesthesia. *Anesthesiology* 39:459–460, 1973

174. Lockhart CH, Jenkins JJ: Ketamine-induced apnea in

patients with increased intracranial pressure. *Anesthesiology* **37**:92–93, 1972

175. Gasser S, Cohen M, Aygen M: The effect of ketamine on pulmonary artery pressure. *Anaesthesia* **29**:141–146, 1974

176. Morray JP, Lynn AM, Stamm SJ, et al: Hemodynamic effects of ketamine in children with congenital heart disease. *Anesth Analg* **63**:895–899, 1984

177. Hickey PR, Hansen DD, Cramolini GM: Pulmonary and systemic hemodynamic responses to ketamine in infants with normal and elevated pulmonary vascular resistance. *Anesthesiology* **61**:A438, 1984

178. Way WL, Costley EC, Way EL: Respiratory sensitivity of the newborn infant to meperidine and morphine. *Clin Pharmacol Ther* **6**:454–459, 1965

179. Kupferberg HJ, Way EL: Pharmacologic basis for the increased sensitivity of the newborn rat to morphine. *J Pharmacol Exp Ther* **141**:105–109, 1963

180. Mirkin BL: Developmental pharmacology. *Ann Rev Pharmacol* **10**:255–272, 1970

181. Hickey PR, Hansen DD: Fentanyl- and sufentanil-oxygen-pancuronium anesthesia for cardiac surgery in infants. *Anesth Analg* **63**:117–124, 1984

182. Hickey PR, Hansen DD, Wessell D: Pulmonary and systemic responses to high dose fentanyl in infants. *Anesth Analg* **64**:483–486, 1985

183. Schieber RA, Stiller RL, Cook DR: Cardiovascular and pharmacodynamic effects of high-dose fentanyl in newborn piglets. *Anesthesiology* **63**:166–171, 1985

184. Koren G, Goresky G, Crean P, et al: Pediatric fentanyl dosing based on pharmacokinetics during cardiac surgery. *Anesth Analg* **63**:577–582, 1984

185. Yaster M: The dose response of fentanyl in neonatal anesthesia. *Anesthesiology* **66**:433–435, 1987

186. Ellis DJ, Steward DJ: Fentanyl dosage is associated with reduced blood glucose in pediatric patients after hypothermic cardiopulmonary bypass. *Anesthesiology* **72**:812–815, 1990

187. Anand KJS, Hickey PR: Halothane-morphine compared with high-dose sufentanil for anesthesia and postoperative analgesia in neonatal cardiac surgery. *N Engl J Med* **326**:1–9, 1992

188. Koehntop DE, Rodman JH, Brundage DM, et al: Pharmacokinetics of fentanyl in neonates. *Anesth Analg* **65**:227–232, 1986

189. Singleton MA, Rosen JI, Fisher DM: Pharmacokinetics of fentanyl for infants and adults. *Anesthesiology* **61**:A440, 1984

190. Johnson KL, Erickson JP, Holley FO, Scott JC: Fentanyl pharmacokinetics in the pediatric population. *Anesthesiology* **61**:A441, 1984

191. Collins G, Koren G, Crean P, et al: The correlation between fentanyl pharmacokinetics and pharmocodynamics in preterm infants during PDA ligation. *Anesthesiology* **61**:A442, 1984

192. Collins G, Koren G, Crean P, et al: Fentanyl pharmacokinetics and hemodynamic effects in preterm infants during ligation of patent ductus arteriosus. *Anesth Analg* **64**:1078–1080, 1985

193. Koren G, Goresky G, Crean P, et al: Unexpected alterations in fentanyl pharmacokinetics in children undergoing cardiac surgery: Age related or disease related? *Dev Pharmacol Ther* **9**:183–191, 1986

194. Nesson PS, Streisand JB, Mulder SM, et al: Comparison of oral transmucosal fentanyl citrate and an oral solution of meperidine, diazepam, and atropine for premedication in children. *Anesthesiology* **70**:616–621, 1989

195. Streisand JB, Stanley TH, Hague B, et al: Oral transmucosal fentanyl citrate premedication in children. *Anesth Analg* **69**:28–34, 1989

196. Goldstein-Dresner MC, Davis PJ, Kretchman E, et al: Comparison of oral transmucosal fentanyl citrate with meperidine, diazepam, and atropine as in children with congenital heart disease. *Anesthesiology* **74**:28–33, 1991

197. Niemegeers CJ, Schellenkens KH, VanBever WF, Janssen PA: Sufentanil, a very potent and extremely safe intravenous morphine-like compound in mice, rats and dogs. *Arzneimittelforschung* **26**:1551–1556, 1976

198. Reddy P, Liu W, Port D, et al: Comparison of haemodynamic effects of anaesthetic doses of alphaprodine and sufentanil in the dog. *Can Anaesth Soc J* **27**:345–356, 1980

199. Meuldermans W, Hurkmans R, Heykants J: Plasma protein binding and distribution of fentanyl, sufentanil, alfentanil and lofentanil in blood. *Arch Int Pharmacodyn Ther* **25**:4–19, 1982

200. deLange S, Boscoe M, Stanley T, Pace N: Comparison of sufentanil-oxygen and fentanyl-oxygen for coronary artery surgery. *Anesthesiology* **56**:112–118, 1982

201. Howie M, Rietz J, Reilley T, et al: Does sufentanil's shorter half-life have any clinical significance? *Anesthesiology* **59**:A146, 1983

202. Sanford TJ, Smith NT, Dec-Silver H, Harison WK: A comparison of morphine, fentanyl and sufentanil anesthesia for open-heart surgery, induction, emergence, and extubation. *Anesth Analg* **65**:259–266, 1986

203. Sebel P, Bovill J: Cardiovascular effects of sufentanil anesthesia. *Anesth Analg* **61**:115–119, 1982

204. deLange S, Boscoe M, Stanley T, et al: Antidiuretic and growth hormone response during coronary artery surgery with sufentanil-oxygen and alfentanil-oxygen anesthesia in man. *Anesth Analg* **61**:434–438, 1982

205. Bovill J, Sebel P, Blackburn C, Heykants J: The pharmacokinetics of alfentanil (R39209): A new opiate analgesic. *Anesthesiology* **57**:439–443, 1982

206. Rosow C, Philbin D, Moss J, et al: Sufentanil vs. fentanyl: I. Suppression of hemodynamic responses. *Anesthesiology* **59**:A323, 1983

207. Bovill J, Sebel P. Fiolet J, et al: The influence of sufentanil on endocrine and metabolic responses to cardiac surgery. *Anesth Analg* **62**:391–397, 1983

208. Hickey P, Hansen D: Fentanyl and sufentanil-oxygen-pancuronium anesthesia for cardiac surgery in infants. *Anesth Analg* **63**:117–124, 1984

209. Henderson JM, Brodsky DA, Fisher DM, et al: Pre-induction of anesthesia in pediatric patients with nasally administered sufentanil. *Anesthesiology* **68**:671–675, 1988

210. Helmers JHJH, Noorduin H, Van Peer A, et al: Comparison of intravenous and intranasal sufentanil absorption and sedation. *Can J Anaesth* **36**:5; 494–497, 1989

211. DeCastro J, Van De Weter A, Wouter L, et al: Comparative study of cardiovascular, neurological and metabolic side-effects of 8 narcotics in dogs. *Acta Anaesth Belg* **30**:5–99, 1979

212. Camu F, Gepts E, Rucquoi M, Heykants J: Pharmaco-

kinetics of alfentanil (R39709) in man. *Anesth Analg* **61**: 657–661, 1982

213. Hug C: *Alfentanil: Pharmacology and Uses in Anaesthesia.* Langhorne, PA, Adis Press, 1984

214. Davis PJ, Stiller RL, Cook DR, et al: Effects of cholestatic hepatic disease and chronic renal failure on alfentanil pharmacokinetics in children. *Anesth Analg* **68**:579–83, 1989

215. Meistelman C, Saint-Maurice C, Lepaul M, et al: A comparison of alfentanil pharmacokinetics in children and adults. *Anesthesiology* **66**:13, 1987

216. Roure P, Jean N, Leclerc A-C, et al: Pharmacokinetics of alfentanil in children undergoing surgery. *Br J Anaesth* **59**:1437, 1987

217. Davis PJ, Killian A, Stiller RL, et al: Pharmacokinetics of alfentanil in newborn premature infants and older children. *Dev Pharmacol Ther* **13**:21–27, 1989

218. Killian A, Davis PJ, Stiller RL, et al: Influence of gestational age on pharmacokinetics of alfentanil in neonates. *Dev Pharmacol Ther* **15**:82–85, 1990

219. McDonnell T, Bartkowski R, Williams J: ED_{50} or alfentanil for induction of anesthesia in unpremedicated young adults. *Anesthesiology* **60**:136–140, 1984

220. Nauta J, Delange S, Koopman D, et al: Anesthetic induction with alfentanil, a new short acting narcotic analgesic. *Anesth Analg* **61**:267–272, 1982

221. deLange S, Boscoe M, Stanley T, Pace N: Comparison of sufentanil-oxygen and alfentanil-oxygen for coronary artery surgery. *Anesthesiology* **56**:112–118, 1982

222. Leysen J, Commern W, Niemegers C: Sufentanil a superior ligand for u-opiate receptors: Binding properties and regional distribution in rat brain and spinal cord. *Eur J Pharmacol* **87**:209–225, 1983

223. Kay B, Pleuvry B: Human volunteer studies of alfentanil (R39209), a new short-acting narcotic analgesic. *Anaesthesia* **35**:952–956, 1980

224. Kay B, Stephenson D: Alfentanil (R39209): Initial clinical experiences with a new narcotic analgesic. *Anaesthesia* **35**:1197–1201, 1980

225. Kramer M, Kling D, Walter P, et al: Alfentanil, a new, short acting opioid. Haemodynamic and respiratory aspects. *Anaesthesist* **32**:265–271, 1983

226. Stanley T, Pace N, Liu W, et al: Alfentanil-N_2O vs fentanyl-N_2O balanced anesthesia: Comparison of plasma hormonal changes, early postoperative respiratory function and speed of postoperative recovery. *Anesth Analg* **62**:285, 1983

227. deLangre S, Boscoe M, Stanley T, et al: Catecholamine and cortisol response to sufentanil-oxygen and alfentanil-oxygen anaesthesia during coronary artery surgery. *Can Anaesth Soc J* **30**:248–254, 1983

228. Ecobichon DJ, Stephen DS: Perinatal development of human blood esterases. *Clin Pharmacol Ther* **14**:44–46, 1973

229. Blankenbaker WL, DiFazio CA, Berry FA Jr: Lidocaine and its metabolites in the newborn. *Anesthesiology* **42**:325–330, 1975

230. Moore RG, Thomas J, Triggs DB, et al: The pharmacokinetics and metabolism of anilide local anesthetics in neonates. *Eur J Clin Pharmacol* **14**:203–212, 1978

231. Morgan D, McQuillan D, Thomas J: Pharmacokinetics and metabolism of the anilide local anesthetics in neonates. *Eur J Clin Pharmacol* **13**:365–371, 1981

232. Finholt DA, Stirt JA, DiFazio CA, Moscicki JC: Lidocaine pharmacokinetics in children. *Anesthesiology* **63**: A467, 1985 (abstr)

233. Eyres RL, Kidd J, Oppenheim R, Brown TCK: Local anaesthetic plasma levels in children. *Anaesth Intensive Care* **6**:243–247, 1978

234. Ecoffey C, Desparmet J, Berdeaux A, et al: Pharmacokinetics of lidocaine in children following caudal anaesthesia. *Br J Anaesth* **56**:1399–1401, 1984

235. Bokesch PM, Castaneda AR, Ziemer G, Wilson JM: The influence of a right-to-left cardiac shunt on lidocaine pharmacokinetics. *Anesthesiology* **67**:739–744, 1987

236. Dauchot P, Gravenstein JS: Effects of atropine on the electrocardiogram in different age groups. *Clin Pharm Exp Ther* **12**:274–280, 1971

237. Gaviotaki A, Smith RM: Use of atropine in pediatric anesthesia. *Int Anesthesiol Clin* **1**:97–114, 1962

238. Harris WS, Goodman PM: Hyperreactivity to atropine in Down's syndrome. *N Engl J Med* **279**:407, 1968

239. Priest JH: Atropine response of the eyes in mongolism. *Am J Dis Child* **100**:869–872, 1960

240. Berg JM, Brandom MWG, Kirwan BH: Atropine in mongolism. *Lancet* **2**:441–442, 1959

241. Cook DR, Fischer CG: Neuromuscular blocking effects of succinylcholine in infants and children. *Anesthesiology* **42**:662–665, 1975

242. Cook DR, Fischer CG: Characteristics of succinylcholine neuromuscular blockade in infants. *Anesth Analg* **57**:63–66, 1978

243. Goudsouzian NG, Liu LMP: The neuromuscular response of infants to a continuous infusion of succinylcholine. *Anesthesiology* **60**:97–101, 1984

244. Walts LF, Dillon JB: The response of newborns to succinylcholine and d-tubocurarine. *Anesthesiology* **31**:35–38, 1969

245. Churchill-Davidson HC, Wise RP: The response of the newborn infant to muscle relaxants. *Can Anaesth Soc J* **11**:1–5, 1964

246. Donlon JV, Ali HH, Savarese JJ: A new approach to the study of four non-depolarizing relaxants in man. *Anesth Analg* **53**:924–939, 1974

247. Goudsouzian NG, Liu LMP, Coté CJ: Comparison of equipotent doses of non-depolarizing muscle relaxants in children. *Anesth Analg* **60**:862–866, 1981

248. Goudsouzian NG, Liu LMP, Savarese JJ: Metocurarine in infants and children: Neuromuscular and clinical effects. *Anesthesiology* **49**:266–269, 1978

249. Goudsouzian NG, Ryan JF, Savarese JJ: The neuromuscular effects of pancuronium in infants and children. *Anesthesiology* **41**:95–98, 1974

250. Goudsouzian NG, Donlon JV, Savarese JJ, Ryan JF: Reevaluation of dosage and duration of action of d-tubocurarine in the pediatric age group. *Anesthesiology* **43**:416–425, 1975

251. Goudsouzian NG, Martyn JJA, Liu LMP: The dose response effect of long-acting non-depolarizing neuromuscular blocking agents in children. *Can Anaesth Soc J* **31**: 246–250, 1984

252. Cook DR: Sensitivity of the newborn to tubocurarine. *Br J Anaesth* **53**:320, 1981

253. Fisher DM, O'Keefe C, Stanski DR, et al: Pharmacokinetics and pharmacodynamics of d-tubocurarine in in-

fants, children, and adults. *Anesthesiology* **57**:203–208, 1982

254. Pittet JF, Tassonyi E, Morel DR, et al: Neuromuscular effect of pipecuronium bromide in infants and children during nitrous oxide-alfentanil anesthesia. *Anesthesiology* **72**:432–435, 1990

255. Sarner, JB, Brandom BW, Cook DR, et al: Clinical pharmacology of doxacurium chloride (BW A938U) in children. *Anesth Analg* **67**:303–306, 1988

256. Sarner JB, Brandom BW, Dong ML, et al: Clinical pharmacology of pipecuronium in infants and children during halothane anesthesia. *Anesth Analg* **71**:362–366, 1990

257. Cook DR, Freeman JA, Lai AA, et al: Pharmacokinetics and pharmacodynamics of doxacurium in normal patients and those with hepatic or renal failure. *Anesth Analg* **72**:145–150, 1991

258. Caldwell JE, Canfell PC, Castagnoli KP, et al: The influence of renal failure on the pharmacokinetics and duration of action of pipecuronium bromide in patients anesthetized with halothane and nitrous oxide. *Anesthesiology* **70**:7–12, 1989

259. Stiller RL, Cook DR, Chakravorti S: *In vitro* degradation of atracurium in human plasma. *Br J Anaesth* **57**:1085–1088, 1985

260. Stiller RL, Brandom BW, Cook DR: Determinations of atracurium by high-performance liquid chromatography. *Anesth Analg* **64**:58–62, 1985

261. Brandom BW, Woelfel SK, Cook DR, et al: Clinical pharmacology of atracurium in infants. *Anesth Analg* **63**:309–312, 1984

262. Brandom BW, Rudd GD, Cook DR: Clinical pharmacology of atracurium in pediatric patients. *Br J Anaesth* **55**:117s–121s, 1983

263. Brandom BW, Cook DR, Woelfel SK, et al: Atracurium infusion in children during halothane, isoflurane, and narcotic anesthesia. *Anesth Analg* **64**:471–476, 1985

264. Goudsouzian NG, Liu L, Coté CJ, et al: Safety and efficacy of atracurium in adolescents and children anesthetized with halothane. *Anesthesiology* **39**:459–462, 1983

265. Goudsouzian NG, Liu LMP, Gionfriddo M, Rudd GD: Neuromuscular effects of atracurium in infants and children. *Anesthesiology* **62**:75–79, 1985

266. Brandom BW, Cook DR, Stiller RL, et al: Pharmacokinetics of atracurium in anesthetized infants and children. *Br J Anaesth* **58**:1210–1213, 1986

267. D'Hollander AA, Luyckx C, Barvais L, DeVille A: Clinical evaluation of atracurium besylate requirement for a stable muscle relaxation during surgery: Lack of age-related effects. *Anesthesiology* **59**:237–240, 1983

268. Durant NN: Norcuron, a new nondepolarizing neuromuscular blocking agent. *Semin Anesth* **1**:47–56, 1982

269. Fisher DM, Miller RD: Neuromuscular effects of vecuronium (ORG NC45) in infants and children during N_2O, halothane anesthesia. *Anesthesiology* **58**:519–523, 1983

270. D'Hollander AA, Massaux F, Nevelsteen M, Agoston S: Age-dependent dose-response relationship of ORG NC45 in anaesthetized patients. *Br J Anaesth* **54**:653–657, 1982

271. Goudsouzian NG, Martyn J, Liu LMP, Gioffrido M: Safety and efficacy of vecuronium in adolescents and children. *Anesth Analg* **62**:1083–1088, 1983

272. Rupp SM, Miller RD, Gencarelli PJ: Vecuronium-induced neuromuscular blockade during enflurane, halothane, and isoflurane in humans. *Anesthesiology* **60**:102–105, 1984.

273. Miller RD, Rupp SM, Fisher DM, et al: Clinical pharmacology of vecuronium and atracurium. *Anesthesiology* **61**:444–453, 1984

274. Fisher DM, Castagnoli K, Miller RD: Vecuronium kinetics and dynamics in anesthetized infants and children. *Clin Pharm Ther* **37**:402–406, 1985

275. Foldes FF, Nagashima H, Nguyen HD, et al: The neuromuscular effects of ORG9426 in patients receiving balanced anesthesia. *Anesthesiology* **75**:191–196, 1991

276. Brandom BW, Sarner JB, Woelfel SK, et al: Mivacurium infusion requirements in pediatric surgical patients during nitrous oxide-halothane and during nitrous oxide–narcotic anesthesia. *Anesth Analg* **71**:16–22, 1990

277. Digby-Leigh M, McLoyd D, Belton MK, et al: Bradycardia following intravenous administration of succinylcholine in anesthetized children. *Anesthesiology* **18**:698–702, 1957

278. Craythorne NWB, Turndorf H, Dripps RD: Changes in pulse rate and rhythm associated with the use of succinylcholine in anesthetized children. *Anesthesiology* **21**:465–471, 1960

279. Cook DR, Westman H, Rosenfeld L, Hendershot RJ: Pulmonary edema in infants: Possible association with intramuscular succinylcholine. *Anesth Analg* **60**:220–223, 1981

280. Fisher DM, Cronnelly R, Miller RD, Sharma M: The neuromuscular pharmacology of neostigmine in infants and children. *Anesthesiology* **59**:220–225, 1983

281. Fisher DM, Cronnelly R, Sharma M, Miller RD: Clinical pharmacology of edrophonium in infants. *Anesthesiology* **61**:428–433, 1984

282. Meakin G, Sweet PT, Bevan JC, Bevan DR: Neostigmine and edrophonium as antagonists of pancuronium in infants and children. *Anesthesiology* **59**:316–321, 1983

Chapter 10 | Extracorporeal Circulation and Circulatory Assist Devices in the Pediatric Patient

Frank H. Kern, Willis G. Gieser, David M. Farrell

Cardiopulmonary bypass (CPB) began in the early 1950s when creative young surgeons recognized that performing complex open-heart surgery required a heart-lung machine. Gibbon developed the first heart-lung machine, and he was the first physician to repair successfully an atrial septal defect using his machine in 1953.[1] The machine was large, cumbersome, and required 14 U of blood to prime.

One year later, at the University of Minnesota, Lillehei performed the first closure of a ventricular septal defect using the technique of cross circulation. Cross circulation used a human donor (usally a parent) as a "heart-lung machine." A venous cannula was placed into the heart patient's superior vena cava and blood coursed through a pump head and into the femoral vein of the donor. A second cannula was placed into the donor's femoral artery, and flow from the femoral artery was returned to the heart patient's carotid artery. Cross circulation was first used in 1954. Forty-five patients, mostly children, were operated on using this technique, with an overall survival rate of 63%, a result that was quite outstanding by mid-1950s standards.[2,3]

Kirklin, then at the Mayo Clinic, began developing a pump oxygenator based on the original Gibbon device in the early 1950s. After 2 years of successful laboratory work, eight children underwent open-heart surgery using the Gibbon-Mayo pump oxygenator, with a 50% survival rate. The Gibbon-Mayo pump oxygenator required 5–11 U of freshly drawn blood to prime. Blood flow through the oxygenator had to be slow and controlled to prevent foaming of blood, which was lethal because of the lack of defoaming agents.[4]

Since the 1950s, pediatric CPB has evolved from a high-risk technology with a 50% mortality to a safe and effective procedure performed at many hospitals throughout the world. Yet, despite the successful application of the technology and nearly 50 years of investigation, the effect of CPB on the patient remains poorly understood. This is particularly true in children, in whom CPB substantially alters normal physiology.

ANATOMY OF THE EXTRACORPOREAL CIRCUIT

A schematic diagram of the extracorporeal circuit is presented in Fig 10–1. The circuit consists of an oxygenator (bubble or membrane), pumps (roller or centrifugal), tubing, filters (fluid and gas), cardiotomy circuit, cannulas (venous and arterial), and priming solution. Each of these components will be discussed in detail.

Oxygenators
In the pediatric population, oxygenators must provide efficient gas exchange over a wide range of temperatures (10–40°C), pump flow rates (0–200 mL/kg/min), hematocrit (15–30%), circuit pressures, and gas flow rates. Most commercially available oxygenators (both bubble and membrane) achieve effective gas exchange under these diverse conditions.

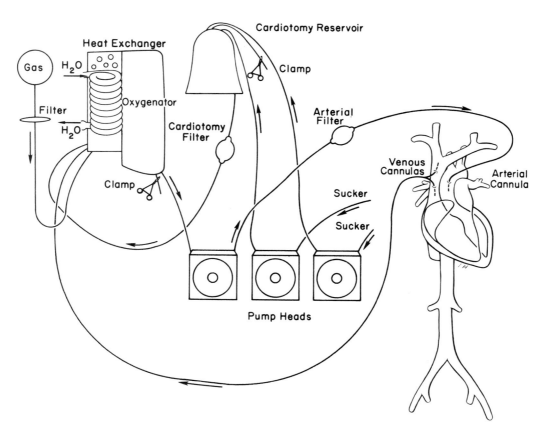

Figure 10–1. A schematic drawing of the extracorporeal circuit.

Bubble Oxygenators. In a bubble oxygenator, fresh gas is passed through a dispersing plate (diffuser, sparger), producing bubbles of varying size. The bubbled gas passes into an oxygenating column where the blood and gas mix, producing a froth of gas and blood. It is within this froth that gas exchange occurs. The efficiency of gas exchange is dependent on the surface area of the gas bubbles and the transit time through the oxygenating column. Multiple small bubbles provide a greater surface area than large gas bubbles. Small bubbles improve gas exchange within the froth and are preferable. Transit time through the oxygenating column depends on the amount of blood in the arterial reservoir.

The oxygenated blood-gas froth passes through a defoaming mesh or sponge that is coated with silicone antifoam. The antifoam decreases the surface tension of the bubbles, causing them to collapse and release trapped gas. Defoamed blood then passes into the arterial reservoir. A high level of blood in the reservoir provides additional time for defoaming and allows residual microbubbles to rise to the surface of the reservoir. Because the arterial outlet is located on the bottom of the oxygenator, the incidence of gaseous microemboli is reduced. Too large a reservoir blood level, however, may limit the area available for gas and blood interaction, reducing the efficiency of the oxygenator.

A major concern with oxygenators, however, is blood trauma. Trauma to blood causes hemolysis, complement activation, thrombocytopenia, and platelet aggregation.[5,6] Complement activation and platelet damage cause pulmonary endothelial damage and contribute to the exaggerated stress response (high levels of circulating catecholamines, hormones, and vasoconstrictors, such as prostaglandin $F_{2\alpha}$ ($PGF_{2\alpha}$) and thromboxane) during CPB.[7] Platelet microaggregates may cause systemic microembolization and neurologic injury. Bubble oxygenators, with a direct blood:gas interface, are more traumatic to the cellular elements of blood. Therefore, they pose a greater overall risk than membrane oxygenators. In one study, a higher incidence of retinal microemboli and neuropsychiatric deficits were seen in adult CPB patients using a bubble oxygenator as compared with a membrane oxygenator.[8] A recent study, utilizing a silicone membrane oxygenator (SciMED, SciMed Life Systems, Inc, Minneapolis, MN), demonstrated no increase in the vasoconstrictors, thromboxane and $PDF_{2\alpha}$, when warm partial cardiopulmonary bypass was initiated as extracorporeal membrane oxygenation (ECMO) therapy for neonates with severe pulmonary disease.[9] This is in marked contrast to hypothermic CPB studies using bubble oxygenators in which thromboxane production, complement, and platelet activation are commonly described.[10–12] Based on these considerations, membrane oxygenators may be preferable for cardiopulmonary bypass in both children and adults.

Membrane Oxygenators. The membrane oxygenator attempts to approximate a human lung. The membrane acts as a synthetic alveolar-capillary membrane, with no direct interface between the blood and gas. There are currently two distinct types of membrane oxygenators: hollow fiber and folded membrane.

Hollow-Fiber Oxygenators. These types of oxygenators consist of a large series of microporous polypropylene tubes. Each tube acts as a series of alveolar-capillary membranes. Gas flows inside and blood flows outside of the tubes. Small pores, approximately 3–5 μm in size, allow some contact between the blood and gas phases at the initiation of bypass. During perfusion, however, protein deposits form along the pores, preventing direct contact between the gas and blood.

Because hollow-fiber membranes are microporous, a slow continuous leakage of protein occurs over time. The protein leak reduces membrane efficiency and patient plasma proteins. For these reasons, hollow-fiber membranes are not recommended for long-term perfusion. An example of a hollow-fiber membrane oxygenator is the D705 Midiflow (Dideco, Italy) that is used exclusively for pediatric bypass. It is small in size and has a low priming volume.

The microporous system is the most common method used for perfusion during bypass. Its advantage is improved gas exchange with a relatively small total membrane surface area. The disadvantages are protein leak and gas emboli. Gas embolization occurs if negative pressure develops on the blood side of the membrane, which entrains gas into the arterial blood to be pumped into the systemic circulation of the patient.

Folded-Membrane Oxygenators. These types of oxygenator are subdivided into plate types and coil types. Plate-type membranes are microporous and their function is similar to the hollow-fiber oxygenators. An example of a plate-type membrane oxygenator is the Variable Prime Cobe Membrane Lung (VPCML®) (Fig 10–2). The membrane of this oxygenator has two separate compartments: a small compartment for infants (surface area of 0.4 m²) and a larger compartment for children (surface area of 0.85 m²). For small adults, both compartments can be used in series for a combined membrane surface area of 1.25 m². The separate compartment structure of the oxygenator allows priming volumes of 220, 290, and 375 mL, respectively (priming volume is defined as the volume of the membrane compartment plus the minimal rated venous reservoir level). An additional advantage of the VPCML® oxygenator is the inclusion of the cardiotomy reservoir and the heat exchanger within the device.

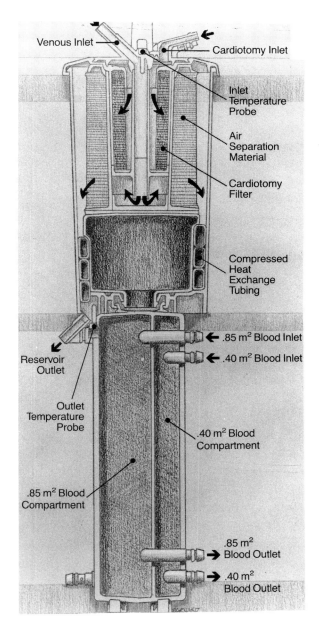

Figure 10–2. The Variable Prime Cobe Membrane Lung (VPCML®) oxygenator is easily adapted to infants, small children, or adolescents by selecting one of three membrane-priming areas, a 0.4-m² membrane compartment for infants, a 0.85-m² membrane compartment for children, and both compartments used together for adolescents (1.25 m²). Blood enters the VPCML from the cardiotomy circuit and the venous inlet. Blood is filtered, warmed, oxygenated, and then pumped back into the patient's arterial circulation.

The coil-type membrane is made of nonporous silicone and is the only nonporous membrane currently available. Nonporous membranes require a larger surface area for gas exchange but do not leak protein. They are the only membranes currently recommended for long-term perfusion. The SciMED membrane that is used for ECMO support is an example of a nonporous silicone membrane.

Pumps

Roller or centrifugal pumps are currently used for CPB. The twin rotary-type roller pump is the most widely used pump in pediatric perfusion (Fig 10–3). This pump consists of two rollers that are oriented 180 degrees from each other. The roller pumps provide continuous blood flow by partially occluding the tubing between the roller and the pump casing. Blood is displaced in a forward direction by the roller generating continuous, nonpulsatile flow. The second roller acts as a valve to minimize back flow. The rollers are never totally occlusive because that would encourage hemolysis. Ideally, the amount of occlusion for each roller is set independently of the other. This is especially true in neonate and infant perfusion where maladjustment of occlusion increases the error in estimating pump flow rate.

Centrifugal pumps are newer devices that have gained increasing popularity because of their use in ECMO and ventricular assist devices. Flow is maintained by the entrainment of blood against spinning impellers (curved blades) or by creating a vortex utilizing a centrifugal cone. The advantages of centrifugal pumps are less damage to formed blood elements, a vortex design that entrains air (minimizing the likelihood of small systemic air emboli), and less damage to pump tubing (reducing the likelihood of particulate emboli from the internal surface of the pump tubing). These pumps are also capable of producing pulsatile blood flow that may improve flow in the microcirculation (see below). An example is the Biomedicus (Biomedicus, Eden Prairie, MN) pump (Fig 10–4).

Tubing

Tubing size should be small to reduce prime volume but large enough to achieve effective flow rates and low cir-

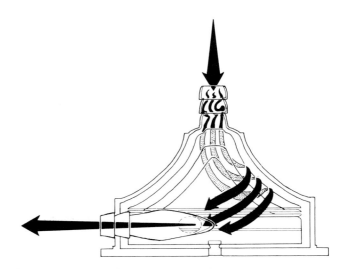

Figure 10–4. The Biomedicus centrifugal pump. Blood is entrained against spinning blades and pumped in a forward direction. This design allows air to be drawn toward the top of the pump, separating air from the pump outlet located at the bottom of the pump.

cuit pressure. Both the length and the diameter of the tubing contribute to prime volume. In neonates, 0.25-inch tubing is used for both the arterial and venous limbs of the circuit. Tube length is kept as short as possible. Positioning the pump as close to the surgical field as is feasible significantly reduces the length of tubing. For example, 0.25-inch tubing requires approximately 30 mL of volume per meter of tube length. Each meter of tubing, therefore, requires a prime volume equal to 10% of the newborn's circulating blood volume.

Cardiotomy Circuit

The cardiotomy circuit consists of a reservoir, roller pumps (distinct from the pump used for circulatory support), and filters. The circuit is used to suction blood from the field and return it to the patient's circulation. Suction tubing from the cardiotomy circuit can be attached to suction cannulas in the surgical field or to aortic, atrial, or ventricular vents. Collected blood is drained into a venous reservoir that can then be added to the oxygenator through the venous inflow port and returned to the patient's circulation.

Filters

All fluids and gas entering the extracorporeal circuit are filtered. The gas inflow line is filtered through a 0.2-μm filter to prevent bacterial contamination or entry of particulate contaminants that may be present in stored gases. Fluids pass through a variety of filters. Crystalloid solutions added to the perfusate are initially passed through a 0.2-μm bacteriostatic filter. This eliminates any particulate matter accumulated during storage in the plastic bag and removes bacteria larger than 0.2 μm in

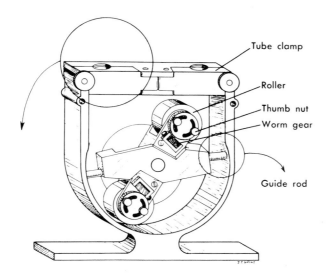

Figure 10–3. A nonocclusive roller pump is the most commonly used pump for CPB. The twin roller design is used to eliminate back flow. (*From Nose Y: The Oxygenator. St. Louis: CV Mosby, 1973, p 171, with permission.*)

Tube clamp

Roller

Thumb nut

Worm gear

Guide rod

size. Once primed with crystalloid, the extracorporeal fluid is again filtered through a second 0.2-μm filter to remove any particulate matter that may dislodge from the oxygenator, venous reservoir, or pump tubing. Blood, filtered through a standard 40-μm transfusion filter, is then added to the perfusate. The mixed crystalloid and blood perfusate passes through a 40-μm filter in the arterial limb of the extracorporeal circuit before entering the patient's circulation. The 40-μm filter is small enough to exclude most microemboli such as fat, platelets, and other debris that may enter from the cardiotomy suction.

Cannulas

Cannulas must be flexible and capable of maintaining their shape and flow characteristics despite rapid changes in temperature during hypothermic CPB. In neonates and infants, the cannula's tip needs to be small enough to insert into tiny aortas and not impede blood flow around the cannula. At the same time, the cannula tip must be large enough to sustain adequate perfusion flow rates at relatively low pressures. Excessive perfusion pressure at the level of the cannula tip may create a powerful jet of blood that could damage the intima of the aorta and blood cells. Modifications of the cannula tip can substantially change flow characteristics. Tables 10–1 and 10–2 list recommended cannula size and special features of pediatric cannulas.

Arterial Cannulation.

The arterial cannula is generally placed into the ascending aorta; however, the child's great vessel anatomy and the type of surgical procedure may influence arterial cannula choice and placement. Cannula choice may be affected by the size of the aorta. For example, in infants with moderately small aortas, an appropriately sized aortic cannula may fit so snugly that it physically obstructs aortic outflow. Biomedicus cannulas have thinner walls and larger internal diameters for a given French size. A smaller Biomedicus catheter can provide effective pump flow without obstructing the aorta in such infants (see Table 10–1).

Cannula placement is also affected by great vessel anatomy. In hypoplastic left heart syndrome, the ascending aorta is extremely small and cannot accept an arterial cannula. The arterial cannula is therefore placed in the main pulmonary artery. Systemic perfusion is maintained from the pulmonary artery through the ductus arteriosus and into the aorta. Infants with interrupted aortic arch require two aortic cannulas, one in the ascending aorta to perfuse the head and one in the descending aorta to perfuse the body.

The surgical procedure may also dictate aortic cannula placement. In newborns with transposition of the great arteries, the arterial cannula is placed in the distal aspect of the ascending aorta because a large portion of the surgery occurs on the aortic root. The distal placement of the aortic cannula may actually alter the distribution of the pump flow away from the head vessels, as discussed later.

Femoral artery cannulation is uncommon in infant heart surgery. The femoral and iliac vessels of infants are relatively small and may not accept an adequately sized cannula to provide effective systemic perfusion. In older children requiring reoperation, sternotomy may pose a high risk of inadvertently entering a conduit or a ventricular chamber. Femoral cannulation and peripheral bypass may prove life saving under these circumstances.

Venous Cannulation.

Venous anatomy can be very complex. Bilateral superior venae cavae (SVC), inferior venae cavae (IVC), which drain into an azygous vein or hemiazygous vein, or hepatic veins, which drain directly into an atrial chamber, are common anatomic variations of the venous system (see Chapter 17). Venous cannulation must consider these variables as well as the type of perfusion planned.

If the repair is going to take place under deep hypothermic circulatory arrest, venous cannulation is simple. A large single venous cannula is placed in the right atrium to achieve effective venous drainage. Once the patient is cooled, the cannulas are removed and surgery proceeds in a cannula-free field (the surgeon may elect to leave the aortic cannula in place if it does not obstruct the surgical field). In contrast, repairs performed during continuous flow must address the complex venous anatomy. This is particularly true in patients with complex venous anatomy requiring surgery within the atrial chambers such as the modified Fontan procedure (see Chapter 19).

In the modified Fontan operation (total cavopulmonary anastomosis), as many as three venous cannulas may be required. A venous cannula must be placed at the SVC/innominate junction because the operation requires a direct anastomosis of the SVC to the right pulmonary artery. Venous drainage is more effective and the cannula is less obstructive to the surgical field if a right-angle venous cannula is used. The IVC is cannulated with a straight venous cannula that is inserted below the pericardial reflection. A cannula with a short tip avoids plac-

TABLE 10–1. RECOMMENDED ARTERIAL CANNULAS FOR CHILDREN

Weight (kg)	Cannula Size (French)	Internal Diameter (in)	
		Bard	Biomedicus
<5	10	0.067	0.079
5.0–7.5	12	0.091	0.105
7.5–15.0	14	0.109	0.131
15–30	16	0.125	0.158
30–50	18	0.148	
>50	20	0.164	

TABLE 10–2. PEDIATRIC VENOUS CANNULAS

Cannula Type	Manufacturer	Special Characteristics	Use
Straight	Bard–William Harvey	Lighthouse tip with closed end; multiple side hole, short tip; wire reinforcement prevents kinking	Standard bicaval cannula
Straight (infant)	Bard–William Harvey	Same as above but smaller, lower-volume cannula	Standard bicaval cannula or single atrial cannula
Straight	Research Medical Inc.	Lighthouse tip with open end plus multiple side holes; wire reinforced	Standard bicaval cannula
Straight	Biomedicus	Thin wall with open end and side holes; better flow with smaller external diameter	Femoral cannula
Straight (infant)	Biomedicus	Thin wall with open end and side holes; better flow with smaller external diameter	VAD, ECMO, or single atrial cannula
Right Angle	DLP	Thin wall with metal tip and open end; metal tip prevents kinking	Direct SVC cannulation
Right Angle	Polystan	Lighthouse tip	Direct SVC cannulation

Abbreviations: VAD, ventricular assist device; ECMO, extracorporeal membrane oxygenation; SVC, superior vena cava.

ing the cannula beyond the hepatic veins and causing hepatic venous obstruction. A third venous cannula may be required if a large left SVC is present. If the left-sided SVC is very small or if it decompresses into a bridging vein draining into the right SVC or azygous, it may be ligated.

In order to meet the surgical requirements, a large assortment of venous cannulas should be available. Table 10–2 lists several types of venous cannulas and their particular characteristics. The type of venous cannula used and the amount of venous return depend on cannula size, patient anatomy, site of insertion, and effective cannula placement by the surgeon.

Impact of Cannula Placement. Appropriate placement of aortic and venous cannulas is important to ensure effective systemic perfusion. A malpositioned venous cannula has the potential for vena caval obstruction. The problems of venous obstruction are magnified during CPB because of low perfusion pressures. This is particularly true in the neonate, in whom large, relatively stiff venous cannulas easily distort very pliable great veins.[13–15]

A cannula in the IVC may obstruct venous return from the splanchnic bed resulting in ascites from increased hydrostatic pressure or directly reduce perfusion pressure across the mesenteric, renal, and hepatic vascular beds. Significant renal, hepatic, and gastrointestinal dysfunction may ensue and should be anticipated in the patient with unexplained ascites after weaning from CPB.

Similar cannulation problems may result in SVC obstruction. This problem may result in elevated jugular venous pressure, decreased cerebral perfusion pressure, and cerebral edema. Reduced cerebral blood flow velocity, using transcranial Doppler monitoring, during transient occlusion of the SVC cannula has been observed

(personal observation). In the operating room, it is advisable either to monitor SVC pressures directly via an internal jugular line or by looking at the patient's face for signs of increased puffiness or venous distension after initiating bypass. Discussions with the perfusionist regarding adequacy of venous return should alert the anesthesiologist and the surgeon to potential venous cannula problems. Patients with anomalies of the large systemic veins (persistent left superior vena cava or azygous continuation of an interrupted IVC) are at particular risk for venous cannulation problems.[16]

Problems with aortic cannula placement are also likely in neonates and infants. The tip of the aortic cannula may be beyond the takeoff of the innominate artery and therefore flow to the right side of the cerebral circulation may be retrograde through the circle of Willis. Similarly, the position of the aortic cannula may promote preferential flow down the aorta or induce a Venturi effect to steal flow from the cerebral circulation. This problem has been suggested during xenon cerebral blood flow (CBF) measurements by noting large discrepancies in CBF between the right and left hemisphere after initiating CPB (personal observation). Placement of the aortic cannula in a more distal location, commonly employed in procedures in which ascending aorta or proximal aortic arch reconstruction is required (arterial switch procedure), may alter CBF. Cooling patterns are substantially different in neonates and infants compared with those commonly observed in the adult or older child. Rectal cooling precedes tympanic membrane cooling, suggesting that a disproportionate amount of pump flow may be directed away from the cerebral circulation.[17]

Differences Between Children and Adults

The physiologic effects of CPB in neonates, infants, and children are grossly different from adults (Table 10–3). Pediatric patients are exposed to biologic extremes, in-

TABLE 10–3. MAJOR PHYSIOLOGIC DIFFERENCES OF CPB IN CHILDREN VS ADULTS

	Adults	Children
Amount of hemodilution of ECF*	13%	60%
Temperature (°C)	28–32	15–20
Pump flow (mL/kg/min)	50	0–200
Mean arterial pressure (mm Hg)	≥30	20?
Paco₂ (mm Hg)	30–45	20–80

*ECF, extracellular fluid.

cluding deep hypothermia (15–20°C), hemodilution (3- to 15-fold greater dilution of circulating blood volume than typically seen in adults), low perfusion pressures (20–20 mm Hg), wide variation in pump flow rates (ranging from highs of 200 mL/kg/min to total circulatory arrest) and alpha-stat versus pH-stat blood pH management. These parameters significantly differ from normal physiology and impact on organ function during and after CPB. In addition to these prominent changes, subtle variations in glucose supplementation, cannula placement, the presence of aortopulmonary collaterals, and patient age may also be important factors that affect organ function during cardiopulmonary bypass.

Adult patients are rarely exposed to these biologic extremes. Temperature is not usually decreased below 25°C, hemodilution is more moderate, perfusion pressure is generally maintained at 50–80 mm Hg (although some centers accept perfusion pressures of 30 mm Hg), flow rates are maintained at 50–65 mL/kg/min, and pH management strategy is less influential because of moderate hypothermic temperatures and the rare use of circulatory arrest. Variables, such as glucose supplementation, are generally not a problem in adult patients owing to large hepatic glycogen stores. Venous and arterial cannulas are larger, produce less deformation of the atria and aorta, and their placement is more predictable. Although superficially similar, the conduct of cardiopulmonary bypass in children is considerably different from adults. Therefore, one would expect marked physiologic differences in the response to CPB in the child.

PHYSIOLOGY OF BYPASS

Prime

The priming solutions used in pediatric cardiopulmonary bypass are of greater importance than in adults because of the large priming to blood volume ratio. In adults, the priming volume is equivalent to 25–33% of the patient's blood volume, whereas in neonates and infants, the priming volume exceeds patient blood volume by 200–300%. Therefore, care must be taken to achieve a physiologically balanced prime.

Most pediatric priming solutions, however, have variable concentrations of electrolytes, calcium, glucose,

and lactate. Electrolytes, glucose, and lactate concentrations may be increased if the prime includes large amounts of bank blood or decreased if minimal amounts of bank blood are added. Calcium concentrations are generally reduced in pediatric prime solutions. Hypocalcemia may contribute to the rapid slowing of the heart with the initiation of bypass. The main constituents of the priming solution include crystalloid, banked blood (to maintain a temperature-appropriate hematocrit), and colloid. Other supplements that may be added are mannitol, a buffer (sodium bicarbonate or tris(hydroxymethyl)aminomethane [THAM]), and steroids. Many institutions add colloid to the pump prime in neonates and small infants or use whole blood in the priming solution. Low concentrations of plasma proteins have been shown experimentally to impair lymphatic flow and alter pulmonary function by increasing capillary leak.[18,19] Although adding albumin to pump prime has not been shown to alter outcome in adults during CPB, one study has suggested that maintaining normal colloid osmotic pressure may improve survival in infants undergoing CPB.[20,21]

For neonates and infants, blood must be added to the priming solution. Most institutions use packed red blood cells (RBCs) in their prime solution. However, some institutions use whole blood. The main disadvantage of whole blood over packed RBCs is a higher glucose load. Hyperglycemia may increase the risk of neurologic injury if brain ischemia occurs. The advantage of adding whole blood to the priming solution is the maintenance of higher concentrations of plasma factors. Circulating clotting factors are significantly diluted in neonates during CPB, as described later.

Mannitol is added to promote an osmotic diuresis and to scavenge oxygen free radicals from the circulation. Steroids are added to stabilize membranes for the theoretical advantage of reducing ion shifts during periods of ischemia. However, steroids may increase blood glucose. Steroids remain one of the more controversial additives in priming solutions.

Hemodilution. Although hemoconcentrated blood has an improved oxygen-carrying capacity, its viscosity reduces efficient flow through the microcirculation. Hypothermia, coupled with the nonpulsatile flow of CPB, impairs blood flow through the microcirculation. Blood sludging, small vessel occlusion, and multiple areas of tissue hypoperfusion may result. Therefore, hemodilution is an important consideration during hypothermic CPB. The appropriate level of hemodilution for a given hypothermic temperature, however, is not well defined.

Experimental evidence suggests that reducing hematocrits to as low as 15% provides a sufficient quantity of oxygen delivery to the myocardium at normothermia (provided intravascular volume, colloid osmotic pressure, and normotension are maintained).[22] At hypothermic temperatures, animal studies and observations in patients who belong to the Jehovah's Witnesses religious sect suggest hematocrits reduced to as low as 10% provide adequate oxygen delivery during CPB as long as flow rates and perfusion pressure are maintained.[23,24]

Most centers maintain hematocrit levels at 20 ± 2% during deep hypothermia (15–20°C) and will allow the hematocrit to drift as low as 15% before transfusing additional red blood cells. Although this is an arbitrary limit, lower hematocrit values have not been systematically evaluated to ensure adequate oxygen delivery to tissues. Cerebral oxygen delivery is an especially important consideration because cerebral autoregulation is impaired at deep hypothermic temperatures and after total circulatory arrest.

In order to achieve an hematocrit of 20 ± 2% in neonates and infants, banked blood is added to the priming solution. A calculation of the mixed hematocrit on CPB (the hematocrit of the total priming volume [TPV] plus the patient's blood volume) can be calculated by the formula:

$$Hct_{CPB} = \frac{(BV_{pt})(Hct_{pt})}{(BV_{pt}) + TPV}$$

where Hct_{CPB} = the mixed Hct (TPV + BV_{pt}), BV_{pt} = patient's blood volume (weight [kg] × estimated blood volume [mL/kg]), TPV = total priming volume, and Hct_{pt} = starting hematocrit of the patient.[25] This calculation estimates the patient hematocrit using an asanguineous prime and is useful for older children and adolescents. In neonates and infants, the perfusionist must add blood to the pump prime in order to achieve a desired hematocrit during hypothermic CPB. The following formula estimates the amount of red blood cells that must be added to achieve this hematocrit.

$$\begin{aligned} \text{Added RBCs (mL)} = {} & (BV_{pt} + TPV)(Hct_{desired}) \\ & - (BV_{pt})(Hct_{pt}) \end{aligned}$$

where added RBCs = milliliters of packed RBCs added to the prime volume, BV_{pt} = patient's blood volume, TPV = total priming volume, $Hct_{desired}$ = the desired hematocrit on CPB, and Hct_{pt} = starting hematocrit of the patient.

Currently, no evidence exists for defining the optimal hematocrit after weaning from CPB. Decisions about hematocrits are based on cardiac function and anatomy after the repair. Palliated patients or patients with moderate to severe myocardial dysfunction benefit from the improved oxygen-carrying capacity of hematocrit levels of 50% or higher. Patients with a physiologic correction and excellent myocardial function should tolerate hematocrit levels of 25% or lower.[22] In children with mild to moderate myocardial dysfunction accepting hematocrit levels between these extremes seems prudent. Therefore, in patients with physiologic correction, moderately good ventricular function, and hemodynamic stability,

the risks associated with blood and blood product transfusion should be strongly considered before transfusion is performed in the immediate postbypass period.

Flow Rates

Recommendations for optimal pump flow rates for children have historically been based on the patient body mass and the maintenance of efficient organ perfusion as determined by arterial blood gases, acid-base balance, and whole-body oxygen consumption during cardiopulmonary bypass (Fig 10–5).[26,27] Table 10–4 lists recommended, albeit arbitrary, normothermic flow rates for children based on body weight. Metabolism is reduced at hypothermic temperatures. Pump flow rates can therefore be reduced and still meet or exceed tissue metabolic needs.

Anticoagulation and Reversal

The contact of blood with the nonendothelialized surfaces of the CPB circuit initiates the coagulation cascade. To prevent coagulation during cardiopulmonary bypass, the patient must be adequately anticoagulated with heparin. In 1975, Bull devised a quantitative method for heparin administration using the activated clotting time (ACT) as an endpoint.[28] By maintaining ACTs of between 300 and 600 seconds, visible clot formation in the operative field and the pump oxygenator were prevented. A more fastidious evaluation using a radioimmunoassay for fibrin monomers demonstrated the presence of fibrin monomers when ACTs were maintained between 300 and 400 seconds.[29] Therefore, it may be preferable to keep ACTs at 400 seconds or greater for prolonged periods of CPB in both the adult and pediatric population.

Although it is now feasible to measure plasma heparin levels, there is generally a poor correlation between heparin levels and activated clotting time.[25] Because it is the effect of heparin on coagulation and not plasma heparin concentration that is important, the activated clotting time remains the preferred monitor of effective coagulation during CPB. However, heparin concentrations may be helpful after heparin reversal with protamine to assess residual heparin activity or the presence of heparin rebound.

Before initiating bypass, heparin is generally administered in an initial bolus dose of 300–400 U/kg (3–4 mg/kg), which produces an ACT level of 400 seconds or greater. Heparin is administered before cannulation of the great vessels either by direct injection into the right atrium or through a functioning central line. In either case, care must be taken to assure that heparin enters the central circulation. Blood should be aspirated before injection, and an ACT of greater than 400 seconds should be documented before initiating CPB. Periodic measurements of the ACT are performed throughout CPB to assure an adequate degree of anticoagulation.

At the end of CPB, heparin activity is antagonized

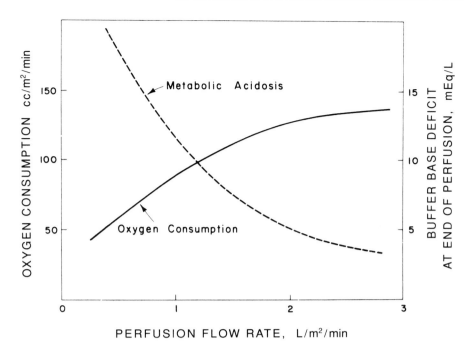

Figure 10–5. Determination of optimum flow rate has traditionally been based on systemic oxygenation and acid-base balance. These data are less useful when deep hypothermia used. At deep hypothermia, metabolism is severely reduced and cerebral autoregulation is lost. (*From Norman JC: Cardiac Surgery, 2nd ed. East Norwalk, CT: Appleton & Lange, 1972, with permission.*)

by protamine in a ratio of 1 mg of protamine for every 100 U (1 mg) of residual heparin ACT effect. Bleeding after heparin reversal remains a common and difficult problem, particularly in neonates and young infants. CPB alters the coagulation system through factor and platelet hemodilution, platelet dysfunction (due to hypothermia and platelet activation by the pump oxygenator), and, to a lesser degree, secondary fibrinolysis (disseminated intravascular coagulation, DIC).[30,31] These problems are magnified in infants and neonates because of the marked degree of hemodilution on CPB, the use of deep hypothermia, high flow rates (resulting in greater shear forces), greater exposure of blood to the nonendothelialized surface of the CPB circuit, the use of prostaglandin E_1 (a platelet inhibitor that is used for ductal patency), and hepatic dysfunction. Hepatic dysfunction reduces factor levels and may be due to organ immaturity (neonate) or systemic hypoperfusion (left-sided obstructive lesion, excessive left-to-right shunting, or primary myocardial failure) resulting in hepatic synthetic dysfunction.[32]

TABLE 10–4. RECOMMENDED PUMP FLOW RATES FOR CPB IN CHILDREN

Weight (kg)	Pump Flow Rate (mL/kg/min)
<3	150–200
3–10	125–175
10–15	120–150
15–30	100–120
30–50	75–100
>50	50–75

Table 10–5 is a coagulation profile from 20 newborn infants undergoing CPB.[33] Prebypass fibrinogen levels and platelet numbers are normal in these newborns. However, the percent activity of factors II, V, VII, VIII, IX, and X is reduced when compared with healthy newborns.[34] During bypass, factor activity is further reduced by hemodilution and fibrinolysis.

Thrombocytopenia occurs to a greater extent than can be accounted for by hemodilution alone and probably reflects platelet activation by the nonendothelialized surfaces of the CPB circuit and pump oxygenator. At the termination of CPB, a diffuse coagulopathy with relatively severe reductions in factor activity (including fibrinogen) and platelet number is present. Fibrinogen deficiency is more striking in newborns with a prebypass fibrinogen level less than 200 mg/dL resulting from decreased hepatic synthesis of fibrinogen. Hepatic immaturity and/or reduced hepatic function due to poor systemic perfusion are the most likely causes. At the end of CPB, fibrinogen levels in such infants are uniformly less than 100 mg/dL, signifying a marked fibrinogen deficiency. Hypofibrinogenemia may be an important factor contributing to postbypass hemorrhage (Table 10–6).

The approach to hemostasis in neonates and infants should reflect these hemostatic problems. Fresh whole blood, which has both factors and active platelets, is a more complete therapy and the preferred blood product for transfusion after heparin reversal with protamine in neonates and infants.[35] Recent studies have shown improved platelet function and a reduced transfusion requirement when fresh whole blood is compared with

TABLE 10–5. COAGULATION PROFILE IN NEONATES DURING CPB

Assay	Pre-CPB	1 min on CPB	Cold CPB	Warm CPB	Post-protamine	ICU
Fibrinogen	200 ± 59*	92 ± 18	94 ± 21	107 ± 24*	142 ± 28*	183 ± 33
Factor 2	56 ± 13	30 ± 7	32 ± 8	33 ± 7§	48 ± 10	60 ± 33
Factor 5	68 ± 20*	15 ± 4	17 ± 5	22 ± 7*	39 ± 11*	46 ± 10
Factor 7	54 ± 11†	26 ± 5	27 ± 6	28 ± 5†	41 ± 8†	53 ± 16
Factor 8	48 ± 20‡	0	0	0	32 ± 15‡	72 ± 45
Factor 9	31 ± 13	20 ± 8	23 ± 5	31 ± 4	31 ± 9	40 ± 12
Factor 10	52 ± 10	31 ± 7	31 ± 7	34 ± 8§	46 ± 10	47 ± 16
Platelets (k/mm³)	225 ± 54*	65 ± 17	45 ± 8	93 ± 28*	120 ± 29*	
Antithrombin 3	49 ± 22	30 ± 12	29 ± 15	32 ± 13§	57 ± 28	68 ± 23
Heparin (units)	0.02 ± 0.03	0.41 ± 0.08	0.42 ± 0.08	0.42 ± 0.08	0.04 ± 0.04	0.07 ± 0.06
ACT (seconds)	168 ± 20	>700	>700	>700	151 ± 31	

Fibrinogen, Factors 2, 5, 7, 8, 9, 10, and antithrombin 3 are in % activity.
* $P < 0.0001$.
† $P < 0.002$.
‡ $P < 0.005$.
§ < 0.05.
(From Kern FH, et al: Coagulation defects in neonates during CPB. Ann Thorac Surg 54:541–546, 1992.)

component therapy.[36,37] The freshness of the blood remains controversial. In a recent study, fresh whole blood (24 and 48 hours old) was of equal value to very fresh whole blood (<6 hours old) in children under 2 years of age. Both products proved superior to component therapy for these young children, but too few neonates were evaluated to determine if very fresh whole blood would be more beneficial in newborns, in whom immature hepatic function and prolonged bypass have a greater impact on coagulation.

Newer approaches to reducing postbypass hemorrhage are preservation of platelet function and prevention of fibrinolysis through drug therapy. Drugs such as desmopressin (DDAVP), ε-aminocaproic acid, and aprotinin have been evaluated. DDAVP, which raises plasma von Willebrand factor, was initially reported to reduce blood loss after CPB.[38] However, two recent studies

TABLE 10–6. NEONATES WITH PREBYPASS LOW FIBRINOGEN LEVELS IN MG/DL

Assay	All Patients ($n = 15$)	Patients with Fibrinogen <200 ($n = 7$)	Patients with Fibrinogen ≥200 ($n = 8$)
Pre-CPB	209 ± 58	160 ± 23†	260 ± 32‡
1 min post-CPB	93 ± 19	86 ± 17	102 ± 21
Cold CPB	95 ± 21	77 ± 8	102 ± 21
Warm CPB	109 ± 23	90 ± 15	127 ± 16
Post-protamine	140 ± 31*	112 ± 11*	163 ± 24‡
2–3 h Post-operative	183 ± 35	175 ± 42	189 ± 32

Fibrinogen is in % activity.
* $P < 0.05$
† $P < 0.001$.
‡ $P < 0.003$.
(From Kern FH, et al: Coagulation defects in neonates during CPB. Ann Thorac Surg 54:541–546, 1992.)

were unable to confirm this.[39,40] ε-Aminocaproic acid, an inhibitor of fibrinolysis, showed a small but significant decrease in postoperative blood loss in one study.[41] More recently, aprotinin, which inhibits fibrinolysis and preserves platelet function through an antifibrinolytic effect, markedly improved postoperative hemostasis in adult patients.[42,43] However, improved hemostasis has not been documented in children.

CONDUCT OF CPB

Initiation of CPB

Once the aortic and venous cannulas are positioned and connected to the arterial and venous limbs of the extracorporeal circuit, bypass is initiated. The arterial pump is slowly started, and once forward flow is assured, venous blood is drained into the oxygenator. Pump flow rate is gradually increased until full circulatory support is achieved. If venous return is diminished and circuit pressure or mean arterial pressure excessive, pump flow rates must be reduced. Increased circuit pressure and inadequate venous return are usually due to malposition or kinking of the arterial and venous cannulas, respectively. The diagnosis and management of serious problems during perfusion such as hypoxia, acute aortic dissection, hypertension, and hypotension are similar in children and adults. The reader is referred to a textbook of adult cardiac anesthesia.

The rate at which venous blood is drained from the patient is determined by the gradient due to the height difference between the patient and the oxygenator inlet and the diameter of the gradient due to the venous cannula and tubing. Venous drainage is enhanced by increasing the height difference between the oxygenator inlet and the patient or by using a larger venous cannula.

Venous drainage is reduced by either decreasing the height difference between the oxygenator and the patient or partially clamping the venous line.

In neonates and infants, some degree of hypothermia is commonly used. For this reason, the pump prime is kept cold (18°–22°C). When the cold prime perfuses the myocardium, the heart rate immediately slows and contraction is impaired. The contribution to total blood flow pumped by the infant's heart rapidly diminishes at the onset of CPB. Therefore, to sustain adequate systemic perfusion at or near normothermic temperatures, the arterial pump must reach full flows quickly. CPB is initiated in neonates and infants by starting arterial inflow first. Once arterial flow is assured, the venous drainage is unclamped and blood is siphoned from the right atrium into the inlet of the oxygenator. Initiation of arterial flow before unclamping the venous drainage prevents the potential problem of exsanguination if aortic dissection or malplacement of the aortic cannula occurs. Neonates and infants have a low blood volume to prime volume ratio and intravascular volume falls precipitously if the venous drainage precedes aortic inflow. Once aortic cannula position is assured, the pump flow rates are rapidly increased to maintain effective systemic perfusion. Because coronary artery disease is not a consideration, the myocardium should cool evenly. When a cold prime is used, caution must be exercised in using the pump to infuse volume prior to initiating CPB. Infusion of cold perfusate may result in bradycardia and impaired cardiac contractility before the surgeon is prepared to initiate CPB.

Once CPB begins, observation of the heart is crucial. Ineffective venous drainage can rapidly result in ventricular distension. This is especially true in infants and neonates, in whom ventricular compliance is low and the heart is relatively intolerant of excessive preload augmentation (a flat Starling curve).[44] If ventricular distension occurs, pump flow must be reduced and the venous cannula repositioned. Alternatively, the heart may be vented by placing a pump sucker into the right atrium and across the right-sided atrioventricular valve.

Monitors of the Oxygenator or Oxygenator-Patient Interface.

Essential monitors of the extracorporeal circuit include pressure, flow, biochemical variables (blood gases, pH, electrolytes, hematocrit), and temperature. Pressure, flow, temperature, and oxygenator reservoir level are monitored continuously, whereas biochemical analyses are performed either continuously with indwelling electrodes or intermittently in a laboratory. The mean arterial pressure of the patient is continuously measured via an indwelling arterial catheter in the radial, femoral, brachial, dorsalis pedis, or other artery. Central venous, left atrial, or pulmonary pressures are also monitored via appropriate catheter-transducer systems.

Arterial Inflow Line Pressure. The pressure required to force blood through the arterial cannula is higher than the patient's mean arterial pressure because the arterial inflow tubing is small compared with the aorta and lung causing a pressure differential between the extracorporeal circuit and the patient. This pressure, often termed the "pump pressure" or "back pressure," is measured in the arterial inflow tubing via a partially occluding clamp. Normal pressures are 250–260 mm Hg at patient mean arterial pressures of 50–60 mm Hg but vary with the system. There are two very important reasons for continuous monitoring of the arterial inflow line pressure: (1) there is a possibility of disruption of the extracorporeal circuit with pressures greater than 300 mm Hg, and (2) correct arterial inflow cannula placement can be assured by observing a pulsatile pressure prior to initiation of bypass.

Flow. Flow is measured using an electromagnetic flowmeter on the arterial inflow tubing or by determining the number of pump revolutions per unit time. Flow rates measured by the latter method are dependent upon the inside diameter of the tubing, the size of the arterial cannula, and the speed of the pump. In addition to monitoring flow, a sensor can be placed on the oxygenator reservoir to indicate when the blood level in the reservoir has decreased to critical levels. The level sensor is particularly critical in an oxygenator with a rigid reservoir because the wall of a collapsible reservoir is sucked onto the arterial outlet when it is empty preventing massive air embolism.

Biochemical Variables. Arterial P_{O_2}, P_{CO_2}, and pH should be measured within 5 minutes of initiation of perfusion and at 30-minute intervals thereafter. More frequent determinations are necessary when clinical events require immediate information. Venous P_{O_2} is measured if arterial P_{O_2} is decreased or there is concern about tissue oxygenation. Current work suggests that correction of the blood gases during bypass to the patient's temperature is unnecessary. Instead, normal blood gases should be maintained in the patient when measured at 37°C in the laboratory.[45–47] Although sampling ports on both arterial and venous inlets of the oxygenator are available, the values obtained from these sites are usually higher than those in the patient.[48] Shunting of blood within the patient accounts for this difference. Therefore, blood samples during bypass should be taken from the patient's arterial catheter rather than the oxygenator. Serum potassium and hematocrit are also determined at similar time intervals as blood gases.

Because transport to a laboratory and performance of the tests in the laboratory setting may take 10–12 minutes, many perfusionists use on-line systems such as the Diamond Gem–6 (Diamond Sensor Systems, Ann Arbor, MI) system, which provides values within 130 seconds of sample introduction. Fluorescence sensors (such as the Cardiovascular Devices Intravascular Blood Gas Monitoring System) in the patient's intra-arterial catheter permit continuous blood gas data. Rapid acquisition of blood gas parameters permits frequent changes in gas/blood flow ratios in the oxygenator to prevent hypoxia, hyperoxia, hypocarbia, or hypercarbia.

Temperature. The temperature of the arterial and venous blood as well as patient esophageal, rectal, nasopharyngeal, and tympanic membrane temperature are continuously monitored using appropriate thermistors. Perfusion cooling and rewarming must be carefully monitored to prevent the occurrence of temperature gradients in excess of 10°C between patient and perfusate during rewarming.

Ventilating Gases. Oxygen, carbon dioxide, and anesthetic vapor concentrations are determined in gases entering and exiting from the oxygenator. Various types of analysis systems may be used, including infrared analysis, mass spectrometers, and Raman scattering techniques. In addition, anesthetic gases must be scavenged from the exhaust part of the oxygenator in a manner similar to that used from the anesthesia machine.[49–51]

Hypothermic CPB

Hypothermic CPB preserves organ function during cardiac surgery. Three distinct methods are used: moderate hypothermia (25–32°C), deep hypothermia (15–20°C), or deep hypothermia with total circulatory arrest (TCA). The choice of methods is based on surgical conditions, patient size, the type of operation, and potential physiologic impact on the patient.

Moderate hypothermia is the principal method used in older children and adolescents. In these patients, venous cannulas are less obtrusive and the heart can easily accommodate superior and inferior venae cavae cannulas. Bicaval cannulation reduces right atrial blood return and improves the surgeon's view of intracardiac anatomy. Moderate hypothermia may also be chosen for less demanding cardiac repairs in infants, such as an atrial or uncomplicated ventricular septal defect.

Deep hypothermic cardiopulmonary bypass is generally reserved for neonates and infants requiring complex cardiac repair. However, certain older children with complex cardiac disease or severe aortic valve regurgitation (where cardioplegia becomes less effective in producing electrical silence) benefit from deep hypothermic temperatures. For the most part, deep hypothermia is selected to allow the surgeon to operate under conditions of low-flow CPB or TCA. Low pump flows improve the operating conditions for the surgeon by providing a near bloodless field. Deep hypothermic CPB with TCA allows the surgeon to remove the atrial and aortic cannulas. Utilizing this technique, surgical repair is more precise because of the bloodless and cannula-free operative

field. Circulatory arrest, even at deep hypothermic temperatures, raises questions about hypothermic preservation of organ function, with the brain being at greatest risk. Extensive clinical experience using TCA suggest that a safe circulatory arrest period is approximately 50–60 minutes.[52] Formal experimental data evaluating the effect of TCA on organ function, however, remains limited.

Physiology of Hypothermic CPB and TCA. The goal of hypothermic CPB is to provide organ protection through a reduction in cellular metabolism and preservation of high-energy phosphate stores. As temperature decreases, both basal and functional cellular metabolism and the rate of adenosine triphosphate (ATP) and phosphocreatine consumption are substantially reduced.[53,54] At deep hypothermia, cellular metabolism is so low that cellular integrity and basal metabolic needs are met by high-energy phosphate stores for a relatively prolonged period of time. Hypoxic/ischemic injury begins when high-energy phosphate stores are depleted. Although all organs are at risk for hypoxic/ischemic injury, the brain is the most sensitive. Therefore, brain ischemia/hypoxia is the limiting factor when using low flow rates and TCA.

Hypothermic CPB and the Brain

MODERATE HYPOTHERMIA. The physiologic impact of CPB with moderate hypothermia (MHCPB) on children is similar to that described for adults.[55,56] The systemic vasculature constricts with temperature reduction and thereby directs a larger proportion of flow toward the brain. Cerebral blood flow (CBF) and metabolism ($CMRO_2$) decrease with cooling and the percentage of total pump flow proportioned to the cerebral circulation increases as temperature decreases.[57] CBF is dependent on brain metabolism. If metabolic needs are high, the cerebral vascular resistance falls, and CBF increases. This relationship, called flow/metabolism coupling, remains intact during moderate hypothermic CPB.[56,58]

Pressure flow autoregulation, or the ability to maintain a constant CBF despite wide ranges in mean arterial pressures, also remains intact during moderate hypothermic CPB. Alterations in perfusion pressure over a range of 15–18 mm Hg do not alter CBF (Fig 10–6). Thus, during moderate hypothermia, the cerebral vasculature remains capable of dilation during low perfusion pressure and constriction when perfusion pressure is high.[59]

DEEP HYPOTHERMIA. During deep hypothermia (using alpha-stat blood gas strategy), the normal vascular responses that are present during MHCPB are lost.[55,58,59] In the brain, the cerebral vasculature cannot dilate in response to low mean arterial pressures and therefore reductions in systemic pressure decrease CBF, ie, a loss

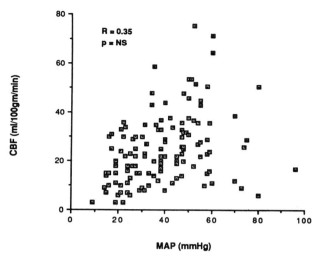

Figure 10–6. At moderate hypothermic temperatures, CBF is independent of mean arterial pressure. This is due to cerebral pressure/flow autoregulation.

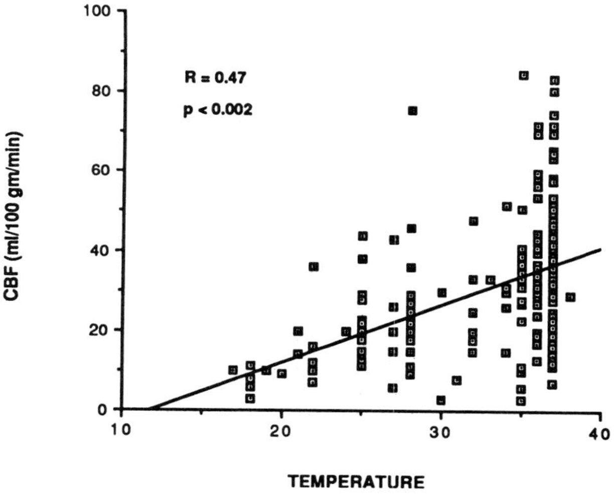

Figure 10–8. CBF decreases linearly with hypothermia.

of pressure flow autoregulation (Fig 10–7). Deep hypothermic temperatures affect CBF and cerebral metabolism differently. CBF decreases with cooling in a linear fashion and cerebral metabolism decreases in an exponential fashion (Figs 10–8 and 10–9). The net result is that CBF becomes more luxuriant at deep hypothermic temperatures and flow/metabolism coupling is lost. At normothermia, the mean ratio of CBF to $CMRO_2$ is 20/1, and at deep hypothermia, the ratio increases to 75/1.[58] This finding becomes important when low-flow CPB is used.

In theory, low-flow CPB could provide an indefinite period of effective cerebral perfusion during hypother-

mia if adequate cerebral oxygen delivery is supplied. Because cerebral blood flow becomes increasingly luxuriant with temperature reduction, pump flow requirements should decrease at lower temperatures.[25,57] Recent evidence suggests that at deep hypothermic temperatures (15–18°C), reductions in pump flow rate to 30–35 mL/kg/min in neonates and infants do not significantly impact on cerebral metabolism. In fact, animal data (supported by a small number of measurements made in human infants) indicate that pump flow rates may be reduced to as low as 10 mL/kg/min at deep hypothermic temperatures before impacting on cerebral metabolic needs.[54,60] At more moderate hypothermic

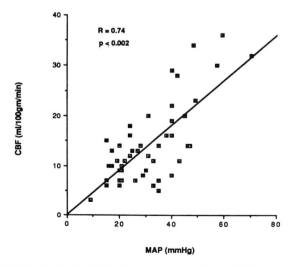

Figure 10–7. At deep hypothermic temperatures, CBF decreases with reductions in mean arterial pressure. Pressure/flow autoregulation is lost at deep hypothermic temperatures.

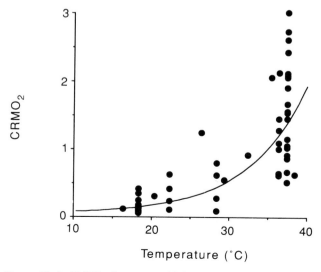

Figure 10–9. $CMRO_2$ decreases with hypothermia. There is an exponential relationship between temperature and hypothermia.

temperatures of 27–28°C, flow reductions to 30–35 mL/kg/min in the neonate and infant appear to impact on the brain's metabolic needs, suggesting that these pump flow rates are at best marginal for CPB using moderate hypothermic temperatures. These findings are consistent with the effect of temperature on CBF/CMRO$_2$ ratios.[60,61]

DEEP HYPOTHERMIC CPB WITH TCA. Figure 10–10 is a diagrammatic representation of the cellular events causing ischemic brain injury. Hypothermia prevents ischemic injury by interrupting this cascade at several levels, including reduction of the cerebral metabolic rate and preservation of high-energy phosphate stores. By reducing the metabolic rate of the brain, ATP stores are preserved, transmembrane ionic gradients are maintained, and the damaging effects of calcium entry and excitatory neurotransmitter release are prevented.[54,62–66]

Extensive clinical experience using TCA has shown the duration of a safe circulatory arrest period to be approximately 50–60 minutes.[52] A more precise method of predicting safe limits for TCA based on brain metabolism has recently been described.[58] For the brain, the metabolic reduction induced by hypothermia is described by the temperature coefficient of Q$_{10}$, which is the ratio of brain metabolism measured at two temperatures separated by 10°C. It has recently been shown that

hypothermia decreases CMRO$_2$ by a mean of 3.6 for every 10°C reduction in temperature in children.[58] If one assumes that the brain can tolerate an ischemic period of 3–5 minutes at normothermia without causing ischemic brain damage, Q$_{10}$ data means that if the brain is thoroughly cooled to 15°C, brain metabolism is sufficiently reduced to allow for a "safe" circulatory arrest period of 53–90 minutes. Similarly, safe arrest periods can be predicted for any temperature based on Q$_{10}$ data for children (Table 10–7). These data are supported by investigators who have examined the protective effect of deep hypothermia by measuring high-energy phosphate compounds with ^{31}phosphorus nuclear magnetic resonance (^{31}P-NMR).[54,63] These investigators report that whereas ATP is rapidly depleted during normothermic arrest, ATP levels are slowly depleted during deep hypothermic arrest (15–20°C). Despite the apparent safety of total circulatory arrest, both transient and permanent neuropsychologic dysfunction have been reported in as many as 25% of all infants undergoing TCA.[67] In palliative surgery, such as stage 1 repair of hypoplastic left heart syndrome, acquired neuropathologic injury has been reported in as many as 45% of patients.[68] Such findings suggest that other factors, such as cardiac function after bypass, may also play important roles in determining neurologic outcome in patients with congenital heart disease.

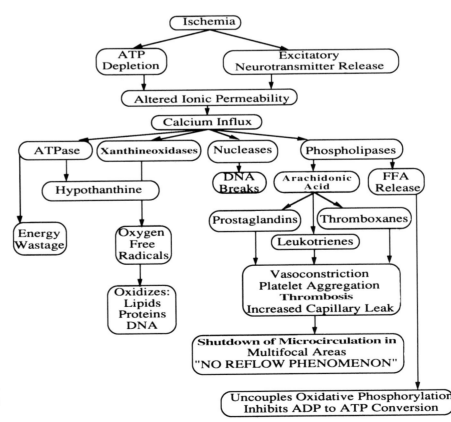

Figure 10–10. A flow chart describing the cellular events occurring during normothermic arrest.

TABLE 10–7. DEFINING SAFE PERIODS OF TCA BASED ON HYPOTHERMIA

NPT	TCA Limits*	
37°C	3.0 min	5.0 min
32°C	5.7 min	9.5 min
30°C	7.3 min	12.5 min
27°C	11.1 min	18.5 min
25°C	14.4 min	24.0 min
20°C	27.9 min	46.5 min
18°C	36.3 min	60.3 min
15°C	53.4 min	89.0 min

Abbreviations: NPT, nasopharyngeal temperature; TCA, total circulatory arrest.

* TCA limits based on an assumed safe normothermic arrest of 3–5 min.

EFFECTS OF CO_2 REGULATION. During CPB, multiple groups have independently shown that CBF increases with increasing arterial carbon dioxide tension.[56,69,70] In children, however, the CBF response to increases in CO_2 tension is diminished by two factors: deep hypothermia and young age.[71] The attenuated response during deep hypothermia is not surprising in view of the effect of hypothermia on the cerebral microcirculation and animal data demonstrating an age-dependent increase in CBF response to CO_2 from fetus to newborn to adults.[72] The role of CO_2 management in CPB has been studied extensively in animals and adult human patients. Based on the effect of CO_2 on arterial and intracellular pH at hypothermic temperatures, two divergent blood gas management strategies have been advocated during CPB: alpha-stat and pH-stat.[73] Alpha-stat strategy maintains a neutral intracellular pH as temperature is lowered. Enzymatic function is most efficient when intracellular electrochemical neutrality is preserved.[73,74] In contrast, pH-stat strategy allows hydrogen ions to accumulate as temperature decreases. At deep hypothermic temperatures, the intracellular pH is increasingly acidotic. With a low intracellular pH, electrochemical neutrality is lost and enzymatic function is impaired.[73] Biologic enzyme systems necessary for ATP generation are perhaps the most sensitive to pH changes. Therefore, the production of high-energy phosphates may be significantly impaired with pH-stat management.

In terms of cell function, it would seem that alpha-stat strategy would be the preferred method for maintaining intracellular enzymatic function at stable hypothermic CPB with or without TCA.[75] During TCA, brain tissue becomes increasingly acidotic throughout the period of no flow. If pH-stat is used with TCA, a greater accumulation of acid occurs in the brain. The resultant severe cerebral acidosis may impair brain function and prevent full brain recovery.

During the rewarming period, the brain is reperfused and must eliminate or correct the low pH toward normal. This may be hampered by a high residual acid load after circulatory arrest and from the increasing metabolic demands of the rewarming brain. Once weaned from CPB, the brain becomes dependent on the postbypass function of the heart to sustain adequate cerebral perfusion and eliminate accrued metabolic debt. If cardiac output is marginal or right atrial filling pressures high, cerebral perfusion may be further impaired. By reducing the brain's acid load before separating from CPB, better enzymatic function and improved ATP synthesis should result. Recent evidence suggests that alpha-stat or the use of a pH more alkaline than alpha-stat may be a better strategy for achieving a more normal brain tissue pH after deep hypothermic CPB with or without total circulatory arrest.[75]

It is important to emphasize that a uniformly hypothermic brain temperature is the most crucial aspect of cerebral protection. If an extremely low $Paco_2$ impairs cooling efficiency through cerebral vasoconstriction, the benefits of an alkaline brain pH become less important. Similarly, if elevated levels of $Paco_2$ increase cerebral blood flow and improve brain cooling, increased $Paco_2$ may be beneficial, especially during active brain cooling. Several studies address the importance of thoroughly cooling the brain.

Bellinger and associates demonstrated that accelerated rates of cooling ($>1°C/min$) during CPB using alpha-stat regulation is associated with a lower developmental quotient in neonates undergoing deep hypothermic circulatory arrest.[76] A recent study[58] describes four patients who, despite having achieved nasopharyngeal and rectal temperatures of 18°C, had significantly higher cerebral oxygen extraction and cerebral metabolic rates than their cohorts. Three of these patients went on to have significant neurologic dysfunction despite a relatively short period of circulatory arrest. The most likely explanation is inadequate cerebral perfusion resulting in inefficient brain cooling and the existence of intracerebral temperature gradients.[58]

During deep hypothermia with or without TCA, the addition of CO_2 during active brain cooling could potentially improve the distribution of the cold perfusate to deep brain structures. Although not proven, enhancing the distribution of extracorporeal perfusate to deep cortical structures may help cool the whole brain and reduce conductive warming during the arrest period.[71] During active cooling, alpha-stat strategy may be counterproductive. Once cool, however, if TCA or deep hypothermia with low flow is planned, converting to an alpha-stat or alkaline-stat strategy may help preserve intracellular brain pH by improving enzymatic function and reducing the postarrest cerebral acidosis. Although this approach is appealing, experimental and clinical studies to demonstrate its validity in a controlled fashion are necessary before general use.

HYPOTHERMIC INJURY TO THE BRAIN. Early experience with deep hypothermia suggested that using extremely low temperatures (esophageal temperatures of >10°C) dramatically increased neurologic and pulmonary injury. Neurologic sequelae, especially choreoathetosis, were commonly reported.[77–79] Neuropathologic examination of the brain of animals undergoing profound levels of hypothermia revealed microvascular lesions compatible with the no reflow phenomenon.[80] Similar histologic brain lesions were observed in children who died after cardiac surgery using circulatory arrest.[77] These early reports diminished the enthusiasm for profound levels of hypothermia and most institutions limited hypothermic temperatures to 18–20°C.

These early reports contrast with current practice and recent studies using more extreme levels of hypothermia. For example, the use of cold cerebroplegia (perfusing the brain with hemodiluted blood cooled to 6–10°C) has been suggested by Bachet et al as an alternative to hypothermic arrest during aortic arch surgery in adults.[81] This group reports reduced neurologic injury using this technique. In many institutions, infants are rapidly cooled to rectal temperatures of 15°C. Using such techniques, it is not uncommon to decrease esophageal temperatures below 10°C and tympanic membrane temperatures to 10 and 12°C. This cooling strategy has not increased the incidence of neurologic sequelae.

The difference between earlier studies and current experience is most likely due to hemodilution. All of the early reports used surface cooling techniques without hemodilution. At low temperatures, the viscosity of blood increases, red cell deformity is reduced, and microvascular sludging results. The result is multifocal cerebral hypoperfusion (the pathologic picture of no reflow) and brain injury. The use of deep hypothermia with hemodilution eliminates these no reflow lesions.[63] The limit at which hypothermia damages the brain is not defined, but recent experience suggests that temperatures of 10°C and below are probably not deleterious as long as appropriate hemodilution is used.

GLUCOSE REGULATION DURING HYPOTHERMIC CPB. In recent years, a substantial amount of the literature on animal and human studies has shown conclusive evidence of the detrimental effect of hyperglycemia during complete, incomplete, and focal cerebral ischemia.[82–85] The role of glucose in potentiating cerebral injury appears to be due to two factors: ATP utilization and lactic acidosis.[86,87]

The anaerobic metabolism of glucose requires phosphorylation and the expenditure of two molecules of ATP before ATP production can occur. This initial ATP expenditure may result in a rapid depletion of ATP and may explain why hyperglycemia worsens neurologic injury.[88,89] Lactic acidosis is also important in glucose-augmented cerebral injury, probably as a glycolytic enzyme inhibitor. Lactate slows anaerobic ATP production by inhibiting glycolysis immediately after ATP is consumed in the phosphorylation of glucose.[90]

Although a strong scientific argument can be made for the detrimental effects of hyperglycemia during ischemia, there is very little evidence supporting worsening neurologic outcome in hyperglycemia during CPB and/or TCA in children. Stewart et al retrospectively reviewed 34 children undergoing deep hypothermic circulatory arrest and suggested a worse neurologic outcome in the hyperglycemic children; however, the results were reported as a nonsignificant statistical trend.[91] A pathologic review of acquired neurologic lesions in patients undergoing the Norwood stage I procedure for hypoplastic left heart syndrome suggested hyperglycemia as a significant associated finding in patients with extensive cerebral necrosis or intraventricular hemorrhage. Although associated, a host of other potentially damaging factors (periods of hypoxia, low diastolic and systolic pressures, and thrombocytopenia) were statistically associated with the observed neuropathology.[68] Therefore, the neuropathologic insult cannot be attributed to hyperglycemia alone.

Hypoglycemia is a frequent concern in neonates during the perioperative period. Reduced hepatic synthetic function coupled with decreased glycogen stores puts the newborn at increased risk for hypoglycemic events. In newborns with congenital heart disease, reduced systemic perfusion (eg, critical coarctation, hypoplastic left heart syndrome, critical aortic stenosis) may compromise hepatic function to impair glucose production further. These patients may be fully dependent on exogenous glucose and may require 20–30% dextrose to maintain euglycemia in the prebypass period.

Older children are not immune to hypoglycemic events and are therefore susceptible to hypoglycemia-induced neurologic injury. Although anesthesiologists are more conscious of hypoglycemia in the neonate, patients with prolonged, low cardiac output states (cardiomyopathies, pretransplant patients, critically ill postoperative patients) requiring reoperation and on substantial inotropic support are at risk for reduced glycogen stores and intraoperative hypoglycemia.[92]

The cerebral impact of hypoglycemia during bypass is further complicated by the consequences of hypothermia, CO_2 management, and other factors that may modify normal cerebral vascular responses during bypass. In a dog model, insulin-induced hypoglycemia to 30 mg/dL does not alter electroencephalographic (EEG) findings. However, after 10 minutes of hypocapnic hypoglycemia, the EEG becomes flat.[93] When regional blood flow is examined in these animals, cortical and hippocampal blood flow remains normal, whereas other regions of the brain have reduced flow. The loss of EEG activity from hypoglycemia alone does not normally occur until glucose levels of 8 mg/dL or less are reached (hypoglycemic coma).[94]

During deep hypothermic CPB and TCA, cerebral blood flow and metabolism are altered. The additive effect of hypoglycemia, even if mild, may cause alterations in cerebral autoregulation and culminate in increased cortical injury.[68,95] The common practice of using hyperventilation to reduce pulmonary artery pressure in neonates and infants during weaning from CPB and in the early postbypass period could further exacerbate hypoglycemic injury. Glucose monitoring and rigid maintenance of euglycemia are an important part of CPB management in the patient with congenital heart disease.

Renal Effects. The combined effects of hypothermia, nonpulsatile perfusion, and reduced mean arterial pressure causes release of angiotensin, renin, catecholamines, and antidiuretic hormones.[96–99] These circulating hormones promote renal vasoconstriction and reduce renal blood flow. The addition of pulsatile perfusion improves renal blood flow by inhibiting renin release and redistributing blood flow to the renal cortex.[100] Urine flow and renal tissue oxygenation are improved.[101]

Despite the negative impact of CPB on renal function, studies have been unable to link low-flow, low-pressure, nonpulsatile perfusion with postoperative renal dysfunction.[102,103] The factors that correlate best with postoperative renal dysfunction are profound post-CPB low cardiac output and preoperative renal dysfunction. Preoperative factors include primary renal disease, low cardiac output, and angiographic dye-related renal injury after cardiac catheterization.[104,105]

Another factor to be considered in pediatric bypass is organ immaturity. Glomerular filtration rate and medullary concentrating ability are substantially reduced in pediatric patients. Therefore, prolonged periods of CPB may result in greater fluid retention than is typically seen in adult patients. The net result may be increased total body water and greater difficulty with postoperative weaning from ventilatory support.

Pulmonary Effects. Pulmonary function after cardiopulmonary bypass is characterized by reduced static and dynamic compliance, reduced functional residual capacity, and an increased A-a gradient.[106,107] Atelectasis and increased capillary leak due to hemodilution and hypothermic CPB are the most likely etiologies.[108] Hemodilution reduces circulating plasma proteins, reduces intravascular oncotic pressure, and favors water extravasation into the extravascular space. Hypothermic CPB causes complement activation and leukocyte degranulation.[109] Leukocytes and complement promote capillary-alveolar membrane injury and microvascular dysfunction through platelet plugging and release of mediators that increase pulmonary vascular resistance.[110] Recent evidence suggests that hypothermia or the combination of hypothermia with nonpulsatile perfusion may be more important than CPB itself in inducing lung injury.[9] Greeley et al suggested that vascular endothelial injury from hypothermic nonpulsatile perfusion is the major factor causing lung injury rather than exposure to the nonendothelialized bypass circuit.[111] This was recently supported by a study comparing ECMO and conventional ventilator therapy for persistent pulmonary hypertension of the newborn (PPHN). Neither conventional ventilator therapy nor the initiation of normothermic bypass (ECMO) increased the level of the circulating plasma vasoconstrictors (thromboxane or $PGF_{2\alpha}$) in patients with PPHN. In fact, vasoconstrictor concentrations decreased as lung function improved in both therapies. Similarly, an increase in concentrations of thromboxane could not be detected across the pump oxygenator in children undergoing cardiopulmonary bypass.[7,111] This suggests that the bypass circuit and oxygenator may not be as important as the effect of nonpulsatile cold perfusion or hypothermia alone in causing lung injury.

Stress Response and CPB. The release of a large number of metabolic and hormonal substances including catecholamines, cortisol, growth hormone, prostaglandins, complement, glucose, insulin, β-endorphins, and other substances characterize the stress response during hypothermic CPB.[6,112,113] The likely causes for the elaboration of these substances include contact of blood with the nonendothelialized surface of the pump tubing and oxygenator (less likely based on ECMO experience),[9] nonpulsatile flow, low perfusion pressure, hemodilution, hypothermia, and decreased depth of anesthesia. Other factors that may contribute to elevations of stress hormones include delayed renal and hepatic clearance during hypothermic CPB, myocardial injury, and exclusion of the pulmonary circulation from bypass. The lung is responsible for metabolizing and clearing many of these stress hormones. The stress response generally peaks during rewarming from cardiopulmonary bypass. There is evidence that the stress response can be blunted by increasing the depth of anesthesia, especially using high-dose narcotics.[114]

It is unclear at what level elevated circulating stress hormones (a normal adaptive response) become detrimental. There is little question that these substances could mediate undesirable effects such as myocardial damage (catecholamines), systemic and pulmonary hypertension (catecholamines), pulmonary endothelial damage (complement, prostaglandins), and pulmonary vascular reactivity (thromboxane). Recently, Anand et al have demonstrated the benefits of ablation of the stress hormones with fentanyl or sufentanil in premature infants undergoing cardiac surgery, and they have also shown that neonates with complex CHD who die in the postoperative period demonstrate much higher hormonal and metabolic responses during the intra- and postoperative periods compared with survivors with similar cardiac defects.[113–115] The measured levels of stress hormones and catecholamines in the neonates are generally an order of magnitude greater than those measured during CPB in the adult. Thus, one assumes that this is a nonphysiologic and probably deleterious response. Although blunting the extremes of the stress response seems warranted, there is additional evidence suggesting that the newborn stress response, especially the endogenous release of catecholamines, may be an adaptive metabolic response necessary for survival at birth.[116] Thus, complete elimination of an adaptive stress response may not be desirable (Table 10–8). To what extent acutely ill neonates with congenital heart disease are dependent on their stress response for maintaining hymodynamic stability is currently unknown.

Nonpulsatile versus Pulsatile Perfusion. Evidence for microcirculatory dysfunction with nonpulsatile perfusion can be found in a large number of studies. Ogata and associates, in 1960, directly observed that capillary flow in the omentum slowed and virtually ceased during nonpulsatile CPB at normothermia.[117] At flow rates of 60 and 75 mL/kg/min, nonpulsatile flow resulted in lower total-body oxygen consumption and pH and the development of base deficits than with pulsatile perfusion. Matsumato et al showed that at $37^{\circ}C$, nonpulsatile perfusion produced capillary sludging, dilation of the postcapillary venules, and increased edema formation in the conjunctival and cerebral microcirculations.[118]

In contrast, pulsatile CPB maintained capillary blood flow in the omentum, eliminated sludging in the conjunctival and cerebral microcirculation, and reduced jugular venous lactate.[117–119] Evidence also suggests that pulsatile perfusion may provide better cerebral perfusion. Studies of hypothermic low-flow cardiopulmonary

bypass in a dog model demonstrate that converting low-flow nonpulsatile CPB at 25 mL/kg/min to pulsatile perfusion improves brain pH, Pco_2, and Po_2.[75] Measurements of $CMRO_2$ in neonates, infants, and children demonstrate that nonpulsatile perfusion accounts for a 9% reduction in brain metabolism.[58] Pulsatile perfusion may, therefore, improve cerebral perfusion at both normothermic and hypothermic temperatures. When low-flow cardiopulmonary bypass is used, the addition of pulsatile flow may provide improved microcirculatory perfusion and allow for better oxygen delivery to tissue at lower flow rates.

REWARMING AND SEPARATION FROM CPB

The rewarming period is initiated by increasing the temperature in the arterial perfusate to approximately $8–10^{\circ}C$ above the venous blood temperature. Larger temperature gradients may increase the risk of gaseous bubbles coming out of solution. Electrical activity usually resumes spontaneously with cardiac warming. In infants and neonates, fibrillation is uncommon owing to the reduced ventricular muscle mass. Spontaneous fibrillation that is difficult to convert during rewarming may signify air in the coronary arteries or, more ominously, poor myocardial preservation during bypass. Increasing mean arterial pressure will improve coronary perfusion and force air out of the coronary arteries. Once tympanic (or nasopharyngeal) and rectal temperatures reach $36^{\circ}C$, the patient is weaned from CPB.

When weaning from CPB, the heart is allowed to fill by clamping the venous return line and reducing the arterial inflow until adequate blood volume is achieved. Blood volume is assessed by direct visualization of the heart and measuring right atrial or left atrial filling pressure. When filling pressures are adequate, the arterial inflow is stopped. The arterial cannula is left in place so that a slow infusion of residual pump perfusate can be used to optimize filling pressures. Myocardial function is assessed by direct cardiac visualization and either placement of a transthoracic left atrial catheter, a percutaneous internal jugular catheter or transthoracic right atrial catheter, or by the use of intraoperative epicardial or transesophageal echocardiography. When cardiac physiology has been normalized, the pulse oximeter can be used to assess the adequacy of cardiac output.[120] Low saturations or the inability of the oximeter to register a pulse may indicate very low cardiac output and increased systemic resistance.[121]

After the repair of complex congenital heart defects, weaning from cardiopulmonary bypass may be difficult. Under these circumstances, a distinction must be made among (1) poor surgical result with a residual defect requiring re-repair, (2) pulmonary artery hypertension, and

TABLE 10–8. REPRESENTATIVE PEAK CATECHOLAMINE LEVELS FOR CPB AND BIRTH

Study (Reference)	Norepine- phrine	Epinephrine
Adults during CPB (Hoar et al, 1977)[156]	6.6 ± 1.5	4.7 ± 2.2
Adults during CPB (Bovill, et al, 1983)[157]	11.5 ± 2.3	5.7 ± 1.8
Neonates during CPB (halothane + MSO_4) (Anand et al, 1992)[115]	39.8 ± 12.2	7.9 ± 2.9
Neonates during CPB (fentanyl) (Anand et al, 1990, 1991)[113,115]	12.7 ± 4.1	?
Neonate at birth (Lagerkrantz, et al, 1984)[116]	≈ 47	?
Asphyxiated at birth (Lagerkrantz et al, 1984[116]	≈ 200	?

All values are nanomoles per milliliter.

(3) right or left ventricular dysfunction. Two general approaches are customarily used either independently or in conjunction. An intraoperative "cardiac catheterization" is done to assess isolated pressure measurements from the various chambers of the heart; catheter pull-back measurements to evaluate residual pressure gradients across valves, repaired sites of stenosis, and conduits; and oxygen saturation data to look for residual shunts.[122] Alternatively, the use of epicardial echocardiography with Doppler color flow or transesophageal echocardiography have been used to provide an intraoperative "picture" of structural or functional abnormalities to assist in the evaluation of the postoperative cardiac repair.[123] If structural abnormalities are found, the patient is returned to CPB and residual defects are repaired prior to leaving the operating room. Leaving the operating room with a significant residual structural defect adversely affects survival and increases patient morbidity[123,124] (see Chapter 6).

Functional as well as structural problems are rapidly identified by these methods and therapy can then be directed toward specific correction. Left ventricular dysfunction can be treated by optimizing preload and heart rate, increasing coronary perfusion pressure, correcting ionized calcium levels, and adding inotropic support. Inotropic support is usually begun with calcium supplementation (10–30 mg/kg) and dopamine (5–15 μg/kg/min). If function remains poor, a second drug is usually added or substituted. For left ventricular dysfunction, a more potent inotrope is begun, such as epinephrine at a dose of 0.03–0.05 μg/kg/min, and titrated to effect. Dobutamine may be used as an alternative second-line drug; however, dobutamine in conjunction with dopamine may produce significant sinus tachycardia in neonates and infants. This may relate to structural similarities between dobutamine and isoproterenol.[125] Amrinone in conjunction with epinephrine may improve left ventricular contractility and reduce systemic afterload.[126,127] This combination is very effective for left ventricular dysfunction. Other combinations of inotropic and dilation drugs may also be used. If very high doses of inotrope are required, consideration for mechanical circulatory support with extracorporeal membrane oxygenation (ECMO) or a left ventricular assist device (LVAD) should be strongly considered. Pulmonary hypertension is best treated with ventilatory manipulations. However, drug therapy as described in Chapter 18 may also be beneficial.

Right ventricular dysfunction can be treated by reducing pulmonary vascular resistance with ventilatory manipulations, increasing coronary perfusion pressure with phenylephrine or epinephrine, and reducing pulmonary artery pressure with amrinone or isoproterenol.[126–128,141] It is important to remember that the right ventricle is mostly dependent on systolic pressure for coronary perfusion. Therefore, drug therapy must maintain systemic perfusion pressure. Prostaglandin E_1 or tolazoline may cause substantial systemic hypotension and be counterproductive.[129]

Mechanical Circulatory Assistance in Pediatric Patients

Mechanical circulatory assistance for the failing adult heart has achieved wide application. Three modalities are currently available for circulatory support in children. These include the intra-aortic balloon pump (IABP), ECMO, and ventricular assist devices (VADs). Selecting the appropriate technology is based on the patient's underlying disease, size, heart rate, and degree of hypoxemia. Indications for mechanical circulatory support in the pediatric patient include (1) an inability to wean from CPB owing to primary ventricular dysfunction (ie, correctable residual anatomic defects have been eliminated); (2) failure of selective surgical interventions used to reduce volume or pressure load on an unaccepting ventricle (ie, placing a small hole in an atrial septal defect [ASD] patch to allow a dysfunctional right ventricle to shunt blood right to left at the atrial level and increase systemic cardiac output.) (3) successful weaning from bypass but escalating inotropic support due to evolving ventricular dysfunction; and (4) severe pulmonary artery hypertension despite maximal ventilatory support, systemic alkalinization, and inotropy. It is important to emphasize that care must be taken to assure that the problem is functional and not anatomic. Inotropic and mechanical ventricular assistance cannot overcome a poor operative result. Echocardiography and/or pressure monitoring should indicate the site of ventricular dysfunction: right, left, or biventricular dysfunction.

Intra-aortic Balloon Pump. The IABP consists of a long narrow balloon that is positioned in the descending aorta just distal to the left subclavian artery. The balloon inflates during diastole and displaces blood from the thoracic aorta. Proximal aortic blood displacement increases aortic root pressure and augments coronary blood flow. Blood that is displaced distally improves systemic perfusion by augmenting mean arterial pressure. During systole, the balloon is deflated allowing the left ventricle to eject blood into a relatively empty, low-resistance descending aorta and systemic afterload is reduced. The net result is a decrease in myocardial wall tension, reduced myocardial oxygen consumption, and augmented coronary perfusion.

Precise function of the IABP depends upon synchronizing inflation and deflation with the cardiac cycle. Either the arterial waveform or the electrocardiogram (ECG) can be used. When timed to the arterial waveform, balloon inflation is set to begin at the dicrotic notch. If inflation begins earlier, left ventricular ejection will be compromised by balloon inflation. Deflation begins when the arterial trace reaches its nadir. If deflation begins too soon, the descending aorta may not fully evacuate its blood volume, decreasing diastolic arterial pressure and coronary augmentation. If deflation is delayed, the left ventricle must pump against an increased resistance (see Chapter 23).

Despite the overwhelming success of balloon counterpulsation in adults, pediatric use of the balloon pump has been disappointing. The IABP has not improved outcome in children under 5 years of age when used for postoperative myocardial dysfunction nor in older patients after Fontan procedures.[130] In children more than 5 years of age undergoing corrective procedures, IABP has successfully treated postoperative LV dysfunction. Several factors contribute to the unfavorable results of IABP in children, including (1) higher heart rates in children, (2) increased aortic elasticity, (3) the presence of aortopulmonary collaterals in cyanotic patients, (4) palliative rather than complete repairs, and (5) a higher incidence of RV and biventricular dysfunction.

Heart Rate. Typically, the heart rate in neonates, infants, and young children after CPB are in the range of 130–180 beats per minute (bpm). At these heart rates, balloon inflation and deflation are not crisp enough to effectively time with the cardiac cycle. In attempts to improve timing, the IABP is usually reduced to augment every other or every fourth beat (1:2 or 1:4 timing). Although timing may improve, the effectiveness of the IABP is reduced 50–80%. In a child with poor myocardial function, this is usually inadequate support.

Increased Aortic Elasticity. In children, the aortic wall is much more compliant than in adults. The lack of aortic rigidity diminishes the pressure gradient generated by balloon inflation during diastole. Afterload reduction and coronary blood flow enhancement are less effective.

Aortopulmonary Collaterals. In cyanotic congenital heart lesions, aortopulmonary collaterals are common. During balloon inflation, proximal aortic pressure is reduced because blood is shunted through these collaterals into the pulmonary circulation. Diastolic augmentation is diminished and balloon counterpulsation becomes less effective.

Palliative Repairs. Patients undergoing shunt procedures or Fontan operation for single ventricle are less likely to benefit from balloon counterpulsation. In the former case, the shunt behaves like a surgically created aortopulmonary collateral, which prevents diastolic augmentation by shunting blood into the pulmonary circulation. In patients undergoing Fontan procedures, maintaining adequate systemic perfusion is critically dependent on single ventricular function and low pulmonary vascular resistance. When ventricular dysfunction is the primary problem, an IABP has generally provided inadequate augmentation and more definitive intervention with ECMO or a VAD is required.

Biventricular or RV Failure. When right ventricular dysfunction occurs alone or in conjunction with LV failure, IABP is not effective. Although some centers have reported placing IABP in the main pulmonary artery for right ventricular failure, the small size of the main pulmonary artery significantly limits balloon size and thus stroke volume.[131,132] Right and biventricular failure are best treated by ECMO or a VAD.

A miniature intra-aortic balloon pump was developed and used successfully in small animals.[133] However, there are no commercially available devices and its clinical efficacy in comparison with ECMO and VADs remains unknown.

Extracorporeal Membrane Oxygenation. In the early 1970s, several case reports of the successful application of prolonged cardiopulmonary bypass in adults with trauma or combined cardiac and respiratory failure appeared.[134–136] These early reports led to an National Institutes of Health–sponsored trial of ECMO for acute respiratory failure in the adult patients.[137] The overall survival rate for both groups was less than 10% and the ECMO trial was considered a failure. This early experience diminished the enthusiasm for this technology, and its application became limited to neonates with acute respiratory failure, in whom a clear improvement in survival was easily demonstrated.[138–140]

ECMO was a profound failure in the adult population because of the strict criteria used for entry into the study. The average patient on ECMO spent more than 9 days on maximal ventilatory support before randomization.[137] Pathologic evaluation demonstrated a high incidence of pulmonary fibrosis and hyaline membrane formation.[141]

These findings are crucial and extremely relevant to patients with congenital heart disease. Mechanical circulatory assistance is used to rest a "stunned" myocardium that is capable of recovery. Therefore, mechanical circulatory assistance should be considered early before irreversible damage occurs. Mechanical circulatory support is not salvage therapy but is a next level of support, just as one would consider a more potent inotrope such as epinephrine if dopamine or dobutamine were insufficient. Complications from prolonged cardiogenic shock in patients unresponsive to extended periods of maximal medical management may not be reversible and increase the likelihood of ECMO-related complications and failure.

Technique. The ECMO circuit is illustrated in Fig 10–11. When ECMO is used for circulatory support, venoar-

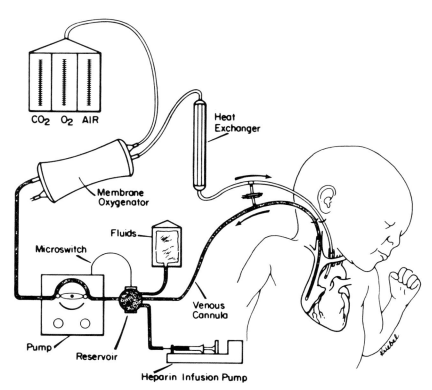

Figure 10–11. A schematic drawing of an ECMO circuit.

terial cannulation is chosen. Venovenous bypass provides gas exchange but does not provide cardiac support. Venous and arterial access may be achieved through a large peripheral artery and vein or by direct chest cannulation. Peripheral sites include the neck (internal jugular vein and carotid artery) or groin (femoral or iliac artery and vein). Chest cannulation is obtained through a median sternotomy, with venous return through a single right atrial cannula (anatomic considerations may necessitate left atrial cannulation) and arterial inflow through an ascending aortic cannula. Although peripheral cannulation is preferred for children with respiratory failure, peripheral sites may not be adequate for children with postbypass circulatory failure. Femoral and iliac vessels of children are small and may not accept large enough cannulas to allow full circulatory support on ECMO.[142] ECMO support using neck cannulation has been successful.[143–145] However, peripheral cannulation techniques that drain only the right side of the circulation may not offer effective decompression of the left side of the heart in children with severe left ventricular or biventricular failure. Experimental evidence suggests that ECMO provides more effective circulatory support in dogs with myocardial infarction if left ventricular drainage is added.[146] Klein and colleagues reported nine children who required ECMO to wean from CPB.[145] The two surviving patients in this series had chest cannulation and a separate left atrial drain. The other advantage of chest cannulation is simplicity. These patients

have recently undergone median sternotomy for their cardiac operation and therefore cannulation is simply a matter of reopening the chest incision. Peripheral cannulation requires a fresh surgical dissection in a hemodynamically unstable child. The disadvantages of chest cannulation include mediastinal bleeding and the risk of mediastinitis.

Circuit Function. The ECMO circuit functions similarly to a CPB circuit. Blood is drained from the right atrial cannula by a gravity siphon to a small distensible bladder (equivalent to the cardiotomy reservoir on a CPB circuit). The bladder serves to regulate flow through the pump. If the bladder collapses owing to inadequate return, a servoregulator shuts down the pump. From the bladder, blood passes through a pump (roller or centrifugal) and enters a silicone rubber membrane oxygenator (SciMED). The size of the membrane oxygenator is based on its "rated flow," which denotes the maximum blood flow rate at which venous blood leaves the membrane oxygenator with a saturation of 95%. The membrane oxygenator must be large enough to provide a rated flow that is greater than the calculated cardiac output required for the patient. After leaving the oxygenator, the blood is warmed through a countercurrent heat exchanger and perfused through the aortic inflow cannula. A bridge is placed between the arterial inflow tubing and the venous drainage tubing to allow the perfusate to recirculate. This is used principally during cannulation and weaning from the circuit. Pump flow rates are similar to those described for normothermic cardiopulmonary bypass. The circuit volume is generally 350–400 mL in young infants.

Before initiating ECMO, the patient must be anticoagulated. Generally 100–150 U/kg of heparin is given and the activated clotting time is maintained between 180 and 220 seconds via a continuous heparin infusion. Relatively large infusions of heparin may be needed because of increased heparin clearance by the extracorporeal circuit and blood components.[147] Once on ECMO, blood products are transfused to maintain a hematocrit of 40–45%, a minimum platelet count of 50,000–70,000, and fibrinogen levels of 150–200 mg/dL are maintained with cryoprecipitate. After initiating ECMO, hemodynamics stabilize and inotropic support can be reduced.

Experience. Table 10–9 is a summary of 71 patients with congenital heart disease requiring ECMO for postoperative circulatory support due to intractable cardiac failure or severe pulmonary vasoreactive crisis; 42 of 71 patients survived, for an overall survival rate of 59%.[142–145] If patients were successfully weaned from CPB and ECMO was begun in the postoperative period, 42 of 57 (74%) of children survived. Mortality was significantly greater if patients could not wean from CPB and ECMO support was instituted in the operating room. In this group, only 2 of 14 patients survived (14%). A left atrial vent was placed in 3 of these 14 patients put on ECMO directly from CPB. Two of these patients (67%) survived.

Complications. Complications from ECMO therapy include hemorrhage (48%), renal insufficiency (29%), neurologic injury (17%), dysrhythmias (17%), infectious complications (10%), and ECMO circuit problems (10%) (Table 10–10). Hemorrhage was a sufficiently significant complication to warrant surgical exploration in 21 patients, discontinuation of ECMO in 5 patients, and

caused death in 1 patient. In children unable to wean from CPB, ECMO successfully supported the circulation, but hemorrhagic complications were extremely common and significantly contributed to morbidity and mortality. Renal insufficiency and neurologic complications were primarily attributed to severe cardiogenic shock in the postbypass (pre-ECMO) period. Intracranial hemorrhage, however, did occur in four patients. ECMO was discontinued in all four and two subsequently died. Sustained cardiac dysrhythmias occurring after institution of ECMO were reflective of severe myocardial injury and implied a poor prognosis. Sepsis from intravascular catheters was the most common infectious complication. Mediastinitis occurred in one patient with disseminated candidiasis.

Although an extremely effective means of support, the high mortality rate associated with weaning directly from CPB to ECMO is of concern. Reasons for excessive mortality include severe ventricular dysfunction and recalcitrant hemorrhage. Recovery from severe ventricular dysfunction is predicated on the concept that the myocardium sustained a transient injury and is capable of recovery with time, ie, "stunned myocardium." ECMO decreases ventricular wall tension, increases coronary perfusion pressure, and maintains systemic perfusion with oxygenated blood. If left ventricular function is severely impaired, left ventricular end-diastolic pressure may remain high and endocardial perfusion may be impaired. Left atrial venting may reduce left ventricular end-diastolic pressure and improve myocardial recovery. Hemorrhage, however, remains a troublesome problem owing to the need for anticoagulation.

Ventricular Assist Devices. An alternative approach is to use a VAD that supports only the circulation. VADs do not include oxygenators and, therefore, require significantly less anticoagulation, which minimizes hemorrhagic complications. Compared with ECMO, VADs

TABLE 10–9. REPORTED SERIES USING ECMO FOR CIRCULATORY SUPPORT

| | | | | | | Reason for Initiating ECMO | | | |
| | | | | | | Failure to Wean from CPB | | Postop Ventricular Failure | |
Series	No. of Patients	Overall Survival	Femoral	Neck	Cardiac	No.	Survival	No.	Survival
Kanter (1987)[142]	13	7 (54%)	5	0	8	1	0 (0%)	12	7 (58%)
Klein (1990)[145]	36	23 (64%)	0	30	6	9	2 (22%)	27	12 (74%)
Rogers (1989)[144]	12	5 (42%)	2	5	5	3	0 (0%)	8	5 (63%)
Weinhaus (1989)[143]	10	7 (70%)	0	4	6	1	0 (0%)	9	8 (89%)
Totals	71	42 (59%)	7	39	25	14	2 (14%)	56	42 (73%)

Abbreviation: ECMO, extracorporeal membrane oxygenation.

TABLE 10–10. ECMO COMPLICATIONS

Series	Hemorrhage (Severe)		Dysrhythmia	Renal Failure	Infectious	Neurologic	ECMO Circuit
Kanter (1987)[142]	9/13	(8)	N/R	5/13	N/R	3/13	2/13
Klein (1990)[145]	17/36	(5)	3/36	NR	3/36	4/36	3/36
Rogers (1989)[144]	3/10	(3)	N/R	1/10	1/10	1/10	N/R
Weinhaus (1989)[143]	5/12	(5)	5/12	4/12	2/12	4/12	N/R
Totals	34/71 (48%)	21 (62%)	8/48 (17%)	10/35 (29%)	6/58 (10%)	12/71 (17%)	5/49 (10%)

Abbreviation: ECMO, extracorporeal membrane oxygenation.

may be a preferred means of circulatory support for children who are unable to wean from CPB owing to primary left ventricular dysfunction. VADs allow direct control of left atrial filling pressure, and therefore left ventricular end-diastolic pressure can be decreased to enhance left ventricular recovery.

There are two types of VADs: pulsatile and nonpulsatile. Pulsatile devices are sophisticated pumps, initially designed as permanent artificial implantable hearts. These pumps are durable, cause minimal blood trauma, and can be used for prolonged periods. Their most common use today is as a bridge to cardiac transplantation. Because of the lack of availability, high cost, and sophistication, these devices are not commonly used for postbypass ventricular support of the stunned myocardium. Typical devices include the Jarvik 7 (Symbion, Inc, Salt Lake City, UT) and the Donachy/Thoratec pump (Thoratec, Berkeley, CA).

Nonpulsatile continuous flow pumps are less expensive and are commercially available. The most widely used device is the centrifugal pump in which blood is moved by its entrainment against spinning blades or cones. An example is the Biomedicus pump. Centrifugal pumps require direct heart cannulation. A left ventricular assist device (LVAD) (Fig 10–12) requires a left atrial venous cannula and an aortic cannula. Wire-reinforced cannulas are preferred because kinking can markedly reduce cardiac output or cause ventricular distension. The cannulas are secured in place and connected via polyvinylchloride tubing to the ports on the pump head.

The LVAD is activated and flow rates increased until the patient is completely weaned from CPB and the LVAD is providing full circulatory support. Left and right atrial cannulas are strongly recommended for monitoring during LVAD. Low left atrial pressures reduce left ventricular end diastolic pressure and may improve left ventricular recovery. In addition, there is no venous reservoir in the centrifugal pump system; therefore, pressure monitoring is essential to ensure adequate intravascular volume to sustain pump flow rates and prevent arterial air embolism. Low left atrial pressures may be due to hypovolemia or right ventricular failure.

A right atrial pressure will differentiate between in-adequate volume and right ventricular dysfunction. If right atrial pressures are increased and left ventricular filling pressures decreased, significant right ventricular failure is present. Supporting the right ventricle with inotropes such as dopamine, amrinone, isoproterenol, or prostaglandin E_1 may be helpful. However, if right ventricular dysfunction is prominent, biventricular support is considered. Right ventricular support is instituted with a right ventricular assist device (RVAD). Wire-reinforced right atrial and main pulmonary artery cannulas are placed. These cannulas are connected to a second centrifugal pump.

Management of a biventricular system (BVAD) is more complicated. Flows need to be adjusted independently to unload the right ventricle, maintain adequate blood return to the left atrium, and ensure effective systemic flows and perfusion pressure. Generally, left atrial pressures are maintained at 5–10 mm Hg and right atrial pressures at 5–12 mm Hg. A pressure of less than 5 mm Hg in the left atrium is treated by increasing patient intravascular volume. Left atrial pressure monitoring is even more critical in neonates and infants because flow through the VAD is measured by an in-line electromagnetic flow probe that is inaccurate at flow rates below 500 mL/m².

Once the patient is stabilized on the VAD, heparin is antagonized and residual coagulopathy treated with blood and blood components. Owing to prolonged CPB, a severe coagulopathy is usually present. Treatment with platelets, fresh frozen plasma, and cryoprecipitate are commonly required. Once bleeding is controlled, low-dose heparin is administered to maintain an ACT at 120–180 seconds.

Published experience with VADs is limited to adults. The overall survival rate from the Combined Registry of the International Society for Heart Transplantation and the American Society for Artificial Internal Organs reports a 24% survival rate in 451 patients receiving a VAD for postcardiotomy cardiogenic shock.[148] This is consistent with the experience at the Cleveland Clinic, which reported an overall 23% survival rate. Survival for RVAD, LVAD, and BVAD were 22, 23, and 25%, respectively, in the Cleveland Clinic series.[149]

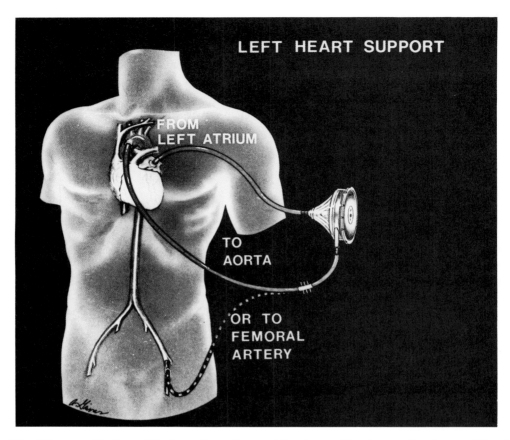

Figure 10–12. Left heart ventricular assist using a Biomedicus centrifugal pump. Usual approaches to cannulation for left ventricular support are shown.

At Boston Children's Hospital, a Biomedicus centrifugal pump has been used in six patients. In two cases, VADs were used preoperatively for stabilization of cardiomyopathy-myocarditis. One patient improved and was successfully weaned from an LVAD and the other went on to transplant. In children with postcardiotomy cardiogenic shock, four patients received a ventricular assist device (two LVAD and two RVAD). All four recovered myocardial function and were weaned from ventricular assistance. Three of the four patients survived. In contrast, ECMO was used in eight patients with postcardiotomy cardiogenic shock, and only two patients (25%) survived more than 30 days. Although this is a small number of patients, it does raise the concern that ECMO may not be as effective as a VAD for a stunned myocardium. Bleeding and the absence of left-sided venting are the most likely causes. By reducing left ventricular end-diastolic pressure, VADs may be more effective in maximizing myocardial recovery.

A recent addition to the mechanical support devices is the hemopump.[150] The hemopump is a catheter-mounted miniature pump that has a distal No. 21 French flexible inflow cannula and a proximal flexible drive shaft. The device is inserted through a femoral artery cutdown and is fluoroscopically guided so the distal inflow cannula lies in the left ventricle. The drive shaft is encased in a double-layered catheterlike sheath and exits the patient at the cutdown site. The distal drive shaft is connected to an external motor and console that provides rotary motion to the pump. Blood is continuously aspirated from the left ventricle and pumped into the aortic root. This miniature pump can generate blood flows of up to 3.8 L/min at speeds of 25,000 rpm. Because this device is placed percutaneously, it has potential for wider applications.[151–155]

Early experience with this device for postcardiotomy left ventricular failure has been encouraging. In one adult series, a hemopump VAD was placed in nine patients with refractory cardiac failure and an inability to wean from CPB.[155] All nine patients successfully weaned from CPB with the hemopump. Six patients improved enough to have the hemopump removed and five survived beyond hospital discharge. The pediatric experience is limited to one 9-year-old child who developed medically refractory biventricular dysfunction 5 months after heart transplantation. Because the catheter was too large to insert through the femoral artery, the hemopump was surgically placed by way of the distal abdominal aorta. Myocardial function improved and the child was weaned from mechanical support on the sixth day.[155] Smaller devices are being developed and may have future application for younger children.[149]

REFERENCES

1. Gibbon JH: Application of a mechanical heart and lung apparatus to cardiac surgery. *Minnesota Med* **37**:171–177, 1954
2. Lillehei CW, Varco RL, Cohen M, Warden HE: The first open-heart repairs of ventricular septal defect, atrioventricularis communis, and tetralogy of Fallot using extracorporeal circulation by cross-circulation: A 30-year follow-up. *Ann Thorac Surg* **41**:4–21, 1986
3. Warden HE: C Walton Lillehei: Pioneer cardiac surgeon. *J Thorac Cardiovasc Surg* **98**:833–845, 1989
4. Kirklin JW: The middle 1950's and C Walton Lillehei. *J Thorac Cardiovasc Surg* **98**:822–824, 1986
5. Sade RM, Bartles DM, Dearing JP, et al: A prospective randomized study of membrane versus bubble oxygenators in children. *Ann Thorac Surg* **29**:502–511, 1979
6. Hindmarsh KW, Sankaran K, Watson VG: Plasma beta-endorphin concentrations in neonates associated with acute stress. *Dev Pharmacol Ther* **7**:198–204, 1984
7. Faymonville ME, Derby-Dupont G, Larbuisson R, et al: Prostaglandin E$_2$, prostacyclin and thromboxane changes during nonpulsatile cardiopulmonary bypass in humans. *J Thorac Cardiovasc Surg* **91**:858–866, 1986
8. Blauth C, Smith P, Newman S, et al: Retinal microembolism and neuropsychiatric deficit following clinical cardiopulmonary bypass: Comparison of a membrane and a bubble oxygenator. *Eur J Cardiothorac Surg* **3**:135–139, 1989
9. Bui KC, Hammerman C, Hirshel RB, et al: Plasma prostanoids in neonates with pulmonary hypertension treated with conventional therapy and with extracorporeal membrane oxygenation. *J Thorac Cardiovasc Surg* **101**:973–983, 1991
10. Ylikorkala O, Saarela E, Viinikka L: Increased prostacyclin and thromboxane production in man during cardiopulmonary bypass. *J Thorac Cardiovasc Surg* **82**:245–247, 1981
11. Zapol WM, Peterson MB, Wonders TR, et al: Plasma thromboxane and prostacyclin metabolites in sheep cardiopulmonary bypass. *Trans Am Soc Artif Intern Organs* **26**:556–560, 1980
12. Pearson DT, McArdle B, Poslad SJ, et al: A clinical evaluation of the performance characteristics of one membrane and five bubble oxygenators: Haemocompatibility studies. *Perfusion* **1**:81–98, 1986
13. Bering EA Jr: Effect of body temperature change on cerebral oxygen consumption during hypothermia. *Am J Physiol* **200**:417, 1961
14. Stow PJ, Burrows FA, McLeod ME, Coles JG: The effect of cardiopulmonary bypass and profound hypothermic circulatory arrest on anterior fontanelle pressure in infants. *Can J Anaesth* **34**:450–454, 1987
15. Friesen RH, Thieme R: Changes in fontanel pressure during cardiopulmonary bypass and hypothermic arrest in infants. *Anesth Analg* **66**:94–96, 1987
16. Hickey PR, Wessel DL: Anesthesia for treatment of congenital heart disease. *J Cardiothorac Anesth* **2**:635–723, 1987
17. Kern FH, Jonas RA, Mayer JE, et al: Conventional temperature monitoring is a poor correlate of efficient brain cooling. *Anesthesiology* **75**:A57, 1991 (abstr)
18. Schupbach P, Pappova E, Schilt W, et al: Perfusate oncotic pressure during cardiopulmonary bypass: Optimum level as determined by metabolic acidosis, tissue edema, and renal function. *Vox Sang* **35**:332–344, 1978
19. Byrick RJ, Kay JC, Noble WH: Extravascular lung water accumulation in patients following coronary artery surgery. *Can Anaesth Soc J* **24**:332–345, 1977
20. Marelli D, Paul A, Sam CP, et al: Does the addition of albumin to the prime solution in cardiopulmonary bypass affect clinical outcome? *J Thorac Cardiovasc Surg* **98**:751–756, 1989
21. Haneda K, Sato S, Ischizawa E, et al: The importance of colloid osmotic pressure during open heart surgery in infants. *Tohoku J Exp Med* **147**:65–71, 1985
22. Leone BJ, Spahn DR, McRae RL, Smith LR: Effects of hemodilution and anesthesia on regional function of compromised myocardium. *Anesthesiology* **73**:A596, 1990 (abstr)
23. Kawashima Y, Yamamoto Z, Manabe H: Safe limits of hemodilution in cardiopulmonary bypass. *Surgery* **76**:391–397, 1974
24. Henling CE, Carmichael MJ, Keaths AS, Cooley DA: Cardiac operation for congenital heart disease in children of Jehovah's Witnesses. *J Thorac Cardiovasc Surg* **89**:914–920, 1985
25. Greeley WJ, Kern FH: Anesthesia for pediatric cardiac surgery. In Miller RD (ed): *Anesthesia*, 3rd ed. New York: Churchill Livingstone, 1990, pp 1653–1692
26. Hickey PR, Wessel DI: Anesthesia for treatment of congenital heart disease. In Kaplan JA (ed): *Cardiac Anesthesia*. Philadelphia: WB Saunders, 1987, pp 635–724
27. Fox LS, Blackstone EH, Kirklin JW, et al: Relationship of whole body oxygen consumption to perfusion flow rate during hypothermic cardiopulmonary bypass. *Thorac Cardiovasc Surg* **83**:239–248, 1982
28. Bull BSJ, Korpman RA, Huse M, Briggs BD: Heparin therapy during extracorporeal circulation. I Problems inherent in existing heparin protocols, II The use of a dose response curve to individualize heparin and protamine dosage. *J Thorac Cardiovasc Surg* **69**:674–689, 1975
29. Young JA, Kisker CT, Doty DB: Adequate anticoagulation during cardiopulmonary bypass determined by activated clotting time and the appearance of fibrin monomer. *Ann Thorac Surg* **26**:321–325, 1978
30. Mohr R, Golan M, Nartinowitz V, et al: Effect of cardiac operation on platelets. *J Thorac Cardiovasc Surg* **92**:434–451, 1986
31. Umlus J: Fibrinolysis and disseminated intravascular coagulation in open heart surgery. *Transfusion* **16**:460–468, 1976
32. Massicotte P, Mitchell L, Andrew M: A comparative study of coagulation systems in newborn animals. *Pediatr Res* **20**:961–965, 1986
33. Kern FH, Morana NJ, Sears J, Hickey PR: Coagulation defects in neonates during CPB. *Ann Thorac Surg* **54**:541–546, 1992

34. Peters M, Ten Cate JW, Jansen E, Breederveld C: Coagulation and fibrinolytic factors in the first week of life in healthy infants. *J Pediatr* **106**:292–296, 1985

35. Manno CS, Hedberg KW, Kim HC, et al: Comparison of the hemostatic effects of fresh whole blood, stored whole blood and components after open heart surgery in children. *Blood* **77**:930–936, 1991

36. Lavee J, Martinowitz U, Mohr R, et al: The effect of transfusion of fresh whole blood versus platelet concentrates after cardiac operations. A scanning electron microscope study of platelet aggregation on extracellular matrix. *J Thorac Cardiovasc Surg* **97**:204–212, 1989

37. Mohr, R, Martinowitz U, Lavee J, et al: The hemostatic effect of transfusing fresh whole blood versus platelet concentrates after cardiac operations. *J Thorac Cardiovasc Surg* **96**:530–534, 1988

38. Saltzman EW, Weinstein MJ, Weintraub RM, et al: Treatment with desmopressin acetate to reduce blood loss after cardiac surgery: A double-blind randomized trial. *N Engl J Med* **314**:1402–1406, 1986

39. Hackmann T, Gascoyne RD, Naiman SC, et al: A trial of desmopressin (1-desamino–8-D-arginine vasopressin) to reduce blood loss in uncomplicated cardiac surgery. *N Engl J Med* **321**:1437–1443, 1989

40. Hedderich GS, Petsikas DJ, Cooper BA, et al: Desmopressin acetate in uncomplicated coronary artery bypass surgery: A prospective randomized clinical trial. *Can J Surg* **33**:33–36, 1990

41. Van der Salm TJ, Ansell JE, Okike ON: The role of epsilon aminocaproic acid in reducing bleeding after cardiac operation: A double-blind randomized study. *J Thorac Cardiovasc Surg* **95**:538–540, 1988

42. Havel M, Teufelsbauer H, Knobel P, et al: Effect of intraoperative aprotinin administration on postoperative bleeding in patients undergoing cardiopulmonary bypass operation. *J Thorac Cardiovasc Surg* **101**:968–972, 1991

43. Alajmo F, Calamai G, Perna AM: High-dose aprotinin: Hemostatic effects in open heart operations. *Ann Thorac Surg* **48**:536–539, 1989

44. Becker AE, Caruso G: Congenital heart disease—A morphologist's view on myocardial dysfunction. In Becker AE (ed): *Paediatric Cardiology*. Edinburgh: Churchill Livingstone, 1986

45. Ream AK, Reitz BA, Silverberg G: Temperature correction of pCO_2 and pH in estimating acid-base status. *Anesthesiology* **56**:41–44, 1982

46. Andritsch RF, Muravchick S, Gold MI: Temperature correction of arterial blood gas parameters. *Anesthesiology* **55**:311–316, 1981

47. Swain JA: Acid-base status, hypothermia and cardiac surgery. *Perfusion* **1**:231–238, 1986

48. Gravenstein N, Rollman JE, Berryessa RG, Slogoff S: The oxygenator sampling port. A potential source of error. *Anesthesiology* **62**:825–826, 1985

49. Annis JP: Scavenging system for the Harvey blood oxygenator. *Anesthesiology* **45**:359–360, 1976

50. Miller JO: A device for removal of waste anesthetic gases from the extracorporeal oxygenator. *Anesthesiology* **44**:181–184, 1976

51. Muravchick S: Scavenging enflurane from extracorporeal pump oxygenators. *Anesthesiology* **47**:468–470, 1977

52. Kirklin JW, Barratt-Boyes BG: *Cardiac Surgery*. New York: John Wiley & Sons, 1986, p 39

53. Michenfelder JD. The hypothermic brain. In Michenfelder JD (ed): *Anesthesia and the Brain*. New York: Churchill Livingstone, 1988, pp 23–34

54. Swain JA, McDonald TJ, Griffith PK, et al: Low flow hypothermic cardiopulmonary bypass protects the brain. *J Thorac Cardiovasc Surg* **102**:76–84, 1991

55. Greeley WJ, Ungerleider RM, Smith LR, Reves JG: Cardiopulmonary bypass alters cerebral blood flow in infants and children during and after cardiovascular surgery. *Circulation* **78**(Pt 4):II356, 1988

56. Govier AV, Reves JG, McKay RD, et al: Factors and their influence on regional cerebral blood flow during nonpulsatile cardiopulmonary bypass. *Ann Thorac Surg* **38**:592–600, 1984

57. Fox LS, Blackstone EH, Kirklin JW, et al: Relationship of brain blood flow and oxygen consumption to perfusion flow rate during profound hypothermic cardiopulmonary bypass: An experimental study. *J Thorac Cardiovasc Surg* **87**:658–664, 1984

58. Greeley WJ, Kern FH, Ungerleider RM, et al: The effect of hypothermic cardiopulmonary bypass and total circulatory arrest on cerebral metabolism in neonates, infants and children. *J Thorac Cardiovasc Surg* **101**:783–794, 1991

59. Greeley WJ, Ungerleider RM, Kern FH, et al: Effects of cardiopulmonary bypass on cerebral blood flow in neonates, infants and children. *Circulation* **80**(suppl I):I209–I215, 1989

60. Kern FH, Ungerleider RM, Reves JG, et al: The effect of altering pump flow rate on cerebral blood flow and cerebral metabolism in neonates, infants and children. *Ann Thorac Surg* 1991 (in press).

61. Henriksen L: Brain luxury perfusion during cardiopulmonary bypass in humans. A study of the cerebral blood flow response to changes in CO_2, O_2 and blood pressure. *J Cereb Blood Flow Metab* **6**:366–378, 1986

62. Rich TL, Langer GA: Calcium depletion in rabbit myocardium: Calcium paradox protection by hypothermia and cation substitution. *Circ Res* **51**:131–151, 1982

63. Norwood WI, Norwood CR, Castaneda AR: Cerebral anoxia: Effect of deep hypothermia and pH. *Surgery* **86**:203–210, 1979

64. Globus MY, Ginsberg MD, Harik ST, et al: Role of dopamine in ischemic striatal injury: Metabolic evidence. *Neurology* **37**:1712–1719, 1987

65. Moskowitz MA, Meyer E, Wurtman RJ, et al: Attenuation of catecholamine antagonists of the hypothermia that follows cerebral infarction in the gerbil. *Life Sci* **293**:332, 1975

66. Rothman SM, Olney JW: Glutamate and the pathophysiology of hypoxic-ischemic brain damage. *Ann Neurol* **19**:105–111, 1986

67. Ferry PC: Neurologic sequelae of open-heart surgery in children. *Am J Dis Child* **144**:369–373, 1990

68. Glauser TA, Rorke LB, Weinberg PM, Clancy RR: Acquired neuropathologic lesions associated with the hypoplastic left heart syndrome. *Pediatrics* **85**:991–1000, 1990

69. Murkin JM, Farrar JK, Tweed WA, et al: Cerebral autoregulation and flow/metabolic coupling during cardiopulmonary bypass. *Anesth Analg* **66**:825–832, 1987

70. Prough DS, Stump DA, Roy RC, et al: Response of cere-

bral blood flow to changes in carbon dioxide tension during hypothermic cardiopulmonary bypass. *Anesthesiology* **64:**576–581, 1986

71. Kern FH, Ungerleider RM, Quill TJ: Cerebral blood flow response to changes in $PaCO_2$ during hypothermic cardiopulmonary bypass in children. *J Thorac Cardiovasc Surg* **101:**618–622, 1991

72. Rosenberg AA, Jones MD, Traystman RJ, et al: Response of cerebral blood flow to changes in PCO_2 in fetal, newborn and adult sheep. *Am J Physiol* **242:**H862–H866, 1982

73. Swan H: The importance of acid-base management for cardiac and cerebral preservation during open heart operations. *Surg Gynecol Obstet* **158:**391–414, 1984

74. Somero GN, White FN: Enzymatic consequences under alpha stat regulation. In Rahn H, Prakash O (eds): *Acid-Base Regulation and Body Temperature.* Boston: Nijhoff, 1985, pp 55–80

75. Watanabe T, Hrita H, Kobayashi M, Washio M: Brain tissue pH, oxygen tension and carbon dioxide tension in profoundly hypothermic cardiopulmonary bypass. *J Thorac Cardiovasc Surg* **97:**396–401, 1989

76. Bellinger PC, Wernovsky G, Rappaport LA, et al: Cognitive development of children following early repair of transposition of the great arteries using deep hypothermic circulatory arrest. *Pediatrics* **87:**701–707, 1991

77. Bjork VO, Hultquist G: Contraindications to profound hypothermia. *J Thorac Cardiovasc Surg* **44:**1–9, 1962

78. Egerton N, Egerton WS, Kay JH: Neurologic changes following profound hypothermia. *Ann Surg* **157:**366–382, 1963

79. Brunberg JA, Doty DB, Reilly EL: Choreoathetosis in infants following cardiac surgery with deep hypothermia and circulatory arrest. *J Pediatr* **84:**232–235, 1974

80. Treasure T, Naftel DC, Conger KA, et al: The effect of hypothermic circulatory arrest on cerebral function, morphology, and biochemistry. *J Thorac Cardiovasc Surg* **86:**761–770, 1983

81. Bachet J, Guilmet D, Goudot B, et al: Cold cerebroplegia. A new technique of cerebral protection during operations of the transverse aortic arch. *J Thorac Cardiovasc Surg* **102:**85–93, 1991

82. Lanier WL, Stangland KJ, Scheithauer BW, et al: The effects of dextrose infusion and head position on neurologic outcome after complete cerebral ischemia in primates: Examination of a model. *Anesthesiology* **66:**39–48, 1987

83. Pulsinelli WA, Waldman S, Rawlinson D, Plum F: Moderate hyperglycemia augments ischemic brain damage: A neuropathologic study in the rat. *Neurology* (*NY*) **32:**1239–1242, 1982

84. Pulsinelli WA, Levy DE, Sigsbee B, et al: Increased damage after ischemic stroke in patients with hyperglycemia with or without established diabetes mellitus. *Am J Med* **74:**540–544, 1983

85. Nakakimura K, Fleischer JE, Drummond JC, et al: Glucose administration before cardiac arrest worsens neurologic outcome in cats. *Anesthesiology* **72:**1005–1011, 1990

86. Farias LA, Willis BS, Gregory GA: Effects of fructose-1,6-diphosphate, glucose, and saline on cardiac resuscitation. *Anesthesiology* **65:**595–601, 1986

87. Plum F: What causes infarction in ischemic brain? *Neurology* (*NY*) **33:**222–233, 1983

88. Magalini SI, Bondoli A, Scrascia E: The action of phosphocreatine and fructose-1,6-diphosphate on blood in vitro. *Resuscitation* **5:**103–110, 1977

89. Perroni L, Ensoli G, Nunziata A, et al: Comparative study of the effects of fructose-1,6-diphosphate, fructose, and physiologic saline on the blood levels of glucose and adenosine-triphosphate after an oral glucose load. *Pharmacol Res Commun* **12:**147–153, 1980

90. Kubler W, Katz AM: Mechanism of early "pump" failure of the ischemic heart: Possible role of adenosine triphosphate depletion and inorganic phosphate accumulation. *Am J Cardiol* **40:**467–471, 1977

91. Steward DJ, Da Silva CA, Flegel T: Elevated glucose levels may increase the danger of neurologic deficit following profound hypothermic cardiac arrest. *Anesthesiology* **68:**653, 1988 (letter to the editor)

92. Auer RN: Progress review: Hypoglycemic brain damage. *Stroke* **17:**699–708, 1986

93. Sieber FE, Derrer SA, Saudek CD, Traystman RJ: Effect of hypoglycemia on cerebral metabolism and carbon dioxide responsivity. *Am J Physiol* **156:**H697–H706, 1989

94. Cilluffo JM, Anderson RE, Michenfelder JD, Sundt TM: Cerebral blood flow, brain pH, and oxidative metabolism in the cat during severe insulin-induced hypoglycemia. *Cereb Blood Flow Metab* **2:**337–346, 1982

95. Siesjo BK, Ingvar M, Pelligrino D: Regional differences in vascular autoregulation in the rat brain in severe insulin-induced hypoglycemia. *J Cereb Blood Flow Metab* **3:**478–485, 1983

96. Taylor KM, Morton IL, Brown JJ, et al: Hypertension and the renin angiotensin system following open heart surgery. *J Thorac Cardiovasc Surg* **74:**840–845, 1977

97. Watkins L Jr, Lucas SK, Gardner TJ, et al: Angiotensin II levels during cardiopulmonary bypass: A comparison of pulsatile and nonpulsatile flow. *Surg Forum* **29:**229–235, 1978

98. Stanley TH, Philbin DM, Coggins CH: Fentanyl-oxygen anesthesia for coronary artery surgery: Cardiovascular and antidiuretic hormone responses. *Can Anaesth Soc J* **26:**168–172, 1979

99. Stanley TH, Berman L, Gren O, et al: Plasma catecholamine and cortisol responses to fentanyl-oxygen anesthesia for coronary artery operations. *Anesthesiology* **55:**250–253, 1980

100. Goodman TA, Gerard DF, Bernstein EF, Dilley RB: The effects of pulseless perfusion on the distribution of renal cortical blood flow and renin. *Surgery* **80:**31–39, 1976

101. German JC, Chalmers GS, Mukherjee D, et al: Comparison of nonpulsatile and pulsatile extracorporeal circulation on renal tissue perfusion. *Chest* **61:**65–68, 1972

102. Hilberman M, Myers BD, Carrie BJ, et al: Acute renal failure following cardiac surgery. *J Thorac Cardiovasc Surg* **77:**880–888, 1979

103. Kron IL, Joob AW, Van Meter C: Acute renal failure in the cardiovascular surgical patient. *Ann Thorac Surg* **39:**590–598, 1985

104. Hilberman M, Derby GC, Spencer RJ, et al: Sequential pathophysiological changes characterizing the progression from renal dysfunction to acute renal failure following

cardiac operation. *J Thorac Cardiovasc Surg* **79**:838–844, 1980

105. Gomez-Campdera FJ, Maroto-Alvaro E, Galinanes M, et al: Acute renal failure associated with cardiac surgery. *Child Nephrol Urol* **9**:139–153, 1988

106. Deal CW, Warden JC, Monk I: Effect of hypothermia on lung compliance. *Thorax* **25**:105–109, 1970

107. Ashmore PG, Wakeford J, Harterre D: Pulmonary complications of profound hypothermia with circulatory arrest in the experimental animal. *Can J Surg* **7**:93–96, 1964

108. Vincent RN, Lang P, Elixson M, et al: Measurement of extravascular lung water in infants and children after cardiac surgery. *Am J Cardiol* **54**:161–165, 1984

109. Howard RJ, Crain C, Franzini DA, et al: Effects of cardiopulmonary bypass on pulmonary leukostasis and complement activation. *Arch Surg* **123**:1496–1501, 1988

110. Royall JA, Levin DL: Adult respiratory distress syndrome in pediatric patients. Clinical aspects, pathophysiology and mechanisms of lung injury. *J Pediatr* **112**:169–180, 1988

111. Greeley WJ, Bushman GA, Kong DL, et al: Effects of cardiopulmonary bypass on eicosanoid metabolism during pediatric cardiovascular surgery. *J Thorac Cardiovasc Surg* **95**:842–849, 1988

112. Greeley WJ, Leslie JB, Su M: Plasma atrial naturetic peptide release during pediatric cardiovascular anesthesia and surgery. *Anesthesiology* **65**:A414, 1986 (abstr)

113. Anand KJS, Hansen DD, Hickey PR: Hormonal-metabolic stress response in neonates undergoing cardiac surgery. *Anesthesiology* **73**:661–670, 1990

114. Anand KJS, Sippell WG, Aynsley-Green A: Randomized trial of fentanyl anesthesia in preterm neonates undergoing surgery: Effects on the stress response. *Lancet* **1**:243–248, 1987

115. Anand KJS, Hickey PR: Halothane-morphine compared with high dose sufentanil for anesthesia and postoperative analgesia in neonatal cardiac surgery. *N Engl J Med* **326**:1–9, 1992

116. Lagerkrantz H, Slotkin TA: The "stress" of being born. *Sci Am* **254**:100–107, 1986

117. Ogata T, Ida Y, Nonoyama A, et al: A comparative study of the effectiveness of pulsatile and nonpulsatile flow in extracorporeal circulation. *Arch Jpn Chir* **29**:59–66, 1960

118. Matsumato T, Wolferth CC Jr, Perlman MH: Effects of pulsatile and non-pulsatile perfusion upon cerebral and conjunctival microcirculation in the dog. *Am Surg* **37**:61–64, 1971

119. Geha AS, Salayemeh MT, Abe T, Baue AE: Effect of pulsatile cardiopulmonary bypass on cerebral metabolism. *J Surg Res* **12**:381–387, 1972

120. Oshita S, Uchimoto R, Oka H, et al: Correlation between arterial blood pressure and oxygenation in tetralogy of Fallot. *J Cardiovasc Anesth* **3**:597–600, 1989

121. Severinghaus JW, Spellman BA: Pulse oximeter failure thresholds in hypotension and vasoconstriction. *Anesthesiology* **73**:532–537, 1990

122. Gold JP, Jonas RA, Lang P, et al: Transthoracic intracardiac monitoring lines in pediatric surgical patients: A ten year experience. *Ann Thorac Surg* **42**:185–191, 1986

123. Ungerleider RM, Greeley WJ, Sheikh KH, et al: The use of intraoperative echo with Doppler color flow imaging to predict outcome after repair of congenital cardiac defects. *Ann Surg* **210**:526–533, 1989

124. Ungerleider RM, Greeley WJ, Sheikh KH, et al: Routine use of intraoperative epicardial echo and Doppler color flow imaging to guide and evaluate repair of congenital heart lesions: A prospective study. *J Thorac Cardiovasc Surg* **100**:297–309, 1990

125. Bohn DJ, Poirer CS, Edmonds JF, et al: Efficacy of dopamine, dobutamine, and epinephrine during emergence from cardiopulmonary bypass in children. *Crit Care Med* **8**:367–372, 1980

126. Lawless S, Burckart G, Diven W, et al: Amrinone pharmacokinetics in neonates and infants. *J Clin Pharmacol* **28**:283–284, 1988

127. Hines R, Barash PG: Right ventricular failure. In Kaplan JA (ed): *Cardiac Anesthesia*. Philadelphia: W.B. Saunders, 1987, pp 995–1020

128. Greeley WJ, Kern FH, Kisslo JA, Ungerleider RM: Intramyocardial air causing right ventricular dysfunction after repair of congenital heart defects. *Anesthesiology* **73**:1042–1046, 1990

129. D'ambra M, LaRaia P, Phellan D, et al: A new therapy for refractory right heart failure and pulmonary hypertension after mitral valve replacement. *J Thorac Cardiovasc Surg* **89**:567–572, 1985

130. Pollock JC, Charlton MD, Williams WG, et al: Intraaortic balloon pumping in children. *Ann Thorac Surg* **29**:552–530, 1980

131. Opravil M, Gorman AJ, Krejcie TC, et al: Pulmonary artery balloon counterpulsation for right ventricular failure I. Experimental results. *Ann Thorac Surg* **38**:242–253, 1984

132. Moran JM, Opravil M, Gorman AJ, et al: Pulmonary artery balloon counterpulsation for right ventricular failure II. Clinical experience. *Ann Thorac Surg* **38**:254–259, 1984

133. Fukumasu F, Blaylock R, Veasy LG, et al: Intra-aortic balloon pumping device for infants. *Clin Cardiol* **2**:348–353, 1979

134. Hill JD, O'Brien TG, Murray JJ, et al: Extracorporeal oxygenation for acute post-traumatic respiratory failure (shock-lung syndrome): Use of the Bramson membrane lung. *N Engl J Med* **286**:629–634, 1972

135. Bartlett RH, Gazzaniga AB, Fong SW, Burns NE: Prolonged extracorporeal support in man. *J Thorac Cardiovasc Surg* **68**:918–932, 1974

136. Pyle RB, Helton WC, Johnson FW, et al: Clinical use of the membrane oxygenator. *Arch Surg* **110**:966–970, 1975

137. Zapol WM, Snider MT, Hill JD, et al: Extracorporeal membrane oxygenation in severe respiratory failure: A randomized prospective study. *JAMA* **242**:2193–2196, 1979

138. Bartlett RH, Andrews AF, Toomasian JM, et al: Extracorporeal membrane oxygenation for newborn respiratory failure: 45 cases. *Surgery* **92**:425–433, 1982

139. Bartlett RH, Roloff DW, Cornell RG, et al: Extracorporeal circulation in neonatal respiratory failure: A prospective randomized study. *Pediatrics* **76**:479–487, 1985

140. Toomasian JM, Snedecor SM, Cornell RG, et al: National experience with extracorporeal membrane oxygenation for newborn respiratory failure: Data from 715 cases. *Trans ASAIO* **34**:140–147, 1988

141. Gille JP, Bagniewski AM: Ten years of use of extracorporeal membrane oxygenation (ECMO) in the treatment of acute respiratory insufficiency. *Trans ASAIO* **22**:102–109, 1976

142. Kanter KR, Pennington G, Weber TR, et al: Extracorporeal membrane oxygenation for postoperative cardiac support in children. *J Thorac Cardiovasc Surg* **93**:27–35, 1987

143. Weinhaus L, Canter C, Noetzel M, et al: Extracorporeal membrane oxygenation for circulatory support after repair of congenital heart defects. *Ann Thorac Surg* **48**:206–212, 1989

144. Rogers AJ, Trento A, Siewers RD, et al: Extracorporeal membrane oxygenation for postcardiotomy cardiogenic shock in children. *Ann Thorac Surg* **47**:903–906, 1989

145. Klein MD, Shaheen KW, Whittlesey GC, et al: Extracorporeal membrane oxygenation for the circulatory support of children after repair of congenital heart disease. *J Thorac Cardiovasc Surg* **100**:498–505, 1990

146. Eugene J, McColgan SJ, Moore-Jefferies EW, et al: Cardiac assist by extracorporeal membrane oxygenation with in-line left ventricular venting. *Trans Am Soc Artific Intern Organs* **30**:98–101, 1984

147. Green TP, Isham-Schopf B, Irmiter RJ, et al: Inactivation of heparin during extracorporeal circulation in infants. *Clin Pharmacol Ther* **48**:148–154, 1990

148. Miller CA, Pae WE Jr, Pierce WS: Combined registry for the clinical use of mechanical ventricular assist devices, postcardiotomy cardiogenic shock. *ASAIO Trans* **36**:43–46, 1990

149. Golding LAR: Postcardiotomy mechanical support. *Semin Thorac Cardiovasc Surg* **3**:29–32, 1991

150. Merhige ME, Smalling RW, Cassidy D, et al: Effect of the hemopump left ventricular assist device on regional myocardial perfusion and function. *Circulation* **80**(suppl III):III158–III166, 1989

151. Phillips SJ, Barker L, Balentine B, et al: Hemopump support for the failing heart. *ASAIO Trans* **36**:M626–632, 1990

152. Loisance D, Deleuze P, Dubois-Rande JL, et al: Hemopump ventricular support for patients undergoing high risk coronary angioplasty. *ASAIO Trans* **36**:M623–M626, 1990

153. Sholtz KH, Tebbe U, Chemnitius M, et al: Transfemoral placement of the left ventricular assist device "hemopump" during mechanical resuscitation. *Thorac Cardiovasc Surg* **38**:69–72, 1990

154. Frazier OH, Macris MP, Wampler RK: Treatment of cardiac allograft failure by use of an intra-aortic axial flow pump. *J Heart Transplant* **9**:508–514, 1990

155. Burnett CM, Vega JD, Radovancevic B, et al: Improved survival after hemopump insertion in patients experiencing postcardiotomy cardiogenic shock during cardiopulmonary bypass. *ASAIO Trans* **36**:M626–M629, 1990

156. Hoar PF, Stone JG, Faltas AN, et al: Hemodynamic and adrenergic responses to anesthesia and operation for myocardial revascularization. *J Thorac Cardiovasc Surg* **80**:242–248, 1977

157. Bovill JG, Sebel PS, Fiolet JWT, et al: The influence of sufentanil on endocrine and metabolic responses to cardiac surgery. *Anesth Analg* **62**:391–397, 1983

Chapter 11 | Myocardial Preservation

John J. McAuliffe III

Congenital heart defects are successfully repaired under satisfactory operating conditions created by cardiopulmonary bypass, and although the outcome is usually favorable, some patients sustain myocardial injury during surgery. Myocardial injury does not always result in death. Postoperative manifestations range from arrhythmias to the need for vigorous inotropic support. The hearts of those patients who succumb have evidence of injury that may vary in severity from subtle subcellular changes to frank necrosis. The cause of this injury was initially ascribed to imbalances between myocardial energy supply and demand. The results of more recent work suggest that the etiology is far more complex. The role of reperfusion-related phenomena in mediating myocardial damage is now a field of intensive investigation. Toxic oxygen-free radicals, a cause of damage at multiple sites within the heart, may be detoxified or inhibited by various means.

The advent of cardiac transplantation in children has created a need for new techniques to preserve myocardium in a viable state for several hours between harvest and reperfusion in the recipient. The problems associated with cardiac preservation for transplant are different from those encountered during repair of congenital cardiac defects.

HISTORY OF MYOCARDIAL PRESERVATION

The history of myocardial preservation begins with hypothermia, initially recognized as a therapeutic modality in the fourth millennium BC by the Egyptians.[1] Interest in hypothermia remained limited until 1950 when Bigelow and co-workers[2,3] reported that dogs could be surface cooled to a body temperature of 25°C with a profound reduction in oxygen requirement. They also reported that inflow of blood to the heart could be arrested for up to 15 minutes with survival. Other groups began to investigate the physiologic effects and ways to control hypothermia. The investigations led to the first successful repair of a congenital heart defect by Lewis and Trauffic[4] using surface cooling–induced hypothermia. Moderate hypothermia (rectal temperatures 28–31°C) could be produced by surface cooling alone. Between 1953 and 1958, surface cooling was popular by virtue of its ease and wide availability.

Induced moderate hypothermia limited the surgeon to 8 minutes of continuous circulatory arrest time. Repair of complex lesions required more time than could be provided by this technique. The Kyoto group led by Hikasa investigated deep hypothermia induced by surface cooling as a means of providing a longer "safe" operating period. With cooling to the 17–22°C range, circulatory arrest times of 15–75 minutes were tolerated.[5] In a series reported in 1969, 71 infants underwent surgery for ventricular septal defect or tetralogy, with a 91.4% survival rate using this technique.[5]

The use of deep hypothermic arrest following surface cooling was championed by Merindino and Mohri in the United States. In 1969, that group[6] reported the successful repair of defects in six of seven patients (weighing 2.2–8.8 kg) with transposition of the great vessels and five of eight patients with total anomalous pulmonary venous return.

The introduction of extracorporeal circulation (ECC) in the 1950s provided an alternate means of inducing hypothermia. Early attempts to use ECC to induce hypothermia were fraught with technical difficulties, especially when attempts were made to apply the technique to small infants.[7,8] In the late 1950s, some success was achieved in the application of ECC to infants. Routine application of the technique to the repair of congenital defects in infants was reported by the Kyoto group[6] and subsequently by Barratt-Boyes and co-workers.[9] These authors reported limited use of ECC for cooling and rewarming. The initial cooling from 37 to 28°C was accomplished using surface cooling. Rewarming was accomplished with ECC alone. Extracorporeal cooling is now widely used to reduce total body oxygen demand and lower myocardial temperatures, so that periods of circulatory arrest up to 1 hour may be tolerated.

During the period when moderate hypothermia was in wide use, other means of extending the "safe" operating period were explored. In 1955, Melrose et al[10] reported the use of a blood cardioplegic solution containing 2.5% potassium citrate as a means of achieving up to 15 minutes of arrest time with full recovery. Clinical use of the "Melrose solution" resulted in reports of myocardial necrosis.[11,12] The use of cardioplegia fell into disfavor and remained a laboratory curiosity for nearly 20 years.

The downfall of cardioplegia generated enthusiasm for other means of myocardial preservation. Surface cooling of the heart by bathing it constantly in ice sludge was tried.[13] It was reasoned that direct cooling of the heart should reduce the metabolic demand below that achieved by body surface cooling and thus allow a greater period of arrest time. The reasoning was correct but the methodology was wrong. Myocardial injury[14] occurred as a direct result of the profound cooling and the technique was all but abandoned in the early 1960s.

New studies advocating the use of cardioplegia appeared in the 1970s.[15,16] The combination of cardioplegia and topical hypothermia reduced long-term myocardial pathology.[17]

At present, myocardial preservation techniques continue in a state of evolution. Techniques used in the past and those now in use are listed in Table 11–1. Recent advances in our understanding of biochemical pathways and mechanisms of injury serve as the guideposts for future developments in the field. Many centers now employ extracorporeal core cooling, cardioplegia, and topical cooling to achieve maximal myocardial protection.

MYOCARDIAL INJURY

Risk Factors

Congenital Lesions. The patient with congenital heart disease is physiologically very different from the patient with coronary artery disease. In most congenital heart lesions, the coronary vasculature is unobstructed. Lesions resulting in mixing of saturated and desaturated blood are common in patients with congenital heart disease and rare in the patient with coronary artery disease. Intracardiac blood flow patterns vary widely among patients with congenital anatomic abnormalities of the heart. As a consequence, myocardial oxygen supply is not generally compromised by obstruction within the coronary vessels but by forward output limitations or by virtue of receiving desaturated blood.

General categories of risk for intraoperative injury can be defined. Patients with anomalous origin of the coronary artery may have evidence of ischemic myocar-

TABLE 11–1. METHODS OF MYOCARDIAL PRESERVATION

Technique		Advantages	Disadvantages
1. Continuous coronary perfusion with fibrillation on CPB	O	Easy, reduces likelihood of air emboli	Cannot achieve bloodless field; high myocardial O_2 consumption
2. Intermittent aortic cross-clamping on CPB	N	Quiet bloodless field	Must interrupt intracardiac procedure to reperfuse heart—prolongs operation time; incomplete protection
3. Surface-induced moderate hypothermia with cross-clamping, *no* CPB	N	Quiet bloodless field; easy, widely available technique	Limited ischemic time 8 min continuous, 24 min total; cardiac massage needed to support circulation to start of rewarming
4. Deep hypothermia with cross-clamping and circulatory arrest (surface cooling, rewarming)	O	Quiet bloodless field; no cannulas in field; useful in tiny infants in whom CPB could be difficult; high success rate; longer ischemic time than item 3	Few people presently familiar with the technique; long cooling and rewarming times; need external massage to support circulation; fibrillation a potential problem
5. Same as item 4 but with core cooling, rewarming.	F	Quiet bloodless field; no cannulas in field; rapid cooling, rewarming; more rapid correction of acidosis than with surface warming; circulatory support without cardiac massage; neurologic problems of low incidence[117,118]	Cannulation can be technically difficult; myocardial ATP stores depleted more quickly than if cardioplegia added to technique
6. Topical hypothermia added to item 5	N	Technically easy to do	Can be difficult to use as sole technique in surgery for congenital defects; uneven cooling; late subendocardial fibrosis
7. Perfusion hypothermia (cardioplegia) added to item 5	F	As in item 5 plus rapid cardiac arrest, better presentation of ATP levels, more uniform myocardial cooling	Potential for air embolism in coronaries; does not fully protect against reperfusion injury; high K^+ can cause arrhythmias in small patients during rewarming

Abbreviations: N, not used or little used technique for correction of congenital defects; O, occasionally used technique for correction of congenital defects; F, frequently used technique for correction of congenital defects.

dial injury at the time of diagnosis. They are very vulnerable to further insult. Recently developed operative techniques used to correct this defect involve elective cardiac arrest. Patients with hypoplastic systemic ventricle syndromes have poor forward output through the aorta. The coronary perfusion is marginal unless there is adequate retrograde perfusion via the ductus arteriosus. Perfusion via the ductus arteriosus can be maintained preoperatively by the use of prostaglandin E. Cannulation of the aorta is technically difficult and placement of the aortic cannula may further compromise a tenuous coronary blood supply.

Myocardial Immaturity. Certain congenital cardiac lesions are severe enough to require correction in the first days or weeks of life. The myocardium is immature and differs from that of an "adult" myocardium. The time of transition from immature to adult human myocardium is unknown. Certain biochemical transitions may be delayed by the physiologic alterations that result from congenital heart defects. Much of the information about the "immature" myocardium is based on animal studies, partly verified in the human newborn or fetus.

The differences between adult and immature myocardium fall into three broad categories: cytoarchitecture, physiology, and biochemistry (Table 11–2).

The cytoarchitecture of the newborn heart is poorly suited to the production of excessive tension. The contractile elements are few in number and not well organized. The mitochondria are not as closely related to the contractile elements as in the adult myocardium. Other differences include decreased sarcoplasmic reticulum with a poorly developed T-tubular system.[18]

The physiologic correlates of the cytoarchitectural differences have been elucidated. The immature myocardium is more dependent upon transarcolemmal Ca^{2+} flux for contraction than is the adult.[19,20] Calcium chan-

nel blockers more profoundly depress the newborn than the adult myocardium.[21] The immature heart is unable to increase output in response to increased preload but dramatically decreases output with decreased preload. Acutely increased afterload is poorly tolerated and decreases cardiac output.[22] The postnatal time course of myocardial adaptation to afterload is unknown at this time.

Biochemically, the immature myocardium has compensatory mechanisms to allow force generation despite the reduced availability of cytosolic Ca^{2+}. The contractile apparatus is composed of thin and thick filaments. The thin filament proteins of the heart exist as isoforms. One of these proteins, troponin T (TNT) undergoes an isoform shift with postnatal age.[23] The shift in TNT isoforms is associated with a change in the Ca^{2+} sensitivity of the myofilament such that in the newborn, activation occurs at a lower Ca^{2+} concentration than in the adult.[23] The thick filament contains four myosin subunits; two light chains and two heavy chains. The heavy chains contain adenosine triphosphatase (ATPase) that hydrolyzes adenosine triphosphate (ATP) to provide the energy for cross-bridge cycling. The heavy myosin isozymes of humans do not change with age. However, the light chains change and modulate the activity of the ATPases.[24] The fetal light chains persist in patients with congenital heart disease, reducing the rate of ATP hydrolysis by the myofilaments and unfavorably altering the force-velocity relationships of the myocardium.

Newborns of several species lack a key isozyme of creatine kinase (CK) involved in energy shuttling.[25] High-energy phosphate is transported as creatine phosphate (CrP). This is formed by conversion of ATP plus creatine to CrP plus adenosine diphosphate (ADP). In the adult, this reaction takes place in the inner mitochondrial membrane and is catalyzed by the mitochondrial isozyme of CK.

TABLE 11–2. IMMATURE VERSUS "ADULT" MYOCARDIUM

	Immature	Adult
Cytoarchitectures	1. Few contractile elements	1. Many contractile elements
	2. Fewer mitochondrial rows along contractile elements	2. Mitochondria form rows along contractile elements
	3. Reduced amount of sarcoplasmic reticulum	3. Abundant sarcoplasmic reticulum in close approximation
	4. Poorly formed T tubules	4. Well formed T tubules
Biochemical	1. Lower myofibrillar ATPase activity	1. Normal myofibrillar ATPase activity
	2. Fetal light chain myosins present	2. No fetal light chains
	3. No mitochondrial CK	3. Mitochondrial CK
	4. More potential for glycolytic ATP generation (tolerates anoxia better than adult)	4. Oxidative metabolism
Physiologic	1. Decreased developed tension	1. Normal developed tension
	2. Decreased CO with increasing of preload	2. Able to maintain CO with increase of preload
	3. Small or no increase in CO with increasing preload	3. Increased CO with increased preload
	4. Ca^{2+} for excitation-contraction coupling transsarcolemma	4. Ca^{2+} for excitation-contraction coupling from sarcoplasmic reticulum

CrP is then transported to the contractile apparatus for reconversion to ATP. The flux through the CK system, or rate of exchange of high-energy phosphate bonds between ATP and CrP, is dependent on the content of mitochondrial CK.[26] The increase in CK flux with workload is reduced in the newborn heart as compared with the adult. The result is potential restriction of high-energy phosphate availability during periods of high demand that could limit mechanical performance.

The immature myocardium would be expected to have an increased susceptibility to ischemic injury during surgical repair. Ischemic contracture occurs in the immature myocardium at higher ATP levels than in the adult.[27] Maintenance of ATP concentrations during surgery is critical in this group of patients if contractures are to be avoided. However, the immature myocardium consistently appears to have greater tolerance for ischemia than adult hearts.[28] In a study of isolated rabbit hearts, there was less release of CK and better recovery of cardiac output in neonatal hearts than in the adult (Fig 11–1).

Myocardial Hypertrophy. Another group at risk are patients with hypertrophic lesions. Subendocardial blood flow is frequently marginal and may be reduced to inadequate levels during the prebypass period if low perfusion pressures occur. Surface myocardial cooling is often uneven[29] but the distribution of cardioplegia solution may be more uniform. If surface cooling alone is used, some areas of the heart are less well protected against ischemic injury than others.

Myocardial Failure. Patients with clinical evidence of cardiac decompensation (low output and increased filling pressures) may be at highest risk for further intraoperative injury. High filling pressures reduce subendocardial perfusion. Any reduction in perfusion pressure causes further deterioration of cardiac performance, a subsequent increase in filling pressures, and a vicious cycle ending in death. Maintenance of forward output and perfusion pressure in the prebypass period is essential in this group of patients.

The decompensating heart is abnormal biochemically.[30–32] Calcium transport mechanisms are impaired, the contractile apparatus cannot generate normal force-velocity relationships, and energy shuttling within the cell is compromised. The Ca^{2+} reuptake capacity of the sarcoplasmic reticulum (SR) is reduced owing to a downregulation of the SR-ATPase.[31] Further, the number and function of β-receptors is also reduced in the failing heart.[32] These marginal systems may be further damaged by reperfusion injury. Intraoperative injury invariably involves the calcium transport systems[33]; the visible result is poor systolic and diastolic function. Myopathic hearts are more prone to reperfusion injury than normal hearts because they are unable to withstand the calcium influx that can accompany reperfusion.[34]

Periods of Vulnerability

Myocardial damage may occur during several different phases of the operation. During the prebypass period, the most common mechanism of injury is inadequate perfusion. The subendocardium is the area most vulnerable to underperfusion.

An "at-risk period" ends with the initiation of cardiopulmonary bypass. The metabolic demands of the heart are greatly decreased by cardiopulmonary bypass. Venting of the left ventricle further reduces cardiac work. At 37°C, the beating empty left ventricle consumes only 30–50% of the oxygen consumed by the working left ventricle (Fig 11–2).[35]

The euthermic, beating, empty heart is vulnerable to injury. Factors contributing to injury are preexisting hypertrophy and low perfusion pressure. Ischemic injury has been noted in the subendocardium of the hypertrophied adult heart if the perfusion pressure decreased below 50 mm Hg.[36,37] Normal infants may have mean pressures only slightly greater than this value; however, in the immature myocardium, the threshold pressure for ischemia is probably lower than 50 mm Hg. Low-perfusion pressures are common during surgery for congenital heart defects. The period of time during which the myocardium is exposed to these low pressures is generally short. Consequently, there is little likelihood of serious damage. However, long periods of hypoperfusion may produce clinically significant injury in a previously hypertrophied heart.

Hypothermia compromises subendocardial blood flow in the nonhypertrophied heart, with patent coronary arteries if perfusion pressure is reduced. At 28°C, reduction of perfusion pressure from 100 to 50 mm Hg reduced subendocardial blood flow in canine hearts (Fig 11–3).[37] ST segment elevation of the intracavitary elec-

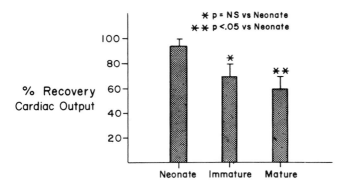

Figure 11–1. After 30 minutes of ischemia in an isolated working rabbit heart, neonatal hearts (8-day-old animals) demonstrated better recovery of cardiac output than either 33-day-old (immature) or adult animals. This suggests that neonatal hearts tolerate hypoxia better, possibly as a result of higher tissue glycogen levels. (*From Bove EL, Stammers AH: Recovery of left ventricular function after hypothermic global ischemia. J Thorac Cardiovasc Surg 91:115– 122, 1986, with permission.*)

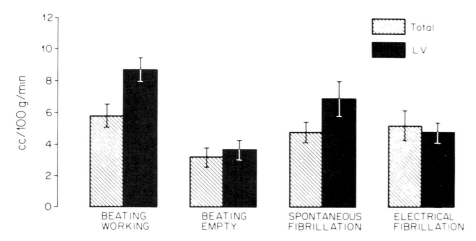

Figure 11–2. Total and left ventricular oxygen consumption in the heart under different working conditions. The oxygen consumption of the beating, empty heart (as on cardiopulmonary bypass) is less than under any other condition. Normal left ventricular oxygen consumption in humans is about 8–10 cc/min/100 g. (*From Hottenrott CE, et al: The hazard of ventricular fibrillation in hypertrophic ventricles during cardiopulmonary bypass. J Thorac Cardiovasc Surg 68:615–625, 1974, with permission.*)

trocardiogram was noted soon after the perfusion pressure was decreased. Gross histologic evidence of ischemia was present if the low-perfusion pressure and hypothermia were maintained for 60 minutes.

No such evidence of injury was found in the nonhypertrophied heart exposed to the lower perfusion pressure if normothermia was maintained. Hypothermia in the presence of lower perfusion pressures is deleterious to the heart by decreasing the diastolic time interval, increasing diastolic wall tension, and distortion of subendocardial vessels due to incomplete diastolic relaxation.

Attempt to prevent the bradycardia associated with hypothermia exacerbates the problem by increasing oxygen demand. Hypothermia increases the per beat oxygen consumption of the heart.[37,38]

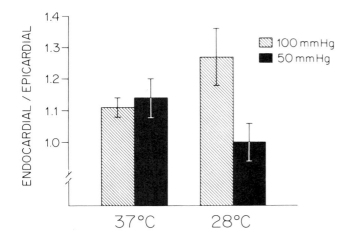

Figure 11–3. Endocardial/epicardial flow ratios at temperatures of 37 and 28°C at perfusion pressures of 50 and 100 mm Hg. Subendocardial flow decreases at a perfusion pressure of 50 under hypothermic conditions. (*From McConnell DH, et al: Studies on the effects of hypothermia on regional myocardial blood flow and metabolism during cardiopulmonary bypass. II. Ischemia during moderate hypothermia in continually perfused beating hearts. J Thorac Cardiovasc Surg 73:95–101, 1977, with permission.*)

Rapid core cooling to low temperature (15°C) on bypass has been implicated as a possible contributor to postischemic myocardial injury. Rebeyka et al noted that isolated perfused juvenile rabbit hearts exposed to cold (15°C) perfusate for 20 minutes prior to cardioplegic arrest for 2 hours had significantly greater loss of both systolic and diastolic function as well as ATP stores compared with hearts that were perfused at 37°C prior to institution of cardioplegic arrest at 10°C.[39] Small infants may be especially prone to rapid myocardial cooling and consequent myocardial contracture.[40] These findings have also been extended to a clinical trial in which cardioplegic arrest was induced with warm-blood cardioplegia. A group of 57 infants weighing less than 6 kg underwent repair of congenital defect following induction of cardioplegia at 37°C with hyperkalemic blood followed by cooling to 15°C with cold blood. Using mortality as an indicator, Williams et al[40] found that this group had a better outcome than a matched control group of 440 infants treated with standard blood cardioplegia.

Cross-clamping the aorta may result in a brief but potentially damaging period of ventricular fibrillation, especially if the left ventricle is inadequately vented. Patients with aortic valvular stenosis are prone to this complication. Fibrillation increases oxygen consumption four- to fivefold compared with the arrested state even in the presence of hypothermia. A fibrillating heart at 22°C requires twice as much oxygen per minute as an arrested heart at 37°C (see Fig 11–2).[41] After cross-clamping the aorta, fibrillation, if it occurs, must be terminated rapidly. ATP stores are significantly reduced by as little as 10 seconds of fibrillation.[42]

Following electromechanical arrest of the heart, the intracardiac repair begins. During this period of time, the heart is quiet, the field bloodless, and operative exposure is optimal. Mechanical quiescence is not synonymous with biochemical quiescence. The heart continues to consume high-energy phosphates even though no mechanical work is done. The rate of consumption is related to temperature. The "safe" operating period is consequently a function of temperature; the cooler the myocardium, the longer the safe period. The safe period is exceeded when ATP levels fall to levels associated with irreversible damage. Factors other than energy stores may also dictate the maximum "safe" period.

After completion of the intracardiac repair, the aortic cross-clamp is removed and reperfusion of the heart occurs. Oxygenated blood and substrate are supplied to a previously ischemic myocardium. The biochemical events that follow are probably the most significant mediators of myocardial injury. The heart is most vulnerable to damage during reperfusion.

Mechanisms of Injury

During the prebypass period, most injury is the result of inadequate perfusion. Hypoxemia alone will not cause injury to the newborn or cyanotic patient. The neonatal heart tolerates hypoxemia if substrate is provided and if metabolic by-products are removed.[27] The heart of the patient with cyanotic congenital heart disease is able to generate sufficient output to meet the resting metabolic demands of the body. It is the reduction of substrate availability and the decrease in washout of toxic by-products that mediate injury.

Ischemia. The ultimate low-perfusion state is ischemia; it is the total absence of blood flow. Ischemia causes irreversible injury if allowed to persist. Periods of ischemia shorter than those required to produce irreversible injury may predispose the heart to reperfusion-related damage.[43] The biochemical changes within the cell resulting from prolonged ischemia are shown in Fig 11–4.

Effects on Myocytes. Ischemia affects both the myocardial muscles and coronary vasculature. Mechanical function decreases dramatically with the onset of ischemia. End-diastolic pressures increase and ventricular compliance decreases. These phenomena are manifestations of ATP depletion. The contractile apparatus is the major consumer of ATP in the beating heart. With substrate limitation, ATP stores are rapidly consumed by mechanical activity. The rise in end-diastolic pressures is a consequence of impaired intracellular calcium uptake and ATP depletion. ATP is required to dissociate the cross bridges between actin and myosin. In the absence of ATP and the presence of Ca^{2+} rigor, cross bridges are formed and an irreversible contracture results.

Ischemia induces changes within the contractile apparatus that reduce the sensitivity of the proteins to calcium and reduce the maximal rate of ATP hydrolysis.[44] The first of these effects is reversible. The sensitivity of the contractile apparatus to Ca^{2+} returns to near normal values on reperfusion. The maximal activity of the myo-

fibrillar ATPase remains depressed. The reduction in the activity is an explanation for the observed decrease in *dp/dt* (change in pressure with time) following ischemic injury.

Endogenous glycogen stores are utilized to generate ATP via glycolysis. This process continues only as long as cytosolic $NADH^+$ levels are below the threshold for inhibition of glycolysis.[45] The ongoing hydrolysis of ATP and glycolysis itself contribute to steadily increasing levels of $NADH^+$. Eventually, glycolysis ceases and ATP production with it. ATP consumption continues until stores are depleted. An ischemic contracture is the manifestation of ATP depletion. The resultant injury may be irreversible. Glycolysis results in the generation of high osmolality, acidosis, and altered redox states within the cell that can slow the generation of free radicals. However, the consensus of opinion is that glycolysis is detrimental to the *ischemic* heart. During hypoxia or anoxic *perfusion* glycolysis can maintain the neonatal heart for variable periods of time.

Ongoing glycolysis generates lactate. Tissue levels of lactate have been inversely correlated with postischemia recovery.[46] High concentrations have been found to produce mitochondrial injury.[47] However, more recent data from isolated cell systems suggest lactate alone is not sufficient to cause anoxic damage or predispose to reperfusion injury.[48]

During ischemia, the mitochondria are unable to generate ATP. The activity of mitochondrial complex I (NADH: ubiquinone reductase) decreases significantly during ischemia and is further reduced on reperfusion. Changes occur within the cytochrome oxidase system that result in a univalent reduction of oxygen rather than the normal tetravalent reduction.[49,50] This change results in the generation of oxygen free radicals upon reperfusion. Oxygen free radicals may also be formed by the mitochondria during periods of ischemia. Postischemic dysfunction can result from the effects of lipid peroxidation caused by these free radicals.

The other organelle affected by ischemia is the SR. The SR actively takes up calcium from the cytosol and thereby terminates contraction. This process consumes ATP (1 μmol/2 μmol Ca^{2+} transported) and is stimulated by calmodulin activity. Ischemia interferes with Ca^{2+} uptake by the SR through (1) ATP depletion, (2) reduction in SR calmodulin activity,[51] and (3) change in intracellular pH. Decreasing intracellular pH decreases Ca^{2+} uptake.[51] The effect of pH change decreases with time, but other factors continue to depress SR function during ischemia.[52]

The consequence of reduced SR calcium uptake is increased cytosolic free Ca^{2+} concentrations. High levels of intracellular calcium in conjunction with calmodulin can activate phospholipases.[52] During ischemia, calmodulin activity remains normal except in the SR.[51] Calcium-calmodulin activation of phospholipase A_2 may

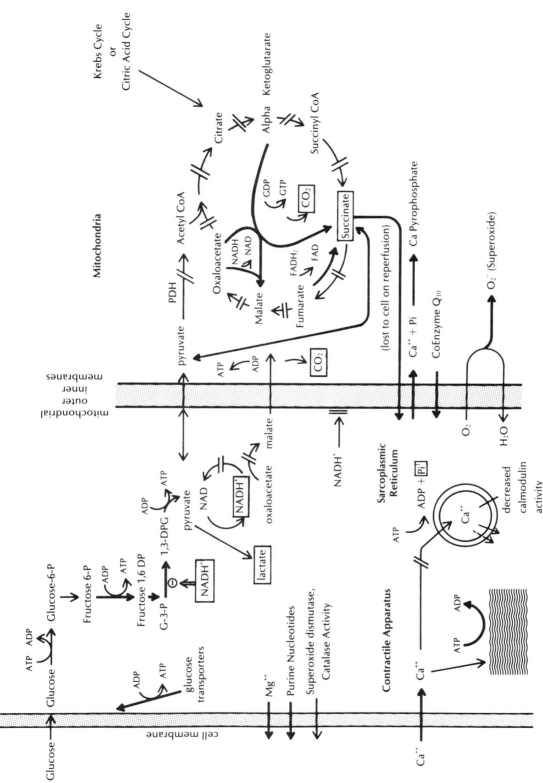

Figure 11–4. During ischemia, ATP must be utilized to recruit glucose transporters. If ATP levels fall too low before enough glucose transporters can be recruited to support glycolysis, ATP depletion results. Anaerobic metabolism results in accumulation of acid metabolites: Pi, lactate, CO_2, reducing equivalents in the cytosol, and $NADH^+$. Accumulation of $NADH^+$ will inhibit glycolysis at the step shown. The oxidation of Krebs cycle intermediates is inhibited. Succinate and pyruvate are produced by anaerobic mitochondrial metabolism. Succinate is lost from the cell on reperfusion, effectively depleting Krebs cycle intermediates. Ca^{2+} enters the cell but the SR is unable to take up the excess Ca^{2+}. The excess Ca^{2+} is taken up by the mitochondria and causes continued activation of the contractile apparatus. This activation will deplete ATP stores. Mg^{2+} and purine nucleotides as well as SOD and catalase activity are lost during ischemia. Mitochondrial coenzyme Q_{10} activity decreases during ischemia. The cytochrome oxidase system univalently reduces O_2 to yield superoxide radicals, O_2^-. Symbols: —— Pathways unique to or enhanced by ischemia; $-|\!\!\rightarrow$ pathways blocked by ischemia; $=\!=\!=$ metabolites accumulating during ischemia; $\ominus$ inhibitor of conversion step.

result in membrane damage with loss of intracellular contents, including creatine kinase. Elevated blood levels of the MB-CK isoform are indicative of myocardial injury.

Adenine nucleotides are found in coronary sinus blood following variable periods of ischemia. Loss of adenine nucleotides from the myocardium results in sustained low cellular ATP levels. Up to 3 days are required for ATP levels to return to normal following only 15 minutes of normothermic ischemia.[54]

Effects on Coronary Vasculature. The changes that occur within the coronary vasculature during ischemia are more subtle but no less deleterious to the heart. The purine metabolisms of the coronary endothelium and the myocytes are closely related. Much of the adenine nucleotide salvage occurs in the vascular endothelium.[55] Ischemic injury affects the endothelium resulting in loss of nucleotides even after short durations of ischemia.

The coronary capillary endothelium is the only site within the myocardium of uric acid production.[56] Uric acid is produced from hypoxanthine and xanthine by the enzyme xanthine dehydrogenase. During ischemia, xanthine dehydrogenase is converted to xanthine oxidase by the action of a Ca^{2+}-dependent protease.[57] Xanthine oxidase converts xanthine and hypoxanthine to uric acid, but it also catalyzes the formation of toxic oxygen radicals. These substances are formed on reperfusion and are capable of mediating "reperfusion injury." This position is not universally accepted. Data acquired from ischemic rat hearts indicate that there is only minimal conversion of xanthine dehydrogenase to xanthine oxidase.[58] Whether this observation is unique to the rat remains to be determined.

Toxic oxygen radicals are formed in low concentrations in the normal heart. They are detoxified by endogenous superoxide dismutase, catalase, and peroxidases. The activity of these free radical scavengers is dramatically reduced by ischemia.[59] Ischemia renders them ineffective during the reperfusion period; consequently free radical–mediated damage ensues. The activity of lytic enzymes is increased during ischemia.

The vascular endothelium is the source of endothelium-dependent relaxing factor (EDRF), which is probably nitric oxide (NO), and prostacyclin. These substances are critical for the maintenance of normal coronary flow. Ischemia and possibly cardioplegia solution themselves alter the responsiveness of the coronary vasculature to 5-hydroxytryptamine, which causes release of EDRF.[60] Loss of normal endothelial function leads to pathologic vasoconstriction by the coronary vessels in response to various biochemical metabolites. Ischemic injury may also leave the endothelium vulnerable to activation of platelets and neutrophils and their adhesion upon reperfusion, resulting in further injury.

Reperfusion. At the cellular level, reperfusion is potentially the most destructive phase during the operative repair of a congenital heart defect. Generation of oxygen radicals and calcium influx both occur during perfusion of the myocardium. Both of these phenomena may injure the heart. There is a "burst" of free radical production that peaks 2–4 minutes after reperfusion and continues for 3 hours or more after reflow. Exogenously supplied superoxide dismutase may have only a transient effect because of its short half-life (6–10 minutes) relative to the long duration of the free radical burst.[61] Much of the damage produced by toxic oxygen radicals is mediated by the hydroxyl radical $OH^{\cdot}$.[62] This entity is formed by the interaction of the superoxide radical, $O_2^{\cdot}$, and hydrogen peroxide via the Haber-Weiss reaction ($O_2^{\cdot}$ + $H_2O_2 \rightarrow O_2$ + OH^- $OH^{\cdot}$). This reaction is usually slow in the absence of metal catalysts. However, ferric iron and other metals can greatly accelerate the rate of this reaction.[63] The reactant $O_2^{\cdot}$ is formed by the conversion of hypoxanthine to xanthine by xanthine oxidase in the presence of oxygen. An alternative pathway for $O_2^{\cdot}$ generation is via one-electron reduction of O_2 catalyzed by the enzyme NADPH-oxidase that is present in neutrophils and is activated by complement C5a. Complement activation is a frequent event during bypass. Subsequent dismutation of $O_2^{\cdot}$ forms H_2O_2. If superoxide dismutase is present in sufficient amounts, the $O_2^{\cdot}$ radical is destroyed rapidly and the Haber-Weiss reaction cannot proceed for lack of reactant.[53] Iron chelators such as deferoxamine can also inhibit the Haber-Weiss reaction directly.

The hydroxyl radical is especially toxic because it has been shown to react with polyunsaturated fatty acids (a common membrane constituent) to form lipid hydroperoxides.[64] Liquid hydroperoxides are capable of causing sustained chain reactions resulting in extensive membrane damage and possible disruption of cellular integrity.

Ultrastructural damage produced by $OH^{\cdot}$ includes vacuolization and edema of the vascular endothelium, severe swelling of the myocardial mitochondria, and myocyte basement membrane blebbing.[52] Membranous cellular debris was found in the vessels of septal preparations exposed to $O_2^{\cdot}$ and $OH^{\cdot}$. The primary damage caused by free radicals is not the generation of "holes" in the cell membrane but rather inactivation of proteins critical to maintenance of cellular homeostasis. A vast array of proteins are involved, including glycolytic enzymes, cation channels, SR-ATPases, and others. Free radical damage to the glycolytic pathway has been postulated to cause increased intracellular Ca^{2+} via impaired Na^+-K^+ exchange with consequent Ca^{2+} for Na^+ exchange.

Functional changes induced by $OH^{\cdot}$ include significant decreases in developed tension and diminished ability of the SR to take up calcium. The diminished calcium uptake is a consequence of the uncoupling of Ca^{2+} transport from ATP hydrolysis[65]; this effect is exacerbated by acidosis. Both radicals and excess Ca^{2+}

have been implicated in the decrease in NADH: ubiquinone oxidase (complex I) activity in mitrochondria on reperfusion with O_2 containing perfusate.[49,66] Loss of complex I activity uncouples oxidative phosphorylation.

Another effect of the generation of oxygen radicals is the production of arachidonic acid metabolites capable of mediating vasoconstriction within the coronary vasculature. This effect, combined with the direct damage to the vascular endothelium could, theoretically, lead to microinfarcts in the areas of involved myocardium.

Calcium Influx. Events during the ischemic period may predispose the myocyte to a massive influx of calcium on reperfusion. The SR is unable to take up Ca^{2+} normally because of depressed ATP stores and OH^--mediated injury. Five to 10 μM or greater intracellular Ca^{2+} concentrations activate lytic enzymes and uncouple substrate oxidation from phosphorylation.[67] The combined effects of mitochondrial respiratory chain damage and Ca^{2+} entry can be significant. "Stunned" reperfused, postischemic hearts have fourfold greater than normal oxygen consumption at a given work load (Fig 11–5). Supraphysiologic calcium concentrations in the reperfusate are undesirable. Recovery of function following ischemia is inversely related to the Ca^{2+} (ionized) concentration of the reperfusate. The lower the intracellular ATP levels following ischemia, the greater the sensitivity of the myocardium to the damaging effects of Ca^{2+}.[46]

Prevention of Myocardial Injury

To achieve a successful operative outcome, the heart of the patient with a congenital cardiac defect must be protected from the injuries just described. Myocardial protection begins with a carefully planned and executed anesthetic technique that prevents prebypass injury by careful maintenance of filling pressures, arterial pressure, and blood gases in order to maintain adequate organ perfusion and oxygenation. Rapid myocardial cooling to low temperatures would be avoided if possible.

Distention of the heart must be avoided during the rewarming period. Overdistention compromises subendocardial flow. Calcium should be used judiciously because overzealous use of Ca^{2+} impairs myocardial recovery by promoting calcium influx.

If low systemic pressures are noted on attempting to discontinue bypass, the patient should be returned to bypass to support the circulation. The addition of an inotropic agent is best accomplished with extracorporeal circulatory support. Troublesome arrhythmias may also necessitate continued bypass while correction is attempted with pacing or pharmacologic intervention.

The anesthetic technique should be tailored to the surgical procedure. For example, if surface cooling to achieve deep hypothermia is to be used, ventilation must be controlled to produce mild to moderate hypocarbia. Hypocarbia prevents the development of ventricular fibrillation and improves cardiac performance during cooling.[67] Hypocarbia during cooling was believed by many

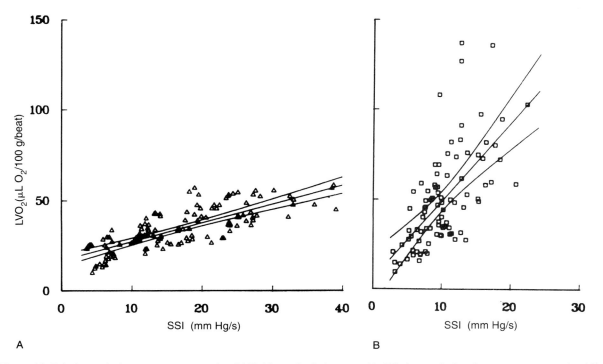

Figure 11–5. Left ventricular oxygen consumption (LVO_2) is markedly increased in (*B*), the postischemic state as compared to (*A*), the preischemic state. (*A, B*) Linear regression plots of LVO_2 against left ventricular systolic circumferential wall stress (SSI). These data indicate a fourfold increase in oxygen consumption in "stunned," postischemic myocardium. (*From Bavaria JE, et al: Myocardial oxygen utilization after reversible global ischemia. J Thorac Cardiovasc Surg 100:210–220, 1991, with permission.*)

workers to compromise cerebral blood flow. However, the studies of Murkin and co-workers[68] and Prough and colleagues[69] suggest that under conditions of hypothermia, the brain enjoys luxury perfusion at a temperature-corrected (37°C) P_{CO_2} of 40. Reduction of cerebral blood flow secondary to hypocarbia is well tolerated during hypothermia. A pH of 7.6–7.8 prior to deep hypothermic arrest results in optimum postreperfusion cerebral recovery.[70]

Equally important is the careful and expeditious execution of the surgical procedure from incision to closure. Long delays in cannulation may result in needlessly lengthened periods of myocardial hypoperfusion. Long intervals between application of the aortic cross-clamp and perfusion of the heart with cold cardioplegia solution can cause excessive consumption of ATP stores.

Attention to detail and careful technique alone will not provide adequate protection from injury. Other modalities are required. The most commonly used is hypothermia. It is also the most effective modality in preventing myocardial damage if careful technique is used.

HYPOTHERMIA

Hypothermia reduces the metabolic rate of the heart. Enzymatic systems obey van't Hoff's law; there is an exponential decrease in reaction rate with decreasing temperature. This relationship applies to oxygen consumption. Oxygen consumption decreases by a factor of 2.8 for each 10-degree fall in temperature. At 17°C, the myocardial oxygen consumption is only 12% of that at 37°C.

Hypothermia has a stabilizing effect on membranes and alters membrane fluidity.[71] Low temperatures also protect the heart from "calcium paradox," a phenomenon due to massive influx of Ca^{2+} on reperfusion with a Ca^{2+}-containing medium.[72] Hypothermia during the period of perfusion with Ca^{2+}-free medium appears to prevent the membrane damage noted during normothermic perfusion with Ca^{2+}-free medium.

Although preventing the development of calcium paradox, hypothermia increases the sensitivity of the myocardium to exogenous calcium. Fibrillation may be easily induced in the hypothermic heart by exogenously administered calcium. This sensitivity may be due in part to potassium loss from the myocytes as a result of hypothermia. Therefore, calcium should be avoided or used with caution during surface cooling of patients to achieve moderate or deep hypothermia.

The ability of hypothermia alone to prevent myocardial ischemic injury is limited. Animal studies provide the best data for evaluating the duration of "safe" ischemia time at various temperatures. The limits of tolerable ischemia time appear to be 30–45 minutes at 22°C

and up to 60 minutes at 15°C.[62] After 96 minutes of ischemia at 15°C, severe myocardial injury was found in canine hearts.[73] The histologic evidence of injury included cellular and interstitial edema, myelin figures, and myofibrillar lysis.[74]

The effects of temperature on the myocardium appear to be age dependent. In the neonatal heart, hypothermia alone may confer more protection than hypothermia plus certain cardioplegia solutions. This finding does not extend to the mature heart.

The safe use of hypothermia as a modality for myocardial preservation is predicated on the user knowing its proper application and limitations. Several strategies have been devised to reduce myocardial temperatures safely. These include surface cooling, core cooling using ECC, topical cooling of the myocardium, and perfusion cooling of the myocardium.

Topical Hypothermia. The heart may be cooled by perfusion cooling or topical cooling. Topical cooling was initially attempted by bathing the heart surface and chambers with ice slush. This practice resulted in myocardial injury as a result of profound myocardial cooling. In 1959, Shumway and Lower reported the effectiveness of continuous topical cooling as a means of myocardial protection.[75] They used a continuous lavage of the pericardial well by iced saline (2–4°C). Using this technique, good myocardial function was noted following 60 minutes of aortic cross-clamping without using cardioplegia. The use of the technique requires the formation of a pericardial well by the surgeon. Iced saline (2–4°C) must flow into the well at a rate of 100–150 mL/min in an adult. The head must be elevated approximately 30 degrees and the patient tilted to the left to keep the heart adequately immersed in the cold saline (Fig 11–6). Systemic temperatures of 28–30°C, low systemic perfusion indices, and venting of bronchial return are required to prevent cavitary warming and cardiac distention. The requirements of submersion of a large fraction of the heart makes the technique difficult, but not impossible, to apply to the repair of congenital cardiac lesions. Shumway and co-workers[76] used topical hypothermia to repair a tetralogy of Fallot in a 14-year-old patient. The patient tolerated 25 minutes of aortic cross-clamp time without serious clinical sequelae.

Topical hypothermia is ineffective in achieving uniform myocardial cooling in hypertrophied hearts. Reliance on topical cooling alone can result in inadequate myocardial protection with consequent postoperative myocardial dysfunction. Electromechanical activity was noted to persist in a high percentage of patients in whom topical myocardial cooling was the sole means of myocardial protection.[77] In such patients, perfusion hypothermia should be used in combination with topical hypothermia. Subendocardial damage, as assessed by fibrosis, was found to be less in hearts protected by the

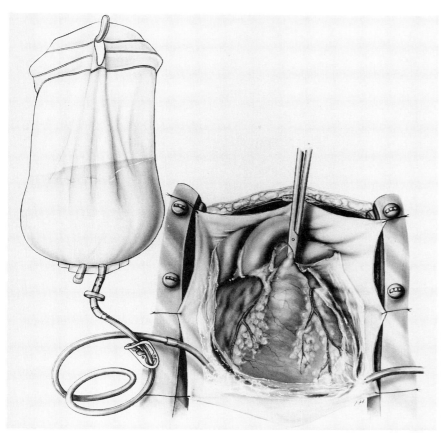

Figure 11–6. A system for the delivery of topical hypothermia to the heart. Normal saline at a temperature of 5°C or less flows into the pericardial well and is suctioned near the cardiac apex to prevent the liquid from overflowing the pericardial space. *(From Lake CL: Cardiovascular Anesthesia. New York: Springer Verlag, 1985, p. 352, with permission.)*

combination of perfusion hypothermia and topical hypothermia than in those hearts protected by topical myocardia alone.

Modifications of the topical hypothermia technique are used in many centers. One modification is the combined use of perfusion cooling and bathing of the myocardial surface with iced saline to achieve initial cooling of the heart. The continuous saline lavage is not used, but the combination of perfusion and topical cooling is repeated every 20 minutes.

Cardioplegia. Myocardial cooling is most effectively achieved by perfusing the coronary vasculature with iced (2–4°C) solution (Fig 11–7). Myocardial temperatures below 20°C are attained within minutes of the initiation of cold perfusion of the coronary arteries.[78] This rapid cooling can produce myocardial standstill as well as protect the myocardium from ischemic damage during the period of aortic cross-clamping. This technique may, however, predispose to later injury.[39,40] Temperatures of 6°C or below produce cardiac arrest[16] but can result in tissue damage.[14] Cardioplegic solutions can be used to induce cardiac arrest at higher temperatures. Other advantages of the use of cardioplegia include a more rapid and reliable onset of electromechanical silence.

In 1955, Melrose and co-workers[10] reported that addition of potassium citrate to cold hypertonic blood reli-

ably produced elective cardiac arrest and permitted up to 15 minutes of ischemia with recovery of function. They used the term *cardioplegia* to describe the solution. However, evidence of myocardial necrosis in laboratory animals and patients after elective cardiac arrest had been produced using Melrose solution resulted in the abandonment of cardioplegic solutions.[11,12] Melrose's original concepts were correct, but the concentrations of the constituents of his cardioplegic solution were incorrect.

There are now almost as many cardioplegic solutions as there are centers using them. Despite the variation in formulation, two broad types of cardioplegic solutions can be defined: blood cardioplegia and crystalloid cardioplegia. At present, there is no overwhelming evidence for one type of cardioplegic solution for myocardial protection during the repair of congenital heart defects.[79,80]

Blood Cardioplegia. The use of blood cardioplegia was based upon the assumption that the oxygen carried by the hemoglobin would provide extra protection against ischemic injury. This assumption has been both verified and refuted by experimental evidence.[80,81]

The reasons for the discrepancy relate to the temperature of the cardioplegic solution infused.[80] The ability of hemoglobin to deliver oxygen to tissue decreased at lower temperatures. At 5°C, more oxygen is available

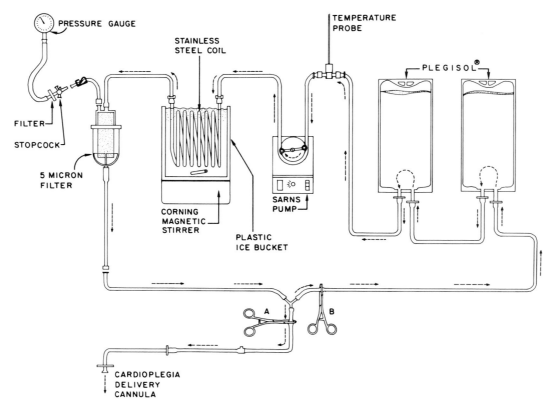

Figure 11–7. A system for the delivery of hypothermic, crystalloid cardioplegia. The solution is cooled in a continuously agitated ice bath. It then passes through a roller pump and filters before entering the aortic root when clamp A is removed. The pressure of the inflow is also measured. When cardioplegia is not in use, the solution is recirculated by replacing the clamp at A and removing clamp B.

to tissue from oxygenated crystalloid solution than oxygenated blood cardioplegic solution. However, if cardioplegic solution is delivered at higher temperatures, such as 20–27°C, then blood cardioplegic solutions will be able to deliver more oxygen to tissues than crystalloid cardioplegic solutions.

Blood contains many other components in addition to hemoglobin, including calcium, magnesium, protein, hormones, and cellular elements. Some studies claiming that blood cardioplegic solutions provided better myocardial protection than crystalloid cardioplegic solutions failed to add divalent cations to the crystalloid solutions used in the comparative studies. The omission of these ions from the crystalloid cardioplegic solutions may have played a significant role in the observed superiority of blood cardioplegia over the asanguineous cardioplegic solutions. If blood and crystalloid cardioplegic solutions have the same ionic constituents added (not that the concentrations of the ionic species are the same as in blood), there is little or no advantage to the use of blood cardioplegic solution in cases for which low infusion temperatures are used[80] (Fig 11–8).

The rheologic properties of blood cardioplegia are worthy of note. The viscosity of blood increases as temperature falls. Because of higher viscosity, cold blood solutions require longer infusion times than does an asanguineous cardioplegic solution. Prolonged infusions may have a beneficial effect on distribution in nonhypertrophied hearts. Distribution of the cardioplegic solution in a nonhypertrophied heart after multiple (14) doses[79] was found to be more uniform with blood than crystalloid. This improvement in perfusion is observed even if the red blood cells have been rendered incapable of O_2 transport. The presence of red blood cells or other microparticles allows perfusion of the entire capillary bed. No flow is seen in the true capillaries if they are perfused with nonparticulate solutions (colloid or crystalloid).[82] Despite this theoretical advantage, blood and calcium-containing crystalloid cardioplegic solutions were found to have identical intracardiac distribution after three doses (40-minute aortic cross-clamp time).

The use of blood cardioplegic solutions requires a delivery system. This is usually part of the cardiopulmonary bypass unit and includes a pump, heat exchanger, and reservoir. A quantity of blood is removed from the bypass circuit and stored in the reservoir. Potassium is added to achieve the desired K^+ concentration. The

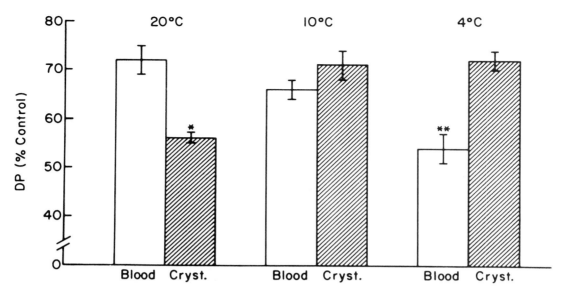

Figure 11–8. The effect of blood or crystalloid cardioplegia on ventricular function at different temperatures. The use of blood cardioplegia is more important in the recovery of ventricular function at temperatures of 20°C than at 4 or 10°C. At lower temperatures, developed pressure (DP) is improved by crystalloid cardioplegia. (*From Magovern GJ Jr, et al: Failure of blood cardioplegia to protect myocardium at lower temperatures. Circulation 66(suppl I):60–67, 1982, with permission.*)

solution is infused by a pump into the aortic root using pressures ranging from 50 to 100 mm Hg.

Care must be taken to avoid excessive intravascular pressure during infusion of the solution. Flows of 400–500 mL/min/m² produce rapid arrest of electromechanical activity and effective myocardial cooling. The pressures needed to yield these flows depend on hematocrit, delivery temperature, coronary vessel patency, and vascular tone. Technical factors such as conduit, coronary, or aortic cannula diameters also affect required infusion pressure.

Blood cardioplegic solution should be infused frequently during the cross-clamp period. It is most often used at delivery temperatures of 20°C or greater and, consequently, does not achieve the same degree of myocardial cooling. Excessive rewarming of the heart can occur if the solution is not reinfused at regular intervals (approximately 20 minutes). Factors that increase the likelihood of excessive myocardial rewarming are a high rate of bronchial return and systemic perfusion temperatures of 27°C or greater. Increased bronchial flow can be troublesome in patients with pulmonary artery atresia. These vessels must frequently be isolated and controlled, if possible, before institution of cardiopulmonary bypass to prevent excessive return to the heart.

Crystalloid Cardioplegia. Complex congenital heart defects are frequently repaired under conditions of moderate to deep hypothermia (25°C or below). If circulatory arrest is planned, deep hypothermia (15–17°C) is frequently used. Maximal cooling of the myocardium is desirable in these cases. This can best be achieved with 2–4°C crystalloid solution infused through the aortic root. Under these conditions, properly formulated crystalloid solutions are as effective as blood cardioplegia in preserving high-energy phosphate stores and preventing ischemic injury.[79]

Crystalloid cardioplegic solutions are formulated to resemble either intracellular (Bretschneider solution) or extracellular (St. Thomas Hospital solution) fluid. The degree of myocardial protection afforded by a solution resembling intracellular fluid is affected by the rate and volume of infusion. Decreased protection is noted if high rates of infusion or large volumes are used. If a solution based on extracellular fluid is used, the degree of protection does not vary with volume or rate of infusion of the cardioplegic solution.[83] However, not all solutions based on extracellular fluid afford the same protection.

COMPONENTS OF CARDIOPLEGIC SOLUTIONS. The formulation of cardioplegic solutions remains a source of great debate. However, potassium, magnesium, calcium, sodium, and buffers appear to be beneficial in preserving myocardial function. The osmolarity of cardioplegic solutions also merits comment (Table 11–3).

Potassium. Melrose's original cardioplegic solution contained potassium citrate. The potassium concentration and increased osmolarity contributed to the myocardial damage during clinical use of the Melrose solution. Excessively high potassium (K^+) concentrations (40 mEq/L or greater) are potentially injurious to the myocardium. Most clinically used solutions employ K^+ concentrations of 15–40 mEq/L.

TABLE 11–3. CARDIOPLEGIA CONSTITUENTS

Constituent	Action
Cold (hypothermia)	Reduced MVO_2, membrane stabilization
Potassium	Produces arrest in diastole; high concentrations result in contractures
Calcium	Membrane stabilization (in low concentration); high concentrations result in contractures
Magnesium	Prevents Mg^{2+} loss from cells; blocks Ca^{2+} entry during ischemia
Sodium	Prevents excessive accumulation of cell water; high Na^+ promotes Ca^{2+} entry during ischemia
Buffer	Phosphate, histidine, THAM can reduce intracellular H^+ (raise pH); permits ongoing ATP generation during ischemia
Substrate	Ribose, adenosine, and hypoxanthine to retard ATP degradation and improve postischemic recovery
Osmolar active	Reduces cell swelling; osmolarity greater than 400 promotes Ca^{2+} influx during reperfusion
Oxygen	Can be extracted from crystalloid at low temperature; allows aerobic metabolism during cross-clamp period
Steroids	Membrane stabilization; prevents lipid peroxidation

A 1970 study found that under conditions of hypothermia (15°C) and ischemia, ATP and creatine phosphate levels are better maintained if electromechanical arrest is produced than in the absence of electromechanical arrest.[84] In 1975, Hearse and co-workers[16] demonstrated that hypothermia and hyperkalemia had additive effects on the preservation of myocardial ATP stores during ischemia. This finding was subsequently confirmed by other investigators.

The major effect of potassium is the production of electromechanical arrest that results from depolarization of the cell membrane. A state of diastole is maintained as long as there is increased extracellular potassium. The potassium concentration needed to produce diastolic arrest is a function of temperature; decreasing as temperature is decreased, (eg, at 37°C, 20 mEq/L of K^+ is required to produce arrest, and at 24°C, only 13 mEq/L needed). The benefit derived from electromechanical arrest is a function of temperature and potassium concentration.

Potassium concentrations greater than 40 mEq/L appear to alter the permeability of the myocyte to calcium.[85] Extracellular calcium may enter the cell and thereby increase energy consumption.

The measured oxygen consumption of hearts exposed to very high potassium concentrations (170 mEq/L) is twice that measured in hearts exposed to lower concentrations (80 mEq/L) of potassium.[86] The left ventricular diastolic pressure of isolated hypothermic

(17°C) perfused neonatal rabbit hearts increases with the onset of potassium-induced arrest. The magnitude and duration of the increase in end-diastolic pressure increases dramatically as potassium concentration exceeded 60 mEq/L (author's unpublished data). Rich and Brady[85] found that myocardial contracture, or "stone heart," could be induced in hearts exposed to solutions containing more than 100 mEq/L of potassium.

There is not unanimous acceptance of hyperkalemia in cardioplegic solutions. Laboratory and clinical studies[87,88] found no improvement in postischemic recovery between groups of hearts treated with either high K^+ (20–30 mEq/L) or low K^+ (4–10 mEq/L) cardioplegic solutions. Data from one of the laboratory studies suggest that in the presence of a strong buffer, high K^+ concentrations (30 mEq/L or greater) are detrimental. Myocardial function was better preserved during the reperfusion period with a 10 mEq/L K^+ buffered cold cardioplegic solution.[87] The cardioplegic solutions used in that study had no calcium, low sodium (27 mEq/L), and a high pH (7.8). The addition of buffer (histidine) and 30 mEq/L of K^+ resulted in extensive damage on reperfusion. The pattern of injury was similar to that produced by massive Ca^{2+} influx. This suggests that there are complex interactions between ionic species that must be investigated before new cardioplegic formulations are used clinically.

Magnesium and Calcium. Divalent cations have profound effects on membrane fluidity and stability.[89] Perfusion of isolated interventricular septum with calcium-free medium results in membrane damage that is not entirely prevented with cadmium (a divalent cation with an ionic radius closer in size to Ca^{2+} than to Mg^{2+}). Hypothermia (18°C) prevents the membrane damage seen with calcium depletion.[71] Tolerance to calcium depletion diminishes with increasing temperature. At 18°C, nearly complete functional recovery is seen in hearts exposed to Ca^{2+}-free medium for 30 minutes then reperfused with Ca^{2+}-containing medium. Recovery is only 70% at 22°C and less than 20% at 28°C for the same duration of exposure to Ca^{2+}-free medium prior to reexposure to Ca^{2+}. The injury responsible for the decreased function is termed calcium paradox. Ca^{2+} concentrations as low as 50 μmol/L prevent the development of calcium paradox.[72]

In a recent study of cardioplegic solutions containing one of three Mg^{2+} concentrations (0, 1.2, and 15 mM) in combination with one of three Ca^{2+} concentrations (0.05, 1.5, and 4.5 mM), Brown and co-workers[90] determined that optimal recovery from ischemia occurred at 0.05 mM Ca^{2+} and 15 mM Mg^{2+}. The functional and metabolic recovery was reduced by decreasing $[Mg^{2+}]$ or by increasing $[Ca^{2+}]$. The decrement in recovery with increasing Ca^{2+} was more pronounced as temperature decreased[90] (Fig 11–9).

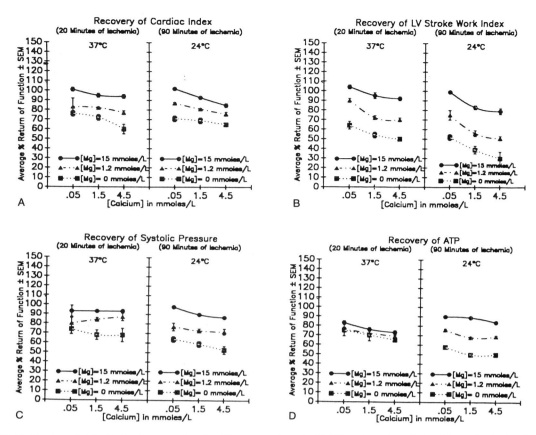

Figure 11–9. The beneficial effects of magnesium in either normothermic (37°C) or hypothermic (24°C) cardioplegia after 20 or 90 minutes of ischemia regardless of calcium concentration are indicated by greater recovery of cardiac index (*A*), left ventricular stroke work index (*B*), systolic pressure (*C*), and myocardial adenosine triphosphate (*D*). (*From Brown PS, et al: Magnesium ion is beneficial in hypothermic crystalloid cardioplegia. Ann Thorac Surg 51:359–367, 1991, with permission.*)

The St. Thomas Hospital solution has a $[Mg^{2+}]$ of 15 mM and a $[Ca^{2+}]$ of 1.2 mM. This solution is optimal in adult hearts as demonstrated by multiple experiments. However, this solution is suboptimal in both neonatal rabbit[91] and neonatal guinea pig[92] myocardium in studies of multidose or continuous infusion of the cardioplegic solutions. In the neonatal rabbit, left ventricular power was 70% of control after 60 minutes of ischemia and less than 65% of control after 90 minutes of ischemia despite infusions of cardioplegic solution every 30 minutes and maintenance of myocardial temperature at 10°C by cooling with saline. At both time intervals, the adult hearts had full recovery despite significant reductions in myocardial ATP content. The neonatal hearts maintained ATP content at control levels but still experienced poor mechanical recovery. Thus, there is a clear dissociation between ATP content and recovery. In addition, coronary perfusion was reduced on reperfusion in the neonatal heart but not in the adult heart.[91]

In the neonatal guinea pig heart, the St. Thomas solution increased resting tension, cell water, and cellular Ca^{2+} content. In addition to these deleterious effects, the recovery of contractile function was significantly less in the neonatal heart than in the adult heart.[92]

These studies and clinical experience indicate that the optimal cardioplegic solution for the neonatal heart has yet to be formulated. The interactions between Na^+, Mg^{2+}, and Ca^{2+} may be different than in the adult heart. The lipid composition of neonatal membranes is also different from the adult, so that divalent cation interactions may alter membrane fluidity-temperature relationships differently from adult myocardium. Cardioplegia studies carried out in neonatal piglet hearts suggest that these hearts may require a "physiologic" Ca^{2+} concentration for optimum protection.[93] This point is still controversial.

There is, however, general agreement that inclusion of Mg^{2+} in cardioplegic solutions is beneficial. Magnesium is lost from the myocardium during ischemic arrest. This loss may result in impairment of cardiac recovery because Mg^{2+} is known to reduce the transsarcolemmal flux of Ca^{2+} and inhibit Na^+ influx into the cell among other effects that are related to its function as a cofactor for many enzymatic reactions.

Magnesium can produce cardioplegia in high concentrations. This observation was the basis for the

"Kirsch solution." Most clinically used solutions have a lower magnesium concentration than the Kirsch solution. Hearse and co-workers[94] found a 15 mmol/L concentration to be optimal. Nuclear magnetic resonance (NMR) spectroscopic studies have found that the addition of magnesium to cardioplegic solutions improved maintenance of high-energy phosphate stores under conditions of hypothermic arrest,[95] yet these same investigators found that the addition of K^+ to a magnesium-based cardioplegic solution failed to protect ATP stores. This is in contrast to the study of Hearse and co-workers,[96] who found that additional protection was conferred by the addition of K^+ to a Mg^{2+} solution. As in the case of comparisons between blood and crystalloid solutions, the temperature involved may be the important factor in the different conclusions.

Sodium. Intracellular sodium and calcium concentrations are interrelated. These two ions can be exchanged via a common channel termed the Na^+-Ca^{2+} exchanger. Interventions that increase intracellular sodium activity may cause a dramatic increase in intracellular Ca^{2+} activity. In the absence of Ca^{2+} and Mg^{2+}, sodium may enter the cell through Ca^{2+} channels.

The effects of changes in extracellular sodium concentrations are more complex than would be predicted by consideration of transcellular Na^+-Ca^{2+} exchange alone. Perfusion of isolated hearts with low sodium perfusate causes calcium-dependent increases in diastolic pressure, energy consumption, and dissociation of oxygen consumption from work. The effect is postulated to be mediated by alterations in SR calcium cycling.[97]

Despite the theoretical considerations, a cardioplegic solution with decreased Na, the Bretschneider "HTK" solution, is used clinically with success. This solution has essentially no Ca^{2+} (15–20 μmol) and a high buffering capacity. Low Na^+ concentrations can arrest the heart by inhibition of the "fast" inward current required for depolarization. If K is added, Na^+ pump activity is stimulated and intracellular Na^+ decreases in response. This effect reduces cell swelling and Ca^{2+} influx on reperfusion.[98]

Hypertonic saline should be avoided because it increases intracellular sodium concentration with a subsequent increase in intracellular Ca^{2+} concentration. The "ideal" sodium concentration for standard cardioplegia is not firmly established but is probably between 90 and 120 mmol/L.[95,99] The St. Thomas solution contains 120 mM Na^{2+} (110 mM as NaCL and 10 mM as $NaHCO_3$).

The action of Na^+ ion is complex. Entry into the cell during ischemia is mediated via Na^+-H^+ exchange. Thus, accumulation of H^+ within the cell can increase Na^+ during the early phases of reperfusion with a consequent rise in Ca^{2+}. If the Na^+-H^+ exchanger is blocked by ameloride, the increases in cell Na^+ and Ca^{2+} seen on reperfusion are blocked.[100]

Buffer. ATP consumption continues during ischemia. Hydrogen ion is generated as a consequence of ATP hydrolysis causing intracellular acidosis unless some provision is made for buffering. The cell has some limited buffering capacity. An important buffer is the amino acid histidine. Histidine has an imidazole group that can exist in a protonated or deprotonated state. The latter can be a proton acceptor and thereby buffer intracellular pH changes. The cost of using histidine residues as buffer is high because the activity of enzymes is reduced or destroyed if histidine residues in active sites undergo protonation.

If ATP stores decrease during ischemia, endogenous glycogen is converted to glucose for metabolism to ATP and lactate.[87] If intracellular levels of ATP are maintained, exogenous glucose is used in preference to glycogen. The problem then is the maintenance of ATP levels during ischemia.

These problems can be mitigated by the use of a buffer in the cardioplegic solution. The choice of buffer may be important. The bicarbonate ion is an inefficient buffer of intracellular pH change and has even been found to cause intracellular acidosis, whereas other species such as phosphate can buffer intracellular pH changes. Adequate intracellular buffering is associated with better functional recovery (Fig 11–10).

Lange and colleagues[101] studied the effects of alkalinity and temperature on the effectiveness of multidose bicarbonate-buffered cardioplegic solutions. The use of 37°C, pH 8.2, bicarbonate-buffered cardioplegic solution failed to alter intracellular pH. The same solution when cooled to 10°C before infusion produced transient increases in intracellular pH. The increases in pH paralleled decreases in myocardial temperature. The magnitude of the intracellular pH change was equal to that pH change that could be predicted on the basis of the temperature change alone. There was no need to invoke buffering of intracellular H^+ by the bicarbonate in the cardioplegic solution to explain the pH change.

Tromethamine (THAM) and histidine are both effective in increasing intracellular pH if supplied in the perfusate.[102] Removal of reducing equivalents from the cytosol by a buffer prevents the inhibition of glycolysis by nicotine adenine dinucleotide hydrogen (NADH). However, THAM is toxic to certain tissues. Histidine has the desirable property of shifting its pKa into the alkaline range with decreasing temperature. The change is in the same direction and of the same magnitude as the change in pH of pure water with temperatures.[103] It has been postulated that the pKa shift of the imidazole group of histidine residues of intracellular proteins accounts for the increase in intracellular pH with hypothermia. This pH change with temperature protects the activity of intracellular enzymes and maintains chemical neutrality. Histidine buffering maintains ATP levels during ischemia and prevents glycogenolysis by promoting utili-

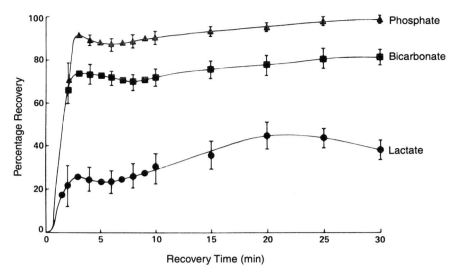

Figure 11–10. Cardioplegic solutions containing phosphate or bicarbonate buffer allow better recovery of aortic flow than lactate buffer in the isolated rat heart model. (*From Hearse DJ, et al: Myocardial protection during bypass and arrest: A possible hazard with lactate-containing infusates. J Thorac Cardiovasc Surg 72:880–884, 1976, with permission.*)

zation of exogenous glucose.[87] Histidine appears, theoretically, to be the ideal buffer for use in cardioplegic solutions; however, in clinical practice, phosphate is very effective.

OSMOLARITY. Melrose's original cardioplegic solution had an osmolarity of greater than 500 mOsm/L, which contributed to the myocardial damage it produced in clinical use. Severe myocardial damage is caused by solutions with osmolarities greater than 400 mOsm. Hyperosmolar solutions cause myocardial injury by several mechanisms, one of which is intracellular water loss, which produces conformation change in protein structures within the cell.

Another mechanism by which hypertonic cardioplegic solutions may cause damage is by raising intracellular sodium ion activity. Lado and co-workers[104] studied the effects of solutions of high osmolarity on the intracellular sodium and calcium ion activity. The solutions were made hyperosmolar by the addition of sucrose while ion concentrations were kept constant. Segments of heart exposed to hypertonic (448 and 610 mOsm/L) solutions developed rapid increases in resting tension and dramatic decreases in contracted size. Intracellular calcium ion activity was increased beyond that expected on the basis of osmolar concentration effects due to osmotic water loss. The increase in calcium activity was thought to be a consequence of Na^+-Ca^{2+} exchange. The hyperosmolar solutions first induced a rise in intracellular sodium ion activity that resulted in a change in the Na^+ electrochemical gradients across the cell membrane. Na^+-Ca^{2+} exchange reduces the intracellular Na^+ load at the cost of increasing myoplasmic Ca^{2+}.

The effects of hypo-osmolar solutions on intracellu-

lar ion activities are opposite to those seen with hyperosmolarity. Intracellular sodium ion activity is reduced to a level predicted on the basis of osmotic dilution. Calcium activity decreases much more than predicted on the same basis. This decrease in intracellular calcium activity is offset by increased cell swelling secondary to water gain. Experimentally, the optimum osmolarity for solutions designed for either cardioplegia or donor organ preservation is between 300 and 320 mOsm/L.

MISCELLANEOUS CONSTITUENTS

Substrates. At one time, glucose was thought to be a desirable component of cardioplegic solution. In theory, glycolysis could be maintained and energy stores preserved. However, few clinically used cardioplegic solutions contain glucose because of the detrimental effects of ongoing glycolysis during hypothermic ischemic arrest.

Provision of other substrates, ie, those involved in purine synthesis, may provide better recovery of both myocardial energy stores and function. In studies of isolated hearts, continuous provision of adenosine in the pre- and postischemic periods improved postischemic function.[105] Hypoxanthine[106] and ribose[107] provided independently also enhanced postischemic function. All three substrates were included in a standard hyperkalemic (16 mMK) crystalloid cardioplegic solution and administered prior to 1 hour of *normothermic* (37°C) global ischemia. The animals receiving the adenosine-, hypoxanthine-, and ribose-supplemented cardioplegic solution (AHR) exhibited significantly better postischemic recovery of both ATP stores and function when compared with a group receiving only the standard cardioplegic solution[108] (Fig 11–11). The mechanisms by

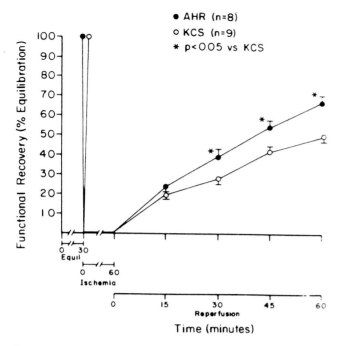

Figure 11–11. Ventricular developed pressure after 20, 45, and 60 minutes of reperfusion was significantly greater in hearts treated during normothermic ischemic arrest with adenosine, hypoxanthine, and ribose (AHR)–containing cardioplegia as compared to 16 mEq/L potassium cardioplegia. (*From Wyatt DA, et al: Purine-enriched asanguineous cardioplegia retards adenosine triphosphate degradation during ischemia and improves postischemic ventricular function. J Thorac Cardiovasc Surg 97:771–778, 1989, with permission.*)

which these substrates improve recovery are complex but include utilization of the salvage pathways in which adenosine is phosphorylated to adenosine monophosphate (AMP) and eventually to ATP. Hypoxanthine is phosphorylated in the presence of phosphoribosyl pyrophosate (in the presence of ribose) to form inosine monophosphate and subsequently AMP. Additionally, provision of these compounds may retard loss of purine metabolites during ischemia and reperfusion.

Steroids. Although not universally accepted to be effective in improving myocardial preservation, steroids are another frequently added component of the cardioplegic solutions. However, a recent study suggests that dexamethasone prevents myocardial injury mediated by peroxidation stimulated by calcium load.[108] Similar protection was provided by α-tocopherol (vitamin E).[109,110]

Calcium Entry Blockers. Calcium channel blockers have been tested as additives to cardioplegic solutions. Initial studies demonstrated that verapamil, diltiazem, and nifedipine protected the normothermic, globally ischemic heart.[111–113] The mechanism of protection was not directly related to preservation of ATP stores but to limitation of mitochondrial Ca^{2+} uptake. The observed protective effect could be masked if the myocardial tem-

perature was reduced to 25°C.[114,115] Following 60 minutes of ischemia at 25°C, there was no significant difference in postischemic recovery between hearts protected with hypothermia alone and those protected with hypothermia plus nifedipine. Nifedipine did, however, confer additional protection if ischemia time was extended to 3 hours. Nifedipine also appears to protect the myocardium from the deleterious effects of profound cooling; ie, temperatures of 5°C. The mechanism of the protective effect is unknown.

Diltiazem added to cardioplegic solution (150 μg/kg) improved recovery after 30 minutes of cold (15–20°C) ischemia compared with standard cardioplegia using segmental shortening and dye indicators as measures of function and injury, respectively.[116] In a clinical trial, patients receiving diltiazem cardioplegia remained asystolic during the reperfusion period and required pacing to be weaned from bypass.[117]

Nicardipine, one of the dihydropyridine calcium channel blockers, has been studied for its ability to reduce central nervous system (CNS) damage following ischemic injury. It has also been found to improve postreperfusion cardiac function in patients aged 6 months to 20 years undergoing cardiac surgery when added to a cardioplegic solution in a concentration of 0.25 mg/L.[118] There were no differences between the nicardipine group and control group in age, bypass or cross-clamp time, temperature (23°C), or rate of spontaneous defibrillation (54–75%). Both groups had a 35–38% use of inotropes, but the nicardipine group had better cardiac indices and left ventricular stroke work index (LVSWI) at lower wedge pressures than did the control group. The experimental group also had less evidence of myocardial injury as judged by MB-CK levels. Nicardipine is less likely than diltiazem or verapamil to cause decreased inotropy or conduction defects. It may be a useful adjunct to standard cardioplegic solutions.

OTHER CONSIDERATIONS. Many conclusions regarding cardioplegic solutions are based on studies carried out in isolated heart preparations. The experience with solutions found to be beneficial in the laboratory may be disappointing in the clinical arena because of poorly controlled factors such as noncoronary collateral flow. Conversely, solutions that are less than optimal in the isolated heart may perform well in a clinical setting. Such findings are probably a consequence of noncoronary collateral flow supplying needed ions or substrate that are absent in the cardioplegic solution. This source of supply is unreliable and unpredictable. Under conditions of deep hypothermic arrest, noncoronary collateral flow is nonexistent. Cardioplegic solutions must be evaluated in models comparable to the clinical settings in which they are used.

Adjuvants to Cardioplegia. The objective of surgical repair of a congenital heart defect is anatomic correction and a fully functional myocardium. Present myocardial preservation techniques fall short of this goal. Certain experimental adjuvants to current preservation methods may eventually improve postoperative myocardial function in the clinical setting. Experimental modalities include the preoperative use of xanthine oxidase inhibitors, the use of intraoperative free radical scavengers, potassium channel agonists, and angiotensin-converting enzyme inhibitors.

Xanthine Oxidase Inhibitors. The enzyme xanthine oxidase is a major producer of toxic oxygen free radicals during reperfusion. Clinical manifestations of free radical generation include arrhythmias following short periods and myofibrillar disruption after longer periods of ischemia and reperfusion.[102] The severity of these untoward events is lessened by inhibition of xanthine oxidase prior to the initiation of reperfusion.

Allopurinol is a clinically used xanthine oxidase inhibitor. It is frequently used to pretreat pediatric (and adult) patients with lymphocytic leukemia prior to the initiation of chemotherapy. This drug has been the subject of a number of recent studies testing its usefulness in preventing postischemic injury. Manning et al[120] studied the effect of allopurinol pretreatment on both ischemia-induced and reperfusion-induced arrhythmias in adult rats. Allopurinol had no effect on the incidence of ischemia-induced arrhythmias. Further studies from the St. Thomas Hospital group[121] indicate that allopurinol pretreatment results in slightly more effective free radical scavenging during reperfusion.

Other groups have documented the effectiveness of allopurinol in limiting the area of myocardium infarcted during normothermic, regional ischemia, and reperfusion in dogs.[122,123] Although the model differs from that of the hypothermic global ischemia present during aortic cross-clamping, the results suggest that reperfusion injury that enhances existing ischemic damage can be prevented.

England and colleagues[124] conducted a prospective study to determine the efficacy of free radical scavenging and allopurinol pretreatment on oxygen free radical generation during cardiopulmonary bypass. They used plasma H_2O_2 as a marker of free radical generation. Hydrogen peroxide levels were significantly lower than control in both the scavenged and allopurinol-treated groups at discontinuation of bypass and following protamine administration. These studies suggest that allopurinol may have a useful role as an adjuvant to currently used myocardial protection schemes. Some of the apparent discrepancies with the early studies of allopurinol are explained by the fact that allopurinol inhibits the xanthine dehydrogenase reaction and its metabolite oxypurinol inhibits the xanthine oxidase reaction. The results of the studies would be biased to the degree that allopurinol was or was not converted to oxypurinol.

Free Radical Scavengers. In addition to xanthine oxidase, free radicals are produced by the auto-oxidation of catecholamines or by previously ischemic but viable mitochondria. Formation by mitochondria occurs during active oxygen consumption via the univalent oxygen reduction pathway. The damage caused by mitochondria-generated oxygen free radicals is limited by the antioxidant coenzyme Q_{10}. Mitochondrial coenzyme Q_{10} levels are reduced during regional and global ischemia. This reduction allows membrane injury and peroxidation of additional coenzyme Q_{10} to occur as a result of the free radicals formed. The ability of the mitochondria to generate ATP is also decreased as a consequence of depletion of coenzyme Q_{10} stores.[50]

Free radicals generated by mechanisms other than xanthine oxidase must be detoxified by exogenously supplied scavengers. Generation by mitochondria presents a problem because the radicals can initiate membrane peroxidation without ever being exposed to the action of scavenging agents. Those radicals generated by cell surface mechanisms such as auto-oxidation of catecholamines can be destroyed by perfusate-supplied free radical scavengers.

Mannitol is an effective scavenger of hydroxyl radical.[125] It is used as a constituent in several different cardioplegic solutions, primarily for its osmotic properties. The washout effect of noncoronary collateral flow may limit the effectiveness of mannitol supplied in cardioplegia as a free radical scavenger. To be effective in this role, mannitol should be supplied during the reperfusion period. Ouriel and co-workers[126] found that hearts reperfused with a mannitol-containing solution following 45 minutes of normothermic global ischemia had more complete recovery than those receiving reperfusate without mannitol. The beneficial effect can be negated if the osmolarity of the solution exceeds 370 mOsm.

Superoxide dismutase (SOD), catalase, and peroxidase are enzymes that are free radical scavengers. Superoxide dismutase catalyzes the conversion of O_2 to H_2O_2, whereas catalase and peroxidase destroy H_2O_2. Numerous studies have shown that these agents are effective in reducing the severity of oxygen free radical-mediated reperfusion injury.[127–129] For reasons that are unclear, the use of peroxidase alone in the preischemia period results in increases in diastolic pressure during hypothermic cardioplegic arrest. This effect is eliminated by addition of deferoxamine (0.05 mM) to the cardioplegic solution.[130]

In an in vitro model, hearts treated with a cardioplegic solution containing SOD and catalase had improved coronary blood flow and ventricular function compared with hearts receiving conventional cardioplegia. In clinical practice, noncoronary collateral flow can reduce or prevent the usefulness of free radical scavengers given in cardioplegic solution. The greater effectiveness of catalase and allopurinol over superoxide dismutase in the maintenance of ventricular function after hypothermic cardioplegia is demonstrated in Fig 11–12.[130]

A study by Chambers and colleagues suggests that SOD and catalase are more effective if given in a reperfusion solution rather than in the cardioplegic solution.[121] The likelihood of SOD having no effect on reducing myocardial damage increases as the reperfusion period increases because the biological half-life of SOD is short (about 6 minutes), whereas the formation of oxygen radicals continues for hours.[61] SOD is more effective if conjugated to polyethylene glycol to extend its half-life to 20 hours.[61]

Deferoxamine, an iron chelator, is both a direct inhibitor of the Haber-Weiss reaction by virtue of its iron-chelating properties and a scavenger of the singlet oxygen radical $O_2^{.}$. Studies of the efficacy of deferoxamine indicate that there is a strong dose and timing dependency to its effect.[131] Deferoxamine improves postischemic myocardial function and coronary flow when given with cardioplegia rather than as a preischemia treatment or during reperfusion.

Potassium Channel Agonists and ACE Inhibitors. Vascular tone is dependent on the membrane potential of the vascular smooth muscle (VSM). Hyperpolarization reduces the influx of Ca^{2+} through the voltage-dependent channels and causes vasodilation. Potassium chan-

nel agonists such as cromakalim and pinacidil cause hyperpolarization of the VSM. These two agents have been investigated for their ability to protect against ischemic injury in the heart. If infused *prior* to either induction of 90 minutes of normothermic regional or 25 minutes of normothermic global ischemia, cromakalim significantly reduces infarct size and reperfusion contracture. In addition, reperfusion function and coronary flow were also significantly better than in control hearts.[132]

Similarly, angiotensin-converting enzyme (ACE) inhibitors have been found to improve postischemic function[133] and reduce electrical instability.[134] The action of these drugs is complex and may involve stimulation of synthesis of "cardioprotective" prostaglandins. Differences in the mechanisms of protection are postulated for sulfhydryl-containing agents such as zofenopril, which may directly scavenge free radicals, and nonsulfhydryl agents such as enalaprilat, which protect by a prostaglandin-mediated mechanism.[133] Studies of these agents in combination with cardioplegic solutions are incomplete. Preliminary data suggests that K-channel agonists and/or ACE inhibitors are promising adjuncts to cardioplegic techniques.

Reperfusion Solutions. Reperfusion solutions are useful for the purpose of replenishing lost intracellular substrate. Key metabolic intermediates lost during ischemia and reperfusion include purine nucleotides, succinate, and pyruvate.[135] NAD^+ is converted to $NADH^+$ during anaerobic glycolysis. The cell has a limited ability to reconvert $NADH^+$ to NAD via cytosolic malate dehydrogenase. The net reaction is $NADH^+$ + malate. In an anaerobic environment, malate cannot be reconverted to oxaloacetate (OAA) by mitochondrial malate dehydrogenase. The result is the depletion of cytosolic OAA and accumulation of $NADH^+$ (Table 11–4).

The provision of glutamate during reperfusion accelerates restoration of normal intracellular levels of NAD^+ and α-ketoglutarate. Glutamate and mitochondrial OAA can undergo transamination to yield ketoglutarate and aspartate. The mitochondrial membrane is freely permeable to aspartate. Aspartate can then be deaminated in the cytosol to yield OAA. Provision of glutamate allows $NADH^+$ to be converted to NAD^+, with repletion of cytosolic OAA levels and regeneration of Krebs cycle intermediates.

The five-carbon sugar ribose is an essential intermediate for both the de novo and the salvage pathway synthesis of purine nucleotides.[136] Ribose can also serve as a source of pyruvate for oxidative phosphorylation if the glycolytic pathway is blocked by metabolites produced during ischemia.[137] Provision of ribose during reperfusion can result in improved function by virtue of its roles in various biochemical pathways. The combination of ribose and glutamate in a potassium blood cardioplegic reperfusion solution are superior to unmodified

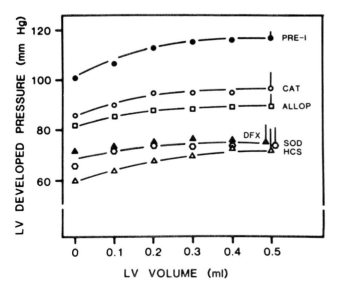

Figure 11–12. The left ventricular developed pressure plotted as a function of left ventricular volume in an isolated rabbit heart demonstrates the functional improvement produced by addition of catalase (CAT) and allopurinol (ALLOP) but not by superoxide dismutase (SOD) or hypothermic cardioplegia solution (HCS) alone. (*From Myers CL, et al: Effects of supplementing hypothermic crystalloid cardioplegia solution with catalase, superoxide dismutase, allopurinol, or deferoxamine on functional recovery of globally ischemic and reperfused isolated hearts. J Thorac Cardiovasc Surg 91:281–289, 1986, with permission.*)

TABLE 11-4. REPERFUSION INJURY

Injury	Site	Manifestations (Biochemical and Clinical)
Washout of Krebs cycle intermediates	Mitochondria	Diminished ATP production; low O_2 consumption
Purine nucleotide washout	Cytosol Mitochondria	Slow ATP regeneration; poor output
Oxygen-free radical damage	Mitochondria	Uncoupled oxidative phosphorylation Decreased ATP production
	SR	Uncoupled ATP hydrolysis from Ca^{2+} transport; high EDP; pump failure; "stone heart"
	Contractile apparatus	Poor tension development for any given Ca^{2+} Reduces cardiac output, pressures, pump failure
Ca^{2+} influx	Mitochondria	Uncoupled oxidative phosphorylation
	Contractile apparatus	Ongoing contracture; high EDP; pump failure; "stone heart"
Ca^{2+} stimulated phospholipases	Membranes	High serum CKs; poor myocardial performance
Loss of EDRF synthesis	Vascular	Decreased coronary flow, poor postischemic cardiac
Neutrophil adhesion	Endothelium	function

pump blood, and other solutions, in restoring postischemic cardiac function in dogs.[138]

Depleted intracellular stores of ATP can be replenished by provision of ATP and magnesium chloride during the reperfusion period.[139] The degree of functional recovery of the heart is sensitive to the amount of ATP provided. Hearts reperfused with excessive amounts of ATP have worse postischemic function than those reperfused with control solution. If ATP and magnesium chloride was provided at a low rate (0.13 mg/kg/min) for the first 30 minutes of reperfusion, nearly 100% recovery of left ventricular ejection function was attained. However, myocardial compliance remained depressed, as did oxygen extraction. The depressed oxygen extraction probably reflected the diminished availability of mitochondrial substrate for oxidative phosphorylation. The alternative explanation is mitochondrial injury.

An asanguineous reperfusion solution has been used clinically with apparent benefit.[140] The solution was designed to maintain electrical silence, reintroduce Ca^{2+} in physiologic concentration, and provide glutamate, buffering, and moderate hyperosmolarity (by adding mannitol). The addition of mannitol protects against free radical damage and reduces cellular edema. This reperfusate was infused via the aortic root just before removal of the cross-clamp. A total of 1000 mL at a rate of 200–300 mL/min was given. Patients receiving this solution had significantly better indices of myocardial function than did those not receiving it. Of patients undergoing mitral valve replacement, those receiving the asanguineous reperfusion required less inotropic support than the control group. The same phenomenon was not observed in the group of patients undergoing aortic valve surgery.

Much research is being directed toward prevention of reperfusion injury. Recognition of the involvement of blood elements in this process has led to new areas of

investigation. A very interesting area of research is the use of neutrophil antibodies as a means of reducing postischemic injury. Endothelial injury, which is postulated as a result of ischemia and reperfusion, promotes neutrophil adhesion and subsequent inflammatory damage. The endothelial injury can be prevented experimentally using antibodies against the neutrophil surface glycoprotein CD18. In a dog model of regional ischemia (at 37°C), the use of the neutrophil antibody anti-Mol reduced the infarcted area (as a percentage of at-risk area) by 46% after 6 hours of reperfusion. If the anti-Mol treatment is continued for 48 hours postischemia, a reduction in infarcted area is noted at 72 hours of reperfusion.[144] Inhibition of neutrophil adhesion to the vascular endothelium in at-risk areas represents a new and potentially promising area in the field of myocardial preservation.

Donor Heart Preservation. The routine repair of congenital cardiac defects does not test the limits of myocardial preservation as does organ preservation for transplantation. The donor heart must be stored for transport in a way that it will not be damaged by preservation technique and will function effectively after 4–6 hours of storage. In early trials of various solutions, infant hearts proved to be more difficult to protect than other organs.

Recent studies have found that hearts protected with an "intracellular" (University of Wisconsin, UW)–type solution were more likely to regain full function after transplant than hearts protected with an "extracellular" solution (Stanford vs St. Thomas II).[142,143] For a given solution, the infusion conditions are extremely important. For the St. Thomas solution, if initial arrest is produced at 37°C followed by infusion of cold (7.5°C) solution, the postischemic function is better than if an initial cold infusion is used.[144] The opposite is true for the UW solution. If initially infused at 20°C with subsequent cooling of the heart to 4°C, function decreases relative to hearts receiving the initial infusion of UW solution at 4°C.[143]

The UW solution used in these studies did not contain Ca^{2+}. Recent studies by the University of Wisconsin group indicate that the addition of 0.5 mM Ca^{2+} greatly enhances the post-transplant survival of kidneys (up to 5-day preservation with continuous perfusion).[145] As in the case of cardioplegic solutions, the optimum solution, technique, or organ preservation for transplant is yet to be developed. However, the current UW solution has been found to protect rabbit hearts for up to 8 hours at 4°C with no decrease in function.[144] The period of time during which hearts are removed from the cold environment and placed in the body and prior to reperfusion must of necessity be minimized to reduce the likelihood of loss of myocardial function. It is during this period that technical factors can either help or hinder the effectiveness of the preservation technique employed at organ harvest (see Chapter 22).

Failure of Myocardial Preservation. The following concepts should guide both present and future myocardial preservation techniques:

1. Preservation of ATP levels does not ensure *adequate* functional recovery, much less optimum function recovery.
2. The optimum Ca^{2+} concentration in cardioplegic solutions varies with age.
3. The interactions between Mg^{2+}, Ca^{2+}, and Na^{2+} are complex and temperature dependent.
4. Extracellular buffering alone is not enough; buffers that protect against intracellular acidosis (which HCO_3 does not) are preferred.
5. Prevention of reperfusion injury by means of antioxidants, free radical scavengers, or other means improves functional recovery.
6. Preservation of vascular endothelial function must be optimized.

Even the most well-formulated cardioplegic solution may fail to provide protection from myocardial injury. There are multiple reasons for this failure and the majority of them are technical (Table 11–5). Cunningham and co-workers[98] found that technical errors during aortic cross-clamping led to inadequate myocardial protection. These errors were failure to reinject the cardioplegic solution frequently enough, allowing electrocardiographic activity to return and myocardial temperatures to exceed 28°C. The surgeon and anesthesiologist must be aware of the time intervals between injections of cardioplegic solution. Ideally, reinfusion should occur every 20 minutes and generally should not be allowed to exceed 30 minutes except if deep hypothermic arrest is

TABLE 11–5. REASONS FOR FAILURE OF MYOCARDIAL PRESERVATION*

Preexisting myocardial injury
Technical factors
    Premature cardiac rewarming
    Myocardial distention
    Prolonged fibrillation
    Premature return of electromechanical activity
    Infrequent use of cardioplegic solution
    Coronary air emboli
Free radical damage
Myocardial substrate depletion
Calcium influx

* As manifested by poor myocardial performance on completion of rewarming, necessitating use of inotropes or continued support on bypass.

used. If cardiac electrical activity is noted, immediate reinfusion of cardioplegic solution is necessary. Despite all precautions, there appears to be a limit to the ischemia time during the surgical repair of congenital lesions. This time limit was 85 minutes in work by Bull and colleagues.[146] After longer times, postoperative mortality increased.

Myocardial rewarming can be a difficult problem. There are multiple contributing factors such as room temperature, heat generated by operating room lights, systemic perfusion temperature, and noncoronary collateral flow. The right atrium appears most susceptible to rapid rewarming to the systemic perfusion temperature. This phenomenon has been implicated as the cause of atrial arrhythmias during the postischemic period.[147]

Noncoronary collateral flow can defeat the best myocardial preservation efforts. It contributes to myocardial distention, rewarming, and washout of cardioplegic solution. Washout is helpful in eliminating poorly formulated cardioplegic solutions but more often prematurely terminates the beneficial effects of well-designed solutions.[148]

High rates of noncoronary collateral flow are seen in patients with well-developed bronchial vessels. Noncoronary collateral flow is related to the systemic perfusion index. Low indices reduce the return to the left heart through these channels, thus reducing myocardial distention and rewarming. Adequate left ventricular venting is necessary to prevent cavity distention and premature subendocardial rewarming. The rate of left ventricular subendocardial rewarming can be slowed by the use of low (20°C) systemic perfusion temperature.

The most carefully conducted procedure cannot prevent all the biochemical events that lead to reperfusion injury. Many clinically used cardioplegic solutions do not contain any ingredients to prevent or slow the generation of free radicals on reperfusion. Therefore, if improvement in survival following surgical correction of congenital heart defects is to be achieved, this problem must be solved.

REFERENCES

1. Swan H: Clinical hypothermia: A lady with a past and some new promise for the future. *Surgery* **73**:736–758, 1973

2. Bigelow WG, Callaghan JC, Hopps JA: General hypothermia for experimental intracardiac surgery: Use of electrophrenic respiration, an artificial pacemaker for cardiac stand-still and radiofrequency rewarming in general hypothermia. *Ann Surg* **132**:531–539, 1950

3. Bigelow WG, Lindsay WK, Harrison RE, et al: Oxygen transport and utilization in dogs at low body temperature. *Am J Physiol* **160**:125–137, 1950

4. Lewis FJ, Trauffic M: Closure of atrial septal defects with the aid of hypothermia; experimental accomplishments and the report of one successful case. *Surgery* **33**:52–59, 1953

5. Okamoto Y: Clinical studies for open heart surgery in infants with profound hypothermia. *Arch Jpn Chir* **38**:188–207, 1969

6. Mohri H, Dillard DH, Crawford EW, et al: Method of surface induced deep hypothermia for open heart surgery in infants. *J Thorac Cardiovasc Surg* **58**:262–270, 1969

7. Cooley DA, Hallman GC: Surgery during the first year of life for cardiovascular anomalies. A review of 500 consecutive operations. *J Cardiovasc Surg* **5**:584–590, 1964

8. Zervini EJ, Verginelli G, Bitencourt D, et al: Surgical treatment of congenital heart defects in patients under two years of age. *J Cardiovasc Surg* **5**:608–618, 1964

9. Barratt-Boyes BG, Simpson M, Neutze J: Intracardiac surgery in neonates and infants using deep hypothermia with surface cooling and limited cardiopulmonary bypass. *Circulation* **43**(suppl I):25–30, 1971

10. Melrose DG, Dreyer B, Bentall HH, Baker JBE: Elective cardiac arrest. *Lancet* **2**:21–22, 1955

11. McFarland JA, Thomas LB, Gilbert JW, Morrow AG: Myocardial necrosis following elective cardiac arrest with potassium citrate. *J Thorac Surg* **40**:200–208, 1960

12. Helmsworth JA, Kaplan S, Clark L C Jr, et al: Myocardial injury associated with asystole induced with potassium citrate. *Ann Surg* **149**:200–206, 1959

13. Hufnagel CA, Conrad P, Schanno J, Pifarre R: Profound cardiac hypothermia. *Ann Surg* **143**:790, 1955

14. Speicher CE, Ferrigan L, Wolfson SK, et al: Cold injury of the myocardium and pericardium in cardiac hypothermia. *Surg Gynecol Obstet* **114**:659–665, 1962

15. Gay WA, Ebert PA: Functional, metabolic and morphologic effects of potassium induced cardioplegia. *Surgery* **74**:284–290, 1973

16. Hearse DJ, Stewart DA, Braimbridge MV: Hypothermic arrest and potassium arrest: Metabolic and myocardial protection during elective cardiac arrest. *Circ Res* **36**:481–489, 1975

17. Myojin K, Mee R, Fishbein M, et al: Long term effects of hyperkalemic cardioplegia and local hypothermia on gross and microscopic structure of the left ventricle. *Surg Forum* **29**:267–269, 1978

18. Hoerter J, Mazet F, Vassort G: Perinatal growth of the rabbit cardiac cell: Possible implications for the mechanism of relaxation. *J Mol Cell Cardiol* **13**:725–740, 1982

19. Maylie JG: Excitation-contraction coupling in neonatal and adult myocardium of cat. *Am J Physiol* **242**:H834–H843, 1982

20. Chin TK, Friedman WF, Klitzner TS: Developmental changes in cardiac myocyte calcium regulation. *Circ Res* **67**:574–579, 1990

21. Boucek RJ, Shelton ME, Artman M, et al: Comparative effects of verapamil, nifedipine and diltiazem on contractile function in the isolated immature and adult rabbit heart. *Pediatr Res* **18**:948–952, 1984

22. Rudolph AM: Distribution and regulation of blood flow in the fetal and neonatal lamb. *Circ Res* **57**:811–821, 1985

23. McAuliffe JJ, Gao L, Solaro RJ: Change in myofibrillar activation and troponin C Ca^{2+} binding associated with troponin T isoform switching in developing rabbit heart. *Circ Res* **66**:1204–1216, 1990

24. Hirzel HO, Thchschmid CR, Schneider J, et al: Relationship between myosin isoenzyme composition, hemodynamics and myocardial structure in various forms of human cardiac hypertrophy. *Circ Res* **57**:729–740, 1985

25. Ingwall JS, Kramer MF, Friedman WF: Developmental changes. In Jacobus WE, Ingwall JS (eds): *Heart Creatine Kinase: The Integration of Isoenzymes for Energy Distribution*. Baltimore: William & Wilkins, 1980, pp 9–17

26. Perry S, McAuliffe JJ, Balschi J, et al: Flux thru the creatine kinase reaction: The role of mitochondrial creatine kinase. Montreal: Society for Magnetic Resonance in Medicine Meeting, Aug 18–22, 1986 (abstr)

27. Jarmakani JM, Takafumi N, Langer GA: The effect of calcium and high energy phosphate compounds on myocardial contracture in the newborn and adult rabbit. *J Mol Cell Cardiol* **10**:1017–1029, 1978

28. Bove EL, Stammers AH: Recovery of left ventricular function after hypothermic global ischemia. *J Thorac Cardiovasc Surg* **91**:115–122, 1986

29. Bleese N, Doring V, Kalmar P, et al: Intraoperative myocardial protection by cardioplegia in hypothermia: Clinical findings. *J Thorac Cardiovasc Surg* **75**:405–413, 1978

30. Ingwall JS: Changes in the creatine kinase system during the transition from compensated to uncompensated hypertrophy in the spontaneously hypertensive rat. In Tarazi RC, Dunbar JB (eds): *Perspectives in Cardiovascular Research*, Vol 8. New York: Raven Press, 1983, pp 145–155

31. Mercadier JJ, Lampre AM, Duc P, et al: Altered sarcoplasmic reticulum Ca^{2+}-ATPase gene expression in the human ventricle during end-stage heart failure. *J Clin Invest* **85**:305–309, 1990

32. Bristow MR, Hershberger RE, Port JD, et al: Beta adrenergic pathways in the non-failing human ventricular myocardium. *Circulation* **82**(suppl I):12–25, 1990

33. Nayler WG, Poole-Wilson PA, Williams A: Hypoxia and calcium. *J Mol Cell Cardiol* **11**:683–706, 1979

34. Karmazyn M: Reduced tolerance to reperfusion associated injury in hearts from myopathic hamsters. *Basic Res Cardiol* **80**:392–398, 1985

35. Hottenrot CE, Towers B, Kurkji HJ, et al: The hazard of ventricular fibrillation in hypertrophied ventricles during cardiopulmonary bypass. *J Thorac Cardiovasc Surg* **66**:742–753, 1973

36. Baird RJ, Dutka F, Okumori M, et al: Surgical aspects of regional myocardial blood flow and myocardial pressure. *J Thorac Cardiovasc Surg* **69**:17–29, 1975

37. McConnell DH, Brazier JR, Cooper N, Buckberg GD: Studies on the effects of hypothermia on regional myocar-

dial blood flow and metabolism during cardiopulmonary bypass. II. Ischemia during moderate hypothermia in continually perfused beating hearts. *J Thorac Cardiovasc Surg* **73**:95–101, 1977

38. Archie JR, Kirklin JW: Effect of hypothermic perfusions on myocardial oxygen consumption and coronary resistance. *Surg Forum* **24**:186–191, 1973
39. Rebeyka IM, Hanan SA, Borges MR, et al: Rapid cooling contracture of the myocardium. The adverse effect of prearrest cardiac hypothermia. *J Thorac Cardiovasc Surg* **100**:240–249, 1990
40. Williams WG, Rebeyka IM, Tibshirani RJ, et al: Warm induction blood cardioplegia in the infant. A technique to avoid rapid cooling myocardial contracture. *J Thorac Cardiovasc Surg* **100**:896–901, 1990
41. Buckberg GD, Brazier JR, Nelson RL, et al: Studies of the effects of hypothermia on regional myocardial blood flow and metabolism during cardiopulmonary bypass. I. The adequately perfused beating, fibrillating and arrested heart. *J Thorac Cardiovasc* **73**:87–94, 1977
42. Levett JM, Kadowaki MH, Ip JH, et al: Rapid depletion of myocardial high energy phosphates by a short period of ventricular fibrillation prior to cardioplegic arrest. *Circulation* **72**(suppl III):375, 1975 (abstr)
43. Bolli R: Mechanisms of myocardial "stunning." *Circulation* **82**:723–738, 1990
44. Hess ML, Warner MF, Robbins AD, et al: Characterization of the excitation-contraction coupling system of the hypothermic myocardium following ischemia and reperfusion. *Cardiovasc Res* **15**:390, 1981
45. Rovetto MJ, Lamberton WF, Neely JR: Mechanisms of glycolytic inhibition in ischemic rat hearts. *Circ Res* **37**:742–751, 1975
46. Neely JR, Grotyohann LW: Role of glycolytic products in damage to ischemic myocardium: Dissociation of adenosine triphosphate levels and recovery of function of reperfused ischemic hearts. *Circ Res* **55**:816–824, 1984
47. Armiger LC, Gavin JB, Herdson PB: Mitochondrial changes in dog myocardium induced by neutral lactate in vitro. *Lab Invest* **31**:29–33, 1974
48. Geisbuhler TP, Rovelto MJ: Lactate does not enhance anoxial reoxygenation damage in adult rat cardiac myocytes. *J Mol Cell Cardiol* **22**:1325–1335, 1990
49. Veitch K, Caucheteux D, Hombroeckx A, Hue L: Mitochondrial damage during cardiac ischaemia and reperfusion: The role of oxygen. *Biochem Soc Trans* **18**:548, 1990
50. Feeney L, Berman ER: Membrane damage by free radicals. *Invest Ophthalmol* **15**:789–792, 1976
51. Turla MB, Gnegy ME, Epps S, Shlafer M: Loss of calmodulin activity in cardiac sarcoplasmic reticulum after ischemia. *Biochem Biophys Res Commun* **130**:617, 1985
52. Krause S, Hess ML: Characterization of cardiac sarcoplasmic reticulum dysfunction during short-term normothermic global ischemia. *Circ Res* **55**:176–184, 1984
53. Nayler WG: The role of calcium in the ischemic myocardium. *Am J Pathol* **102**:262–270, 1981
54. DeBoer LWV, Ingwall JS, Kloner RA, Braunwald E: Prolonged derangements of canine myocardial purine metabolism after a brief coronary artery occlusion not associated with anatomic evidence of necrosis. *Proc Natl Acad Sci* **77**:5471–5475, 1980
55. Gerlach E, Nees S, Becker BF: The vascular endothelium:

A survey of some newly evolving biochemical and physiologic features. *Basic Res Cardiol* **80**:459–474, 1985
56. Jarasch ED, Grund C, Bruder G, et al: Localization of xanthine oxidase in mammary gland epithelium and capillary endothelium. *Cell* **25**:67–82, 1981
57. Jarasch ED, Bruder G, Heid HW: Significance of xanthine oxidase in capillary endothelial cells. *Acta Physiol Scand* **548**(suppl):39–46, 1986
58. Kehrer JP, Piper HM, Sies H: Xanthine oxidase is not responsible for reoxygenation injury in isolated perfused rat heart. *Free Res Commun* **3**:69–71, 1987
59. Otani HF, Engelman RM, Rousou JA, et al: Alteration of antioxidative and lipogenic enzyme activities during ischemia and reperfusion in neonatal pig heart. *Circulation* **72**(suppl III):363, 1985 (abstr)
60. Saldanha C, Hearse DJ: Coronary vascular responsiveness to 5 hydroxytryptamine before and after infusion of hyperkalemic crystalloid cardioplegia in the rat heart. *J Thorac Cardiovasc Surg* **98**:783–787, 1989
61. Lucchesi BR: Modulation of leukocyte-mediated myocardial reperfusion injury. *Annu Rev Physiol* **52**:561–576, 1990
62. Burton KP, McCord JM, Ghai G: Myocardial alterations due to free radical generation. *Am J Physiol* **246**:H776–H783, 1984
63. Fridovich I: The biology of oxygen radicals. *Science* **201**:875–880, 1978
64. Flamm ES, Demopocilas HB, Seligman ML, et al: Free radicals in cerebral ischemia. *Stroke* **9**:445–447, 1978
65. Rowe GT, Manson NH, Caplan M, Hess ML: Hydrogen peroxide and hydroxyl radical mediation of activated leukocyte depression of cardiac sarcoplasmic reticulum. *Circ Res* **55**:584–591, 1983
66. Darley-Usmar VM, Smith DR, O'Leary JJ, et al: Hypoxia-reoxygenation induced damage in the myocardium: The role of the mitochondria. *Biochem Soc Trans* **18**:526–528, 1990
67. Swan H, Zeavin I, Blount SG Jr, Virtue RW: Surgery by direct vision in the open heart during hypothermia. *JAMA* **153**:1081–1085, 1953
68. Murkin JM, Farrer JK, Tweet WA, et al: Cerebral autoregulation and flow metabolism coupling during cardiopulmonary bypass: The influence of $PaCO_2$. *Anesth Analg* **66**:825–832, 1987
69. Prough DS, Stump DA, Roy RC, et al: Response of cerebral blood flow to changes in carbon dioxide tension during hypothermic cardiopulmonary bypass. *Anesthesiology* **64**:576–581, 1986
70. Coles JG, Taylor MJ, Pearce JM, et al: Cerebral monitoring of somatosensory evoked potentials during profoundly hypothermic circulatory arrest. *Circulation* **70**(suppl 1):96–102, 1984
71. Frank JS, Rich TL, Beydler S, Kreman M: Calcium depletion in rabbit myocardium: Ultrastructure of the sarcolemma and correlation with the calcium paradox. *Circ Res* **51**:117–130, 1982
72. Rich TL, Langer GA: Calcium depletion in rabbit myocardium: Calcium paradox protection by hypothermia and cation substitution. *Circ Res* **51**:117–130, 1982
73. Swanson DK, Dufek JH, Kahn DR: Left ventricular function after preserving the heart for 2 hours at 15°C. *J Thorac Cardiovasc Surg* **79**:755–760, 1980

74. Engedal H, Skagseth E, Saetersdal TS, Myklebust R: Cardiac hypothermia evaluated by ultrastructural studies in man. *J Thorac Cardiovasc Surg* 75:548–554, 1978

75. Shumway NE, Lower RR: Topical hypothermia for extended periods of anoxic arrest. *Surg Forum* 10:563–566, 1959

76. Shumway NE, Lower RR, Stofer RC: Selective hypothermia of the heart in anoxic cardiac arrest. *Surg Gynec Obstet* 109:750–754,1959

77. Conti VR, Bertranou EG, Blackstone EH, et al: Cold cardioplegia versus hypothermia for myocardial protection: Randomized clinical study. *J Thorac Cardiovasc Surg* 76:577–589, 1978

78. Reitz BA, Baumgartner WA, Stenson EB: Myocardial protection by topical hypothermia. In Ionescu MI (ed): *Techniques in Extracorporeal Circulation*. Boston: Butterworths, 1981, pp 281–294

79. Heitmiller RF, DeBoer LWV, Geffin GA, et al: Myocardial recovery after hypothermic arrest: A comparison of oxygenated crystalloid to blood cardioplegia: The role of calcium. *Circulation* 72(suppl 2):241–253, 1985

80. Magovern GJ, Flagerty JT, Gott VL, et al: Failure of blood cardioplegia to protect myocardium at lower temperatures. *Circulation* 66(suppl 1):60–67, 1982

81. Bing OHL, La Raia PH, Gaasch WH, et al: Independent protection provided by red blood cells during cardioplegia. *Circulation* 66(suppl 1):81–84, 1982

82. Zweifach BW: The distribution of blood perfusion in capillary circulation. *Am J Physiol* 130:512–520, 1940

83. Jynge P, Hearse DJ, Braimbridge MV: Protection of the ischemic myocardium: Volume-duration relationships and the efficacy of myocardial infusates. *J Thorac Cardiovasc Surg* 76:698–705, 1978

84. Kubler W, Spieckerman PG: Regulation of glycolysis in the ischemic and the anoxic myocardium. *J Mol Cell Cardiol* 1:351–377, 1970

85. Rich TL, Brady AJ: Potassium contracture and utilization of high energy phosphates in rabbit heart. *Am J Physiol* 226:105–113, 1974

86. Bretschneider JH, Hubner G, Knoll, et al: Myocardial resistance and tolerance to ischemia: Physiologic and biochemical basis. *J Cardiovasc Surg* 16:241–260, 1975

87. Del Nido PJ, Wilson GJ, Mickle DAG, et al: The role of cardioplegic solution buffering in myocardial protection: A biochemical and histopathological assessment. *J Thorac Cardiovasc Surg* 89:689–699, 1985

88. Ellis RJ, Mangano DT, Van Dyke DC, Ebert PA: Protection of myocardial function not enhanced by high concentrations of potassium during cardioplegic arrest. *J Thorac Cardiovasc Surg* 78:698–707, 1978

89. Trauble H, Eibl H: Electrostatic effects of lipid phase transition: Membrane structure and ionic environment. *Proc Natl Acad Sci* 71:214–219, 1974

90. Brown PS, Holland FW, Parenteau GL, Clark RE: Magnesium ion is beneficial in hypothermic crystalloid cardioplegia. *Ann Thorac Surg* 51:359–367, 1991

91. Magovern JA, Pae WE, Miller CA, Waldenhausen JA: The immature and the mature myocardium: Responses to multidose crystalloid cardioplegia. *J Thorac Cardiovasc Surg* 95:618–624, 1988

92. Watanabe H, Yokosawa T, Eguchi S, Imai S: Difference in the mechanical response to a cardioplegic solution observed between the neonatal and the adult guinea pig myocardium. *J Thorac Cardiovasc Surg* 97:59–66, 1989

93. Corno AF, Bethencourt DM, Laks H, et al: Myocardial protection in the neonatal heart: A comparison of topical hypothermia and crystalloid and blood cardioplegic solutions. *J Thorac Cardiovasc Surg* 93:163–172, 1987

94. Hearse DJ, Stewart DA, Baimbridge MV: Myocardial protection during ischemic cardiac arrest: Importance of magnesium in cardioplegic infusates. *J Thorac Cardiovasc Surg* 75:877–885, 1978

95. Pernot AC, Ingwall JA, Menasche P, et al: Evaluation of high-energy phosphate metabolism during cardioplegic arrest and reperfusion: A phosphorus-31 nuclear magnetic resonance study. *Circulation* 67:1296–1303, 1983

96. Hearse DJ, Stewart DA, Chain EB: Recovery from cardiac bypass and elective cardiac arrest. The metabolic consequences of various cardioplegic procedures in the isolated rat heart. *Circ Res* 35:448–457, 1974

97. Renlund DG, Lakatta EG, Mellits ED, Gerstenbleth G: Calcium dependent enhancement of myocardial diastolic tone and energy utilization dissociates systolic work and oxygen consumption during low sodium perfusion. *Circ Res* 57:876–888, 1985

98. Jynge P: Calcium and cardioplegia. Proceedings of the Symposium on Cardioplegia, London, 1980

99. Stinner B, Krohn E, Gebhard MM, Bretschneider HJ: Intracellular sodium activity and Bretschneider's cardioplegia: Continuous measurement by ionselective microelectrodes at initial equilibrium. *Basic Res Cardiol* 84:197–207, 1989

100. Meng H, Pierce GN: Involvement of sodium on the protective effect of 5-(N,N-dimethyl)-ameloride on ischemia-reperfusion injury in isolated rat ventricular wall. *J Pharm Exp Ther* 256:1094–1100, 1991

101. Lange R, Cavanaugh AC, Zierler M, et al: The relative importance of alkalinity, temperature, and the washout effect of bicarbonate-buffered multi-dose cardioplegic solution. *Circulation* 70(suppl 1):75–83, 1984

102. Preusse CJ, Gebhard MM, Bretschneider JH: Interstitial pH value in the myocardium as an indicator of ischemic stress of cardioplegically arrested hearts. *Basic Res Cardiol* 77:372–387, 1982

103. Reeves RB, Malan A: Model studies of intracellular acid base temperature responses in ectotherms. *Respir Physiol* 28:49–63, 1976

104. Lado MG, Sheu SS, Fozzard HA: Effects of tonicity on tension and intracellular sodium and calcium activities in sheep heart. *Circ Res* 54:576–585, 1984

105. Ely SW, Mentzer RW, Lasley RD, et al: Functional and metabolic evidence of enhanced myocardial tolerance to ischemia and reperfusion with adenosine. *J Thorac Cardiovasc Surg* 90:549–556, 1985

106. Lasley RD, Ely SW, Berne RM, Mentzer RM: Allopurinol enhanced adenine nucleotide repletion after myocardial ischemia in the isolated rat heart. *J Clin Invest* 81:16–20, 1988

107. Pasque MK, Spray TL, Pellom GL, et al: Ribase-enhanced myocardial recovery following ischemia in the isolated working heart. *J Thorac Cardiovasc Surg* 83:390–398, 1982

108. Wyatt DA, Ely SW, Lasley RD, et al: Purine enriched asanguineous cardioplegia retards adenosine triphosphate

degradation during ischemia and improves post ischemic ventricular function. *J Thorac Cardiovasc Surg* **97:**771–778, 1989

109. Saxon ME: Stabilizing effects of antioxidants and inhibitors of prostaglandin synthesis on after contractions in Ca^{2+}-overloaded myocardium. *Basic Res Cardiol* **80:**345–352, 1985

110. Erin AN, Spirin MM, Tabidze LV, Kagan VE: Formation of alpha-tocopherol complexes with fatty acids: Possible mechanism of biomembrane stabilization by vitamin E. *Biokhimia* **48:**1597–1602, 1983

111. Nayler WG, Ferrari R, Williams A: Protective effect of pretreatment with verapamil, nifedipine and propranolol on mitochondrial function in the ischemic and reperfused myocardium. *J Mol Cell Cardiol* **46:**242–248, 1980

112. Weishaar RE, Bing RJ: The beneficial effect of a calcium channel blocker, diltiazem, on the ischemic-reperfused heart. *J Mol Cell Cardiol* **12:**993–1009, 1980

113. Jolly SR, Menahan LA, Gross GJ: Diltiazem in myocardial recovery from global ischemia and reperfusion. *J Mol Cell Cardiol* **13:**359–372, 1981

114. Nayler WG: Protection of the myocardium against postischemic reperfusion damage: The combined effect of hypothermia and nifedipine. *J Thorac Cardiovasc Surg* **84:**897–905, 1981

115. Hearse DJ, Yamamoto F, Shattock MJ: Calcium antagonists and hypothermia: The temperature dependency of the negative inotropic and anti-ischemic properties of verapamil in the isolated rat heart. *Circulation* **70**(suppl I):54–64, 1984

116. Rebeyka IM, Axford-Gatley RA, Bush BG, et al: Calcium paradox in an in vivo model of multidose cardioplegia and moderate hypothermia. Prevention with diltiazem or trace calcium levels. *J Thorac Cardiovasc Surg* **99:**475–483, 1990

117. Christakis GT, Fremes SE, Weisel RD, et al: Diltiazem cardioplegia. *J Thorac Cardiovasc Surg* **91:**647–661, 1986

118. Mori F, Miyamoto M, Tsuboi H, et al: Clinical trial of nicardipine cardioplegia in pediatric cardiac surgery. *Ann Thorac Surg* **49:**413–418, 1990

119. Cunningham JN, Adams PX, Knopp EA, et al: Preservation of ATP, ultra-structure, and ventricular function after aortic cross-clamping and reperfusion: Clinical use of blood potassium cardioplegia. *J Thorac Cardiovasc Surg* **78:**708–720, 1979

120. Manning AS, Coltart DJ, Hearse DJ: Ischemia and reperfusion induced arrhythmias in the rat: Effects of xanthine oxidase inhibition with allopurinol. *Circ Res* **55:**545–548, 1984

121. Chambers DJ, Braimbridge MV, Hearse DJ: Prevention of production, or scavenging of free radicals enhances myocardial protection with cardioplegia arrest. *Circulation* **72**(suppl 3):376, 1985 (abstr)

122. Akizuki S, Yoshida S, Chamber D, et al: Blockage of the O_2-radical producing enzyme, xanthine oxidase, reduces infarct size in the dog. *Fed Proc* **43:**540, 1984 (abstr)

123. Werns SW, Shea MJ, Mitsos SE, et al: Reduction of the size of infarction by allopurinol in the ischemic-reperfused canine heart. *Circulation* **73:**518–524, 1986

124. England MD, Cavarocchi NC, Pluth JR: Oxygen free radical generation during cardiopulmonary bypass: Use of oxygen derived free radical scavengers. *Circulation* **72**(suppl 3):376, 1985 (abstr)

125. Delmaestro FR, Thaw HH, Bjork J, et al: Free radicals as mediators of tissue injury. *Acta Physiol Scand* **492**(suppl 1):43–57, 1980

126. Ouriel K, Gensberg ME, Patti CS, et al: Preservation of myocardial function with mannitol reperfusate. *Circulation* **72**(suppl 2):254–258, 1985

127. Przyklenk K, Kloner RA: Superoxide dismutase plus catalase improve contractile function in the canine model of the "stunned myocardium." *Circ Res* **58:**148–156, 1986

128. Schlafer M, Kane PF, Kirsch MM: Superoxide dismutase plus catalase enhances the efficacy of hypothermic cardioplegia to protect the globally ischemic, reperfused heart. *J Thorac Cardiovasc Surg* **83:**830–839, 1982

129. Stewart JR, Blackwell WH, Creete SL, et al: Prevention of myocardial ischemic reperfusion injury with oxygen free radical scavengers. *Surg Forum* **33:**317–320, 1982

130. Myers CL, Weiss SJ, Kirsch MM, et al: Effects of supplementary hypothermic crystalloid cardioplegia solution with catalase, superoxide dismutase, allopurinol, or deferoxamine on functional recovery of globally ischemic and perfused isolated hearts. *J Thorac Cardiovasc Surg* **91:**281–289, 1986

131. Menasche P, Grousset C, Gauduel Y, et al: Prevention of hydroxyl radical formation: A critical concept for improving cardioplegia: protective effects of deferoxamine. *Circulation* **76**(suppl 5) 180–185, 1987

132. Grover GJ, Dzwonczyk S, Parham CS, Sleph PG: The protective effects of cromakalim and pinacidil on reperfusion function and infarct size in isolated perfused rat hearts and anesthetized dogs. *Cardiovasc Drugs Ther* **4:**465–474, 1990

133. Przyklenk K, Kloner RA: Angiotensin converting enzyme inhibitors improve contractile function of stunned myocardium by different mechanisms of action. *Am Heart J* **121:**1319–1330, 1991

134. Tio RA, deLangen CD, deGraeff PA, et al: The effect of oral pretreatment with zofenopril, an angiotensin-converting enzyme inhibitor, on early reperfusion and subsequent electrophysiologic stability in the pig. *Cardiovasc Drug Ther* **4:**695–703, 1990

135. Taegtmeyer H: Metabolic responses to cardiac hypoxia: Increased production of succinate by rabbit papillary muscle. *Circ Res* **43:**805–808, 1978

136. Goldthwait DA: Mechanisms of synthesis of purine nucleotides in heart muscle extracts. *J Clin Invest* **36:**1572–1578, 1957

137. Metzler DE: Catabolism of sugars: The pentose phosphate pathways. In *Biochemistry: The Chemical Reactions of Living Cells.* New York: Academic Press, 1977, pp 543–546

138. Haas GS, DeBoer LWV, O'Keefe DD: Reduction of postischemic myocardial dysfunction by substrate repletion during reperfusion. *Circulation* **70**(suppl 1):65–74, 1984

139. McDonagh PF, Laks H, Chaundry IH, Baue AE: Improved myocardial recovery from ischemia: Treatment with low-dose adenosine triphosphate-magnesium chloride. *Arch Surg* **119:**1379–1384, 1984

140. Menasche P, Dunica S, Kural S, et al: An asanguinous

reperfusion solution: An effective adjunct to cardioplegic protection in high risk value operations. *J Thorac Cardiovasc Surg* **88**:278–286, 1984

141. Lucchesi BR, Werns SW, Fantone JC: The role of the neutrophils and free radicals in ischemic myocardial injury. *J Mol Cell Cardiol* **21**:1241–1251, 1989

142. Wicomb WN, Hill JD, Avery J, Collins GM: Comparison of cardioplegia and UW solutions for short-term rabbit heart preservation. *Transplantation* **47**:733–734, 1989

143. Ledingham SJ, Katayama O, Lachno DR, Yacoub M: Prolonged cardiac preservation: Evaluation of the University of Wisconsin preservation solution by comparison with the St. Thomas Hospital cardioplegic solution in the rate. *Circulation* **82**(suppl 4):351–358, 1990

144. Takahashi A, Hearse DJ, Braimbridge MV, Chambers DJ: Harvesting hearts for long-term preservation: Detrimental effects of initial hypothermic infusion of cardioplegic solutions. *J Thorac Cardiovasc Surg* **100**:371–378, 1990

145. McAnultry JF, Plerg RJ, Southard JH, Belzer FO: Successful five-day perfusion preservation of the canine kidney. *Transplantation* **47**:37–41, 1989

146. Bull C, Cooper J, Stack J: Cardioplegic protection of the child's heart. *J Thorac Cardiovasc Surg* **88**:287–293, 1984

147. Chen YF, Lin YT: Comparison of the effectiveness of myocardial preservation in right atrium and left ventricle. *Ann Thoracic Surg* **40**:25–30, 1985

148. Buckberg GD: Intraoperative myocardial protection. In Ionescu MI (ed): *Techniques in Extracorporeal Circulation.* Boston: Butterworths, 1981, pp 231–278

Chapter 12 | Perioperative Care of the Child with Congenital Cardiac Disease

Roger A. Moore

The incidence of congenital heart disease in children is approximately 1%,[1-3] although epidemiologic studies have found occurrence rates as low as 0.24% of live births[4] and as high as 2% of children in the first year of life.[5] Diverse factors such as geography, population makeup, and prenatal care may account for some of the observed variability. However, a significant number of these children require surgical intervention for their congenital cardiac lesion at some time. Without therapeutic intervention, as many as 50% of these children die within the first year of life.[4,6,7]

Acquired cardiac lesions in children and adolescents are increasing because of a resurgence of streptococcal infections leading to rheumatic cardiac disease.[8] In a study performed by the National Center for Health Statistics,[5] as many as 4.6% of adolescents were found to have some form of cardiac disease. These compelling statistics have provided the primary impetus for the development of the subspecialty of pediatric cardiac anesthesiology.

Over the past two decades, the evolution of pediatric cardiac surgery has been toward operating on children at ever younger ages and performing complete cardiac repairs rather than palliative procedures.[9,10] This evolution could not have occurred without technical improvements in both anesthesia and extracorporeal circulation.[11] In order for the anesthesiologist to provide safe and sound perioperative care for these small pediatric cardiac patients, extensive knowledge derived from both pediatric anesthesia and cardiac anesthesia must be merged. The pediatric cardiac anesthesiologist must expertly manage the widely differing physiologic and functional requirements of patients ranging in age from the newborn to the adult. Additionally, the pertinent anat-

omy and physiology of each type of congenital heart defect must be integrated into the total anesthetic management plan. Finally, an in-depth knowledge of the anesthetic ramifications of the extracardiac defects and congenital syndromes is needed. Because of the immense difficulty in integrating the often contradictory requirements of multiple defects in individual patients into safe and rational anesthetic plans, the pediatric cardiac anesthesiologist must actively participate in the patient's care from the initial preoperative visit until the child is discharged from the intensive care unit.

PREOPERATIVE EVALUATION

Because children have a wide spectrum of congenital cardiac diseases, differing physiologic needs at different ages, and ranges of physical decompensation, each child requires individual and thorough preoperative evaluation. The wide variability encountered in pediatric cardiac anesthesia is apparent when contrasting the care of the neonate to that of a teenager. The neonate's increased cardiac index, increased alveolar ventilation, increased ratio of well-perfused tissue to total body mass, increased oxygen consumption, increased volume of distribution, and slower drug metabolism necessitate a much different physiologic and pharmacologic approach compared with the older child.

The pediatric cardiac anesthesiologist's goals during the preoperative visit are to (1) obtain a clinical knowledge of the child's emotional and physical state, (2) gain a detailed understanding of the physiologic and hemodynamic effects of the patient's cardiac lesion, (3) psychologically prepare both the child and the family for the proposed operative procedure, (4) educate the parents concerning the anesthetic management and empathetically obtain informed consent, and (5) formulate a rational anesthetic plan individualized to the needs of each specific patient. Medicolegal and ethical issues such as blood transfusions in children of members of Jehovah's Witnesses religious sect or "do not resuscitate" declarations should be addressed when necessary.

Medical History

The preoperative examination for the child undergoing cardiac surgery should include routine questioning about allergies, medications, past medical history, previous anesthetic experiences, and present illness. In addition, a detailed evaluation of the child's exercise tolerance in comparison with peers assesses the child's physical cardiac compensation. A history of increasing fatigability, increased shortness of breath, more frequent cyanotic episodes, or feeding dysfunctions such as dyspnea, diaphoresis, and irritability in the infant point to a loss of cardiorespiratory reserve. It also is important to develop an in-depth knowledge of the child's cardiac lesion, including previous palliative surgical procedures. The anesthetic ramifications of taking down a Pott's anastomosis between the descending aorta and pulmonary artery are far different from closure of the physiologically similar Blalock-Taussig shunt between the subclavian artery and pulmonary artery. The Blalock-Taussig shunt can usually be ligated before initiating cardiopulmonary bypass, whereas closure of a Pott's anastomosis may require circulatory arrest.

Another key goal of the preoperative visit, aside from obtaining medical information about the physical state of the patient, is to educate and reassure both the child and family.[12] Though infrequently verbalized, many children undergoing cardiac surgery fear awareness or pain during the surgical procedure. The anesthesiologist can effectively alleviate this fear by addressing it directly and by providing a simple, nonthreatening account of the perioperative course. The occasional child who is convinced that the cardiac surgery will end in death is of more concern.[13] Preoperative feelings of doom should not be taken lightly because evidence exists that such patients may have an increased risk of postoperative morbidity.[14,15] Once again, direct and honest confrontation of this fear is necessary with reassurance and stress upon a positive outlook. Consideration should be given to delaying the surgical procedure until professional psychological support can be provided if unreasonable fear of death persists.

Physical Examination

The child with a poorly compensated congenital cardiac lesion shows evidence of failure to thrive. Important information can be obtained by observing the position of the child's height, weight, and head circumference on routine pediatric growth grids. A comparison of the child's vital signs with those of the normal child in the appropriate age range (Tables 12–1 and 12–2; also see Table 5–1) is also of value in determining the child's cardiorespiratory reserve. Relative bradycardia in an infant dependent on heart rate for maintenance of cardiac output indicates the need for immediate medical intervention even before initiating the anesthetic plan. Similarly, tachypnea is one of the earliest signs of developing congestive heart failure.

The physical examination should seek to discover other signs of congestive heart failure such as irritability, diaphoresis, rales, jugular venous distension, and hepatomegaly.[16] Other than noting the presence of clubbing of the digits, evaluation of the extremities should include assessment of pulse volume and equality and blood pressures in all four extremities. The finding of a variation in blood pressure between extremities suggests the presence of an unexpected coarctation of the aorta or an anomalous origin of an extremity's arterial blood supply. Without previous knowledge of this defect, misinterpretation of intraoperative blood pressures could occur if that extremity was used. In addition, in children with Blalock-Taussig shunts, the pulse will be absent or reduced in the arm in which the subclavian artery to pulmonary artery anastomosis was constructed.

The higher metabolic requirements of children, compared with adults, combined with their relatively smaller functional residual capacity requires that a patent airway be maintained.[17] The cyanotic child with a lower oxygen reserve and one with hyperresponsive pulmonary vasculature are particularly at risk in the presence of a compromised airway. Certain children such as those with the Pierre Robin syndrome or the Treacher Collins syndrome can be extremely difficult intubation problems and may require surgical availability for tracheostomy. All children undergoing cardiac surgery deserve careful examination of their upper airway. The presence of a narrow palate, enlarged tonsils, large tongue, or mandib-

TABLE 12–1. THE RELATIONSHIP OF AGE TO RESPIRATORY AND HEART RATES

Age	Respiratory Rate (breaths/min)	Mean Heart Rate (beats/min)
0–24 hr	40–50	120
1–7 d	30–50	135
8–30 d	30–50	160
3–12 mo	25–35	140
1–3 yr	25–35	125
3–5 yr	25–30	100
8–12 yr	20–25	80
12–16 yr	16–25	75

(Adapted from Todres D: Growth and development. In Ryan T, Todres D, Cote C, and Goudsouzian N [eds]: A Practice of Anesthesia for Infants and Children. New York: Grune & Stratton, 1986, p 11, with permission.)

**TABLE 12–2. THE RELATIONSHIP OF AGE TO
BLOOD PRESSURE**

Age	Normal Blood Pressure Mean Systolic	Mean Diastolic (mm Hg)
0–12 hr (Preterm)	50	35
0–12 hr (Full-term)	65	45
4 d	75	50
6 wk	95	55
1 yr	95	60
2 yr	100	65
9 yr	105	70
12 yr	115	75

(From Todres D: Growth and development. In Ryan T, Todres D, Cote C, Goudsouzian N (eds): A Practice of Anesthesia for Infants and Children. New York: Grune & Stratton, 1986, p 11, with permission.)

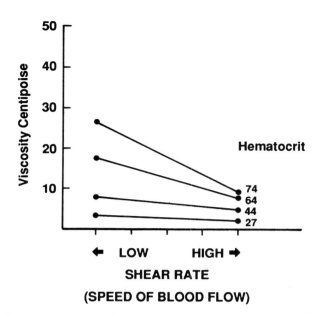

Figure 12–1. The relationship between the shear rate or speed of blood in blood vessels and the viscosity of the blood is shown for a variety of hematocrits. In low-flow vessels where shear rates are low, increased hematocrit causes exponential increases in viscosity. In high-flow vessels, increases in hematocrit lead to a more linear increase in viscosity. *(Adapted from Kontras S, Bodenbender J, Craenen J, et al: Hyperviscosity in congenital heart disease. J Pediatr 76:214–220, 1970, with permission.)*

ular hypoplasia alerts the anesthesiologist to potential airway management problems.

Because 8.5% of children with symptomatic congenital heart disease can be identified as a specific congenital syndrome and 25% have some extracardiac anomaly, the physical examination should establish the presence of any other defects that might alter anesthetic management.[18–20] For example, children with the Down syndrome frequently have endocardial cushion defects,[21] but their anesthetic management is complicated by increased anticholinergic sensitivity,[22] cervical spine dislocation,[23,24] enlarged tongue, and lax pharyngeal muscles.

Laboratory Studies

Hemoglobin. The hemoglobin concentration is determined preoperatively because the presence of anemia may require priming of the extracorporeal circuit with red blood cells. If the child has prior exposure to blood products, blood typing and cross matching should be performed early to ensure availability of compatible blood if serum antibodies are present. On the other hand, the hypoxemia of cyanotic congenital heart disease induces erythropoiesis that can produce hematocrits of 70% or greater. The increased red blood cell mass leads to expansion of the intravascular volume and a relative hypervolemia.[25]

Polycythemia increases blood viscosity, especially in the small peripheral, low-flow vessels, to such an extent that significant impairment of peripheral tissue perfusion occurs. The increase in shear forces is more pronounced in the low-flow blood vessels, such as capillary beds and veins[26,27] (Fig 12–1), than in the high-flow, arterial systems. In the high-flow vessels, such as the arteries, viscosity increases linearly with increases in hematocrit, but in the low-flow vessels, the increase in viscosity is exponential. Because a hematocrit more than

70% may lead to poor tissue perfusion and metabolic acidosis, consideration should be given to preoperative erythrophoresis in these children. This problem becomes critically important in the context of limited preoperative oral hydration and exposure of the child to a cold operating room environment, both of which can significantly increase blood viscosity. Without erythrophoresis in these children, the danger of end-organ thrombosis and infarction becomes acute.[28,29]

The level of hematocrit and, therefore, the blood viscosity, might be expected to affect the relative shunting of blood in patients with intracardiac lesions. When infants with ventricular septal defects with left-to-right shunting are provided isovolemic red blood cell exchange transfusions to increase their hematocrits from 30 to 40%, they sustain significant drops in pulmonary blood flow while maintaining systemic blood pressure.[30] The result is a decrease in the left-to-right shunting. Intracardiac shunting in children with cyanotic heart disease is also affected by changing the hematocrit. In patients with tetralogy of Fallot, decreasing hematocrit from 70 to 60% did not improve pulmonary blood flow, whereas in patients with D-transposition of the great arteries, shunting increased between the pulmonary and systemic circulations improving peripheral oxygenation.[31] Therefore, the optimal preoperative hematocrit varies with the patient's cardiac lesion. In acyanotic patients with left-to-right shunting, a higher hematocrit improves the balance between pulmonary and systemic blood flow.[30] However, in cyanotic congenital heart disease, the optimal hematocrit is dependent upon whether the pulmonary blood flow is dependent (tetralogy of Fallot) or independent (transposition of the great vessels) of the systemic circuit.[31]

The choice of the optimal hematocrit must be balanced not only against its effect on shunting but upon many other factors. Serum 2,3-diphosphoglycerate (DPG) increases with increasing hematocrit.[32,33] The increased DPG level, as well as the presence of acidosis, shifts the oxyhemoglobin dissociation curve to the right to decrease the affinity between hemoglobin and oxygen and to increase peripheral unloading of oxygen.

Hemostasis. All children with congenital heart disease undergoing open-heart surgical procedures are at risk for perioperative hemostatic derangements. Because hemostatic abnormalities are commonly found in children with congenital heart disease,[34–36] every child should have a preoperative evaluation, including a platelet count, prothrombin time, partial thromboplastin time, and fibrinogen level. These tests allow the anesthesiologist to identify and prepare for any preexisting coagulation problems.

Coagulopathy of Polycythemia. Children with severe polycythemia commonly have a number of hemostatic derangements. The proposed mechanism for these derangements is that peripheral sludging of blood secondary to increased blood viscosity leads to a low-grade, intravascular coagulation with activation of fibrinolysis, degranulation of platelets, and consumption of coagulation factors.[37–40] In the situation where a normal preoperative platelet count is observed, the platelets may still be functionally abnormal. Also, the absolute platelet count must be evaluated in the context of the individual patient. In children with severe polycythemia, the serum volume is relatively constricted in spite of an expanded intravascular volume. Therefore, the absolute platelet count may be misleadingly increased, especially when the serum volume may have been further depleted by diuretic therapy or dehydration. A good rule is to have platelets available for transfusion of all children undergoing open-heart surgical procedures when a high probability of usage exists, such as (1) preoperative platelet counts less than 120,000 platelets/mm^3, (2) children with cyanotic congenital heart disease associated with significant polycythemia, (3) children undergoing repeat operative procedures on the heart, and (4) children who have taken medications containing acetylsalicylic acid within 1 week of the surgical procedure.

The hemostatic derangements found in association with the polycythemia of cyanotic congenital heart disease can be partially corrected preoperatively by the use of erythrophoresis. A volume exchange transfusion of 20 mL/kg of fresh frozen plasma for an equal volume of red blood cells removed from the patient immediately improves hemostasis and normalizes platelet function within 3 days.[40] Similarly, following repair of a patient's cyanotic congenital heart disease, coagulation abnormalities return to normal as the red blood cell mass decreases.[37]

Neonatal Coagulopathy. Another problem in hemostasis is presented by the newborn undergoing open-heart surgery. Owing to the immaturity of hepatic function, these children often have inadequate liver-dependent coagulation factors. Early preoperative treatment with intramuscular or intravenous vitamin K will help restore hemostatic function in these children.

Glucose, Electrolytes, and Arterial Blood Gases. Children on diuretic therapy are at risk for hypokalemia, particularly if they are digitalized. Therefore, serum electrolytes should be evaluated preoperatively in these children. All infants, particularly those in congestive heart failure, are at risk for both hypoglycemia[41,42] and hypocalcemia.[9] The signs of reduced serum glucose and calcium can be quite subtle and nonspecific, such as the presence of jitteriness, tachypnea, and tachycardia. Because of this, laboratory evaluation should be performed preoperatively on all infants, and continued monitoring should be undertaken throughout the operative procedure and postoperative period.

Preoperative arterial blood gases indicate the amount of respiratory reserve a particular child might have. Arterial P_{O_2} values of 30–40 mm Hg and peripheral O_2 saturations less than 70% indicate a severe reduction of cardiorespiratory reserve to the point where progressive metabolic acidosis can be expected. Early or emergent intervention may well be necessary to stabilize these children in the preoperative period. In any case, such reductions in oxygenation indicate the need for meticulous management of the child's airway during induction of anesthesia.

Chest Radiograph and Electrocardiogram. The principal value of the preoperative chest radiograph is its comparison with previous chest radiographs. An enlarged heart, development of pulmonary edema, or the appearance of new infiltrates are indicators that a delay in surgery may be necessary in order to optimize the child's respiratory state. In addition, an assessment of collateral blood flow in coarctation of the aorta, based upon the severity of rib notching; determination upon which side a Blalock-Taussig shunt will be performed, based on the location of the aortic arch; and quantitation of the pulmonary blood flow, based upon the pulmonary vascular prominence, can all be accomplished.

The electrocardiogram is best evaluated in conjunction with a pediatric cardiologist owing to the wide range of "normal values" in children and the changing definition of "normal" with differing age ranges (see Table 5–2). For each congenital heart lesion, there is normally a spectrum of electrocardiographic features depending upon the severity of the lesion, the extent to which the lesion has affected cardiac chamber size, and the age of the child. For the anesthesiologist, the greatest value of the preoperative electrocardiogram is to evaluate preexisting arrythmias and to serve as a baseline for postoperative comparative purposes.

Cardiac Catheterization. The cardiac catheterization data, combined with information from echocardiographic studies, is extremely valuable when formulating the anesthetic plan. Whether a patient with tetralogy of Fallot has isolated valvular pulmonic stenosis, or a combination of infundibular and valvular pulmonic stenoses, completely alters the anesthetic management. In addition, the change in the pulmonary vascular resistance of children with pulmonary hypertension on exposure to 100% oxygen or isoproterenol infusions during cardiac catheterization helps to direct important anesthetic considerations both perioperatively and during the period following the definitive repair.[43] Although much information can be derived from the written catheterization report, direct evaluation of the angiogram is preferred. Such an evaluation is most helpful when performed in the presence of both the pediatric cardiologist and cardiac surgeon, thus allowing interdisciplinary interaction during the formulation of the anesthetic plan (see Chapter 7).

PREMEDICATION

An important goal of the anesthesiologist is to have the child arrive in the operating room calm and quiet with intact cardiorespiratory reflexes. An important first step in obtaining a cooperative, trusting child is to provide a reassuring and thorough preoperative visit.[12,44] Taking objects that will be used during the operation, such as a face mask, on the preoperative visit in order to familiarize the child with them in a nonthreatening environment and "acting out" the use of the face mask help to reduce the child's fears.[45] Also, allowing the child to take a familiar or favorite toy to the operating room adds to the child's security and cooperation. In addition, most children undergoing open-heart surgical procedures receive pharmacologic premedication. Agents used should be viewed as the first step in developing an anesthetic foundation and may include (1) an anticholinergic, (2) a sedative-hypnotic, and (3) an analgesic.

Anticholinergics

Anticholinergic drugs are primarily used to reduce airway secretions that might predispose the child to laryngo-spasm and to prevent bradycardia mediated by vagal receptors during induction and intubation. Because the younger child is dependent upon heart rate for maintenance of cardiac output, prevention of bradycardia has added significance for preservation of cardiovascular stability. One of the most commonly used anticholinergics is atropine, which can be given either intramuscularly or orally (0.02 mg/kg, with a minimum dose of 0.15 mg and a maximum dose of 0.4 mg).[46,47] Within 15 minutes of an intramuscular injection, significant antisialagogic effects are observed, although cardiac vagolytic effects are already disappearing and may require supplementation during the anesthetic induction. Scopolamine can be substituted for atropine (0.01 mg/kg IM with a minimum dose of 0.1 mg and a maximum dose of 0.4 mg[48]), although scopolamine has less effect on vagally mediated cardiac responses.[49] An advantage of scopolamine is a more intense antisialagogic effect as well as central nervous system sedative effects that are reversible with physostigmine (0.035 mg/kg). Glycopyrrolate (0.01 mg/kg IM with a minimum of 0.1 mg and a maximum of 0.4 mg) also has intense antisialogic activity but reduced cardiac vagolytic activity compared to atropine.[50] Of interest, when glycopyrrolate is given in conjunction with an acetylcholinesterase inhibitor, such as neostigmine, it may be more protective against bradyarrhythmias than atropine.[51] Also gastric volume and gastric acidity are reduced to a greater extent by glycopyrrolate than by the other anticholinergics.[52]

Sedative, Hypnotic, and Analgesic Drugs

The choice of sedative and analgesic agents must be directed by the patient's clinical state and cardiac lesion. Preexisting debilitating illness, respiratory compromise, congestive heart failure, and cyanosis are important considerations factored into premedicant choice. Children with cyanotic congenital heart disease can experience transient, significant oxygen desaturation following premedication.[48] The purpose of providing premedication for these children is to decrease patient anxiety, thereby decreasing total body oxygen consumption and avoiding a hyperdynamic cardiovascular state that, in the presence of infundibular pulmonary stenosis, could lead to spasm and systemic desaturation. On the other hand, desaturation might also be caused by oversedation that obtunds respiratory reflexes.[53]

Numerous sedative-hypnotics have been used as premedications. Pharmacologic agents commonly used include secobarbital[48] (2–3 mg/kg, with maximum 100 mg intramuscularly), phenobarbital[46] (2–4 mg/kg intramuscularly or orally, with maximum dose of 100 mg), methohexital (25 mg/kg rectally),[54–56] diazepam (0.2–0.6 mg/kg orally, with maximum 10 mg),[47,57,58] and midazolam (intranasally 0.2–0.3 mg/kg,[59,60] rectally 0.5–1.0 mg/kg,[55,61] orally 0.5–0.75 mg/kg,[62] and intramuscularly 0.08 mg/kg).[63] Many of the recent studies on premedication dosages have been performed in healthy pediatric outpatients, so consideration should be given to decreasing the suggested dosages in the child with cardiovascular compromise, especially with agents having cardiac-depressant effects such as the barbiturates.

Analgesic agents are often combined with sedative-hypnotics to produce a child who is sleeping quietly on arrival in the operating room.[46–48,57] These pharmacologic agents include morphine (0.1–0.2 mg/kg intramuscularly with a maximum dose of 10 mg),[46,48] meperidine (1.5–3.0 mg/kg orally or 1 mg/kg intramuscularly, with a maximum dose of 100 mg),[46,47,57] fentanyl (15–20 μg/kg orally transmucosally),[57,64] and sufentanil (1.2–3.0 μg/kg nasally).[65] Because all narcotics produce dose-related respiratory depression, particularly when given in combination with a sedative,[66] special care must be used when any evidence of airway obstruction or lack of respiratory reserve exists. The type of premedication has an important effect in determining preinduction stability, including the occurrence of hypoxic episodes.[47] In addition, the route of administration must be considered. Evidence exists that oxygen saturation transiently decreases more frequently after intramuscular than after oral or rectal premedication.[67]

Controversy continues about whether a child with congenital heart disease should receive a light premedication that allows preservation of airway reflexes and physiologic stability or heavy premedication that reduces preinduction stress.[48,53] For children over 1 year of age, most pediatric anesthesiologists prefer a heavy premedication. Suggested oral and intramuscular premedications are presented in Table 12–3. Replacement of diazepam by midazolam is likely in the future because of the better intramuscular and gastrointestinal absorption of midazolam. However, owing to respiratory depressant effects when midazolam is combined with a narcotic,[66] the appropriate dose of midazolam in pediatric cardiac patients is unclear.

Other Medications

The child with a cardiac lesion may be taking a variety of cardiovascular drugs prior to undergoing corrective cardiac surgery. Digitalis may be used for arrhythmia control or congestive heart failure, diuretics for congestive heart failure, and β-blockers to control pulmonary infundibular spasm in tetralogy of Fallot or subaortic spasm in idiopathic hypertrophic subaortic stenosis. As a general rule, if a child requires a medication for cardiovascular stability during the preoperative period, that medication should be continued up to the time of surgery. An exception to this rule is the use of digitalis in children who will undergo cardiac surgery requiring cardiopulmonary bypass. For these children, digitalis is normally discontinued 24 hours prior to the surgical procedure because serum digitalis levels can increase to potentially toxic levels in the postoperative period.[68,69] The increase in digitalis level is of particular concern in the pediatric population and is most pronounced in children who have undergone recent digitalization.[70] If digitalis therapy is essential to control superventricular tachycardia, careful attention to maintaining adequate postcardiopulmonary bypass potassium levels is essential.

Preoperative Fasting

In the general pediatric outpatient setting, an in-depth reevaluation of preoperative fasting orders has occurred.[71,72] The previous philosophy was to avoid oral intake for at least 8 hours prior to surgical procedure. The approach has now liberalized to the point of allowing oral hydration with clear fluids up to 2 hours prior to the surgical procedure.[71] The advantage of this policy change for the polycythemic congenital cardiac patient is obvious because the need for preoperative placement of an intravenous catheter for hydration is eliminated. However, conclusions drawn from the studies on healthy outpatient pediatric patients cannot be extrapolated to the debilitated cyanotic cardiac patient, especially in regard to the risk for aspiration of residual gastric contents. Some liberalization of the previous restrictive 8-hour NPO (nothing by mouth) rule can be adopted. A rational approach to NPO orders in children scheduled for open-heart surgery is provided in Table 12–4.

TABLE 12–3. PREMEDICATION FOR PEDIATRIC OPEN-HEART SURGERY

Intramuscular Premedication for Children Undergoing Open Heart Surgery*	
0–6 mo	Atropine, 0.02 μg/kg (minimum 0.15 μg)
6–12 mo	Atropine, 0.02 μg/kg (minimum 0.15 μg) Pentobarbital, 2 mg/kg
>12 mo	Scopolamine, 0.01 μg/kg (maximum 0.4 μg) Pentobarbital, 2 mg/kg (maximum 100 mg) Morphine, 0.2 mg/kg (maximum 10 mg)
Oral Premedication for Children Undergoing Open-Heart Surgery*	
> 2 yr	Atropine, 0.02 μg/kg (maximum 0.4 μg) Meperidine, 1.5 mg/kg (maximum 100 mg) Diazepam, 0.2 mg/kg (maximum 5 mg)

Modification of these suggested dosages is mandated by the child's clinical condition.

TABLE 12–4. NPO ORDERS

0–12 mo	Offer milk, formula, and solids up to 8 hr before scheduled procedure; then offer only clear liquids up to 4 hr before scheduled procedure.
12 mo to 2 yr	Offer solids and nonclear liquids up to 8 hr before procedure; then offer only clear liquids up to 6 hr before procedure.
2 yr or older	Make NPO 8 hr prior to procedure.
If severe polycythemia is present or if surgery is delayed, consider intravenous hydration.	

ANESTHETIC MANAGEMENT

After the complete evaluation of the child's medical history, physical examination, and laboratory findings, an anesthetic plan based on each child's specific needs should be formulated. The development of the anesthetic plan is aided by formulating a physiologic profile or cardiac grid[73] for each child that considers optimization of various hemodynamic elements in order to establish and maintain intraoperative stability.

Physiologic Profile—Cardiac Grid

The elements of the cardiac grid include preload, afterload, heart rate, pulmonary vascular resistance, and myocardial contractility. Suggested guidelines are provided in Table 12–5 for a variety of commonly encountered cardiac lesions, but it should be understood that the ultimate cardiac grid produced for each patient must incorporate additional factors such as the patient age, severity of illness, associated medical problems, and combination of cardiac lesions.[73,74] Not infrequently, the optimal physiologic situation for one factor is contrary to the needs dictated by other factors. The anesthesiologist's job is to weigh the importance of each factor before determining the final anesthetic plan. Additionally, flexibility must be incorporated into the plan because changing intraoperative conditions as well as unexpected or undesirable responses to manipulations of the various

parameters may require modifications of the anesthetic. Finally, once the cardiac surgical procedure, whether total repair or palliative procedure, is completed, the cardiac grid for the child changes to the physiologic state produced by the surgical intervention. The child's new physiologic needs after surgery should be anticipated and appropriate adjustments in the anesthetic plan made.

A cardiac grid is only a tool to help to develop a rational approach to the anesthetic. The reasoning and thought necessary to develop each grid creates a better understanding of the overall and often contradictory needs of the child's disease processes and provides a more comprehensive approach to the child's intraoperative management.

Anesthetic and Monitoring Preparations

Before the child enters the operating room suite, extensive preparation should have already occurred. In addition to routine preparations for any anesthetic that include the presence of a working suction apparatus, a functional anesthetic machine with appropriate ventilatory tubing, and an assortment of endotracheal tubes and laryngoscopic equipment, additional preparation must be made for the child undergoing an open-heart surgical procedure. A working defibrillator with appropriately sized paddles must be present. Appropriate blood products should be readily available in the event an emer-

TABLE 12–5. CARDIAC GRID—DESIRED PHYSIOLOGIC CHANGES FOR COMMON CONGENITAL CARDIAC LESIONS

Lesion	Preload	Pulmonary Tone	Systemic Tone	Heart Rate	Contractility
Left-to-Right Shunts					
ASD	↑	↑	↓	N	N
VSD	↑	↑	↓	N	N
PDA	↑	↑	↓	N	N
Waterston, Potts, or Blalock-Taussig	↑	↓	↑	N	N
Right-to-Left Shunts					
Tetralogy with infundibular pulmonic stenosis	↑	↓	↑	N-↓	N-↓
Truncus	↑	N	↑	↑	↑
Transposition	N	↓	N	↑	N
Tetralogy without infundibular pulmonic stenosis	↑	↓	↑	↑	N-↑
Total anomalous pulmonary venous return	↑	↑	↓	N	N
Obstructive					
Aortic stenosis	↑	N	↑	↓	N
Idiopathic hypertrophic subaortic stenosis	↑	N	N-↑	↓	↓
Pulmonic stenosis, valvular	↑	↓-N	N	↑	N
Pulmonic stenosis, infundibular	↑	↓	N	↓	↓
Mitral stenosis	↑	↓	N	↓	N
Coarctation	↑	N	↓	N	N
Tricuspid stenosis	↑	N	↑	↓-N	N
Pulmonary artery band	↑	↓-N	N	↑	N
Regurgitant					
Aortic	↑	N	↓	↑	N
Mitral	↓ or N	↓	↓	↑-N	N
Ebstein's	↑	↓	N	↑-N	N

Abbreviations: N, normal; ASD, atrial septal defect; VSD, ventricular defect; PDA, patent ductus arteriosus.

gency transfusion is necessary. During assembly of intravenous and pressure transducer tubing, extreme caution must be taken to remove all air bubbles. The reason for such a precaution in the child with right-to-left intracardiac shunting is obvious because of the risk for direct systemic embolization of air. However, even a child with left-to-right shunting or only a probe patent foramen ovale is at risk for brain, kidney, or other organ infarction due to air embolization occurring during transient reversal of shunt flow.[75] Some precautions to prevent the inadvertent introduction of air into a patient's vascular system are listed in Table 12–6.

Pharmacologic Preparation. In addition to the anesthetic drugs that are selected based upon the physiologic requirements dictated by the cardiac grid, a variety of other pharmacologic agents should be prepared in advance in the proper concentrations based upon the child's weight. Drugs that should be prepared for all patients as well as drugs that should be immediately available are listed in Table 12–7.

Monitoring. Prior to the child's arrival into the operating room, the extent, type, and location of intraoperative monitoring modalities must be determined. For openheart surgical procedures, monitoring includes an electrocardiogram, peripheral and central temperatures, invasive blood pressure monitoring, central venous pressure cannula, urine volume measurement, arterial oxygenation saturation, and end-expiratory capnography. It must be realized that each of these monitoring modalities has potential pitfalls that can provide misleading information to the unwary practitioner.

Oxygen Monitors. Pulse oximetry and percutaneous oxygen evaluation are valuable for the early identification of intraoperative hypoxic events.[76,77] However, the site chosen for placement of these devices is important because the use of an extremity that has reduced blood flow, either from a previous palliative shunt or from compression during the operative procedure, causes false interpretations of intraoperative events. Such events occur during repair of coarctation of the aorta when the blood supply to the left arm may be significantly compromised. Also, although hypoxemia can usually be identified relatively well using these modalities, neither avoids hyperoxic states in neonates. For this reason, although noninvasive determinations of oxygen saturation or oxygen tension are valuable for continuous monitoring of clinical trends, the measurements should be correlated with arterial blood gas measurements. Pulse oximetry is particularly valuable during pulmonary arterial banding.[78,79]

Capnography. Information obtained from capnography in children with congenital heart disease must also be interpreted in conjunction with an understanding of the child's disease process. In children with acyanotic cardiac disease, a relatively good correlation exists between the end-expiratory CO_2 and the arterial $Paco_2$. However, in the presence of a right-to-left shunt, the end-expiratory carbon dioxide consistently underestimates the true arterial carbon dioxide level.[80,81] The reason for the observed arterial to end-tidal carbon dioxide difference is the relatively larger dead space in cyanotic heart disease due to right-to-left shunting and its attendant decrease in alveolar CO_2 tension.

End-tidal carbon dioxide monitoring is inaccurate in children under 8 kg in weight when a continuous flow, time-cycled ventilator is used on account of dilution of the expired CO_2 with ventilation gases. A decrease in the end-expiratory to arterial carbon dioxide gradient can be accomplished by using a ventilator that interrupts the flow of fresh gas at the end of each expiration, allowing sampling of undiluted end-expiratory gas.[82] Distal sampling at the tip of the endotracheal tube compared with a proximal site does not significantly improve the reliability of the carbon dioxide sampling.[83]

Intravascular Monitors. Invasive monitoring also has pitfalls, particularly in infants at risk for the development of retrolental fibroplasia. In the presence of a patent ductus arteriosus, arterial catheters placed in the left radial or femoral locations may underestimate the Pao_2 reaching the retina. This can lead to the inadvertent use of inspired oxygen concentrations at levels that may increase the risk of retrolental fibroplasia.[84] For this reason, the use of the right radial or temporal artery for blood gas sampling is recommended in neonates. However, the choice of the arterial catheter site will be partially dictated by the operative procedure. In addition, flushing of arterial cannulas both in the radial and temporal arteries should be done gently to avoid retrograde

TABLE 12–6. PRECAUTIONS FOR PREVENTION OF INTRAVASCULAR AIR BUBBLES

1. Thoroughly remove all air from intravenous and monitoring tubing before the child enters the operating room.
2. Just prior to child entering operating room, inspect all plastic tubing again.
3. When connecting fluid-filled tubing to cannulas, have a free flow of fluid from both tubing and cannulas.
4. Before injecting a drug from a syringe intravenously, eject a small amount of drug from syringe to clear air from the needle and syringe hub.
5. Do not inject the last milliliter of drug from syringe because of microbubbles on plunger.
6. Use air traps on intravenous tubing whenever possible.
7. Avoid nitrous oxide whenever possible.
8. Never leave a central venous pressure cannula open to air when the possibility of a negative intrathoracic pressure exists.

TABLE 12–7. NONANESTHETIC DRUGS USED IN PEDIATRIC CARDIAC SURGERY

Drugs to be prepared in advance for bolus administration:

Atropine sulfate*	0.2	mg/kg
Calcium chloride or	10	mg/kg
calcium gluconate	30	mg/kg
Epinephrine*	1–10	μg/kg
Heparin	400	μg/kg for systemic anticoagulation
Lidocaine*	1	mg/kg
Phenylephrine	1–2	μg/kg (double second dose to effect)
Protamine sulfate	1	mg/100 U heparin
Sodium bicarbonate	$0.3 \times \dfrac{\text{body weight (kg)} \times \text{base deficit}}{2}$	
Trimethaphan	10	μg/kg (double second dose to effect)

Drugs to be prepared in advance for infusion administration:

One of the following:

Epinephrine	0.1	μg/kg/min
Dopamine	5	μg/kg/min
Isoproterenol	0.1	μg/kg/min
Dobutamine	5	μg/kg/min
Amrinone	5	μg/kg/min

Drugs to have readily available but not prepared:

Bretylium	5	mg/kg slowly
Chlorpromazine	0.1	mg/kg slowly
Decadron	1	mg/kg
Diphenylhydantoin	4	mg/kg slowly
Digoxin	40	μg/kg for children between 2 months and 2 years; otherwise 30 μg/kg (give 50% of this dose initially and 25% of this dose every 6 h × 2 for digitalization)
Diphenhydramine	0.3	mg/kg
Edrophonium	0.01	mg/kg
Esmolol	100	μg/kg/min
ε-Aminocaproic acid	70	mg/kg
Ethacrynic acid	0.5	mg/kg
Furosemide	0.5	mg/kg
Glucagon	0.05	mg/kg
Glucose (50%)	1	mL/kg
Glycopyrrolate	0.01	mg/kg
Hydrocortisone	20	mg/kg
Insulin	0.1–0.3	μg/kg
Labetalol	0.25	mg/kg
Mannitol	0.5	g/kg
Naloxone*	0.01	mg/kg
Neostigmine	0.07	mg/kg
Nitroglycerin	0.5	μg/kg (increase to effect)
Procainamide	2	mg/kg slowly
Propranolol	10–50	μg/kg slowly
Potassium chloride (mEq)	$0.3 \times \dfrac{\text{body weight (kg)} \times [\text{desired K}^+ \text{ (mEq)} - \text{serum K}^+ \text{ (mEq)}]}{2}$	
Scopolamine	0.01	mg/kg
Sodium nitroprusside	0.1	μg/kg/min (increase to effect but do not exceed 8 μg/kg/min)
Theophylline	4	mg/kg slowly
Verapamil	0.05	mg/kg slowly (maximum 2.5 mg, repeated to effect)
Vitamin K	0.5–2	mg (infants)
	5–10	μg/kg (children)

* Endotracheal administration acceptable.

embolization to the brain.[85] If a shunt using a subclavian artery has been performed, or is to be performed, the arteries of the ipsilateral arm should obviously be avoided. For ligation of a patent ductus arteriosus or repair of coarctation of the aorta, the arteries supplied by the left subclavian artery should not be used for monitoring because compression or partial clamping of the left subclavian artery frequently occurs during surgery. In addition, 7–8% of children with coarctation of the aorta have an anomalous origin of the right subclavian artery from the descending aorta, which may necessitate using the temporal artery for intraoperative monitoring.

In addition to the commonly used radial artery, femoral,[87,88] brachial,[86] or axillary[89] arterial cannulation sites can be used in children. Long-term percutaneous arterial monitoring postoperatively in neonates has been effectively performed using the radial, posterior tibial, or temporal artery with few complications.[90]

In the postcardiopulmonary bypass period, radial arterial pressures underestimate the central aortic pressure.[86,87] If radial arterial pressures are monitored, an extra pressure transducer should be readily available that can be connected with high-pressure tubing to a needle that is directly placed by the surgeon into the central aorta.

The central veins are cannulated through either the internal or external jugular venous vessels,[91–93] although the femoral[94] and axillary veins[95] are alternative sites. Cannulation of the external jugular vein has a high success rate and low incidence of complications. However, there is a relatively high incidence of the catheter tip curving retrograde into the neck through an ipsilateral cervical vein leading to venous thrombosis.[96]

No matter what site is chosen for central venous cannulation, the catheter should be inserted by an experienced anesthesiologist who is knowledgeable about the anatomic venous variations that can be encountered in congenital heart disease. Flow-directed pulmonary artery catheters are rarely used in children, although some centers advocate their use in selected cases.[97]

During cardiac surgery, transthoracic vascular cannulas are placed directly by the surgeon during or after cardiopulmonary bypass. These cannulas can include a 2.5 to 5.0 French thermistor probe for pulmonary artery placement in order to perform cardiac output determinations.[99] Transthoracic cannulas are associated with a low, but potentially fatal, incidence of cardiac tamponade or cardiac arrest. Severe bleeding can also occur after catheter removal. In addition, migration of the catheter during the operative procedure can lead to misinterpretation of hemodynamic data[100] (see Chapter 8).

Other Monitors. A new modality for intraoperative monitoring that has gained increased acceptance during pediatric cardiac surgery is transesophageal echocardiography. Pediatric transducers now allow the transesophageal evaluation of pediatric patients with congenital heart disease.[101,102] The use of epicardial transducers directly on the heart[103,104] provides additional information. Two-dimensional echocardiography with color flow Doppler not only allows real time evaluation of cardiac function but is also valuable for assessing the adequacy of the operative repair.[102,105] In addition, postcardiopulmonary bypass myocardial dysfunction secondary to coronary artery air embolization can be evaluated,[106] and debubbling of the heart prior to weaning from cardio-

pulmonary bypass can be directed by transesophageal evaluation of intracavitary air (see Chapter 6).

Measurement of anterior fontanelle pressure in combination with visual evoked potentials[107] and more recently transcranial Doppler sonography,[108] have been suggested for the intraoperative monitoring of neurologic function, especially after profound hypothermic circulatory arrest in neonates. Before these modalities can be recommended for routine monitoring, further evaluation of their ability to predict accurately the risk of neurologic damage and to direct effective therapeutic interventions in neonates is necessary.

Anesthetics. The choice of anesthetic agents is based upon a variety of factors, including the severity of the child's disease, the physiologic requirements dictated by the cardiac grid, the age of the child, the presence of venous access, the child's level of anxiety on entrance into the operating room, and other associated problems, such as the presence of a compromised airway. Because there is a spectrum for each of these variables, no single induction technique or anesthetic agent can be recommended. The pediatric cardiac anesthesiologist must weigh the advantages and disadvantages of each approach to decide the best method for any particular patient. The primary goal for each child is to provide the least physiologically and psychologically stressful conditions.

Induction Techniques

For the most part, induction techniques for pediatric cardiac anesthesia include inhalational, intravenous, intramuscular, and rectal. Heavy premedication allows the use of a "steal" inhalation technique. In this situation, the child arrives in the operating room sleeping, and prior to movement from the stretcher onto the operating room table, a combination of 50% nitrous oxide and 50% oxygen, with incremental increases of a potent inhalational agent, is provided to the child via a face mask without ever awakening the child. As induction of anesthesia proceeds, the child is moved onto the operating room table and precordial stethoscope, electrocardiograph, pulse oximeter, capnograph, and noninvasive sphymomanometry applied. After an intravenous catheter is started, an intubating dose of neuromuscular blocking drug is given. Nitrous oxide is discontinued to prevent expansion of any air bubbles that might enter the venous circulation, and the potent inhalational agent is decreased to approximately one quarter MAC to allow blood pressure to increase to facilitate the insertion of the percutaneous arterial cannula. Use of an automated blood pressure cuff is then discontinued. After insertion of the arterial cannula, the inspired concentration of the inhalation anesthetic is once again increased in preparation for intubation. Following intubation, a central venous cannula and an esophageal echocardiographic transducer or esophageal stethoscope are inserted.

If the child arrives in the operating room awake, which is usually the case in children less than 1 year of age, the electrocardiograph, precordial stethoscope, pulse oximeter, and noninvasive sphygmomanometer are placed prior to induction of anesthesia. Induction is performed with a combination of 50% nitrous oxide in 50% oxygen, with incremental increases of a potent inhalational agent, usually halothane. Occasionally, an awake child will not tolerate a mask induction without severe restraint because of intense anxiety or mental retardation. The options for these circumstances are the use of intramuscular ketamine or rectal methohexital or the placement of an intravenous cannula specifically for parenteral induction of anesthesia. Once induction is accomplished, a larger-bore intravenous cannula can be inserted.

Effects of Congenital Heart Disease on Anesthetic Uptake and Distribution.
The speed of anesthetic induction in children with congenital heart disease is affected by such factors as intracardiac shunts, functional residual capacity, minute ventilation, cardiac output, cerebral blood flow, and anesthetic blood gas solubility. Each of these factors must be considered when choosing the anesthetic agent for a particular child.

Effect of Ventilation and Cardiac Output.
The adequacy of ventilation has important effects on the speed of an inhalational induction. As anesthetic vapor is taken up from the alveoli, alveolar anesthetic concentration decreases until the vapor is replaced by the next inspiration. The relative anesthetic gas concentration in the alveoli is greater with rapid alveolar ventilation. Blood-anesthetic concentration increases faster resulting in a more rapid induction of anesthesia.

The solubility of the anesthetic agent is as important as alveolar ventilation. The more soluble the anesthetic agent, the greater the speed of induction with hyperventilation.[109] The blood gas solubility of commonly used inhalation agents, ordered from the lowest to the highest solubility, are nitrous oxide (0.47), isoflurane (1.41), enflurane (1.78), and halothane (2.36). Therefore, the speed of induction with a relatively insoluble agent, such as nitrous oxide, is less affected by hyperventilation than that of a more soluble agent, such as halothane. The decrease in functional residual capacity occurring during anesthesia in children is similar in patients with congenital heart disease.[109]

Hyperventilation may slow anesthetic induction by decreasing cerebral blood flow secondary to decreased blood carbon dioxide levels causing cerebral vasoconstriction. A decrease in cerebral blood flow limits the rise in the brain tissue concentration of anesthetic gas, thereby delaying the onset of anesthesia. However, in the case of the more soluble anesthetics, the effect of hyperventilation, increasing alveolar concentration of the inhaled agent, predominates to induce anesthesia more rapidly.[110,111] However, direct cerebral vascular effects of the anesthetics may modify the effects produced by ventilatory changes.

Hyperventilation is also one of the most reliable and efficient ways to decrease pulmonary vascular resistance in children with pulmonary hypertension.[112] The resultant increase in pulmonary blood flow allows more rapid pickup of alveolar anesthetic, which paradoxically results in a faster fall in alveolar anesthetic concentration and may slow the speed of induction. The pulmonary vasodilating effect of hyperventilation is secondary to changes in pH rather than to absolute partial pressure of carbon dioxide in the blood.

Increased heart rate increases cardiac output in children causing more rapid uptake of anesthetic gases from the alveoli and a relative decrease in alveolar anesthetic concentrations. In spite of the greater total amount of anesthetic agent absorbed in this situation, peak anesthetic concentrations in the blood going to the brain are slightly lower, reducing the speed of induction. Blood gas solubility also determines the slowing of anesthesia induction with tachycardia. More soluble anesthetic agents are most affected by changes in heart rate.[109,110] Because heart rate is directly related to cardiac output in younger children, who are unable to increase their stroke volume, tachycardia speeds the delivery of the intravenous anesthetic agent to the child's brain. Induction time with intravenous agents is faster with increased cardiac outputs.

Effect of Intracardiac Shunting.
Anesthesia uptake and distribution are significantly affected by intracardiac shunts. The direction of shunt flow can transiently reverse because of changing pressure relationships throughout the cardiac cycle and positive pulmonary pressures during mechanical ventilation. For this discussion, pure right-to-left or left-to-right shunts will be considered, but it must be realized that most children with congenital heart disease have bidirectional shunting.

Children with right-to-left shunting of blood have deoxygenated blood bypassing the pulmonary circuit. The result is that blood from the pulmonary circuit carrying oxygen and anesthetic agent is diluted by unoxygenated blood without anesthetic vapor that bypassed the pulmonary circulation. Lower blood anesthetic concentrations reach the brain, slowing anesthetic induction with inhalation agents.[109] The delay of inhalational induction is particularly evident when soluble anesthetic agents are used.[113,114] Where mixed shunts are present, as in tetralogy of Fallot with a Blalock-Taussig shunt, the slowing of inhalation induction is blunted[114] because more effective pulmonary blood flow is available to pick up anesthetic agent. Intravenous agents theoretically would have a slightly more rapid onset of action because some of the anesthetic would bypass the pulmonary circuit to reach the brain slightly faster.

In children with left-to-right intracardiac shunts, blood that has circulated through the lungs picking up anesthetic agent is recycled through the lungs once again picking up additional agent.[109] The slightly higher anesthetic concentration in blood would theoretically speed the induction time for inhaled anesthetic agents in patients with left-to-right shunts.

Clinically, induction speed changes insignificantly unless cardiac output decreases concurrently to cause proportionally more of the cardiac output to go to the brain.[114] Theoretically, intravenous agents would have a slower onset of action with left-to-right shunts owing to the delay in the agent reaching the brain because of pulmonary recirculation. Clinically, this effect is minimal. In fact, no difference in the onset of action of pancuronium was found in children with acyanotic and cyanotic heart disease. However, the onset time for muscle relaxation was delayed compared with children without heart disease.[115] Proposed reasons for this delay, at least in children with right-to-left shunting, include an increased volume of distribution, decreased cardiac output, and increased protein binding of the muscle relaxant.[115]

Anesthetic Choice

A variety of agents have been effectively used to anesthetize children with congenital heart disease.[116] Matching the anesthetic agent to the particular physiologic needs of a child is a more rational approach.

Intravenous Agents.

All intravenous induction agents require the preinduction placement of an intravenous cannula. Because one goal of anesthesia induction is to maintain a physiologically stress-free state, the stress and anxiety surrounding the placement of an intravenous cannula may negate the possibility of a smooth preoperative period. Therefore, intravenous induction techniques are usually reserved for children with an existing intravenous cannula, children who will not tolerate mask inductions, or children whose severity of illness mandates the need for an intravenous induction technique. Thiopental sodium (4 mg/kg) has been used extensively as an intravenous induction agent for general anesthetics. However, owing to the direct myocardial depressant effect in combination with the dilation of systemic vascular beds resulting in hypotension, the use of thiopental sodium in pediatric cardiac anesthesia has been limited, usually to older children or those with cardiovascular stability.[117] Ketamine (1–4 mg/kg intravenously or 2–10 mg/kg intramuscularly) provides a relatively stable hemodynamic state during induction[118] owing to the compensatory central sympathetic activation that ketamine provides. In severely compromised children, ketamine can produce myocardial depression.[119]

Theoretically, the increase in heart rate and myocardial contractility produced from sympathetic stimulation might have adverse effects in patients with infundibular pulmonic stenosis. However, clinical usage has not substantiated this potential risk.[120,124] Other advantages of ketamine include the ability to induce anesthesia in the presence of a high inspired oxygen concentration, bronchodilator properties in patients with bronchospastic disease,[125] and antiarrhythmogenic actions.[118,126] Of concern are reports that ketamine may increase pulmonary vascular resistance, especially in patients with pulmonary vascular obstructive disease.[127] The use of ketamine during diagnostic cardiac catheterizations while trying to make therapeutic decisions about proposed surgical intervention may result in erroneous hemodynamic data. However, not all studies have found increased pulmonary vascular resistance with ketamine, especially when the child is adequately ventilated.[124]

High-dose narcotic for pediatric cardiac anesthesia was first introduced after Lowenstein's report of high-dose intravenous morphine (1–2 mg/kg) as an acceptable anesthetic for adult cardiac patients.[128] However, for patients with congenital cardiac disease, high-dose morphine has several disadvantages, primarily the decrease in systemic vascular resistance secondary to histamine release. In patients with cyanotic heart disease, decreased systemic vascular resistance can cause severe cardiovascular decompensation. At the present time, morphine has been virtually supplanted by newer narcotics with fewer adverse hemodynamic effects.

Fentanyl (50 μg/kg intravenously) became popular for pediatric cardiac anesthesia after its effectiveness was demonstrated in premature infants undergoing ligation of patent ductus arteriosus.[129] Pharmacokinetic studies indicate that premature infants undergoing closed cardiac procedures,[130] as well as children requiring extracorporeal circulation,[131] have higher than expected requirements of fentanyl, which can be provided by either intermittent bolus or continuous infusion techniques.[131,132] Fentanyl anesthesia minimizes hormonally mediated stress responses resulting in attenuation of catecholamine hemodynamic reactivity[133] and hyperglycemia.[134] The importance of modifying the stress response in neonates with complex congenital cardiac lesions has been demonstrated by higher mortality rates when stress responses are unattenuated.[135,136] One additional concern is that fentanyl markedly depresses baroreceptor control of the heart rate in term neonates.[137] Generally, however, fentanyl is a safe agent for both the induction and maintenance of anesthesia for children with congenital heart disease.

Sufentanil (5–10 μg/kg) is also used as the sole anesthetic in children undergoing cardiac surgery.[138,139] Hemodynamic stability and blunting of the hormonal stress response by sufentanil is similar to fentanyl. However, unpredictable hemodynamic hyperreactivity has been observed during sufentanil anesthesia, suggesting the need for supplemental anesthesia.[139] Alfentanil (50 μg/kg bolus with 1 μg/kg/min infusion) has also been used during pediatric cardiac surgery to supplement inhalation anesthesia.[140] Computerized continuous infusions of intravenous anesthetic drugs has been proposed as an alternative to using inhalation anesthetics for children undergoing cardiac surgery.[141]

Inhalation Agents. Because mask induction of anesthesia circumvents the need for preinduction intravenous cannulation, inhalation agents hold a prominent place as induction agents for pediatric cardiac anesthesia. Nitrous oxide is frequently used as an adjunct to other inhalation and intravenous agents.[142–144] Owing to the potential increase in the size of embolized air bubbles that get into the vascular circuit, the use of nitrous oxide in children with intracardiac shunts is primarily limited to the induction period. In addition, nitrous oxide has a direct cardiac depressant effect that is more pronounced in infants and children than in adults.[142,145] Although the predicted MAC for nitrous oxide is 105 volume percent, the fractional MAC, when lower percentages of nitrous oxide are delivered, is additive to the MAC of other inhalational agents.[146] The uptake of nitrous oxide as well as other inhalation agents is faster in infants compared with adults because of their higher cardiac output, greater alveolar ventilation, and proportionally larger compartment of well-perfused tissue relative to total body mass.[147] Nitrous oxide can increase systemic vascular resistance, pulmonary vascular resistance, central venous pressure, and peak inspiratory pressure while decreasing heart rate, stroke volume, and mean arterial pressure.[148–150] These hemodynamic effects could cause cardiovascular deterioration in a child with borderline myocardial decompensation.[148] The increase in pulmonary vascular resistance associated with nitrous oxide may be secondary to a relative decrease in inspired oxygen tension owing to the replacement of oxygen by nitrous oxide rather than direct vasoconstriction.[151,152] Patients with preexisting pulmonary hypertension demonstrate greater increases in pulmonary vascular resistance on exposure to nitrous oxide.[153,154]

Halothane remains one of the most frequently used inhalational induction agents for pediatric cardiac anesthesia in spite of many potential negative features. Its primary advantage is easy acceptability, allowing smooth "steal" inductions. The primary disadvantage of halothane is dose-dependent β-blocking action[155,156] that can lead to cardiovascular collapse in children with a compromised myocardium.[155,156] The depressant effect is more pronounced on the newborn than on the adult myocardium.[157–161] This finding is of particular concern because higher halothane concentrations are required in the younger children in order to reach equipotent MAC levels.[162,163] The overall result is potentially severe my-

ocardial depression at anesthetic concentrations.[164] Under certain circumstances, the β-blocking actions may actually be beneficial in maintaining a child's hemodynamic stability, such as for idiopathic hypertrophic subaortic stenosis or infundibular pulmonic stenosis. Atropine premedication may attenuate some of the myocardial depression produced by halothane.[165] Halothane's predilection for increasing myocardial sensitivity to catecholamines that, in turn, predisposes to arrythmogenesis is also of concern.[166] Because of increased myocardial sensitivity to catecholamines and the dose-dependent myocardial depression, halothane concentrations should be regulated with great care. For children with significant congenital heart lesions, exposure should be limited to peak inspired concentrations of 2%. Although reductive metabolism of halothane is greater in patients with cyanotic congenital heart disease, these children do not seem to be at increased risk for hepatic damage from halothane exposure.[167] Advantages of halothane usage include the ability to use high inspired oxygen concentrations, easy regulation of β-blockade, bronchodilation, stability of both pulmonary and systemic vascular resistances,[156,168] and the potential for early extubation.

Isoflurane has also been used as a primary anesthetic agent for children undergoing cardiac surgery.[169,170] Like halothane, isoflurane produces a dose-dependent depression of the myocardium[158,169] that is minimized with atropine pretreatment.[171] There is evidence that isoflurane depresses the myocardium, which is based upon echocardiographic measurements of left ventricular shortening fraction and mean velocity of circumferential fiber shortening, to a lesser extent than halothane at equal MAC concentrations.[160] However, the baroreflex control of heart rate is significantly impaired, which limits its use in neonates in whom adequate cardiac output depends upon compensatory chronotropic changes.[172,173] Myocardial sensitization to catecholamines by isoflurane occurs to a lesser extent than with halothane.[166] An important reason isoflurane has not replaced halothane as an anesthesia induction agent is its pungent odor, which is poorly tolerated by children.

Neuromuscular Blocking Drugs. These drugs are selected on the basis of their hemodynamic effects and duration of action. In the newborn, the immature myoneural junction has less neuromuscular reserve to tetanic stimulation,[174,175] which might suggest an increased or prolonged neuromuscular blocking effect compared with the older child. However, paradoxically, the younger child requires a higher milligrams per kilogram dose[175,176] owing to the relatively larger extracellular volume and, thus, the volume of distribution for the muscle relaxant. Neonatal respiratory muscles are not resistant to paralysis, as is observed in older children and adults. Instead, respiratory muscle paralysis parallels peripheral muscle relaxation.[177] Succinylcholine (1–2 mg/kg intravenously or 3–4 mg/kg intramuscularly), the only depolarizing muscle relaxant presently available, has limited use in pediatric cardiac anesthesia because of its short duration of action. It produces severe bradycardia in infants and small children, which limits its use in children with cardiovascular compromise.[178,179] In the older child, muscular fasciculations may significantly increase serum potassium, which would be of concern in children with existing hyperkalemia.[180] Except for the occasional need for urgent neuromuscular blockade provided by an intramuscular injection of succinylcholine, there is little reason for using succinylcholine during cardiac surgery in children.

Pancuronium (0.1 mg/kg) is a long-acting nondepolarizing neuromuscular blocker that increases heart rate through vagolysis and increased atrioventricular conduction.[181,182] However, tachycardia does not always occur in pediatric patients with cardiac disease.[183,184] If tachycardia is undesirable, a shorter-acting nondepolarizing muscle relaxant such as vecuronium (0.1 mg/kg)[185,186] or atracurium[187] is a possible alternative, either in bolus form or as a continuous infusion. In addition, longer-acting nondepolarizing relaxants such as pipecuronium (0.05–0.08 mg/kg)[188,189] or doxacurium (0.05–0.08 mg/kg)[190,191] can be given in bolus doses. The newer nondepolarizing muscle relaxants provide complete hemodynamic stability, and the choice between agents is primarily made on the basis of the expected duration of the surgical procedure.

The variety of physiologic and pharmacologic differences of the anesthetic agents and neuromuscular blockers allows the pediatric cardiac anesthesiologist to match closely a particular child's physiologic requirements to the specific pharmacologic agents. However, more important than the specific anesthetic agent used is the experience and adaptability of the anesthesiologist. There is increasing evidence that a variety of anesthetic techniques and agents can be used with equally acceptable outcomes[116,192] as long as the anesthesiologist providing the care understands the potential dangers of each of the selected agents and is prepared to respond immediately when adverse conditions dictate the need.

PREBYPASS CONSIDERATIONS

Ventilation

After an adequate period of mechanical ventilation, a baseline arterial blood gas determination should be obtained in the prebypass period. The decision to hyperventilate a child to produce an end-tidal carbon dioxide in the 20–mm Hg range or to provide normocarbia should have been decided prior to induction of anesthesia based upon the physiologic requirements determined during formulation of the cardiac grid. Metabolic acidosis is often present on the initial arterial blood gas sample, especially in children with cyanotic congenital heart disease and can be corrected early in the surgical procedure to help reverse any related increase in pulmonary vascular resistance or depression in myocardial contractility. Humidification of inhaled gases is recommended[193,194] in order to maintain respiratory tract integrity, to decrease insensible fluid losses, and to preserve thermal homeostasis.

Exposure to high inspired oxygen concentrations can cause deterioration of pulmonary function; however, most children undergoing open-heart surgery receive increased inspired concentrations of oxygen throughout the operative procedure. The primary exceptions are infants at risk for retrolental fibroplasia. Between the gestational ages of 36 and 42 weeks, neonatal retinal vessels undergo maturation, Until maturation is complete, exposure to increased arterial partial pressures of oxygen constricts the peripheral retinal vessels causing formation of fibrotic membranes—retrolental fibroplasia. In newborns of less than 44 weeks' gestation, partial pressures of oxygen of 70 mm Hg or less are considered safe,[195] although the critical oxygen tension and length of exposure are unknown.[196] Of some concern is a report of retrolental fibroplasia developing in an infant with cyanotic congenital heart disease,[197] the least likely situation for retrolental fibroplasia to occur. It is known that a single short, intraoperative exposure to high partial pressures of oxygen is sufficient to produce retrolental fibroplasia,[84] so great care must be taken to control inspired oxygen concentrations for infants at risk. At all times, the anesthesiologist must balance the danger of producing retrolental fibroplasia against the danger of causing hypoxemic brain damage. All children at risk for retrolental fibroplasia should receive a preoperative ophthalmologic evaluation and weekly evaluations postoperatively to a gestational age of 44 weeks.

Fluid and Electrolyte Balance

Fluid management for each child depends on the differing preload requirements of the specific cardiac lesion and the age-based fluid requirements. Aside from hemodynamic stability, the primary objective of fluid management is to maintain an adequate urine output of at least 0.5–1.0 mL/kg/h. A urinary catheter is essential for the intraoperative management of fluid therapy during cardiac surgery. If adequate urine flow cannot be maintained with fluid challenges and adequate cardiovascular function, pharmacologic intervention with mannitol (0.5–1.0 g/kg bolus) or furosemide (0.25–1.0 mg/kg bolus) should be considered.

The choice of the intravenous fluid in the prebypass period depends largely on the child's age. Evidence is accumulating that dextrose solutions given at rates that are even less than maintenance levels can lead to relative hyperglycemia.[198,199] In addition, elevations in blood glucose can occur in children undergoing hypothermic circulatory arrest whether or not glucose-containing solutions have been utilized.[200] The elevation of glucose is of particular concern in light of the fact that postoperative neurologic outcome can be adversely affected when high serum glucose levels have been maintained.[201,202] At present, glucose-containing infusions should be reserved for children at high risk for hypoglycemia and in children less than 1 year of age.[203] In the young child, the potential risk for neurologic damage from exposure to hyperglycemia must be weighed against the known risk of neurologic damage with hypoglycemia. The use of 10% dextrose and 0.25% saline in newborns and 5% dextrose and 0.25% saline in children between 1 month and 1 year of age provides appropriate maintenance intravenous fluid therapy. Children over 1 year of age should receive only Ringer's lactate solution without glucose supplementation. Additional fluid for all ages can be provided in the form of Ringer's lactate to make up for third-space losses, which may exceed 4 mL/kg/h during intrathoracic surgery, and for measured blood losses.

In addition to evaluation of arterial blood gas, baseline calcium, magnesium, and potassium levels should be drawn prior to bypass, especially in infants in whom derangement in these electrolytes are frequent. Periodic monitoring of the hemoglobin level is also necessary.

Hypercyanotic Spells

Prior to initiation of cardiopulmonary bypass, children with tetralogy of Fallot are prone to develop hypercyanotic spells secondary to increased right-to-left shunting of blood across the ventricular septal defect. Two primary mechanisms can be responsible for this acute hypoxemia.[204] One is a decrease in systemic vascular resistance resulting in systemic hypotension and producing increased right-to-left shunting and increased arterial desaturation. This mechanism particularly comes into play when the systemic mean arterial pressure falls below 60 mm Hg.[205] The standard treatment to reverse the hypercyanotic condition is a bolus of an α-adrenergic agonist such as phenylephrine (1–2 μg/kg). In small children, direct abdominal aortic compression can also reverse a hypercyanotic crisis.[206] Early treatment is recommended to prevent the development of refractory acidosis with the attendant myocardial depression.[207]

Another mechanism for hypercyanotic episodes is increased sympathetic stimulation or direct mechanical stimulation to the right ventricular outflow tract leading to spasm of the pulmonary infundibulum.[204] In this situation, phenylephrine may help by increasing systemic resistance, thereby forcing more blood through the pulmonary outflow tract. However, a more rational approach is β-adrenergic blockade to relax the pulmonary in-

fundibulum. Propranolol has traditionally been the β-blocker of choice.[204,208] However, esmolol (100 μg/kg/min infusion) may be more advantageous owing to rapid onset of action, rapid metabolism, and short duration of negative inotropy.[209]

Anticoagulation Prior to cannulation of the aorta and right atrium during preparation for initiation of cardiopulmonary bypass, systemic anticoagulation must be assured. Because a linear relationship exists for each patient between the activated clotting time and the dosage of heparin (in units/kilogram),[39,210] a plot of the heparin dose-response curve can be made prior to initiation of cardiopulmonary bypass in order to provide the desired level of anticoagulation. However, there may not be enough time between giving the heparin and initiating bypass to produce a heparin dose-response curve. In this case, a single bolus dose of heparin (400 U/kg) can be given through the central venous cannula, and the activated clotting time checked to assure it is over 400 seconds before initiation of cardiopulmonary bypass.[211] Overanticoagulation is always preferred to underanticoagulation.

On insertion of the aortic cannula, the equality of carotid pulses should be checked. Rarely, the aortic cannula may obstruct or even enter the right bracheocephalic artery resulting in significant neurologic damage during bypass.[212] At the time of cannulation, an additional dose of neuromuscular blocker should be given to ensure continued paralysis following hemodilution occurring on initiation of cardiopulmonary bypass. Complete blockade is required at this time to prevent air entry into the heart during attempted inspiration when the heart is still beating and the right atrium is open.

BYPASS CONSIDERATIONS

The management of cardiopulmonary bypass is discussed in detail in Chapter 10. However, the primary objective of the anesthesiologist during bypass is to ensure continued homeostasis of the arterial blood gases, electrolytes, anticoagulation, hemoglobin, temperature, urine output, analgesia, and perfusion pressure. As soon as the child is placed on extracorporeal circulation, the face should be evaluated for venous congestion and distension that can occur with obstruction of venous return through the superior vena cava cannula. The optimal perfusion pressure during bypass is controversial and directly related to the child's temperature-dependent metabolic state, but mean perfusion pressures ranging between 30 and 80 mm Hg are generally acceptable as long as urinary flow remains adequate and metabolic acidosis does not develop. The primary concern is to ensure that adequate perfusion pressures are provided in order to avoid postbypass neurologic sequelae and cognitive deficits.[213–215] Typically, the child's metabolic needs and oxygen requirements decrease about 9% for each 1°C decrease in temperature. However, the lower temperature also increases blood viscosity, which limits peripheral perfusion. An exceptionally low perfusion pressure obtained from a peripheral arterial cannula during bypass should be compared with the central arterial pressure (aorta or femoral) before initiating aggressive therapy.

Following the surgical repair of the cardiac lesion and removal of the aortic cross clamp, occasionally there is a spontaneous return of normal sinus rhythm. Frequently, however, ventricular fibrillation is present requiring electrical conversion. In order to establish a heart rate between 90 and 100 beats per minute, atrial or atrioventricular sequential pacing is required. By the time the core temperature is 34°C and the nasal temperature is 37°C, normal arterial blood gases and electrolytes should be present. Ventilation of the patient is reinstituted at prebypass settings. An early indication of a need for inotropic support is increased intracardiac filling pressures without the concurrent appearance of aortic ejection during partial occlusion of venous return to the extracorporeal circuit. The choice of inotropic support is variable, but the frequent occurrence of right heart failure following cardiopulmonary bypass in congenital heart disease increases the value of inotropic agents with pulmonary vascular dilating effects, such as amrinone[216,217] or isoproterenol. Dopamine is also an effective inotropic agent, especially when urinary output is reduced.[218] When using positive inotropic drugs, it is important to ensure normalization of the pH because inotropic activity is significantly depressed by metabolic acidosis.[219] Hypertensive children can be treated with nitroprusside infusions with favorable results.[220] The importance of maintaining the cardiac index at greater than 2 L/min/m^2 has been shown by the exponential increase in acute cardiac failure and death in children with lower postoperative cardiac indices[221] (Fig 12–2). Anesthesia with myocardial depressant properties should not be reinstituted until the patient has been weaned from cardiopulmonary bypass and hemodynamically stability reestablished. A checklist of important factors to evaluate before weaning from bypass is presented in Table 12–8.

POSTBYPASS CONSIDERATIONS

Heparin Antagonism

After discontinuation of cardiopulmonary bypass, heparin is antagonized with protamine sulfate. Protamine is administered slowly through a peripheral intravenous cannula because calcium chelation by protamine causes peripheral dilation, negative inotropy, and hypotension. Calcium chloride (administered via the central venous

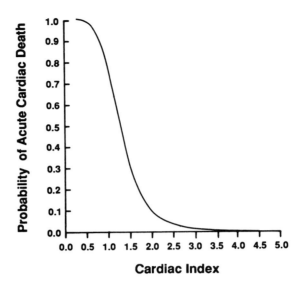

Figure 12–2. There is a direct relationship between postoperative cardiac output and mortality in children following open-heart surgery. As cardiac output falls below 2 L/m^2/min, mortality increases significantly. (*Adapted from Parr G, Blackstone E, Kirklin J: Cardiac performance and mortality early after intracardiac surgery in infants and young children. Circulation 51:867–874, 1975, with permission.*)

cannula) will typically reverse a hypotensive episode secondary to advertent rapid administration of protamine. Some evidence exists that this hypotensive response may be avoided by administration of protamine through the left atrium or through the aorta.[222] Occasionally, anaphylactoid[223] or anaphylactic[224] reactions to protamine are encountered that may necessitate reinstitution of anticoagulation and return to cardiopulmonary bypass.

Protamine alone may be insufficient to provide adequate postoperative hemostasis, especially in children with cyanotic congenital heart disease with preexisting hemostatic derangements.[37,38,225] Dilution of coagula-

TABLE 12–8. CHECKLIST PRIOR TO WEANING FROM CARDIOPULMONARY BYPASS

1. Sinus heart rate of 90–100 beats/min—possible atrial or AV pacing
2. Absence of cardiac arrhythmia (suppression of atrial fibrillation with procainamide infusion or ventricular arrythmia with lidocaine infusion)
3. Reestablishment of ventilation—ensure peak airway pressures are at prebypass levels
4. Nasal temperature over 27° C and core temperature over 34° C
5. Normal electrolytes (especially potassium)
6. Normal arterial blood gases (especially pH and base deficit)
7. Hematocrit greater than 21%
8. Inotropic infusion ready or running depending on the trial of volume loading of the heart
9. Transducers recalibrated and extra transducers ready for direct monitoring from the surgical field
10. Blood and blood products readily available

tion factors by the extracorporeal circuit, platelet destruction by the perfusion apparatus, pulmonary or splenic sequestration of platelets, and initiation of fibrinolytic pathways due to vascular endothelial damage contribute to postbypass hemostatic derangements. Platelet infusions and, occasionally, fresh frozen plasma are necessary. In addition, inhibition of fibrinolysis with ε-aminocaproic acid decreases postbypass blood loss.[226–228]

Temperature Stabilization

In the postbypass period, all children are at risk for developing hypothermia, which leads to acidosis,[229] increased oxygen consumption,[230] and cardiorespiratory depression.[231] Meticulous attention and aggressive intervention should be used to prevent hypothermia. Owing to the larger surface area to body mass ratio, the smaller child is at the greatest risk for significant intraoperative heat loss.[232] The easiest method for ensuring thermal neutrality is to increase the ambient temperature in the operating room, thereby reducing convective heat loss.[230,233] In addition, the use of plastic drapes and blankets conserves heat.[234] Evaporative losses are reduced by humidification of inspired gases. Humidification from a saturation of 25–75% reduces respiratory tract evaporative heat losses by as much as 50%.[231] The use of heating blankets[234] and prewarming of infused intravenous solutions and blood[235] significantly reduces conductive heat loss. Intravenous fluid volumes of 100 mL infused at 5°C reduce the temperature of a 3-kg child by 1°C. Finally, radiant heat losses are controlled both by increasing the ambient temperature[236] and by wrapping the child's head in reflective material. In the intensive care unit, overhead radiant warmers and infrared lamps are very helpful in maintaining normothermia.[237]

Extubation

The decision to extubate a child who has undergone open-heart surgery has to be individualized for each patient based upon the child's age, hemodynamic stability, respiratory reserve, type of operative procedure performed, adequacy of hemostasis, and general medical condition (see Chapter 24). Early extubation, including removal of the endotracheal tube in the operating room, has been advocated,[238,239] but the potential value of early extubation must be weighed against the morbidity asso-

ciated with the stress of another induction and intubation if the child must return to the operating room in the early postoperative period.[240] The first few hours following open-heart surgery are critical for determining cardiac and respiratory stability, as well as the adequacy of hemostasis. A conservative method for extubation at least 2 hours after an open-heart surgical procedure and for timing extubation by specific extubation criteria (Table 12–9) may be the most prudent approach.

REFERENCES

1. Nora J: Etiologic aspects of congenital heart diseases. In Adams FH, Emmanouilides GC, Riemenschneider TA (eds): *Moss' Heart Disease in Infants, Children and Adolescents,* 4th ed. Baltimore: Williams & Wilkins, 1989, pp 15–23
2. Editor: Congenital heart-disease; incidence and aetiology. *Lancet* 2:692–693, 1975
3. Mitchell S, Korones S, Berendes H: Congenital heart disease in 56,109 births. Incidence and natural history. *Circulation* 43:323–332, 1971
4. Fyler D: Report on the New England regional infant cardiac program. *Pediatrics* 65(suppl):376–461, 1980
5. Roberts J: Cardiovascular conditions of children 6–11 years and youth 12–17 years. National Center for Health Survey, U.S. Department of Health, Education, and Welfare, Publication No. (PHS) 78–1653, Series 11, No. 166:1–47, 1978
6. Mehrizipo A, Hirsch M, Taussig H: Congenital heart disease in the neonatal period. Autopsy study of 170 cases. *Pediatrics* 65:721–726, 1964
7. Miller G: Congenital heart disease in the first week of life. *Br Heart J* 36:1160–1166, 1974
8. Veasy LG, Wiedmeier S, Orsmond GS, et al: Resurgence of acute rheumatic fever in the intermountain area of the United States. *N Engl J Med* 316:421–427, 1987
9. Bove E, Behrendt D: Open heart surgery in the first week of life. *Ann Thorac Surg* 29:130–134, 1980
10. Castaneda A, Lamberti J, Sade R, et al: Open heart surgery during the first three months of life. *J Thorac Cardiovasc Surg* 68:719–731, 1974
11. Hickey P, Andersen N: Deep hypothermic circulatory arrest: A review of pathophysiology and clinical experience as a basis for anesthetic management. *J Cardiothorac Anesth* 1:137–155, 1987
12. Egbert L, Battit G, Turndorf H, et al: Value of the preoperative visit by an anesthetist. *JAMA* 185:553–555, 1963
13. Barnes C, Kenny F, Call T, et al: Measurement in management of anxiety of children for open heart surgery. *Pediatrics* 49:250–259, 1972
14. Kilpatrick D, Miller W, Allain A, et al: The use of psychological test data to predict open-heart surgery outcome. A prospective study. *Psychosomat Med* 37:62–73, 1975
15. Kimball CP: Predictive study of adjustment to cardiac surgery. *J Thorac Cardiovasc Surg* 58:891–896, 1969
16. Nadas A, Hauck A: Pediatric aspects of congestive heart failure. *Anesth Analg* 39:466–472, 1960
17. Motoyama E, Cook C: Respiratory physiology. In Smith R (ed): *Anesthesia for Infants and Children,* 4th ed. St Louis: CV Mosby, 1980, pp 38–66

TABLE 12–9. EXTUBATION CRITERIA AFTER OPEN-HEART SURGERY

1. Awake and responsive
2. Good muscle tone with inspiratory pressure of at least −20 mm Hg
3. Cardiac index over 2 L/min/m² on minimal inotropic support
4. Pao₂ over 150 mm Hg on Fio₂ of <0.5
5. Rectal temperature over 36° C
6. Chest drainage less than 1 mL/kg/h

18. Greenwood R, Rosenthal A, Nadas A: Cardiovascular malformation associated with omphalocele. *J Pediatr* **85**:818–821, 1974

19. Greenwood R, Rosenthal A, Nadas R: Cardiovascular abnormalities associated with congenital diaphragmatic hernia. *Pediatrics* **57**:92–97, 1976

20. Friedman S, Saraclar M: The high frequency of congenital heart disease in oculo-auriculovertebral dysplasia (Goldenhar's syndrome). *J Pediatr* **85**:873–874, 1974

21. Rowe R, Uchida I: Cardiac malformation in mongolism. *Am J Med* **31**:726–735, 1961

22. Harris W, Goodman R: Hyper-reactivity to atropine in Down's syndrome. *N Engl J Med* **279**:407–410, 1968

23. Moore R, McNicholas K, Warran S: Atlantoaxial subluxation with symptomatic spinal cord compression in a child with Down's syndrome, *Anesth Analg* **66**:89–90, 1987

24. Shaffer T, Dyment P, Luckstead E, et al: Atlantoaxial instability in Down's syndrome. *Pediatrics* **74**:152–153, 1984

25. Rosenthal A, Button L, Nathan D, et al: Blood volume changes in cyanotic congenital heart disease. *Am J Cardiol* **27**:162–167, 1971

26. Kontras S, Bodenbender J, Craenen J, et al: Hyperviscosity in congenital heart disease. *J Pediatr* **76**:214–220, 1970

27. Replogle R, Meisselman H, Merrill E: Clinical implications of blood rheology studies. *Circulation* **36**:148–160, 1967

28. Gordon R, Ravin M: Rheology and anesthesiology. *Anesthesiology* **57**:252–261, 1978

29. Phornphutkul C, Rosenthal A, Nadas A, et al: Cerebrovascular accidents in infants and children with cyanotic congenital heart disease. *Am J Cardiol* **32**:329–334, 1973

30. Lister G, Hellenbrand W, Kleinman C, et al: Physiologic effects of increasing hemoglobin concentration in left-to-right shunting in infants with ventricular septal defects. *N Engl J Med* **306**:502–506, 1982

31. Rosenthal A, Fyler D: Effect of red cell volume reduction on pulmonary blood flow in polycythemia of cyanotic congenital heart disease. *Am J Cardiol* **33**:410–414, 1974

32. Ravin M, Drury W, Keitt A, et al: Red cell 2,3-diphosphoglycerate in surgical correction of cyanotic congenital heart disease. *Anesth Analg* **52**:599–604, 1973

33. Rosenthal A, Mentzer W, Eisenstein E, et al: The role of red blood cell organic phosphates in adaptation to congenital heart disease. *Pediatrics* **47**:537–547, 1971

34. Goldschmidt B: Fibrinolysis in children with congenital heart-disease (letter). *Lancet* **1**:677, 1969

35. Kontras S, Sirak H, Newton W: Hematologic abnormalities in children with congenital heart disease. *JAMA* **195**:611–615, 1966

36. Colon-Otero G, Gilchrist G, Holcomb G, et al: Preoperative evaluation of hemostasis in patients with congenital heart disease. *Mayo Clin Proc* **62**:379–385, 1987

37. Ekert H, Sheers M: Preoperative and postoperative platelet function in cyanotic congenital heart disease. *J Thorac Cardiovasc Surg* **67**:184–190, 1974

38. Komp D, Sparrow A: Polycythemia in cyanotic heart disease—A study of altered coagulation. *J Pediatr* **76**:231–236, 1970

39. Bull B, Huse W, Brauer F, et al: Heparin therapy during extracorporeal circulation, Part II. *J Thorac Cardiovasc Surg* **69**:685–689, 1975

40. Maurer H, McCue C, Robertson L, et al: Correction of platelet dysfunction and bleeding in cyanotic congenital heart disease by simple red cell volume reduction. *Am J Cardiol* **35**:831–835, 1975

41. Benzing G III, Schubert W, Hug G, et al: Simultaneous hypoglycemia and acute congestive heart failure. *Circulation* **40**:209–216, 1969

42. White R, Moffitt E, Feldt R, et al: Myocardial metabolism in children with heart disease. *Anesth Analg* **51**:6–10, 1972

43. Burrows F, Rabinovitch M: The pulmonary circulation in children with congenital heart disease: Morphologic and morphometric considerations. *Can J Anaesth* **32**:364–373, 1985

44. Jackson K: Psychologic preparation as a method of reducing the emotional trauma of anesthesia in children. *Anesthesiology* **12**:293–300, 1951

45. Naylor D, Coates T, Kan J: Reducing distress in pediatric cardiac catheterization. *Am J Dis Child* **138**:726–729, 1984

46. Nicolson S, Betts E, Jobes D, et al: Comparison of oral and intramuscular preanesthetic medication for pediatric inpatient surgery. *Anesthesiology* **71**:8–10, 1989

47. Goldstein-Dresner M, Davis P, Kretchman E, et al: Double-blind comparison of oral transmucosal fentanyl citrate with oral meperidine, diazepam, and atropine as preanesthetic medication in children with congenital heart disease. *Anesthesiology* **74**:28–33, 1991

48. DeBock T, Davis P, Tome J, et al: Effect of premedication on arterial oxygen saturation in children with congenital heart disease. *J Cardiothorac Anesth* **4**:425–429, 1990

49. Freeman A, Bachman L: Pediatric anesthesia: An evaluation of preoperative medication. *Anesth Analg* **38**:429–432, 1959

50. Cozanitis D, Dundee J, Khan M: Operative study of atropine and glycopyrrolate on suxamethonium induced changes in cardiac rate and rhythm. *Br J Anaesth* **52**:291–293, 1980

51. Wong A, Salem M, Mani M, et al: Glycopyrrolate as a substitute for atropine in reversal of curarization in pediatric cardiac patients. *Anesth Analg* **53**:412–418, 1974

52. Salem M, Wong A, Mani M, et al: Premedicant drugs and gastric juice pH and volume in pediatric patients. *Anesthesiology* **44**:216–219, 1976

53. Hensley F: Premedication for children with congenital heart disease—beneficial or harmful? *J Cardiothorac Anesth* **4**:423–424, 1990

54. Forbes R, Dull D, Murray D, et al: Cardiovascular effects of rectal methohexital in children. *Anesthesiology* **69**:A752, 1986

55. Pilato M, Everts E, Yemen T, et al: Premedication in pediatric outpatient surgery: Comparison of oral midazolam to rectal methohexital. *Anesth Analg* **72**:S214, 1991 (abstr)

56. Maguire H, Webb G, Rees A, et al: Noninvasive evaluation of cardiovascular effects of preoperative sedation in children. *Can J Anaesth* **26**:29–33, 1979

57. Nelson P, Streisand J, Mulder S, et al: Comparison of oral transmucosal fentanyl citrate and an oral solution of meperidine, diazepam and atropine for premedication in children. *Anesthesiology* **70**:616–621, 1989

58. Root B, Loveland J: Pediatric premedication with diazepam or hydroxyzine: Oral vs. intramuscular route. *Anesth Analg* **52**:717–723, 1973

59. Wilton N, Leigh J, Rosen D, et al: Preanesthetic sedation of preschool children using intranasal midazolam. *Anesthesiology* **69**:972–975, 1988

60. Walbergh E, Wills R, Eckhert J: Plasma concentrations of midazolam in children following intranasal administration. *Anesthesiology* **74**:233–235, 1991

61. Spear R, Yaster M, Berkowitz I, et al: Preinduction of anesthesia in children with rectally administered midazolam. *Anesthesiology* **74**:670–674, 1991

62. Feld L, Negus J, White P: Oral midazolam preanesthetic medication in pediatric outpatients. *Anesthesiology* **73**:831–834, 1990

63. Rita L, Seleny F, Muzurek A, et al: Intramuscular midazolam for pediatric preanesthetic sedation: A double-blind controlled study with morphine. *Anesthesiology* **63**:528–531, 1985

64. Feld L, Champeau M, Steennis A, et al: Preanesthetic medication in children: A comparison of oral transmucosal fentanyl citrate versus placebo. *Anesthesiology* **71**:374–377, 1989

65. Henderson J, Brodsky D, Fisher D, et al: Pre-induction of anesthesia in pediatric patients with nasally administered sufentanil. *Anesthesiology* **68**:671–675, 1988

66. Bailey P, Pace N, Ashburg M, et al: Frequent hypoxemia and apnea after sedation with midazolam and fentanyl. *Anesthesiology* **73**:826–830, 1990

67. Stow P, Burrows F, Lerman J, et al: Arterial oxygen saturation following premedication in children with cyanotic congenital heart disease. *Can J Anaesth* **35**:63–66, 1988

68. Carruthers S, Cleland T, Kelly T, et al: Plasma and tissue digoxin concentrations in patients undergoing cardiopulmonary bypass. *Br Heart J* **37**:313–320, 1975

69. Morrison J, Killip T: Serum digitalis and arrhythmia in patients undergoing cardiopulmonary bypass. *Circulation* **47**:341–352, 1973

70. Krasula R, Hastreiter A, Levitsky S, et al: Serum, atrial, and urinary digoxin levels during cardiopulmonary bypass in children. *Circulation* **49**:1047–1052, 1974

71. Schreiner M, Triebwasser A, Keon T: Ingestion of liquids compared with preoperative fasting in pediatric outpatients. *Anesthesiology* **72**:593–597, 1990

72. Cote C: NPO after midnight for children—A reappraisal. *Anesthesiology* **72**:589–592, 1990

73. Moore R: Anesthesia for the pediatric congenital heart patient for noncardiac surgery. *Anesth Rev* **8**:23–29, 1981

74. Moore R: Anesthesia considerations for patients undergoing palliative or reparative operations for congenital heart disease. In Swedlow D, Raphaely R: (eds): *Cardiovascular Problems in Pediatric Critical Care*. New York: Churchill Livingstone, 1986 pp 176–177

75. Jaffe R, Pinto F, Schnittger I, et al: Intraoperative ventilator-induced right-to-left intracardiac shunt. *Anesthesiology* **75**:153–155, 1991

76. Rolf N, Cote C, Liu L, et al: A single-blind study of combined pulse oximetry and capnography in children. *Anesthesiology* **73**:A1125, 1990 (abstr)

77. Patel K, Venus B, Pratap K, et al: Cutaneous PO$_2$ monitoring during pediatric cardiac surgery. *Anesthesiology* **53**:S343, 1980 (abstr)

78. Casthely P, Redko V, Dluzneski J, et al: Pulse oximetry during pulmonary artery banding. *J Cardiothorac Anesth* **1**:297–299, 1987

79. Warnecke I, Bein G, Bucherl E: The relevance of intraoperative pressure and oxygen saturation monitoring during pulmonary artery banding in infancy. *J Cardiothorac Anesth* **3**:31–36, 1989

80. Lindahl S, Yates A, Hatch D: Relationship between invasive and noninvasive measurements of gas exchange in anesthetized infants and children. *Anesthesiology* **66**:168–175, 1987

81. Beusch M, Lenz G, Kottler B: Arterial to end-tidal CO$_2$-gradients in infants and children with cyanotic and acyanotic congential heart disease during cardiac surgery. *J Cardiothorac Anesth* **4**:S128, 1990

82. Badgwell J, Heavner J, May W, et al: End-tidal PCO$_2$ monitoring in infants and children ventilated with either a partial rebreathing or a non-rebreathing circuit. *Anesthesiology* **66**:405–410, 1987

83. Rich G, Sullivan M, Adams M: Is distal sampling of end-tidal CO$_2$ necessary in small subjects? *Anesthesiology* **73**:265–268, 1990

84. Betts E, Downes J, Schaffer D, et al: Retrolental fibroplasia and oxygen administration during general anesthesia. *Anesthesiology* **47**:518–520, 1977

85. Lowenstein E, Little J, Lo H: Prevention of cerebral embolization from flushing radial-artery cannulas. *N Engl J Med* **285**:1414–1415, 1971

86. Gravlee G, Wong A, Adkins T, et al: A comparison of radial, brachial, and aortic pressures after cardiopulmonary bypass. *J Cardiothorac Anesth* **3**:20–26, 1989

87. Gallagher J, Moore R, McNicholas K, et al: Comparison of radial and femoral arterial blood pressures in children after cardiopulmonary bypass. *J Clin Monit* **1**:168–171, 1985

88. Glenski J, Beynen F, Brady J: A prospective evaluation of femoral artery monitoring in pediatric patients. *Anesthesiology* **66**:227–229, 1987

89. Lawless S, Orr R: Axillary arterial monitoring of pediatric patients. *Pediatrics* **84**:273–275, 1989

90. Randel S, Tsang B, Wung J, et al: Experience with percutaneous indwelling peripheral arterial catheterization in neonates. *Am J Dis Child* **141**:848–851, 1987

91. Mitto P, Barankay A, Spath P, et al: Central venous catheterization in infants and children with congenital heart diseases—Experiences with 400 consecutive punctures. *J Cardiothorac Anesth* **3**(suppl 1): 53, 1989

92. Verghese S, Patel R, Hannallah R: Evaluation of two central venous catheterization techniques in children. *Anesthesiology* **71**:A1041, 1989 (abstr)

93. Cote C, Jobes D, Schwartz A, et al: Two approaches to cannulation of a child's internal jugular vein. *Anesthesiology* **50**:371–373, 1979

94. Kanter R, Zimmerman J, Strauss R, et al: Central venous catheter insertion by femoral vein: Safety and effectiveness for the pediatric patient. *Pediatrics* **77**:842–847, 1986

95. Metz R, Lucking S, Chaten F, et al: Percutaneous catheterization of the axillary vein in infants and children. *Pediatrics* **85**:531–533, 1990

96. Moore R, McNicholas K, Naidech H, et al: Clinically silent venous thrombosis following internal and external jugular central venous cannulation in pediatric cardiac patients. *Anesthesiology* **62**:640–643, 1985

97. Introna R, Martin D, Pruett J, et al: Percutaneous pulmonary artery catheterization in pediatric cardiovascular anesthesia. Insertion techniques and use. *Anesth Analg* **70**:562–566, 1990

98. Gold J, Jonas R, Lang P, et al: Transthoracic intracardiac monitoring lines in pediatric surgical patients: A ten-year experience. *Ann Thorac Surg* **42**:185–191, 1986

99. Freed M, Keane J: Cardiac output measured by thermodilution in infants and children. *J Pediatr* **92**:39–42, 1978

100. Moore R, McNicholas K, Gallagher J, et al: Migration of pediatric pulmonary artery catheters. *Anesthesiology* **58**:102–104, 1983

101. Muhiudeen I, Roberson D, Silverman NH, et al: Intraoperative echocardiography in children with congenital cardiac shunt lesions: Comparison of transesophageal and epicardial echocardiography. *Anesthesiology* **73**:A103, 1990 (abstr)

102. Muhiudeen I, Roberson D, Silverman NH, et al: Intraoperative echocardiography in infants & children with regurgitant valvar lesions: Comparison of TEE and epicardial echocardiography. *Anesthesiology* **73**:A104, 1990 (abstr)

103. Greeley W, Ungerleider R, Stanley T, et al: Intraoperative echocardiography and color flow imaging during pediatric cardiovascular anesthesia and surgery. *Anesthesiology* **60**:A778, 1988

104. Ungerleider R, Greeley W, Sheikh K, et al: The use of intraoperative echo with Doppler color flow imaging to predict outcome after repair of congenital cardiac defects. *Ann Surg* **210**:526–534, 1989

105. Jureidini S, Alpert B, Durant R, et al: Two-dimensional echocardiographic assessment of adequacy of pulmonary artery banding. *Pediatr Cardiol* **6**:239–244, 1986

106. Greeley W, Kern F, Ungerleider R, et al: Intramyocardial air causes right ventricular dysfunction after repair of a congenital heart defect. *Anesthesiology* **73**:1042–1046, 1990

107. Burrows F, Hillier S, Mcleod M, et al: Anterior fontanel pressure and visual evoked potentials in neonates and infants undergoing profound hypothermic circulatory arrest. *Anesthesiology* **73**:632–636, 1990

108. Hillier S, Burrows F, Bissonnette B, et al: Cerebral hemodynamics in neonates and infants undergoing cardiopulmonary bypass and profound hypothermic circulatory arrest: Assessment by transcranial doppler sonography. *Anesth Analg* **72**:723–728, 1991

109. Thorsteinsson A, Jonmarker C, Larsson A, et al: Functional residual capacity in anesthetized children: Normal values and values in children with cardiac anomalies. *Anesthesiology* **73**:876–881, 1990

110. Munson E, Bowers D: Effects of hyperventilation on the rate of cerebral anesthetic equilibrium. *Anesthesiology* **28**:377–381, 1967

111. Eger E II: *Anesthetic Uptake and Action.* Baltimore: Williams & Wilkins, 1974, pp 122–145, 146–159.

112. Wessel D, Hickey P, Hansen D: Pulmonary and systemic hemodynamic effects of hyperventilation in infants after repair of congenital heart disease. *Anesthesiology* **67**:A526, 1987 (abstr)

113. Stoelting R, Longnecker D: The effect of right-to-left shunt on the rate of increase of arterial anesthetic concentration. *Anesthesiology* **36**:352–356, 1972

114. Tanner GE, Angers DG, Barash PG, et al: Effect of left-to-right, mixed left-to-right, and right-to-left shunts on inhalational anesthetic induction in children: A computer model. *Anesth Analg* **64**:101–107, 1985

115. Lucero V, Lerman J, Burrows F: Onset of neuromuscular blockade with pancuronium in children with congenital heart disease. *Anesth Analg* **66**:788–790, 1987

116. Laishley R, Burrows FA, Lerman J, Roy WL: Effect of anesthetic induction regimens on oxygen saturation in cyanotic congenital heart disease. *Anesthesiology* **65**:673–677, 1986

117. Seelye E: Anaesthesia for children with congenital heart disease. *Anaesth Intensive Care* **1**:512–516, 1973

118. White P, Way W, Trevor A: Ketamine—Its pharmacology and therapeutic uses. *Anesthesiology* **56**:119–136, 1982

119. Waxman K, Shoemaker W, Lippmann M: Cardiovascular effects of anesthetic induction with ketamine. *Anesth Analg* **59**:355–358, 1980

120. Greeley W, Buchman G, Davis D, et al: Comparative effects of halothane and ketamine on systemic arterial oxygen saturation in children with cyanotic heart disease. *Anesthesiology* **65**:666–668, 1986

121. Hollister G, Burn J: Side effects of ketamine in pediatric anesthesia. *Anesth Analg* **53**:264–267, 1974

122. Levin R, Seleny F, Streczyn M: Ketamine-pancuronium-narcotic technic for cardiovascular surgery in infants—A comparative study. *Anesth Analg* **54**:800–805, 1975

123. Radnay P, Arai T, Nagashima H: Ketamine-gallamine anesthesia for great-vessel operations in infants. *Anesth Analg* **53**:365–369, 1974

124. Hickey P, Hansen D, Cramolini M, et al: Pulmonary and systemic hemodynamic responses to ketamine in infants with normal and elevated pulmonary vascular resistance. *Anesthesiology* **62**:287–293, 1985

125. Aviado D: Regulation of bronchomotor tone during anesthesia. *Anesthesiology* **42**:68–80, 1975

126. Dowdy E, Kaya K: Studies of the mechanism of cardiovascular responses to CI–581. *Anesthesiology* **29**:931–943, 1968

127. Wolfe R, Loehr J, Schaffer M, et al: Hemodynamic effects of ketamine, hypoxia and hyperoxia in children with surgically treated congenital heart disease residing > 1200 meters above sea level. *Am J Cardiol* **67**:874–887, 1991

128. Lowenstein E, Hallowell P, Levine F, et al: Cardiovascular response to large doses of intravenous morphine in man. *N Engl J Med* **281**:1389–1393, 1969

129. Robinson S, Gregory G: Fentanyl-air-oxygen anesthesia for ligation of patent ductus arteriosus in preterm infants. *Anesth Analg* **60**:331–334, 1981

130. Collins C, Koren F, Crean P, et al: Fentanyl pharmacokinetics and hemodynamic effect in preterm infants during ligation of patent ductus arteriosus. *Anesth Analg* **64**:1078–1080, 1985

131. Koren G, Goresky G, Crean P, et al: Pediatric fentanyl dosing based on pharmacokinetics during cardiac surgery. *Anesth Analg* **63**:577–582, 1984

132. Newland M, Leuschen P, Sarafian L: Fentanyl intermittent bolus technique for anesthesia in infants and children undergoing cardiac surgery. *J Cardiothorac Anesth* **3**:407–410, 1989

133. Hickey P, Hansen D, Wessel D, et al: Blunting of stress responses in the pulmonary circulation of infants by fentanyl. *Anesth Analg* **64**:1137–1142, 1985

134. Ellis D, Steward D: Fentanyl dosage is associated with reduced blood glucose in pediatric patients after hypothermic cardiopulmonary bypass. *Anesthesiology* **72**:812–815, 1990

135. Anand K, Hansen D, Hickey P: Hormonal-metabolic stress responses in neonates undergoing cardiac surgery. *Anesthesiology* **73**:661–670, 1990

136. Anand KJS, Hickey PR: Halothane-morphine compared with high dose sufentil for anesthesia and postoperative analgesia in neonatal cardiac surgery. *N Engl J Med* **326**:1–9, 1992

137. Murat I, Levron J, Berg A, et al: Effects of fentanyl on baroreceptor reflex control of heart rate in newborn infants. *Anesthesiology* **68**:717–722, 1988

138. Hickey P, Hansen D: Fentanyl- and sufentanil-oxygen-pancuronium anesthesia for cardiac surgery in infants. *Anesth Analg* **63**:117–124, 1984

139. Moore R, Yang S, McNicholas K, et al: Hemodynamic and anesthetic effects of sufentanil as the sole anesthetic for pediatric cardiovascular surgery. *Anesthesiology* **62**:725–731, 1985

140. Hollander J, Hennis P, Burm A, et al: Alfentanil in infants and children with congenital heart defects. *J Cardiothorac Anesth* **2**:12–17, 1988

141. Kern F, Ungerleider R, Jacobs J, et al: Computerized continuous infusion of intravenous anesthetic drugs during pediatric cardiac surgery. *Anesth Analg* **72**:487–492, 1991

142. Murray D, Forbes R, Murphy K, et al: Nitrous oxide: Cardiovascular effects in infants and small children during halothane and isoflurane anesthesia. *Anesth Analg* **67**:1059–1064, 1988

143. Hensley F, Larach D, Martin D, et al: The effect of halothane/nitrous oxide/oxygen mask induction on arterial hemoglobin saturation in cyanotic heart disease. *J Cardiothorac Anesth* **1**:289–296, 1987

144. Barankay A, Spath P, Mitto P, et al: Sufentanil–nitrous oxide/oxygen versus halothane–nitrous oxide/oxygen anesthesia in children undergoing cardiac surgery. Hemodynamics and plasma catecholamines. *Anaesthesist* **38**:391–396, 1989

145. Goldberg A, Sohn Y, Phear W: Direct myocardial effects of nitrous oxide. *Anesthesiology* **37**:373–380, 1972

146. Murray D, Mehta M, Forbes R, et al: Additive contribution of nitrous oxide to halothane MAC in infants and children. *Anesth Analg* **71**:120–124, 1990

147. Salanitre E, Rackow H: The pulmonary exchange of nitrous oxide and halothane in infants and children. *Anesthesiology* **30**:388–394, 1969

148. Lappas D, Buckley M, Laver M, et al: Left ventricular performance and pulmonary circulation following addition of nitrous oxide to morphine during coronary-artery surgery. *Anesthesiology* **43**:61–69, 1975

149. Wong K, Martin W, Hornbein T, et al: Cardiovascular effects of morphine sulfate with oxygen and with nitrous oxide in man. *Anesthesiology* **38**:542–549, 1973

150. Thorburn J, Smith G, Vance J, et al: Effect of nitrous oxide on the cardiovascular system and coronary circulation of the dog. *Br J Anaesth* **51**:937–942, 1979

151. Haggendal O, Linder E, Nordstrom G: The haemodynamic effects of nitrous oxide anaesthesia on systemic and pulmonary circulation in dogs. *Acta Anaesth Scand* **20**:429–436, 1976

152. Heerdt P, Caldwell R: The mechanism of nitrous oxide-induced changes in pulmonary vascular resistance in a dog model of left atrial outflow obstruction. *J Cardiothorac Anesth* **3**:568–573, 1989

153. Schulte-Sasse U, Hess W, Tarnow J: Pulmonary vascular responses to nitrous oxide in patients with normal and high pulmonary vascular resistance. *Anesthesiology* **57**:9–13, 1982

154. Hilgenberg J, McCammon R, Stoelting R: Pulmonary and systemic vascular responses to nitrous oxide in patients with mitral stenosis and pulmonary hypertension. *Anesth Analg* **59**:323–326, 1980

155. Barash P, Glanz S, Katz J, et al: Ventricular function in children during halothane anesthesia. *Anesthesiology* **49**:79–85, 1978

156. Merin R, Kumazawa M, Luka N: Myocardial function and metabolism in the conscious dog and during halothane anesthesia. *Anesthesiology* **44**:402–415, 1976

157. Krane E, Su J: Comparison of the effects of halothane on newborn and adult rabbit myocardium. *Anesth Analg* **66**:1240–1245, 1987

158. Lerman J, Oyston J, Gallagher T, et al: The minimum alveolar concentration (MAC) and hemodynamic effects of halothane, isoflurane, and sevoflurane in newborn swine. *Anesthesiology* **73**:717–721, 1990

159. Brandom B, Brandom R, Cook D: Uptake and distribution of halothane in infants: In vivo measurements and computer simulations. *Anesth Analg* **62**:404–410, 1983

160. Wolf W, Neal M, Peterson M: The hemodynamic and cardiovascular effects of isoflurane and halothane anesthesia in children. *Anesthesiology* **64**:328–333, 1986

161. Boudreaux P, Schieber R, Cook D: Hemodynamic effects of halothane in the newborn piglet. *Anesth Analg* **63**:731–737, 1984

162. Gregory G, Eger E II, Munson E: The relationship between age and halothane requirement in man. *Anesthesiology* **30**:488–491, 1969

163. Nicodemus H, Nassiri-Rahimi C, Bachman L, et al: Median effective doses (ED_{50}) of halothane in adults and children. *Anesthesiology* **31**:344–348, 1969

164. Friesen R, Lichtor J: Cardiovascular depression during halothane anesthesia in infants: A study of three induction techniques. *Anesth Analg* **61**:42–45, 1982

165. Miller B, Friesen R: Oral atropine premedication in infants attenuates cardiovascular depression during halothane anesthesia. *Anesth Analg* **67**:180–185, 1988

166. Johnston R, Eger E II, Wilson C: Comparative interaction of epinephrine with enflurane, isoflurane and halothane in man. *Anesth Analg* **55**:709–712, 1976

167. Moore R, McNicholas K, Gallagher J, et al: Halothane metabolism in acyanotic and cyanotic patients undergoing open heart surgery. *Anesth Analg* **65**:1257–1262, 1986

168. Eger E II, Smith N, Stoelting R, et al: Cardiovascular effects of halothane in man. *Anesthesiology* **32**:396–409, 1970

169. Morgan P, Lynn A, Parrot C, et al: Hemodynamic and metabolic effects of two anesthetic techniques in children undergoing surgical repair of acyanotic congenital heart disease. *Anesth Analg* **66**:1028–1030, 1987

170. Lindahl S, Dyke R, Abel M, et al: Congenital heart malformations and uptake of isoflurane. *Anesthesiology* **69**:A737, 1988 (abstr)

171. Friesen R, Lichtor J: Cardiovascular effects of inhalation induction with isoflurane in infants. *Anesth Analg* **62**:411–414, 1983

172. Murat I, Lapeyre G, Saint-Maurice C: Isoflurane attenuates baroreflex control of heart rate in human neonates. *Anesthesiology* **70**:395–400, 1989

173. Palmisano B, Clifford P, Coon R, et al: Depression of the heart rate component of the arterial baroreflex by halothane and isoflurane in growing piglets. *Anesthesiology* **71**:A1029, 1989 (abstr)

174. Goudsouzian N: Maturation of neuromuscular transmission in the infant. *Br J Anaesth* **52**:205–214, 1980

175. Churchill-Davidson H, Wise R: Neuromuscular transmission in the newborn infant. *Anesthesiology* **24**:271–278, 1963

176. Goudsouzian N, Donlon J, Savarese J, et al: Reevaluation of dosage and duration of action of d-tubocurarine in the pediatric age group. *Anesthesiology* **43**:416–425, 1975

177. Churchill-Davidson H, Wise R: Response of the newborn infant to muscle relaxants. *Can J Anaesth* **11**:1–5, 1964

178. Craythorne N, Turndorf H, Dripps R: Changes in pulse rate and rhythm associated with the use of succinylcholine in anesthetized children. *Anesthesiology* **21**:465–470, 1960

179. Leigh M, McCoy D, Belton M, et al: Bradycardia following intravenous administration of succinylcholine chloride to infants and children. *Anesthesiology* **18**:698–702, 1957

180. Weintraub H, Heisterkamp D, Cooperman L: Changes in plasma potassium concentration after depolarizing blockers in anaesthetized man. *Br J Anaesth* **41**:1048–1052, 1969

181. Bennett E, Bowyer D, Giesecke A, et al: Pancuronium bromide: A double blind study in children. *Anesth Analg* **52**:12–18, 1973

182. Geha D, Rozelle B, Raessler K, et al: Pancuronium bromide enhances atrioventricular conduction in halothane-anesthetized dogs. *Anesthesiology* **46**:342–345, 1977

183. Maunuksela E, Gattiker R: Use of pancuronium in children with congenital heart disease. *Anesth Analg* **60**:798–801, 1981

184. Cohen N: Hemodynamic effects of pancuronium in critically ill children. *Anesthesiology* **53**:S159, 1980 (abstr)

185. Sloan M, Lerman J, Bissonnette B: Pharmacodynamics of high-dose vecuronium in children during balanced anesthesia. *Anesthesiology* **74**:656–659, 1991

186. Eldadah M, Newth C: Vecuronium by continuous infusion for neuromuscular blockade in infants and children. *Crit Care Med* **17**:989–992, 1989

187. Fisher D, Canfell P, Spellman M, et al: Pharmacokinetics and pharmacodynamics of atracurium in infants and children. *Anesthesiology* **73**:33–37, 1990

188. Pittet J, Tassonyi E, Morel D, et al: Pipecuronium-induced neuromuscular blockade during nitrous oxide-fentanyl, isoflurane, and halothane anesthesia in adults and children. *Anesthesiology* **71**:210–213, 1989

189. Sarner J, Brandom B, Dong M, et al: Clinical pharmacology of pipecuronium in infants and children during halothane anesthesia. *Anesth Analg* **71**:362–366, 1990

190. Emmott R, Bracey B, Goldhill DR, et al: Cardiovascular effects of doxacurium, pancuronium and vecuronium in anaesthetized patients presenting for coronary artery bypass surgery. *Br J Anaesth* **65**:480–486, 1990

191. Stoops C, Curtis C, Kovach D, et al: Hemodynamic effects of doxacurium chloride in patients receiving oxygen sufentanil anesthesia for coronary artery bypass grafting or valve replacement. *Anesthesiology* **69**:365–370, 1988

192. Glenski J, Friesen R, Berglund N, et al: Comparison of the hemodynamic and echocardiographic effects of sufentanil, fentanyl, isoflurane, and halothane for pediatric cardiovascular surgery. *J Cardiothorac Anesth* **2**:147–155, 1988

193. Epstein R: Humidification during positive-pressure ventilation of infants. *Anesthesiology* **35**:532–536, 1971

194. Bissonnette B, Sesser D, LaFlamme P: Passive and active inspired gas humidification in infants and children. *Anesthesiology* **71**:350–354, 1989

195. Committee on retrolental fibroplasia: Retrolental fibroplasia. *Pediatrics* **57** (suppl):591–642, 1976

196. Friesen R, Lichtor J: Cardiovascular depression during halothane anesthesia in infants; a study of three induction techniques. *Anesth Analg* **61**:42–45, 1982

197. Kalina R, Hodson A, Morgan B: Retrolental fibroplasia in a cyanotic infant. *Pediatrics* **50**:765–768, 1972

198. Robertie P, Butterworth J, Dudas L, et al: Impaired calcium mobilization in children undergoing cardiopulmonary bypass. *Anesthesiology* **73**:A1137, 1990 (abstr)

199. Mikawa K, Maekawa N, Goto R, et al: Effects of exogenous intravenous glucose on plasma glucose and lipid homeostasis in anesthetized children. *Anesthesiology* **74**:1017–1022, 1991

200. Zuker H, Nicolson S, Steven J, et al: Blood glucose concentrations during anesthesia in children undergoing hypothermic circulatory arrest. *Anesthesiology* **69**:A739, 1988 (abstr)

201. Lanier W, Strangland K, Scheithauer B, et al: The effects of dextrose infusion and head position on neurologic outcome after complete cerebral ischemia in primates: Examination of a model. *Anesthesiology* **66**:39–48, 1987

202. Stewart D, DaSilva C, Flegel T: Elevated blood glucose levels may increase the danger of neurological deficit following profoundly hypothermic cardiac arrest. *Anesthesiology* **68**:653, 1988 (letter to editor)

203. Sieber F, Smith D, Traystman R, et al: Glucose: A reevaluation of its intraoperative use. *Anesthesiology* **67**:71–81, 1987

204. Greeley W, Stanley T, Ungerleider R, et al: Intraoperative hypoxemic spells in tetralogy of Fallot: An echocardiographic analysis of diagnosis and treatment. *Anesth Analg* **68**:815–819, 1989

205. Oshita S, Uchimoto R, Oka H, et al: Correlation between arterial blood pressure and oxygenation in tetralogy of Fallot. *J Cardiothorac Anesth* **3**:597–600, 1989

206. Baele P, Rennotte M, Veyckemans F: External compression of the abdominal aorta reversing tetralogy of Fallot cyanotic crisis. *Anesthesiology* **75**:146–149, 1991

207. Shaddy R, Judd V, McGough E: Continuous intravenous phenylephrine infusion for treatment of hypoxemia spells in tetralogy of Fallot. *J Pediatr* **114**:468–470, 1989

208. Ponce F. Williams L, Webb H, et al: Propranolol palliation of tetralogy of Fallot: Experience with long term drug treatment in pediatric patients. *Pediatrics* **52**:100–108, 1973

209. Nussbaum J, Zane E, Thys D: Esmolol for the treatment of hypercyanotic spells in infants with tetralogy of Fallot. *J Cardiothorac Anesth* **3**:200–202, 1989

210. Bull B, Korpman R, Huse W, et al: Heparin therapy during extracorporeal circulation, Part I. *J Thorac Cardiovasc Surg* **69**:674–684, 1975

211. Young J, Kisker C, Doty D: Adequate anticoagulation during cardiopulmonary bypass determined by activated clotting time and the appearance of fibrin monomer. *Ann Thorac Surg* **26**:231–240, 1978

212. Ross W, Lake C, Wellons H: Cardiopulmonary bypass complicated by inadvertent carotid cannulation. *Anesthesiology* **54**:85–86, 1981

213. Ferry P: Neurologic sequelae of cardiac surgery in children. *Am J Dis Child* **141**:309–312, 1987

214. Newburger J, Silbert A, Buckley L, et al: Cognitive function and age at repair of transposition of the great arteries in children. *N Engl J Med* **310**:1495–1499, 1984

215. Bellinger D, Wernovsky G, Rappaport L, et al: Cognitive development of children following early repair of transposition of the great arteries using deep hypothermic circulatory arrest. *Pediatrics* **87**:701–707, 1991

216. Hess W: Effects of amrinone on the right side of the heart. *J Cardiothorac Anesth* **3**:38–44, 1989

217. Goenen M, Pedemonte O, Baele P, et al: Amrinone in the management of low cardiac output after open heart surgery. *Am J Cardiol* **56**:33B–38B, 1985

218. Lang P, Williams R, Norwood W, et al: The hemodynamic effects of dopamine in infants after corrective cardiac surgery. *J Pediatr* **96**:630–634, 1980

219. Friedman W: The intrinsic physiologic properties of the developing heart. *Prog Cardiovasc Dis* **15**:87–111, 1972

220. Appelbaum A, Blackstone E, Kouchoukos N, et al: Afterload reduction and cardiac output in infants early after intracardiac surgery. *Am J Cardiol* **39**:445–451, 1977

221. Parr G, Blackstone E, Kirklin J: Cardiac performance and mortality early after intracardiac surgery in infants and young children. *Circulation* **51**:867–874, 1975

222. Aris A, Solanes H, Bonnin J, et al: Intraaortic administration of protamine: Method for heparin neutralization after cardiopulmonary bypass. Cardiovascular diseases. *Bull Texas Heart Inst* **8**:23, 1981

223. Ullman D, Bloom B, Danker P, et al: Protamine-induced hypotension in a two-year-old child. *J Cardiothorac Anesth* **2**:497–499, 1988

224. Moorthy S, Pond W, Rowland R: Severe circulatory shock following protamine (an anaphylactic reaction). *Anesth Analg* **59**:77–78, 1980

225. Colon-Otero G, Gilchrist G, Holcomb G, et al: Preoperative evaluation of hemostasis in patients with congenital heart disease. *Mayo Clin Proc* **62**:379–385, 1987

226. Brodsky I, Gill D, Lusch C: Fibrinolysis in congenital heart disease. Preoperative treatment with ε-aminocaproic acid. *Am J Clin Pathol* **51**:51–57, 1969

227. Lambert C, Marengo-Rowe A, Leveson J, et al: Treatment of postperfusion bleeding using ε-aminocaproic acid, cryoprecipitate, fresh frozen plasma, and protamine sulfate. *Ann Thorac Surg* **28**:440–444, 1979

228. McClure P, Izsak J: Use of epsilon-aminocaproic acid to reduce bleeding during cardiac bypass in children with congenital heart disease. *Anesthesiology* **40**:604–608, 1974

229. Gandy G, Adamson K, Cunningham N, et al: Thermal environment and acid-base homeostasis in human infants during the first few hours of life. *J Clin Invest* **43**:751–758, 1964

230. Hey E, Katz G: The optimum thermal environment for naked babies. *Arch Dis Child* **45**:328–335, 1970

231. Berry F, Hughes-Davies D, DiFazio C: A system for minimizing respiratory heat loss in infants during operation. *Anesth Analg* **52**:170–175, 1973

232. Adamsons K, Towell M: Thermal homeostasis in the fetus and newborn. *Anesthesiology* **26**:532–548, 1965

233. Adamsons K, Gandy G, James L: Influence of thermal factors upon oxygen consumption of the newborn human infant. *J Pediatr* **66**:495–508, 1965

234. Goudsouzian N, Morris R, Ryan J: The effects of a warming blanket on the maintenance of body temperatures in anesthetized infants and children. *Anesthesiology* **39**:351–353, 1973

235. Roe C, Stantulli T, Blair C: Heat loss in infants during general anesthesia and operations. *J Pediatr Surg* **1**:266–274, 1966

236. Bennett E, Patel K, Grundy E: Neonatal temperature and surgery. *Anesthesiology* **46**:303–304, 1977

237. Shimn W, Halford P: Method for maintaining the neonate's intraoperative core temperature. *Surgery* **75**:416–420, 1974

238. Barash P, Lescovich F, Katz J: Early extubation following pediatric cardiothoracic operation: A viable alternative. *Ann Thorac Surg* **29**:228–233, 1980

239. Schuller J, Bovill J, Nijveld A, et al: Early extubation of the trachea after open heart surgery for congenital heart disease. *Br J Anesth* **56**:1101–1108, 1984

240. Glenn J, Don H, Ebert P, et al: Tracheal extubation after cardiac surgery in children. *Anesthesiology* **53**:S158, 1980 (abstr)

Chapter 13 | Septal and Endocardial Cushion Defects

John R. Cooper, Jr.

Pathologic communications between the atria, ventricles, or both result from defects in the interatrial (ASD) or interventricular (VSD) septa or endocardial cushions. Although the lesions are discussed here as isolated defects, these anomalies often accompany other congenital cardiac lesions resulting in pathophysiology different from that of isolated defects.

ATRIAL SEPTAL DEFECTS

Anatomic Types

Ostium secundum, patent foramen ovale, and sinus venosus are the anatomic types of ASDs. The interatrial septum can also be entirely absent. The embryology of these defects is discussed in Chapter 3.

Patent Foramen Ovale. In most patients, this type of ASD is an incidental finding, although its incidence is quite high. For example, in 40% of patients undergoing repair of VSD, a patent foramen ovale (PFO) was found.[1] PFO results from lack of fusion between the septum primum and secundum and has pathophysiologic significance in only two instances: (1) it may provide a route for air in the right atrium to enter the left atrium, and (2) it may allow significant right-to-left shunting in postoperative patients with high right-sided pressures such as after right ventriculotomy.[2] For this reason, many surgeons routinely examine the atrial septum during intracardiac operations and close a PFO if found (see Fig 13–1).

Ostium Secundum. Ostium secundum is the most common type (80%) of ASD[3](Fig 13–1). It results from resorption of the septum primum either in an abnormal manner, producing a fenestrated opening, or on the dorsal edge, producing a short septum primum that

cannot close the foramen ovale. In addition, defective (short) septum secundum development will not allow a normal septum primum to close the foramen ovale. Very large ASDs may result from a combination of both processes.[4]

Sinus Venosus. This rare defect is located high in the atrial septal wall above the fossa ovalis close to the junction of the superior vena cava and right atrium (see Fig 13–1). It results from (1) abnormal development of the septum secundum; (2) failure of the sinus venosus, the primitive venous collecting chamber, to be absorbed into the atrial wall; (3) a combination of both. Sinus venosus defects are almost always accompanied by partial anomalous pulmonary venous return with the right superior pulmonary vein entering the right atrium at the junction of the superior vena cava and right atrium.

Common Atrium. Failure of the atrial septum to develop entirely or a confluence of different types of ASDs will produce a single atrial chamber. At times, a single atrium is also associated with endocardial cushion defects.

Pathophysiology

The primary pathologic process present in all septal defects is the shunting of blood from one cardiac chamber to another. The degree and direction of shunting depends on two factors: (1) the relative compliance of the two cardiac chambers involved and (2) the area of the defect. Compliance of the atria or ventricles is the more important factor because it represents the filling resistance of each chamber. In the first few weeks of life, wall thickness and chamber compliance are essentially equal, so little shunting occurs. As the infant ages, pulmonary vascular resistance decreases, the right ventricular wall thins, and blood tends to shunt from left to right. Obvi-

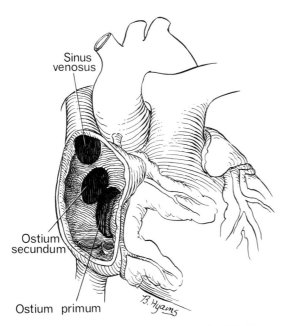

Figure 13–1. Atrial septal defects. (*From Cooley DA, Norman JC: Techniques in Cardiac Surgery. Houston: Texas Medical Press, 1975, p 19 with permission.*)

ously, the larger the area of the defect, the greater the volume of shunted blood.

As a result of left-to-right shunt, pulmonary blood flow increases. Small to moderate increases in pulmonary flow are usually well tolerated (pulmonary flow/systemic flow ratio (Qp/Qs <1.5). When Qp/Qs is greater than 3, symptoms of fatigue, dyspnea, and right heart failure due to volume overload appear. This process is usually insidious in onset and may not be manifest until adulthood. With large defects, symptoms occur in early infancy. Increased pulmonary blood flow increases pulmonary artery pressure and pulmonary vascular resistance (PVR) gradually increases. When PVR increases, right ventricular hypertrophy develops with a further increase in pulmonary pressures and decrease in the volume of the left-to-right shunt. Eventual equalization of ventricular pressures occurs with bidirectional shunting, and, finally, with severe pulmonary vascular hypertension, the shunt reverses to right-to-left pattern leading to cyanosis. The cyanotic phase of this process is called the Eisenmenger syndrome and is considered inoperable.

Surgical closure of septal defects is intended to halt this progression. In patients with elevated pulmonary artery pressures, the increased pulmonary vascular resistance may be primarily flow dependent and hence reversible by surgical therapy. However, in patients with fixed (irreversible) pulmonary vascular resistance, closure of the defect may precipitate acute right heart failure and death. The process of shunt reversal is basically the same for all isolated septal defects, although the rate

of progression varies. Progression is slow in patients with ASDs and rapid in those with complete AV canal. The rate of progression in patients with VSDs varies directly with the size of the defect.

Natural History

Unlike VSDs, ASDs do not often close spontaneously. Small, hemodynamically insignificant ASDs have no effect on life span, although there is a small increase in the risk of bacterial endocarditis and paradoxical embolization. Larger defects are usually well tolerated into adulthood, although an occasional infant with a large ASD will develop significant congestive failure. The effects of left-to-right shunting and right ventricular volume overload do not usually manifest themselves until the third decade of life. Similarly, pulmonary vascular changes do not develop early. About 14% of adult patients will develop congestive heart failure and another 20% will have dysrhythmias[3] and may have significantly shortened life spans.[5] With increasing age, the incidence of significant pulmonary vascular disease gradually increases, with a rare patient progressing to the Eisenmenger syndrome. Conversely, some elderly patients with large defects may not develop elevated pulmonary vascular resistance, yet very young patients may. This suggests that processes other than elevated pulmonary blood flow may be operative in these patients.[6]

Diagnostic Features

Patients with uncomplicated ASD are relatively asymptomatic. Young children may have frequent respiratory infections, whereas older children and adults complain of fatigue and dyspnea. On physical examination, heart size and rhythm are normal, but there is a systolic murmur, maximal at the pulmonic area, and fixed splitting of the second heart sound. A tricuspid flow murmur results from relative tricuspid stenosis secondary to the increased tricuspid valve flow accompanying left-to-right shunting.

Incomplete right bundle branch block is often present on the electrocardiogram (ECG). If pulmonary hypertension is present, the ECG may present evidence of right ventricular hypertrophy. Increased peripheral pulmonary vascularity and cardiac enlargement may be present on the chest radiograph of patients with large defects and left-to-right shunting. Echocardiography provides a noninvasive means of detecting ASDs and assessing accompanying physiologic changes. Transthoracic echocardiography has at least an 89% sensitivity for primum and secundum defects but is less helpful for sinus venosus types.[7]

On cardiac catheterization, intracardiac pressures are usually normal, but an increase in oxygen saturation occurs at the atrial level. A small systolic gradient across the pulmonary outflow tract results from increased shunt flow (Table 13–1). Additional evidence for shunting can be obtained by hydrogen catheter or dye dilution

TABLE 13–1. CARDIAC CATHETERIZATION FINDINGS IN SEPTAL DEFECTS

	Chamber	Pressure (mm Hg)	Oxygen Saturation (96)
Atrial septal defects	SVC	2	63
	RA	2	83
	RV	26/3	83
	PA	23/8	83
	PWP	3	98
	SA	108/66	95
Ventricular septal defects	SVC	2	63
	RA	2	62
	RV: High	60/2	75
	Low	60/2	85
	PA	55/25	88
	PWP	8	90
	SA	90/60	95

Abbreviations: SVC, superior vena cava; RA, right atrium; RV, right ventricle; PA, pulmonary artery; PWP, pulmonary wedge pressure; SA, systemic artery.

methods. The site of the defect is demonstrable by angiography, but increasing numbers of patients with secundum defects undergo surgery based on diagnostic echocardiography if no additional defects are apparent.[8]

The diagnostic features change dramatically when patients develop right-to-left shunting through an ASD. These patients have cyanosis and clubbing. Because of pulmonary hypertension, the pulmonic component of the second sound is increased and a decrescendo diastolic murmur of pulmonic regurgitation may be present. Right ventricular hypertrophy, enlargement of the main pulmonary artery, and increased lung markings are present on the chest radiograph. Cardiac catheterization documents the increased right ventricular and pulmonary artery pressures.

Anesthesia and Perioperative Care

The guidelines for premedication, monitoring, induction, and intraoperative management are applicable to all types of septal defects.

Premedication. The goal of premedication in patients with septal defects is no different from premedication for other cardiac or general surgery patients—a well-sedated, cooperative patient with maintenance of cardiovascular and respiratory stability. Oral, rectal, or intramuscular drugs may be used depending upon patient condition, patient preference, degree of patient cooperation, and proposed surgical procedure. Pentobarbital, 2–4 mg/kg, by mouth or per rectum, 2 hours before operation plus meperidine, 2 mg/kg, or morphine, 0.1 mg/kg, and scopolamine, 0.1 mg, intramuscularly, 1 hour before oper-

ation produce reliable sedation and hypnosis. In patients under 1 year of age, and in patients with significant degrees of heart failure or low cardiac output, dosage is reduced or, at times, eliminated. Cyanosis in patients with an isolated septal defect indicates shunt reversal, a late stage of the disease, a potentially inoperable lesion, and the necessity for caution with premedication.

Induction Techniques. Most patients with septal defects have a left-to-right shunt that tends to decrease induction time of moderately soluble inhalation agents such as halothane. Because shunted blood recirculated through the lungs will be partially saturated with the anesthetic agent, alveolar concentration will increase more rapidly, speeding induction. Concentration of insoluble agents such as nitrous oxide are little influenced by this mechanism and induction is not accelerated. Intravenous agents are said to have a slower onset of effect because of the additional dilution by recirculating blood. The anesthesiologist can compensate for the shunt by increasing the concentration of intravenous agent, albeit at the risk of overdosage. These factors, although real, have little clinical importance during induction of anesthesia when compared with other factors such as adequacy of premedication and maintaining adequate ventilatory volume.

The induction technique in patients with left-to-right shunts is not critical and can be guided by patient's desires, degree of cooperation, or presence of a preinduction intravenous infusion. Patients with infusions in place or who prefer intravenous induction can be safely induced with thiopental, 2–4 mg/kg, or other intravenous induction drugs followed by succinylcholine or pancuronium for neuromuscular blockade prior to intubation. In patients with more advanced disease (pulmonary hypertension with right heart failure), fentanyl, 5–10 μg/kg, or ketamine, 1–2 mg/kg, can be substituted for thiopental for intravenous induction. After induction, inhalational agents are added as the clinical situation warrants.

Smaller children usually require an inhalational induction and halothane remains the most widely used and satisfactory agent for this purpose. Adequate premedication in these patients facilitates induction without struggling. After placement of ECG leads and a blood pressure cuff, 50% N$_2$O and oxygen is begun followed by the addition of halothane 0.5%. Halothane is increased in 0.5% increments every three breaths up to 3–4% if the clinical response permits, although 2% or less is usually sufficient with spontaneous respiration. Once assisted ventilation is started, inspired concentration should be decreased to prevent overdosage. After induction, an intravenous infusion can be started and a muscle relaxant administered before tracheal intubation. If securing intravenous access is difficult, as may be the case in infants, intramuscular administration of succinyl-choline (4 mg/kg) plus atropine (0.005 mg/kg) is useful. After intubation, a further decrease in the inspired concentration allows blood pressure to increase to facilitate arterial cannula insertion. Most patients for elective repair of septal defects are anesthetized in this fashion because operation usually occurs before school age.

Infants are also anesthetized with an inhalational technique if stable. However, most infants presenting for correction have moderate heart failure and an intravenous infusion preoperatively, so an intravenous induction technique is utilized.

Inhalation techniques with potent agents have a theoretical disadvantage of decreasing cardiac output and systemic vascular resistance and potentially reversing the left-to-right shunt. Shunt reversal usually does not occur in the absence of marked pulmonary hypertension and right ventricular hypertrophy. If pulmonary vascular obstructive disease and/or right heart failure are present, an intravenous technique or intramuscular ketamine, 8 mg/kg, are substituted to allow intravenous cannulation.

Monitoring. Basic monitoring for ASD or VSD repair is the same as for most other major cardiovascular procedures: electrocardiogram, blood pressure (invasive and noninvasive), pulse oximetry, capnography, central venous pressure, temperature, urine output, and laboratory analysis of arterial blood gases and electrolytes. Central venous pressure is a good guide to fluid therapy. However, it can be misleading in at least two circumstances: (1) after right ventriculotomy, right heart pressures tend to be high because of compromised right ventricular function and normal left ventricular function, and (2), after closure of an ASD, left atrial pressures are temporarily higher than right atrial pressures. Left atrial cannulas may be useful in some instances but are not needed routinely. Pulmonary artery catheters for measurement of pressure or cardiac output are used in some centers but have not gained wide acceptance because of problems with insertion in small children, displacement during cannulation or repair, the possibility of crossing the septal defect, cost, and an unknown value in affecting outcome.

Use of intraoperative echocardiography has increased in popularity recently and is routine in some centers for specific operations. Both transesophageal and epicardial probes are employed. Its primary purpose in repair of septal defects is to detect significant residual shunting, as well as assessment of ventricular and/or valvular function.[9]

Management of Cardiopulmonary Bypass. The prebypass and extracorporeal circulation considerations in patients with septal defects are no different from those for patients undergoing repair of other types of congenital heart defects. In infants or small children, the surgeon may elect to use deep hypothermia with circulatory arrest to repair an AV canal or a large VSD. Preparation for deep hypothermia and circulatory arrest involves extra pharmacologic preparations and equipment for surface and core cooling.

Air Embolism. In any patient with abnormal communication between the right and left heart, there is always a hazard of an embolus, air or particulate, reaching the left heart and being ejected into the systemic circulation, particularly to the cerebral circulation. Because the volume of air required to produce cerebral infarction is unknown, avoidance of all air is the goal.

The most common source of air is the intravenous tubing, including side ports, tubing connections, and stopcocks. Bubbles tend to adhere to sites where there is a change in lumen diameter. Before starting the infusion, the tubing should be rechecked because small bubbles may come out of solution and coalese during no flow, especially in a warm operating room for a pediatric patient. Meticulous care prevents introduction of bubbles during attachment of tubing to catheters and injection of drugs.

A second potential source of air emboli is cannulation of the right atrium for cardiopulmonary bypass. If the central venous pressure is low, air may be entrained into the atrium when the venous cannula is inserted. Positive airway pressure during insertion may help to prevent air entrainment. After venous cannulas are in place and filled with blood and attached to the common venous inflow, air may appear in the "Y" connector. Before bypass, this air can flow back to the patient if the caval cannulas are not clamped. If an inexperienced surgical assistant removes the caval clamps while the common venous line is still clamped, air will be sucked back into the right atrium if central venous pressure is low and a "paradoxical" embolus may occur. Close observation during cannulation of the great vessels by the anesthesiologist and surgical team prevents this surgical misadventure.

Air is always present in the cardiac chambers when any one cardiac chamber has been opened for surgical repair of a septal defect. Many methods are used to remove this air before natural circulation is restored but no method completely removes all air.[2]

SURGICAL THERAPY

Because of the late sequelae of ASD, operative closure is recommended, preferably at 4 or 5 years before the patient starts to school. Closure is also recommended for older patients, but repair after age 41 is associated with a decrease in long-term survival compared with those repaired prior to this age.[10]

The surgical approach is through a standard midline sternotomy with conventional ascending aorta and selective caval cannulation for extracorporeal circulation. The right atrium is opened longitudinally and the defect closed with a synthetic plastic or pericardial patch. Simple suture closure is used if the opening is small. In patients with sinus venosus defects, the anomalous pulmonary venous drainage is corrected by placing the patch so that the opening of the pulmonary vein is on the left atrial side.

Results of operation are uniformly good with very low mortality in uncomplicated cases.[8, 11] The major postoperative complication is supraventricular dysrhythmia related perhaps to atriotomy, with the incidence of dysrhythmia increasing with the age of the patient. Conduction disturbances may occur, especially if suturing was near the coronary sinus and bundle of His. If the patient also has pulmonary vascular disease, surgical morbidity and mortality is increased.

After closure of ASD, overtransfusion may be a special problem in the early postoperative period and can lead to pulmonary edema. Typically, an acute increase in left atrial pressure and a decrease in right atrial pressure follows closure of ASD.[12] These disparate pressures can make transfusion based on central venous pressure hazardous and consideration should be given to left atrial pressure monitoring in patients at special risk. Residual defects are an infrequent complication.

Transcatheter ASD Closure

Closure of ASDs with devices delivered by a cardiac catheter, although still experimental, are becoming more successful. Because of the relatively large delivery system, application is limited by the size and location of the defect and size of the patient.[13–15] General anesthesia may or may not be utilized, but the potential for embolization of the device demands full surgical team availability.

Postoperative Care

Prosthetic or pericardial patch closure of an uncomplicated ASD is usually curative. Extubation can be performed in the operating room or early postoperative period. However, transient, or occasionally permanent, conduction system abnormalities may be present.

ATRIOVENTRICULAR CANAL DEFECTS

Anatomic Types

Atrioventricular canal defect lesions consist of two types: partial AV canal, or ostium primum (see Fig 13–1), and complete AV canal, or atrioventricularis communis (Fig 13–2). A high incidence of the Down syn-

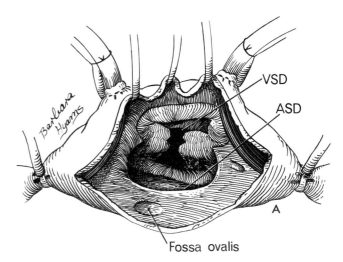

Figure 13–2. Views of complete atrioventricular canal from right atrium. (*From Cooley DA, Norman JC: Techniques in Cardiac Surgery. Houston: Texas Medical Press, 1975, with permission.*)

drome is associated with both partial and complete AV canal.

Partial AV Canal. Partial AV canal results from failure of the septum primum to fuse with the endocardial cushions. This is usually associated with a cleft in the anterior leaflet of the mitral valve causing mitral regurgitation and increasing left-to-right shunting. The jet of blood from the incompetent valve is usually directed into the right atrium, predisposing to early development of cardiac failure. The basal (upper) portion of the ventricular septum is also absent but no interventricular communication exists because the AV valves are fused to the lower portion of the ventricular septum. Some patients with low-volume shunts may remain asymptomatic for decades and are similar to patients with secundum ASDs. Few of these patients develop pulmonary hypertension. Patients with large shunts develop significant pulmonary hypertension early in life and a large number are symptomatic in infancy. These children need early surgical intervention.

Complete AV Canal. Complete AV canal is caused by failure of fusion of the septum primum with the cushions and in addition failure of the cushions themselves to fuse. The result is an interatrial communication, an interventricular communication, a cleft in the mitral valve, and an abnormal tricuspid valve. Further classification on the basis of specific valvular anomalies is beyond the scope of this chapter. Systemic pressures in both ventricles, large left-to-right shunts, and early onset of pulmonary hypertension with symptoms of cardiac failure are present. Significant pulmonary vascular changes tend to develop quickly but are usually reversible up to age 2 years.

Pathophysiology

The pathophysiology of atrioventricular canal defects is shunting at atrial, ventricular, or both sites with or without associated atrioventricular valvular regurgitation (see earlier discussion of shunting).

Natural History

The course of patients with AV canal defects depends on the degree of valvular incompetence, the shunt volume, and the rapidity of onset of pulmonary vascular changes. In Kirklin's series, 5% of patients with partial AV canals required surgical intervention by 1 year, 30% by 4 years, and 50% by age 10.[16] By contrast, 30% of patients with complete AV canals required operation by 1 year and 70% by 2 years. In the past, surgical therapy for complete AV canal consisted of early pulmonary artery banding followed by total correction at an older age. Because of improved results with primary repair in infants and small children compared with the staged operation,[17] most centers currently favor primary correction, although banding still has its advocates.[18]

Diagnostic Features

In primum ASD, there is widely fixed splitting of the second heart sound. Both systolic and diastolic murmurs may be present resulting from the septal defect, mitral regurgitation, and excessive flow. On chest radiograph, the heart is enlarged with left atrial enlargement in primum ASD or mitral regurgitation. Right atrial and ventricular enlargement are present on ECG. Echocardiography may be used to diagnose canal-type lesions with high accuracy, but cardiac catheterization is almost always performed to identify the defect more specifically and to assess pulmonary vascular resistance.

In ostium primum defect, the low-lying position of the catheter as it passes from the right to left atrium is pathognomonic. With complete AV canal, a catheter easily passes into all four cardiac chambers. An increase in oxygen saturation is present at atrial and/or ventricular levels. The left ventricular angiogram is particularly helpful in the diagnosis because the outflow tract is narrow and elongated (the gooseneck deformity), whereas the right ventricular border appears ragged owing to the cleft mitral valve.

Anesthesia and Perioperative Management

The principles of anesthetic management of patients with AV canal defects are similar to those with atrial or ventricular septal defects. Avoidance of air embolism or shunt alteration are the primary goals in the prebypass period. Deep hypothemia with low pump flow or profound hypothermia with circulatory arrest are used by some surgeons during intracardiac repair. Postbypass maneuvers to reduce pulmonary vascular resistance and reduce left ventricular afterload if mitral regurgitation is present may be required.

Surgical Therapy

The surgical approach is by right atriotomy during cardiopulmonary bypass. The valve defects are repaired by suturing the cleft and then the ASD and VSD (if present) are closed by a patch. The repaired valves often need to be suspended from the patch.[19]

Mortality after surgical therapy in recently operated patients was less than 1% in uncomplicated ostium primum defects and 4% in patients with associated mitral valve incompetence.[20] In patients with complete AV canals, surgical mortality ranged from 5% to 13%,[20,21] again depending on the degree of valvular dysfunction.

Postoperative Care

Prominent problems after repair include conduction disturbances, valvular incompetence, and low cardiac output requiring vasoactive drug support. Contributing to the low cardiac output is persistent pulmonary hypertension or intermittent pulmonary vasospasm with right ventricular failure. Patients with postoperative pulmonary hypertension are difficult management problems and experience increased mortality rates.

VENTRICULAR SEPTAL DEFECTS

Anatomic Types

Ventricular septal defect (VSD) is the most common isolated congenital heart defect, constituting 20% of all such defects. One common classification is based on anatomic location.[22] Type I (Fig 13–3), or supracristal defects (5% of all VSDs),[23] are located above the crista supraventricularis just under the annulus of the aorta. Because of this location, the right coronary cusp of the aortic valve may lack support and prolapse into the defect causing aortic regurgitation that may be hemodynamically significant. Type II, or infracristal defects (80% of all VSDs)[23], are lower in the membranous septum beneath the crista supraventricularis.[23] Both type I and II defects result from partial or complete failure of fusion of the endocardial cushion to the aorticopulmonary septum and muscular ventricular septum. Type III, or "canal-type," defects (11% incidence)[23] are equivalent to the VSD that accompanies complete AV canal. They result from partial failure of the endocardial cushions to fuse. Type IV, or muscular, defects (2–7% incidence),[4,23] probably result from excessive resorption of septal tissue during the muscular septal formation. They may be located anywhere in the muscular septum and may be multiple ("Swiss cheese" defect).

Pathophysiology

Like the lesions discussed earlier, pathophysiologic effects of VSD include shunting, pulmonary hypertension, and heart failure due to volume overload.

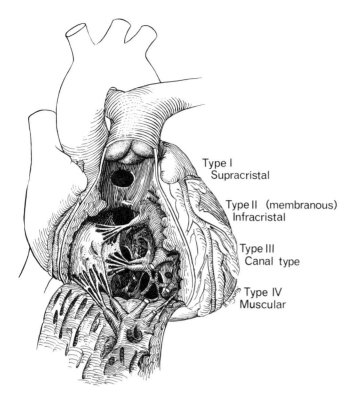

Figure 13–3. Classification of ventricular septal defects. (*From Cooley DA, Norman JC: Techniques in Cardiac Surgery. Houston: Texas Medical Press, 1975, with permission.*)

Natural History

The natural course of patients with VSDs varies largely with the size of the defect, the magnitude of the resultant shunt, and the age of the patient at onset, and degree of pulmonary hypertension. In 20 to 50% of patients, the defects close spontaneously, especially if the defect is small and in the muscular septum. This usually occurs by age 5.[24]

If the VSD is small (restrictive) with low shunt flow, there is thought to be no decrease in life expectancy except in patients who contract bacterial endocarditis. Closure of VSDs for the sole purpose of preventing endocarditis is controversial and many physicians do not recommend it. Larger VSDs with high left-to-right shunt (nonrestrictive) lead to symptoms from pulmonary hypertension and early congestive failure. If mild, symptoms may be controlled medically and may decrease with increasing age if the VSD decreases in size relative to the rest of the heart or closes spontaneously. Severely symptomatic patients may require surgical treatment in infancy. In the past, because of a high surgical mortality in small patients, pulmonary artery banding was often done initially to reduce pulmonary artery flow and "protect" the pulmonary circulation followed by closure of the VSD at age 3 or 4.[23] Although staged operation is still done in patients with VSD accompanied

by other defects, such as aortic coarctation or pulmonary disease, definitive repair of the defect in infancy is preferred when patients with isolated defects are symptomatic. Surgical closure of septal defects prevents the progression of pulmonary vascular disease to the stage of shunt reversal. Even in patients with elevated pulmonary artery pressures, the increased pulmonary vascular resistance may be reversed with surgical therapy. However, in patients with fixed pulmonary vascular resistance, closure of the defect may precipitate acute right heart failure and death.

Diagnostic Features

Patients with small VSDs have a systolic murmur at the third or fourth left intercostal space. The second heart sound is normally split but is accentuated only with large defects. Cyanosis is absent unless left-to-right shunting is present. Although the chest radiograph is normal with small defects, large defects cause left atrial enlargement, cardiomegaly, right ventricular hypertrophy, and increased pulmonary vascularity. The ECG is normal with small defects, but there are signs of right or biventricular hypertrophy with large defects. Left atrial enlargement causes broad P waves on ECG. Except for small muscular defects, echocardiography has good sensitivity and specificity for the detection of VSDs, especially with employment of color flow Doppler techniques. However, cardiac catheterization remains an integral part of a complete evaluation in selected patients. Shunting at the ventricular level is apparent on catheterization with a step-up in oxygen saturation at the ventricular level. Left ventricular angiography is usually the definitive portion of the examination. Measurement of pulmonary artery pressures and calculation of resistance and changes in either shunting or pulmonary vascular resistance to intervention are also important. Typical catheterization findings are in Table 13–1.

Anesthesia and Perioperative Management

Care of patients with ventricular septal defects follows the principles previously outlined. The presence of heart failure or the use of right ventriculotomy for repair may preclude the use of volatile anesthetics with myocardial depressant properties.

Surgical Therapy

The operation may be performed through the right atrium, the right ventricle, or the left ventricle. The right atrial approach through the tricuspid value is commonly used for membranous defects. Supracristal lesions usually require a right ventriculotomy, and muscular defects, especially if low in the septum and multiple, are best approached through a left apical ventriculotomy.

Infant mortality after VSD closure ranges from 5 to 10%[1] and is lower than the mortality following the two-stage approach with initial pulmonary artery banding. In older patients with isolated uncomplicated defects, mortality now approaches 1%.[25]

Recently, transcatheter closure of VSDs has been attempted with some success as a substitute for surgical therapy[26] or in conjunction with it for repair of complex defects.[27] The impact of these techniques on patient management, which are restricted by delivery system and patient size, is unknown.

Postoperative Care

The major postoperative complication of VSD repair is heart block from injury to conduction tissue. Either the AV node or bundle of His may be injured depending on the location of the defect. Transient block from edema secondary to suturing may appear later in intensive care and temporary atrial and ventricular pacing electrodes should be placed in all patients. In patients with ventriculotomies, temporary inotropic support may be required postoperatively.

Hemodynamically significant residual shunting occurs in 6–10% of patients and may result from an additional undetected defect, especially in the muscular septum, or a leak in the suture line.[28] These events can be diagnosed by intraoperative color flow Doppler or contrast echocardiography.

In most children with uncomplicated ventricular septal defects, endotracheal extubation can be performed in the operating room or early in the intensive care unit. More complicated septal defects or patients with pulmonary hypertension should not be extubated early. Many of these patients require vasoactive drugs for treatment of right ventricular failure or conduction defects. Isoproterenol, sodium nitroprusside, nitroglycerin, or other vasodilators are used to decrease pulmonary artery pressure and to reduce the mitral regurgitation occurring after repair of clefts in the mitral leaflets. Intravenous isoproterenol is also useful to convert heart block occurring after bypass to sinus or atrial rhythm.

ACKNOWLEDGMENT

The author is indebted to Arthur S. Keats, M.D., for his review of this manuscript.

REFERENCES

1. Doty DB, Lamberth WC: Repair of ventricular septal defects. *World J Surg* **9**:516–521, 1985
2. Rodigas PC, Meyer FJ, Haasler GB, et al: Intraoperative 2-dimensional echocardiography: Ejection of microbubbles from the left ventricle after cardiac surgery. *Am J Cardiol* **50**:1130–1132, 1982
3. Behrendt DM: Atrial septal defect. In Arciniegas E (ed): *Pediatric Cardiac Surgery*. Chicago: Year Book Medical, 1985, p 133
4. Moore KL: *The Developing Human*. Philadelphia: WB Saunders, 1982, p 320–323
5. Campbell M: Natural history of atrial septal defects. *Br Heart J* **32**:820–926, 1970
6. Vick WG, Titus JL: Defects of the atrial septum including the atrioventricular canal. In Garson A, Bricker JT, McNamara DG (eds): *The Science and Practice of Pediatric Cardiology*. Philadelphia: Lea & Febiger, 1990, p 1028
7. Shub C, Dimopoulos IN, Seward JB, et al: Sensitivity of 2-dimensional echocardiography in the direct visualization of atrial septal defect utilizing the subcostal approach: Experience with 154 patients. *J Am Coll Cardiol* **2**:127–135, 1983
8. Freed MD, Nadas AS, Norwood WI, et al: Is routine preoperative cardiac catheterization necessary before repair of secundum and sinus venosus atrial septal defects? *J Am Coll Cardiol* **4**:333–336, 1984
9. Ungerleider RM, Greeley WJ, Sheikh KH, et al: The use of intraoperative echo with Doppler color flow imaging to predict outcome after repair of congenital cardiac defects. *Ann Surg* **210**:526–534, 1989
10. Murphy JG, Gersh BJ, McGoon MD, et al: Long-term outcome after surgical repair of isolated atrial septal defect. *N Engl J Med* **323**:1645–1650, 1990
11. Shub C, Tajik AJ, Seward JB, et al: Surgical repair of uncomplicated atrial septal defect without "routine" preoperative cardiac catheterization. *J Am Coll Cardiol* **6**:49–54, 1985
12. Sondergard T, Paulsen PK: Some immediate consequences of closure of atrial septal defects of the secundum type. *Circulation* **69**:905–913, 1984
13. Mullins CE. Therapeutic cardiac catheterization. In Garson A, Bricker JT, McNamara DG (eds): *The Science and Practice of Pediatric Cardiology*. Philadelphia: Lea & Febiger, 1990, pp 2207–2208
14. Mills NW, King TD: Nonoperative closure of left to right shunts. *J Thorac Cardiovasc Surg* **72**:371–378, 1976
15. Borow KM, Karp R: Atrial septal defect. *N Engl J Med* **323**:1698–1700, 1990
16. Kirklin JW, Barratt-Boyes BG: *Cardiac Surgery*. New York: John Wiley & Sons, 1986, p 567
17. Berger TJ, Kirklin JW, Blackstone EH, et al: Primary repair of complete antrioventricular canal in patients less than 2 years old. *Am J Cardiol* **41**:906–913, 1978
18. Silverman N, Levitsky S, Fisher E, et al: Efficacy of pulmonary artery banding in infants with complete atrioventricular canal. *Circulation* **68**(suppl II): II-148–II-153, 1983
19. Cooley DA, Norman JC: *Techniques in Cardiac Surgery*. Houston, Texas Medical Press, 1975 pp 77, 89
20. Studer M, Blackstone EH, Kirklin JW, et al: Determinants of early and late results of repair of atrioventircular septal (canal) defects. *J Thorac Cardiovasc Surg* **84**:523–542, 1982
21. Castaneda A, Mayer JE, Jonas RA: Repair of complete atrioventricular canal in infancy. *World J Surg* **9**:590–597, 1985
22. Becu LM, Fontana RS, DuShave JW, et al: Anatomic and pathologic studies in ventricular septal defect. *Circulation* **14**:649, 1956
23. Hallman GL, Cooley DA: *Surgical Treatment of Congenital Heart Disease*. Philadelphia: Lea & Febiger, 1975, p 108

24. Wells WJ, Lindesmith GG: Ventricular septal defect. In Arciniegas E (ed): *Pediatric Cardiac Surgery*. Chicago: Year Book Medical, 1985, p 144

25. Rizzoli G, Blackstone EH, Kirklin JW, et al: Incremental risk factors in hospital mortality after repair of ventricular septal defect. *J Thorac Cardiovasc Surg* **80**:494–500, 1980

26. Lock JE, Block PC, McKay RG, et al: Transcatheter closure of ventricular septal defects. *Circulation* **78**:361–368, 1988

27. Bridges ND, Perry SB, Keane JF, et al: Preoperative transcatheter closure of congenital muscular ventricular septal defects. *N Engl J Med* **324**:1312–1317, 1991

28. Vincent RN, Lang P, Chipman CW, et al: Assessment of hemodynamic status in the intensive care unit immediately after closure of ventricular septal defect. *Am J Cardiol* **55**:526–529, 1985

Chapter 14 | Tetralogy of Fallot

Paul N. Samuelson and William A. Lell

Tetralogy of Fallot occurs in approximately 15% of infants with congenital heart disease. There is about an equal incidence in females and males and no specific correlation as to genetic etiology or associated causative conditions except perhaps a slightly greater incidence in offspring of parents having tetralogy of Fallot (1.5% versus those without [0.1%]) of all live births.[1,2]

ANATOMY

The tetralogy of Fallot is a name applied to a complex of anatomic malformations characterized by underdevelopment of the right ventricular infundibulum and displacement of the infundibular septum resulting in right ventricular outflow stenosis or atresia and a large ventricular septal defect (VSD) usually in the subaortic position, and with the aortic origin overriding the right ventricle (Fig 14–1).[3,4] However, there is a wide variation in this basic anatomic morphology, diverse and variable pathophysiology, clinical signs and symptoms, and multiple surgical methods of therapy.

The multiple structural variations from the classic anatomic description of the tetralogy of Fallot create a spectrum of pathophysiologic sequelae and clinical presentations. The critical determinant is the degree of obstruction to pulmonary blood flow (Fig 14–2).

Although almost all patients with tetralogy of Fallot have right ventricular infundibular narrowing, obstruction may also occur at the pulmonary valve, the pulmonary valve annulus, the main pulmonary artery, the bifurcation of the pulmonary artery, the proximal branches of the pulmonary artery, and the distal branches of the pulmonary artery. Pulmonary atresia with absence of the main pulmonary artery is considered by Kirklin and others to be a variant of the tetralogy of Fallot, whereas others would consider it to be type IV truncus arteriosus.[5] This semantic controversy does not influence the technique of surgical repair.[5]

Narrowing of the right ventricular infundibulum may occur at low, intermediate, or high positions in the infundibular chamber. The infundibulum may also be diffusely narrowed or, in a few instances, of normal size. The pulmonary valve is stenotic in about 75% of the cases of tetralogy and bicuspid in approximately two thirds.[6] In addition, the leaflets of the pulmonary valve are often thickened and the commissures fused. The pulmonary valve may, in fact, be atretic in up to 25% of autopsy patients and 7% of surgical patients.[1] The pulmonary valve annulus is at times the major site of obstruction and in tetralogy of Fallot is most commonly smaller than the aortic annulus. The main pulmonary artery trunk is frequently smaller than the aorta. Both of these relationships are reversed from normal.

In tetralogy of Fallot with pulmonary stenosis, the combination of infundibular and valvular stenosis occurs in the majority of cases (74%), with isolated infundibular stenosis in 26% of the cases.[4] When pulmonary atresia exists, there must be collateral circulation to the lungs provided by systemic to pulmonary artery anastomoses such as the ductus arteriosus or bronchopulmonary collaterals.

Narrowing and malformations at the pulmonary artery bifurcation or at the origins of the right and left pulmonary arteries are more common in patients with tetralogy of Fallot with pulmonary atresia than those with pulmonary stenosis; however, they may occur in both conditions and must be recognized preoperatively.[5] Extreme variations of pulmonary artery anatomy may result in the absence of the pulmonary artery, discontinuity of the right and left pulmonary arteries, or discontinuity of the origin of either of the pulmonary arteries. In some rare instances, there may be complete absence of a left or right pulmonary arterial system, with the lung totally perfused by collateral circulation.

The VSD in classic tetralogy of Fallot is subaortic and usually large. It is separated from the pulmonary valve by the crista supraventricularis and the common atrioventricular bundle of the conduction system lies

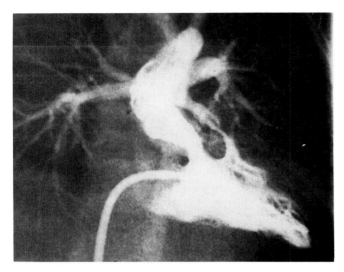

Figure 14–1. Classic tetralogy of Fallot with severe infundibular and annular stenosis. (*Courtesy of L.M. Bargeron, MD*)

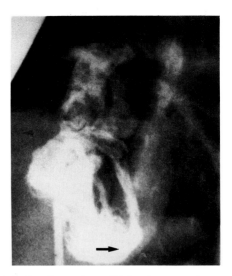

Figure 14–3. Classic tetralogy of Fallot demonstrating an additional apical ventricular septal defect on angiogram with injection into the right ventricle. (*Courtesy of L.M. Bargeron, MD*)

along its inferior margin. In 3–15% of patients with tetralogy of Fallot, there may be additional VSDs, usually of the muscular type (Fig 14–3).[7] The aorta arises from both ventricles and is more anterior than normal, usually with about 50% of the orifice overriding the right ventricle. The terminology of "double-outlet right ventricle" with pulmonary stenosis is used by some when aortic overriding exceeds 50–80%. Partial "transposition of the great arteries" implies continuity between the anterior leaflet of the mitral valve and the aortic valve.

A right aortic arch is present in 25% of patients with tetralogy of Fallot. This influences the ability to perform early palliative systemic-pulmonary artery anastomoses. Furthermore, in 10% of the cases of right aortic arch, there is an aberrant left subclavian artery arising from the distal aorta and passing anterior to the esophagus.[4]

The right ventricular wall thickness is similar to that of the left ventricle unless the VSD is restrictive. The coronary arteries are usually large, tortuous, and with a large infundibular branch of the right coronary artery. There is anomalous origin of the anterior descending coronary artery from the right coronary artery in about 5% of the patients. More rarely, the right coronary artery may originate from the left coronary artery passing across the right ventricular outflow tract. Thus, coronary artery anatomy influences the surgical repair of tetralogy of Fallot.[7]

ASSOCIATED ANOMALIES

Patent ductus arteriosus (4.0%), multiple VSDs (2.4%), complete atrioventricular canal (2.2%), partial anomalous pulmonary venous drainage (1.0%), and dextrocardia (1.0%) are the major associated cardiac anomalies occurring in patients undergoing surgical repair of tetralogy of Fallot.[4] Aortic incompetence occurs infrequently in young patients with tetralogy of Fallot, but may be related to cardiomyopathy, endocarditis, or coexisting natural or surgical systemic-pulmonary artery shunts in older patients. Minor associated cardiac disorders include atrial septal defect (9%), persistent left superior vena cava (8%), and anomalous origin of the left anterior de-

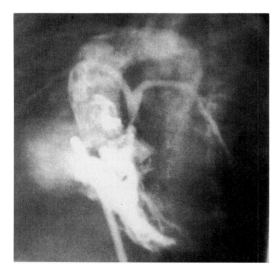

Figure 14–2. Tetralogy of Fallot with diffusely hypoplastic pulmonary arteries in an infant. (*Courtesy of L.M. Bargeron, MD*)

scending coronary artery from the right coronary artery (4%). All of the above anatomic variations may influence in one way or another the pathophysiologic presentation and surgical repair.

PATHOPHYSIOLOGY

The most frequent consequence of the combination of obstruction to pulmonary blood flow and a large VSD is right-to-left shunting and thus systemic desaturation presenting as cyanosis. Except when there is a restrictive VSD, the right and left ventricles work at essentially identical pressure during systole. The left ventricular output is determined by the pulmonary venous return and the right-to-left shunted blood. The degree of right-to-left shunting is determined by the amount of obstruction to pulmonary blood flow at the infundibulum, pulmonary valve annulus, and pulmonary vasculature. Although this obstruction is relatively "fixed," there are "reactive" factors that can alter the amount of right-to-left shunting. A decrease in pulmonary vascular resistance lowers the right ventricular pressures reducing right-to-left shunting.[8,9] Decreases in systemic vascular resistance may increase right-to-left shunting and cyanosis. Cyanosis is detected earlier and to a greater degree in patients with pulmonary atresia as opposed to those with pulmonary stenosis. The presence of native systemic-pulmonary collateral blood flow may ameliorate the cyanosis.

The body compensates for the hypoxemia secondary to the obstruction to pulmonary blood flow primarily by pulmonary collateral circulation and polycythemia. Except in patients with pulmonary atresia, hypoxia is usually not a problem early in infancy. However, with closure of the ductus arteriosus or with increasing "spasm" of the infundibulum, hypoxic "spells" may occur. Hyperviscosity is not generally a problem until the hematocrit exceeds 65%.

"Tet Spells"

"Spells" or episodes of paroxysmal hyperpnea occur in 20–70% of patients with a peak frequency at age 2–3 months of age. The spells are usually initiated by crying, feeding, or defecation. Although the etiology is uncertain, spells are probably initiated by events that result in increased oxygen demand associated with decreasing arterial PaO and pH and increasing Paco. This leads to hyperventilation, increased venous return, increased right-to-left shunting, and further decreases in PaO and pH.[10] As the hypoxia continues, systemic vascular resistance further decreases and the right-to-left shunt increases. Some suggest that, in fact, the spells may be initiated or exacerbated by infundibulum hypercontractility or "spasm." There is some support for this in certain patients who seem to benefit from propranolol therapy.[11,12] Episodes of paroxysmal hyperpnea have been successfully terminated with intravenous sodium bicarbonate presumably owing to correction of the peripheral metabolic acidosis and thus a return to more normal systemic vascular resistance. Phenylephrine has been successful in treating these episodes by increasing the systemic vascular resistance and decreasing the right-to-left shunt. Also, morphine and general anesthesia have been associated with improvement in arterial oxygen saturation, presumably by central depression of the hyperpneic response. Squatting, characteristically exhibited by children with tetralogy of Fallot, results in a decrease in arterial blood flow to the legs and thus an effective increase in systemic vascular resistance. There is also a decrease in venous blood return from the legs and therefore a lesser amount of desaturated blood returned to the heart and less right-to-left shunting.[13,14] Interestingly, the natural history of spells is that of a decrease in frequency and severity after 2–3 years whether or not surgery is performed. Presumably this is due to anatomic and physiologic adaptation of the patient to chronic hypoxia.

NATURAL HISTORY

The natural history of patients with tetralogy of Fallot is variable and mainly determined by the degree of right ventricular and pulmonary artery outflow obstruction. Twenty-five percent of untreated infants born with tetralogy of Fallot and pulmonary stenosis die in the first year of life, 40% by four years, 70% by 10 years, and 95% by 40 years of age.[4] It is interesting that approximately 25% of patients born with tetralogy of Fallot and pulmonary stenosis are acyanotic for a number of weeks until the obstruction to pulmonary blood flow increases, usually as a result of hyperactivity of the infundibular area and/or closure of the ductus arteriosus. Increasing arterial oxygen desaturation, cyanosis, and polycythemia occur. There is a gradual increase in the incidence of pulmonary artery thrombosis, cerebral artery thrombosis, and cerebral abscesses increasing with age. Late deaths in adulthood in untreated tetralogy of Fallot are usually the result of chronic congestive heart failure secondary to cardiomyopathy following chronic right ventricular hypertrophy and hypoxia and/or anatomically and functionally induced aortic valve insufficiency.[5,15–18]

Infants born with tetralogy of Fallot and pulmonary *atresia* have a greater likelihood of dying than those with pulmonary stenosis. Early deaths are usually the result of hypoxia related to spontaneous closure of the ductus arteriosus, and 50% of the untreated patients die in the first year, 75% by 3 years, and 92% by 10 years.[4,5]

There is a special subset of patients with tetralogy

of Fallot who have naturally occurring large pulmonary blood flow via collaterals and, although not completely palliative, these patients remain less cyanotic and live longer. Later deaths are usually due to congestive heart failure with or without aortic insufficiency.

DIAGNOSTIC FEATURES

In order to formulate and conduct a safe, smooth, and efficient anesthetic in patients with tetralogy of Fallot, a thorough knowledge of the patients' anatomic defects and their pathophysiologic responses to those defects must be obtained. It is necessary to know which compensatory mechanisms, including pharmacotherapy, the patients are utilizing to deal with their pathologic lesions. Knowledge of the above as well as the cardiovascular effects of the anesthetic and adjuvant agents will allow the anesthesiologist to care for these patients safely.[19]

History, Physical Examination, and Laboratory Findings

The history of the patient's illness with regard to frequency and severity of cyanotic episodes will help to quantify the degree of pulmonary outflow obstruction present. Physical appearance of the patient as well as laboratory data, peripheral oxygen saturation, and hematocrit will add to this knowledge. Polycythemia will be present in the cyanotic patient. The platelet count may also be decreased. The chest radiograph shows a small or normal-sized heart with a dominant right ventricle and concave pulmonary artery segment (see Fig 5–3). Right ventricular hypertrophy and right axis deviation are seen on electrocardiogram. Of course, a thorough knowledge of the planned surgical procedure will allow one to tailor the anesthetic approach appropriately.

Cardiac Catheterization

Data obtained at cardiac catheterization, including angiocardiography and echocardiography, are essential in guiding the surgical and anesthetic management of the patient with tetralogy of Fallot. The measured peripheral oxygen saturation aids in the assessment of the degree of obstruction of pulmonary blood flow. Calculation of the pulmonary vascular resistance during administration of oxygen, tolazoline, or nitroglycerin indicates whether the pulmonary vascular resistance is "fixed" or, in fact, "reactive." The ratio of the pulmonary blood flow to systemic blood flow, or at least some angiographic documentation of the right-to-left and left-to-right shunting, will help to quantify the degree of pulmonary outflow obstruction. The pressure in the right ventricle will usually be similar to that in the left ventricle. However, the systolic pressure gradient across the right ventricular infundibulum to the pulmonary artery is useful in assessing the postoperative "capacity" of the pulmonary vasculature.

Angiography and Echocardiography. Extensive and exacting angiographic and echocardiographic representation of the cardiac and vascular anatomy is essential to the handling of patients with tetralogy of Fallot.[20,21] It is very important to know the site(s) of pulmonary outflow obstruction (any combination of pulmonary infundibulum, pulmonary valve, pulmonary annulus, proximal and distal pulmonary arteries). VSDs must be documented. The source and amount of pulmonary blood flow (ie, bronchopulmonary collaterals, patent ductus arteriosus, surgically created systemic pulmonary artery shunts) must be defined. Angiography should demonstrate the patency and any potential problems with previously created shunts. If narrowing or kinking of the native pulmonary artery exists, extensive surgical correction may be necessary. Angiography is also useful in documenting and quantifying concomitant anomalies (see above) that may change the surgical repair of the tetralogy of Fallot from "simple" to "complex." In addition, angiography should document the position and structure of the aortic arch as well as potential abnormal origins or distribution of the subclavian or coronary arteries. The possibility of aortic regurgitation, especially in older patients with tetralogy, can be evaluated as well as contractility of the ventricles, both right and left. Although tricuspid regurgitation is unusual, it may be present in patients older than 10–15 years of age.

ANESTHETIC AND PERIOPERATIVE MANAGEMENT

Interventional Catheterization

During interventional catheterization procedures, general anesthesia with ketamine may be used in the pediatric cardiac catheterization laboratory.[22–24] The patients are premedicated with pentobarbital, 6–8 mg/kg, morphine, 0.1 mg, and scopolamine, 0.01 mg/kg. The patients are induced with either intramuscular ketamine, 4 mg/kg, or intravenous ketamine, 1–2 mg/kg. In the older patients, ketamine is supplemented with intravenous midazolam as required.[25] In infants (< 1 month, weighing <4 kg) or seriously ill children, elective oral tracheal intubation is carried out with the aid of vecuronium. Patients are ventilated with air unless they are extremely cyanotic. This allows appropriate oxygen saturation data to be obtained during the catheterization. During the closed palliative procedure, patients are ventilated with 100% oxygen. If the closed procedure is potentially difficult, elective endotracheal intubation may be utilized even in the older patients.

Palliative Procedures

Anesthetic management for these closed surgical procedures is similar to that for the "open" surgical repairs.[26] In the severely cyanotic infant, anesthetic induction is with intramuscular or intravenous ketamine, fentanyl, or sufentanil. In less severely cyanotic patients, an inhalation induction with halothane is carried out. When an intravenous route is obtained, supplemental small doses of fentanyl or sufentanil are utilized. Intra-arterial monitoring is not routinely employed in patients for closed surgical procedures unless they are severely acidotic, unstable preoperatively, or a need for prolonged postoperative ventilation is anticipated. The overall goal of the anesthetic management is for early extubation in the operating room or in the intensive care unit, mobilization, and feeding of the infant. Monitoring of the peripheral oxygen saturation with a pulse oximeter as well as end-tidal carbon dioxide measurement aids in the management of these patients. An automated blood pressure monitoring device is utilized in the absence of a radial artery catheter. If the efficacy of the shunting procedure is questioned, an intra-arterial catheter will be used to monitor postoperative oxygen saturation. Because a small number of patients develop unilateral pulmonary edema following a systemic to pulmonary artery shunt, one must be alert to this complication at the end of the anesthetic and in the early hours in the intensive care unit. This complication is presumably related to increased blood flow to a previously inadequately perfused lung and necessitates, in most instances, return to the operating room and narrowing of the shunt. This is a much less frequent complication with the classic Blalock-Taussig shunt as well as the Gore-Tex (W.L. Gore Associates, Elkton, MD) tube graft than with the larger Waterston and Potts shunts.[4]

Anesthesia for the so-called "open" palliative procedures, utilizing cardiopulmonary bypass, such as placement of an outflow patch across the infundibulum to the pulmonary artery with or without a perforated patch closure of the VSD is described below.

Weaning from bypass is facilitated by maintaining the highest oxygen concentration possible in the blood, a slightly low carbon dioxide concentration, and an elevated pH through vigorous ventilation.[27] As during definitive surgical repairs, the pulmonary vascular resistance may need to be manipulated using drugs such as nitroglycerin, phentolamine, tolazoline, and/or prostaglandin E.[28] In addition, any deficiency in left or right ventricular function is treated with positive inotropic drugs.

One must be alert to the fact that the peripheral oxygen saturation of these patients will *not* be markedly improved by open palliative procedures. In addition, the continuous concern of air emboli must persist into the postoperative period because a right-to-left shunt of significant magnitude is present. These patients are frequently the most seriously ill in the early postoperative period. Patients selected for these open palliative procedures are those with deficient pulmonary vasculature and preoperatively estimated poor or inadequate right ventricular size and function.

Definitive Procedures

The younger patients are premedicated with intramuscular pentobarbital, 5 mg/kg, morphine, 0.1 mg/kg, and scopolamine, 0.01 mg/kg. Older patients may have oral benzodiazepine substituted for the pentobarbital. The anesthetic induction in smaller patients with difficult venous access is with intramuscular ketamine, 4 mg/kg, or halothane and oxygen inhalation followed by placement of an intravenous catheter and pancuronium or vecuronium, 0.1 mg/kg, to facilitate endotracheal intubation.[29] Extreme care is used to eliminate all air from intravenous lines to avoid systemic emboli across the right-to-left shunt.[30,31] In patients with a preexisting intravenous catheter, induction of anesthesia is performed with either ketamine, 1–2 mg/kg, intravenously, or inhalation with halothane and oxygen followed by muscle relaxant. Of note, ketamine does not appear to increase pulmonary vascular resistance in these patients.[32,33] Although the induction of anesthesia with an inhalation agent in a patient with a right-to-left shunt may be delayed,[34,35] it is an effective and safe technique in these patients with tetralogy of Fallot.[36] One must, however, be alert to decreases in systemic vascular resistance manifesting as decreases in blood pressure. These should be treated with a decrease in inhalation agent as well as prompt use of vasoconstrictor such as phenylephrine to minimize right-to-left shunting.[8,37] Continuous monitoring of the peripheral oxygen saturation with a pulse oximeter and end-tidal carbon dioxide measurement are helpful as a rough measure of right-to-left shunting and pulmonary blood flow. Intraoperative "tet spells" are treated by increased administration of intravenous fluids, phenylephrine, β-adrenergic blockade, oxygen, direct aortic compression, or manual abdominal compression.[38,39]

Following anesthetic induction, peripheral intravenous catheters, a radial artery catheter, and a single- or double-lumen catheter in the right internal jugular vein are placed. The internal jugular catheter must be short enough so it does not interfere with the superior vena cava cannula used during cardiopulmonary bypass. When there is a persistent left superior vena cava, a catheter may be placed in the left internal jugular vein to evaluate the adequacy of drainage of this system during cardiopulmonary bypass.

Anesthesia is maintained with fentanyl (25–50 μg/kg) or sufentanil (5–10 μg/kg) with the addition of inhalation agent as tolerated and usually without nitrous oxide.[40] In some instances, high-dose narcotic-oxygen is utilized without the inhalation agent and with or without a ketamine induction. This has been shown to be a highly successful technique intra- and postoperatively, particularly in small cyanotic infants, presumably by minimizing paroxysmal increases in a "labile" pulmonary circulation.[26,41] During cardiopulmonary bypass, anesthesia is maintained with intravenous narcotic and pancuronium with or without benzodiazepine.

Cardiopulmonary Bypass. Cardiopulmonary bypass is performed with a membrane oxygenator with a prime calculated for a mixed machine-patient hematocrit of approximately 22%. Systemic hypothermia to a temperature of nasopharyngeal 24–26°C is used. If a period of total circulatory arrest is anticipated, the patient is cooled to a nasopharyngeal temperature of 18–20°C. Cold potassium cardioplegic solution is infused into the root of the aorta for myocardial protection. If there is a preexisting systemic to pulmonary artery shunt, it is dissected out prior to going on cardiopulmonary bypass and clamped or ligated upon initiation of cardiopulmonary bypass.

A prior Potts anastomosis is handled by placing the patient head down and perfusing the aorta through the femoral artery. Upon initiation of cardiopulmonary bypass, the Potts anastomosis is digitally occluded through the pulmonary artery by the surgeon, the patient cooled, and a clamp placed across the aortic arch vessels. The Potts anastomosis is closed from the inside of the left pulmonary artery and air evacuated from the aortic arch before the clamp is removed and circulation is restored.[42]

Perfusion pressure may be decreased in these patients during cardiopulmonary bypass in part secondary to flow through aortopulmonary artery collaterals. Vasoconstrictors may be ineffective in raising perfusion pressure. In fact, the shunt flow, and therefore blood return to the left heart, may be aggravated by peripheral constriction (eg, with phenylephrine).

Prior to weaning from cardiopulmonary bypass but after the heart has been reperfused and has a stable cardiac rhythm and rate, a measurement of the ratio of right ventricular pressure to left ventricular pressure ($P_{RV:LV}$) at left and right atrial pressures of 12–14 mm Hg is made. This ratio is used to judge the adequacy of the repair of the pulmonary outflow obstruction. If the ratio is greater than approximately 0.8 and an infundibular outflow patch has not been placed, one must be placed before discontinuation of bypass. If the ratio is 0.8 and an infundibular patch has been placed and it is thought to be adequate, progressive weaning from bypass continues. If the right ventricular pressure is higher than the left ventricular pressure, serious consideration is given to further correction of the outflow tract obstruction. Transesophageal echocardiography may be useful to evaluate the anatomy.[21,43,44] If further correction is impossible, perforation of the VSD patch may be necessary to reduce pressure in the right ventricle.[4,5,45,46]

Postbypass Period. With surgical hemostasis, adequate rate and rhythm, and the above right ventricular pressure data, "weaning" from cardiopulmonary bypass is attempted. One must be alert to the factors that can alter the "reactive" pulmonary vasculature. One such factor is ventilation. Controlled ventilation with the lowest possible airway pressures should be used to optimize arterial oxygen tension while maintaining an arterial carbon dioxide tension of 30–35 mm Hg and a pH of approximately 7.5.[27] If these criteria are satisfied and pulmonary artery pressure or right atrial pressure relative to left atrial pressure remains increased, pharmacotherapy is initiated to decrease pulmonary vascular resistance.[8,47–50] Numerous agents can alter the pulmonary vascular resistance. It is difficult to predict which one will work best in a given situation. Nitroglycerin is tried initially, often in combination with dopamine to augment ventricular contractility. Amrinone may be dramatically helpful.[51] If this combination is unsuccessful, pulmonary vasodilators such as phentolamine, tolazoline, or prostaglandin E_1 should be tried. In addition, other inotropes such as dobutamine or epinephrine may be required. These interventions are rarely required following "simple" repair of tetralogy of Fallot. However, they are used more frequently in patients who are severely ill with pulmonary atresia and borderline pulmonary hypertension or right ventricular function. Right ventricular failure may occur after right ventriculotomy.

Arrhythmias are uncommon. The presence of heart block alerts one to possible AV conduction system injury during closure of the VSD. This is particularly true if the VSD is not in the standard location. A residual shunt with systemic desaturation may be due to a leak through or around the VSD patch. The leak through the patch usually resolves over the early postoperative days. Repeat catheterization may be necessary to define the origin of the persistent right-to-left shunt.

Patients are then transported to the intensive care unit where they are initially maintained on any vasodilator with or without inotropic drugs begun in the operating room. Weaning from these medications occurs as tolerated with close observations of the right and left atrial pressure, pulmonary artery pressure, and dye dilution cardiac output measurements. In the majority of simple repairs, the patient is extubated on the evening of or morning after surgery. Transfer from the intensive care unit often occurs on the first postoperative day.

INTERVENTIONAL CATHETERIZATION, PALLIATIVE PROCEDURES, AND DEFINITIVE SURGERY

The traditional two-stage repair of tetralogy beginning with a palliative shunt in infancy and later total repair was challenged by Barratt-Boyes in 1969 when he performed total repair in infants using surface cooling, deep hypothermia, and circulatory arrest.[52,53] Surgical techniques include closure of the VSD and infundibular enlargement with or without outflow patch enlargement of the right ventricle, pulmonary artery conduits, and valved extracardiac conduits.

Interventional Catheterization

"Closed" palliative procedures are applicable in some patients with tetralogy of Fallot. Catheterization procedures, including balloon catheter dilation of the pulmonary valve and/or pulmonary vessels as well as embolic occlusion of bronchopulmonary collaterals, are discussed in Chapter 7.

Palliative Surgical Procedures

Additional "closed" palliative procedures include the surgical creation of systemic to pulmonary artery shunts. Some surgical teams use a Gore-Tex interposition graft between the subclavian artery and the pulmonary artery.[54] This type of graft is most frequently utilized in the small infant with inadequate pulmonary blood flow or those with tetralogy and pulmonary atresia. The Gore-Tex graft is also applicable in older patients with smaller than optimal pulmonary arteries with the hope of obtaining an increase in pulmonary artery size and vascularity to facilitate subsequent complete repair.[51,55–57] Other shunts that are occasionally performed are the classic and modified Blalock-Taussig (subclavian artery to pulmonary artery anastomosis),[55] the Waterston shunt[36] (ascending aorta to right pulmonary artery), the Potts shunt[59] (descending aorta to left pulmonary artery), or a central shunt creating an aorta to pulmonary artery "window" with or without a Gore-Tex graft. Problems associated with palliative shunts include (1) too much shunt flow causing failure or pulmonary vascular disease; (2) too little shunt flow with no improvement in oxygen saturation; (3) unilateral shunting; ie, to one lung (as in the Waterston and Blalock-Taussig shunts).

Definitive Surgery

Surgical repair is categorized as "simple" for patients with tetralogy of Fallot with pulmonary stenosis or atresia requiring closure of the VSD through the right atrium or right ventricle with or without an infundibular outflow patch or pulmonary valvotomy. Included in this group are patients with a classic Blalock-Taussig shunt or a subclavian artery to pulmonary artery Gore-Tex shunt. The surgical procedure is termed "complex" if it involves the placement of an extracardiac conduit and/or reconstruction of a small or distorted main pulmonary artery, bifurcation of the pulmonary arteries, or right or left proximal pulmonary arteries. Also included in this complex group is any patient with a preexisting Potts anastomosis or, in some cases, a Waterston shunt. However, the likelihood of right ventricular dysfunction and/or high pulmonary vascular resistance is greater in the complex procedures and will be addressed subsequently.

POSTOPERATIVE CARE

Early reoperation following definitive surgical repair of tetralogy of Fallot may be necessary for excessive bleed-ing, persistent right-to-left shunting, right ventricular failure, or for previously undiagnosed anatomic defects. Early reoperation following palliative shunt procedures is rare, although it may be necessary for excessive bleeding, or unilateral pulmonary edema may necessitate narrowing of the systemic to pulmonary artery shunt.

Results following operation for tetralogy of Fallot are influenced by the heterogeneity of anatomic and clinical presentations. The hospital mortality has decreased markedly over the last 30 years and is now 1–5% whether the repair is done primarily or secondarily following a classic Blalock-Taussig or Gore-Tex shunt procedure. In the subset of patients less than 2 years old for routine repair of uncomplicated tetralogy of Fallot, the mortality is 6–8%. This mortality is increased if the tetralogy of Fallot is complicated by pulmonary artery hypoplasia or by other pulmonary artery problems, increased age, or increased preoperative disability. Whether there is a difference between primary versus two-stage repair in these complex situations remains uncertain. Of those patients dying in the hospital following repair of the tetralogy, approximately 50% of deaths are due to acute cardiac failure and 25% to acute or chronic pulmonary dysfunction.[60] The hospital mortality following 141 shunt procedures at the University of Alabama at Birmingham (1967–1984) was less than 1% for tetralogy of Fallot with pulmonary stenosis and 12% for tetralogy with pulmonary atresia.[5,60] There is a higher mortality with Waterston and Potts anastomoses as well as palliative right ventricular to pulmonary artery anastomic operations performed on cardiopulmonary bypass.

The major incremental risk factors associated with hospital death following complete repair are pulmonary artery pathology, major associated cardiac anomalies, increased hematocrit, very young age, more than one palliative operation, placement of outflow conduit, and an elevated $P_{RV:LV}$ in the operation room (especially if >1).[60] Incremental risk factors for hospital deaths following classic shunt procedures include pulmonary atresia and young age.[60] Events occurring in this population other than hospital deaths include a 7% incidence of shunt closure within 30 days postoperatively, 1% incidence of sudden death, 1% incidence of brain abscess, and 1% incidence of gangrene of the hand. Progressive pulmonary vascular disease is unlikely following classic Blalock-Taussig shunts until more than 7 years postoperatively.

LONG-TERM RESULTS

Long-term survival statistics are available for tetralogy of Fallot and include a 96% 10-year survival rate.[61] The risk factors for premature late death include high $P_{RV:LV}$ in the operating room (ratio >0.85 resulting in a two and a half times greater death rate than a ratio of 0.5), a Potts anastomosis, increased age, and perhaps transannular patch if greater than 25 years postoperatively.[61] Studies report that greater than 95% of totally repaired tetralogy patients are "fully active" at a mean of 10 years postoperatively.[61]

Residual defects include pulmonary hypertension, VSD (1% of patients); tricuspid regurgitation (64% of patients), aortic regurgitation and pulmonic regurgitation (75% of patients); right ventricular dysfunction and RVOT obstruction (11–15% of patients), of which subvalvular obstruction is most common and annular or main PA stenosis less common; and right bundle branch block and ventricular arrhythmias (20–58% of patients).[62–64] Late reoperation has been required in 2–3% of patients for some of these defects.[62]

The severity of the pulmonic regurgitation correlates with RV cavity area. The severity of tricuspid regurgitation is unrelated to either pulmonic stenosis or regurgitation. Both tricuspid and pulmonic regurgitation increase ventricular volume and pressure leading to ventricular dysfunction.

In a large series of children undergoing complete correction of tetralogy at a mean age of 7 months, 24 of 203 patients were found to have RV outflow track obstruction at infundibular, valvular, or supravalvular levels with gradients in excess of 40 mm Hg.[63] The most common outflow track obstruction is subvalvular pulmonic stenosis, but annular or main pulmonary artery stenosis may also be present. In Kirklin's series, the long-term probability of death was inversely related to pulmonary artery size.[64] The size of the pulmonary arteries, as well as the postrepair peak RV/peak LV pressure ratio correlate with outcome.[64]

Early age at repair minimizes ventricular dysfunction. Gradients over 40 mm Hg are associated with decreased right and left ventricular ejection fractions.[65] In addition to gradients, pulmonary regurgitation and preoperative hypoxia contribute to RV dysfunction.

Common complex dysrhythmias include ventricular tachycardia and PVCs. In Chandar's series, spontaneous VPCs were found in 48% of patients after tetralogy repair. Inducible ventricular tachycardia was noted in 17% of patients.[66] Older age at time of repair, longer follow-up time, pulmonic insufficiency, biventricular dysfunction (particularly RV enlargement and low LV ejection fraction), and residual outflow obstruction with RV systolic hypertension have been suggested as causes of postoperative dysrhythmias leading to late sudden death in 5% of patients.[66–68] Arrhythmias may be due to ventricular scar surrounded by cells with increased automaticity that serves as a site for reentry of VT. However, Vaksman and co-workers reported no increased mortality in patients with ventricular dysrhythmias not receiving antiarrhythmic therapy, but the incidence of poor hemodynamic results was only 9%.[69] Ambulatory ECG monitoring for 24 hours and exercise testing to elicit arrhythmias should be performed in patients after tetralogy of Fallot repair.

Abnormalities in both the respiratory and cardiovascular response to exercise have been noted in patients after repair of tetralogy. In Rowe's series, vital capacity was decreased to less than 80% predicted, respiratory rate increased at peak exercise, and breathing reserve decreased with increased pulmonic regurgitation. Fifteen percent of Rowe's patients had outflow track gradients greater than 15 mm Hg. Ventricular dysrhythmias did not affect exercise performance in Rowe's series.[70] Perrault et al[71] compared teen-aged patients who had undergone repair of tetralogy of a VSD before the age of 5 with age-matched controls. Maximal exercise tolerance was normal in all subjects. They noted that although there were no significant differences in oxygen consumption among the groups, maximum heart rate and cardiac index were reduced in all postcardiac patients.[70] Other studies suggest that decreased exercise tolerance may be inversely related to age at correction (worsened in older children and older age at correction). Possible etiologies of the impaired cardiorespiratory response to exercise include impaired reflex control of heart rate, autonomic dysfunction, abnormal right ventricular function (endocardial fibroelastosis), RV outflow obstruction increasing with exercise, exercise-induced ectopy, or pulmonic regurgitation increasing RV area.

REFERENCES

1. Guntheroth G, Kawabori I, Baum D: Tetralogy of Fallot. In Adams FH, Emmanouilides GC (eds): *Moss' Heart Disease in Infants, Children, and Adolescents*, 3rd ed. Baltimore: Williams & Wilkins, 1984, pp 215–228
2. Sanchez Cascos A: Genetics of Fallot's tetralogy. *Br Heart J* 33:899–904, 1971
3. Kirklin JW, Karp RB: *The Tetralogy of Fallot from a Surgical Viewpoint.* Philadelphia: WB Saunders, 1970
4. Kirklin JW, Barratt-Boyes BG: Ventricular septal defect and pulmonary stenosis or atresia. In Kirklin JW, Barratt-Boyes BG (eds): *Cardiac Surgery*, 2nd ed. New York: John Wiley and Sons, 1993, pp 749–824
5. Fallot's tetralogy. In Anderson RH, McCartney FJ, Shinebourne EA, Tynan M: *Pediatric Cardiology.* New York: Churchill Livingstone, 1987, pp 765–798
6. Lev M, Eckner FAO: The pathologic anatomy of tetralogy of Fallot and its variations. *Dis Chest* 45:251–261, 1964
7. Fellows KE, Freed MK, Keane JR, et al: Results of routine preoperative coronary angiography in tetralogy of Fallot. *Circulation* 51:561–566, 1975
8. Samuelson PN: Pulmonary hypertension and systemic desaturation. In Reves JG (ed): *Common Problems in Cardiac Anesthesia.* New York: Year Book Medical, 1987, pp 90–96
9. Hansen DD, Hickey PR: Anesthesia for hypoplastic left heart syndrome. *Anesth Analg* 65:127–132, 1986
10. Morgan BC, Guntheroth WG, Bloom RS, Fyler DC: A clinical profile of paroxysmal hyperpnea in cyanotic congenital heart disease. *Circulation* 31:66–69, 1965
11. Garson A Jr, Gillettee PC, McNamara DG: Propranolol: The preferred palliation for tetralogy of Fallot. *Am J Cardiol* 47:1098–1104, 1981

12. Ponce FE, Williams LC, Webb HM, et al: Propranolol palliation of tetralogy of Fallot: Experience with long-term treatment in pediatric patients. *Pediatrics* **52**:100–108, 1973
13. Guntheroth WG, Morgan BC, Mullins GL, et al: Venous return with knee-chest position and squatting in tetralogy of Fallot. *Am Heart J* **75**:313–318, 1968
14. O'Donnell TV, McIlroy MB: The circulatory effects of squatting. *Am Heart J* **64**:347–356, 1962
15. Borow KM, Green LH, Castaneda AR, Keane IF: Left ventricular function after repair of tetralogy of Fallot and its relationship to age at surgery. *Circulation* **61**:1150–1158, 1980
16. Calder AI, Barratt-Boyes BG, Brandt PWT, Neutze JM: Postoperative evaluation of patients with tetralogy of Fallot repaired in infancy. *J Thorac Cardiovasc Surg* **77**:704–720, 1979
17. Rygg III, Olesen K, Boesen I: The life history of tetralogy of Fallot. *Dan Med Bull* **18**:25–30, 1971
18. Bertranou EG, Blackstone EH, Hazelrig JB, et al: Life expectancy without surgery in tetralogy of Fallot. *Am J Cardiol* **42**:458–466, 1978
19. Lell WA, Reves JG: Anesthesia for cardiovascular surgery. In Kirklin JW, Barratt-Boyes BG (eds): *Cardiac Surgery*, 2nd ed. New York: John Wiley and Sons, 1993, pp 167–194
20. Bargeron LM Jr, Elliott LP, Soto B, et al: Axial cineangiography in congenital heart disease. Section I. Concept, technical and anatomic considerations. *Circulation* **58**:1075–1083, 1977
21. Hillel Z, Thys D, Ritter S, et al: Two-dimensional color flow Doppler echocardiography for intraoperative monitoring of cardiac shunt flows in patients with congenital heart disease. *J Cardiothorac Anesth* **1**:142–147, 1987
22. Perry SB, Keane JF, Lock JE: Interventional catheterization in pediatric congenital and acquired heart disease. *Am J Cardiol* **61**:109G–117G, 1988
23. Bridges ND, Perry SB, Keane JF, et al: Preoperative transcatheter closure of congenital muscular ventricular septal defects. *N Engl J Med* **324**:1312–1317, 1991
24. Malviya S, Burrows FA, Johnston AE, Benson LN: Anaesthetic experience with paediatric interventional cardiology. *Can J Anaesth* **36**:320–324, 1989
25. White PF, Vasconez LO, Mathes S, et al: Comparison of midazolam and diazepam for sedation during plastic surgery. *Plast Reconstr Surg* **81**:703–710, 1988
26. Hickey PR, Hansen DD: Fentanyl- and sufentanil-oxygen-pancuronium anesthesia for cardiac surgery in infants. *Anesth Analg* **63**:117–124, 1984
27. Marshall C, Lindgren L, Marshall BE: Metabolic and respiratory hydrogen ion effects on hypoxic pulmonary vasoconstriction. *J Appl Physiol* **57**:545, 1984
28. D'Ambra, LaRaia P, Phellen D, Lappas D: Prostaglandin E: A new therapy for refractory right heart failure and pulmonary hypertension after mitral valve replacement. *J Thorac Cardiovasc Surg* **89**:567–572, 1985
29. Greeley WJ, Bushman GA, Davis DP, Reves JG: Comparative effects of halothane and ketamine on systemic arterial oxygen saturation in children with cyanotic heart disease. *Anesthesiology* **65**:666–668, 1986
30. Gronert GA, Messick J, Cucchiara R: Paradoxical air embolism from a patent foramen ovale. *Anesthesiology* **50**:548–549, 1979
31. Hickey PR, Hansen DD, Norwood WI, Castaneda AR: Anesthetic complications in surgery for congenital heart disease. *Anesth Analg* **63**:657–664, 1984
32. Hickey PR, Hansen DD, Cramolini GM, et al: Pulmonary and systemic hemodynamic responses to ketamine in infants with normal and elevated pulmonary vascular resistance. *Anesthesiology* **62**:287–293, 1985
33. Topkins MG: Anesthetic management of cardiac catheterization. *Int Anesthesiol Clin* **15**:59–69, 1980
34. Stoelting RK, Longnecker DE: The effect of right-to-left shunt on the rate of increase in arterial anesthetic concentration. *Anesthesiology* **36**:352–356, 1972
35. Tanner GE, Angers DG, Barash PG, Mulla A, et al: Effect of left-to-right, mixed right-to-left, and right-to-left shunts on inhalational anesthetic induction in children. A computer model. *Anesth Analg* **64**:101–107, 1985
36. Laishley RS, Burrow FA, Lerman J, Roy WL: Effect of anesthetic induction regimens on oxygen saturation in cyanotic congenital heart disease. *Anesthesiology* **65**:673–677, 1986
37. Nudel DB, Berman MA, Talner NS: Effects of acutely increasing systemic vascular resistance on oxygen tension in tetralogy of Fallot. *Pediatrics* **58**:248–251, 1976
38. Nolan SP, Kron IL, Rheuban K: Simple method for treatment of intraoperative hypoxic episodes in patients with tetralogy of Fallot. *J Thorac Cardiovasc Surg* **85**:796–797, 1983
39. Baele PL, Rennotte M-T, Veyckmans FA: External compression of the abdominal aorta reversing tetralogy of Fallot cyanotic crisis. *Anesthesiology* **75**:146–149, 1991
40. Hickey PR, Hansen DD, Strafford M, et al: Pulmonary and systemic hemodynamic effects of N_2O in infants with normal and elevated pulmonary vascular resistance. *Anesthesiology* **65**:374–378, 1986
41. Hickey PR, Hansen DD, Wessel D, et al: Blunting of stress responses in the pulmonary circulation of infants by fentanyl. *Anesth Analg* **64**:1137–1142, 1985
42. Kirklin JW, Devloo RA: Hypothermic perfusion and circulation arrest for surgical correction of tetralogy of Fallot with previously constructed Potts' anastomosis. *Dis Chest* **39**:87–91, 1961
43. Ritter SB, Thys D: Pediatric transesophageal color flow imaging: Smaller probes for smaller hearts. *Echocardiography* **6**:431–440, 1989
44. Ritter SB: Pediatric transesophageal color flow imaging 1990: The long and short of it. *Echocardiography* **7**:713–725, 1990
45. Blackstone EH, Kirklin JW, Pacifico AD: Decision-making in repair of tetralogy of Fallot based on intraoperative measurements of pulmonary arterial outflow tract. *J Thorac Cardiovasc Surg* **77**:526–532, 1979
46. Blackstone EH, Kirklin JW, Bertranou EG, et al: Preoperative prediction from cineangiograms of postrepair right ventricular pressure in tetralogy of Fallot. *J Thorac Cardiovasc Surg* **78**:542, 1979
47. Hoffman JIE, Heymann MA: Pulmonary arterial hypertension secondary to congenital heart disease. In Weir EK, Reeves JT (eds): *Pulmonary Hypertension*. Mt Kisco, NY: Futura, 1984, pp 93–114
48. Rabinowitch M: Pulmonary hypertension. In Adams FH, Emmanouilides GC (eds): *Moss' Heart Disease in Infants,*

Children, and Adolescents, 3rd ed. Baltimore: Williams & Wilkins, 1984, pp 669–691

49. Drummond WH, Gregory GA, Heymann MA, Phibbs RA: The independent effects of hyperventilation, tolazoline, and dopamine on infants with persistent pulmonary hypertension. *J Pediatr* **98**:603–611, 1981

50. Rubin LF: Cardiovascular effects of vasodilator therapy for pulmonary artery hypertension. *Clin Chest Med* **4**:309–319, 1983

51. Wynands JE: Amrinone: Is it the inotrope of choice? *J Cardiothorac Anesth* **3**:47–57, 1989

52. Barratt-Boyes BG, Neutze JM: Primary repair of tetralogy of Fallot in infancy using profound hypothermia with circulatory arrest and limited cardiopulmonary bypass: A comparison with conventional two-stage management. *Ann Surg* **178**:406–411, 1973

53. Kirklin JW, Blackstone EH, Pacifico A, et al: Routine primary repair vs two-stage repair of tetralogy of Fallot. *Circulation* **60**:373–386, 1979

54. Di Benedetto G, Tiraboschi R, Vanini V, et al: Systemic-pulmonary artery shunt using PTFE prosthesis (Gore-Tex). Early results and long-term follow-up on 105 consecutive cases. *Thorac Cardiovasc Surg* **29**:143–147, 1981

55. Blalock A, Taussig HB: The surgical treatment of malformations of the heart in which there is pulmonary stenosis or pulmonary atresia. *JAMA* **128**:189–202, 1945

56. Kirklin JW, Bargeron LM Jr, Pacifico AD: The enlargement of small pulmonary arteries by preliminary palliative operations. *Circulation* **56**:612–617, 1977

57. Gale AW, Arciniegas E, Green WE, et al: Growth of the pulmonary annulus and pulmonary arteries after the Blalock-Taussig shunt. *J Thorac Cardiovasc Surg* **77**:459–465 1979

58. Waterston DJ: Treatment of Fallot's tetralogy in children under one year of age. *Rozhl Chir* **41**:181–183 1962

59. Potts WJ, Smith S, Gibson S: Anastomosis of the aorta to a pulmonary artery. *JAMA* **132**:627–631, 1946

60. Kirklin JW, Blackstone EH, Kirklin JK, et al: Surgical results and protocols in the spectrum of tetralogy of Fallot. *Ann Surg* **198**:251–265, 1983

61. Katz NM, Blackstone EH, Kirklin JW, et al: Late survival and symptoms after repair of tetralogy of Fallot. *Circulation* **65**:403–410, 1982

62. Ebert PA: Second operations for pulmonary stenosis or insufficiency after repair of tetralogy of Fallot. *Am J Cardiol* **50**:637–640, 1982

63. Walsh EP, Rockenmacher S, Keane JF, et al: Late results in patients with tetralogy of Fallot repaired in infancy. *Circulation* **77**:1062–1067, 1988

64. Kirklin JW, Blackstone EH, Shimezaki Y, et al: Survival, functional status, and reoperations after repair of tetralogy of Fallot with pulmonary atresia. *J Thorac Cardiovasc Surg* **96**:102–116, 1988

65. Sunakawa A, Shirotani H, Yokoyama T, Oku H: Factors affecting biventricular function following surgical repair of tetralogy of Fallot. *Jpn Circ J* **52**:401–410, 1988

66. Chandar JS, Wolff GS, Garson A, et al: Ventricular arrhythmias in postoperative tetralogy of Fallot. *Am J Cardiol* **65**:655–661, 1990

67. Kavey REW, Thomas FD, Byrum CJ, et al: Ventricular arrhythmias and biventricular dysfunction after repair of tetralogy of Fallot. *J Am Coll Cardiol* **4**:126–131, 1984

68. Zahka KG, Horneffer PJ, Rowe SA, et al: Long-term valvular function after total repair of tetralogy of Fallot. Relation to ventricular arrhythmias. *Circulation* **76**:III-14–III-19, 1988

69. Vaksman G, Fournier A, Davignon A, et al: Frequency and prognosis of arrhythmias after operative correction of tetralogy of Fallot. *Am J Cardiol* **66**:346–349, 1990

70. Rowe SA, Zahka KG, Manolio TA, et al: Lung function and pulmonary regurgitation limit exercise capacity in postoperative tetralogy of Fallot. *J Am Coll Cardiol* **17**:461–466, 1991

71. Perrault H, Drblik SP, Montigny M, et al: Comparison of cardiovascular adjustments to exercise in adolescents 8 to 15 years of age after correction of tetralogy of Fallot, ventricular septal defect, or atrial septal defect. *Am J Cardiol* **64**:213–217, 1989

Chapter 15 | Transposition of the Great Vessels

James A. DiNardo

Complete transposition of the great vessels (TGV) is a common congenital heart lesion accounting for 5–7% of all congenital cardiac defects, second in frequency only to isolated ventricular septal defects.[1] Without intervention, TGV has a high mortality rate: 45% of patients will die within the first month and 90% within the first year of life.[2] This is particularly unfortunate because infants with complete TGV rarely have other extracardiac defects. Advancements in medical and surgical therapy in the past 20 years have greatly improved the outlook for these infants. In particular, the use of prostaglandin E₁ to maintain ductal patency, the Rashkind-Miller balloon septostomy, and early corrective surgery, rather than multiple palliative procedures, have significantly improved long-term outcome for infants with complete TGV. The necessity for early surgical intervention in the care of these infants requires that the anesthesiologist fully understand the pathophysiology of this lesion, the goals of the proposed surgical procedures, and the postoperative sequelae.

ANATOMY

Transposition of the great vessels refers specifically to the anatomic discordance of the ventriculoarterial connections such that the aorta arises from the right ventricle and the pulmonary artery arises from the left ventricle. The embryologic development of the defect is discussed in Chapter 3. The designation D-TGV refers to the situation where the aorta is situated anterior and to the right of the pulmonary artery, whereas in L-TGV, the aorta is anterior and to the left of the pulmonary artery. The physiologic consequences of ventriculoarterial discordance depend on whether there is atrioventricular concordance (complete TGV) or atrioventricular discordance (congenitally corrected TGV).

As in normally related great vessels, the coronary arteries in TGV arise from the aortic sinuses that face the pulmonary artery. In normally related vessels, the sinuses of Valsalva are located on the anterior portion of the aorta, whereas in TGV, they are located posteriorly. In the majority of TGV patients (60%), the right sinus is the origin of the right coronary artery, whereas the left sinus is the origin of the left main coronary artery.[3] In the remainder of cases, there is considerable variability, with the most common variations being shown in Fig 15–1.

In patients with complete TGV, the most commonly associated cardiac anomalies are patent foramen ovale (PFO), patent ductus arteriosus (PDA), ventricular septal defect (VSD), and subpulmonic stenosis, or left ventricular outflow tract obstruction (LVOTO). Approximately 50% of patients with TGV will present with a PDA prior to prostaglandin E₁ administration. The foramen ovale is almost always patent, but a true secundum atrial septal defect (ASD) exists in only about 5% of patients. Although angiographically detectable VSDs may occur in 30–40% of patients, only about one third of these defects are hemodynamically significant.[3] Thus, for practical purposes, 75% of patients have an intact ventricular septum (IVS).[4] LVOTO is present in about 30% of patients with VSD and is most often due to an extensive subpulmonary fibromuscular ring or mechanical obstruction from malposition of the outlet portion of the ventricular septum.[3] Only 5% of patients with IVS have significant LVOTO. In these patients, there is a dynamic obstruction of the LV outflow tract during systole due to leftward bulging of the ventricular septum and anterior movement of the anterior leaflet of the mitral valve.[5] Valvular pulmonary stenosis is rare in patients with TGV.[3] Other less commonly seen lesions are functionally important tricuspid or mitral regurgitation (4% of each) and coarctation of the aorta (5%).[3]

Bronchopulmonary collateral vessels (aorta to pul-

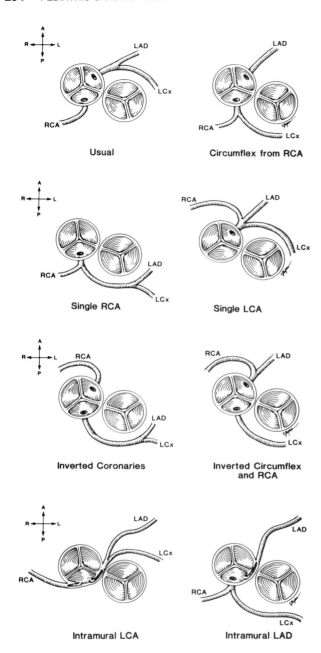

Figure 15–1. Depiction of the most common coronary artery patterns in transposition of the great vessels. The aorta is depicted anterior and to the right of the pulmonary artery. RCA, right coronary artery; LCA, left coronary artery; LAD, left anterior descending coronary artery; LCx, left circumflex coronary artery. (*From Mayer JE, Sanders SP, Jonas RA, et al: Coronary artery pattern and outcome of arterial switch operation for transposition of the great arteries. Circulation 82(suppl 4):144, 1990, with permission.*)

monary artery proximal to the pulmonary capillaries) are visible angiographically in 30% of patients with complete TGV and the functional patency of these vessels has been conclusively demonstrated.[6] The larger and more extensive collaterals generally involve the right lung. These collaterals provide a site for intercirculatory mixing and have been implicated in the accelerated devel-opment of pulmonary vascular occlusive disease in patients with TGV.

Congenitally Corrected TGV

In corrected transposition, blood circulates physiologi-cally because transposition of the great vessels is associ-ated with discordance of the atria and ventricles.[8] Mitral and tricuspid valves remain associated with the ap-propriate atria. Although the circulation is correct, asso-ciated abnormalities are clinically important. These de-fects include VSD with or without pulmonic stenosis, left AV valvular insufficiency, but occasionally stenosis, and disturbances of AV conduction (primarily AV block). Congestive heart failure is a frequent presenting com-plaint.

Cardiomegaly is present on chest radiograph and the pulmonary artery is more medially placed because it lies to the right of the aorta. Although cardiac catheterization is essential to establish the diagnosis and associated anom-alies, it is frequently complicated by dysrhythmias.[8]

Surgical repair of these defects is difficult, particu-larly when ventriculotomy is necessary because of aber-rant coronary arteries. Shunt procedures are often necessary when pulmonic stenosis is present. Surgical procedures are often complicated by dysrhythmias. How-ever, more recent surgical series demonstrated a 78% 5-year survival after closure of VSD, insertion of pulmo-nary artery conduit, and atrioventricular valve repair.[9] Modifications of surgical technique to avoid the conduct-ing system maintain sequential atrioventricular conduc-tion.[10]

PATHOPHYSIOLOGY

In complete TGV atrioventricular concordance (right atrium [RA] to right ventricle [RV]; and ventriculoarte-rial discordance (RV to aorta; LV to left atrium [LA] to left ventricle [LV]) to pulmonary artery) produce a par-allel rather than a normal series circulation (Fig 15–2A). In congenitally corrected TGV, atrioventricular discor-dance (RA to LV; LA to RV) and ventriculoarterial dis-cordance (RV to aorta; LV to pulmonary artery) produce a series circulation. In the parallel arrangement of com-plete TGV, deoxygenated systemic venous blood recir-culates through the systemic circulation without reaching the lungs to be oxygenated. This recirculated systemic venous blood represents a physiologic right-to-left shunt. Likewise, oxygenated pulmonary venous blood recircu-lates uselessly though the pulmonary circulation. This recirculated pulmonary venous blood represents a phys-iologic left-to-right shunt. Thus, in a parallel circulation, the physiologic shunt or the percentage of venous blood from one system that recirculates in the arterial outflow of the same system is 100% for both circuits.[7] Unless there are one or more communications between the par-allel circuits to allow *intercirculatory mixing*, the parallel arrangement is not compatible with life.

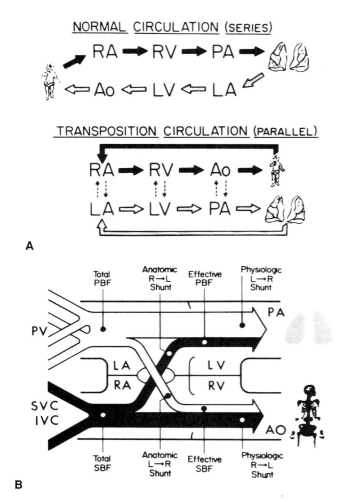

NORMAL CIRCULATION (SERIES)

TRANSPOSITION CIRCULATION (PARALLEL)

A

B

Figure 15–2. The circulation in transposition of the great vessels. (*A*). Schematic of normal series circulation and of transposition parallel circulation. Potential sites for intercirculatory mixing are indicated by dashed arrows. (*B*). Detailed schematic of blood flow and shunts in complete transposition of the great arteries. Blood recirculated from the pulmonary veins to the pulmonary artery represents a physiologic left-to-right shunt. Blood recirculated from the systemic veins to the aorta represents a physiologic right-to-left shunt. Effective pulmonary blood flow (systemic veins to pulmonary artery—PBF) is the result of an anatomic right-to-left shunt. Effective systemic blood flow (pulmonary veins to aorta—SBF) is the result of an anatomic left-to-right shunt. The majority of total systemic and total pulmonary blood flow comprises recirculated blood. SVC, superior vena cava; IVC, inferior vena cava; PV, pulmonary veins; LA, left atrium; RA, right atrium; LV, left ventricle; RV, right ventricle; PA, pulmonary artery; Ao, AO, aorta. (*From Paul MH: Complete transposition of the great arteries. In Adams FH, Emmanouilides GG (eds): Moss' Heart Disease in Infants, Children, and Adolescents. 4th ed. Baltimore: Williams and Wilkins, 1989, p 382, with permission.*)

The sites available for intercirculatory mixing in complete TGV can be intracardiac (PFO, ASD, VSD) or extracardiac (PDA, bronchopulmonary collaterals). Several factors affect the amount of intercirculatory mixing. The number, size, and position of anatomic communications is important.[11,12] One large, nonrestrictive communication provides better mixing than two or three restrictive communications. Reduced ventricular compliance and elevated systemic and pulmonary vascular resistance tend to reduce intercirculatory mixing by impeding flow across anatomic communications. The position of the communication is also important. Poor mixing occurs even with large anterior muscular VSDs owing to their unfavorable position.[11] Finally, in the presence of adequate intercirculatory mixing sites, the extent of intercirculatory mixing is directly related to total pulmonary blood flow.[11–13] Patients with reduced pulmonary blood flow secondary to subpulmonary stenosis or pulmonary vascular occlusive disease (PVOD) have reduced intercirculatory mixing.

Intercirculatory mixing is the result of anatomic right-to-left and anatomic left-to-right shunts that are equal in magnitude. The anatomic right-to-left shunt produces *effective pulmonary blood flow*, which is the volume of systemic venous blood reaching the pulmonary circulation. The anatomic left-to-right shunt produces *effective systemic blood flow*, which is the volume of pulmonary venous blood reaching the systemic circulation. Effective pulmonary blood flow, effective systemic blood flow, and the volume of intercirculatory mixing are always equal. Total systemic blood flow is the sum of recirculated systemic venous blood plus effective systemic blood flow. Likewise, total pulmonary blood flow is the sum of recirculated pulmonary venous blood plus effective pulmonary blood flow. Recirculated blood makes up the largest portion of total pulmonary and systemic blood flow, with effective blood flows contributing only a small portion of the total flows. The net result is the *transposition physiology* where the pulmonary artery oxygen saturation is greater than the aortic oxygen saturation. Figures 15–2*B* and 15–3 further elucidate these concepts.

Arterial saturation (Sao_2) will be determined by the relative volumes and saturations of the recirculated systemic and effective systemic blood flows reaching the aorta. This is summarized in the following equation: aortic saturation = ([systemic venous saturation] [recirculated systemic blood flow] + [pulmonary venous saturation] [effective systemic blood flow]) / (total systemic blood flow). This is illustrated in Figure 15–3, where $Sao_2 = ([50][1.2] + [99][1.1]) / 2.3 = 73\%$. Obviously, the greater the effective systemic blood flow (intercirculatory mixing) relative to the recirculated systemic blood flow, the greater the aortic saturation. For a given amount of intercirculatory mixing and total systemic blood flow, a decrease in systemic venous or pulmonary venous saturation decreases arterial saturation.

NATURAL HISTORY

The natural history of complete TGV without intervention is death in 90% of patients within the first year of life.[2] Anoxia and intractable congestive heart failure (CHF) are the two primary causes of death. The early

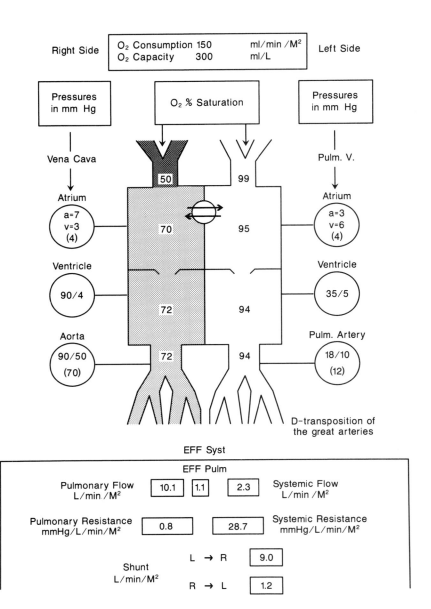

Figure 15–3. Depiction of saturations, pressures, and blood flows in complete transposition of the great vessels with intercirculatory mixing at the atrial level and a small left ventricular outflow tract gradient. It is apparent that total pulmonary blood flow (10.1 L/min/ m²) is almost five times total systemic blood flow (2.3 L/min/m²). Effective (EFF) pulmonary and effective systemic blood flow are equal (1.1 L/min/m²) and are the result of an anatomic shunt at the atrial level. The physiologic left-to-right shunt is 9 L/min/ m²; this represents blood recirculated from the pulmonary veins to the pulmonary artery. The physiologic right-to-left shunt is 1.2 L/min/m²; this represents blood recirculated from the systemic veins to the aorta. In this depiction, pulmonary vascular resistance is low (approximately 1/35 of systemic vascular resistance) and there is a small (17-mm peak to peak) gradient from the left ventricle to the pulmonary artery. These findings are compatible with the high pulmonary blood flow depicted. (*Modified from Freed MD, Keane JF: Profiles in congenital heart disease. In Grossman W (ed): Cardiac Catheterization and Angiography. Philadelphia: Lea and Febiger, 1986, p 463, with permission.*)

onset and progression of pulmonary vascular occlusive disease (PVOD) plays a major role in the dismal outlook in these patients.

Normally, pulmonary vascular resistance decreases progressively in the days and weeks following birth. The normal process of postnatal pulmonary maturation is altered by the development of PVOD in infants with TGV. In fact, compared with other forms of congenital heart disease, infants with TGV are at particular risk for accelerated development of PVOD. Systemic hypoxemia, the presence of bronchopulmonary collaterals which deliver deoxygenated blood to precapillary pulmonary arterioles, platelet aggregation in the lung, [11] and polycythemia have all been implicated.[6,14] Infants with TGV and large VSD without LVOTO are at even higher risk for early development of PVOD owing to exposure of the pulmonary vascular bed to high flows and systemic pressures.

In contrast, the presence of LVOTO affords some protection from the early development of PVOD by protecting the pulmonary vasculature from high pressures and flows.[15] Histologic evidence of advanced PVOD (histologic grade 3; see Chapter 18) is found in 20% of patients with TGV and large VSD without LVOTO before 2 months of age and in 78% after after 12 months of age. For patients with TGV and IVS, advanced PVOD occurs in only 1 and 34%, respectively, of patients at the same time intervals.[16]

The development of PVOD increases pulmonary vascular resistance and pulmonary hypertension that, in turn, decreases pulmonary blood flow. The reduction in pulmonary blood flow decreases intercirculatory mixing and worsens systemic hypoxemia. Furthermore, advanced irreversible pulmonary hypertension reduces the corrective surgical options available to the patient. Definitive surgical intervention must occur before the development of irreversible PVOD.

Four clinical subsets based on anatomy, pulmonary blood flow, and intercirculatory mixing are commonly used to characterize patients with complete TGV. These are summarized in Table 15–1. Management of patients in each of the groups will differ.

TGV WITH IVS

The majority of neonates with TGV and IVS manifest marked cyanosis within the first day of life.[17] In addition, metabolic acidosis evolves secondary to the poor tissue oxygen delivery accompanying the hypoxemia. Once a diagnosis of this clinical subset is made, balloon atrial septostomy is performed in the catheterization laboratory and prostaglandin E_1, at a dose of 0.05–0.1 μg/kg/min, is administered. Prostaglandin E_1 is used to dilate and maintain patency of the ductus arteriosus.[18] The combination of ductal patency and atrial septostomy improves intercirculatory mixing, systemic oxygenation, and systemic oxygen delivery. In instances in which the metabolic acidosis is severe, sodium bicarbonate administration may be necessary in addition to these measures. Hypothermia and blood loss occurring during catheterization may also complicate stabilization of these infants. In some centers, these stabilized neonates are brought promptly to the operating room for an arterial switch or atrial switch procedure. In other centers, prostaglandin E_1 is discontinued after creation of the atrial septostomy. If the neonate remains stable without prostaglandin E_1, definitive surgical therapy, in the form of an atrial switch procedure, may be delayed. If the neonate cannot be stabilized without prostaglandin E_1, immediate surgical therapy is indicated.

TGV AND VSD

Infants in this subset are mildly cyanotic with symptoms of congestive heart failure. Pulmonary blood flow is increased and there is extensive intercirculatory mixing. Reducing pulmonary vascular resistance (PVR) to further augment pulmonary blood flow and intercirculatory mixing will not greatly influence systemic oxygenation. Reducing PVR in these patients may increase the recirculated volume of the pulmonary circuit by increasing circuit compliance. Maintaining systemic blood flow will then necessitate an increase in cardiac output from a failing heart. These patients are commonly stable enough not to require immediate surgical or catheterization laboratory intervention. They are candidates for an arterial switch procedure before intractable congestive heart failure (CHF) or advanced PVOD occur.

TGV WITH VSD AND LVOTO

The degree of cyanosis in these infants will depend on the extent of LVOTO. LVOTO reduces pulmonary blood flow and intercirculatory mixing and protects the pulmonary vasculature from the increased pressures and volumes that accelerate the development of PVOD. The more severe the LVOTO, the less effective will be efforts to increase pulmonary blood flow by decreasing PVR. When LVOTO is severe, the infant is severely cyanotic and progressively develops polycythemia. These infants may require a palliative aortopulmonary shunt to increase pulmonary blood flow. Definitive treatment for these patients is a Rastelli procedure.

TGV WITH PVOD

The goal of diagnosis and treatment of infants with TGV is to intervene surgically before development of PVOD. As PVOD advances, the infant becomes progressively cyanotic and polycythemic. Efforts to reduce PVR will increase pulmonary blood flow and intercirculatory mixing in infants where PVR is not fixed. Infants with advanced PVOD (PVR > 10 Wood units; histologic grade 4) are generally candidates only for palliative therapy. In particular, closure of a VSD in the presence of advanced pulmonary hypertension carries a high mortality owing to afterload mismatch and the resultant pulmonary ventricular (LV) dysfunction. These patients are candidates for a palliative atrial switch procedure without closure of the VSD.

DIAGNOSTIC FEATURES

Cyanosis and CHF are the most consistent signs associated with complete TGV. In patients in whom intercirculatory mixing is limited, cyanosis is severe with little evidence of CHF. CHF is a more common finding in patients with increased pulmonary blood flow, a large amount of intercirculatory mixing, and mild cyanosis.

TABLE 15–1. CLASSIFICATION OF TGV ANATOMY AND PHYSIOLOGY

Anatomy	PBF	ICM
1. TGV with IVS	Increased	Small
1a. TGV with IVS, atrial septostomy, or PDA	Increased	Large
2. TGV with VSD	Increased	Large
3. TGV with VSD and LVOTO	Reduced	Small
4. TGV and PVOD	Reduced	Small

Abbreviations: TGV, PBF, transposition of the great vessels; pulmonary blood flow; ICM, intercirculatory mixing; IVS, intact ventricular septum; PDA, patent ductus arteriosus; VSD, ventricular septal defect; LVOTO, left ventricular outflow tract obstruction; PVOD, pulmonary vascular occlusive disease.

Chest radiographs may appear normal in the first few weeks of life in infants with TGV and IVS. Eventually, the triad of an enlarged egg-shaped heart (large right atrium and ventricle), narrow superior mediastinum, and increased pulmonary vascular markings evolves. In patients with TGV and VSD without LVOTO, an enlarged cardiac silhouette and prominent pulmonary vascular markings are seen at birth. Right axis deviation and right ventricular hypertrophy (RVH) are the electrocardiographic (ECG) findings in TGV with IVS, whereas right axis deviation, left ventricular hypertrophy (LVH), and RVH are seen with TGV and VSD.

Two-dimensional echocardiography is a valuable tool in the assessment of infants with TGV. It accurately establishes the diagnosis of TGV and reliably identifies associated abnormalities such as VSD, mitral and tricuspid valve abnormalities, and LVOTO.[19,20] Echocardiographic analysis of ventricular septal position[21,22] or LV geometry[23,24] is also used to noninvasively assess the LV to RV pressure ratio and LV mass in neonates with TGV and IVS being evaluated as candidates for an arterial switch procedure.

Cardiac catheterization is the gold standard for preoperative assessment of coronary anatomy, the LV outflow tract, the pulmonic valve, pulmonary pressures, and the LV to RV pressure ratio in patients considered for an arterial switch procedure. Typical findings are in Fig 15–3. During catheterization of infants with PVOD, a trial of ventilation at an F_{IO_2} of 1 may be used to determine whether PVR is fixed or remains responsive to oxygen-induced pulmonary vasodilatation. After establishment of the diagnosis, balloon atrial septostomy is performed in neonates.

ANESTHETIC AND PERIOPERATIVE MANAGEMENT

The anesthetic goals for the patient with TGV are summarized in Table 15–2. In infants older than 6–8 months of age, premedication may be necessary to facilitate separation from the parents. In infants with tenuous cardiovascular status, premedication under supervision of the anesthesiologist is preferred. A combination of ketamine (2–3 mg/kg intramuscularly) and atropine (0.01 mg/kg intramuscularly) or oral midazolam (0.3–0.5 mg/kg orally) are both useful. Older, better compensated children such as those presenting for a Rastelli repair with a functioning aortic to pulmonary artery shunt may require a more substantial oral or intramuscular premedication.

In infants with TGV over 6–9 months of age, advanced polycythemia may be present. Spontaneous cerebral vascular accidents may rarely occur in infants with hematocrits greater than 65% owing to high blood viscosity. In order to reduce the risk of this disastrous complication, preoperative intravenous hydration should be

TABLE 15–2. ANESTHETIC GOALS IN THE PATIENT WITH TGV

1. Maintain heart rate, contractility, and preload to maintain cardiac output. Decreases in cardiac output decrease systemic venous saturation with a resultant decrease in arterial saturation.
2. Maintain ductal patency with prostaglandin E₁ (0.05–0.1 μg/kg/min) in ductal-dependent patients.
3. Avoid increases in PVR relative to SVR. Increases in PVR decrease pulmonary blood flow and reduce intercirculatory mixing. In patients with PVOD, ventilatory interventions should be used to reduce PVR. In patients with LVOTO that is not severe, ventilatory interventions to reduce PVR increase pulmonary blood flow and intercirculatory mixing.
4. Reductions in SVR relative to PVR should be avoided. Decreased SVR increases recirculation of systemic venous blood and decreases arterial saturation.
5. In patients with TGV and VSD with symptoms of CHF, ventilatory interventions to reduce PVR are not warranted. They will produce small improvements in arterial saturation at the expense of systemic perfusion.

Abbreviations: TGV, transposition of the great vessels; SVR, systemic vascular resistance; PVR, pulmonary vascular resistance; PVOD, pulmonary vascular occlusive disease; LVOTO, left ventricular outflow tract obstruction; VSD, ventricular septal defect; CHF, congestive heart failure.

undertaken in polycythemic infants. Chronically cyanotic infants are also prone to coagulopathies that are multifactorial in nature.[25] Qualitative and quantitative platelet defects, hypofibrinogenemia, low-grade disseminated intravascular coagulopathy (DIC), and factor deficiencies have all been implicated.[26] Polycythemia, by reducing plasma volume and coagulation factor levels, may also contribute to the development of a coagulopathy.[26] In cases of severe polycythemia, erythropheresis with whole blood removed and replaced with fresh frozen plasma or isotonic saline is indicated.[27] Prostaglandin E₁ infusions should be continued until initiation of cardiopulmonary bypass to assure an adequate intercirculatory mixing site in prostaglandin-dependent neonates.

In patients with reduced pulmonary blood flow or poor intercirculatory mixing, efforts should be made to reduce PVR and increase pulmonary blood flow or intercirculatory mixing. As no pharmacologic or anesthetic agents exist that preferentially reduce PVR, the most reliable method to reduce PVR is through ventilatory interventions. An increased F_{IO_2},[28] a P_{CO_2} in the 20–30 mm Hg range,[29] and a pH in the 7.50–7.56 range[30] effectively reduce PVR in infants. In patients with PVOD, ventilatory measures to reduce PVR are useful if PVR is not fixed. Hypercarbia, acidosis, and hypoxemia further increase PVR and should be avoided. Anesthetic agents that depress contractility should be avoided because of the limited myocardial reserve of neonates and infants. This is particularly true in neonates with TGV and IVS in whom systemic oxygen delivery is tenuous and in infants with TGV and VSD in whom left ventricular volume overload is present. In addition, reactive increases in PVR are commonly seen in the immature pulmonary vasculature and may severely compromise pulmonary blood flow.[31]

Ideally, preinduction monitoring should include a blood pressure cuff, ECG, pulse oximeter, end-tidal CO_2 monitor, and a precordial stethoscope. In reality, a pulse oximeter and a precordial stethoscope may be all that is practical in the early stages of induction. The other monitors are then quickly added as induction progresses. Pulse oximetry sensors should be placed on a number of sites to ensure measurement of SpO_2 at all critical times during the procedure. An intra-arterial catheter is placed during or just after induction. Many infants presenting for emergent surgery will have an umbilical artery or femoral artery catheter in place. A central venous pressure/drug infusion catheter is placed after intubation and stabilization. Double-lumen central venous catheters are preferred. Nasopharyngeal and rectal temperature probes are also placed following induction.

A narcotic-based anesthetic (fentanyl, 50–100 μg/kg, or sufentanil, 10–15 μg/kg) induction and maintenance is recommended. The narcotic dose is infused over a period of 5–10 minutes. High-dose narcotics provide hemodynamic stability, do not depress the myocardium, and blunt reactive pulmonary hypertension.[31] In order to avoid bradycardia, pancuronium (0.1 mg/kg) is administered as the narcotic infusion commences; its vagolytic activity offsets the vagotonic activity of the narcotics.[32] Reductions in heart rate invariably reduce cardiac output in infants owing to their limited preload reserve.[33] Surgical stimulation (skin incision, sternotomy, sternal spreading, or aortic manipulation) may induce hypertension. At the above-recommended doses of narcotics, attempts to treat hypertension with additional narcotic are unlikely to be successful.[34] A benzodiazepine may be titrated (midazolam, 0.025–0.05 mg/kg), keeping in mind that narcotic-benzodiazepine combinations are synergistic in reducing peripheral vascular resistance.[35] Alternatively, a small quantity of an inhalation agent may be used.

In instances in which intravenous access is difficult, ketamine (2–3 mg/kg intramuscularly) and atropine (0.02 mg/kg intramuscularly) can be given while the airway is managed and an IV started. Low concentrations of inspired halothane can be used to accomplish the same end, but it must be remembered that these infants are extremely prone to anesthetic-induced myocardial depression. In situations in which more rapid intubating conditions are desirable without an intravenous line, ketamine (4–5 mg/kg), atropine (0.02 mg/kg), and succinylcholine (4–5 mg/kg) can be given together intramuscularly in the same syringe. Ketamine does not increase PVR as long as normocarbia is maintained and hypoxemia avoided.[36] Atropine is added to reduce the secretions produced by ketamine.

SURGICAL TECHNIQUES

Palliative Procedures

Blalock-Hanlon Atrial Septectomy. This procedure, described in 1950, surgically creates an ASD to serve as a site for intercirculatory mixing in the infant with TGV.[37] The procedure is performed via a right thoracotomy without cardiopulmonary bypass. A clamp is placed across a small portion of both atria and the right pulmonary veins in the area of the interatrial sulcus. Parallel incisions are made in the right and left atria and a portion of the posterior atrial septum is then excised. The resulting atrial incision is then closed leaving behind an ASD. The temporary occlusion of the right pulmonary veins may cause transient hemodynamic decompensation and arterial desaturation as well as hemorrhage in the right lung secondary to pulmonary venous obstruction. This procedure has been largely replaced by the less invasive Rashkind-Miller balloon atrial septostomy.[38] In the catheterization laboratory, a balloon-tipped catheter is advanced across the foramen ovale from the right atrium into the left atrium. The balloon is inflated in the left atrium and the catheter pulled back across the atrial septum into the right atrium creating an ASD (see Chapter 7).

Systemic to Pulmonary Artery Shunts. In patients with TGV, VSD, and severe LVOTO, pulmonary blood flow and intercirculatory mixing is very limited. A procedure to increase pulmonary blood flow has to involve the pulmonary artery distal to the obstruction. In these patients, a Blalock-Taussig shunt, central shunt, or Waterston shunt (see Chapter 2) may be used for palliation in children thought to be too small (less than 2 years old) for a definitive Rastelli procedure.

Mustard Procedure. The Mustard procedure, to be described in detail later in this chapter, is an atrial switch procedure used as a definitive repair. In patients with TGV, VSD, and advanced PVOD, the Mustard procedure has been used for palliation.[39] In this setting, the Mustard procedure is performed without closure of the VSD. Systemic oxygenation improves secondary to improved intercirculatory mixing. Maintenance of the VSD avoids the high mortality associated with pulmonary ventricular (LV) dysfunction associated with VSD closure in patients with PVOD. Although this procedure improves arterial saturation and exercise tolerance, it does nothing to reverse or prevent progression of PVOD.[39]

Definitive Procedures

Intra-atrial Physiologic Repairs: Mustard and Senning Procedures. Both the Mustard and the Senning procedures are atrial switch procedures that surgically create discordant atrioventricular connections in the presence of the preexisting discordant ventriculoarterial connections. Thus, following repair, systemic venous blood is routed to the LV, which is connected to the pulmonary artery. Likewise, pulmonary venous blood is routed to the RV, which is connected to the aorta. This arrangement results in physiologic, but not anatomic, correction of TGV.

Mustard Procedure. The Mustard procedure, described in 1964, is summarized in Fig 15–4 A–C.[40] The interatrial septum is excised creating a large ASD. A baffle made of native pericardium or synthetic material is then used to redirect pulmonary and systemic venous blood.

Pulmonary venous blood flows over the baffle and is directed across the tricuspid valve into the RV. Systemic venous blood flows on the underside of the baffle to be directed across the mitral valve into the LV.

Senning Procedure. In the Senning procedure (Fig 15–5 A–D), autologous tissue from the right atrial wall and interatrial septum is used in place of pericardium or synthetic material.[41] Pulmonary venous and systemic venous blood is routed in the same fashion as in the Mustard procedure.

Both procedures are done with hypothermic car-

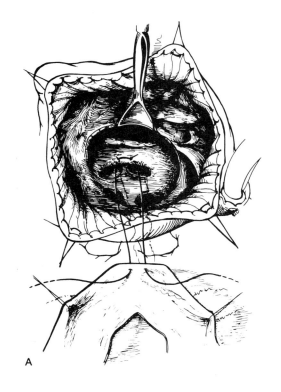

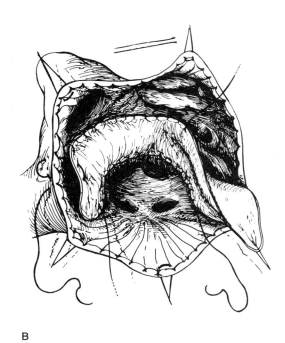

A

B

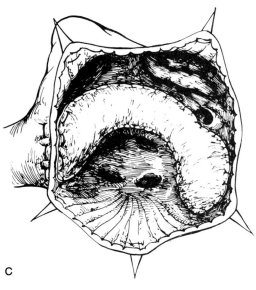

C

Figure 15–4. Details of the Mustard operation. (*A*). View into the right and left atria from an incision into the right atrium. The retractor is on the lip of the surgically excised interatrial septum. The coronary sinus is seen draining into the right atrium just to the right of the retractor. Just above and to the left of the coronary sinus is the tricuspid valve orifice. The SVC is seen in the lower left corner of the right atrium, whereas the IVC is seen in the lower right corner. The four pulmonary veins and the mitral valve orifice are seen in the floor of the left atrium. The pericardial baffle is seen being attached just above the left pulmonary veins. (*B*). Same orientation as in (*A*). The baffle is sutured along the lip of the atrial septum, the floor of the left atrium, and the orifices of the IVC and SVC. As a result, the orifice of the SVC and the orifice of the IVC are enclosed by the baffle such that systemic venous blood is directed through the mitral valve. (*C*) Same orientation as in (*A*). The completed baffle is seen. When the right atrium is closed, pulmonary venous and coronary sinus blood will flow over the baffle through the tricuspid valve. The small right-to-left shunt created by directing coronary sinus blood into the systemic circulation is of no clinical consequence. (*From Stark J: Mustard's operation for transposition of the great arteries. In Jamieson SW, Shumway NE (eds): Rob and Smith's Operative Surgery. 4th ed. London: Butterworth, 1986, p 307, with permission.*)

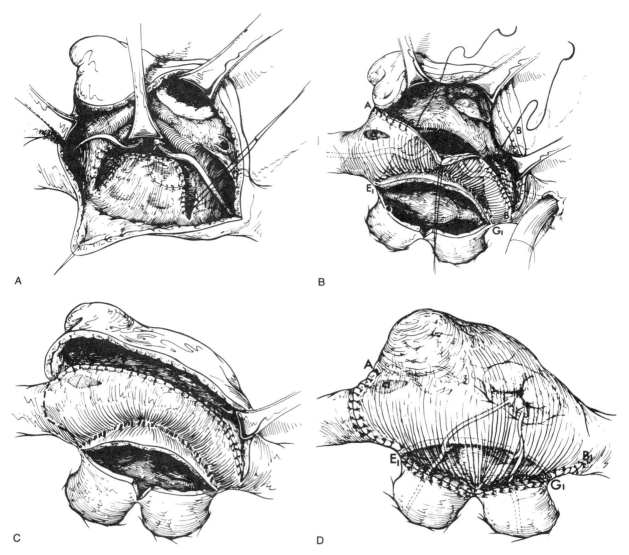

Figure 15–5. Details of the Senning operation. (*A*) View into the right and left atria from an incision into the right atrium. The upper retractor is seen in the orifice of the tricuspid valve. The lower retractor is seen on the lip of the surgically excised interatrial septum. The coronary sinus is seen to the far right. A flap of tissue from the excised interatrial septum has been sutured in front of the left pulmonary veins and along the floor of the left atrium. (*B*) Same orientation as in (*A*). An incision (point E$_1$ to G$_1$) has been made into the left atrium. The boundaries of the right atriotomy are labeled A, B, and B$_1$. The sinus node is labeled A. The four pulmonary veins are seen in the floor of the left atrium. The inferior free wall of the right atrium is sutured to the lip of the interatrial septum such that systemic venous blood is directed through the mitral valve. (*C*) Same orientation as in (*A*). Completed suture line for redirection of systemic venous blood through the mitral valve. (*D*) Same orientation as in (*A*). Completion of the procedure. The superior free wall of the right atrium and the free wall of the left atrium are joined. The free wall of the right atrium is closed over the top of the SVC in the area of the dotted line seen in (*C*). The white arrows depict redirection of pulmonary venous blood through the tricuspid valve. As with the Mustard operation, coronary sinus blood is directed across the tricuspid into the systemic circulation. (*From Brom AG, Quagebeur JM, Rohmer J: Cardiac surgery. In Jamieson SW, Shumway NE (eds): Rob and Smith's Operative Surgery, 4th ed. London: Butterworth, 1986, p 316, with permission.*)

diopulmonary bypass with aortic cross-clamping and cardioplegic arrest. Some centers use intervals of low-flow cardiopulmonary bypass, whereas others use deep hypothermic circulatory arrest (DHCA), particularly in small infants. In both procedures, the area of the sinus node must be avoided to reduce dysrhythmia complications. The Mustard and the Senning procedures for patients with TGV and IVS are generally performed in early infancy (6–9 months), but recently the trend has been toward repair in the neonatal period.[42,43] For patients with TGV and VSD, the atrial switch procedures carry a high operative mortality and poor long-term results.[44,45] These patients are generally treated with the arterial switch procedure to be described below.[46]

Arterial Anatomic Repair: Arterial Switch (Jatene) Procedure.

The arterial switch procedure anatomically corrects the discordant ventriculoarterial connections. Following repair, the right ventricle is connected to the pulmonary artery and the left ventricle to the aorta. Clinical success with the Jatene procedure, summarized in Fig 15–6, was achieved in 1975.[47] In brief, the pulmonary artery and the aorta are transected distal to their respective valves. The coronary arteries are initially explanted from the ascending aorta with 3–4 mm of surrounding tissue. The explant sites are repaired either with pericardium or synthetic material. The coronary arteries are reimplanted into the proximal pulmonary artery (neoaorta). The great arteries are then switched with the distal pulmonary artery brought anterior (Lecompte maneuver) to be reanastomosed to the old proximal aorta (right ventricular outflow) and the distal aorta reanastomosed to the old proximal pulmonary artery (left ventricular outflow).

The majority of patients with TGV have coronary anatomy that is suitable for the coronary reimplantation necessary in the arterial switch procedure[48,49] (see Fig 15–1). Patients with certain types of coronary anatomy (inverted coronaries, single right coronary artery) are at risk for postoperative myocardial ischemia and death because reimplantation causes distortion of the coronary ostia or narrowing of the artery itself.[23,49] The emergence of two parallel coronary arteries above but in contact with the posterior valve commissure or the intramural origin of the coronaries (see Fig 15–1; intramural LCA, intramural LAD) also presents a technical challenge. These patients may require resuspension of the neo–pulmonary valve once the coronaries and a surrounding tissue cuff are excised.[23,49]

In order for the arterial switch procedure to be successful, the original pulmonary ventricle (LV) must have sufficient mass to be capable of becoming the systemic ventricle following the switch. Patient selection and the timing of the surgical procedure are therefore important variables in determining the success of this procedure. The Jatene procedure was originally described in patients with TGV and a large VSD or a large PDA.[47] In these patients, the pulmonary ventricle (LV) remains exposed to systemic pressures and the LV mass remains sufficient to support the systemic circulation. For this subset of patients, the arterial switch procedure is generally performed within the first 2–3 months of life before intractable CHF or irreversible PVOD intervene.[50]

In patients with TGV and IVS, there is progressive reduction in LV mass as the physiologic pulmonary hypertension present at birth resolves progressively over the first days following birth. Adequate LV mass to support the systemic circulation exists in these patients for only the first 2 or 3 weeks following birth.[51,52] In patients with TGV and IVS, the arterial switch procedure can be performed primarily or as the second phase of a staged procedure. A successful primary arterial switch procedure must generally be performed within the first 20 days of life.[4]

Favorable candidates for the procedure in the neonatal period must have a left ventricular to right ventricular pressure ratio of at least 0.6 by catheterization. Alternatively, two-dimensional echocardiography can be used to assess noninvasively the LV to RV pressure ratio.[21] Three types of ventricular septal geometry have been described.[21] Patients in whom the ventricular septum bulges to the left (type 3), indicating a low pressure

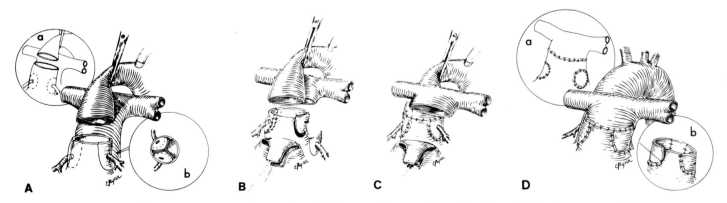

A   **B**   **C**   **D**

Figure 15–6. Details of the arterial switch procedure. (*A*). The aorta is transected and the left and right main coronary arteries are excised using (a) either a button of aortic wall or (b) a segment of aortic wall extending from the rim of the aorta. (*B*). The pulmonary artery is transected. An equivalent segment of the pulmonary arterial wall is excised and the coronary arteries are sutured to the proximal pulmonary artery. (*C*). The distal pulmonary artery is brought anterior to the ascending aorta (Lecompte maneuver) and the proximal pulmonary artery is anastomosed to the distal aorta. (*D*). The sites of the explanted coronary arteries are repaired using either (a) a patch of prosthetic material or (b) a segment of pericardium. Finally, an anastomosis between the proximal aorta and the distal pulmonary artery is constructed. (*From Castenda AR, Norwood WI, Jonas RI et al: Transposition of the great arteries and intact ventricular septum: Anatomical repair in the neonate. Ann Thorac Surg 38:440, 1984, with permission.*)

in the pulmonary ventricle (LV), are not candidates for a neonatal arterial switch procedure. Patients with septal bulging to the right (type 1), indicating a high pressure in the pulmonary ventricle (LV), and those patients with an intermediate septal position (type 2) are considered good candidates. Most neonates with TGV and IVS who are suitable candidates for an arterial switch procedure have type 2 septal geometry. Two-dimensional echocardiographic analysis of the ratio of the lateral to the anteroposterior LV diameter has also been used successfully to assess LV systolic pressure.[24]

In the staged arterial switch procedure, the LV is "prepared" to accept the systemic workload by placement of a pulmonary artery band within the first 2 months of life.[53] In addition, an aortopulmonary shunt with entry to the pulmonary artery distal to the band is necessary to prevent hypoxemia. The band must be tight enough to increase pressure in the pulmonary ventricle (LV) to approximately one half to two thirds that in the systemic ventricle (RV).[54] This will increase afterload sufficiently to prevent regression of LV mass. However, if the band is too tight, there may be LV decompensation secondary to afterload mismatch. At 3–6 months of age, the pulmonary artery is debanded, the shunt taken down, and an arterial switch procedure performed. Currently there is less enthusiasm for the staged arterial switch procedure than for the primary procedure. Placement of the pulmonary artery band to the proper tightness is not an easy task. Furthermore, the pulmonary artery band and systemic to pulmonary artery shunt may result in distortion of the pulmonary artery making the definite arterial switch procedure difficult. Whether the staged arterial switch procedure results in better long-term outcome than an atrial switch procedure for patients with TGV and IVS remains to be seen.

The arterial switch procedure is generally not done in patients where mechanical LVOTO exists. Correction of the LVOTO is difficult, and without complete correction of the LVOTO, these patients will be left with aortic or subaortic stenosis.[55] On the other hand, patients with dynamic LVOTO have been shown to have no gradient across the LV outflow tract following the arterial switch procedure.[56]

The arterial switch procedure is done using hypothermia cardiopulmonary bypass with aortic cross-clamping and cardioplegic arrest. Deep hypothermia and periods of circulatory arrest (DHCA) or intervals of low-flow cardiopulmonary bypass are customarily used as well. Closure of a VSD is preferentially done transatrially through the tricuspid valve. It is desirable to avoid approaching a VSD through the RV because an incision in the RV may contribute substantially to postoperative RV dysfunction.

Rastelli Procedure. The Rastelli procedure was described in 1969 as a method of anatomically correcting TGV with VSD and LVOTO.[57] The procedure is summarized in Fig 15–7. The pulmonary artery is transected and ligated distal to the pulmonary valve. A right ventriculotomy is performed and the VSD is closed with a patch-tunnel such that the LV is in continuity with the aorta. The VSD may have to be enlarged in some cases to prevent subaortic stenosis. The right ventriculotomy site is then used as the proximal end of an external RV to pulmonary artery valved conduit. The result is LV to aortic continuity and RV to pulmonary artery continuity with bypass of the subpulmonic stenosis. This procedure is performed with hypothermic cardiopulmonary bypass, aortic cross-clamping, and cardioplegic arrest. The majority of these patients will have had a palliative systemic to pulmonary artery shunt that is taken down prior to beginning the Rastelli procedure.

Patients are generally greater than 2–3 years of age at the time of the Rastelli procedure. This delay allows adequate growth of the RV and pulmonary arteries topermit placement of a valved conduit of adequate size to accommodate further patient growth. In addition, a right ventriculotomy is very poorly tolerated by infants with immature myocardium and limited contractile elements. Despite delay of the operative procedure, many of these

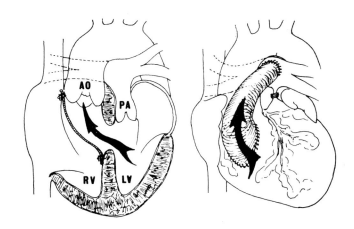

Figure 15–7. Schematic of the Rastelli procedure for repair of transposition of the great vessels with ventricular septal defect and left ventricular outflow tract obstruction. (*A*). The VSD is closed with a patch such that left ventricular outflow is directed across the aortic valve. (*B*). The proximal pulmonary artery is ligated and a valved conduit is placed from the right ventricle to the main pulmonary artery.

patients require reoperation for conduit stenosis and larger conduits as they grow. The current use of pulmonary artery homograft conduits in place of woven Dacron valved conduits or aortic homograft conduits appears to reduce the incidence of conduit stenosis.[58,59]

Damus-Stansel-Kaye Procedure. An alternative to the arterial switch procedure for TGV and VSD is the Damus-Stansel-Kaye procedure described independently by Damus, Stansel, Kay, and Alverez. This procedure can be used where coronary anatomy precludes an arterial switch procedure.[60] It is illustrated in Fig 15–8. A right ventriculotomy is performed and the VSD is closed. The pulmonary artery is transected just proximal to its bifurcation and the proximal end of the pulmonary artery is reanastomosed end to side to the aorta. This establishes LV to aorta continuity. Right ventricular to pulmonary artery continuity is established via a valved conduit from the ventriculotomy to the distal end of the pulmonary artery.

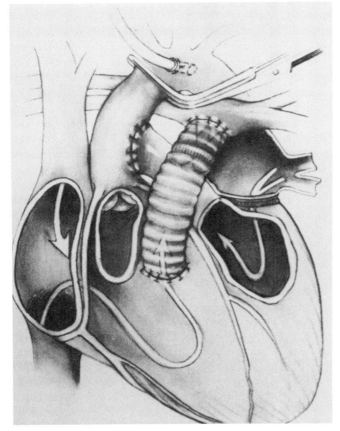

Figure 15–8. Schematic of the Damus-Stansel-Kaye procedure. The proximal pulmonary artery has been anastomosed end to side to the aorta. A valved conduit has been placed from the right ventricle to the main pulmonary artery. The resulting pressure gradient keeps the aortic valve closed and permits right ventricular to pulmonary artery continuity via the conduit. (*From Ceithaml EL, Puja FJ, Danielson GK et al: Results of the Damus-Stansel-Kaye procedure for transposition of the great arteries and for double outlet right ventricle with subpulmonary ventricular septal defect. Ann Thorac Surg 38: 435, 1984, with permission.*)

With LV pressure greater than RV pressure, the pressure gradient is such that the native aortic valve (located in continuity with the RV) remains closed and ejection from the RV is via the conduit. This procedure is performed with hypothermic cardiopulmonary bypass, aortic cross-clamping, and cardioplegic arrest.

Reparation A L'Etage Ventriculaire Procedure. A recently described alternative to the arterial switch procedure for TGV with VSD and to the Rastelli procedure for TGV and VSD with LVOTO is the reparation a l'etage ventriculaire (REV) procedure.[61,62] This procedure has the advantage of requiring neither coronary reimplantation nor use of an external valved conduit. A right ventriculotomy is performed and the VSD enlarged by septal resection. LV to aortic continuity is created by means of a VSD patch-tunnel closure. The pulmonary artery is transected just above the valve and the proximal stump is ligated. The distal pulmonary artery segment is fitted with a valved prosthesis and reanastomosed to the right ventriculotomy site creating RV to pulmonary artery continuity. This procedure is performed with hypothermic cardiopulmonary bypass, aortic cross-clamping, and cardioplegic arrest.

POSTOPERATIVE CARE

The care of patients following palliative or definite surgical therapy for TGV must be tailored to the preoperative condition of the patient and the type of surgical procedure performed.

Mustard and Senning Procedures

The placement of intra-atrial baffles may result in systemic and/or pulmonary venous obstruction in the immediate postbypass period. Systemic venous obstruction produces a low cardiac output state and, in the extreme, a superior vena cava syndrome. Pulmonary venous obstruction produces a low output state and pulmonary edema. The anesthesiologist should be prepared to recognize these problems and communicate them to the surgeon. Treatment will require reinstitution of bypass for baffle revision.

Dysrhythmias immediately following atrial switch procedures may be problematic. Atrial pacing may be required for sinus bradycardia, whereas atrioventricular sequential pacing will be needed for slow junctional rates. Rate control for rapid atrial flutter may require pharmacologic intervention with digoxin or attempts at cardioversion. Atrial flutter with block may be tolerated by some patients owing to the slower ventricular response rate.

Right (systemic) ventricular dysfunction may be exacerbated in the postbypass period. Patients undergoing right ventriculotomy to close a VSD or those with poor right ventricular protection during the aortic cross-clamp period are particularly at risk. Both mechanical and functional tricuspid regurgitation may be seen after discontinuation of bypass. Disruption of the tricuspid valve apparatus can occur during transatrial closure of a VSD. Functional tricuspid regurgitation often results from the right ventricular dilation that accompanies ventricular dysfunction. Inotropic support of the RV may be required. Dobutamine (5–10 µg/kg/min) or dopamine (5–10 µg/kg/min) are useful to provide potent inotropic support without increasing PVR.

Arterial Switch Procedure

Bleeding from the extensive suture lines in the postbypass period may be problematic. Efforts to reduce aortic blood pressure combined with aggressive blood component therapy is often required. As a general rule, 1 U of platelets per 10 kg of body weight will increase the platelet count by 50,000–70,000/mm^3. In instances in which 1.5–2.0 blood volumes are lost, procoagulant replacement may require that as much as 30% of the blood volume be replaced with fresh frozen plasma.

Myocardial ischemia following reimplantation of the coronary arteries is a potential problem following the arterial switch procedure. In some circumstances, the ischemia is transient secondary to coronary air emboli. Maintenance of high perfusion pressures on cardiopulmonary bypass (CPB) after aortic cross-clamp removal will facilitate distal migration of air emboli. In other instances, kinking of the reimplanted artery or compromise of the implanted coronary ostia may require immediate surgical intervention. In both instances, pharmacologic intervention with nitroglycerin and β-blockade may be necessary in the immediate management.

Despite comprehensive preoperative evaluation, the LV of patients undergoing an arterial switch procedure may be marginal in its ability to support the systemic circulation in the post-CPB period (see Table 15–3). This may occur as the result of myocardial ischemia, inadequate LV mass, inadequate myocardial preservation of the LV during aortic cross-clamping, or a combination of these variables. Inotropic support of the LV and afterload reduction may be necessary to terminate bypass successfully. This can be accomplished with a dobutamine (10–20 µg/kg/min) and nitroprusside (0.15–0.5 µg/kg/min) combination. In instances in which LV failure is severe, epinephrine (0.25–1.0 µg/min) may have to be used in combination with nitroprusside. Alternatively, amrinone (10–20 µg/kg/min following a loading dose of 1.5 mg/kg) can be used. It is advisable to administer the loading dose of amrinone while on bypass to minimize its vasodilatory effects.

Rastelli Procedure

Right (pulmonary) ventricular dysfunction may occur in the post-CPB period. These patients are at risk because a right ventriculotomy is used to close the VSD and to

TABLE 15–3. POST-CPB MANAGEMENT

1. Maintain heart rate (preferably sinus rhythm) at an age-appropriate rate. Cardiac output is likely to be more heart rate dependent in the post-CPB period. In patients having undergone atrial switch procedures, antidysrhythmia therapy or pacing may be necessary.
2. Aggressive treatment of myocardial ischemia is necessary when it occurs following coronary reimplantation.
3. Reductions in aortic and pulmonary artery pressures may be necessary to help prevent suture line bleeding following the arterial switch procedure. Aggressive blood component therapy is often necessary as well.
4. Systemic ventricular (RV after atrial switch procedure and LV after arterial switch procedure) dysfunction may necessitate use of inotropic and vasodilator therapy to terminate CPB.

create the new pulmonary outflow tract. In some instances, inotropic support of the RV may be required. Dobutamine (5–10 µg/kg/min) or dopamine (5–10 µg/kg/min) is useful in this instance as either provides potent inotropic support without increasing PVR. Stenosis at the anastomosis of the pulmonary conduit to the pulmonary artery will increase RV afterload and exacerbate RV dysfunction. In cases in which the stenosis is severe, revision of the anastomosis may be necessary.

IMMEDIATE AND LONG-TERM RESULTS

Atrial Switch Procedures

The immediate and long-term results of the Mustard and Senning procedures in patients with TGV and IVS are good, with an actuarial survival rate of approximately 95% at 1 year and approximately 80% at 20 years.[63–65] The immediate and long-term results of atrial switch procedures in patients with TGV and VSD are less favorable, with an actuarial survival rate of 80% at 1 year and only 60–70% at 5 years.[44] The majority of patient deaths in this subgroup are due to RV dysfunction, often in association with tricuspid insufficiency.[44,45] Morbidity after atrial switch procedures results from systemic or pulmonary venous obstruction, arrhythmias, and ventricular failure (systemic).

Pulmonary venous obstruction is rare, occurring in approximately 2% of patients.[64] Although pulmonary venous obstruction is most likely to appear within 1 year of operation, it has been reported as late as 14 years after the procedure. Percutaneous balloon dilation of the pulmonary venous pathway has been used successfully after both Mustard and Senning repairs.[66,67] Superior vena caval obstruction (approximately 5%) is more common than inferior vena caval obstruction (approximately 1%).[64] A higher incidence of asymptomatic superior vena caval obstruction (approximately 15%) has been detected in late catheterization studies.[64] Percutaneous balloon dilation has been used to treat this complication as well.[68]

Dysrhythmias in the immediate and late postoperative period following Mustard and Senning procedures are well recognized complications.[69,70] Although there was hope that the use of autologous atrial tissue in the Senning procedure might reduce the incidence of dysrhythmias compared with the Mustard procedure, this has not been the case.[70,71]

In the immediate postoperative period, approximately 80% of patients will be in sinus rhythm.[72] Improvements in surgical technique are largely responsible for the decrease in early postoperative dysrhythmias that has been seen over the years.[73] The most common dysrhythmias are sinus bradycardia, ectopic atrial beats, slow junctional rhythm, and supraventricular tachycardia, especially atrial flutter.[69,70] The dysrhythmias appear to be due to abnormalities in sinus node function, delayed intra-atrial conduction, and prolonged atrial refractory periods secondary to the operative procedure.[69] Atrioventricular node dysfunction also occurs but less commonly.

Unfortunately, late dysrhythmias continue to be a problem. There is progressive loss of sinus rhythm following both the Mustard and Senning operations. Actuarial analysis of several recent series reveals that by 8–10 years after operation, only 60–70% of patients will be in sinus rhythm at rest.[63,71–74] The majority of patients not in sinus rhythm are in a junctional rhythm. Late sudden death has been noted in patients following atrial switch surgery and is thought to be secondary to dysrhythmias.[63]

A major concern in patients having undergone atrial switch procedures is the fact that the right ventricle is not physiologically adapted to support the systemic circulation. Systemic (RV) ventricular ejection fraction is reduced in the majority of atrial switch patients and RV end-diastolic volume is elevated.[75–77] Furthermore, systemic ventricular response to increased afterload is abnormal, demonstrating an inability to increase ventricular work in the face of increased afterload.[75] Systemic (RV) ventricular systolic function appears to be better preserved at late follow-up in patients who undergo repair early as opposed to late in infancy.[78,79] Despite these abnormalities, the vast majority (80–90%) of long-term survivors of atrial switch operations for TGV with IVS are in New York Heart Association (NYHA) functional class 1 or 2.[71,80] Right ventricular dysfunction leading to death or functional class 3 or 4 status is much more likely in patients with TGV and VSD who undergo atrial switch procedures.

The exercise response of patients having undergone an atrial switch procedure is clearly abnormal. Asymptomatic children have a normal increase in cardiac output in response to submaximal exercise. However, they clearly have a reduced maximal aerobic capacity and oxygen consumption.[81–83] In contrast to normal children, systemic ventricular ejection fraction and stroke volume remain unchanged, whereas end-diastolic volume increases

during exercise in TGV patients.[84–86] Furthermore, following atrial switch procedures, patients have an impaired chronotropic response to exercise that exacerbates the increase in right ventricular end-diastolic volume.[82]

Arterial Switch Procedure

Immediate results for the arterial switch in experienced institutions is excellent, with an actuarial survival at 1 year of 90% for patients with TGV and IVS and 83% for patients with TGV and VSD.[87] Owing to the relative newness of the arterial switch procedure, long-term follow-up is less complete than for the atrial switch procedure. Results from six institutions experienced in the arterial switch procedure revealed an actuarial 2.5-year survival rate of 90% for patients with TGV and IVS and 83% for patients with TGV and VSD.[87] Similar results have been reported by other experienced groups.[88–90]

Supravalvular pulmonary stenosis is probably the most common complication of the arterial switch procedure. Mild to moderate supravalvular stenosis may occur in 10–44% of patients.[91–93] In the majority of patients, this stenosis is not progressive and is due to the sacrifice of tissue necessary to ensure an adequate cuff of tissue around the explanted coronaries. Supravalvular stenosis severe enough to require reoperation (generally a gradient greater than 60–70 mm Hg) occurs in 2–10% of patients depending on the series.[87–90,94] Balloon dilation has been unsuccessful in the treatment of supravalvular pulmonary stenosis after the Jatene procedure.[95]

Trivial or mild aortic regurgitation is a frequent finding after the arterial switch procedure, occurring in 7–40% of patients at midterm follow-up.[88,90,93,94,96] There is some evidence that this complication is more prevalent in patients having undergone the two-stage arterial switch procedure.[88,96] To date, aortic insufficiency has not been a source of morbidity or required reoperation. Long-term follow-up is needed to assess the significance of this finding.

In contrast to the atrial switch procedure, electrophysiologic abnormalities are uncommon after the arterial switch procedure. The most common abnormalities are rare, asymptomatic, atrial and ventricular premature beats. Right bundle branch block is more common in patients after the arterial switch procedure with closure of a VSD.[97,98]

The long-term status of the coronary circulation has been a concern following the arterial switch procedure. Concern has centered around kinking of the reimplanted coronaries and failure of the reimplanted coronary ostia to grow. In the vast majority of patients followed to date, these problems have not materialized.[99] The overwhelming majority of patients have patent coronary arteries seen on postoperative coronary angiography. However, reversible perfusion defects following both dipyridamole[100] and isoproterenol[101] stress thallium scintigraphy suggest that stress-induced myocardial ischemia secondary to reduced coronary flow reserve is present after the arterial switch procedure. In one study of patients following two-stage repair, these perfusion defects were associated with echocardiographic wall motion abnormalities.[102] Despite these findings, the patients in these studies are clinically well. The significance of these defects is presently unclear and clarification will require additional studies and long-term follow-up.

One of the potential advantages of the arterial switch procedure over atrial switch procedures is the use of the native LV as the systemic ventricle. Follow-up data to date indicate that patients after arterial switch procedures have higher systemic ventricular ejection fractions than patients after atrial switch procedures.[76,77] In fact, patients with TGV and IVS repaired in infancy[103] and patients with TGV and VSD with later repair have LV end-diastolic dimensions and contractile indices similar to normal subjects.[89] There is some suggestion that systemic ventricular systolic function following the two-stage arterial switch is reduced compared with that after neonatal primary repair.[77,103,104] This issue remains to be resolved.

Rastelli Procedure

Recent experience with the Rastelli procedure for TGV with VSD and LVOTO is excellent, with 100% survival at 1 year postsurgery in one series.[105] Actuarial survival at 12 years is 60–75%.[105,106] However, this figure reflects an increased hospital mortality rate (20–30%) seen in the early days of the procedure. Late survival is better in patients undergoing the procedure in the current era.[105,107] At mid- and long-term follow-up, patients after the Rastelli procedure have increased LV end-diastolic and end-systolic volumes and diminished LV contractile function compared with normal subjects.[108] Despite these findings, the majority (90%) of patients are in NYHA functional class 1 or 2 following the Rastelli procedure.[105]

As discussed previously, the incidence of conduit stenosis has diminished with the use of cryopreserved pulmonary homograft. When reoperation for conduit stenosis is required, it can be accomplished at a low risk of mortality.[105]

REFERENCES

1. Fyler DC: Report of the New England Regional Infant Cardiac Program. *Pediatrics* **65**(suppl):375–461, 1980.
2. Liebman J, Cullum L, Belloc NB: Natural history of transposition of the great arteries. Anatomy and birth and death characteristics. *Circulation* **40**:237–262, 1969
3. Paul MH: Complete transposition of the great arteries. In Adams FH, Emmanoulides GC, Riemenschneider TA (eds): *Moss' Heart Disease in Infants, Children, and Adolescents*. Baltimore: Williams & Wilkins, 1989, pp 371–423
4. Castaneda AR, Mayer JE: Neonatal repair of transposition of the great arteries. In Long WA (ed): *Fetal and Neonatal Cardiology*. Philadelphia: WB Saunders, 1990, pp 789–795
5. Aziz KU, Paul MH, Idriss FS, et al: Clinical manifestations of dynamic left ventricular outflow tract stenosis with D-transposition of the great arteries with intact ventricular septum. *Am J Cardiol* **44**:290–297, 1979
6. Aziz KU, Paul MH, Rowe RD: Bronchopulmonary circulation in D-transposition of the great arteries: Possible role in genesis of accelerated pulmonary vascular disease. *Am J Cardiol* **39**:432–438, 1977
7. McGoon DC, Mair DD: On the unmuddling of shunting, mixing, and streaming. *J Thorac Cardiovasc Surg* **100**:77–82, 1990
8. Friedberg DZ, Nadas AS: Clinical profile of patients with congenitally corrected transposition of the great arteries. *N Engl J Med* **282**:1053–1059, 1970
9. Hwang B, Bowman F, Malm J, Krongrad E: Surgical repair of congenitally corrected transposition of the great arteries: Results and followup. *Am J Cardiol* **50**:781–785, 1982
10. Doty DB, Truesdell SC, Marvin WJ: Techniques to avoid injury of the conduction tissue during surgical treatment of corrected transposition. *Circulation* **68**(suppl 2):63–69, 1983
11. Mair DD, Ritter DG: Factors influencing intercirculatory mixing in patients with complete transposition of the great arteries. *Am J Cardiol* **30**:653–658, 1972
12. Mair DD, Ritter DG: Factors influencing systemic arterial oxygen saturation in complete transposition of the great arteries. *Am J Cardiol* **31**:742–748, 1973
13. Mair DD, Ritter DG, Ongley PA, Helmholz HF: Hemodynamics and evaluation for surgery of patients with complete transposition of the great arteries and ventricular septal defect. *Am J Cardiol* **28**:632–640, 1971
14. Terai M, Nakazawa M, Takao A, et al: Thrombocytopenia in patients with aortopulmonary transposition and an intact ventricular septum. *Br Heart J* **57**:371–374, 1987
15. Newfield EA, Paul MH, Mustger AJ, Idriss FS: Pulmonary vascular disease in complete transposition of the great arteries: A study of 200 patients. *Am J Cardiol* **34**:75–82, 1974
16. Clarkson PM, Neutze JM, Wardhill JC, et al: The pulmonary vascular bed in patients with complete transposition of the great arteries. *Circulation* **53**:539–542.
17. Levin DL, Paul MH, Muster AJ, et al: The clinical diagnosis of D-transposition of the great vessels in the neonate. *Arch Intern Med* **137**:1421–1425, 1977
18. Freed MD, Heymann MA, Lewis AB, et al: Prostaglandin E$_1$ in infants with ductus arteriosus-dependent congenital heart disease. *Circulation* **64**:899–905, 1981
19. Daskalopoulos DA, Edwards WD, Driscoll DJ, et al: Correlation of two-dimensional echocardiography and autopsy findings in complete transposition of the great arteries. *J Am Coll Cardiol* **2**:1151–1157, 1983
20. Chin AJ, Yeager SB, Sanders SP, et al: Accuracy of prospective two-dimensional echocardiographic evaluation of left ventricular outflow tract in complete transposition of the great arteries. *Am J Cardiol* **55**:759–764, 1985
21. Castenada AR, Norwood WI, Jonas RA, et al: Transposition of the great arteries and intact ventricular septum: Anatomical repair in the neonate. *Ann Thorac Surg* **38**:438–443, 1984
22. van Doesburg NH, Bierman FZ, Williams RG: Left ven-

tricular geometry in infants with D-transposition of the great arteries and intact ventricular septum. *Circulation* **68**: 733–739, 1983

23. Planche C, Bruniaux J, Lacour-Gayet F, et al: Switch operation for transposition of the great arteries in neonates: A study of 120 patients. *J Thorac Cardiovasc Surg* **96**:354–363, 1988

24. Sidi D, Planche C, Kachaner J, et al: Anatomic correction of simple transposition of the great arteries in 50 neonates. *Circulation* **75**:429–435, 1987

25. Colon-Otero G, Gilchrist GS, Holcomb GR, et al: Preoperative evaluation of hemostasis in patients with congenital heart disease. *Mayo Clin Proc* **62**:379–385, 1987

26. Milam JD, Austin SF, Nihill MR, et al: Use of sufficient hemodilution to prevent coagulopathies following surgical correction of cyanotic heart disease. *J Thorac Cardiovasc Surg* **89**:623–629, 1985

27. Perloff JK, Rosove MH, Child JS, Wright GB: Adults with cyanotic congenital heart disease: Hematologic management. *Ann Intern Med* **109**:406–413, 1988

28. Abman, SH, Wolfe RR, Accurso FJ: Pulmonary vascular response to oxygen in infants with severe bronchopulmonary dysplasia. *Pediatrics* **75**:80–84, 1985

29. Morray JP, Lynn AM, Mansfield PB: Effect of pH and pCO$_2$ on pulmonary and systemic hemodynamics after surgery in children with congenital heart disease and pulmonary hypertension. *J Pediatr* **113**:474–479, 1988

30. Schreiber MD, Heyman MA, Soifer SJ: Increased arterial pH, not decreased PaCO$_2$ attenuates hypoxia-induced pulmonary vasoconstriction in lambs. *Pediatr Res* **20**:113–117, 1986

31. Hickey PR, Hansen DD: Fentanyl- and sufentanil-oxygen-pancuronium anesthesia for cardiac surgery in infants. *Anesth Analg* **63**:117–124, 1984

32. Savarese JJ, Lowenstein E: The name of the game: No anesthesia by cookbook. *Anesthesiology* **62**:703–705, 1985

33. Friedman WF: Intrinsic physiologic properties of the developing heart. *Prog Cardiovasc Dis* **15**:87–111, 1972

34. Philbin DM, Rosow CE, Schneider RC, et al: Fentanyl and sufentanil anesthesia revisited: How much is enough? *Anesthesiology* **73**:5–11, 1990

35. Heikkila H, Jalonen J, Arola M: Midazolam as adjunct to high-dose fentanyl anesthesia for coronary artery bypass grafting operation. *Acta Anaesthesiol Scand* **28**:683–689, 1984

36. Hickey, PR, Hansen, DD, Cramolini GM, et al: Pulmonary and systemic vascular responses to ketamine in infants with normal and elevated pulmonary vascular resistance. *Anesthesiology* **62**:287–293, 1985

37. Blalock A, Hanlon CR: The surgical treatment of complete transposition of the aorta and pulmonary artery. *Surg Gynecol Obstet* **90**:1–15, 1950

38. Rashkind WJ, Miller WW: Creation of an atrial septal defect without thoracotomy: A palliative approach to complete transposition of the great arteries. *JAMA* **196**:991–992, 1966

39. Dhasmana JP, Stark J, DeLeval M, et al: Long-term results of the "palliative" Mustard operation. *J Am Coll Cardiol* **6**:1138–1141, 1985

40. Mustard WT: Successful two-stage correction of transposition of the great vessels. *Surgery* **55**:469–472, 1964

41. Senning A: Surgical correction of transposition of the great vessels. *Surgery* **45**:966–980, 1959

42. Matherne GP, Razook JD, Thompson WM, et al: Senning repair for transposition of the great arteries in the first week of life. *Circulation* **72**:840–845, 1985

43. DeLeon VH, Hougen TJ, Norwood WI, et al: Results of the Senning operation for transposition of the great arteries with intact ventricular septum in neonates. *Circulation* **70**(suppl 1):21–25, 1984

44. Penkoske PA, Westerman GR, Marx GR, et al: Transposition of the great arteries and ventricular septal defect: Results with the Senning operation and closure of the ventricular septal defect in infants. *Ann Thorac Surg* **36**:281–288, 1983

45. George BL, Laks H, Klitzner TS, et al: Results of the Senning procedure in infants with simple and complex transposition of the great arteries. *Am J Cardiol* **59**:426–430, 1987

46. Corno A, George B, Pearl J, Laks H: Surgical options for complex transposition of the great arteries. *J Am Coll Cardiol* **14**:742–749, 1989

47. Jatene AD, Fontes VF, Paulista PP, et al: Anatomic correction of transposition of the great vessels. *J Thorac Cardiovasc Surg* **72**:364–370, 1976

48. Yacoub MH, Radley-Smith R: Anatomy of the coronary arteries in transposition of the great arteries and methods for their transfer in anatomical correction. *Thorax* **33**:418–424, 1978

49. Mayer JE, Sanders SP, Jonas RA, et al: Coronary artery pattern and outcome of the arterial switch operation for transposition of the great arteries. *Circulation* **82**(suppl 5): 139–145, 1990

50. Bove EL, Beckman RH, Snider AR, et al: Arterial repair for transposition of the great arteries and large ventricular septal defect in early infancy. *Circulation* **78**(suppl 3):26–31, 1988

51. Bano-Rodrigo A, Quero-Jimenez M, Moreno-Granado F, Gamallo-Amat C: Wall thickness of ventricular chambers in transposition of the great arteries: Surgical implications. *J Thorac Cardiovasc Surg* **79**:592–597, 1980

52. Danford D, Huhta J, Gutgesell H: Left ventricular wall stress and thickness in complete transposition of the great arteries: Implications for surgical intervention. *J Thorac Cardiovasc Surg* **89**:610–615, 1985

53. Yacoub MH, Radley-Smith R, MacLaurin R: Two-stage operation for anatomical correction of transposition of the great arteries with intact ventricular septum. *Lancet* **1**:1275–1278, 1977

54. Ilbawi MN, Idriss FS, DeLeon SY, et al: Preparation of the left ventricle for anatomical correction in patients with simple transposition of the great arteries. *J Thorac Cardiovasc Surg* **94**:87–94, 1987

55. Idriss FS, DeLeon SY, Nikaidoh H, et al: Resection of left ventricular outflow obstruction in D-transposition of the great arteries. *J Thorac Cardiovasc Surg* **74**:343–351, 1977

56. Yacoub MH, Arensman FW, Keck E, Radley-Smith R: Fate of dynamic left ventricular outflow tract obstruction after anatomic correction of transposition of the great arteries. *Circulation* **68**(suppl 2):56–62, 1983

57. Rastelli GC, McGoon DC, Wallace RB: Anatomic correction of transposition of the great arteries with ventricular

septal defect and subpulmonary stenosis. *J Thorac Cardiovasc Surg* **58**:545–552, 1969
58. Livi U, Abdulla A-K, Parker R, et al: Viability and morphology of aortic and pulmonary homografts. A comparative study. *J Thorac Cardiovasc Surg* **93**:755–760, 1987
59. McGrath LB, Gonzalez-Lavin L, Graf D: Pulmonary homograft implantation for ventricular outflow tract reconstruction: Early phase results. *Ann Thorac Surg* **45**:273–277, 1988
60. Ceithaml EL, Puga FJ, Danielson GK, et al: Results of the Damus-Stansel-Kaye procedure for transposition of the great arteries and for double-outlet right ventricle with subpulmonary ventricular septal defect. *Ann Thorac Surg* **38**:433–437, 1984
61. Sakata R, Lecompte Y, Batisse A, et al: Anatomic repair of anomalies of ventriculoarterial connection associated with ventricular septal defect. 1. Criteria of surgical decision. *J Thorac Cardiovasc Surg* **95**:90–95, 1988
62. Borromee L, Lecompte Y, Batisse A, et al: Anatomic repair of anomalies of ventriculoarterial connection associated with ventricular septal defect. 2. Clinical results in 50 patients with pulmonary outflow tract obstruction. *J Thorac Cardiovasc Surg* **95**:96–102, 1988
63. Williams WG, Trusler GA, Kirklin JW, et al: Early and late results of a protocol for simple transposition leading to an atrial switch (Mustard) repair. *J Thorac Cardiovasc Surg* **95**:717–726, 1988
64. Turina M, Siebenmann R, Nussbaumer P, Senning A: Long-term outlook after atrial correction of transposition of great arteries. *J Thorac Cardiovasc Surg* **95**:828–835, 1988
65. Merlo M, DeTommasi SM, Brunelli F, et al: Long-term results after atrial correction of complete transposition of the great arteries. *Ann Thorac Surg* **51**:227–231, 1991
66. Coulson JD, Jennings RB, Johnson DH: Pulmonary venous atrial obstruction after the Senning procedure: Relief by balloon dilation. *Br Heart J* **64**:160–162, 1990
67. Cooper SG, Sullivan ID, Bull C, Taylor JFN: Balloon dilatation of pulmonary venous pathway obstruction after Mustard repair for transposition of the great arteries. *J Am Coll Cardiol* **14**:194–198, 1989
68. Benson LN, Yeatman L, Laks H: Balloon dilatation for superior vena caval obstruction after the Senning procedure. *Cathet Cardiovasc Diagn* **11**:63–68, 1985
69. Vetter VL, Tanner CS, Horowitz LN: Electrophysiologic consequences of the Mustard repair of D-transposition of the great arteries. *J Am Coll Cardiol* **10**:1265–1273, 1987
70. Byrum CJ, Bove EL, Sondheimer HM, et al: Hemodynamic and electrophysiologic results of the Senning procedure for transposition of the great arteries. *Am J Cardiol* **58**:138–142, 1986
71. Bender HW, Stewart JR, Merrill WH, et al: Ten years' experience with the Senning operation for transposition of the great arteries. Physiological results and late follow-up. *Ann Thorac Surg* **47**:218–223, 1989
72. Deanfield J, Camm J, Macartney F, et al: Arrhythmia and late mortality after Mustard and Senning operation for transposition of the great arteries. An eight-year prospective study. *J Thorac Cardiovasc Surg* **96**:569–576, 1988
73. Campbell DN, Clarke DR: Transposition of the great arteries. The atrial switch (baffle) procedure. In *Cardiac Surgery: State of the Art Reviews*, Vol 3, No. 1, Philadelphia: Hanley and Belfus, 1989, pp 241–256.
74. Turley K, Hanley FL, Verrier ED, et al: The Mustard procedure in infants (less than 100 days of age). Ten-year follow-up. *J Thorac Cardiovasc Surg* **96**:849–853, 1988
75. Borow KM, Keane JF, Castenada AR, Freed MD: Systemic ventricular function in patients with tetralogy of Fallot, ventricular septal defect and transposition of the great arteries repaired during infancy. *Circulation* **64**:878–885, 1981
76. Okuda H, Nakazawa M, Imai Y, et al: Comparison of ventricular function after Senning and Jatene procedures for complete transposition of the great arteries. *Am J Cardiol* **55**:530–534, 1985
77. Martin RP, Qureshi SA, Ettedgui JA, et al: An evaluation of right and left ventricular function after anatomical correction and intra-atrial repair operations for complete transposition of the great arteries. *Circulation* **82**:808–816, 1990
78. Graham TP, Burger J, Bender HW, et al: Improved right ventricular function after intra-atrial repair of transposition of the great arteries. *Circulation* **72**(suppl 2):45–51, 1985
79. Schmidt KG, Cloez JL, Silverman NH: Assessment of right ventricular performance by pulsed Doppler echocardiography in patients after intraatrial repair of aortopulmonary transposition in infancy or childhood. *J Am Coll Cardiol* **13**:1578–1585, 1989
80. Ashraf MH, Cotroneo J, DiMarco D, Subramanian S: Fate of long-term survivors of Mustard procedure (inflow repair) for simple and complex transposition of the great arteries. *Ann Thorac Surg* **42**:385–289, 1986
81. Musewe NN, Reisman J, Benson LN, et al: Cardiopulmonary adaptation at rest and during exercise 10 years after Mustard atrial repair for transposition of the great arteries. *Circulation* **77**:1055–1061, 1988
82. Paridon SM, Humes RA, Pinsky WW: The role of chronotropic impairment during exercise after the Mustard operation. *J Am Coll Cardiol* **17**:729–732, 1991
83. Ensing GJ, Heise CT, Driscoll DJ: Cardiovascular response to exercise after the Mustard operation for simple and complex transposition of the great vessels. *Am J Cardiol* **62**:617–622, 1988
84. Peterson RJ, Franch RH, Fagman WA, Jones RH: Comparison of cardiac function in surgically corrected and congenitally corrected transposition of the great arteries. *J Thorac Cardiovasc Surg* **96**:227–236, 1988
85. Benson LN, Bonet J, McLaughlin P, et al: Assessment of right ventricular function during supine bicycle exercise after Mustard's operation. *Circulation* **65**:1052–1059, 1982
86. Parrish MD, Graham TP, Bender HW, et al: Radionuclide angiographic evaluation of right and left ventricular function during exercise after repair of transposition of the great arteries. Comparison with normal subjects and patients with congenitally corrected transposition. *Circulation* **67**:178–183, 1983
87. Norwood WI, Dobell AR, Freed MD, et al: Intermediate results of the arterial switch procedure. A 20-institution study. *J Thorac Cardiovasc Surg* **96**:854–863, 1988
88. Yamaguchi M, Hosokawa Y, Imai Y, et al: Early and midterm results of the arterial switch operation for transposition of the great arteries in Japan. *J Thorac Cardiovasc Surg* **100**:261–269, 1990

89. Quaegebuer JM, Rohmer J, Ottenkamp J, et al: The arterial switch operation. An eight-year experience. *J Thorac Cardiovasc Surg* **92**:361–384, 1986

90. Losay J, Planche C, Gerardin B, et al: Midterm surgical results of arterial switch operation for transposition of the great arteries with intact ventricular septum. *Circulation* **82**(suppl 4):146–150, 1990

91. Martin MM, Snider AR, Bove EL, et al: Two-dimensional and Doppler echocardiographic evaluation after arterial switch repair in infancy for complete transposition of the great arteries. *Am J Cardiol* **63**:332–326, 1989

92. Paillole C, Sidi D, Kachaner J, et al: Fate of the pulmonary artery after anatomical correction of simple transposition of the great arteries in newborn infants. *Circulation* **78**:870–876, 1988

93. Gleason MM, Chin AJ, Andrews BA, et al: Two-dimensional and Doppler echocardiographic assessment of neonatal arterial repair for transposition of the great arteries. *J Am Coll Cardiol* **13**:1320–1328, 1989

94. Wernovsky G, Hougen TJ, Walsh EP, et al: Midterm results after the arterial switch operation for transposition of the great arteries with intact ventricular septum: clinical, hemodynamic, echocardiographic, and electrophysiologic data. *Circulation* **77**:1333–1344, 1988

95. Saxena A, Fong LV, Ogilvie BC, Keeton BR: Use of balloon dilatation to treat supravalvular pulmonary stenosis developing after anatomical correction for complete transposition. *Br Heart J* **64**:151–154, 1990

96. Martin RP, Ettedgui JA, Quereshi SA, et al: A quantitative evaluation of aortic regurgitation after anatomic correction of transposition of the great arteries. *J Am Coll Cardiol* **12**:1281–1284, 1988

97. Vetter VL, Tanner CS: Electrophysiologic consequences of the arterial switch repair of D-transposition of the great arteries. *J Am Coll Cardiol* **12**:229–237, 1988

98. Villafane J, White S, Elbl F, et al: An electrocardiographic midterm follow-up study after anatomic repair of transposition of the great arteries. *Am J Cardiol* **66**:350–354, 1990

99. Arensman FW, Sievers HH, Lange P, et al: Assessment of coronary and aortic anastomoses after anatomic correction of transposition of the great arteries. *J Thorac Cardiovasc Surg* **90**:597–604, 1985

100. Losse B, Mecklenbeck W, Kramer HH, Krian A: Thallium myocardial imaging after anatomical correction of D-transposition of the great arteries. *Circulation* **78**(suppl 2):293, 1988

101. Vogel M, Smallhorn JF, Gilday D, et al: Assessment of myocardial perfusion in patients after arterial switch operation. *J Nucl Med* **32**:237–241, 1991

102. Vogel M, Smallhorn JF, Trusler CA, Freedom RM: Echocardiographic analysis of regional left ventricular wall motion in children after the arterial switch operation for complete transposition of the great arteries. *J Am Coll Cardiol* **15**:1417–1423, 1990

103. Colan SD, Trowitzsch E, Wernovsky G, et al: Myocardial performance after arterial switch operation for transposition of the great arteries with intact ventricular septum. *Circulation* **78**:132–141, 1988

104. Sievers HH, Lange PE, Onnasch DGW, et al: Influence of the two-stage anatomic correction of simple transposition of the great arteries on left ventricular function. *Am J Cardiol* **56**:514–519, 1985

105. Kirklin JW, Barratt-Boyes GB: Complete transposition of the great arteries. In Kirklin JW, Barratt-Boyes BG (eds): *Cardiac Surgery*. New York: John Wiley & Sons, 1986, pp 1129–1217

106. Kececioglu D, Vogt J, de Vivie ER: Late results following Rastelli corrective operations in transposition of great vessels. *Z Kardiol* **77**:432–435, 1988

107. Moulton AL, de Leval MR, MacCartney FJ, et al: Rastelli procedure for transposition of the great arteries, ventricular septal defect, and left ventricular outflow tract obstruction. *Br Heart J* **45**:20–28, 1981

108. Graham TP, Franklin RCG, Wyse RKH, et al: Left ventricular wall stress and contractile function in transposition of the great arteries after the Rastelli operation. *J Thorac Cardiovasc Surg* **93**:775–784, 1987

Chapter 16 | Hypoplastic Left Heart Syndrome

Susan Craig Nicolson and David R. Jobes

In hypoplastic left heart syndrome (HLHS) there is only one fully developed ventricle. It is the most common congenital cardiac malformation involving a single ventricle and is the fourth most common congenital cardiac lesion presenting in infancy. HLHS accounts for 25 and 15% of the cardiac deaths within the first week and month of life, respectively.[1] Males are affected slightly more often than females. The recurrence risk for siblings of patients with this syndrome has been reported to be 0.5%, with a 2.2% risk for other congenital heart lesions. The vast majority of neonates with HLHS are born at term and few have noncardiac anomalies. Two rare chromosomal abnormalities (duplication of the short arm of chromosome 12 and trisomy 18) as well as Turner's syndrome are reported to have a high incidence of HLHS. A karyotype should be included in the preoperative evaluation in any female neonate with HLHS and males who have any somatic abnormality.

Prior to 1970, all forms of HLHS were considered fatal with or without operation, and frequently no intervention was recommended. Successful surgical treatments that offer long-term survival are cardiac allotransplantation or a series of reconstructive procedures. Heart transplantation is a single surgical intervention providing a structurally and physiologically normal heart for neonates with HLHS.[2,3] Reconstructive procedures produce a circulatory system with Fontan physiology.[4] Fontan originally described a surgical procedure for physiologic correction of tricuspid atresia, another form of single ventricle (see Chapter 19). This procedure results in separation of the pulmonary and systemic circulations and is predicated on the concept that the pulmonary circulation can be maintained without a pumping chamber if pulmonary vascular resistance (PVR) is low. The improved understanding of neonatal physiology, coupled with Fontan's success, renewed interest in surgical intervention in infants with other forms of single ventricle.

Although virtually all newborns with HLHS can be stabilized by ensuring patency of the ductus arteriosus and a pulmonary blood flow (Qp) to systemic blood flow (Qs) ratio of unity, prolonged association of the pulmonary circulation with the systemic circulation will ultimately result in either intractable congestive heart failure or development of pulmonary vascular obstructive disease. Because the native anatomy prohibits long-term survival, neonates with HLHS require surgical intervention early in life before a decrease in the physiologically increased PVR of the newborn occurs precluding a Fontan procedure as the primary repair. Thus, a temporary initial stage is needed that prevents death,[5,6] and prepares the anatomy for a Fontan procedure later in life.

Anesthesiologists must clearly understand the anatomic and physiologic components of the syndrome because the effects of drugs and techniques that are used successfully in managing nearly all other patients with congenital heart disease produce adverse hemodynamic effects, even cardiac arrest, in these patients. There are very narrow margins for either hypocarbia or hyperoxia causing profound hemodynamic compromise even before surgery can begin. No matter which surgical option is chosen initially, the management of these patients is the same up to the institution of cardiopulmonary bypass. When transplantation is chosen, subsequent management follows that of other infants, as discussed in Chapter 22.

ANATOMY

HLHS describes a spectrum of congenital cardiac malformations that have in common varying degrees of underdevelopment of left-sided heart structures. The syndrome was initially described in 1952 by Lev[7] and later termed HLHS by Noonan and Nadas.[8] The central anatomic feature in the most common form of HLHS is aortic valve atresia with resultant hypoplasia of the ascending aorta. As a consequence of limited outflow, the left ventricle develops abnormally and is hypoplastic or absent. In virtually all patients with aortic atresia, there coexists atresia or stenosis of the mitral valve. Nearly one quarter of children with HLHS have either a double-outlet right ventricle or a complete common atrioventricular canal malaligned over the right ventricle with associated left ventricular hypoplasia and aortic valve atresia. The anatomic lesions that are categorized as HLHS are varied; however, the physiologic similarity of this collection of lesions has resulted in persistence of the term.

PATHOPHYSIOLOGY AND NATURAL HISTORY

The left ventricle is a nonfunctional structure in the child with HLHS. Pulmonary venous return must be routed to the right atrium through an atrial septal defect, a stretched foramen ovale, or rarely by total anomalous pulmonary venous connection. Systemic and pulmonary venous blood mixes in the right atrium. The systemic and pulmonary circulations are supplied in a parallel fashion from the right ventricle, and patency of the ductus arteriosus ensures systemic flow. Perfusion to the transverse arch and ascending aorta is retrograde through the ductus arteriosus. Lower body flow is antegrade via the descending aorta. With the pulmonary arteries connected in parallel with the ductus and descending aorta, the proportion of flow through each depends upon pulmonary (PVR) and systemic vascular resistances (SVR). Neonatal survival is dependent not only on patency of the ductus arteriosus but on adequate mixing of blood at the atrial level and on maintaining a balance between PVR and SVR that results in a Qp:Qs ratio close to unity. Ductal closure, the most common cause of patient demise, results in inadequate systemic and coronary perfusion leading to progressive metabolic acidosis, ischemia, and death. An infant in whom the ductus remains patent will survive beyond the normal period for ductal closure. However, the PVR will progressively decrease physiologically in infants with HLHS as it does in the normal newborn. As both circulations are supplied in a parallel fashion, the decrease in PVR results in ever-increasing pulmonary blood flow. Eventually, acidosis, high-output failure, and ultimately death will result from inadequate systemic and coronary perfusion despite the increase in arterial oxygenation.

DIAGNOSTIC FEATURES

Neonates with HLHS typically exhibit tachypnea, tachycardia, and mild cyanosis within the first few days of life. Peripheral pulses may be normal, diminished, or absent depending upon the degree of patency of the ductus arteriosus at the time of presentation. The majority of patients have a nonspecific soft systolic murmur at the left sternal border and one third have a gallop rhythm at the apex.

The electrocardiogram is frequently reflective of the pathology, including right atrial enlargement and right ventricular hypertrophy. In patients with a malaligned common atrioventricular canal defect, the QRS axis is to the left and superior. The findings on the chest radiograph in neonates with HLHS are nonspecific but often include cardiomegaly and increased pulmonary vascular markings. In the rare patient with an absent or severely restrictive interatrial communication, the lung fields have a reticular pattern that resembles those seen in infants with total anomalous pulmonary venous connection with pulmonary venous obstruction.

Two-dimensional echocardiography alone is sufficient to delineate the anatomy in infants with HLHS making routine cardiac catheterization no longer necessary. After the anatomic details are determined by echocardiography, color flow imaging and pulsed- and continuous-wave Doppler are used to evaluate physiology. Of primary concern is the assessment of the tricuspid or common atrioventricular valve for regurgitation as severe tricuspid insufficiency is usually a contraindication to reconstructive surgery. Fifty-six percent of patients with HLHS have tricuspid regurgitation (35% mild, 16% moderate, 5% severe).[9] As some degree of pulmonary venous obstruction is beneficial by helping prevent pulmonary overcirculation, balloon atrial septostomy (Rashkind procedure) may result in hemodynamic destabilization and is best avoided. Patients with severe arterial desaturation secondary to a restrictive or absent interatrial communication, who might theoretically benefit from balloon atrial septostomy, have a thick muscular septum primum that will require open septectomy.

SURGICAL INTERVENTION—STAGE I

Preoperative Management

Prenatal ultrasound diagnosis and the awareness of potential for survival with surgical intervention has resulted in most patients with HLHS presenting for surgery within the first week of life. Because all patients with HLHS have a ductal-dependent systemic blood flow, continuous infusion of prostaglandin (PG) E_1 (0.05–0.1 μg/kg/min) or oral PGE_2 should be initiated once the diagnosis has been made. The preoperative goal is to maintain Qp:Qs at or close to 1 to ensure hemodynamic and metabolic stability. A Qp:Qs greater than 1 results in metabolic acidosis secondary to systemic hypoperfusion and Qp:Qs much below 1 results in instability from hypoxemia. Management is based on the relative amounts of systemic and pulmonary blood flow of the individual patient. Patients can be divided into three groups: (1) those with adequate pulmonary blood flow and mild pulmonary venous hypertension without congestion as a consequence of relative restriction of the interatrial communication; (2) those with torrential pulmonary blood flow as a result of an unrestrictive, widely patent atrial septal defect; and (3) those with insufficient pulmonary blood flow as a consequence of left atrial outlet obstruction.

Group 1: Qp:Qs At or near 1. Fortunately, the vast majority of patients fall into this group, those with a Qp:Qs at or close to unity. These neonates will have adequate systemic perfusion as evidenced by a normal systemic blood pressure, warm extremities with good peripheral pulses, and the absence of a metabolic acidosis. Although these infants are breathing room air via a natural airway, "ideal" arterial blood gases (pH 7.40, Pao_2 40 mm Hg) will be obtained. Preoperative management is directed at maintaining this homeostatic state. The only anticipated alteration in this group of infants is apnea necessitating tracheal intubation as an adverse effect of PGE_1 administration. Placement of an endotracheal tube must be done carefully as drugs and techniques (hyperventilation with supplemental oxygen) frequently used to facilitate intubation of the trachea can easily disrupt the balance between the two circulations favoring pulmonary blood flow.

Group 2: Qp:Qs Greater than 1. Patients with widely patent atrial septal defects frequently have a Qp:Qs well in excess of 1 resulting in systemic hypoperfusion and a metabolic acidosis. Most neonates will attempt to compensate for acidosis by acutely hyperventilating, which results in a lowering of PVR and further increasing pulmonary blood flow and worsening the acidosis. An occasional patient can be managed by administering sufficient sodium bicarbonate to correct fully the metabolic acidosis. In most patients, the pulmonary to systemic flow ratio is adjusted toward unity by altering the $Paco_2$. Increasing the $Paco_2$ increases PVR and reduces pulmonary blood flow. Control of the $Paco_2$ is accomplished by tracheal intubation and mechanical ventilation. If the $Paco_2$ is maintained at or above 40 mm Hg by reducing the tidal volume and/or respiratory rate at and Fio_2 of 0.21, unacceptable arterial oxygen desaturation often occurs. It is hypothesized that this finding results from declining functional residual capacity (FRC), retained secretions, closure of small airways, atelectasis, and alveolar hypoxemia. The duration of tracheal intubation is directly related to the increasing likelihood of the phenomenon. Alternatively, such desaturation can be avoided without progressively increasing the Fio_2 by maintaining the FRC with an appropriate tidal volume and respiratory rate and adding sufficient carbon dioxide

to the fresh gas flow to keep the arterial Pco_2 at the desired level.

Group 3: Qp:Qs Less than 1. The rare infant in the third group with a markedly restrictive or absent atrial septal defect manifests profound hypoxemia as a consequence of a low pulmonary to systemic blood flow ratio. Emergency surgical intervention is the only rational plan for these neonates. Interventions should be undertaken to intubate the child's trachea using neuromuscular blocking agents and anesthetic agents as tolerated, hyperventilating using an Fio_2 of 1, and ensuring adequate intravascular volume in the interim between diagnosis and institution of cardiopulmonary bypass.

Infrequently, a neonate with HLHS may require inotropic support for low cardiac output and reduced systemic perfusion. Caution should be taken in administering inotropic drugs to these neonates. Experience indicates that dopamine in a dose of 3–5 μg/kg/min can be efficacious. Higher doses of dopamine and other inotropic agents are likely to be counterproductive by further increasing systemic vasoconstriction. Those infants who have had a period of circulatory collapse associated with sepsis or ductal closure should be stabilized, evaluated for central nervous system dysfunction, and observed until renal and hepatic insufficiency if present resolve.

Venous access via a peripheral or umbilical vein is obtained to administer drugs and maintenance fluids. Preferably, an umbilical artery or left radial artery (initial surgical intervention may include a right modified Blalock-Taussig shunt) is used preoperatively to monitor systemic pressure and adequacy of ventilation, oxygenation, and acid-base balance. Infants with indwelling endotracheal tubes prior to surgery should have pulmonary toilet performed taking precautions to avoid acute increases in PVR with passage of the suction catheter.

Transport to the Operating Room

No indication exists for preanesthetic medication in neonates with HLHS. Infants are ideally transported to the operating room in their intensive care unit isolette. The patient's electrocardiogram and arterial pressure, when a catheter is in place, are displayed on a portable monitor. The long effective half-life of PGE_1 allows for discontinuation of the infusion before transport. Intubated infants are connected to either a Mapleson system delivering the same Fio_2 in use in the intensive care unit or a self-inflating bag and valve system using room air to maintain a $Paco_2$ at the pretransport level. Appropriate airway equipment and resuscitative drugs should accompany the infant to the operating room. Caution must be observed to avoid hyperventilation during transport.

Anesthetic Considerations. The anesthetic considerations are identical regardless of whether the child is coming for stage I palliation or heart transplantation. Anesthetic agents should be chosen to induce and maintain anesthesia while at the same time preserving the delicate balance between SVR and PVR and minimizing myocardial depression. In these infants, like all other patients, no anesthetic agent has an effect on PVR without also influencing SVR, and vice versa. Those factors that decrease PVR or increase SVR will promote pulmonary blood flow at the expense of the systemic and coronary circulations. This undesirable situation will be reflected in an increase in the child's Pao_2 and a decrease in systemic arterial blood pressure. Because the arterial saturation is normally less than 100%, alterations in pulmonary blood flow will cause similar directional changes in peripheral oximetry reading provided alveolar oxygen availability is maintained.

Induction of Anesthesia. On arrival in the operating room and preferably prior to induction of anesthesia, electrocardiogram, precordial stethoscope, pulse oximeter, and either an invasive or noninvasive blood pressure device are applied. The anesthesia goals can be met using either a narcotic (fentanyl or sufentanil) and/or an inhalational agent in conjunction with neuromuscular blockade provided ventilation is carefully adjusted. The lowest dose of fentanyl that usually results in minimal or no change in heart rate or blood pressure with laryngoscopy, intubation, or surgical incision prior to cardiopulmonary bypass seems to be 10 μg/kg. Larger doses have been used but appear not to be more efficacious and have a tendency to decrease systemic blood pressure. Additional fentanyl or inhalation agent can be given if the initial dose appears inadequate. Sufentanil has been advocated but no conclusive benefits to a particular narcotic or other anesthetic technique have been demonstrated. Pancuronium is used because of its vagolytic property that reduces the likelihood of vagally stimulated bradycardia and because its rapid onset blunts or eliminates the chest wall rigidity often seen with bolus fentanyl administration. However, these infants often demonstrate adequate neuromuscular blockade only after larger (0.2 mg/kg) than usual (0.1 mg/kg) doses within the expected time interval. Infants of a similar gestational and postconceptual age not receiving PGE_1 do not appear to exhibit this phenomenon. Great care must be taken to avoid excessive minute ventilation, which is enhanced by the increased chest compliance that follows anesthesia and neuromuscular blockade. During this transitional period, it is convenient to incorporate 1–2% CO_2 into the fresh gas flow of a nonrebreathing system. This technique permits a more usual pattern of mechanical ventilation that maintains alveolar and small airway patency while maintaining the arterial $Paco_2$ $\geq$40 mm Hg.

Following induction of anesthesia, an existing endotracheal tube is changed to a clean nasotracheal tube to minimize the potential for tube obstruction from inspissated secretions. Infants with a natural airway have a nasotracheal tube passed primarily. Any additional necessary vascular access is achieved. Three temperature probes (nasopharyngeal, rectal, and esophageal as a component of an esophageal stethoscope), a Foley catheter, and a nasogastric tube are inserted. Precautions are taken during positioning to avoid tissue damage from the combined effects of pressure, hypothermia, and hyperthermia during rewarming.

Precardiopulmonary Bypass. The single most important variable in preserving Qp:Qs at or near 1 during the prebypass period is adjustment of ventilation to keep the arterial Pco_2 at or above 40 mm Hg. During the surface cooling instituted before bypass (keeping the ambient temperature at 20°C, placing the infant on a thermal blanket set at 15°C, and placing ice bags around the head), the resultant decrease in CO_2 production must be appreciated. The $Paco_2$ is maintained at the desired level by adding sufficient CO_2 to the fresh gas flow while FRC is assured by appropriate constant tidal volume and respiratory rate. The inspired concentration of carbon dioxide will increase to 4–5% before bypass as the core temperature falls to 30–32°C. When managed in this way, there is rarely any evidence of pulmonary overcirculation (arterial oxygen saturation in excess of 90% and unacceptably low systemic arterial blood pressure). Should this occur, positive end-expiratory pressure or temporary occlusion of the right pulmonary artery may be used to reduce pulmonary blood flow and preserve systemic perfusion until institution of cardiopulmonary bypass.

Cardiopulmonary Bypass. Pancuronium (0.2 mg/kg) and fentanyl to result in a precirculatory arrest dose of 40 μg/kg is incorporated into the pump priming volume. These doses are intended to provide adequate maintenance levels and effect while on bypass and during circulatory arrest. On institution of bypass, all infusions are stopped, and the patient is cooled for 12 minutes or until the rectal temperature reaches 20°C. Blood is drained from the patient, cannula removed, and for the staged procedure cardioplegic solution is given.

The three goals of stage I are (1) to maintain systemic perfusion, (2) to preserve function of the only ventricle, and (3) to allow normal maturation of the pulmonary vasculature. The first two goals are accomplished with creation of an unobstructed communication from the right ventricle to the systemic circulation. This is achieved by transection of the main pulmonary artery and construction of a neoarta using the proximal pulmonary artery, ascending aorta, and adult pulmonary artery homograft. A central systemic to pulmonary artery shunt (inferior aspect of augmented aortic arch to the confluence of the branch pulmonary arteries) or modified right Blalock-Taussig shunt, of sufficient size to maintain pulmonary blood flow and pressure at normal levels, is created. Limitation of pulmonary blood flow and the establishment of a large nonrestrictive interatrial communication enables the physiologically [8] high PVR of the neonate to fall postoperatively (Fig 16–1)

The atrial septectomy, creation of the neoaorta, and placement of the central shunt are completed during hypothermic arrest. If a modified Blalock-Taussig shunt rather than a central shunt is planned, bypass is reinstituted after completion of the proximal shunt anastomosis and the distal anastomosis is completed during rewarming. Prior to termination of bypass, the following are prepared for immediate use: warmed 24- to 48- hour old whole blood, protamine sulfate, calcium gluconate, an infusion of dopamine, and a transducer for atrial pressure monitoring. Before attempting to wean from bypass, the child's endotracheal tube is suctioned followed by vigorous reexpansion of the lungs.

Immediate Postbypass Period. After stage I, both circulations continue to be supplied from the single ventricle in a parallel fashion. In the majority of patients, termination of bypass is uneventful and requires no unique intervention. Less than 5% of neonates will have

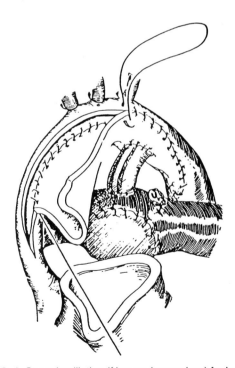

Figure 16–1. Stage I palliation (Norwood procedure) for hypoplastic left heart syndrome. Procedure includes atrial septectomy, followed by division of the main pulmonary artery. The ascending aorta and aortic arch are augmented in size with pulmonary artery allograft. Pulmonary blood flow is provided by a 4-mm central shunt (as shown) or a modified Blalock-Taussig shunt. (*From Norwood WI: Hypoplastic left heart syndrome. Cardiol Clin 7:377–385, 1989, with permission.*)

inadequate pulmonary blood flow through the newly created systemic to pulmonary artery shunt as evidenced by a Pao_2 less than 20–22 mm Hg. The differential diagnosis of inadequate postbypass pulmonary blood flow includes inadequate shunt (anastomotic stricture, kinked, too small), elevated PVR (intrinsic pulmonary disease, arterial hypoxemia, hypercarbia, hypothermia, acidosis), and inadequate systemic pressure secondary to myocardial dysfunction (preoperative injury, inadequate myocardial protection, coronary ischemia, hypocalcemia). Assuming that the technical aspects of the surgery are adequate and that the child is sufficiently warm, efforts to improve pulmonary blood flow include augmentation of intravascular volume, inotropic support to assure adequate systemic pressure, and reducing PVR by lowering the $PaCo_2$ and increasing Fio_2.

A greater number of patients will show signs of pulmonary overcirculation (Pao_2 >45 and widened pulse pressure) in the immediate postbypass period. Once established, this situation is difficult to reverse and can result in death due to inadequate systemic perfusion if not rapidly corrected. Ventilatory manipulations to increase PVR (increase $Paco$, reduce Fio_2) should be instituted. Reestablishing and maintaining the $Paco_2$ at or above 40 mm Hg can be facilitated by using inspired carbon dioxide. Shunt revision to limit pulmonary blood flow is rarely required.

Once assured that the hemodynamics and oxygenation are adequate, the cannulas are removed and protamine sulfate is given to neutralize the heparin. No blood from the extracorporeal circuit is infused after protamine is given at the Children's Hospital of Philadelphia. Initial blood loss can be large owing to extensive suture lines and dilutional coagulopathy. It is essential to restore hemostasis rapidly to limit hemorrhage and its hemodynamic consequences. In a recent study comparing the effects of very fresh whole blood (<6 hours old, never refrigerated), 24- to 48-hour whole blood, and component therapy (packed red blood cells, platelets, fresh frozen plasma) on 24-hour postbypass blood loss, significantly less blood was lost when either of the whole blood products was given to children under 2 years of age undergoing a complex repair.[10] Given there was no difference in the losses between the very fresh and the 24- to 48-hour whole blood groups and the myriad of problems associated with providing very fresh blood (supply, time needed for requisite testing), 24- to 48-hour old whole blood appears to be the ideal product to use to replace losses in these neonates immediately following bypass. A large volume of citrated blood delivered rapidly acutely decreases the ionized calcium resulting in decreased systemic pressure while atrial pressure remains stable or increases. Experience indicates that between 50 and 100 mg of calcium gluconate is needed for each 50 mL of blood replaced, particularly if the rate of replacement exceeds 1.5 mL/kg/min.

Inotropic support is infrequently required. Dopamine, 2–5 μg/kg/min, is useful for its positive inotropic effects. Indications for additional anesthetic in the post-bypass period are seldom observed. This may be due to the previously administered fentanyl or to depressed cerebral function immediately after deep hypothermic circulatory arrest.

Postoperative Care. Following surgery, the patient is transferred to an intensive care unit. Transport is accomplished with electrocardiogram and systemic arterial pressure monitoring, the chest tube is placed on constant portable suction and, when necessary, dopamine is continued by a battery-powered infusion pump.[12] The patient is manually ventilated during transport using the same F_{IO_2} and ventilatory pattern found appropriate following bypass in the operating room. Resuscitative drugs and warmed blood (in syringes after passage through a warming unit) accompany the child to the intensive care unit. When bleeding is ongoing, the intensive care unit must have blood-warming capability ready in advance.

Immediate postoperative management continues the methods established for the individual patient in the operating room. Currently, in patients with a Qp:Qs above unity carbon dioxide is added to the ventilator fresh gas flow to keep the arterial P_{CO_2} at or just above 40 mm Hg, and to modulate changes in PVR seen the first postoperative night. In the vast majority of patients, prevention of hypocarbia is sufficient to maintain the Qp:Qs near 1. Infrequently, the systemic flow is inadequate (low systemic arterial blood pressure, decreased peripheral pulses, cool extremities, persistent metabolic acidosis) despite an F_{IO_2} of 0.21 and a $P_{CO_2} \geq 40$ mm Hg. Provided intravascular volume is judged to be adequate, consideration should be given to augmenting systemic perfusion by lowering the SVR with sodium nitroprusside. In most infants, an attempt is undertaken to wean from positive pressure ventilation within 24 hours of completion of surgery. Extubation is successful in 60–70% of patients on the first postoperative day. The judicious use of negative pressure ventilators has been helpful in limiting prolonged intubation of the airway and barotrauma in those patients in whom weaning is more difficult.

Long-term Outcome. On completion of stage I, the single ventricle is subjected to both a volume and pressure load greater than normal. With a view to long-term preservation of ventricular function, early assessment for suitability for a second and final procedure, a modified Fontan, is undertaken when the children reached 12–18 months of age. The operative mortality following Fontan's procedure in these patients ranges between 20 and 40%. Death is attributed in many to an abrupt change in ventricular geometry as evidenced by a small, thick-walled cavity with a low diastolic volume and compliance

following removal of the volume load associated with the systemic to pulmonary arterial shunt. The anatomic and physiologic consequences of this rapid decrease in end-diastolic volume are an apparent increase in wall thickness because muscle mass does not change as rapidly and impaired diastolic function of the ventricle resulting in increased end-diastolic pressure, increased central venous pressure, and decreased cardiac output. Examination of all the data available preoperatively in these patients was not able to predict those patients who would develop rapid contraction of end-diastolic volume. In an attempt to minimize the physiologic significance of such a rapid geometric change, an intermediate procedure is currently performed in early infancy interposed between the initial palliation (stage I) and the modified Fontan procedure.

SURGICAL INTERVENTION—STAGE II

Options for the intermediate procedure include either a bidirectional cavopulmonary shunt or a hemi–Fontan procedure. The bidirectional cavopulmonary shunt, which connects the SVC to both pulmonary arteries, can be accomplished without the use of cardiopulmonary bypass.[12]

Pathophysiology

The physiology following a hemi–Fontan procedure is similar to that following a bidirectional cavopulmonary anastomosis; its execution, however, requires cardiopulmonary bypass.[13,14] It differs in that all sources of pulmonary blood flow other than that from the SVC are interrupted, thus maximally unloading the ventricle of volume work, and includes the necessary pulmonary arterial reconstruction and correction of associated intracardiac lesions. It is postulated that performing either of these procedures that obligate half the systemic venous return to flow passively through the pulmonary vascular bed will allow for a decrease in end-diastolic volume and a commensurate decrease in muscle mass. Each of these interventions is followed ultimately by the final procedure, a modified Fontan, that directs inferior vena caval blood to the pulmonary arteries and completes the separation of the pulmonary and systemic circulations.

Preoperative Evaluation

Four to 8 months after stage I, patients return electively for a hemi–Fontan procedure. The majority of these infants, although cyanotic, demonstrate appropriate growth and development for their chronologic age. Cardiac catheterization is usually performed prior to the second surgical intervention to evaluate (1) pulmonary vascular resistance, (2) anatomy of the pulmonary arteries and neoaorta, (3) ventricular function, (4) function of the tricuspid or common atrioventricular valve, and (5) size of the interatrial communication. Recent data indicate that children with congenital heart defects can safely ingest clear liquids close to the time of induction of general anesthesia.[15] Attention is given to avoiding preload depletion by preoperative orders to give clear liquids 2–3 hours before induction of anesthesia. Routine preanesthetic medication for age is well tolerated. Oral atropine (0.02 mg/kg) is given to infants under 6 months of age. Children between 6 and 12 months of age receive, in addition, oral pentobarbital (4 mg/km) 90 minutes before arrival in the operating room, which results in a sleeping infant prior to induction of anesthesia.

Anesthetic Considerations

Because both pulmonary and systemic circulations are supplied in a parallel fashion from the single ventricle, theoretically the same considerations apply for the induction of anesthesia for the hemi–Fontan procedure during the first perioperative period. However, the tendency to develop pulmonary overcirculation rapidly during controlled ventilation is blunted, probably because of maturation of the pulmonary vasculature and decreased sensitivity to hypocarbia. Hemodynamic stability is maintained within a wider range of $Paco_2$ and Fio_2. Before induction of anesthesia, a minimum of a precordial stethoscope, pulse oximeter, and blood pressure cuff (on left arm if a right Blalock-Taussig shunt is present) are applied. Most of these children do not have an intravenous catheter in place at the time of induction. Experience indicates that these patients tolerate a routine mask induction with halothane in nitrous oxide and oxygen. Soon after an adequate plane of anesthesia is achieved, nitrous oxide is discontinued and arterial and venous cannulations are accomplished. Nasotracheal intubation, using an endotracheal tube with a leak greater than or equal to 30 cm H_2O to allow maximal ventilatory manipulation following bypass, is facilitated using pancuronium or other neuromuscular blocking drugs. Anesthesia is maintained in the prebypass period with fentanyl (10–20 μg/kg) and inhalational agent as needed. Supplemental fentanyl and pancuronium are added to the pump priming volume. Given the need for reentry into the chest via a median sternotomy, blood should be available before incision. The prebypass procedures for surface cooling and hypothermic circulatory arrest are the same as during stage I.

Surgical Technique for Hemi–Fontan Procedure (Stage II)

The systemic to pulmonary artery shunt is ligated on institution of cardiopulmonary bypass. Details of the surgical procedure during hypothermic circulatory arrest include (1) inspection of the interatrial communication and enlargement as necessary; (2) augmentation of the pulmonary artery confluence with allograft; (3) anastomosis of the superior vena cava (SVC) with the augmented pulmonary arteries; and (4) placement of a patch (dam)

to separate the common atrium from the atriopulmonary anastomosis (Fig 16–2). On completion of this procedure, the systemic venous return from the SVC flows directly through the lungs. The systemic venous return from the inferior vena cava (IVC) mixes with the pulmonary venous return in the common atrium and is ejected by the single ventricle into the neoaorta.

Immediate Postbypass Period

The preparations for terminating cardiopulmonary bypass are the same as following stage I. An additional pressure transducer is prepared to monitor pulmonary artery pressure as well as common atrial pressure. Because pulmonary blood flow depends upon passive perfusion, the physiologic considerations are the same as after modified Fontan procedures. SVC–pulmonary artery pressure should be sufficient to drive blood through the pulmonary circulation. Factors that influence PVR should be manipulated to minimize PVR. These include tracheal toilet, reexpansion of atelectatic lung, correction of any metabolic acidosis, and warming the patient adequately prior to weaning from bypass. Ventilatory parameters after bypass include Fio_2 of 1, large tidal volume, slow respiratory rate, short inspiratory and long expiratory time, and low peak and mean airway pressures to decrease $Paco_2$ and PVR. Not infrequently, these infants will show signs of light anesthesia (tachycardia, hypertension) in the postbypass period, which respond to supplemental doses of narcotic or low-dose inhalational agent. Nitrous oxide is not used because of concern for expansion of possible intravascular air bubbles.

Postoperative Care

The hemi–Fontan procedure not only reduces the volume and pressure load on the single ventricle early in life but addresses any other existing intracardiac (atrial septectomy, atrioventricular valve) and extracardiac (architecture of pulmonary arteries and neoaorta) pathophysiology to optimize cardiac physiology for the third and final intervention, ie, a modified Fontan procedure. This procedure is usually well tolerated, as evidenced by the fact that greater than 95% of patients are extubated on the first postoperative day and the average length of hospital stay is 5 days.

SURGICAL INTERVENTION—STAGE III

The final surgical intervention, a modified Fontan procedure, is undertaken when the ventricular end-diastolic volume and wall thickness have normalized, usually 6–12 months after stage II, the intermediate procedure. Cardiac catheterization evaluates the child's pulmonary arterial anatomy, pulmonary vascular resistance, and ventricular function. A satisfactory functional result after completion of the modified Fontan procedure can be

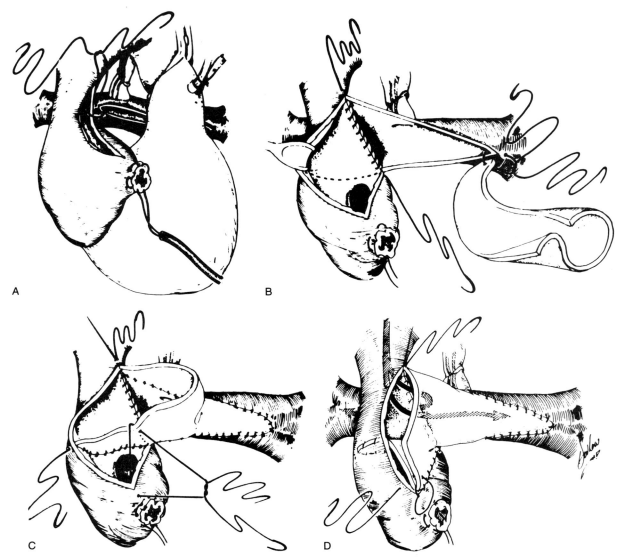

Figure 16–2. Hemi-Fontan procedure. Incisions made in the pulmonary artery, right atrium, and superior vena cava are in (*A*). After ensuring that the interatrial communication is adequate, the pulmonary artery confluence is augmented with allograft (*B*). The superior vena cava is associated with the augmented pulmonary arteries (*C*) and a patch (dam) is positioned to separate the common atrium from the atriopulmonary anastomosis (*D*). (*From Norwood WI, Jacobs ML, Murphy JD. Fontan procedure for hypoplastic left heart syndrome. Ann Thorac Surg. 54:1025–1030, 1992, with permission.*)

expected when the pulmonary artery architecture is close to normal, the PVR is that of a normal mature lung (<2.5 Wood units/m^2) and ventricular function is well preserved (end-diastolic pressure <8–10 mm Hg).

Anesthetic Considerations

The child's pulmonary blood flow depends on right-sided preload and PVR. Children receive the same oral premedication given prior to stage II but to which is added meperidine (3 mg/kg). Before induction, a minimum of a precordial stethoscope, pulse oximeter, and blood pressure cuff are applied. Most of these children do not have an intravenous cannula in place at the time

of induction. However, these children tolerate a routine mask induction with halothane in nitrous oxide and oxygen. When an adequate plane of anesthesia is achieved, nitrous oxide is discontinued. Arterial and venous cannulation is performed remembering that this operation entails a third median sternotomy. Nasotracheal intubation, using an endotracheal tube with a leak greater than or equal to 30 cm of H$_2$O to enable maximal ventilatory adjustments, is facilitated with pancuronium or other neuromuscular blocking drug. The ventilatory requirements are identical to those previously discussed following the hemi–Fontan procedure. Anesthesia is maintained in the prebypass period with fentanyl (10–50 μg/

kg) and inhalational agent as needed. Scopolamine (0.007 mg/kg) is given to children over 18 months of age to minimize postoperative recall of intraoperative awareness. Supplemental narcotic and neuromuscular blocking drugs are incorporated in the pump priming volume. Surface cooling and preparations for hypothermic circulatory arrest are carried out as previously described.

Surgical Technique for Modified Fontan Procedure

After institution of hypothermic circulatory arrest, the right atrium is opened and the patch placed at the time of the hemi–Fontan procedure to separate the atrium from the atriopulmonary anastomosis is excised (see Fig 16–2D). An intra-atrial patch is positioned to direct blood from the IVC to the atriopulmonary anastomosis directing all systemic venous return to the pulmonary bed.

In the rare child considered to be at increased risk of an adverse outcome because of transient or reversible elevation of PVR or ventricular dysfunction, several options exist. One option is the fenestrated Fontan procedure in which an opening of a few millimeters in diameter is left in the interatrial septum.[16] Right-to-left shunting through this fenestration allows cardiac output to be maintained, albeit at the expense of systemic oxygenation, while limiting the elevation in right atrial pressure. Transcatheter closure of the communication offers the advantage of a test closure prior to permanent closure that can be done in the early or late postoperative period depending on the child's hemodynamic variables and oxygenation. A variation on the theme is the snare-adjusted atrial septal defect (ASD), which provides the ability to regulate the size of the communication at the atrial level.[17]

Recently performed modified Fontan procedures permanently exclude part of the hepatic venous drainage from the systemic venous return–pulmonary arterial connection in an attempt to minimize or eliminate the effusions that can plague children after this procedure.

Postbypass Period

After a modified Fontan procedure, all the systemic venous return must flow through the pulmonary capillary bed; thus cardiac output is determined by pulmonary blood flow. The goals of postbypass and postoperative care include maintenance of adequate right-sided preload and low PVR.[18] When both PVR and the right ventricular end-diastolic pressure remain low, the immediate postoperative period is uncomplicated. If PVR fluctuates or increases, aggressive treatment is needed. A combination of inotropic support (dopamine, isoproterenol), peripheral vasodilation (sodium nitroprusside), pulmonary vasodilation (hypocarbia, alkalosis, high F_{IO_2}), a ventilatory pattern designed to minimize peak and mean airway pressures, and augmentation of right-sided preload are used (see Chapter 18).

Long-term Outcome

A number of patients have required major and minor surgery, both elective and emergency, both before and in between the reconstructive stages. Although there is not a large series of patients in any one category, it appears that a carefully administered anesthetic similar to any usually used for age and surgical procedure in patients with palliated or repaired congenital cardiac lesions is tolerated provided the unique ventilatory and circulatory requirements of the reconstructed hypoplastic left heart are consistently met. Because the definitive reconstruction is still evolving, it is important to know the actual procedure performed on a given patient. The expected range of arterial oxygenation and the significance of both increases and decreases to avoid potentially disastrous manipulations of ventilation must be appreciated.[19] Similarly, in patients following both the hemi–Fontan procedure and the modified Fontan procedure, intravascular volume may be larger and venous pressures may need to be maintained higher than in other patients without Fontan physiology. The results for reconstructive surgery for HLHS to continue to improve as knowledge of the anatomy, physiology, and the surgical procedures for this complex group of infants and children increases. The survival rate for the staged repair is now at least as good as that reported for surgery in other neonates with complex congenital heart disease such as pulmonary atresia with intact ventricular septum and truncus arteriosus.

The choice of surgical procedure for infants with HLHS (multistage reconstruction or cardiac transplantation) is unclear. The success of transplantation in neonates depends on the neonatal immune response favoring successful engraftment, normal growth and development of host and graft, and the existence of a donor pool. The Children's Defense Fund reports that each

TABLE 16–1. OUTCOME FOR INFANTS WITH HLHS PRESENTING BETWEEN JANUARY 1989 AND DECEMBER 1990*

Procedure	No. of Patients (%)
Neonates undergoing stage I	149
Hospital mortality (%)	42 (28)
Late mortality (%)	5 (3)
Infants undergoing hemi-Fontan	90
Hospital mortality (%)	9 (0)†
Late mortality	1 (1)
Children undergoing Fontan	43
Hospital mortality	2 (5)
Late mortality (%)	1 (2)
Children undergoing transplant	1
Mortality	0

* Data as of May 1, 1992.
† Among the nine patients who died in the early postoperative period, six presented for hemi-Fontan when they were less than 5 months of age because of ventricular dysfunction or shunt failure that may have adversely impacted on their postoperative physiology.

day in the United States, 72 babies die in the first month of life, and 110 die before their first birthday.[20] If just 10% of these were suitable donors and if they were referred to procurement agencies, most infant heart transplant demands, including replacement hearts for newborns with HLHS, in North America could be met. Data indicates that the donor pool falls well below the required 10%, so much so that neonates with HLHS alone outstrip the donor heart supply. Recent data from the Loma Linda University (Loma Linda, California) experience, which focuses on transplantation, suggests an overall mortality rate of about 47%.[21] This estimate includes deaths while awaiting transplant, as well as postoperative mortality, but does not include deaths before referral to Loma Linda. The one year survival rate of patients actually transplanted was 84%. Similar data from The Children's Hospital of Philadelphia experience that focuses on staged reconstruction suggests an overall mortality of about 40% (Table 16–1).[21,22]

While the comparison of the results of the two treatments appear to be similar, they are based on a number of assumptions and lack a controlled context. For example, transplant patients are highly selected, while virtually all patients referred for reconstruction required only the diagnosis of HLHS. The consequences of either approach have also been observed for a relatively short period of time, and new difficulties are emerging, as are the solutions to recognized problems. A crossover in surgical strategy may be necessary to save more infants. Survivors of the first- and second-stage palliative procedures with less than optimal cardiac function may become candidates for heart transplantation. Conversely, infants who await transplantation may die waiting for an organ, unless the option of reconstruction is made available and exercised. Only time will reveal which surgical option(s) achieves the best quality of life in the greatest number of infants with HLHS.

REFERENCES

1. Fyler DC: Report of the New England regional infant cardiac program. *Pediatrics* **65**:376–471, 1980
2. Bailey LL, Nehlsen-Cannarella SL, Doroshow RW, Jacobson JG, et al: Cardiac allotransplantation in newborns as therapy for hypoplastic left heart syndrome. *N Engl J Med* **315**:949–951, 1986
3. Bailey LL, Gundry SR: Hypoplastic left heart syndrome. *Pediatr Clin North Am* **37**:137–150, 1990
4. Fontan F, Baudet E: Surgical repair of tricuspid atresia. *Thorax* **26**:240–248, 1971
5. Pigott JD, Murphy JD, Barber G, Norwood WI: Palliative reconstructive surgery for hypoplastic left heart syndrome. *Ann Thorac Surg* **45**:122–128, 1988
6. Norwood WI: Hypoplastic left heart syndrome. *Cardiol Clin* **7**:377–385, 1989
7. Lev M: Pathologic anatomy and interrelationship of hypoplasia of the aortic complexes. *Lab Invest* **1**:61–70, 1952
8. Noonan JA, Nadas AS: The hypoplastic left heart syndrome: An analysis of 101 cases. *Pediatr Clin North Am* **5**:1029–1056, 1958
9. Barber G, Helton JG, Aglira BA, et al: The significance of tricuspid regurgitation in hypoplastic left heart syndrome. *Am Heart J* **116**:1563–1567, 1988
10. Manno CS, Hedberg KW, Kim HC, et al: Comparison of the hemostatic effects of fresh whole blood, stored whole blood and components after open heart surgery in children. *Blood* **77**:930–936, 1991
11. Jobes DR, Nicolson SC, Pigott JD, Norwood WI: An enclosed system for continuous postoperative mediastinal aspiration. *Ann Thorac Surg* **45**:101–102, 1988
12. Bridges ND, Jonas RA, Mayer JE, et al: Bidirectional cavopulmonary anastomosis as interim palliation for high-risk Fontan candidates. *Circulation* **82**(suppl IV): IV-170–IV-176, 1990
13. Douville EC, Sade RM, Fyfe DA: Hemi-Fontan operation in surgery for single ventricle: A preliminary report. *Ann Thorac Surg* **51**:893–900, 1991
14. Lamberti JJ: Palliation of univentricular heart without increasing ventricular work. *Ann Thorac Surg* **51**:882–883, 1991
15. Nicolson SC, Dorsey AT, Schreiner MS: Shortened preanesthetic fasting interval in pediatric cardiac surgical patients. *Anesth Analg* **74**:694–697, 1992
16. Bridges ND, Lock JE, Castaneda AR: Baffle fenestration with subsequent transcatheter closure. *Circulation* **82**: 1681–1689, 1990
17. Laks H, Haas GS, Pearl JM, et al: The use of an adjustable intra-atrial communication in patients undergoing the Fontan and other definitive procedures. *Circulation* **78**(Suppl II):357–361, 1988
18. Fyman PN, Goodman K, Casthely PA, et al: Anesthetic management of patients undergoing Fontan procedure. *Anesth Analg* **65**:516–519, 1986
19. Karl HW, Hensley FA, Cyran SE, et al: Hypoplastic left heart syndrome: Anesthesia for elective noncardiac surgery. *Anesthesiology* **72**:753–757, 1990
20. *US News and World Report*, November 7, 1988
21. Norwood WI, Jacobs ML, Murphy JD. Fontan procedure for hypoplastic left heart syndrome. *Ann Thorac Surg* **54**: 1025–1030, 1992
22. Jacobs ML, Norwood WI: Hypoplastic left heart syndrome. In Jacobs ML, Norwood WI (eds): *Pediatric Cardiac Surgery: Current Issues.* Stoneham, UK: Butterworth-Heinemann, 1992, pp 182–192

Chapter 17 | Anomalies of Systemic and Pulmonary Venous Return

Carol L. Lake

Both of the pulmonary and systemic veins are subject to malformation during embryonic development. These alterations result in absence, duplication, transposition, or malposition of these veins. Most of the systemic venous abnormalities are not life threatening. However, completely anomalous pulmonary venous drainage is incompatible with life without the presence of an arteriovenous shunt.

ANOMALIES OF SYSTEMIC VENOUS DRAINAGE

Anomalies of the Inferior Vena Cava

Anatomy When the inferior vena cava (IVC) is formed abnormally during embryogenesis (see Chapter 3), it can be completely absent or one of four anatomic anomalies can occur: (1) transposition or left-sided IVC, (2) retroaortic left renal vein, (3) circumaortic left renal vein, or (4) duplication of the IVC.[1] Chuang and colleagues classified these anomalies with respect to their relationship to the kidneys[2] (Fig 17–1). Both transposition and duplication of the IVC are associated with renal vein anomalies.

Absence of the IVC (Azygous Continuation or Infrahepatic Interruption of the IVC). This anomaly results from failure of union between the hepatic and right cardinal vessels. With absence of the IVC, the hepatic veins join the right atrium directly, whereas other abdominal veins connect to the azygous or hemiazygous system. If there is no connection to the azygous system, blood from the IVC drains through the lumbar and vertebral venous plexuses.[3] A large right superior vena cava (SVC) suggests the presence of azygous connection. Other cardiac anomalies, including malrotation, total anomalous pulmonary venous drainage, atrial septal defect (ASD), pulmonic stenosis or atresia, and levocardia are associated with absent inferior vena cava.

Transposition of the IVC. Transposition of the IVC results in a mirror image of the normal right-sided IVC. The IVC crosses to the right side anterior to the aorta, usually at the level of the renal arteries. Thrombosis of the anomalous left IVC has been reported to mimic a retroperitoneal mass.[4] The incidence of transposition is 0.2–0.5% in large series of anatomic dissections or radiographic clinical material.[1]

Retroaortic Left Renal Vein. With a retroaortic left renal vein, the left renal vein crosses posteriorly to the aorta to join the IVC. The anomaly results during embryologic development when the vein anterior to the aorta regresses, whereas the posterior vein persists. The incidence of retroaortic left renal vein is 1.2–2.4% in the general population.[1]

Circumaortic Left Renal Vein. A circumaortic left renal vein forms a venous collar around the aorta. It results from failure of regression of the vein posterior to the aorta, so that the preaortic and retroaortic left renal veins join before entering the IVC. The retroaortic vein descends one or two vertebral levels caudally and crosses the spine behind the aorta to connect the preaortic vein to the IVC[5]; the preaortic portion receives adrenal, gonadal, and phrenic veins. Lumbar and hemiazygous veins drain into the retroaortic portion. The reported incidence is 1.5–8.7% in a large series of humans.[1]

Double IVC. A duplication anomaly, or double IVC, has an incidence of 0.2–3.0% in humans.[1] It results from failure of regression of the left supracardinal vein. The anomaly consists of large veins on both sides of the aorta below the level of the renal veins. After the left IVC

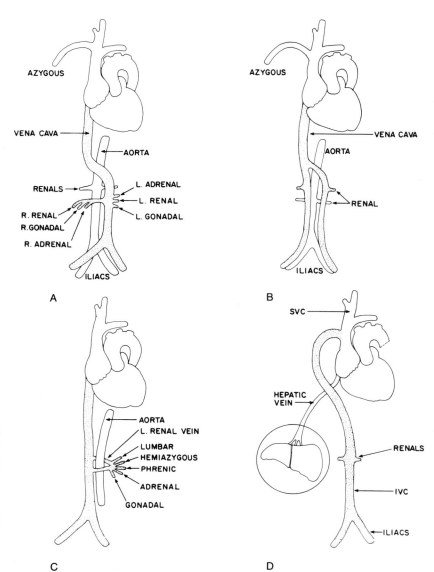

Figure 17–1. Anomalies of the inferior vena cava. (*A*) Anomalies of the postrenal segment. Left IVC. (*B*) Double IVC resulting from persistence of right and left supracardiac veins. The iliac veins continue as separate IVCs. Each renal vein drains into the IVC on its particular side. The left IVC crosses to join the right just after receiving the left renal vein. (*C*) Anomaly of renal segment. Circumaortic left renal vein. (*D*) Anomaly of the prerenal segment. Azygous continuation results when the suprarenal portion of the IVC fails to develop. Hepatic veins drain into the right atrium via a short connection.

receives the left renal vein, it joins with the right IVC either anterior or posterior to the aorta to become the suprarenal IVC.

Pathophysiology. These anomalies have no pathophysiologic effects.

Natural History. Normally, these anomalies cause little problem to the human and become important only during periaortic surgery, when obtaining blood samples from renal veins in the diagnosis of renovascular hypertension, or during insertion of inferior vena caval filters. However, they may be associated with other congenital cardiac or visceral anomalies.[6]

Diagnostic Features. Abdominal computed tomographic scans,[5,7] magnetic resonance imaging,[8] or sonograms will demonstrate the vascular anomalies as tubular

structures on both sides or to the left of the aorta. Inferior venacavograms via the femoral route confirm the precise anatomy. Occasionally, patients with azygous continuation of the IVC or other anomalies will have coronary sinus rhythm on electrocardiography (ECG) when the abnormal P wave originates from the lower right atrium or orifice of the coronary sinus.[9] An interrupted IVC is recognized on the lateral chest radiograph by the absent shadow of the supradiaphragmatic IVC and a prominent azygos-SVC confluence on the posterior-anterior chest radiograph.[10]

Anomalies of the Superior Vena Cava

Anatomy. The most common anomaly is the persistence of the left SVC with a normal right SVC (duplication of the vena cava) occurring in 2–4.3% of patients with congenital cardiac anomalies[10,11] and 0.5% of the normal population. The left SVC drains to the right atrium or coronary sinus, the left atrium, left pulmonary veins, or into the coronary sinus with a window into the left atrium.[12] Sometimes both right and left venae cavae drain to the left atrium.[13] Occasionally, the right SVC is absent.

Drainage to the Right Atrium.

In persistence of the left SVC with normal right SVC, the left arm and left half of the head and neck are drained by the left SVC, if present. The left SVC drains into the right SVC via a brachiocephalic interconnection that crosses in front of the aortic arch, left pulmonary artery, and pulmonary veins in many cases. In about 75% of cases, the left innominate vein is hypoplastic or absent.[11] However, about one half of the reported cases drain into an enlarged coronary sinus that opens into the right atrium at the usual location.[12] The size of the two SVCs are complementary, with the left one large and the right one smaller.

A persistent left SVC with a normal right SVC can be associated with other congenital cardiac malformations such as AV canal, tetralogy of Fallot, or transposition of the great vessels, or septal defects may be present. Anomalies of the IVC also are common, including absence of the hepatic portion of the IVC.[14] When this occurs, blood from the IVC drains via the azygous or hemiazygous system to enter either the normal right SVC or the anomalous left SVC.

Less common is the persistence of left SVC without a right SVC, originally reported in 1862,[15] with a 0.5% or less incidence in the general population (only 67 reported cases as of 1984).[16]

Drainage to the Left Atrium.

When the right SVC,[17] left SVC,[18] or both right and left venae cavae drain to the left atrium, arterial desaturation and other intracardiac pathology (atrial or ventricular septal defects, AV canal, tetralogy of Fallot, or double-outlet right ventricle) are present. Schick and colleagues reported a single acyanotic patient with right SVC drainage to the left atrium who had no evidence of aortic coarctation,[13] atrial septal defect,[19] innominate bridge, or extrathoracic systemic venous collateralization[13] to shunt blood from the right to the left SVC. A similar acyanotic patient was reported by Meadows.[20] The asplenia or polysplenia syndrome may be associated with a left SVC and left atrium connection. Persistent left SVC drainage into the left atrium is usually associated with an atrial septal defect and absence of the coronary sinus.[10] The absence of the coronary sinus may actually be an "unroofed coronary sinus" or a dilated coronary sinus orifice producing a "coronary sinus atrial septal defect."[10]

Unusual Systemic Drainage Sites.

An unusual arrangement, of which only 11 cases have been reported in the literature, is the presence of normal right SVC and IVC with left superior and inferior caval veins draining into the left atria.[11,21,22] Another unusual case, of which there are only seven in the world's literature, involves the entrance of the right superior vena cava into both atria.[23,24] In the reported cases, there were stenosis at the right atrial entry and an aneurysmal dilatation at the left atrial opening. Another exceptional anomaly is IVC drainage into the left atrium with or without an atrial septal defect.[10] Combinations of several systemic venous anomalies produce total anomalous systemic venoatrial connection, an extremly rare condition.[10] Anomalies of systemic venous drainage are occasionally associated with abnormalities of pulmonary venous return.

Pathophysiology.

A right atrial systemic venous connection presents little problem because there is no functional disturbance but only an abnormality in the site of connection. Drainage of the right SVC, left SVC, or both venae cavae into the left atrium increases blood flow to the left heart, decreases blood flow to the right heart, and partially bypasses the pulmonary circulation. Patients with SVC drainage to the left atrium have systemic arterial desaturation secondary to right-to-left shunting as one third of venous return occurs through the SVC. However, cases of left SVC drainage to the left atrium with only large left-to-right shunts and normal arterial saturation have been reported.[13,20]

Natural History.

Persistence of the left SVC is usually of little consequence. However, its persistence may complicate attempted catheterization of the heart from the left arm or cardiac surgery.

Patients with persistent left SVC without a right SVC are generally asymptomatic but may have coronary sinus rhythm or tachyarrhythmias. Coronary sinus rhythm is a low atrial rhythm or left axis deviation of the P wave that has been noted in these patients.[25] These dysrhythmias were previously thought to result from stretching of the AV node and bundle of His due to dilation of the coronary sinus opening into which the entire SVC flow drains. However, more recent study indicates abnormalities (hypoplasia and limited atrial connection) of the sinus node itself without a change in its position or a relation to the size of the coronary sinus.[26] Sinus node dysfunction requiring an epicardial pacing system (because of difficulty in establishing stable right ventricular pacing from the left SVC through the coronary sinus) has been reported.[27] Congenital atrioventricular conduction abnormalities (Mahaim fibers, Kent bundles) are noted 10 times more frequently in patients with persistent left SVC than in the normal population.[28]

Because arterial desaturation occurs in patients with SVC drainage to the left atrium, the complications of cyanosis or paradoxical embolism may occur. Likewise, the increased cardiac work associated with volume overload may lead to heart failure.

Diagnosis. A persistent left SVC causes leftward deviation of the P axis on the ECG and a vertical shadow at the left upper border on the chest radiograph.[10] It can also be recognized as a notch on the inferior border of the left atrial angiogram.[29] When the left SVC connects to the coronary sinus, the echocardiogram demonstrates an echo-free space localized to the left atrioventricular groove that fills with echoes during saline contrast injection into the left arm.[30] Complications of catheterization, including supraventricular tachycardia, occur with greater frequency in patients with left SVC[31] when catheterized through the anomalous vessel.

Persistence of the left SVC in the absence of the right SVC can be demonstrated during cardiac catheterization and angiography, or when difficulties in the placement of pulmonary artery[32] or pacemaker catheters[33] are noted. A catheter in the subclavian or internal jugular vein makes a sharp bend as it enters the right atrium, particularly if inserted from the right-sided veins. Two-dimensional echocardiography also demonstrates the enlarged coronary sinus, particularly in the parasternal long axis view.[34] The injection of saline contrast into a left arm vein will demonstrate the left SVC to coronary sinus connection.

Diagnostic features of SVC drainage to the left atrium include a hyperactive left ventricle, normal first and second heart sounds, and no associated murmurs. Soft systolic murmurs at the left sternal border are heard in some patients.[18] There may be a left supracardiac shadow on the chest radiograph but pulmonary vascularity is normal. Because the left ventricle has greater volume work, left ventricular hypertrophy may be seen on electrocardiogram. Although there is right-to-left shunting, there is no right ventricular hypertrophy on either ECG or radiography. Contrast echocardiography or radionuclide scans (with saline or radionuclide injections in the upper, but not lower, extremities) demonstrate opacification of the left atrium and ventricle without visualization of the right ventricle indicating an anomalous connection of a right SVC to the left atrium.[34–36] If a left SVC connects to the left atrium, radionuclide angiography or contrast echocardiography demonstrates the anomaly with injection in the left arm only.[37] Differential shunting of right and left arm venous return can be demonstrated with total body scanning after injection of radioactive microspheres.[37] The specific diagnosis is confirmed by venous angiography and cardiac catheterization. However, the anomalous connection to the left atrium will be missed when catheterization is performed via the femoral route instead of the brachial veins.

Anesthesia and Perioperative Management. No specific anesthetic problems are present with SVC anomalies except potential difficulties with central venous catheterization from the femoral route. Drainage of the SVC to the right atrium in patients with persistent left SVC with or without a right SVC does not complicate anesthetic care except for the unusual course of central venous catheters and the dysrhythmia potential in patients with persistent left SVC and absent right SVC.

For patients with SVC drainage to the left atrium, no specific anesthetic technique can be recommended. Obviously, care should be taken to avoid air bubbles in intravenous solutions administered in the upper extremities because these would readily pass to the systemic circulation. Intravenous induction of anesthesia would be rapid because any uptake in the pulmonary circulation during the first pass would be precluded. Likewise, administration of an intravenous bolus of drug with cardiodepressant effects would be disadvantageous because high concentrations would occur in the coronary circulation. For these reasons, it would appear advantageous to place intravenous cannulas in the lower extremities.[35]

Surgical Technique. Surgical therapy to correct anomalous SVC is not indicated. However, a knowledge of the variants of the SVC is essential to the surgeon performing aortic, renal, ureteral, or other retroperitoneal surgery.

Usually, a persistent left SVC with otherwise normal venous anatomy (an adequate innominate bridge connecting the left and right SVC) is simply ligated during intracardiac repair of other congenital defects (Fig 17–2). During cardiopulmonary bypass, the right heart is distended with blood and a right atrial or ventricular surgical field obscured if the left SVC is not clamped or separately cannulated. The anomalous left SVC can be occluded with a balloon during catheterization to determine whether or not the collateral channels can handle the venous drainage without an increase in venous pressure (over 15–30 mm Hg) distal to the occlusion.[25,38]

When there is no right SVC or other interconnecting vessel for venous drainage,[39] the left SVC must be cannulated directly or via the coronary sinus during cardiac surgery requiring cardiopulmonary bypass. Another approach to complicated venous cannulation is deep hypothermia with circulatory arrest, particularly during intracardiac surgery in small infants. If an anatomically correct repair is necessary because of additional venous anomalies, three methods are possible: division of the persistent left SVC and reimplantation into the right atrium (Fig 17–3), division and reimplantation into the pulmonary artery, or creation of a tunnel from the anomalous opening into the right atrium.[39] (Fig 17–4).

Because of the effects on oxygenation and cardiac work, relocation to the right atrium of abnormal vena caval drainage to the left atrium is essential. The repair involves actual transfer of the vena cava to the right atrium or left pulmonary artery, transposition of the interatrial septum with a pericardial baffle or patch, or creation of a posterior left atrial tunnel or coronary sinus[40] to join the left vena cava to the systemic venous side of the heart, or ligation of the left SVC[10] (see Fig 17–4).

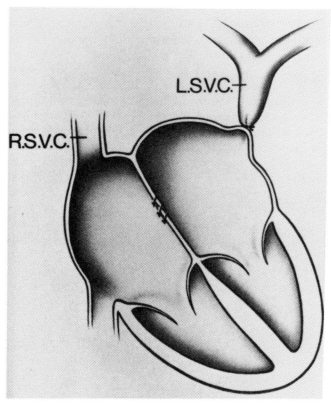

Figure 17–2. Ligation of a persistent left superior vena cava is performed when there is adequate flow through the right superior vena cava. (*From Arciniegas E: Pediatric Cardiac Surgery. Chicago: Year Book Medical, 1985, with permission.*)

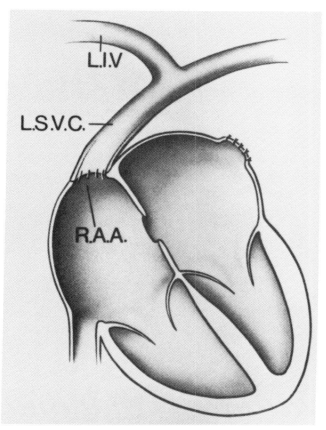

Figure 17–3. Direct anastomosis of the left superior vena cava to the right atrium. (*From Arciniegas E: Pediatric Cardiac Surgery. Chicago: Year Book Medical, 1985, with permission*)

Postoperative Care and Long-term Outcome. Specific postoperative problems after connection of anomalies of systemic venous drainage have not been reported.

Anomalies of Pulmonary Venous Drainage

Anatomy. Anomalous connections of pulmonary venous drainage, which can be either partial (PAPVD) or total (TAPVD), comprise about 1% of congenital heart defects. The embryologic development of the pulmonary venous system has a dual origin from the left atrium and the splanchnic plexus.[41] (see Chapter 3). Several classifications of anomalous pulmonary venous return have been proposed, including those of Neill,[42] Darling,[42] and Smith.[44] The classification of Neill[43] was based on embryologic deviation of the connection between the pulmonary veins and the heart. Four embryologic origins for anomalous pulmonary veins have been described: (1) the umbilicovitelline system of the portal vein and ductus venosus, (2) the right cardinal system via superior vena cava and azygous vein, (3) the left cardinal system via left innominate vein and coronary sinus, and (4) the right atrium with malpositioning of the interatrial septum.[42]

Anomalous pulmonary venous drainage results from atresia or malformation of the common pulmonary veins with persistence of abnormal venous connections. Four types of TAPVD have also been described based on anatomic connections: supracardiac, cardiac, infracardiac, or mixed connections[43] (Fig 17–5). The supracardiac type (type I) with venous return to either the right (via a short connecting vein in 10–15% of cases) or left SVC (as a single trunk in 25–40% of cases) or to the left innominate vein via an anomalous vertical vein is most common. A single case of four anomalous pulmonary veins draining into the right SVC has been reported.[45] Cardiac connections (type II), usually to the coronary sinus, occur in 23% of cases.[46] However, the pulmonary veins may also drain directly and separately into the right atrium in 2–15% of cases. Infracardiac connections to the IVC, portal veins, hepatic veins, or ductus venosus via a common trunk passing through the esophageal hiatus of the diaphragm are least common, occurring in only 21% of cases.[46] Mixed connections in which there is independent drainage of different pulmonary segments to separate sites in the systemic venous system[47] may include multiple pulmonary venous connections,[48] multiple channels,[43] or double levels of drainage.[47,49] Double

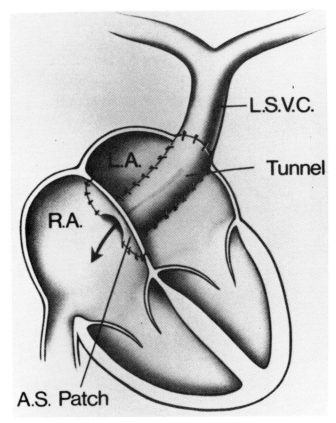

Figure 17–4. Intracardiac transposition of a persistent left superior vena cava is performed by creation of a tunnel with pericardium or prosthetic material along the posterior left atrium. (*From Arciniegas E: Pediatric Cardiac Surgery. Chicago: Year Book Medical, 1985, with permission.*)

connections occur in TAPVD to the right cardinal system if a left SVC (left vertical vein) is present[47] (Fig 17–6). Pulmonary sequestration (bronchial and pulmonary arterial) and other congenital cardiac anomalies (patent ductus arteriosus, single ventricle, coarctation, transposition of the great vessels, pulmonic atresia/stenosis) may be associated with TAPVD or PAPVD.

Supracardiac, infracardiac, and mixed connections are subject to obstruction of the pulmonary venous drainage. Classification of anatomy by the presence or absence of pulmonary venous obstruction at the supra- or infradiaphragmatic connection was attempted by Smith and colleagues.[44] However, Smith's and other classifications have fallen into disuse, with the anatomic classification of Darling as the principal current one.[43] There are several sources of extrinsic obstruction to the anomalous veins. These include the coronary sinus ostium (coronary sinus connections), pulmonary vein–right atrial junction (right atrial connections), diaphragm or ductus venosus (infracardiac connections), pulmonary venous trunk–right SVC junction (right SVC), left main bronchus or left SVC–innominate junction (left SVC).

Pathophysiology. Total anomalous pulmonary venous return is incompatible with life unless there is communication between the left and right sides of the heart, usually through a patent foramen ovale or atrial septal defect. The size of the interatrial communication is the initial determinant of mixed venous blood distribution. If the communication is small, left atrial blood flow is limited, cardiac output reduced, and right atrial and pulmonary pressures increased. With large interatrial communications, blood flow is determined by the resistance in the pulmonary and systemic vasculature. If anomalous pulmonary venous pathways are unobstructed, increased proportions of mixed right atrial blood are directed into the pulmonary circulation as pulmonary vascular resistance decreases in the neonatal period. Although arterial oxygen saturation is 85–90% in these patients, right heart failure develops early. Pulmonary hypertension is a later development in unobstructed TAPVD than in obstructed venous drainage.

Thus, three major problems are associated with anomalous pulmonary venous return. First, the total left-to-right shunt must be compensated by a right-to-left shunt through the atrial septal defect. Second, there may be stenosis at the junction of the anomalous trunk with the vena cava or other vessel resulting in severe pulmonary hypertension. Pulmonary congestion is unlikely with the coronary sinus type. Unexplained pulmonary hypertension and increased pulmonary vascular resistance can be present in the absence of pulmonary venous obstruction. Third, if the right-to-left shunt is small, the right heart has a volume overload causing dilatation and failure, whereas the left atrium is small because of the absence of pulmonary venous return.

Natural History. Patients with pulmonary hypertension, pulmonary venous obstruction, and decreased pulmonary blood flow are most likely to present in early infancy with tachypnea and cyanosis. Those without pulmonary hypertension or venous obstruction and increased pulmonary blood flow have only minimal cyanosis and limited signs or symptoms. As the infant grows, the demands for systemic output increase causing the interatrial septal defect, which provided adequate arteriovenous mixing at birth, to become restrictive.[50] For these reasons, an infant with TAPVD may not become symptomatic until 2–3 months of age. As the decreased left ventricular filling reduces systemic output, cyanosis, metabolic acidosis, and heart failure develop. Without surgery, most infants with TAPVD are dead by 12 months of age.

However, a recent series of 19 patients with TAPVD and large atrial septal defects who underwent corrective surgery as adults was reported by Rodriguez-Collado.[51] Longer survival (to adulthood) requires the presence of a nonrestrictive atrial septal defect, minimal obstruction to pulmonary venous return, and the absence of pulmonary vascular disease.

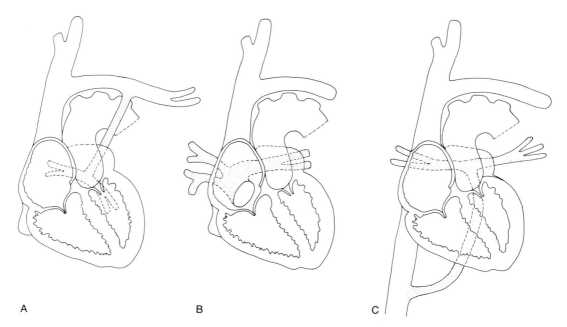

Figure 17–5. Type of TAPVD. (*A*) Supracardiac type in which the pulmonary veins connect to the superior vena cava via a left vertical vein (persistent left superior vena cava). (*B*) Cardiac type in which the pulmonary veins drain into the coronary sinus. (*C*) Infracardiac type in which the pulmonary veins drain into a common pulmonary vein that passes through the diaphragm to enter the inferior vena cava. (*Modified from Darling RC, et al: Total pulmonary venous drainage into the right side of the heart: Report of 17 autopsied cases not associated with major cardiovascular anomalies. Lab Invest 6:44–64, 1957, with permission.*)

Diagnostic Features

Signs and Symptoms. Cyanosis is always present in patients with TAPVD with its severity being dependent upon the amount of mixing of systemic and venous blood, the size of the atrial septal defect, and pulmonary vascular resistance. The amount of pulmonary venous blood depends on pulmonary and systemic vascular re-

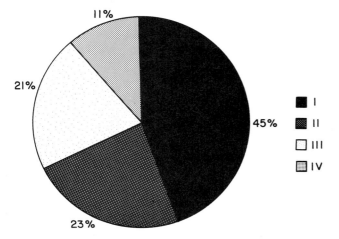

Figure 17–6. The incidence of various types of TAPVD. (*Modified from Gathman GE, et al: Total anomalous pulmonary venous connection. Clinical and physiologic observations of 75 pediatric patients. Circulation 42:143–154, 1970, with permission.*)

sistance. Because left atrial blood flow is limited, reduced cardiac output compromises systemic perfusion. Other physical findings depend on the presence or absence of pulmonary venous obstruction. Hyperactive precordium, normal to loud S_1, wide, fixed splitting of S_2, and a systolic ejection murmur of relative pulmonic stenosis are present when there is no pulmonary venous obstruction. Half of these infants develop symptoms within the first month of life, whereas the remainder become symptomatic between 1 and 12 months of age. Failure to thrive and repeated respiratory infections are common features.

Tachypnea, cyanosis, and other signs of right-sided failure are present in the first few days of life if the pulmonary venous connection is obstructed. The cardiac auscultatory findings are similar to those in patients without obstructed pulmonary veins. Right axis deviation, right atrial enlargement, and right ventricular hypertrophy are seen on ECG in both obstructed and unobstructed types.[44,46] The majority of these infants present within the first month of life and the rest by 12 months of age.

Radiographic Findings. The chest radiograph shows a large cardiac silhouette with conspicuous pulmonary vascularity if there is large pulmonary flow. Pulmonary edema and a granular appearance of the lung fields are present. The cardiac silhouette is often described as a "figure-of–8" or "snowman" when the anomalous vein drains into a persistent left SVC. This finding is usually not present in early infancy.[43] Another radiographic finding is a convexity on the right atrial border when the anomalous connection is at the right atrial level. When there is partial or complete drainage of the right pulmonary veins into the inferior vena cava, the anomalous vein produces a vertical, gently curved scimitar shape on the chest radiograph, prompting the name "scimitar syndrome."[52]

Echocardiographic Findings. Although the anomalous venous channel can be identified as an echo-free space behind the left atrium on echocardiography in some patients,[53] it is generally difficult to visualize the total course of the pulmonary veins. However, intrauterine diagnosis of TAPVD has been reported despite the limited pulmonary blood flow.[54] A small left atrium with a large right ventricle are present on echocardiography, but these findings are nonspecific. Pathologic examination of hearts with TAPVD reveals a large fossa ovalis and a normal-sized elongated left ventricle due to flattening of the interventricular septum.[55] The enlargement of the coronary sinus and the pulmonary veins can be visualized echocardiographically as the body and "tail of a whale" using the parasagittal subxiphoid approach.[56] The dilated vertical vein descending into the liver and dilated intrahepatic veins can be seen on echocardiography of infracardiac TAPVD.[57] If a satisfactory echocardiogram can be obtained, cardiac catheterization and angiography can be avoided.[58,59] Recent studies suggest that two-dimensional echocardiography can be the definitive diagnostic method for TAPVD if no other congenital cardiac abnormalities are present.[59,60] Doppler color flow imaging facilitates diagnosis of the sites of drainage, the presence or absence of obstruction, and coexisting lesions decreasing pulmonary blood flow.[61]

Cardiac Catheterization and Angiography. Cardiac catheterization with measurement of oxygen saturations (Fig 17–7) and pulmonary arteriography is essential for accurate diagnosis of TAPVD with other cardiac anomalies. Right atrial and right ventricular pressures are often increased, particularly when the venous connection is obstructed. Oxygen saturation increases at the site of the anomalous connection. This can result in saturation being higher in the right heart and pulmonary artery than in the left heart with the supracardiac connection because IVC blood is directed across the ASD to the left heart. The converse is true with infracardiac connections in which the left heart saturations will be higher. In general, the oxygen saturations in the right ventricle, pulmonary artery, left atrium, left ventricle, and aorta are similar to those in the right atrium because of the mixing of oxygenated and unoxygenated blood. The levophase of the pulmonary angiogram, enhanced by digital substraction techniques, clearly demonstrates the anomalous connections[60] (Fig 17–8).

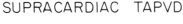

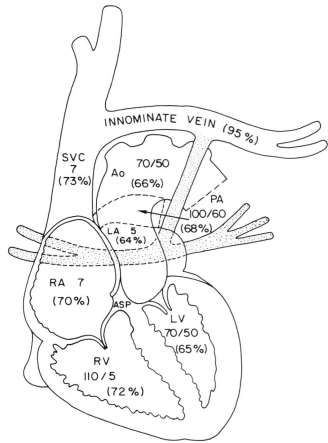

Figure 17–7. Typical cardiac catheterization data in a patient with the supracardiac type of TAPVD. Oxygen saturations are given in parentheses. The right heart saturations are higher than in the left heart in supracardiac TAPVD. Right ventricular pressures are often suprasystemic and also higher than pulmonary artery pressures.

Interventional Cardiac Catheterization. The interatrial communication is restrictive if it is less than 3 mm on echocardiography, an 8-mm balloon does not easily cross the interatrial septal defect, or right atrial mean pressure is greater than left atrial mean pressure.[50] Balloon or blade atrial septostomy is performed during catheterization to increase flow into the left atrium if the interatrial opening is adequate.[50] Percutaneous balloon angioplasty can be used to dilate an obstructed common pulmonary venous trunk at its entrance into the SVC. However, these are only temporary measures until definitive surgical therapy can be instituted.[50]

Anesthesia and Perioperative Management. Patients with anomalous pulmonary venous drainage, usually infants, are severely cyanotic, often acidotic, and subject to rapid cardiovascular deterioration when they require surgery within the first few days of life. If pul-

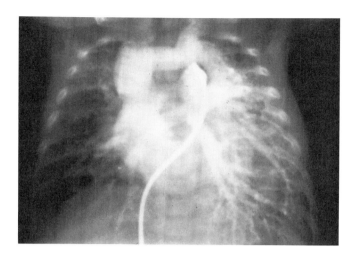

Figure 17–8. The levo phase of a pulmonary angiogram demonstrating the anomalous (supracardiac) drainage of the pulmonary veins. (*Photograph courtesy of Dr. Karen Rheuban.*)

monary venous obstruction is present in addition to the anomalous venous drainage, pulmonary edema, pulmonary hypertension, and right heart failure will be present.

The anesthetic begins with a small dose of neuromuscular blocking agent such as pancuronium or vecuronium and fentanyl if an intravenous (IV) catheter is present. If there is no IV, intramuscular ketamine, 1 mg/kg, can be given to facilitate placement of an intravenous catheter. It is unlikely that a potent inhalation anesthetic such as halothane or isoflurane will be tolerated in these very ill infants or during surgical manipulation to verify the anomalous connections in TAPVD. However, in patients with PAPVD, an inhalation induction prior to placement of intravenous catheters can be used. Maintenance of anesthesia with narcotics in oxygen provides satisfactory anesthesia without myocardial depression. An increase in the inspired oxygen concentration is unlikely to improve arterial oxygenation significantly because the amount of shunting is relatively fixed. However, the institution of controlled ventilation after induction often somewhat improves oxygenation, thus reducing the pulmonary vasoconstriction resulting from hypoxia and improving the patient's general condition.

Invasive monitoring including intra-arterial and central venous catheters should be placed immediately after induction if they have not been placed during the preoperative period. A pulse oximeter, oscillometric blood pressure, and capnograph also are used. Frequent determinations of arterial blood gases should be made to verify the infant's acid-base status and permit rapid correction of acidosis.

If surface cooling is planned, the infant should be placed on a cooling mattress; fluids and inspired gases

are not warmed after vascular cannulation and endotracheal intubation have been performed. Active cooling by immersion in an ice bath is utilized by some groups,[58] although its necessity is unclear. Cardiopulmonary bypass is instituted in the usual fashion and core cooling is used by most surgeons.[62] Continuous low-flow bypass is used by some surgical teams.[63] In other institutions,[58,62,64] when a core temperature of 10–15°C is reached, the extracorporeal circulation is terminated, the intracardiac cannulas removed, and the surgical repair begun. When the repair is finished, cannulas are reinserted, extracorporeal warming commenced, and cardiopulmonary bypass discontinued when the patient is completely rewarmed (rectal temperature >35°C) and vigorous cardiac activity is present.

Inotropic and vasodilator drugs are often necessary to ensure an adequate cardiac output after discontinuation of bypass in these patients. The left ventricle is often unable to support the circulation adequately, probably because it has been relatively underfilled and underutilized prior to surgical correction of TAPVD. Abnormalities of left atrial (small-capacity) and left ventricular architecture have been reported. The capacity of the left ventricle may also be decreased by septal displacement. A hypoplastic aortic valve is sometimes present.

Dobutamine or dopamine may improve the general cardiac decompensation. Placement of left atrial catheters and maintenance of low left atrial pressures prevents fluid overload in patients whose right ventricular compliance is greater than the left because of increased pulmonary blood flow preoperatively. Right atrial pressures should be maintained at 10–12 mm Hg or less. Temporary pacemaker leads should be placed to assure an adequate heart rate (usually 140 beats/min or greater in infants) and in the event that the atrial and AV nodal conducting system have been damaged.

The pulmonary vasculature of patients with TAPVD often has a thickened medial layer, so that pulmonary vascular resistance does not decrease normally after repair. Intraoperative placement of a pulmonary artery catheter allows early recognition of pulmonary hypertensive episodes requiring therapy with vasodilators such as prostaglandin E_1, tolazoline, nitroprusside, isoproterenol, or nitroglycerin. Unfortunately, none of these drugs is a specific pulmonary vasodilator. Occasionally, it may be necessary to fenestrate the atrial patch to allow the right heart to decompress into the left heart when severe pulmonary hypertension is present.

Surgical Technique. Surgical therapy is the only means for survival of patients with anomalous pulmonary venous drainage. One of the early attempts at correction was the use of a closed anastomosis between the left upper pulmonary vein and left atrial appendage.[65] Prior to the development of extracorporeal circulation, inflow occlusion[66] or repair within the atrium without circulatory diversion (atrial well technique)[67] was used to correct TAPVD. Cooley described the right atrial open anastomotic approach using extracorporeal circulation in 1956.[68] Today, extracorporeal circulation with either deep hypothermic low-flow or total circulatory arrest is used for a transatrial, right atrial, or other surgical approach to divert the anomalous flow to the left atrium.[69] However, successful relocation of infradiaphragmatic pulmonary veins to a common atrium in two infants with asplenia syndrome without cardiopulmonary bypass has been reported.[70]

The transatrial approach minimizes the possibility of anatomic distortion of the anastomosis of the anomalous vein with the left atrium. With a cardiac connection, an interatrial patch can be fashioned to divert the flow from the coronary sinus to the left atrium while closing the ASD. Care must be taken to avoid damage to the AV node and bundle of His (Fig 17–9). In the supracardiac type, the common pulmonary trunk is anastomosed to the posterior left atrium directly, the atrial septal defect is closed, and the vertical vein ligated. An atrioseptoplasty technique can also be used. However, creation of a channel in the superior vena cava and atrium risks SVC obstruction and venous thrombosis.[71] An alternative technique for middle or high superior vena caval connections is the division of the SVC proximal to the entry site of the anomalous veins. The cephalad end of the SVC is reanastomosed to the right atrial appendage while a pericardial patch diverts blood from the anomalous vein across an atrial septal defect to the left atrium.[72,73] A similar approach is used for infracardiac connections (Fig 17–10): direct anastomosis to the left atrium, ligation of the descending vertical vein at the diaphragm, and direct or patch closure of the ASD. Some surgical groups[58,61] do not ligate the ascending or descending vertical vein because Appelbaum and colleagues[74] noted hepatic necrosis after ligation of either of the veins. It is possible that the unligated vein acts as a left atrial vent during the immediate postoperative period when left ventricular compliance may be decreased. Combinations of these techniques are used to repair the mixed type of anomalous venous drainage.

Surgical therapy for partial anomalous pulmonary venous return may require any of the previously described techniques for total anomalous drainage. Reimplantation into the left atrium, atrioseptopexy, and intracardiac tunneling have been used successfully. Pulmonary resection is useful instead of reconstruction when severe pulmonary parenchymal disease is present.

Postoperative Care. Some degree of arterial desaturation will often be present after repair if the coronary sinus is still draining into the left atrium. Other causes of arterial desaturation include pulmonary edema and low

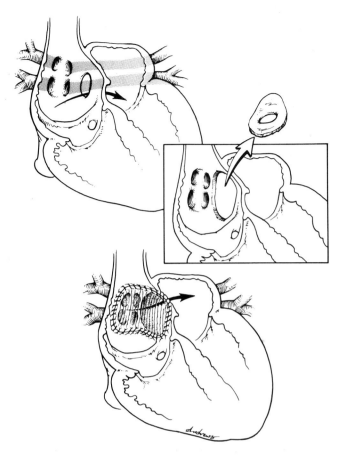

Figure 17–9. Surgical therapy for a cardiac connection of anomalous pulmonary veins. The atrial septal defect is enlarged and a patch sutured to divert the pulmonary veins to the left side of the heart while closing the septal defect. (*From Reardon MJ, et al: Total anomalous pulmonary venous return: Report of 201 patients treated surgically. Texas Heart Inst J 12:131–141, 1985, with permission.*)

cardiac output. Postoperative respiratory support, often for several days in patients with preoperative pulmonary venous obstruction, is mandatory.

Immediate and Long-term Results. Operative mortality is high owing to increased pulmonary vascular resistance causing right heart failure. Although the size and number of pulmonary arteries are normal, the medial wall thickness is increased as in prenatal life and muscle extends into normally nonmuscular alveolar ductal arteries. Surgical series note mortality rates of 2–57%.[64,75,76] Factors that increase mortality are age (<1 month), pulmonary venous obstruction, depressed left ventricular function, poor preoperative condition, and the presence of other cardiac anomalies.[58,63] Surgical technique (transatrial versus posterior approach with cardiac displacement) and more recent surgical series (after 1975) also contribute to lower mortality.[58,69] Wilson and co-workers report that transatrial exposure at the common venous

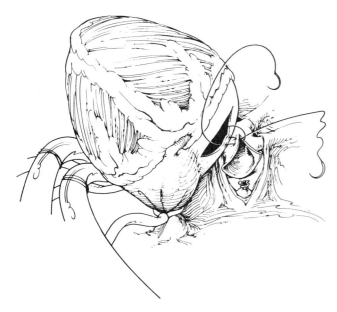

Figure 17–10. Surgical therapy for an infracardiac connection of anomalous pulmonary veins. The cardiac apex is elevated to allow access to the posterior left atrium. The common pulmonary vein is sutured to the left atrium. The atrial septal defect is repaired through a right atriotomy. Whether it is necessary or desirable to ligate the anomalous vertical vein descending through the diaphragm is unclear at present (see text). (*From Reardon MJ, et al: Total anomalous pulmonary venous return: Report of 201 patients treated surgically. Texas Heart Inst J 12:131–141, 1985, with permission.*)

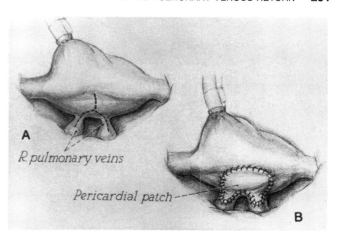

Figure 17–11. The repair of an area of restenosis of the pulmonary veins involves incisions across the stenotic area (*A*) and closure of the resulting defect with a pericardial or polytetrafluoroethylene (Gore Tex) patch (*B*). (*From Wilson WR, et al: Technical modifications for improved results in total anomalous pulmonary venous drainage. J Thorac Cardiovasc Surg 103:861–871, 1992, with permission.*)

chamber, pericardial patch augmentation of the atrium, and interrupted suturing of the common vein to the atrium improved survival.[77] Higher operative mortality has been reported with infracardiac TAPVD into the azygous veins or right SVC resulting from pulmonary venous obstruction.[64,78] The adult series of Rodriguez-Collado reported only a 10% surgical mortality and satisfactory results (reduction of pulmonary artery pressure, normal left ventricular ejection fraction) in 19 patients with supracardiac, cardiac, or mixed connections and large atrial septal defects.[51]

Long-term Results. Stenosis at the anastomotic site or at the orifice of individual veins occurs in 6–16% of patients within the first 6–12 months after repair and may require surgical revision with patch augmentation[75,76,80] (Fig 17–11). It occurs more commonly in infracardiac TAPVD but may occur in other types.[63] If surgical repair is successful in infancy, the long-term prognosis for these patients is excellent.[79] Left atrial reservoir function remains compromised secondary to decreased compliance, so that left atrium acts principally as a conduit.[79] However, pulmonary hypertension is reversible and the small left heart chambers grow and function with only slightly reduced ejection fractions and outputs in most patients.

CONGENITAL PULMONARY VENOUS STENOSIS OR ATRESIA

Congenital pulmonary vein stenosis is a rare malformation that causes a dynamic pulmonary venous obstruction at the site of entry into the left atrium. The etiology is unknown, although Edwards[81] postulated an overgrowth in venous intima and secondary changes in the media, a process similar to that which occurs embryologically in TAPVD. In infants with transposition of the great vessels, left-sided pulmonary vein stenosis becomes progressive because of preferential postnatal flow to the right lung.[82] Congenital atresia of one or more of the pulmonary veins, resulting from defective incorporation of the common pulmonary vein into the left atrium, represents the most severe form of this anomaly.[83]

Diagnosis

Infants with congenital pulmonary venous stenosis or atresia may have other congenital anomalies, such as ventricular septal defects or transposition of the great vessels. If only one or two veins are involved, the patients may be asymptomatic and the lesion undetected during life. However, with more severe involvement, patients are symptomatic. Pulmonary hypertension, hemoptysis, congestive heart failure, and frequent respiratory infections are common. The stenosis may be dynamic in nature but can be demonstrated by pulmonary angiography.

Surgical Repair

A conservative approach of medical management is warranted if only minor symptoms are present. Venoplasty and creation of atrial flaps have been unsuccessful in relieving the obstruction in symptomatic patients. Progressive restenosis occurs when the obstruction is patched with polyethylene or Dacron or direct excision of the stenotic area, suggesting a progressive process.[84] However, the use of autologous material from the atrium itself (atrial appendage) has been recently reported to provide lasting relief of obstruction.[85] With complete stenosis, lobectomy or pneumonectomy may be the procedure of choice for symptomatic patients with unilateral disease.[83]

Anesthetic Management

Because the stenosis can be dynamic in nature, maneuvers likely to increase myocardial contractility are relatively contraindicated. Light anesthesia, hypoxia, hypercarbia, or nitrous oxide, which further worsen pulmonary hypertension, should be avoided. In one patient, the pulmonary artery pressure was inversely related to the depth of anesthesia.[85] Thus, the surgical repair must be adequate even in the presence of vasospasm that may occur in the unanesthetized state.

REFERENCES

1. Giordano JM, Trout HH: Anomalies of the inferior vena cava. *J Vasc Surg* 3:924–928, 1986
2. Chuang VP, Mena CE, Hoskins PA: Congenital anomalies of the inferior vena cava. Review of embryogenesis and presentation of a simplified classification. *Br J Radiol* 47:206–213, 1974
3. van der Horst RL, Hastreiter AR: Congenital interruption of the inferior vena cava. *Chest* 80:638–640, 1981
4. Kumar D, Kumar S, Lounsbury DE: Anomalous inferior vena cava with idiopathic thrombosis simulating a mass. *Computerized Radiol* 7:223–227, 1983
5. Royal SA, Callen PW: CT evaluation of anomalies of the inferior vena cava and left renal vein. *AJR* 132:759–763, 1979
6. Tuma S, Samanek M, Voriskova M, et al: Anomalies of the systemic venous return. *Pediatr Radiol* 5:193–197, 1977
7. Webb WR, Gamsu G, Speckman JM, et al: Computed tomographic demonstration of mediastinal venous anomalies. *AJR* 139:157–161, 1982
8. Fisher MR, Hricak H, Higgins CB: Magnetic resonance imaging of developmental venous anomalies. *AJR* 145:705–709, 1985
9. van der Horst RL, Gotsman MS: Abnormalities of atrial depolarization in infradiaphragmatic interruption of inferior vena cava. *Br Heart J* 34:295–300, 1972
10. Mazzucco A, Bortolotti U, Stellin G, Gallucci V: Anomalies of the systemic venous return: A review. *J Cardiac Surg* 5:122–133, 1990
11. Winter FS: Persistent left superior vena cava, survey of world literature and report of thirty additional cases. *Angiology* 5:90–132, 1954
12. Goor DA, Lillehei LW: *Congenital Malformations of the Heart.* New York: Grune & Stratton, 1975, pp 400–404

13. Schick EC, Lekakis J, Rothendler JA, Ryan TJ: Persistent left superior vena cava and right superior vena cava drainage into the left atrium without arterial hypoxemia. *J Am Coll Cardiol* 5:374–378, 1985
14. Lembo CM, Latte S: Persistence of the left superior vena cava: A case report. *Angiology* 35:58–62, 1984
15. Karnegis JN, Wang Y, Winchell P, Edwards JE: Persistent superior vena cava, fibrous remnant right superior cava and ventricular defect. *Am J Cardiol* 14:573–577, 1964
16. Yarnal JR, Smiley WM, Schwartz DA: Unusual course of a Swan-Ganz catheter. *Chest* 76:585, 1979
17. Park H-M, Summerer MH, Preuss K, et al: Anomalous drainage of the right superior vena cava into the left atrium. *J Am Coll Cardiol* 2:358–362, 1983
18. Vasquez-Perez J, Frontera-Izquierdo P: Anomalous drainage of the right superior vena cava into the left atrium as an isolated anomaly. Rare case report. *Am Heart J* 97:89–91, 1979
19. Singh A, Doyle E, Danilowicz D, Spencer FC: Masked abnormal drainage of the inferior vena cava into the left atrium. *Am J Cardiol* 38:261–264, 1976
20. Meadows WR, Sharp JT: Persistent left superior vena cava draining into the left atrium without atrial oxygen unsaturation. *Am J Cardiol* 16:273–279, 1965
21. deLaval MR, Ritter DG, McGoon DC, Danielson GK: Anomalous systemic venous connection. Surgical considerations. *Mayo Clin Proc* 50:599–610, 1975
22. van Tellingen C, Verzijbergen F, Plokker HWM: A patient with bilateral superior and inferior caval veins. *Int J Cardiol* 5:366–373, 1984
23. Shapiro EP, Al-Sadir J, Campbell NPS, et al: Drainage of right superior vena cava into both atria. *Circulation* 63:712–717, 1981
24. Bharatti S, Lev M: Direct entry of the right superior vena cava into the left atrium with aneurysmal dilatation and stenosis at its entry into the right atrium with stenosis of the pulmonary veins: A rare case. *Pediatr Cardiol* 5:123–126, 1984
25. Lenox CC, Zuberbuhler JR, Park SC, et al: Absent right superior vena cava with persistent left superior vena cava: Implications and management. *Am J Cardiol* 45:117–122, 1980
26. Lenox CC, Hashida Y, Anderson RH, Hubbard JD: Conduction tissue anomalies in absence of the right superior caval vein. *Int J Cardiol* 8:251–260, 1985
27. Camm AJ, Dymond D, Spurrell RAJ: Sinus node dysfunction associated with absence of right superior vena cava. *Br Heart J* 41:504–507, 1979
28. Davis D, Pritchett ELC, Klein GJ, et al: Persistent left superior vena cava in patients with congenital atrioventricular preexcitation conduction abnormalities. *Am Heart J* 101:677–679, 1981
29. Owen JP, Urquhart W: The left atrial notch: A sign of persistent left superior vena cava draining to the right atrium. *Br J Radiol* 52:855–861, 1979
30. Cohen BE, Winer HE, Kronzon I: Echocardiographic findings in patients with left superior vena cava and dilated coronary sinus. *Am J Cardiol* 44:158–161, 1979
31. Fraser RS, Dvorkin J, Rossall RE, Eidem R: Left superior vena cava. A review of associated congenital heart lesions,

catheterization data and roentgenologic findings. *Am J Med* **31**:711–716, 1961

32. Boyes R, Puri VK: Absent right superior vena cava. *Intensive Care Med* **10**:45–46, 1984

33. Harthorne JW, Dunsmore RE, Desanctis RW: Superior vena caval anomaly preventing venous pacemaker implantation. *Br Heart J* **31**:809–810, 1969

34. Snider AR, Ports TA, Silverman NH: Venous anomalies of the coronary sinus: Detection by M-mode, two-dimensional and contrast echocardiography. *Circulation* **60**: 721–727, 1979

35. Ezekowitz MD, Alderson PO, Bulkley BH, et al: Isolated drainage of the superior vena cava into the left atrium in a 52 year old man. *Circulation* **58**:751–756, 1978

36. Truman AT, Rao PS, Kulangara RJ: Use of contrast echocardiography in diagnosis of anomalous connection of right superior vena cava to left atrium. *Br Heart J* **44**:718–723, 1980

37. Konstam MA, Levine DW, Strauss HW, McKusick KA: Left superior vena cava to left atrial communication diagnosed with radionuclide angiocardiography and with differential right to left shunting. *Am J Cardiol* **43**:149–153, 1979

38. Freed MD, Rosenthal A, Bernhard WF: Balloon occlusion of a persistent left superior vena cava in the preoperative evaluation of systemic venous return. *J Thorac Cardiovasc Surg* **65**:835–839, 1973

39. Pugliese P, Murzi B, Aliboni M, Eufrate S: Absent right superior vena cava and persistent left superior vena cava. *J Cardiovasc Surg* **25**:134–137, 1974

40. Alpert BS, Rao PS, Moore HV, Covitz W: Surgical correction of anomalous right superior vena cava to the left atrium. *J Thorac Cardiovasc Surg* **82**:301–305, 1981

41. Rammos S, Gittenberger-deGroot AC, Oppenheimer-Dekker A: The abnormal pulmonary venous connexion: A developmental approach. *Int J Cardiol* **29**:285–295, 1990

42. Neill CA: Development of the pulmonary veins. With reference to the embryology of anomalies of pulmonary venous return. *Pediatrics* **18**:880–886, 1956

43. Darling RC, Rothney WB, Craig JM: Total pulmonary venous drainage into the right side of the heart. *Lab Invest* **6**:44–64, 1957

44. Smith B, Frye TR, Newton WA: Total anomalous pulmonary venous return: Diagnostic criteria and classification. *Am J Dis Child* **101**:41–49, 1961

45. Zoltie N, Walker DR: Total anomalous pulmonary venous drainage into the right superior vena cava. *J Cardiovasc Surg* **24**:537–539, 1983

46. Gathman GE, Nadas AS: Total anomalous pulmonary venous connection: Clinical and physiologic observations of 75 pediatric patients. *Circulation* **42**:143–154, 1970

47. Arciprete P, McKay R, Watson GH, et al: Double connections in total anomalous pulmonary venous connection. *J Thorac Cardiovasc Surg* **92**:146–152, 1986

48. Burroughs JT, Edwards JE: Total anomalous pulmonary venous connection. *Am Heart J* **59**:913–931, 1960

49. Blake HA, Hall RJ, Manion WC: Anomalous pulmonary venous return. *Circulation* **32**:405–414, 1965

50. Ward KE, Mullins CE, Huhta JC, et al: Restrictive interatrial communication in total anomalous pulmonary venous connection. *Am J Cardiol* **57**:1131–1136, 1986

51. Rodriguez-Collado J, Attie F, Zabal C, et al: Total anomalous pulmonary venous connection in adults. *J Thorac Cardiovasc Surg* **103**:877–880, 1992

52. Halasz NA, Halluran KH, Liebow AA: Bronchial and arterial anomalies with drainage of the right lung into inferior vena cava. *Circulation* **14**:826–846, 1956

53. Paquet M, Gutgesell H: Echocardiographic features of total anomalous pulmonary venous connection. *Circulation* **51**:599–605, 1975

54. DeSessa TG, Emerson DS, Felker RE, et al: Anomalous systemic and pulmonary venous pathways diagnosed in utero by ultrasound. *J Ultrasound Med* **9**:311–317, 1990

55. Rosenquist GC, Kelly DJ, Chandra R, et al: Small left atrium and change in contour of the ventricular septum in total anomalous pulmonary venous connection: A morphometric analysis of 22 infant hearts. *Am J Cardiol* **55**:777–782, 1985

56. Williams RG: Echocardiography in the infant. *J Am Coll Cardiol* **5**:30S–36S, 1985

57. Del Torso S, Goh TH, Venables AW: Echocardiographic findings in the liver in total anomalous pulmonary venous connection. *Am J Cardiol* **57**:374–375, 1986

58. Stark J: Anomalies of pulmonary venous return. *World J Surg* **9**:532–542, 1985

59. Huhta JC, Gutgesell HP, Nihill MR: Cross sectional echocardiographic diagnosis of total anomalous pulmonary venous connection. *Br Heart J* **53**:525–534, 1985

60. Van der Velde ME, Parness IA, Colan SD, et al: Two-dimensional echocardiography in the pre- and postoperative management of totally anomalous pulmonary venous connection. *J Am Coll Cardiol* **18**:1746–1751, 1991

61. Sreeram N, Walsh K: Diagnosis of total anomalous pulmonary venous drainage by Doppler color flow imaging. *J Am Coll Cardiol* **19**:1577–1582, 1992

62. Katz NM, Kirklin JW, Pacifico AD: Concepts and practices in surgery for total anomalous pulmonary venous connection. *Ann Thorac Surg* **25**:479–487, 1978

63. Turley K, Tucker WY, Ullyot DL, Ebert PA: Total anomalous pulmonary venous connection in infancy: Influence of age and type of lesion. *Am J Cardiol* **45**:92–97, 1980

64. Reardon MJ, Cooley DA, Kubrusly L, et al: Total anomalous pulmonary venous return: Report of 201 patients treated surgically. *Texas Heart Inst J* **12**:131–141, 1985

65. Muller WH: The surgical treatment of transposition of the pulmonary veins. *Ann Surg* **134**:683–693, 1951

66. Lewis FJ, Varco RL, Tanfic M, Niazi FA: Direct vision repair of triatrial heart and total anomalous pulmonary venous drainage. *Surg Gynecol Obstet* **102**:713–720, 1956

67. Burroughs JT, Kirklin JW: Complete correction of total anomalous pulmonary venous connections: Report of three cases. *Proc Mayo Clin* **31**:182–188, 1956

68. Cooley DA, Ochsner A: Correction of total anomalous pulmonary venous drainage. *Surgery* **42**:1014–1021, 1957

69. Hawkins JA, Clark EB, Doty DB: Total anomalous pulmonary venous connection. *Ann Thorac Surg* **36**:548–560, 1983

70. Lamberti JJ, Waldman JD, Mathewson JW, Kirkpatrick SE: Repair of subdiaphragmatic total anomalous pulmonary venous connection without cardiopulmonary bypass. *J Thorac Cardiovasc Surg* **88**:627–630, 1984

71. Long DM, Rios MV, Elais DO, et al: Parietal and septal

atrioplasty for total correction of anomalous pulmonary venous connection with superior vena cava. *Ann Thorac Surg* **18**:466–471, 1974

72. Vargas FJ, Kreutzer GO: A surgical technique for correction of total anomalous pulmonary venous drainage. *J Thorac Cardiovasc Surg* **90**:410–413, 1985

73. Williams WH, Zorn-Chelton S, Raviele AA, et al: Extracardiac atrial pedicle conduit repair of partial anomalous pulmonary venous connection to the superior vena cava in children. *Ann Thorac Surg* **38**:345–355, 1984

74. Appelbaum A, Kirklin JW, Pacifico AD, Bargeron LM: The surgical treatment of total anomalous pulmonary venous connection. *Isr J Med Sci* **11**:89–96, 1975

75. Lamb RK, Qureshi SA, Wilkinson JL, et al: Total anomalous pulmonary venous drainage. *J Thorac Cardiovasc Surg* **96**:368–375, 1988

76. Oelert H, Schafers HJ, Stegfmann T, et al: Complete correction of total anomalous pulmonary venous drainage: Experience with 53 patients. *Ann Thorac Surg* **41**:392–394, 1986

77. Wilson WR, Ilbawi MN, DeLeon SY, et al: Technical modifications for improved results in total anomalous pulmonary venous drainage. *J Thorac Cardiovasc Surg* **103**:861–871, 1992

78. El Said G, Mullins CE: Management of total anomalous pulmonary venous return. *Circulation* **45**:1240–1250, 1972

79. Mathew R, Thilenius OG, Replogle RL, Arcilla RA: Cardiac function in total anomalous pulmonary venous return before and after surgery. *Circulation* **55**:361–370, 1977

80. Sano S, Brawn WJ, Mee RBB: Total anomalous pulmonary venous drainage. *J Thorac Cardiovasc Surg* **97**:886–892, 1989

81. Edwards J: Congenital stenosis of pulmonary veins. *Lab Invest* **9**:46–66, 1960

82. Vogel M, Ash J, Rowe RD, et al: Congenital unilateral pulmonary vein stenosis complicating transposition of the great arteries. *Am J Cardiol* **54**:166–171, 1984

83. Cabrera A, Vasquez C, Lekuona I: Isolated atresia of the left pulmonary veins. *Int J Cardiol* **7**:298–302, 1985

84. Bini RM, Cleveland D, Ceballos R, et al: Congenital pulmonary venous stenosis. *Am J Cardiol* **54**:369–375, 1984

85. Pacifico AD, Mandke NV, McGrath LB, et al: Repair of congenital pulmonary venous stenosis with living autologous atrial tissue. *J Thorac Cardiovasc Surg* **89**:604–609, 1985

Chapter 18 | Anomalies of the Pulmonary Valve and Pulmonary Circulation

Desmond Bohn

The pulmonary circulation and the right heart are often referred to as "lesser" circulation. From the perspective of heart disease in the adult, where ischemia frequently results in disordered function of the left ventricle, there may be some justification for this statement. In congenital heart disease, however, abnormalities of the right ventricle and pulmonary circulation assume much more prominence and make the designation of the term *lesser* inappropriate. From the time of birth, great changes take place in the pulmonary circulation in order to adapt it for a role that it was never required to perform during fetal life—the pumping of the total cardiac output through the lungs. Nor is the right ventricle morphologically designed to perform as a high-pressure pumping chamber, and consequently, abnormalities of the pulmonary valve or pulmonary vascular bed, which place increased resistive loads on the right ventricle, cause problems early in neonatal life. In order to understand the changes in the pulmonary circulation that occur with congenital heart disease, it is necessary to trace the development of the pulmonary vascular bed during fetal life and the adaptation that occurs in the neonatal period and childhood.

ADAPTATION FROM FETAL TO NEONATAL CIRCULATION

During fetal life, although approximately 67% of cardiac output is ejected by the right ventricle, only 7% of total output is pumped through the lungs.[1] Because pressures in the pulmonary artery (PA) and aorta are approximately the same during fetal life, owing to the increased muscularity of the pulmonary vasculature and the noninflated state of the lungs, the remainder of the output passes through the ductus arteriosus. This structure is highly contractile and its patency is maintained by prostaglandin and hypoxia, whereas closure is stimulated by normoxia and prostaglandin inhibitors. Immediately after birth, a number of profound changes must occur in the lung and pulmonary circulation in order to adapt the infant for extrauterine existence (see Chapter 4). The infant's first breath, which may produce a negative intrathoracic pressure of up to -70 cm H_2O, together with the increase in Pao_2, immediately results in a decrease in pulmonary vascular resistance and an increase in pulmonary blood flow. At the same time, an increase in systemic vascular resistance results in a reversal of the right-to-left flow at the ductal level. During the first 15–20 hours of life, 30–50% of left ventricular output passes from left to right through the ductus.[2] The increase of pulmonary venous return to the left side of the heart distends the left atrium and promotes closure of the foramen ovale. However, functional closure of the foramen ovale rarely occurs immediately after birth, and up to 50% of infants have a demonstrable patent foramen ovale (PFO) at 8 days postdelivery.[3] Probe patency of the foramen ovale can be demonstrated in 50% of children up to 5 years of age and in more than 25% of individuals at over 20 years of age.[4]

Closure of the ductus occurs in two stages. First, contraction of smooth muscle in the vessel wall results in protrusion of the intima into the vessel lumen,[5] which will occur within the first 10–15 hours of life in full-term infants.[6] This does not represent a permanent closure. Closure is delayed or the ductus may reopen in congenital heart disease or neonatal lung disease associated with hypoxemia. A second, more permanent closure occurs by 2–3 weeks of life, when changes in the endothelial lining together with connective tissue formation and fibrosis result in the formation of the vestigial ligamentum arteriosum.[7]

The effects of prostaglandins on ductal tissue have been clearly defined. Prostaglandin E_2 (PGE_2) and prostacyclin or prostaglandin I_2 (PGI_2), are produced endogenously in the wall of the ductus. Endogenous PGI_2 production is 10 times as high as PGE_2, but its potency in terms of dilation of ductal tissue is only a third of that of PGE_2.[11,12] Prostaglandins are also produced by placental tissue and rapidly metabolized in the lungs. In the fetus, levels are much higher than in adults owing to the limited pulmonary blood flow in utero. Postnatally, prostaglandin levels rapidly decline owing to both decreased production associated with removal of the placenta and increased metabolism due to the rapid increase in pulmonary blood flow.

CONGENITAL ANOMALIES OF THE PULMONARY VALVE

Obstructive lesions of the right ventricle and pulmonary circulation, including pulmonary valve stenosis and lesions involving the pulmonary arterial tree, account for 25–30% of all congenital heart lesions.[13] Where these lesions are associated with an intact intraventricular septum, there is no route for decompression of the right ventricle (RV), and consequently, the characteristic feature common to all these anomalies is increased impedance and hypertrophy of the right ventricle. During fetal life, obstructive lesions of this type result in hyperplasia and hypertrophy of the myocardium, which is different from that seen in adult life. Obstructive lesions of either ventricle in the adult result in hypertrophy of cardiac muscle without hyperplasia. Because it is only hyperplasia that results in a simultaneous increase in capillaries, the hypertrophy of the myocardium will rapidly outstrip its blood supply.[13] Biochemical evidence of RV ischemia has been demonstrated in adults in the presence of an acquired increase in RV afterload.[14]

In the fetus and neonate, however, obstructive lesions result in the formation of a capillary supply that keeps pace with the hyperplasia of cardiac muscle, so that there is an adequate blood supply to the hypertrophied muscle. Without this, the newborn infant would be unable to generate the increased intraventricular pressures necessary to maintain blood flow across a fixed obstruction.

Pulmonary Stenosis

Anatomy. Pulmonary valve stenosis (PS) with intact intraventricular septum accounts for 8–10% of all congenital heart defects.[13] The site of obstruction may be purely valvular, valvular obstruction associated with infundibular narrowing, or merely a discrete infundibular stenosis with a normal pulmonic valve (Fig 18–1). In its classic severe form, presenting in the neonatal period, the stenosis takes the form of a conical lesion projecting into the main pulmonary artery frequently with complete fusion of the valve leaflets, with as little as a 1–2-mm opening during systole. Less severe forms of PS occur where only the edges of the cusps are fused leaving the central portions free. Consequently, these lesions may be unnoticed until later in childhood or even adult life.[13]

The other characteristic anatomic changes are right ventricular hypertrophy and poststenotic dilation of the pulmonary artery, which may extend as far as the left pulmonary artery. The degree of dilation does not correspond to the severity of the stenosis and is not seen with isolated infundibular stenosis or in PS associated with pulmonary artery stenosis.

Pathophysiology. In severe PS, right ventricular pressures exceed those of the left ventricle and the signs of cardiac failure manifest themselves shortly after birth. Where the degree of valve stenosis is less severe, or remains fixed while the individual grows, the right ventricle dilates more gradually and cardiac failure occurs later in life. In experimental animals, right heart failure occurs only when the pulmonary valve orifice is reduced to one third of its original diameter.[13]

Although in fetal life there is an increase in capillary supply to the increased myocardial muscle mass associated with pulmonary stenosis, this situation may change

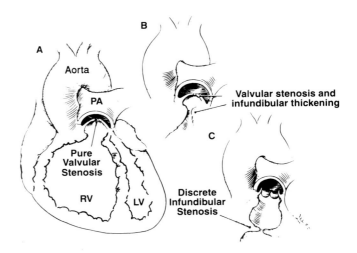

Figure 18–1. The anatomic variations of pulmonary stenosis. (*A*) Pulmonary stenosis with intact intraventricular septum. (*B*) Valvular stenosis with infundibular thickening. (*C*) Primary infundibular stenosis with discrete narrowing in the proximal part of the infundibulum. (*From Emmanouilides GC, Baylen BG: Pulmonary stenosis. In Adams FH, Emmanouilides GC, (eds): Heart Disease in Infants, Children and Adolescents. Baltimore; Williams & Wilkins, 1983, pp 234–262, with permission.*)

in the neonate with severe unrelieved valve obstruction.[14] Becu and colleagues[15] reported coronary artery occlusive lesions and myocardial necrosis at postmortem in infants dying from severe PS. Similarly, Franciosi and Blanc[16] described right ventricular and papillary muscle subendocardial infarction in patients dying of severe PS with massive ventricular hypertrophy.

Natural History. Children with moderate PS are usually asymptomatic for the first 2–3 years of life and later present with fatigue and dyspnea. The severity of symptoms is related to the reduction in cardiac output and pulmonary blood flow consequent to RV outflow obstruction. Moderate or severe PS produces few symptoms at rest, but with exercise, outflow obstruction limits the increase in cardiac output and pulmonary blood flow resulting in cyanosis secondary to increased tissue oxygen extraction. This is compounded by right-to-left shunting through a PFO or ASD because the diastolic pressure in the right ventricle may exceed that in the left ventricle.

Diagnostic Features. The severity of symptoms in pulmonary stenosis varies from infants presenting shortly after birth with severe right heart failure to the older asymptomatic child with mild PS. The clinical features of PS include a loud ejection murmur at the upper left sternal border associated with an early ejection sound (click) in mild or moderate PS. As a general rule, the longer the murmur and the earlier the click occurs in systole, the more severe the PS.[13]

The ECG findings in PS vary with the degree of stenosis. The ECG may be normal in 30–40% of children with mild PS and 10% with moderate PS[13] but is usually abnormal in severe PS. The characteristic findings are a dominant R wave in AVR and the right precordial leads and qR, rS, or an R wave of greater than 20 mm. The T waves may be negative or upright.

Chest radiographs show a prominent main pulmonary artery shadow in 80–90% of children with PS, which is due to poststenotic dilatation of the PA.[13] This finding may be absent in infants and small children. In 50% of cases, the chest radiograph shows some prominence of the right atrium. Cardiomegaly is present only in patients with severe PS. Pulmonary vascular markings are usually normal except in children with right ventricular failure, in whom pulmonary vascularity may be decreased. The clinical diagnosis of PS can be confirmed by two-dimensional and M-mode echocardiography, and an estimation of severity can be made by physical signs, ECG changes, and chest radiography. However, an accurate measurement of the gradient between RV and PA can only be obtained by cardiac catheterization together with angiography to accurately locate the site of obstruction. A right heart catheterization is performed with pressures measured while crossing the right ventricular outflow tract and pulmonary valve. Right ventricular

peak systolic pressures of greater than 30–35 mm Hg and gradients of 10–15 mm Hg across the valve are considered significant.[13]

The classification of PS into mild, moderate, and severe is on the basis of the pressure gradient across the pulmonary valve combined with clinical findings. A gradient of less than 25 mm Hg indicates trivial PS, 25–49 mm Hg mild, 50–79 mm Hg moderate, and greater than 80 mm Hg indicates severe or critical PS.[17] Peak resting RV systolic pressures of 50 mm Hg are recorded in mild stenosis, RV pressures similar to or equal to LV pressures occur in moderate PS, and exceed systemic pressures in severe PS. Resting RV systolic pressures of 250–300 mm HG have been recorded with severe RV outflow track obstruction.[13] Resting cardiac output is usually normal when measured at catheterization even in severe PS. With exercise or intravenous isoproterenol, the systolic gradient across the valve increases.[18–20] Stroke volume is unchanged with exercise and the increase in cardiac output is purely rate dependent.[21–24] In severe PS, an increase in heart rate, by shortening the diastolic filling time, may actually reduce cardiac output. When cardiac output is decreased, an artificially low peak systolic RV pressure is measured during cardiac catheterization. Ventricular systole is prolonged in an attempt to overcome RV outflow tract obstruction. Impedance to diastolic filling increases owing to the hypertrophied, noncompliant right ventricle.[13] This combination of outflow obstruction and impedance to filling may be well tolerated at normal heart rates, where there is adequate time in diastole for right ventricular filling. Tachycardia, however, increases outflow obstruction and reduces RV filling. Measurement of oxygen saturations in various cardiac chambers demonstrates the presence of shunting.[13] Follow-up studies in pulmonary stenosis show that patients with moderate to severe pulmonary stenosis tend to increase their gradients and the stenosis becomes more severe with time, whereas those in the mild category tend to remain the same. Younger patients (<1–2 years old) have a greater tendency to progress from the moderate to severe category.[17]

Surgical Treatment. Surgical treatment for PS with intact intraventricular septum has changed in recent years. In the early days of cardiac surgery, a closed valvotomy was performed through a right ventriculotomy with unpredictable results. Subsequently this was replaced by an open valvotomy under direct vision through an incision in the pulmonary artery, combined with inflow occlusion, with excellent results. Mistrot and co-workers[25] reported a 3.6% mortality in 110 patients with PS repaired using the inflow occlusion technique. However, the mortality rate in the neonatal group was 40% in infants under 10 days of age. Miller and colleagues[26] reported no deaths in five patients less than 1 month old with severe PS who underwent open pulmonary valvotomy. However, there is little doubt that critical pulmonary stenosis with an intact intraventricular septum presenting in the newborn period is a lethal disease. A recent large neonatal series reported a mortality of 42%.[27] With advances in cardiopulmonary bypass, most pulmonary valvotomies are now performed under direct vision. In extremely ill neonates presenting within the first few days of life with severe outflow tract obstruction, an open valvotomy with inflow occlusion or the closed technique via a ventriculotomy, where there is a coincident ventricular septal defect (VSD), is still the preferred approach. Pulmonary valvotomy is often combined with a systemic to pulmonary shunt and/or IV prostaglandin in the pre- and postoperative period.[27]

The persistence of a systolic gradient between RV and PA is an indication to reestablish cardiopulmonary bypass to perform additional resection of the infundibulum. If the gradient persists despite adequate resection, the likely cause is functional infundibular stenosis due to contraction of the infundibular muscle. The pressure gradient across the pulmonary valve decreases 50% within the first 24 hours of surgery in such instances.[28] Intravenous propranolol has been advocated to distinguish between fixed and functional RV outflow tract obstruction, a reduction in RV pressure denoting a dynamic obstruction.[29] However, caution should be exercised in using negative inotropic drugs when cardiac output is decreased.

Balloon Pulmonary Valvuloplasty. In the past 5 years, balloon pulmonary valvuloplasty has increasingly become the preferred method of treatment of children with isolated pulmonary stenosis. However, until recently, the technique could not be applied to infants with pulmonary stenosis who were less than 1 year of age because the smallest balloon catheter was 5 mm in diameter and complete obstruction of the RV outflow tract by the catheter during the procedure is very hazardous in the hypoxic newborn with critical pulmonary stenosis. The technique has now been modified with the use of balloon catheters as small as 2 mm in diameter to dilate the pulmonary valve and allow the passage of the larger catheters across the outflow tract.

The procedure is performed under general anesthesia in children and infants. The femoral artery as well as the vein are catheterized for hemodynamic pressure measurements and right-sided angiography performed. The femoral venous catheter is then changed to a balloon catheter over a guidewire that is positioned across the pulmonary valve. This is carefully de-aired and then hand inflated with a mixture of contrast and saline until the waistline in the balloon caused by the stenotic valve disappears. This inflation is held for 10–15 seconds, during which time there is no RV ejection into the pulmonary artery. Complications of the procedure include catheter rupture, bleeding from the catheter site, brady-

cardia during balloon inflation, and catheter induced-tachydysrhythmias, especially in sick newborns with critical pulmonary stenosis and a small noncompliant right ventricle.[30] Despite this, the procedure has a high rate of success with minimal complications. Khan[31] has reported a series of 17 infants less than 1 year of age in whom the pulmonary systolic pressure gradient was reduced by a mean of 105 mm Hg following balloon valvuloplasty with no mortality. It has been recommended that the indication for balloon valvuloplasty should be a pulmonary systolic pressure gradient of greater than 50 mm Hg.[17]

Peripheral Pulmonary Artery Stenosis
Pulmonary arterial stenosis, either in isolation or in combination with other defects, is found in 2–3% of congenital heart disease.[32] It is most commonly associated with pulmonary valve stenosis and VSD, but it is also common for tetralogy of Fallot to be associated with hypoplasia or stenosis of the pulmonary arteries.

Anatomy. Gay and colleagues[33] classified pulmonary artery stenosis into four types:

Type 1: Stenosis of the main pulmonary artery, right or left PA
Type 2: Stenosis of the bifurcation of the PA extending into both branches
Type 3: Multiple peripheral PA stenosis
Type 4: A combination of main and peripheral artery stenosis

Two thirds of cases are either type 1 or 2. Where the stenosis is discrete, it is associated with poststenotic dilation of the vessel. Where there are long segments of constriction or the vessels are genuinely hypoplastic, poststenotic dilatation is absent.

Pathophysiology. Severe obstruction at the pulmonary arterial level results in right ventricular hypertrophy and increased right ventricular ejection time similar to that seen in pulmonary valvular stenosis. The PA pressure proximal to the stenosis is the same as that in the right ventricle and results in the delayed closure of the pulmonary valve. In unilateral pulmonary artery stenosis, PA pressure is usually normal because the capacity of the pulmonary vessels on the normal side is capable of accommodating the right ventricular stroke volume. This situation may change with exercise, when increasing pulmonary blood flow may cause an increase in PA pressure.[13]

Diagnostic Features. In cases of mild or moderate peripheral pulmonary artery stenosis, symptoms are minimal. Patients with severe PA stenosis may present with dyspnea on exertion, fatigability, and clinical evidence of right ventricle hypertrophy.

The chest radiographic findings differ from those in valvular PS by the absence of the enlarged PA shadow. Pulmonary vascular markings are normal even in unilateral pulmonary artery stenosis.[13] Echocardiography shows hypertrophy of the RV wall and stenosis of the PA as far as the bifurcation. Definitive diagnosis must be made at cardiac catherization, where hemodynamic measurements made while withdrawing the catheter from peripheral branches toward the main PA and right ventricle establish the exact location of the pressure gradient. In severe stenosis, where RV pressure is suprasystemic, there may be right-to-left shunting at the atrial level. Increased main PA pressure suggests the predominance of the peripheral pulmonary artery lesion. When valve stenosis is the major site of obstruction, RV pressure is increased but main pulmonary artery pressure is relatively normal. Angiography is mandatory in order to define precisely the exact location of the obstruction and the extent of the stenosis and to exclude other commonly associated congenital heart lesions such as VSD.

Surgical Treatment. Pulmonary arterioplasty is indicated in severe stenosis of the main pulmonary artery or bifurcation, but results of surgery are by no means always successful, especially where there is associated peripheral artery stenosis.[34,35] Plastic repair of the stenotic area is performed on cardiopulmonary bypass and involves enlarging the caliber of the vessel with a pericardial or prosthetic patch. The prognosis is not as good as with pulmonary valve stenosis. Where there are multiple stenotic lesions in peripheral pulmonary arteries, the prognosis is poor and probably similar to that in primary pulmonary hypertension.[13]

In many instances, the pressure gradient across the stenosis increases with age owing to either disproportionate growth between normal and stenotic segments or increases in cardiac output. However, other investigators note a reduction in pressure gradients with aging.[36,37]

Pulmonary Atresia with Ventricular Septal Defect

Pulmonary valve atresia and ventricular septal defect represent the most severe end of the spectrum of tetralogy of Fallot. What differentiates this lesion from tetralogy, apart from the complete atresia of the pulmonary valve, are the severe abnormalities in size and distribution of the pulmonary arterial tree and the frequent finding of systemic to pulmonary collateral vessels supplying the lung parenchyma, something rarely seen in tetralogy. The anomaly accounted for approximately 2% of all congenital heart defects in one large series.[38]

Anatomy. Pulmonary atresia with VSD is characterized by the absence of any direct continuity between the right ventricle and the central pulmonary arteries (those out-

side the lung). Most commonly, the pulmonary valve and trunk are involved and 75% of cases the atretic arterial segment is recognizable as a solid elastic cord, whereas in the remainder, there is no identifiable connection.[39] The pulmonary arteries are described as being confluent when the right and left pulmonary artery are in communication, whereas the term *nonconfluence* is applied when the atresia extends beyond the main trunk through the bifurcation and interrupts the continuity between the right and left pulmonary arteries.[40] This distinction has important implications for surgical treatment. The blood supply to the lungs is derived entirely from the systemic arterial circulation either through the ductus arteriosus, systemic to pulmonary collateral arteries, or plexuses of bronchial or pleural arteries. A single systemic arterial source to a lung is termed a unifocal blood supply, whereas multiple vessels constitute a multifocal blood supply.[39]

Pathophysiology. The caliber of the central pulmonary arteries depends upon the amount of blood flow through the ductus or collateral vessels. The presence of a patent ductus arteriosus in pulmonary atresia is associated with confluence of the pulmonary arteries in 80% of cases. Ductal and collateral blood supply to the lungs may exist in the same patient but are very rarely found in the same lung. When the ductus arteriosus is widely patent at at birth, the central pulmonary arteries are of normal caliber. However, with postnatal ductal narrowing, the ductus frequently becomes stenosed and the diminished flow results in progressive hypoplasia of the pulmonary arteries. Collateral arteries arise most commonly from the descending thoracic aorta or occasionally from the subclavian artery and number between one and six.[39] In 60% of cases, the collateral arteries enter the lung through the hilum and travel with the bronchi as pulmonary arteries supplying a variable number of bronchopulmonary segments, whereas in the remaining 50%, there is an anastomosis between the central pulmonary arteries or their branches at the hilum or within the lung. The ductus is a precarious source of pulmonary blood supply owing to its tendency to narrow after birth. In this situation, a systemic to pulmonary shunt is frequently required to provide a secure source of pulmonary blood flow. Those infants with a collateral blood supply, on the other hand, tend to have an adequate pulmonary blood flow and do not require a shunt, although stenosis of the collateral arteries is a not uncommon finding. Occasionally, the presence of large collaterals causes hyperfusion of some lung segments and the development of hypertensive pulmonary vascular disease.[39]

The presence of a large, malaligned ventricular septal defect with an overriding aorta in this lesion results in dextro position of the aorta, which arises predominantly from the right ventricle. The right atrium is dilated and hypertrophied and an ASD is present in 50% of cases.[41]

Coronary artery abnormalities are occasionally seen in pulmonary atresia with VSD. There is also an association with other congenital heart defects, including transposition, A-V septal defect, anomalous pulmonary venous connection, and tricuspid stenosis or atresia.[41]

Natural History. Hypoxia and cyanosis are present in the newborn period, commonly after the first 2 days of life when the ductus narrows. In the absence of collateral vessels, pulmonary blood flow is completely duct dependent and must be restored with an intravenous prostaglandin E_1 (PGE_1) infusion prior to placement of a surgical shunt. A significant number of infants do not present with hypoxia in the newborn period because the ductus remains patent or because they have collateral vessels supplying the lung. They eventually develop cyanosis when they outgrow their pulmonary blood supply. Congestive heart failure due to excessive pulmonary blood flow through a large ductus or collateral vessels occurs rarely. Early surgical intervention may be necessary to control heart failure. In patients with a large ductus, the central pulmonary arteries are sufficiently well developed to permit definitive surgical repair. Where heart failure is due to high flow through collaterals, the pulmonary arteries are frequently hypoplastic and unsuitable for total repair. Banding of the collaterals is the only option.

Clinical and Diagnostic Features. The diagnosis of pulmonary atresia with VSD can be made by echocardiography in the newborn period without requiring cardiac catheterization. However, catheterization is required in older patients presenting for definitive repair to assess the size and configuration of the pulmonary arteries and to assess the extent of the collateral supply. Typical findings are systemic pressures in the RV due to the VSD and an inability to enter the pulmonary artery. However, the catheter will pass easily into the aorta across the VSD. The amount of aortic desaturation depends upon the adequacy of pulmonary blood flow. The pulmonary arteries can be entered from the left heart either crossing the VSD or by direct arterial catheterization and then entering the venous side by a previously created surgical shunt or collateral vessels. This is necessary in order to determine whether the right and left pulmonary arteries are confluent or nonconfluent and to identify and trace the source of all systemic to pulmonary collaterals. The chest radiograph shows a boot-shaped heart due to enlargement of the right ventricle producing a prominent upturned cardiac apex. There is a concavity in the region of the pulmonary artery due to failure of the infundibular development. Pulmonary vascular markings will be prominent where there are large systemic to pulmonary collaterals, whereas the lung fields will appear oligemic where the collaterals are small.

Surgical Treatment. The timing and type of surgical treatment in pulmonary atresia with VSD depends on the size and confluency of the pulmonary arteries. Patients with confluent pulmonary arteries of good size with normal distribution may not require a shunting procedure and may undergo a primary repair to establish continuity between the right ventricle and pulmonary artery with a conduit and close the VSD. In instances in which the pulmonary arteries are confluent but hypoplastic or abnormally distributed, staged surgical procedures are necessary. The first stage is the creation of a systemic to pulmonary shunt, usually a right Blalock-Taussig (B-T) anastomosis, to improve oxygenation and promote pulmonary artery growth. If this is successful, the second stage is the establishment of the connection between the RV and the pulmonary arteries. Because the creation of a B-T shunt frequently creates distortion and scarring of the pulmonary artery, some centers have opted for a two-stage surgical repair. The first stage establishes continuity between the RV and the confluence with a conduit or a patch angioplasty.[42] Increased blood flow through the confluence promotes pulmonary artery growth allowing the second stage to be successfully performed 2–3 years later. The second stage consists of closure of the VSD (and ASD when present), replacement of the RV conduit, and ligation of collaterals. Patients who have inadequate peripheral branching of central pulmonary arteries also are unsuitable for a single-stage complete repair as a large number of pulmonary arterial segments are not supplied from the confluence but come from systemic collaterals. These patients require unifocalization procedures to exclude these collaterals and restore pulmonary lobar confluence before a complete repair can be undertaken.

Patients who have nonconfluence of the pulmonary arteries require restoration of the confluence for successful surgical repair. In an infant, a surgical shunt should be placed and, where possible, confluence restored surgically at the same time. A shunt by itself would only result in growth of one pulmonary artery.[39] Patients with hypoplastic nonconfluent pulmonary arteries may need multiple palliative surgical procedures and may never be suitable for surgical repair.

Pulmonary Atresia with Intact Ventricular Septum

Pulmonary atresia with intact intraventricular septum is one of the rarer lesions, accounting for approximately 1–3% of all forms of congenital heart disease.[43] Although, by definition, the pulmonary valve is atretic, this is a highly complex and lethal anomaly with associated abnormalities of right ventricular morphometry, the tricuspid valve, and the coronary circulation. Mortality is increased both with and without surgical treatment.

Anatomy. In 80% of patients, atresia is caused by fusion of the pulmonary valve cusps and probably represents the extreme form of pulmonary valvular atresia. Unlike pulmonary atresia with a ventricular septal defect, the pulmonary arteries and branches are usually well developed and bronchial collateral vessels are rarely present.

Associated tricuspid valve abnormalities affect the long-term outlook and the type of surgical treatment in pulmonary atresia and intact septum. A small tricuspid valve annulus, the most common abnormality, has been linked to the morphologic development of the right ventricle in one classification.[45] The valve leaflets may be hypoplastic or dysplastic, frequently with very abnormal chordae tendinae attached to hypoplastic papillary muscles. Ebstein's anomaly of the tricuspid valve leaflets occurs in 25% of patients and, when present, results in massive right atrial enlargement, tricuspid regurgitation, and ventricular obstruction.[43]

Pathophysiology. The size and configuration of the right ventricle in pulmonary atresia with intact intraventricular septum varies and determines the capacity for ventricular growth and the approach to definitive or palliative surgical treatment. Previous assessments of the degree of RV development were based on size and showed that over half the patients had a severely hypoplastic chamber, whereas a significant proportion of patients had a normal or minimally diminished chamber size. This somewhat imprecise classification has been largely replaced by a classification based on RV configuration.[45] It describes the RV as tripartite with an inlet and trabecular and outlet portions. Pulmonary atresia is defined on the basis of the presence or absence of the components of this tripartite chamber and the size of the tricuspid valve. Patients are classified into three groups: (1) those with generalized hypoplasia of all three components (53%), (2) those without a trabecular portion (19%), and (3) those without trabecular or infundibular components (28%). The second group is further subdivided according to the adequacy of size of the tricuspid valve. The decision regarding the type of surgical approach is then based on this classification.[46]

In addition to these differences in size and configuration, the myocardium of the right ventricle is frequently hypertrophied and shows changes of endocardial fibroelastosis. Within the myocardium, fistulous connections are frequently found between the right ventricular endocardium and the right or left coronary arteries. These vascular channels, which are frequently referred to as sinusoids, form during fetal life secondary to the suprasystemic pressures generated in the very small RV cavity. The ventriculocoronary connections formed by these channels can result in retrograde perfusion of coronary circulation with desaturated blood from the RV or a coronary artery steal where there is run-off of fully

saturated blood into the RV during diastole. The communicating coronary arteries are frequently very abnormal with intimal proliferation, endocarditis, fibrosis, and thrombotic obliteration. The anatomic configuration of the coronary arteries themselves may also be abnormal, with well-documented cases of either single coronary arteries or loss of proximal continuity with the aorta.[47] In a detailed angiographic and postmortem study of 16 newborn infants with pulmonary atresia and intact intraventricular septum, 12 had ventriculocoronary connections (7 of whom had coronary arterial interruption), whereas the remaining 4 had sinusoids without communication to the RV.[47] Three of the infants in the group with ventriculocoronary connections had only a single coronary artery, and if there was no continuity between this artery and the aorta, there was a right ventricular–dependent coronary circulation. In view of these extensive abnormalities in the coronary circulation, it is not surprising that histopathologic studies of infants dying with this anomaly frequently show severe ischemic changes in the myocardium.[47]

The right atrium is dilated, especially when triscupid incompetence is present. There is always a communication between the right and left sides of the circulation at the atrial level either through a patent foramen ovale or an ASD. The ductus arteriosus, which becomes vital as a channel for pulmonary blood flow, is usually smaller than normal at birth. This finding has been ascribed to the limited or absent output from the RV (because of the atretic pulmonic valve) passing through the ductus, which inhibits its development.

Natural History. Although there is complete obstruction to RV outflow, the fetus will survive as long as there is free interatrial communication. Venous return bypasses the RV and enters the systemic circulation via the PFO (Fig 18–2). There is backflow from the RV to the RA when there is associated tricuspid regurgitation. Blood flow to the lungs passes from the aorta to PA through the PDA. Of interest is the observation that although the pulmonary arteries may be hypoplastic, the muscularity of the medial wall of small pulmonary vessels is thinner than normal.[48,49] The mechanism postulated for this is that the increased P_{O_2} of the blood reaching the lungs through the PDA results in less muscularization of the media of the pulmonary arterioles.[50] The maintenance of a venous to systemic communication after birth is of prime importance to the survival in infants with pulmonary atresia. Immediately after birth there is no impedance to right atrial output; however, as pulmonary blood flow (PBF) increases, left atrial pressure increases and, with it, right atrial pressure and size increase to maintain return to the left atrium. Because these infants are usually entirely dependent on the ductus for pulmonary blood flow, the increase in Pa_{O_2} after

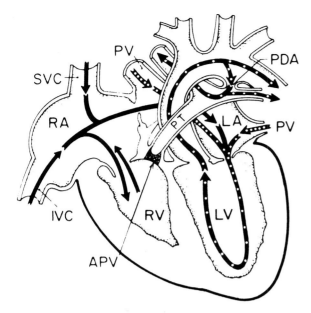

Figure 18–2. The circulation in pulmonary atresia with intact intraventricular septum. Venous return drains into the right atrium and from there to the right ventricle through the tricuspid valve, which may be incompetent. Pulmonary blood flow comes entirely through the ductus and mixes in the left atrium with systemic venous blood shunted across the PFO. APV, atretic pulmonary valve, IVC, inferior vena cava, LV, left ventricle, RV, right ventricle, RA, right atrium, LA, left atrium, PV, pulmonary veins, SVC, superior vena cava, PDA, patent ductus arteriosus, PFO, patent foramen ovale. (*From Emmanouilides GC, Baylen BG, Nelson RJ. Pulmonary atresia with intact intraventricular septum. In Adams FH, Emmanouilides GC (eds): Heart Disease in Infants, Children and Adolescents. Baltimore: Williams & Wilkins, 1983, pp 263–270, with permission.*)

birth, which constricts the ductus, decreases PBF and causes profound hypoxemia. This, in turn, tends to dilate the ductus and increase PBF. However, in most instances, urgent measures to increase PBF are required, either by maintaining duct patency with prostaglandin or by surgical creation of a systemic to pulmonary shunt.

Clinical and Diagnostic Features. Infants with pulmonary atresia usually present shortly after birth with cyanosis and tachypnea. Hypoxemia may be profound and associated with a metabolic acidosis when the duct narrows or closes prematurely. Those patients with a large right ventricle and tricuspid regurgitation commonly have signs of right heart failure.[51,52] There may be no heart murmur initially, but it develops later if the ductus remains patent. ECG shows right axis deviation and right atrial enlargement. As the right ventricle is commonly hypoplastic, left ventricular forces predominate. Although LV dominance also occurs in tricuspid atresia, the right axis deviation in pulmonary atresia helps to distinguish between these two lesions.[43]

Chest radiographs taken in the first 2–3 days of life may be normal in up to 50% of cases.[43] Cardiomegaly

with prominence of the right atrium and left ventricle is commonly seen in infants with right ventricular failure and tricuspid regurgitation. Pulmonary vascular markings are reduced.[53] Two-dimensional echocardiography establishes the diagnosis as it clearly defines the atretic pulmonary valve, the size of the right ventricular cavity, and abnormalities of the tricuspid valve. An estimate of the size of the ASD can also be obtained.[43]

Although the lesions can be well defined on two-dimensional echocardiography, cardiac catheterization may be required to define the anatomy precisely. It is essential that intravenous prostaglandin be given during catheterization to maintain ductal patency. The catheter is introduced via the femoral vein and advanced via the right atrium through the PFO into the left atrium and left ventricle. Difficulty encountered in entering the right ventricle from the right atrium may be due to severe RV hypoplasia or tricuspid atresia.

Pressures in the RV chamber are at suprasystemic levels, with end-diastolic pressures of 10–15 mm Hg associated with a normal LV pressure. Right atrial pressure is 2–3 mm Hg higher than the left. The only catheter access to the PA is through the DA, but caution must be exercised as hypoxemia may result from a decrease in PBF due to impedance of ductal flow.

Venous saturation is often as low as 30% (Pao_2 15 mm Hg) with no difference between RA and RV. Systemic Pao_2 is between 20 and 40 mm Hg depending on ductal flow. Pulmonary venous saturation is usually normal. Left atrial saturation may be lower than LV owing to incomplete mixing of blood shunted from the right atrium.[43]

Angiography will help to define the exact site of atresia and the size of the right ventricle and pulmonary arteries. The first two objectives are accomplished by injection of contrast into the RV, but definition of the pulmonary arteries requires a left ventricular injection, with the dye entering the PA via the ductus. If PA filling is inadequate, a second catheter may be advanced into the aorta from the femoral artery and contrast injected at the origin of the ductus.[43] A balloon atrial septostomy is invariably performed during the procedure to improve atrial mixing.

Preoperative priorities in the management of pulmonary atresia with intact septum are (1) the correction of hypoxia and acidosis by establishing blood flow to the lungs through the ductus arteriosus, and (2) the provision of an adequate outflow for systemic venous return from the right atrium across the foramen ovale, enlarging the foramen with a balloon atrial septostomy if the defect is restrictive. The place of the intravenous infusion of PGE_2 in maintaining duct patency in pulmonary atresia is now well established.[54–58] The drug works equally well with either umbilical artery or peripheral venous infusions. An oral preparation of PGE_2 has been used successfully in neonates with ductus-dependent pulmonary blood flow.[58]

Surgical Treatment. Surgical treatment is based on a two-stage approach; the first stage is palliative treatment in the newborn period to establish adequate pulmonary blood flow either by forward flow through the RV (pulmonary valvotomy), through a systemic to pulmonary artery shunt, or a combination of both. The definitive second stage surgical treatment is either biventricular repair when there is mild hypoplasia of the right ventricle (definitive correction) or a Fontan procedure when moderate or severe RV hypoplasia is present (definitive palliation).[59,60]

Palliative Surgical Treatment. Formerly, the basis of surgical treatment was to increase pulmonary blood flow by a pulmonary valvotomy, using an open or closed technique, when the right ventricular cavity was of adequate size.[61,64] If the RV was hypoplastic, the PBF was increased by a systemic to pulmonary anastomosis,[65,66] which was either a Blalock-Taussig, Potts, or Waterston shunt. Although the Blalock-Taussig shunt is still widely used, an aorta to main pulmonary artery (central) shunt or aorta to left pulmonary artery shunts have been used more recently. The object of these procedures, which are purely palliative, is not only increased pulmonary blood flow, but also growth and development of the right ventricle, in order that these patients become suitable candidates for definitive correction in later life. Several series claim that better results are achieved by a combination of pulmonary valvotomy and a modified Blalock-Taussig shunt, especially in terms of growth of the right ventricle and tricuspid valve.[46,67-70] In the series reported by deLaval et al,[46] the tripartite classification devised by Bull[45] determined the surgical option. Patients with an infundibular cavity had transpulmonary valvotomy combined with a left modified Blalock-Taussig shunt performed with excellent survival and tricuspid valve growth. Laks and colleagues[68,71] use a classification of pulmonary atresia based on whether there is mild, moderate, or severe hypoplasia of the right ventricle. Patients with mild or moderate RV hypoplasia undergo a valvotomy combined with a central shunt or occasionally a valvotomy alone in cases of mild hypoplasia. When severe RV hypoplasia is present, a right modified Blalock-Taussig shunt without a pulmonary valvotomy is performed. A third surgical option is to perform a right ventricular outflow reconstruction with a pericardial patch without a shunt and maintain ductal patency and pulmonary blood flow with intravenous prostaglandin in the expectation that with improving RV compliance, sufficient RV output would make an aortopulmonary shunt redundant.[70]

The surgical option is influenced by the presence of ventriculocoronary connections. Coles[72] showed that 56% had such connections in a series of 99 surgical patients with pulmonary atresia and intact septum. When ventriculocoronary connections were associated with obstruction or narrowing of the left anterior descending coronary artery, there was very high mortality. These patients should have a systemic to pulmonary shunt performed without decompression of the RV by a valvotomy or an outflow patch in order to avoid ischemic injury to the myocardium caused by a decrease in RV pressure.

Definitive Surgical Treatment. Successful palliative surgical treatment for pulmonary atresia and intact septum results in variable growth of the right ventricle, and more children are now presenting for definitive surgical repair. The surgical options are biventricular repair for those with mild RV hypoplasia (definitive correction) and a Fontan procedure for those with severe RV hypoplasia (definitive palliation). The biventricular repair entails the takedown of the systemic to pulmonary shunt, closure of the ASD, transannular patching of the outflow tract, and enlargement of the RV cavity by resection of trabecular muscle. Insertion of a pulmonary valve homograft and a tricuspid valvuloplasty may also be necessary. In patients with a moderately hypoplastic RV, valvuloplasty is feasible if the tricuspid valve is of greater than 70% of normal size.[46] In patients with moderate or severe RV hypoplasia and a small tricuspid annulus, the option most commonly chosen is a Fontan procedure,[46,69,71] although a biventricular repair together with a Glenn shunt to decompress the RV has also been successfully used.[59] The Fontan option is the only choice for those patients with ventriculocoronary connections associated with interruption of the coronary artery.

Pulmonary Valve Insufficiency

Anatomy. Pulmonary insufficiency results from failure of development of mature pulmonary valvular tissue, with only a small rim of primitive connective tissue developing in the RV outflow tract. There are two variants of this anomaly: pulmonary insufficiency with intact intraventricular septum and the more common variation, absence of the pulmonary valve associated with a VSD, obstructive pulmonary valve annulus, overriding aorta, and massive dilation of the pulmonary arteries, which classifies the lesion as tetralogy of Fallot with absent pulmonary valve. This variant is present in 3–6% of children with tetralogy.[73,74]

Pathophysiology. The pathologic features of pulmonary insufficiency are a dilated right ventricle with massive dilation of the main pulmonary artery and its branches. In most instances, this is associated with the classic features of tetralogy of Fallot. The pulmonary valve annulus is frequently constricted and somewhat hypoplastic.

Natural History. The prognosis is poor in the tetralogy variant with death frequently resulting from pulmonary complications secondary to compression of the bronchi by the aneurysmal dilation of the pulmonary arteries.[75] Pulmonary insufficiency with intact ventricular septum is frequently asymptomatic and compatible with prolonged survival. Rabinovitch and co-workers[75] have performed a detailed postmortem analysis of three infants with absent pulmonary valve syndrome: two in association with tetralogy and one with TGA.[75] They demonstrated that, in addition to compression of the main stem bronchi by the dilated pulmonary artery, there was a bizarre pattern of branching in the small pulmonary arteries (Fig 18–3). The normal organized branching of single segmental arteries was replaced by irregular networks of vessels that intertwined with and compressed the intrapulmonary bronchi. They also found that one infant had a reduction in the number of bronchial branches and another a reduction in the total number of alveoli. Consequently, there is extensive intrapulmonary pathology compounding the underlying cardiac defect.

Clinical and Diagnostic Features. Infants with tetralogy of Fallot with an absent pulmonary valve frequently present at birth with respiratory distress, tachypnea, and wheezing secondary to bronchial compression. Respiratory symptoms are improved by placing the infant in the prone position, but death in early neonatal life is not uncommon.[76,77] Patients with isolated pulmonary insufficiency and an intact ventricular septum are typically asymptomatic. In the tetralogy variant, there is a characteristic to-and-fro murmur, hyperinflation of the chest, and inspiratory and expiratory wheezing. The ECG shows right ventricular hypertrophy. Characteristic chest radiographic findings in tetralogy with an absent pulmonary valve include cardiomegaly, dilated right and left main pulmonary arteries, and normal pulmonary vascular markings. Unilateral hyperinflation or atelectasis are common. Two-dimensional echocardiography demonstrates the enlarged right ventricle and the aneurysmal dilation of the pulmonary arteries, although the pulmonary valve itself may be difficult to visualize.[78]

Catheterization of these infants is difficult because of the degree of respiratory distress and should only be performed after endotracheal intubation and institution of mechanical ventilation. In the newborn period, the RV pressure is usually at systemic levels and the shunt through the VSD is from right to left. However, when there is no obstruction to RV outflow, the decrease in pulmonary vascular resistance after birth results in the development of a left-to-right shunt at ventricular level.[78] There is usually a systolic gradient between RV and PA, as there is invariably some narrowing of the PA valve annulus. The diastolic pressure in the pulmonary artery is the same as in the RV. Accurate pressures may be difficult to measure owing to turbulence in the pulmonary artery.

Angiography precisely defines the abnormal anatomy. Injection of contrast into the PA demonstrates both the degree of valvular insufficiency and dilatation of the pulmonary arteries. Estimates of right ventricular end-diastolic volume (RVEDV) and the size of the pulmonary artery are useful in indicating prognosis. Sicker infants have larger RVEDV and greater dilatation of the pulmonary arteries compared with older surviving children.[79]

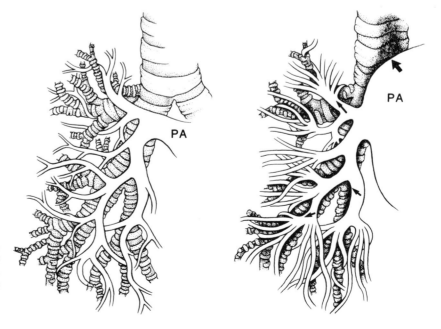

Figure 18–3. Diagrammatic representation of the normal relationship between the pulmonary artery and the left bronchus (*left*) and the compression of the left main bronchus by the aneurysmal pulmonary artery (*right*) in the absent pulmonary valve syndrome. Note also the compression of smaller bronchi, which are entwined by tufts of abnormal vessels. (*From Rabinovitch M, et al: Compression of intrapulmonary bronchi by abnormally branching pulmonary arteries associated with absent pulmonary valves. Am J Cardiol 50:804–813, 1982, with permission.*)

Surgical Treatment. The principal cause of morbidity and mortality in tetralogy with an absent pulmonary valve is the lung pathology that develops secondary to bronchial compression and the underlying broncho- and tracheomalacia.[80] Recurring atelectasis and respiratory infections often progress to a terminal respiratory event. The results of surgical attempts to reduce the caliber of the dilated pulmonary arteries by resecting the aneurysm and/or suspending the PA from the sternum without repair of tetralogy in younger children have been disappointing.[75,81,82]

In older children who have resection of the aneurysm together with correction of the tetralogy, the results are much better.[76,82–85] The prognosis is significantly improved if the patients can be managed with medical treatment until they are old enough to undergo total repair. Arensman and colleagues,[84] who reported on early surgical correction (newborn period) in the treatment of two severely affected infants, stressed the importance of nursing these infants in the prone position in order to relieve the compression of the bronchi by the dilated pulmonary arteries.

Definitive surgical repair consists of closure of the VSD, resection of the aneurysmal dilatation of the PA, and either placing a transannular patch or a conduit across the RV outflow tract during cardiopulmonary bypass. Mavroudis and co-workers[85] use a pulmonary valve prosthesis to reduce peak pulmonary artery pressures and dilatation of the pulmonary artery.

Anesthesia and Perioperative Management of Patients With Abnormalities of the Pulmonary Valve.

Patients with abnormalities of the pulmonary valve present with special problems in perioperative management that are distinct from other forms of congenital heart defects. With the widespread use of intravenous prostaglandin to establish ductal patency prior to surgery, sick, hypoxic infants are a much less frequent occurrence than in past years. It is obviously vitally important that prostaglandins are infused intravenously for the duration of the shunt procedure for pulmonary atresia. The patient's oxygen saturation should also be continuously monitored throughout the procedure.

Postoperative ventilation and prostaglandin infusion are performed after either pulmonary valvotomy or RV outflow tract patching. These maneuvers maintain pulmonary blood flow through the ductus until the compliance of the hypoplastic RV increases for sufficient pulmonary blood flow to be ejected across the outflow tract and through the pulmonary arteries. When a central shunt is placed between the aorta and pulmonary artery in pulmonary atresia, the situation may arise where the systemic and pulmonary circulations behave as two circuits in parallel, analogous to the situation that exists after a stage I Norwood procedure for hypoplastic left heart syndrome. With a large, centrally placed shunt,

diastolic blood pressure may be low and pulse pressure widens with a large runoff of blood across the ductus arteriosus. Decreased diastolic blood pressure is likely to cause further myocardial ischemia in a heart compromised by abnormal circulation through ventriculocoronary connections. In such situations, careful ventilatory adjustments increase P_{CO_2} and decrease pH increasing pulmonary vascular resistance, reducing shunting across the ductus arteriosus, and improving systemic circulation. The long-term use of intravenous prostaglandin in the setting of pulmonary atresia and intact septum may also cause complications. De Moor et al[86] reported the development of necrotizing enterocolitis and renal failure in infants maintained on long-term prostaglandin infusions after palliative surgery.

Infants with critical pulmonary stenosis that present for surgical valvotomy in the newborn period are frequently very labile in the perioperative period. These patients have small, poorly compliant right ventricles and are prone to develop tachyarrhythmias during the surgical procedure. Relieving the valvular obstruction rarely improves the hemodynamics immediately and right ventricular pressures are increased into the postoperative period. These patients are frequently in severe right heart failure with poor ventricular contractility, elevated right atrial pressures, tricuspid regurgitation and occasionally develop hepatic and renal failure. Because of the small capacity of the poorly compliant right ventricle, even small amounts of volume expansion can alarmingly increase right atrial pressure. Inotropic support is frequently required in the postoperative period.

Children with pulmonary valve insufficiency (tetralogy of Fallot with absent pulmonary valve syndrome) may be extremely difficult to manage in the perioperative period. With the dilatation of the pulmonary valve, trunk, and branches, there is frequently compression of the main airways. Affected patients present with episodes of recurrent wheezing and cyanosis, and in its worst form, these patients require nursing in the prone position in order to relieve the vascular compression of the bronchi.[84] If the patient is too symptomatic to be turned into the supine position for the induction of anesthesia, induction is performed in the prone position and the infant turned supine after tracheal intubation.[87]

THE PULMONARY CIRCULATION

Primary Pulmonary Hypertension

Primary or idiopathic pulmonary hypertension occurs infrequently in children, being most commonly seen in young women, although it can affect all ages and sexes. It is defined as increased pulmonary artery pressure and vascular resistance with right ventricular hypertrophy occurring in the absence of known causes, although there is a known association with collagen vascular diseases.

Symptoms include dyspnea, fatigue, chest pain, and syncope.[88] The pathophysiologic process is that of progressive right heart failure. The cross-sectional area of the pulmonary vascular bed is decreased. Exertional dyspnea and fatigue result from fixed cardiac output in response to exercise.[89] Diagnostic evaluation includes echocardiography, cardiac catheterization with measurement of PAP, and pulmonary angiography, although this carries the risk of inducing pulmonary vasospasm. Evaluation should also include a lung perfusion scan and pulmonary function tests to exclude lung disease as a cause of the pulmonary hypertension. On a chest radiograph, the width of both the descending branch of the right pulmonary artery and the left main pulmonary artery are increased.[89] An ECG demonstrates right ventricular hypertrophy, as does the echocardiogram. Arterial blood gases should always be performed to establish the degree of hypoxia. Lung biopsy helps to distinguish primary pulmonary hypertension, but general anesthesia is associated with significant mortality. Death from right heart failure occurs within 3–5 years after diagnosis.[88] Although numerous vasodilator drugs have been tried in an attempt to dilate the pulmonary vascular bed, there is no convincing evidence that any of these have been successful in the long term, and the only option in may patients is the possibility of a heart-lung or lung transplant.

The Pulmonary Circulation and Congenital Heart Disease

Extensive changes occur in the pulmonary circulation secondary to congenital heart disease that have a direct bearing on morbidity and mortality, both before and after corrective cardiac surgery. The pulmonary circulation normally undergoes considerable adaptive change in childhood, particularly in the neonatal period, and this normal adaptation is dramatically altered by the presence of congenital heart disease. Defects associated with excessive pulmonary blood flow result in secondary changes in the peripheral pulmonary circulation that determine not only operability but also may lead to serious and unpredictable changes in right heart pressures and PVR in the postoperative period. Because these changes in the pulmonary vascular bed may originate in utero, it is important to understand the adaptive changes that normally take place in the peripheral pulmonary circulation from fetal to adult life in order to understand the changes that occur with congenital heart defects.

Pulmonary Vascular Development and Anatomy.

The pulmonary arteries in the fetus develop in tandem with the conducting airways, and by 16 weeks of gestation, the full complement of preacinar (above the level of the respiratory bronchiole) vessels are formed.[90] After 16 weeks, these vessels increase in size secondary to changes in diameter and length, whereas intra-acinar

arteries begin to form side by side with the respiratory bronchioles and alveolar saccules. In late gestation, arteries are seen accompanying alveolar ducts and alveoli, but the number of arteries per unit area of lung tissue is less than that in neonatal period and childhood (Fig 18–4).

The distribution of smooth muscle within the vessel wall is radically different in the fetus compared with the older child and adult. In adults, arteries of over 200 μm contain elastic tissue, those between 100 and 150 μm contain a full coat of smooth muscle tissue, and arteries of less than 150 μm are mixed, some being fully muscularized, some partially, and some completely nonmuscular.[91] In the fetus, however, vessels less than 1700 μm in diameter down to 180 μm are fully muscularized, whereas in those between 180–100 μm, only a partial

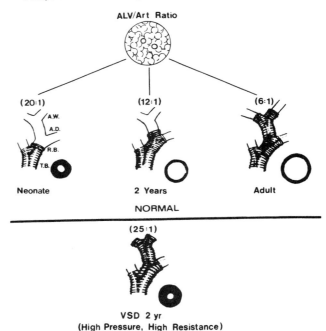

Peripheral Pulmonary Arterial Development

Figure 18–4. Diagrammatic representation of the development of the pulmonary vascular bed through morphometric changes in the vessels: Extension of muscle to peripheral vessels, percent wall thickness (medial hypertrophy), and the ratio of alveoli to arteries. The upper panel represents the normal adaptation through childhood into adult life, whereas the lower shows the typical changes that occur with the congenital heart defects associated with increased pulmonary blood flow. Note that with normal adaptation vascular smooth muscle extends more peripherally with increasing age, but that the vessels increase in diameter and increase in number relative to alveoli. T.B., artery accompanying a terminal bronchiolus; R.B., artery accompanying a respiratory bronchiolus; A.D., artery accompanying an alveolar duct; A.W., artery accompanying an alveolar wall. (*From Rabinovitch M, et al: Lung biopsy in congenital heart defects: A morphometric approach to pulmonary vascular disease. Circulation 58:1107–1122, 1978, with permission.*)

spiral of smooth muscle is present.[90,92] Vessels of less than 100 μm in diameter (intra-acinar vessels) are completely free of smooth muscle. In the fetus, wall thickness of small arteries relative to external diameter is twice that of the equivalent size adult vessel.[92]

Major changes occur in the pulmonary vascular bed in the first 3 years of life. First, there is a decrease in wall thickness in normally muscularized arteries during the first few months of life, so that wall thickness is comparable to that found in adults by 4 months of age. From then on, new muscle only forms as the vessel grows in size. The external artery diameter at each airway level increases throughout childhood. In terms of the degree of muscle extension into vessels in the periphery of the lung, there is gradual extension of smooth muscle further into intra-acinar vessels throughout childhood. By 2 years of age, there is smooth muscle present in vessels down to the level of the respiratory bronchiole, reaching alveolar duct level by 3 years of age (Fig 18–4). The adult pattern of smooth muscle extending out to the alveolar wall level is seen by 19 years of age.[91] The ratio of vessels to alveoli also changes throughout childhood, increasing from 20 alveoli to 1 artery in the newborn to 12:1 at 2 years and 6:1 in the adult (Fig 18–4).

The embryologic development of the pulmonary veins can be distinguished by the fifth week of gestation as an outgrowth from the left atrial chamber. By the eleventh week, there are four separate venous entries to the atrium. The pulmonary venous system within the lung develops in tandem with the arterial system. In contrast to the arteries, veins are less muscular than in the adult, but by 28 weeks' gestation, muscle bundles have appeared.[93] There is little change in these structures during the neonatal period and infancy.

Physiology and Pathophysiology of the Pulmonary Circulation.

The pulmonary circulation has the ability to constrict rapidly and dilate in response to stimuli owing to the fact that its arterial walls are well endowed with smooth muscle, which is sensitive to hypoxia and hydrogen ion, especially in the newborn.[94] The ability of the pulmonary circulation to alter its caliber depends not only on the presence of this smooth muscle but, more importantly, its location within vessels of larger or small diameter (extension of smooth muscle into peripheral vessels). Two other factors also contribute to resistance within the pulmonary vascular bed: (1) the lumen size as determined by the amount of medial hypertrophy of the vessel wall, and (2) the ratio of alveoli to vessels (see Fig 18–4).

The increased arterial oxygenation that occurs at the time of birth relaxes pulmonary vascular smooth muscle with dilation of muscular pulmonary arteries. This process occurs in vessels of less than 200 μ diameter in the first 3 days of life and in larger vessels by the first 3 months.[95] Pulmonary vasodilatation is responsible for the decrease in pulmonary vascular resistance occurring in the early perinatal period. There is further thinning of the wall of larger arteries secondary to both dilatation of the vessels and regression of smooth muscle during the neonatal period.

Natural History of Pulmonary Vascular Changes in Congenital Heart Disease.

The presence of a congenital heart defect profoundly influences the orderly adaptation of the pulmonary circulation from fetal to adult life. Where the defect causes alterations in pulmonary blood flow in utero, profound changes will have taken place in the morphometric configuration of the pulmonary vasculature at the time of birth. Reduced intrauterine pulmonary blood flow, as seen in pulmonary atresia with intact intraventricular septum, decreases pulmonary artery size, number, and muscularity, whereas the degree of extension of smooth muscle toward the periphery is normal (Fig 18–5). Where there is increased intrauterine pulmonary blood flow, such as total anomalous venous connection, the vessel size and number may be normal but the muscularity is increased and smooth muscle extends further into the periphery.

In congenital heart defects that only become hemodynamically significant after birth (eg, VSD, AV septal defect) abnormal pulmonary blood flow profoundly affects the adaptation that takes place between birth and early childhood. If the abnormal blood flow is not reversed by the correction of the congenital defect, a fixed increase in PVR develops (see Fig 18–4). This condition is termed the Eisenmenger syndrome after V. Eisenmenger, who described pulmonary hypertension secondary to congenital heart disease in a 32-year-old with a ventricular septal defect in 1897.[96]

IN UTERO PULMONARY HEMODYNAMIC ABNORMALITY

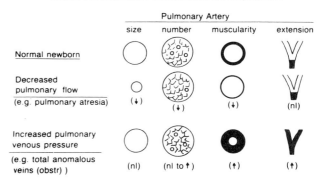

Figure 18–5. Morphometric changes that occur with congenital heart defects that result in hemodynamic abnormalities in utero. Increased venous pressure results in increased muscularity, whereas decreased pulmonary blood flow results in vessel hypoplasia. (*From Rabinovitch M: Morphology of the developing pulmonary bed: Pharmacologic implications. Pediatr Pharmacol 5:31–48, 1985, with permission.*)

Pulmonary hypertension occurs in those lesions associated with an increase in pulmonary blood flow but the frequency and severity depends upon the lesion (Table 18–1). Fifteen percent of infants with a large unrestrictive VSD develop a progressive increase in pulmonary vascular resistance in late infancy or early childhood.[97–99] If the defect is closed within the first 2 years of life, the pulmonary vascular changes regress. If surgery is delayed longer, the changes are fixed and pulmonary artery pressure increases with time.[100–102] In addition, if surgical closure is delayed, these children demonstrate an abnormal increase in pulmonary artery pressure and vascular resistance in response to exercise.[103,104]

Although a large body of information exists in relation to VSD and pulmonary vascular changes, the frequency and severity of pulmonary vascular changes is similar in patients with a previously undiagnosed large PDA.[105] Patients with a secundum ASD do not usually develop pulmonary hypertension until the third decade of life. Severe pulmonary hypertension will develop only in 8% of patients with TGA and intact intraventricular septum,[106] whereas the incidence increases to 40% in the first year of life in TGA and VSD or PDA.[107,108] Pulmonary hypertension invariably develops in infants with atrioventricular septal defect by 2 years of age and in some as early as the first year of life.[109] Truncus arteriosus with unrestricted pulmonary blood flow causes a permanent increase in pulmonary vascular resistance by the end of the second year of life.[110] Surgically created systemic to pulmonary shunts may also result in pulmonary hypertension, especially after the Waterston shunt (ascending aorta to right PA)

or the Potts shunt (descending aorta to left PA), where a frequency of 30% is reported 5 years after creation of the shunt.[111]

Diagnostic Evaluation of Patients with Congenital Heart Disease and Pulmonary Hypertension. Congenital heart defects that increase pulmonary blood flow result in changes in the pulmonary vascular bed that, if advanced, directly influence the feasibility of surgical correction. Therefore, it is important to make an accurate assessment of the extent of these pulmonary vascular changes in order to determine not only if they are reversible but also to anticipate the behavior of the pulmonary vascular bed in the immediate postoperative period. The high degree of pulmonary vascular reactivity associated with defects such as VSD and endocardial cushion defects leads to abrupt changes in pulmonary vascular resistance (PVR) and the development of postoperative pulmonary hypertensive crises.[112,113] An evaluation of the pulmonary vascular bed includes clinical findings, cardiac catheterization data, and in special instances, pulmonary wedge angiogram and lung biopsy data.

Clinical and Catheterization Data. The clinical features of pulmonary hypertension associated with congenital heart defects are subtle and not readily detectable until the condition is advanced. Shortening and softening of the murmur, splitting of the pulmonic second heart sound, and enlargement of the PA or chest radiograph are signs of advanced disease.[114] ECG evidence of right ventricular hypertrophy is a late sign and not a good indicator of pulmonary hypertension.

The only truly accurate information on the degree of pulmonary hypertension and pulmonary vascular resistance comes from right heart catheterization with the measurement of pulmonary artery pressure, the ratio of pulmonary to systemic blood flow (QP:QS), and PVR derived from the Fick principle. Criteria have been established to distinguish those patients whose PVR may decrease after surgery from those in whom pulmonary hypertension will persist.[115,116] A difference in saturation between pulmonary arteries and veins of greater than 2.5 volumes percent or a level of PVR greater than 10 Wood units/m^2 indicate irreversible pulmonary hypertension; PVR measurements of 8–10 U/m^2 are borderline.[117] Although the pulmonary hypertension may be advanced, the potential for reversibility is enhanced if the pulmonary vascular bed is responsive to vasodilators. A decrease in PVR to 6 units or less with the inhalation of 100% oxygen and intravenous tolazoline or isoproterenol demonstrates reversible changes. Although cardiac catheterization yields valuable information, it is important to bear in mind that this is only one "snapshot" of the pulmonary circulation and may be profoundly influenced by such things as sedation, general anesthesia,[118]

TABLE 18–1. MORPHOMETRIC CHANGES IN THE PULMONARY VASCULATURE WITH CONGENITAL HEART DISEASE ASSOCIATED WITH INCREASED AND DECREASED PULMONARY BLOOD FLOW

Lesion	Artery Size	Artery No.	Extension of Muscle	Medial Wall Thickness
Ventricular septal defect	↓	↓	↑	↑
Hypoplastic left heart	N	↑	↑	↑
Coarctation	N	N	↑	↑
TAPVD	N	N	↑	↑
Tetralogy of Fallot	↓	↑ or N	N	↓ or ↑
Pulmonary atresia	↓	↓	N	↓

(*From Rabinovitch M, Reid LM: Quantitative structural analysis of the pulmonary vascular bed in congenital heart defect. In Engle MA (ed): Pediatric Cardiovascular Disease. Philadelphia: FA Davis, 1981, pp 149–170, with permission.*)

polycythemia,[119] and coincident lung disease associated with hypoxemia.[120] More definitive information on the pulmonary vessels themselves can be obtained from a pulmonary wedge angiogram, especially where the hemodynamic changes are borderline.

Pulmonary Wedge Angiogram Data. The injection of contrast material into the pulmonary artery produces a very typical appearance in patients with severe pulmonary hypertension. Rabinovitch and colleagues[121] detailed a pulmonary wedge angiogram technique for a quantitative assessment of abnormalities in the pulmonary vascular bed. A catheter is directed into the posterior basal segment of the right lower lobe and the rate of tapering, as determined by the length of the segment over which the arterial lumen diameter narrows from 2.5 to 1.5 mm, is measured. The more abrupt the tapering, the more severe the degree of pulmonary hypertension (Table 18–2). Other changes in the pulmonary angiogram include diminished pulmonary artery branching, abrupt termination of vessels, tortuosity and narrowing of small arteries, and the absence of the normal background "blush" that results from contrast material filling the pulmonary capillaries.

Lung Biopsy Changes. The definitive description of the lesions in the vessels in pulmonary vascular disease was made by Heath and Edwards in 1958.[122] They classified the changes into grades I–VI (Table 18–3). Grades I–III were considered to be potentially reversible, whereas in grades IV–VI, pulmonary vascular resistance is fixed and irreversible. This classification has been further refined by Rabinovitch and co-workers,[123] who have used morphometric techniques to analyze the vessels in the pulmonary vascular bed and graded the changes depending on (1) the extension of muscle into peripheral arteries (grade A), (2) increased percentage wall thickness (grade B), and (3) decreased alveolar to arterial ratio (grade C) (Table 18–3). In their original study, using

TABLE 18–3. HEATH-EDWARDS GRADING OF PULMONARY VASCULAR DISEASE

Grade	Structural Changes
I	Medial hypertrophy
II	Intimal hyperplasia
III	Occlusive intimal hyperplasia
IV	Arterial dilatation
V	Angiomatoid formation
VI	Fibrinoid necrosis

this morphometric analysis of lung biopsy material in children with congenital heart defects combined with preoperative hemodynamic data in 50 patients undergoing corrective cardiac surgery, they demonstrated that all patients with increased pulmonary blood flow had at least grade A changes, whereas 76% had grade B changes, which were associated with increased preoperative PA pressure. Twenty percent had grade C changes associated with an elevation of PVR. In a subsequent study, the same group[124] combined the morphometric grading system together with the Heath-Edwards classification. They found that increased PAP was uncommon, or at most mild, in patients with grade A or B morphometric changes without structural changes on the Heath-Edwards classification. On the other hand, mean PAP was commonly elevated on those with grade B or C morphometric changes and Heath-Edwards grade I or II changes. Moderate to severe elevation of PAP was found in patients with grade III changes regardless of morphometric grade. When these patients were recatheterized 1 year after surgical repair, the majority had normal PAP and PVR except for those who had grade III Heath-Edwards changes, especially where these were associated with grade B and C morphometric changes.

This technique of assessing the severity of pulmonary vascular changes by open lung biopsy is now used in borderline instances where preoperative hemody-

TABLE 18–2. MORPHOMETRIC GRADING OF LUNG BIOPSY CHANGES COMBINED WITH HEMODYNAMIC AND WEDGE ANGIOGRAM FINDINGS IN CONGENITAL HEART DISEASE WITH INCREASED PULMONARY BLOOD FLOW

Morphometric Grade	Pathologic Change	Cardiac Catheterization Data			Wedge Angiogram
		Hemodynamics			
		Q_p	P_{pa}	R_p	
A	Abnormal muscle extension ± mild medial hypertrophy	↑	N	N	Slow tapering of axial arteries
B	"A" + severe medial hypertrophy	↑	↑	N	Abrupt tapering
C	"B" ↓ artery number and size	± ↑	↑	↑	Very abrupt tapering

(*From Rabinovitch M, Reid LM: Quantitative structural analysis of the pulmonary vascular bed in congenital heart defect. In Engle MA (ed): Pediatric Cardiovascular Disease. Philadelphia: FA Davis, 1981, pp 149–170, with permission.*)

namic measurements suggest that raised pulmonary artery pressure may not regress and that PVR may remain elevated postoperatively making correction of the defect hazardous. The biopsy specimen is taken at the start of surgery, before vessel cannulation, and the decision to proceed is based on changes seen on the frozen-section specimen.

Perioperative Management of Patients with Congenital Anomalies of the Pulmonary Circulation.
General anesthesia in patients with abnormalities of the right heart and pulmonary circulation may profoundly affect hemodynamic variables through the effects of anesthetic drugs, positive pressure ventilation, and systemic output. The anesthetic management of these patients is based on principles similar to those that apply to patients with diseases of the left ventricle, namely, the maintenance of an adequate preload in the RV and minimizing afterload. Assessment of preload requires the use of a central venous or right atrial catheter. Normally, the RV has a relatively high diastolic compliance, and consequently, changes in volume are associated with only small increases in right atrial pressure (RAP). Despite this, manipulation of RV preload plays a vital role in maintaining cardiac output in right-sided lesions, especially where the initiation of positive pressure ventilation can reduce RV preload.

Pulmonary Function and Lung Mechanics.
The changes in the pulmonary vascular bed in congenital heart disease have been previously described. Less well recognized, but equally important, especially in the preoperative period, are alterations in lung function and pulmonary mechanics that contribute to the abnormal oxygenation and CO_2 exchange frequently seen in these disorders. Airway compression by the PA trunk or major branches has been graphically described by Stranger and co-workers.[125] Dilated pulmonary arteries can compress either the left upper lobe or right middle lobe bronchus in lesions associated with left-to-right intracardiac shunts or pulmonary venous obstruction. The left main stem bronchus may also be compressed by an enlarged left atrium in ventricular septal defect associated with a high pulmonary blood flow. Infantile lobar emphysema has also been described in association with pulmonary stenosis.[125] Rabinovitch and co-workers[76] described compression of large bronchi by dilated main pulmonary arteries and compression of intrapulmonary bronchi by tufts of abnormal pulmonary vessels in the absent pulmonary valve syndrome. Any of these abnormalities can result in lobar atelectasis, emphysema, intermittent attacks of wheezing, and blood gas abnormalities. More subtle but equally important is obstruction of the peripheral airways secondary to increased pulmonary blood flow (PBF) in left-to-right intracardiac shunts. Hordof and co-workers[126] have described clinical and radiologic manifes-

tations of peripheral airway obstruction in infants with VSD associated with increased pulmonary to systemic flow ratios, which regressed with closure of the defect. In a later study, Motoyama and colleagues[127] measured expiratory flows (FEF_{75}) in children under general anesthesia at the time of corrective cardiac surgery. They found that increased PBF, secondary to left-to-right shunts, was associated with a decrease in FEF_{75}. Furthermore, when they performed a morphometric analysis on lung biopsy material taken at the time of surgery, they observed that patients with grade B morphometric changes[123] showed prominent smooth muscle hypertrophy and narrowing of the lumen of alveolar ducts and respiratory bronchioles. These observations may explain the finding of a sudden increase in airway resistance commonly seen in patients whose pulmonary artery pressures increase after corrective cardiac surgery for lesions such as VSD and AV septal defects. It is likely that this bronchoconstrictor response may be mediated, at least in part, by the leukotriene products of arachidonic acid metabolism. Leukotrienes C_4 and D_4, previously known as the slow-reacting substance of anaphylaxis (SRS-A), a mediator of bronchoconstriction in asthma, have recently been shown to be present in large quantities in the lung lavage fluid of infants with persistent pulmonary hypertension (PPHN).[128]

There are also changes in lung compliance seen in congenital cardiac disease. Bancalari and co-workers[129] have found that both total and specific lung compliance was significantly lower in children with congenital heart disease (CHD) where there was increased PBF compared with lesions with a normal or decreased PBF. When PBF was increased but PAP was normal, compliance was unchanged, suggesting that it was the pressure level rather than the increased flow within the lung that actually caused the alteration in compliance. Decreased pulmonary compliance has also been described in newborn infants with PPHN.[130]

The other compounding factor in pulmonary vascular disease is the underlying abnormality within the lung parenchyma itself in some children with congenital cardiac defects. In this respect, children with the Down syndrome are particularly at risk for developing both pulmonary vascular changes and pulmonary parenchymal damage secondary to cardiac disease. Cooney and Thurlbeck[131] noted that these children have a significant degree of pulmonary hypoplasia, although the severity of this was unaffected by the presence or absence of a cardiac defect. Pulmonary vascular changes analyzed using morphometric techniques by Yamaki and colleagues[132] in children with CHD and the Down syndrome were noted earlier and were more severe when compared with a group of controls with similar heart disease. TzehPing and co-workers[133] have also observed that pulmonary artery pressures in children with the Down syndrome and CHD were significantly higher than in children with only CHD. Extensive pulmonary damage, with overdistention of peripheral air spaces and interstitial emphysema, has also been described in a large series of patients with the Down syndrome and CHD dying postoperatively[134] (see also Chapter 25).

Blood Gas Changes. Changes in oxygen tension, CO_2, and hydrogen ion concentration have profound effects on pulmonary vascular resistance, especially in the presence of pulmonary vascular disease. The classic studies of Rudolph and Yuan[90] showed that the pulmonary artery pressure and vascular resistance increase sharply when arterial oxygen tension decreases below 50 mm Hg, with an exaggerated response at a pH below 7.4. Both alveolar hypoxia and hypoxemia are potent vasoconstrictors, and acidosis, either respiratory or metabolic, induces pulmonary vasoconstriction both independently and, more particularly, when superimposed on hypoxia.[135] Although there is little doubt that alevolar hypoxia triggers the increase in pulmonary vascular resistance,[136,137] the exact mechanism causing vasoconstriction remains unclear. Currently favored is the theory that vasoconstriction is mediated by the products of arachidonic acid metabolism, in particular the leukotrienes.[138,139] The vasoconstrictor response is at the level of the small pulmonary arterioles or alveolar vessels, but it remains to be resolved whether vasoconstriction is due to the direct effect of a reduced oxygen tension on smooth muscle or indirectly by inhibition of release of vasoconstrictor substances.

The effect of CO_2 on the pulmonary vascular bed is more difficult to determine owing to the problem of separating the effect of CO_2 from that of hydrogen ion concentration. Rudolph's original observations on the effects of pH on pulmonary vascular resistance attempted to address this by examining the effects of changing both CO_2 and hydrogen ion but did not hold one variable constant while changing the other.[90] Scheiber[140] has studied the effects of independent changes in Pa_{CO_2} and pH in the setting of hypoxia-induced pulmonary vasoconstriction in newborn animals. They found that respiratory and metabolic acidosis were equally effective in attenuating hypoxia-induced pulmonary vasoconstriction but that hypocapnia independent of pH (low Pa_{CO_2} with a normal pH) was ineffective. The primary of pH effect on the pulmonary vascular bed in the newborn has also been confirmed by Lyrene.[141]

Positive Pressure Ventilation and the Pulmonary Vascular Bed. The precise response of the pulmonary vascular bed to mechanical ventilation, independent of changes in blood gases, is difficult to determine because of the differing effects of positive pressure on intra- and extra-alveolar pulmonary vessels. Extra-alveolar vessels, which include the small vessels within the lung parenchyma, are directly affected by changes in lung volume. Lung expansion exerts traction on the vessel wall tend-

ing to increase the diameter and reduce the resistance. Intra-alveolar vessels located in the corners of alveolar walls are exposed directly to changes in intra-alveolar pressure whether from spontaneous or positive pressure ventilation. With large negative intrapleural pressures, vascular pressures fall and alveolar pressures can exceed intravascular pressures within the capillary causing vascular compression and an increase in PVR. Similarly, with positive pressure ventilation, alveolar pressure may exceed capillary pressures and PVR increase. The net effect of these changes on intra- and extra-alveolar pressures is that PVR is lowest at lung volumes around functional residual capacity (FRC).[142,143]

The effect of positive end-expiratory pressure (PEEP) on PVR is somewhat variable and is known from studies in patients with the adult respiratory distress syndrome and increased pulmonary artery pressures. In this situation, high levels of PEEP may have an adverse effect on PVR, but the routine use of 5 cm H_2O PEEP to maintain FRC while on positive pressure ventilation has a beneficial effect on PVR.[143] Whatever theoretical considerations apply to the effect of PEEP on PVR, they are definitely of minor importance compared with the positive benefits of PEEP in recruiting lost lung volume and correcting hypoxemia in situations of low lung compliance. The beneficial effect of PEEP on maintaining FRC may be partially mediated by release of PGE_2 and PGI_2 from the lung, both of which are potent bronchodilators. Berend and co-workers[144] showed that the increase in FRC secondary to the application of PEEP is blocked by indomethacin, suggesting that the change in FRC is mediated by prostaglandins. Prostaglandins may also play an important role in the decrease in PVR seen with hyperventilation, especially in PPHN. Cyclical stretching of the lung releases PGE_2, which is a potent pulmonary vasodilator.[145,146] The importance of this mechanism in decreasing pulmonary artery pressure has been questioned in a study in newborn lambs by Morin.[147] He showed that although hyperventilation with decreased CO_2 decreased PAP and PVR and increased measured metabolites of prostaglandin, the effect on the pulmonary circulation was the same when the animals were treated with indomethacin compared with controls.

Cardiac Output Changes in Pulmonary Hypertension. The pulmonary circulation and the right heart cannot be considered in isolation but rather in the context of events that take place in the systemic circulation. Changes in cardiac output and LV performance have major effects on the pulmonary vascular bed. As cardiac output and pulmonary blood flow decrease, PVR increases even though PAP may be unchanged or even increased. Changes in PAP should always be referenced to changes in systemic pressure and cardiac output to accurately assess events in the pulmonary vascular bed. In this respect, the ratio between mean pulmonary artery pressure

(PAP) and mean systemic pressure (SAP), as well as measurements of PVR, are particularly important. One of the cardinal objectives in treating abnormalities of the right heart and pulmonary circulation is the maintenance of adequate output from the right ventricle and, therefore, LV preload. Acute increases in PVR in patients with a reactive pulmonary vasculature initiate a devastating cycle of events resulting in acute right heart failure (increased right ventricular end-diastolic volume and pressure) (Fig 18–6). The thin-walled RV normally compensates poorly for increased impedance to outflow in the acute situation. Where more gradual elevations of impedance occur, such as in chronic outflow obstruction (PS, pulmonary atresia), the ventricular free wall hypertrophies and the chamber is able to generate systemic pressures.

Coronary blood flow to the right ventricle, which normally occurs during diastole, is compromised by acute increases in PVR causing subendocardial ischemia and RV dysfunction.[148,149] Biochemical evidence of RV ischemia has been demonstrated in the presence of increased RV afterload. Right ventricular dysfunction may damage the triscupid valve apparatus resulting in tricuspid insufficiency and/or damage to the sinoatrial or AV nodes producing arrhythmias.[150] In addition to effects on the RV free wall, changes in impedance frequently result in alterations in LV geometry. Increases in RV end-diastolic volume shift the intraventricular septum toward the LV cavity and decrease LV compliance and LVEDV. Cardiac output decreases and left atrial pressure increases as a consequence.[151]

Anesthetic Drugs and the Pulmonary Circulation. Many studies detail the effect of anesthetic agents, both

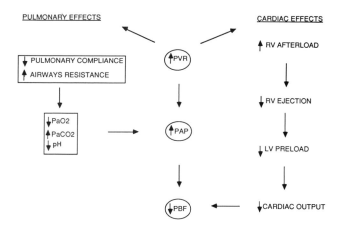

Figure 18–6. Cardiopulmonary effects of increases in pulmonary artery pressure (PAP) and pulmonary vascular resistance (PVR). The cycle of events leads to decreased cardiac output and pulmonary blood flow (PBF), which further aggravates the changes in respiratory mechanics and blood gases. This in turn tends to increase PAP and PVR.

intravenous and inhalational, on the pulmonary vascular bed. Unfortunately, most of these studies investigate the effects of the drug itself on PVR, neglecting the other coincidental effects of changes in Pao_2, pH, $Paco_2$, and lung volumes.

INTRAVENOUS ANESTHETIC AGENTS

Barbiturates. There are a few studies on the effect on barbiturates on pulmonary vascular tone. Thiopentone has been shown to increase tone in isolated pulmonary artery rings but also to block the contractile response to norepinephrine partially, so the effect in humans could not be clearly established.[152] In the intact dog, thiamylal increases PVR, whereas pentobarbital has little effect.[153] Dolar and Sun[154] showed that thiopentone, 10 mg/kg, in healthy adults causes a greater decrease in PAP than could be accounted for by a reduction in cardiac output alone and, therefore, concluded that thiopentone reduces PVR. The most logical explanation for these rather confusing results seems to be that thiopentone, which is well known to cause vasodilation in the systemic circulation, has a similar action in the pulmonary vascular bed, and this, coupled with a reduction in cardiac output, changes PAP. It is highly unlikely that barbiturates have any selective action on the pulmonary vascular bed.

Ketamine. Ketamine was initially considered to increase PVR in patients with pulmonary vascular disease.[155–157] More recent studies in pediatric patients with both normal and elevated PVR have shown no increase in PVR when ventilation was controlled to keep $Paco_2$ and Pao_2 within the normal range.[158,159] Consequently, the use of ketamine in children with abnormal pulmonary vascular reactivity is not contraindicated.

Narcotics. Relatively minor changes in hemodynamics occurring with very high doses of narcotics recommend their use in pediatric patients with abnormalities of the right heart and pulmonary circulation.[160–163] No significant changes in right heart hemodynamics were seen in adults with coronary artery disease given 2 mg/kg of morphine.[164] Similar hemodynamic stability was noted in another group of cardiac patients anesthetized with high-dose fentanyl and oxygen.[165] DeLange and co-workers[166] have reported minor changes in PAP with the induction of anesthesia using fentanyl and sufentanil, but they do not provide data on changes in $Paco_2$ and Pao_2, which are more likely to be responsible for the changes in PAP. Some studies using fentanyl anesthesia in infants have suggested beneficial effects on the pulmonary circulation,[160–162] especially in blunting the response of the pulmonary vascular bed to the stress of endotracheal suctioning.[162] However, in a more recent study by Hickey and colleagues,[167] where 25 µg/kg was used for anesthesia in 12 infants with congenital heart defects, no significant changes in PAP were found. It can be concluded that although high-dose narcotics do not change pulmonary artery pressure and vascular resistance, they may have important benefits in blunting the sympathetically mediated pulmonary hypertensive responses.

INHALATIONAL ANESTHETICS

Nitrous Oxide. Nitrous oxide (N_2O) causes myocardial depression and peripheral vasoconstriction owing to α-adrenergic stimulation.[168–175] However, its effects on the pulmonary circulation have not been as extensively investigated. The addition of nitrous oxide to halothane oxygen anesthesia in healthy subjects or in patients with aortic or mitral valve disease does not change PVR.[176–178] Hilgenberg and co-workers[178] have shown that nitrous oxide has no effect on the pulmonary circulation when added to diazepam in adults undergoing anesthesia for coronary artery grafting. Lunn and colleagues[174] reported a significant increase in PVR in patients with coronary artery disease during high-dose fentanyl anesthesia but the values were still within normal limits. The most conclusive study is that of Schulte-Sasse and co-workers,[179] who studied the pulmonary vascular responses to inhalation of 50% nitrous oxide in 32 adult patients anesthetized and ventilated to normocarbia. In 16 patients with normal PVR, there was a significant increase in pulmonary vascular resistance with the addition of N_2O, regardless of whether fentanyl or halothane was used as the background anesthetic, but PVR did not exceed the normal range.[179] The remaining 16 patients with an elevated PVR due to mitral valve disease had marked increases in pulmonary vascular resistance well beyond the normal range that were unattenuated by either halothane or fentanyl.[165] These findings strongly suggest that nitrous oxide should be avoided in anesthetizing patients with abnormal pulmonary vascular reactivity.

Volatile Agents. Studies on the effects of volatile agents on the pulmonary vascular bed have tended to concentrate on their influence on hypoxic pulmonary vasoconstriction and intrapulmonary shunting. These studies produced conflicting results, some suggesting that hypoxic vasoconstriction was abolished by volatile agents[180] and others suggesting that the vasoconstrictor response is preserved.[181,182] As with intravenous induction agents, many of these studies are difficult to interpret owing to failure to control for other variables, which may profoundly affect PVR. Other studies in humans, however, have shown that halothane and isoflurane do not inhibit hypoxic pulmonary vasoconstriction.[183,184]

Aside from hypoxic vasoconstriction, the other major consideration is the effect of volatile agents on PVR. Studies in animals and humans would suggest that in the presence of normal oxygenation and Pa_{CO_2}, halothane and isoflurane, in clinical concentrations, have little or no effect on PAP and PVR unless there are changes in PBF secondary to decreased cardiac output.[185–193] The potent inhalation agents produce no significant selective changes on pulmonary vessels independent of their effects on systemic vascular tone, myocardial contractility, and cardiac output.

Cardiopulmonary Bypass. Although the initiation of cardiopulmonary bypass (CPB) does not change the pulmonary vasculature, significant events during bypass may change PVR upon discontinuation of CPB. Heinonen and co-workers[194] documented significant increases in PVR for up to 3 hours postbypass in a group of adult patients undergoing coronary artery bypass grafting anesthetized with high-dose fentanyl. Several factors may contribute to the increased PVR, including lung injury caused by complement activation with intrapulmonary sequestration of neutrophils[195,196] and damage to blood constituents by the extracorporeal circulation at the gas-blood interface. Byrick and Noble[197] demonstrated that it is more likely to occur after bubble oxygenation than with membrane oxygenation. The extravascular lung water accumulation following CPB[198] may also contribute to the increase in PVR in the postoperative period.

The reversal of heparin with protamine at the discontinuation of bypass occasionally causes catastrophic rises in PAP and PVR.[199,200] Lowenstein and colleagues[200] reported five cases of abruptly increasing PAP associated with systemic hypotension after protamine. Three of these patients had mitral valve disease with an abnormal pulmonary vascular bed, and the authors caution against the rapid intravenous administration of protamine in patients with increased PVR.

Postoperative Management of Patients with Pulmonary Vascular Disease. Successful management of patients with abnormalities of the right heart and pulmonary circulation is based on the understanding that there are changes not only in the right ventricle and pulmonary vascular bed but also within the systemic circulation, that may profoundly influence cardiac output and pulmonary blood flow. Such patients should be identified by catheterization data, pulmonary wedge angiogram, and lung biopsy preoperatively (see Table 18–2). In the patient with a highly reactive pulmonary vascular bed, alterations in hemodynamics in the immediate perioperative and postoperative periods can catastrophically increase PAP[112,113] just at the time when the myocardial function is at its worst. The cycle of events outlined in Fig 18–6 leads to an abrupt rise in PAP and decrease in cardiac output and, occasionally, a dramatic increase in airway resistance. These events, in turn, result in hypoxemia, hypercarbia, and acidosis and a spiral of further increases in PAP and PVR. Preventing the increase in PAP before the cycle of pulmonary and hemodynamic changes occurs is infinitely preferable to cure.

Postoperative Monitoring. The pulmonary artery pressure of patients with a reactive pulmonary vasculature must be continuously monitored postoperatively. For that reason, a pulmonary artery catheter should be placed during weaning from cardiopulmonary bypass or prior to sternal closure. Additional monitoring includes right atrial or CVP, left atrial pressure, systemic pressure, and dye or thermodilution cardiac output measurements. Pulse oximetry has proved to be a reliable and accurate method of continuously monitoring oxygen saturations in the postoperative period[201] and identifying factors leading to decreased arterial oxygen saturation and increased PAP.

Respiratory Management: Blood Gas Changes. The abnormal pulmonary vascular bed is highly susceptible to changes in both blood gases and lung mechanics. Mechanical ventilation to a $Paco_2$ of 35 is mandatory. The use of neuromuscular blocking drugs may be necessary to achieve optimal ventilation and PVR. Drummond and co-workers[202] noted that hyperventilation to a $Paco_2$ of less than 25 mm Hg and a pH greater than 7.6 resulted in marked increases in $Paco_2$ secondary to a reduction in the PAP:SAP ratio. Similarly, Peckham and Fox[203] demonstrated a reduction in PAP with hyperventilation to a $Paco_2$ of less than 30 mm Hg in a group of newborn infants with PPHN. Although hyperventilation is widely accepted as a method of treating increased PAP in infants, until recently little information was available on the response of the pulmonary vascular bed outside the newborn period. Salmenpera and Heinonen[204] have shown that after CPB the pulmonary vascular bed in the adult may respond in a similar fashion; PAP increased significantly with a rise in $Paco_2$ and decreased during hypocarbia. The effect of CO_2 occurred independently of any change in tidal volume or FRC. They subsequently extended these observations to see if this responsiveness of the pulmonary vascular bed differed before and after cardiopulmonary bypass. They found that there was no change in PVR when hypercarbia occurred before bypass, whereas postoperatively, PVR increased by 50% when a slight respiratory acidosis (pH7.32) was induced by adding CO_2 and by 40% when a similar pH was produced by hypoventilation.[205] Morray[206] demonstrated the marked response of the pulmonary vascular bed to CO_2-mediated changes in pH in children with reactive pulmonary vasculature after corrective cardiac surgery (AVSD and VSD). When the $Paco_2$ was increased from less than 30 mm Hg to 40–45 mm Hg (pH 7.56–7.35), there was a 50% increase in PAP. Positive pressure also has a beneficial effect on lung mechanics, which helps to control PAP. By stretching the lung, mechanical ventilation releases prostaglandins,[145,146] which cause pulmonary vasodilation and may explain the rapid reduction in PAP seen immediately after the onset of hyperventilation before Pco_2 has changed.

Changes in lung volume may also account for the abrupt increases in PAP during weaning from mechanical ventilation to CPAP. Jenkins and co-workers[143] showed that during weaning from low IMV to CPAP in a group of children following cardiac surgery, FRC decreases while PAP and PVR increase, especially in children with underlying pulmonary hypertension. For these reasons, manipulation of PAP and PVR through changes in blood gases and lung mechanics is of primary importance in the management of patients with reactive pulmonary vasculature. Consequently, neuromuscular blockade and mild hyperventilation should be maintained for at least the first 12 hours postoperatively and no attempt at weaning from mechanical ventilation should be made in the first 24 hours unless the PAP is less than 50% of systemic levels and there is no hypoxemia (Fig 18–7). An acute rise in PVR and RV afterload in this period when the myocardium is recovering from the ischemic injury of bypass can result in acute RV failure. After 24 hours postoperatively, the right ventricle should be better able to tolerate an increase in PAP occurring during weaning. In some children with high preoperative PAP and a high postoperative baseline pulmonary artery pressure, a PAP of 50–75% systemic may have to be accepted beyond the first 24- to 48-hour period. It is unrealistic to expect the abnormal muscularization of the pulmonary vascular bed to regress in the first few days after surgery, and a degree of tolerance may be necessary for levels of PAP in this range after the immediate postoperative period. Increases in pulmonary artery pressure that occur despite neuromuscular blockade and mild hyperventilation during the first 12 hours can be treated with additional hyperventilation and possibly vasodilator therapy. When the PAP is less than 50% of systemic arterial pressure, weaning to CPAP and IMV can begin. Should the PAP increase, except during transient episodes of suctioning or coughing, neuromuscular blockade and hyperventilation are reintroduced. If PAP still fails to decrease, pharmacologic support with vasodilators is indicated.

Cardiovascular Management. The other aspect of patient management with increased pulmonary vascular reactivity is manipulation of cardiac output. An adequate preload and augmentation of ventricular performance with the use of inotropes and systemic vasodilators maintain optimum cardiac output with low PVR.

INOTROPIC DRUGS. Certain misconceptions exist about the use of inotropic drugs in diseases of the right heart and pulmonary circulation, of which the principal one is that these drugs increase PAP and PVR. The source of this confusion is the consideration of the pulmonary circulation in isolation from the systemic circulation. Changes in the systemic circulation have a great influence on PAP and PVR. Decreased LV output decreases PBF and increases both PVR and the PAP:SAP ratio. An improve-

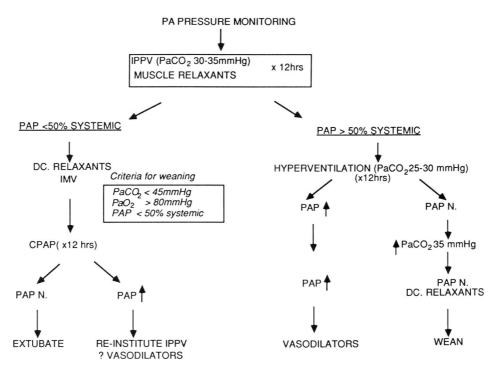

Figure 18–7. An outline plan for the rational approach to the management of patients with increased pulmonary reactivity in the postoperative period. DC, discontinue; PAP, pulmonary artery pressure; N, normal.

ment in LV performance increases PBF and decreases PVR and the PAP:SAP ratio.

The pulmonary circulation is invested with both α and β receptors,[207] and it would be foolhardy to use an inotropic drug with pronounced α effects in patients with a reactive pulmonary bed. Of the inotropes currently in use, isoproterenol has exclusively β-sympathomimetic properties, decreasing both PVR and SVR while augmenting cardiac output.

The situation with dopamine is less clear. There is evidence that dopamine causes a mild degree of pulmonary vasoconstriction when its effect is studied independently from changes in cardiac output.[208,209] However, when its inotropic effects on ventricular performance are examined in patients with pulmonary vascular disease, there is no evidence that dopamine increases PVR. Indeed, Holloway and co-workers[210] studied the effect of dopamine (2–16 μg/kg/min) in 10 adult patients with pulmonary hypertension and found that although PAP increased, it did so in tandem with SAP, so that the PAP:SAP ratio was unchanged. Furthermore, cardiac output increased and PVR and RV pressure decreased, for an overall improvement. Stephenson[211] studied the effect of 8 μg/kg/min of dopamine in a group of children after corrective cardiac surgery and found that PAP and PVR were unchanged and cardiac output increased. Similarly, Williams and colleagues[212] found no change in PVR with dopamine, 7.5 μg/kg/min, in patients after

Fontan procedures. Thus, there is no evidence that dopamine, in doses that primarily produce β-adrenergic stimulation (5–10 μg/kg/min), has adverse effects on the pulmonary circulation; on the contrary, dopamine decreases PVR and the PAP:SAP ratio by its beneficial effect on ventricular performance and cardiac output. When combined with a systemic vasodilator (nitroprusside or nitroglycerin), the beneficial effect is further enhanced.[211–213]

Amrinone, a drug with inotropic and vasodilator properties, effectively increases cardiac output after cardiac surgery in adults and children.[214–216] Fita and co-workers, in a study in adults following open heart surgery, has shown that pulmonary artery pressure decreases as cardiac output increases without any change in heart rate.[214] However, the vasodilator properties predominate over inotropic properties. Berner and colleagues,[217] in a study of amrinone in children after cardiopulmonary bypass, demonstrated a pronounced effect on systemic vascular resistance without any change in stroke volume. Beneficial effects on the pulmonary vascular bed with intravenous amrinone have also been reported in the treatment of patients with heart failure awaiting heart-lung transplantation because of primary pulmonary hypertension in both children[218] and adults.[219]

VASODILATOR DRUGS. The value of vasodilators in the treatment of pulmonary hypertension is debatable. Most of our information about these drugs comes from the treatment of adults with primary pulmonary hypertension and infants with PPHN. Unless invasive hemodynamic data have been monitored, the suggested benefit is questionable. Information regarding potential long-term benefits is limited. Improvement with vasodilators has been claimed to occur in 10–25% of patients with primary pulmonary hypertension.[220] Vasodilators that have been used (Table 18–4) include hydralazine,[219–225] isoproterenol,[22,226–228] diltiazem,[229] nifedipine,[225,230–236] nitroprusside,[224] nitroglycerin,[224,237] and converting enzyme inhibitors.[220] The number of vasodilators that have been tried attests to the fact that there is no genuine pulmonary vasodilator (ie, a drug that consistently dilates the pulmonary vascular bed in preference to the systemic circulation). Of the drugs most commonly used to treat pulmonary hypertension in children, tolazoline is perhaps best known.[112,113,202,203] Although claims have been advanced for its selective action on the pulmonary vascular bed, particularly in infants with PPHN, it also has a pronounced systemic effect. In addition, tolazoline has sympathomimetic properties,[229] which increase systemic output. For these reasons, its effect as a selective pulmonary vasodilator is often variable. Reports of its use in infants with PPHN consist of small series with unpredictable responses. Both Peckham[203] and Drummond[202] reported small numbers of favorable responders in their series, as well as infants whose condition deteriorated with the use of the drug. Although both Wheller[112] and Jones[113] have used the drug successfully to ablate acute pulmonary hypertensive crises during and after cardiac surgery, the drug does have significant serious side effects, namely, gastrointestinal hemorrhage, which cautions against its use. Other drugs that have been successfully used in the treatment of acute pulmonary hypertension in children are prostaglandin E$_1$[235] and prazosin.[239]

TABLE 18–4. VASODILATORS USED IN THE TREATMENT OF PULMONARY HYPERTENSION

Route	Dosage
Intravenous	
Tolazoline	1 mg/kg IV bolus
	1–2 mg/kg/hr
Hydralazine	0.25 mg/kg q4h
Isoproterenol	0.1–1.0 μg/kg/min
Salbutamol	0.5–3.0 μg/kg/min
Nifedipine	0.1–1.0 μg/kg/min
Phentolamine	0.5–5.0 μg/kg/min
Nitroprusside	1–5 μg/kg/min
Nitroglycerin	1–5 μg/kg/min
Phenoxybenzamine	1–2 mg/kg/24 h q6h
Prostacyclin (PGI$_2$)	1–40 μg/kg/min
Amrinone	5–20 μg/kg/min
Oral	
Nifedipine	5–10 mg q6h
Captopril	0.5 mg/kg/d
Diltiazem	15 mg q6h

Responses to vasodilator therapy of pulmonary hypertension are variable. Even oxygen has been reported to decrease pulmonary artery pressure, but not PVR, by decreasing cardiac output secondary to an increase in systemic resistance.[240] Right ventricle performance, a prime determinant of outcome in primary pulmonary hypertension, may decrease with calcium entry blockade.[241] Hydralazine increases both right and left ventricular performance while decreasing pulmonary vascular resistance.[242] Pulmonary artery pressure also decreases in response to venodilation and reduced pulmonary blood flow (as after nitroglycerin). If significant systemic vasodilation occurs without concomitant pulmonary vasodilation, hypotension predominates.[241] Decreased coronary perfusion secondary to hypotension further exacerbates right ventricular failure. Another possibility is worsening of pulmonary hypertension, particularly by drugs with positive inotropic or sympathomimetic properties and an unresponsive pulmonary circulation. Acute deterioration due to the development of LV failure and occasionally death have been associated with the use of calcium channel blockers.[243] With severe RV hypertrophy in primary pulmonary hypertension, leftward septal shift may encroach on the opposite chamber, compromising LV function.

A promising drug in the treatment of pulmonary hypertension is intravenous prostacyclin (PGI$_2$). Compared with other vasodilators, it is the most selective in its action on the pulmonary vascular bed. Its rapid metabolism in one circulation time provides a wide margin of safety if systemic vasodilation occurs. Prostacyclin has been widely used in the treatment of primary pulmonary hypertension, where it has been shown to decrease PVR and increase cardiac output independent of whether it reduces pulmonary artery pressure.[243–245] The marked symptomatic improvement experienced by some patients on prostacyclin has led to its use as a long-term infusion in patients awaiting heart-lung transplantation.[246] Although experience in the use of prostacyclin in the pediatric age group is less extensive, there are reports of significant reductions in PAP in children with primary pulmonary hypertension[245,247] and infants with PPHN.[248] Bush et al[249] have studied the effect of prostacyclin in children with pulmonary vascular disease secondary to congenital heart disease. After baseline studies when breathing room air, they found that intravenous prostacyclin caused the same reduction in PVR as oxygen and a further reduction when infused when breathing on F$_{IO_2}$ of 1.0. In a second study, they found that prostacyclin had similar pulmonary and systemic vasodilator effects to tolazoline.[250]

The most promising new drug for pulmonary hypertension is inhaled nitric oxide. Nitric oxide, an endothelium-derived relaxing factor, has been studied in animals and infants with PPHN.[251,252] Pulmonary artery pressure and vascular resistance decrease within minutes of nitric oxide inhalation without a change in systemic vascular resistance. Additional studies are in progress to determine the effectiveness and toxicity of nitric oxide in perioperative pulmonary hypertension.

Immediate and Long-term Results. Repairs of congenital cardiac lesions that reduce shunting and excessive pulmonary blood flow will improve pulmonary hypertension if the pulmonary vasculature is still reactive. However, the reversibility of pulmonary hypertension is variable depending upon the potential for growth of new pulmonary vessels (reduced after 2 years of age) and the extent of intimal hyperplasia and scarring (arterial muscular hypertrophy is reversible).

REFERENCES

1. Heymann MA, Rudolph AM: Control of the ductus arteriosus. *Physiol Rev* **55**:62–78, 1975
2. Adams FH: Fetal and neonatal circulations. In Adams FH, Emmanouilides GC (eds): *Heart Disease in Infants, Children and Adolescents*. Baltimore: Williams & Wilkins, 1983, pp 11–17
3. Prec KF, Cassels DE: Dye dilution curves and cardiac output in newborn infants. *Circulation* **11**:789–798, 1955
4. Scammon RE, Norris EH: On the time of obliteration of the fetal blood passages (foramen ovale, ductus arteriosus, ductus venosus). *Anat Rec* **15**:165–180, 1918
5. Gittenberger-DeGroot AC, Van Ertbrugen I, Moulaert AJM, et al: The ductus arteriosus in the preterm infant: Histological and clinical observations. *J Pediatr* **96**:88–93, 1980
6. Moss AJ, Emmanouilides GC, Duffie ER: Closure of the ductus arteriosus in the newborn infant. *Pediatrics* **32**:25–30, 1963
7. Fay FS, Cooke PH: Guinea pig ductus arteriosus. II. Irreversible closure after birth. *Am J Physiol* **222**:841–849, 1972
8. Koch G: Lung function and acid-base balance in the newborn infant. *Acta Paediatr Scand* **181**(suppl):7–44, 1969
9. McMurphy DM, Heymann MA, Rudolph MA, et al: Developmental change in the constriction of the ductus arteriosus: Response to oxygen and vasoactive substances in the isolated ductus arteriosus of the fetal lamb. *Pediatr Res* **6**:231–238, 1972
10. Oberhansli-Weiss I, Heymann AM, Rudolph MA, et al: The pattern and mechanisms of response to oxygen by the ductus arteriosus and umbilical artery. *Pediatr Res* **6**:693–700, 1972
11. Clyman RI: Ontogeny of the ductus arteriosus response to prostaglandin and inhibitors of their synthesis. *Semin Perinatol* **4**:115–124, 1980
12. Clyman RI, Heymann MA: Pharmacology of the ductus arteriosus. *Pediatr Clin North Am* **28**:77–93, 1981
13. Emmanouilides GC, Baylen BG: Pulmonary stenosis. In Adams FH, Emmanouilides GC (eds): *Heart Disease in Infants, Children and Adolescents*. Baltimore: Williams & Wilkins, 1983, pp 234–262
14. Vlahakes GJ, Turley K, Hoffman JIE: The pathophysiology of failure in acute right ventricular hypertension: Hemodynamic and biochemical correlations. *Circulation* **63**: 87–95, 1981
15. Becu L, Somerville J, Gallo A: "Isolated" pulmonary valve stenosis as part of more widespread cardiovascular disease. *Br Heart J* **38**:472–482, 1976
16. Franciosi RA, Blanc WA: Myocardial infarcts in infants and children. I. A necropsy study in congenital heart disease. *J Pediatr* **73**:309–319, 1968
17. Rao SR: Indications for balloon pulmonary valvuloplasty *Am Heart J* **116**:1661–1662, 1988
18. Moss AJ, Quivers WW: Use of isoproterenol in the evaluation of aortic and pulmonic stenosis. *Am J Cardiol* **11**:734–737, 1963
19. Neal WA, Lucas RV, Rao S, et al: Comparison of the hemodynamic effects of exercise and isoproterenol infusion in patients with pulmonary valve stenosis. *Circulation* **49**:948–951, 1974
20. Trucone NJ, Steeg C, Dell R, et al: Comparison of the cardiocirculatory effects of exercise and isoproterenol in children with pulmonary and aortic valve stenosis. *Circulation* **56**:79–82, 1977
21. Stone FM, Bessinger FB, Lucas RV, et al: Pre- and postoperative rest and exercise hemodynamics in children with pulmonary stenosis. *Circulation* **49**:1102–1106, 1974
22. Howitt G: Haemodynamic effects of exercise in pulmonary stenosis. *Br Heart J* **28**:152–160, 1966
23. Ikkos D, Jonsson B, Linderholm H: Effect of exercise in pulmonary stenosis with intact ventricular septum. *Br Heart J* **28**:316–330, 1966
24. Johnson B, Lee SJK: Hemodynamic effects of exercise in isolated pulmonary stenosis before and after surgery. *Br Heart J* **30**:60–66, 1968
25. Mistrot J, Neal W, Lyons G, et al: Pulmonary valvotomy under inflow stasis for isolated pulmonary stenosis. *Ann Thorac Surg* **21**:30–37, 1976
26. Miller GAH, Restifo M, Shinebourne EA, et al: Pulmonary atresia with intact ventricular septum and critical pulmonary stenosis presenting in the first month of life. Investigation and surgical results. *Br Heart J* **35**:9–16, 1973
27. Coles JG, Freedom RM, Olley PM, et al: Surgical management of critical pulmonary stenosis in the neonate. *Ann Thorac Surg* **38**:458–465, 1984
28. Mohr R, Milo S, Smolinsky A, et al: Right ventricular pressure drop 24 hours after open heart surgery for isolated pulmonary valve stenosis: The phenomenon and its surgical implication. *Circulation* **64**(suppl 4):127, 1981 (abstr)
29. Moulaer AJ, Buis-Liem TN, Geldoff WC, et al: The postvalvulotomy propranolol test to determine reversibility of the residual gradient in pulmonary stenosis. *J Thorac Cardiovasc Surg* **71**:865–868, 1976
30. Chaffe A, Fairbrass MJ, Chatrath RR: Anaesthesia for valvuloplasty. *Anaesthesia* **43**:359–361, 1988
31. Ali Khan MA, Al-Yousef S, Huhta JC, et al: Critical pulmonary valve stenosis in patients less than 1 year of age: Treatment with percutaneous gradational balloon pulmonary valvuloplasty. *Am Heart J* **117**:1008–1014, 1989
32. Mudd CM, Walter KF, Willman VL: Pulmonary artery stenosis: Diagnostic and therapeutic consideration. *Am J Med Sci* **249**:125–134, 1965
33. Gay BB, Franch RH, Shuford WH, et al: Roentgenologic features of simple and multiple coarctation of the pulmo-

nary artery and branches. *Am J Roentgenol Rad Ther Nucl Med* **90**:599–613, 1963

34. McGoon DC, Kincaid OW: Stenosis of branches of the pulmonary artery: Surgical repair. *Med Clin North Am* **48**: 1083–1088, 1964

35. Thrower WB, Abelmann WH, Harken DE: Surgical correction of coarctation of the main pulmonary artery. *Circulation* **21**:672–678, 1960

36. Hartmann AF, Ellitt LP, Goldrin D: The course of peripheral pulmonary artery stenosis in children. *J Pediatr* **73**:212–216, 1968

37. Wasserman MP, Varghesse PJ, Rowe RD: The evolution of pulmonary arterial stenosis associated with congenital rubella. *Am Heart J* **76**:638–644, 1968

38. Nadas AS, Fyler DC: *Pediatric Cardiology*, 3rd ed. Philadelphia: WB Saunders, 1972, pp 574–577

39. Mair DD, Edwards WD, Julsrud PR, et al: Pulmonary atresia and ventricular septal defect. In Adams FH, Emmanouilides GC, Riemenschneider TA (eds): *Moss' Heart Disease in Infants, Children and Adolescents*, 4th ed. Baltimore: Williams & Wilkins, 1989, pp 289–301

40. Edwards JE, McGoon DC: Absence of anatomic origin from the heart of the pulmonary arterial supply. *Circulation* **47**:393–398, 1973

41. Bharati S, Paul MH, Idriss FS, et al: The surgical anatomy of pulmonary atresia with ventricular septal defect: Pseudotruncus. *J Thorac Cardiovasc Surg* **69**:713–721, 1975

42. Millikan JS, Puga FJ, Danielson GK, et al: Staged surgical repair of pulmonary atresia, ventricular septal defect and hypoplastic, confluent pulmonary arteries. *J Thorac Cardiovasc Surg* **91**:818–825, 1986

43. Emmanouilides GC, Baylen EG, Nelson RJ: Pulmonary atresia with intact intraventricular septum. In Adams GH, Emmanouilides GC (eds): *Moss' Heart Disease in Infants, Children and Adolescents*, Baltimore: Williams & Wilkins, 1983, pp 263–270

44. Rowe RD, Freedom RM, Mehrizi A, et al: *The Neonate with Congenital Heart Disease*, 3rd ed. Philadelphia: WB Saunders, 1981, pp 328–349

45. Bull C, De Leval MR, Mercanti C, et al: Pulmonary atresia and intact ventricular septum: A revised classification. *Circulation* **66**:266–272, 1982

46. De Leval M, Bull C, Stark J, et al: Pulmonary atresia and intact ventricular septum: Surgical management based on a revised classification. *Circulation* **66**:272–280, 1982

47. Gittenberger-de Groot AC, Sauer U, Bindl L, et al: Competition of coronary arteries and ventriculo-coronary arterial communications in pulmonary atresia with intact ventricular septum. *Int J Cardiol* **18**:243–258, 1988

48. Haworth SG, Sauer U, Buhlmeyer K: Effect of prostaglandin E on pulmonary circulation in pulmonary atresia. A quantitative morphometric study. *Br Heart J* **43**:306–314, 1980

49. Wagenvoort CA, Edwards JE: The pulmonary arterial tree in pulmonary atresia. *Arch Pathol* **71**:646–653, 1961

50. Rudolph AM: *Congenital Diseases of the Heart*. Chicago: Year Book Medical, 1974, pp 360–397

51. Cole RB, Muster AJ, Lev M, et al: Pulmonary atresia with intact intraventricular septum. *Am J Cardiol* **21**:23–31, 1968

52. Elliott LP, Adams P, Edwards JE: Pulmonary atresia with intact ventricular septum. *Br Heart J* **25**:489–501, 1963

53. Desilets DT, Marcano BA, Emmanouilides GC, et al: Severe pulmonary valve stenosis and atresia. *Radiol Clin North Am* **6**:367–382, 1968

54. Coceani F, Olley P: The response of the ductus arteriosus to prostaglandins. *Can J Physiol Pharmacol* **51**:220–225, 1973

55. Elliott RB, Starling MB, Neutze JM: Medical manipulation of the ductus arteriosus. *Lancet* **1**:140–142, 1975

56. Heymann MA, Rudolph AM: Ductus arteriosus dilation by prostaglandin E in infants with pulmonary atresia. *Pediatrics* **59**:325–329, 1977

57. Neutze JM, Starling MB, Elliott RB, et al: Palliation of cyanotic congenital heart disease in infancy with E-type prostaglandins. *Circulation* **55**:238–241, 1977

58. Silove ED, Coe JY, Shiu MF, et al: Oral prostaglandin E2 in ductus-dependent pulmonary circulation. *Circulation* **63**: 682–688, 1981

59. Billingsley AM, Laks H, Boyce SW, et al: Definitive repair in patients with pulmonary atresia and intact ventricular septum. *J Thorac Cardiovasc Surg* **97**:746–754, 1989

60. Alboliras ER, Julsrud PR, Danielson GK, et al: Definitive operation for pulmonary atresia with intact ventricular septum. *J Thorac Cardiovasc Surg* **93**:454–464, 1987

61. Moller JH, Girod D, Amplatz K, et al: Pulmonary valvotomy in pulmonary atresia with hypoplastic right ventricle. *Surgery* **68**:630–634, 1970

62. Bowman FO, Malm JR, Hayes CF, et al: Pulmonary atresia with intact ventricular septum. *J Thorac Cardiovasc Surg* **61**:85–95, 1971

63. Dobell AR, Grignon A: Early and late results of pulmonary atresia. *Ann Thorac Surg* **24**:264–274, 1977

64. Rigby ML, Silove ED, Astley R, et al: Pulmonary atresia with intact ventricular septum. Open heart surgical correction at 32 hours. *Br Heart J* **39**:573–575, 1977

65. Trusler GA, Yamamoto N, Williams WG, et al: Surgical treatment of pulmonary atresia with intact ventricular septum. *Br Heart J* **38**:957–960, 1976

66. Moulton AL, Bowman FO, Edie RN, et al: Pulmonary atresia with intact ventricular septum. Sixteen year experience. *J Thorac Cardiovasc Surg* **78**:527–536, 1979

67. DeLeval MR, McKay R, Jones M, et al: Modified Blalock-Taussig shunt. Use of subclavian artery orifice as flow regulator in prosthetic systemic-pulmonary artery shunts. *J Thorac Cardiovasc Surg* **81**:112–119, 1981

68. Laks H, Billingsley AM: Advances in the treatment of pulmonary atresia with intact ventricular septum: Palliative and definitive repair. *Cardiol Clin* **7**:387–398, 1989

69. Joshi SV, Brawn WJ, Mee RBB: Pulmonary atresia with intact ventricular septum. *J Thorac Cardiovasc Surg* **91**:192–199, 1986

70. Foker JE, Braunlin EA, St. Cyr JA, et al: Management of pulmonary atresia with intact ventricular septum. *J Thorac Cardiovasc Surg* **97**:706–715, 1986

71. Milliken JC, Laks H, Hellenbrand W, et al: Early and late results in the treatment of patients with pulmonary atresia and intact ventricular septum. *Circulation* **72**:II61–II69, 1985

72. Coles JG, Freedom RM, Lightfoot NE, et al: Long-term results in neonates with pulmonary atresia and intact ventricular septum. *Ann Thorac Surg* **47**:213–217, 1989

73. Pouget JM, Kelly CE, Pilz CG: Congenital absence of

pulmonic valve: Report of case in a 73 year old man. *Am J Cardiol* 19:732–734, 1969

74. Lev M, Eckner FAD: The pathologic anatomy of tetralogy of Fallot and its variants. *Dis Chest* 45:251–261, 1964
75. Rabinovitch M, Grady S, David I, et al: Compression of intrapulmonary branching pulmonary arteries associated with absent pulmonary valves. *Am J Cardiol* 50:804–813, 1982
76. Lakier JB, Stranger P, Heymann MA, et al: Tetralogy of Fallot with absent pulmonary valve: Natural history and hemodynamic considerations. *Circulation* 50:167–175, 1974
77. Emmanouilides GC, Thanopoulus B, Siassi B, et al: "Agenesis" of the ductus arteriosus associated with the syndrome of tetralogy of Fallot and absent pulmonary valve. *Am J Cardiol* 37:403–409, 1976
78. Emmanouilides GC, Baylen BG: Congenital absence of the pulmonary valve. In Adams FH, Emmanouilides GC (eds): *Heart Disease in Infants, Children and Adolescents.* Baltimore: Williams & Wilkins, 1983, pp 228–233
79. Hiraishi S, Bargeon LM, Emmanouilides GC, et al: Right and left ventricular volume characteristics in infants and children with absent pulmonary valve. *Am J Cardiol* 49: 963, 1982 (abstr)
80. Stellin G, Jonas G, Goh TH, et al: Surgical treatment of absent pulmonary valve syndrome in infants: Relief of bronchial obstruction. *Ann Thorac Surg* 36:468–475, 1983
81. Bove EL, Shaher RM, Alley RM, et al: Tetralogy of Fallot with absent pulmonary valve and aneurysm of the pulmonary artery: Report of two cases presenting as obstructive lung disease. *J Pediatr* 81:339–343, 1972
82. Osman Z, Meng CCL, Girdany BR: Congenital absence of the pulmonary valve: Report of eight cases with review of the literature. *Am J Roentgenol Radium Ther Nucl Med* 106: 58–69, 1969
83. Stafford EG, Mair DD, McGoon DC, et al: Tetralogy of Fallot with absent pulmonary valve: Surgical considerations and results. *Circulation* 47–48(suppl III):24–30, 1973
84. Arensman FW, Francis PD, Helmsworth JA, et al: Early medical and surgical intervention for tetralogy of Fallot with absence of pulmonic valve. *J Thorac Cadiovasc Surg* 84:430–436, 1982
85. Mavroudis C, Turley K, Stranger P, et al: Surgical management of tetralogy of Fallot with absent pulmonary valve. *J Cardiovasc Surg* 24:603–609, 1983
86. De Moor MMA, Human DG, Reichart B: Management of pulmonary atresia or critical pulmonary stenosis and intact ventricular septum with a small or hypoplastic right ventricle. *Int J Cardiol* 19:245–253, 1988
87. Hosking MP, Beynen F: Anesthetic management of tetralogy of Fallot with absent pulmonary valve. *Anesthesiology* 70:863–865, 1989
88. Rich S, Dantzker DR, Ayres SM, et al: Primary pulmonary hypertension: A national prospective study. *Ann Intern Med* 107:216–223, 1987
89. Michael JR, Summer WR: Pulmonary hypertension. *Lung* 163:65–82, 1985
90. Hislop A, Reid L: Intrapulmonary arterial development during fetal life: Branching pattern and structure. *J Anat* 113:35–48, 1972

91. Reid L: The lung: Its growth and remodeling in health and disease.   *AJR* 129:777–778, 1977
92. Hislop A, Reid LM: Growth and development of the respiratory system—Anatomical development. In Davis JA, Dobbin J (eds): *Scientific Foundations of Pediatrics* Baltimore: University Park Press, 1982, pp 390–432
93. Rabinovitch M: Morphology of the developing pulmonary bed: Pharmacological implications. *Pediatr Pharmacol* 5: 31–48, 1985
94. Rudolph AM, Yuan S: Response of the pulmonary vasculature to hypoxia and H + ion concentration changes. *J Clin Invest* 45:399–411, 1966
95. Hislop A, Reid LM: Pulmonary arterial development during childhood: Branching pattern and structure. *Thorax* 28:129–135, 1973
96. Eisenmenger V: Die angeborenen Defecte Kammerschiedewand des Herzens. *Z Kin Med* 132(suppl):1, 1897
97. Dushane JW, Krongrad E, Ritter DG, et al: The fate of raised pulmonary vascular resistance after surgery in ventricular septal defect. In Rowe RD, Kidd BSL (eds): *The Child with Congenital Heart Disease After Surgery.* M Kisco, NY: Futura, 1976, pp 299–312
98. Hallidie-Smith KA, Hollman A, Cleland WP, et al: Effects of surgical closure of ventricular septal defects upon pulmonary vascular disease. *Br Heart J* 31:246–260, 1969
99. Hoffman JIE, Rudolph AM: The natural history of ventricular septal defects in infancy. *Am J Cardiol* 16:634–653, 1965
100. Cartmill TB, DuShane JW, McGoon DC, et al: Results of repair of ventricular septal defect. *J Thorac Cardiovasc Surg* 52:486–501, 1966
101. Castaneda AR, Lamberti J, Sade RM, et al: Open heart surgery during the first three months of life. *J Thorac Cardiovasc Surg* 68:719–731, 1974
102. Friedli B, Kidd BS, Mustard WT, et al: Ventricular septal defect with increased pulmonary vascular resistance. *Am J Cardiol* 33:403–409, 1974
103. Hallidie-Smith KA, Wilson RSE, Hart Z, et al: Functional status of patients with large ventricular septal defect and pulmonary vascular disease 6–16 years after surgical closure of their defect in childhood. *Br Heart J* 39:1093–1101, 1977
104. Maron BJ, Redwood DR, Hirschfeld FW, et al: Postoperative assessment of patients with ventricular septal defect and pulmonary hypertension. Response to upright exercise. *Circulation* 48:864–874, 1973
105. Reid LM, Stevenson JG, Coleman EN et al: Moderate to severe pulmonary hypertension accompanying patent ductus arteriosus. *Br Heart J* 26:600–605, 1964
106. Viles PM, Ongley PM, Titus JL: The spectrum of pulmonary vascular disease in transposition of the great arteries. *Circulation* 40:31–41, 1969
107. Newfeld EA, Paul MH, Muster AJ et al: Pulmonary vascular disease in complete transposition of the great arteries. A study of 200 patients. *Am J Cardiol* 34:75–82, 1974
108. Waldman JD, Paul MH, Newfeld EA, et al: Transposition of the great arteries with intact interventricular septum and patent ductus arteriosus. *Am J Cardiol* 39:232–238, 1977
109. Newfeld EA, Sher M, Paul MH, et al: Pulmonary vascular disease in complete atrio-ventricular canal defect. *Am J Cardiol* 39:721–726, 1977

110. Marcelletti C, McGoon DC, Mair DD: The natural history of truncus arteriosus. *Circulation* **54**:108–111, 1976

111. Paul MH, Millert RA, Potts WJ: Long-term results of aortic pulmonary anastomosis in tetralogy of Fallot: An analysis of the first 100 cases eleven to thirteen years after operation. *Circulation* **23**:525–533, 1961

112. Wheller J, George BL, Mulder DG, et al: Diagnosis and management of postoperative pulmonary hypertensive crisis. *Circulation* **60**:1640–1644, 1979

113. Jones ODH, Shore DF, Rigby ML, et al: The use of tolazoline hydrochloride as a pulmonary vasodilator in potentially fatal episodes of pulmonary vasoconstriction after cardiac surgery in children. *Circulation* **64**:(suppl 2): 134–139, 1981

114. Iverson RE, Linde LE, Kegel S: The diagnosis of progressive pulmonary vascular disease in children with ventricular septal defects. *J Pediatr* **68**:594–600, 1966

115. Mair DD, Ritter DG, Ongley PA, et al: Hemodynamics and evaluation for surgery of patients with complete transposition of the great arteries and ventricular septal defect. *Am J Cardiol* **28**:632–640, 1971

116. Vogel JHK, Grover RF, Jamieson G, et al: Long term physiologic observation in patients with ventricular septal defect and increased pulmonary vascular resistance. *Adv Cardiol* **11**:108–122, 1974

117. Rabinovitch M: Pulmonary hypertension. In Adams FH, Emmanouilides GC (eds): *Heart Disease in Infants, Children and Adolescents.* Baltimore: Williams & Wilkins, 1983, pp 669–691

118. Burrows FA, Rabinovitch M: The pulmonary circulation in children with congenital heart disease: Morphologic and morphometric considerations. *Can Anaesth Soc J* **32**: 364–373, 1985

119. Rosenthal A, Nathan DG, Marty AT, et al: Acute hemodynamic effects of red cell reduction in polycythemia of cyanotic congenital heart disease. *Circulation* **42**:297–308, 1970

120. Vogel JHK, McNamara DC, Blount SG: Role of hypoxia in determining pulmonary vascular resistance in infants with ventricular septal defect. *Am J Cardiol* **20**:346–349, 1967

121. Rabinovitch M, Keane JK, Fellows KE, et al: Quantitative analysis of the pulmonary wedge angiogram in congenital heart defects. Correlation with hemodynamic data and morphometric findings in lung biopsy tissue. *Circulation* **63**:152–164, 1981

122. Heath D, Edwards JE: The pathology of pulmonary vascular disease. *Circulation* **18**:533–547, 1958

123. Rabinovitch M, Haworth SG, Casteneda AR, et al: Lung biopsy in congenital heart disease: A morphometric approach to pulmonary vascular disease. *Circulation* **58**: 1107–1122, 1978

124. Rabinovitch M, Keane JF, Norwood WI, et al: Vascular structure in lung tissue obtained at biopsy correlated with pulmonary hemodynamic findings after repair of congenital heart defects. *Circulation* **69**:655–667, 1984

125. Stranger P, Lucas RV, Edwards JE: Anatomic factors causing respiratory distress in cyanotic congenital heart disease: Special reference to bronchial obstruction. *Pediatrics* **43**:760–769, 1969

126. Hordof AJ, Mellins RB, Gersony WM, et al: Reversibility of chronic obstructive lung disease in infants following repair of ventricular septal defect. *J Pediatr* **90**:187–191, 1977

127. Motoyama EK, Tanaka T, Fricker FJ, et al: Peripheral airway obstruction in children with congenital heart disease and pulmonary hypertension. *Am Rev Respir Dis* **133**: A10, 1986 (abstr)

128. Stenmark KR, James SL, Voelkel NF, et al: Leukotriene C4 and D4 in neonates with hypoxemia and pulmonary hypertension. *N Engl J Med* **309**:77–80, 1983

129. Bancalari E, Jesse MJ, Gelband H, et al: Lung mechanics in congenital heart disease with increased and decreased pulmonary blood flow. *J Pediatr* **90**:192–195, 1977

130. Yeh TF, Lilien LD: Altered lung mechanics in neonates with persistent fetal circulation syndrome. *Crit Care Med* **9**:83–84, 1981

131. Cooney TP, Thurlbeck WT: Pulmonary hypoplasia in Down's syndrome. *N Engl J Med* **307**:1170–1173, 1982

132. Yamaki S, Horiuchi T, Sekino Y: Quantitative analysis of pulmonary vascular disease in simple cardiac anomalies with Down's syndrome. *Am J Cardiol* **51**:1502–1506, 1983

133. TzehPing KC, Krovetz J: The pulmonary vascular bed in children with Down's syndrome. *J Pediatr* **86**:533–538, 1975

134. Yamaki S, Horiuchi T, Takahashi T: Pulmonary changes in congenital heart disease with Down's syndrome: Their significance as a cause of postoperative respiratory failure. *Thorax* **40**:380–386, 1985

135. Fishman A: Hypoxia on the pulmonary circulation: How and where it acts. *Circulation Res* **38**:221–231, 1976

136. Hauge A: Hypoxia and pulmonary vascular resistance: The relative effects of pulmonary arterial and alveolar PO_2. *Acta Physiol Scand* **76**:121–130, 1969

137. Sylvester JT, Harabin AL, Peake ME, et al: Vasodilator and constrictor responses to hypoxia in isolated pig lungs. *J Appl Physiol* **49**:820–825, 1980

138. Ahmed T, Oliver W: Does slow-reacting substance of anaphylaxis mediate hypoxic pulmonary vasoconstriction? *Am Rev Respir Dis* **127**:566–571, 1983

139. Reeves JT, Stemark KR, Voelkel NF: Possible role of leukotrienes in the pathogenesis of pulmonary hypertensive disorders. In Said SI (ed): *The Pulmonary Circulation and Acute Lung Injury.* M Kisco, NY: Futura, 1985

140. Schreiber MD, Heymann MA, Soifer SJ: Increased arterial pH, not decreased $PaCO_2$, attenuates hypoxia-induced pulmonary vasoconstriction in newborn lambs. *Pediatr Res* **20**:113–117, 1986

141. Lyrene RK, Welch KA, Godoy G, Philips JB: Alkalosis attenuates hypoxic pulmonary vasoconstriction in neonatal lambs. *Pediatr Res* **19**:1268–1271, 1985

142. West JE: *Blood Flow: Respiratory Physiology—The Essentials.* Baltimore: Williams & Wilkins, 1979

143. Jenkins J, Lynn A, Edmonds J, et al: Effects of mechanical ventilation on cardiopulmonary function in children after open-heart surgery. *Crit Care Med* **13**:77–80, 1985

144. Berend N, Christopher KL, Voelkel NF: The effect of positive end-expiratory pressure on functional residual capacity: Role of prostaglandin production. *Am Rev Respir Dis* **126**:646–647, 1982

145. Berry EM, Edmonds JF, Wyllie JH: Release of pros-

taglandin E2 and unidentified factors from ventilated lungs. *Br J Surg* **58**:189–192, 1971

146. Said SI: Pulmonary metabolism of prostaglandin and vasoactive peptides. *Ann Rev Physiol* **44**:257–268, 1982

147. Morin F: Hyperventilation, alkalosis, prostaglandins, and pulmonary circulation of the newborn. *J Appl Physiol* **61**:2088–2094, 1986

148. Sibbald WF, Driedger AA: Right ventricular function in acute disease states: Pathophysiologic considerations. *Crit Care Med* **11**:339–345, 1983

149. Laver MB, Strauss W, Pohost GM: Right and left ventricular geometry: Adjustments during acute respiratory failure. *Crit Care Med* **7**:509–519, 1979

150. Donnelly WH, Bucciarelli RL, Nelson RM: Ischemic papillary muscle necrosis in stressed newborn infants. *J Pediatr* **96**:295–300, 1980

151. Prewitt RM, Ghignone M: Treatment of right ventricular dysfunction in acute respiratory failure. *Crit Care Med* **11**:346–352, 1983

152. Andreasen F, Christensen JH: Thiopentone induced changes in the contraction pattern of vascular smooth muscle: The influence of albumin. *Br J Pharmacol* **82**:643–650, 1984

153. Goldberg SJ, Linde LM, Gaal PG, et al: Effects of barbiturates on pulmonary and systemic haemodynamics. *Cardiovasc Res* **2**:136–142, 1968

154. Dolar D, Sun S: The effects of thiopentone on the pulmonary circulation. In Prys-Roberts C, Vickers MD (eds): *Cardiovascular Measurement in Anesthesiology*. New York: Springer-Verlag, 1981, pp 251–255

155. Tweed WA, Minuck M, Mymin D: Circulatory responses to ketamine anesthesia. *Anesthesiology* **37**:613–619, 1972

156. Gooding JM, Dimick AR, Tavakoli M, et al: A physiologic analysis of cardiopulmonary response to ketamine anesthesia in noncardiac patients. *Anesth Analg* **56**:813–816, 1977

157. Spotoft H, Horshin JD, Sorensen MB, et al: The cardiovascular effects of ketamine used for induction of anaesthesia in patients with valvular heart disease. *Can Anaesth Soc J* **26**:463–467, 1979

158. Morray JP, Lynn AM, Stamm SJ, et al: Hemodynamic effects of ketamine in children with congenital heart diseases. *Anesth Analg* **63**:895–899, 1984

159. Hickey PR, Hansen DD, Cramolini GM, et al: Pulmonary and systemic hemodynamic responses to ketamine in infants with normal and elevated pulmonary vascular resistance. *Anesthesiology* **62**:287–293, 1985

160. Hickey PR, Hansen DD: Fentanyl and sufentanil-oxygen-pancuronium anesthesia for cardiac surgery in infants. *Anesth Analg* **63**:117–124, 1984

161. Vacanti JP, Crone RK, Murphy J, et al: Treatment of congenital diaphragmatic hernia with chronic anesthesia to control pulmonary artery hypertension. *Anesthesiology* **59**:A436, 1983 (abstr)

162. Hickey PR, Hansen DD, Wessel D, et al: Blunting of stress responses in the pulmonary circulation of infants by fentanyl. *Anesth Analg* **64**:1137–1142, 1985

163. Koren G, Goresky G, Crean P, et al: Pediatric fentanyl dosing based on pharmacokinetics during cardiac surgery. *Anesth Analg* **63**:577–582, 1984

164. Lappas DG, Geha D, Fischer JE, et al: Filling pressures of the heart and pulmonary circulation of the patient with coronary-artery disease after large intravenous doses of morphine. *Anesthesiology* **42**:153–159, 1975

165. Wynands JE, Wong P, Whalley DG, et al: Oxygen-fentanyl anesthesia in patients with poor left ventricular function: Hemodynamics and plasma fentanyl concentration. *Anesth Analg* **62**:476–482, 1983

166. De Lange S, Boscoe MJ, Stanley TH, et al: Comparison of sufentanil–O$_2$ and fentanyl–O$_2$ for coronary artery surgery. *Anesthesiology* **56**:112–118, 1982

167. Hickey PR, Hansen DD, Wessel DL, et al: Pulmonary and systemic hemodynamic responses to fentanyl in infants. *Anesth Analg* **64**:483–486, 1985

168. Eisele JH, Smith NT: Cardiovascular effects of 40 percent nitrous oxide in man. *Anesth Analg* **51**:956–962, 1972

169. Stoelting RK, Gibbs PS: Hemodynamic effects of morphine and morphine-nitrous oxide in valvular heart disease and coronary artery disease. *Anesthesiology* **38**:45–52, 1973

170. Wong KC, Martin WE, Hornbein TF et al: The cardiovascular effects of morphine sulphate with oxygen and with nitrous oxide in man. *Anesthesiology* **38**:542–549, 1973

171. Lappas DG, Buckley MJ, Laver MB, et al: Left ventricular performance and pulmonary circulation following addition of nitrous oxide to morphine during coronary artery surgery. *Anesthesiology* **43**:61–69, 1975

172. McDermott RW, Stanley TH: The cardiovascular effects of low concentrations of nitrous oxide during morphine anesthesia. *Anesthesiology* **41**:89–91, 1974

173. Eisele JR, Reitan JA, Massumi RA et al: Myocardial performance and N$_2$O analgesia in coronary artery disease. *Anesthesiology* **44**:16–20, 1976

174. Lunn JK, Stanley TH, Eisele J, et al: High dose fentanyl anesthesia for coronary artery surgery: Plasma fentanyl concentrations and influence of nitrous oxide on cardiovascular responses. *Anesth Analg* **58**:390–395, 1979

175. Smith NT, Eger EI II, Stoelting RK, et al: The cardiovascular and sympathomimetic responses to the addition of nitrous oxide to halothane in man. *Anesthesiology* **32**:410–421, 1970

176. Price HL, Cooperman LH, Warden JC, et al: Pulmonary hemodynamics during general anesthesia in man. *Anesthesiology* **30**:629–636, 1969

177. Stoelting RK, Reis RR, Longnecker DE: Hemodynamic responses to nitrous oxide-halothane and halothane in patients with valvular heart disease. *Anesthesiology* **37**:430–435, 1972

178. Hilgenberg JC, McCammon RL, Stoelting RK: Pulmonary and systemic vascular responses to nitrous oxide in patients with mitral stenosis and pulmonary hypertension. *Anesth Analg* **59**:323–326, 1980

179. Schulte-Sasse U, Hess W, Tarnow J: Pulmonary vascular responses to nitrous oxide in patients with normal and high pulmonary vascular resistance. *Anesthesiology* **57**:9–13, 1982

180. Bjertnaes LJ: Intravenous versus inhalation anesthesia-pulmonary effects. *Acta Anaesthesiol Scand* **26**:(suppl 75):18–31, 1982

181. Sykes MK, Gibbs JM, Loh L, et al: Preservation of the pulmonary vasoconstrictor response to alveolar hypoxia

during the administration of halothane to dogs. *Br J Anesth* **50**:1185–1196, 1978

182. Fargas-Babjak A, Forrest JB: Effect of halothane on the pulmonary vascular response to hypoxia in dogs. *Can Anaesth Soc J* **26**:6–14, 1979

183. Rogers SN, Benemof JL: Halothane and isoflurane do not decrease Pa_{O_2} during one-lung ventilation in intravenously anesthetised patients. *Anesth Analg* **64**:946–954, 1985

184. Augustine SD, Benumof JL: Halothane and isoflurane do not impair oxygenation during one-lung ventilation in patients undergoing thoracotomy. *Anesthesiology* **61**:A484, 1984

185. Philbin DM, Lowenstein E: Lack of beta-adrenergic activity of isoflurane in the dog: A comparison of circulatory effects of halothane and isoflurane after propranolol administration. *Br J Anaesth* **48**:1165–1170, 1976

186. Horan BF, Prys-Roberts C, Roberts JG, et al: Haemodynamic responses to isoflurane anaesthesia and hypovolaemia in the dog, and their modification by propranolol. *Br J Anaesth* **49**:1179–1187, 1977

187. Steffey EP, Howland D: Isoflurane potency in the dog and cat. *Am J Vet Res* **38**:1183, 1977

188. Steffey EP, Howland D: Comparison of circulatory and respiratory effects of isoflurane and halothane anesthesia in horses. *Am J Vet Res* **41**:821–825, 1980

189. Marshall C, Lindgren L, Marshall BE: Effects of halothane, enflurane, and isoflurane on hypoxic pulmonary vasoconstriction in rat lungs in vitro. *Anesthesiology* **60**:304–308, 1984

190. Klide AM: Cardiopulmonary effects of enflurane and isoflurane in the dog. *Am J Vet Res* **37**:127–131, 1976

191. Tarnow J, Eberlein HJ, Oser G: Hamodynamik, Myokardkontraktilitat, Ventrikelvolumina und Sauerstoffversorgung des Herzens unter verschiedenen Inhalationsanaesthetika. *Anesthesist* **26**:220–230, 1977

192. Tarnow J, Bruckner JB, Eberlein HJ, et al: Haemodynamics and myocardial oxygen consumption during isoflurane (Forane) anesthesia in geriatric patients. *Br J Anaesth* **48**:669–675, 1976

193. Nicholas JF, Lam AM: Isoflurane-induced hypotension does not cause impairment in pulmonary gas exchange. *Can Anaesth Soc J* **31**:352–358, 1984

194. Heinonen J, Salmenpera M, Takkunen O: Increased pulmonary artery diastolic-pulmonary wedge pressure gradient after cardiopulmonary bypass. *Can Anaesth Soc J* **32**:165–170, 1985

195. Chenoweth DE, Cooper SW, Hugli TE, et al: Complement activation during cardiopulmonary bypass. Evidence for generation of C3a and C5a anaphylatoxins. *N Engl J Med* **304**:497–503, 1981

196. Stimler NP, Hugli TE, Bloor CM: Pulmonary injury induced by C3a and C5a anaphylatoxins. *Am J Pathol* **100**:327, 1980

197. Byrick RJ, Noble WH: Postperfusion lung syndrome. Comparison of Travenol bubble and membrane oxygenators. *J Thorac Cardiovasc Surg* **76**:685–693, 1978

198. Byrick RJ, Kay JC, Noble WH: Extravascular lung water accumulation in patients following coronary artery surgery. *Can Anaesth Soc J* **24**:332–345, 1977

199. Jastrzebski J, Sykes MK, Woods DG: Cardiorespiratory effects of protamine after cardiopulmonary bypass in man. *Thorax* **29**:534–539, 1974

200. Lowenstein E, Johnston WE, Lappas DG: Catastrophic pulmonary vasoconstriction associated with protamine reversal of heparin. *Anesthesiology* **59**:470–473, 1983

201. Fanconi S, Doherty P, Edmonds JF, et al: Pulse oximetry in pediatric intensive care: Comparison with measured saturations and transcutaneous oxygen tension. *J Pediatr* **107**:362–366, 1985

202. Drummond WH, Gregory GA, Heymann MA, et al: The independent effects of hyperventilation, tolazoline, and dopamine on infants with persistent pulmonary hypertension. *J Pediatr* **98**:603–611, 1981

203. Peckam GH, Fox WW: Physiologic factors affecting pulmonary artery pressure in infants with persistent pulmonary hypertension. *J Pediatr* **93**:1005–1010, 1978

204. Salmenpera M, Heinonen J: Pulmonary vascular responses to moderate changes in Pa_{CO_2} after cardiopulmonary bypass. *Anesthesiology* **64**:311–315, 1986

205. Viitanen A, Salmenpera M, Heinonen J, et al: Pulmonary vascular resistance before and after cardiopulmonary bypass: The effect of Pa_{CO_2}. *Chest* **95**:773–778, 1989

206. Morray JP, Lynn AM, Mansfield PB: Effect of pH and P_{CO_2} on pulmonary and systemic hemodynamics after surgery in children with congenital heart disease and pulmonary hypertension. *J Pediatr* **113**:474–479, 1988

207. Hayman AL, Lippton HL, Ignarro LJ, et al: Analysis of autonomic response in the pulmonary vascular bed. In Said SI (ed): *The Pulmonary Circulation and Acute Lung Injury*. Mt Kisco, NY: Futura, 1985

208. Mentzer RM, Alegre CA, Nolan SP: The effects of dopamine and isoproterenol on the pulmonary circulation. *J Thorac Cardiovasc Surg* **71**:807–814, 1976

209. Lejeune P, Naeije R, Leeman M, et al: Effects of dopamine and dobutamine on pulmonary circulation in normoxic and hypoxic dogs. *Am Rev Respir Dis* **133**:A227, 1986 (abstr)

210. Holloway EL, Polumbo RA, Harrison DC: Acute circulatory effects of dopamine in patients with pulmonary hypertension. *Br Heart J* **37**:482–485, 1975

211. Stephenson LW, Edmunds LH, Raphaely R, et al: Effects of nitroprusside and dopamine on pulmonary arterial vasculature in children after cardiac surgery. *Circulation* **60**:I-104–I-110, 1979

212. Williams DB, Kiernan PD, Schaff HV, et al: The hemodynamic response to dopamine and nitroprusside following right atrium-pulmonary artery bypass (Fontan procedure). *Ann Thorac Surg* **34**:51–57, 1982

213. Benson L, Bohn DJ, Edmonds JF, et al: Nitroglycerine therapy in children with low cardiac index after heart surgery. *Cardiovasc Med* **4**:207–215, 1979

214. Fita G, Gomar C, Jiminez J, et al: Amrinone in perioperative low output syndrome. *Acta Anaesthesiol Scand* **34**:482–485, 1990

215. Lawless S, Burckart G, Diven W, et al: Amrinone in neonates and infants after cardiac surgery. *Crit Care Med* **17**:751–754, 1989

216. Wessel A, Seiffert P, Runger T, et al: Amrinone in children with heart defects. *Z Kardiol* **75**(1):14, 1986 (abstr)

217. Berner M, Jaccard C, Oberhansli I, et al: Hemodynamic effects of amrinone in children after cardiac surgery. *Intensive Care Med* **16**:85–88, 1990

218. Kulik TJ, Lock JE: Amrinone for pulmonary hyperten-

sion in infants and children. *Pediatr Res* **18**:125A, 1984 (abstr)

219. Deeb GM, Bolling SF, Guynn TP, et al: Amrinone versus conventional therapy in pulmonary hypertensive patients awaiting cardiac transplantation. *Ann Thorac Surg* **48**:665–669, 1989

220. Packer M: Vasodilator therapy for primary pulmonary hypertension. *Ann Intern Med* **103**:258–270, 1985

221. Rubin LJ, Peter RH: Oral hydralazine therapy for primary pulmonary hypertension. *N Engl J Med* **302**:69–73, 1980

222. Hermiller JB, Bamback D, Thompson MJ, et al: Vasodilators and prostaglandin inhibitors in primary pulmonary hypertension. *Ann Intern Med* **97**:480–489, 1982

223. Packer M, Greenberg B, Massie B, et al: Deleterious effects of hydralazine in patients with primary pulmonary hypertension. *N Engl J Med* **306**:1326–1331, 1982

224. Brend BN, Berger HJ, Matthy RA, et al: Contrasting acute effects of vasodilators (nitroglycerin, nitroprusside and hydralazine) on right ventricular performance in patients with chronic obstructive lung disease and pulmonary hypertension: A combined radionuclide-hemodynamic study. *Am J Cardiol* **51**:1682–1689, 1983

225. Rich S, Brundage BH, Levy PS: The effect of vasodilator therapy on the clinical outcome of patients with primary pulmonary hypertension. *Circulation* **71**:1191–1196, 1985

226. Daoud FS, Reeves JT, Kelly DB: Isoproterenol as a potential pulmonary vasodilator in primary pulmonary hypertension. *Am J Cardiol* **42**:817–822, 1978

227. Lupi-Herrera E, Bialostozky D, Sobrino A: The role of isoproterenol in pulmonary hypertension of unknown etiology (primary). *Chest* **79**:292–296, 1981

228. Pietro DR, LaBresh KA, Shulman RM, et al: Sustained improvement in primary pulmonary hypertension during six years of treatment with sublingual isoproterenol. *N Engl J Med* **310**:1032–1037, 1984

229. Rich S, Brundage BH: High-dose calcium channel-blocking therapy for primary pulmonary hypertension: Evidence for long-term reduction in pulmonary arterial pressure and regression of right ventricular hypertrophy. *Circulation* **76**:135–141, 1987

230. McLeod AA, Jewitt DE: Drug treatment of primary pulmonary hypertension. *Drugs* **31**:177–184, 1986

231. Rubin LJ, Nicod P, Hillis LD, et al: Treatment of primary pulmonary hypertension with nifedipine. A hemodynamic and scintigraphic evaluation. *Ann Intern Med* **99**:433–438, 1983

232. Wood BA, Tortoledo F, Luck JC, et al: Rapid attenuation of response to nifedipine in primary pulmonary hypertension. *Chest* **82**:793–794, 1982

233. Weiner N: Drugs that inhibit adrenergic nerves and block adrenergic receptors. In Gilman AG, Goodman LS, Rall TW, Murad F (eds): *The Pharmacological Basis of Therapeutics.* New York: Macmillan, 1985, pp 181–214

234. Camerini F, Alberti E, Klugman S, et al: Primary pulmonary hypertension: Effects of nifedipine. *Br Heart J* **44**:352–356, 1980

235. Simonneau G, Escourrou P, Duroux P, et al: Inhibition of hypoxic vasoconstriction by nifedipine. *N Engl J Med* **304**:1582–1585, 1981

236. Sturani C, Bassein L, Schiavina M, et al: Oral nifedipine in chronic or pulmonale secondary to severe chronic obstructive lung disease (COPD). *Chest* **84**:135–142, 1983.

237. Pearl RG, Rosenthal MH, Schroeder JS, et al: Acute hemodynamic effects of nitroglycerin in pulmonary hypertension. *Ann Intern Med* **99**:9–13, 1983

238. Swan PK, Tibballs J, Duncan AW: Prostaglandin E$_1$ in primary pulmonary hypertension. *Crit Care Med* **14**:72–73, 1986

239. Powers K, Fyfe DA, Taylor AB et al: Treatment of pulmonary vasospasm with prazosin after atrial septal defect closure in a child. *J Thorac Cardiovasc Surg* **97**:802–803, 1989 (letter)

240. Packer M, Lee WH, Yushak M: Systemic vasoconstrictor effects of oxygen administration in obliterative pulmonary vascular disorders. *Am J Cardiol* **57**:853–858, 1986

241. Packer M, Medina N, Yushak M: Adverse hemodynamic and clinical effects of calcium channel blockage in pulmonary hypertension secondary to obliterative pulmonary vascular disease. *J Am Coll Cardiol* **4**:890–901, 1984

242. Palevsky HI, Fishman AP: Vasodilator therapy for primary pulmonary hypertension. *Ann Rev Med* **36**:563–578, 1985

243. Weir EK, Rubin LJ, Ayres SM et al: The acute administration of vasodilators in primary pulmonary hypertension. Experience from the National Institutes of Health Registry on Primary Pulmonary Hypertension. *Am Rev Respir Dis* **140**:1623–1630, 1989

244. Higenbottam T: The place of prostacyclin in the clinical management of primary pulmonary hypertension. *Am Rev Respir Dis* **136**:782–785, 1987

245. Barst RJ. Pharmacologically induced pulmonary vasodilatation in children and young adults with primary pulmonary hypertension. *Chest* **89**:497–503, 1986

246. Higenbottam T, Wells F, Wheeldon D, et al: Long-term treatment of primary pulmonary hypertension with continuous intravenous epoprostenol (prostacyclin). *Lancet* **1**:1046–1047, 1984

247. Scott JP, Higenbottam TW, Smyth RL, Wallwork J: Acute pulmonary hypertensive crisis in a patient with primary pulmonary artery hypertension treated by both epoprostenol (prostacyclin) and nitroprusside. *Chest* **99**:1284–1285, 1991

248. Kaapa P, Koivisto M, Ylikorkaia O, et al: Clinical and laboratory observations: Prostacyclin in the treatment of neonatal pulmonary hypertension. *J Pediatr* **107**: 951–953, 1985

249. Bush A, Busst C, Booth K, et al: Does prostacyclin enhance the selective pulmonary vasodilator effect of oxygen in children with congenital heart disease? *Circulation* **74**:135–144, 1986

250. Bush A, Busst CM, Knight WB, et al: Comparison of the haemodynamic effects of epoprostenol (prostacyclin) and tolazoline. *Br Heart J* **60**:141–148, 1988

251. Roberts JD, Polaner DM, Todres ID, et al: Inhaled nitric oxide (NO): A selective pulmonary vasodilation for the treatment of persistent pulmonary hypertension (PPHN). *Circulation* **84**(suppl II):II–322, 1991 (abstr)

252. Frostell C, Fratacci MD, Wain JC, et al: Inhaled nitric oxide. *Circulation* **83**:2038–2047, 1991

Chapter 19 | Abnormalities of the Atrioventricular Valves

David A. Lowe and Stephen A. Stayer

The anesthetic management of a child with tricuspid atresia (TA), Ebstein's anomaly, or a malformation of the mitral valve begins with a clear understanding of the anatomy and hemodynamic consequences of the lesion. This may be difficult to achieve because of the considerable anatomic and functional variability within each of these lesions, as well as the frequency of coexisting cardiac anomalies. However, from this understanding will emerge an individualized approach based on the fundamentals of pediatric and cardiac anesthesia that makes the child's response to anesthetic and surgical intervention more predictable.

Figure 19–1 illustrates the normal morphology of the atrioventricular (AV) valves consisting of leaflets that originate from an annulus and attach distally by chordae tendineae to papillary muscles. The tricuspid valve has a large anterior leaflet, a large septal leaflet, and a small posterior leaflet. The mitral valve has an anterior (aortic) leaflet and a posterior (mural) leaflet. In a normal heart, the aortic valve is deeply wedged between the tricuspid and mitral valves, the AV node is bounded by the coronary sinus and the septal annulus of the tricuspid valve, and the circumflex artery sits in the left AV groove adjacent to the mitral annulus.

TRICUSPID ATRESIA

Tricuspid atresia is a condition in which there is no communication between the right atrium and the right ventricle. It is the third most common cause of cyanotic congenital heart disease, after tetralogy of Fallot and D-transposition of the great arteries (D-TGA). In the normal embryo, the tricuspid valve forms from portions of the interventricular septum and endocardial cushions. TA results when the AV canal migrates incompletely to the right. Because the tricuspid valve may be completely absent or represented by an atretic dimple, survival depends on an obligatory interatrial communication to decompress the right atrium (either a patent foramen ovale in two thirds of cases or a secundum atrial septal defect [ASD]) and a systemic to pulmonary shunt. The ASD is usually large and nonrestrictive, allowing the systemic venous return to mix with the pulmonary venous return in the left atrium and pass into a large left ventricle. There is usually a ventricular septal defect (VSD) that permits blood flow into a rudimentary right ventricle, the size of which generally correlates with the size of the VSD. When the ventricular septum is intact or when there is pulmonary atresia, a patent ductus arteriosus (PDA) or other systemic to pulmonary shunt is necessary for survival.

Anatomy

When Kuhne first described the malformation of tricuspid atresia in 1906, he divided his cases into those without transposition of the great arteries (type I) and those with transposition of the great arteries (type II). This classification system was later modified and popularized by Edwards and Burchell[1] depending upon the presence of pulmonary stenosis or atresia and the size of the VSD. Keith et al[2] later described another subgroup composed of patients with L-transposition of the great arteries (type III). Table 19–1 summarizes the different types of TA, their effect on pulmonary blood flow, and their approximate frequency.[2–4]

Type I. The great arteries are normally related (ventriculoarterial concordance) in about 70% of patients with TA (type I). Type I is further subdivided into three subsets depending on the size of the VSD and the presence or absence of pulmonic stenosis (Fig 19–2). In type IA, there is reduced pulmonary blood flow because of the absence of a VSD, the absence of a right ventricular

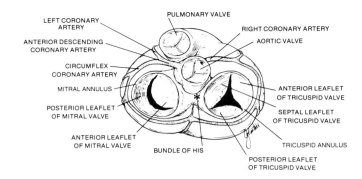

Figure 19–1. Normal heart (coronal section).

cavity, pulmonary atresia, and a main pulmonary artery that is either small or atretic. Here, pulmonary flow is dependent on a PDA. Half of all cases of TA and about 75% of patients with normally related great arteries are classified type IB. In type IB, pulmonary blood flow is obstructed by a small restrictive VSD and a small right ventricular cavity with infundibular pulmonary stenosis. Although the pulmonic valve and the pulmonary arteries are small, they rarely cause obstruction. As in type IA, adequate pulmonary blood flow is ductal dependent. In type IC, the pulmonary blood flow is either normal or increased because of a large VSD and a pulmonary artery that is either normal or enlarged.

Type II. About 30% of patients with TA have D-TGA (ventriculoarterial discordance) and are classified as type II (Fig 19–3). Type IIA is an uncommon form in which pulmonary blood flow depends on a PDA because the main pulmonary artery, arising from the left ventricle, is atretic. Another uncommon form is type IIB, associated with a large VSD, a right ventricular cavity that is generally larger than in type I, and subpulmonary stenosis and/or pulmonary valve stenosis

that equalizes the pulmonary blood flow with that of the systemic circulation.

Over 70% of patients with TA and D-TGA are type IIC. Affected children usually have severe heart failure because of excessive pulmonary blood flow. The majority of the left ventricular output is delivered to the pulmonary artery, which is either normal or enlarged, without the protection of subpulmonic or valvular obstruction. Neonates with type IIC may not present with congestive failure until their high pulmonary vascular resistance (PVR) falls unless their VSD is restrictive. Coarctation of the aorta, hypoplasia of the aortic arch, and PDA are frequently present in patients with type IIC.

Type III. Type III is a very rare combination of TA and L-TGA in which the aorta is anterior and to the left and the pulmonary artery is posterior and to the right (Fig 19–4). There may be normal positioning of the ventricles with pulmonary or subpulmonary stenosis (type IIIA) or ventricular inversion with subaortic stenosis (type IIIB). As with any patient with L-transposition, there is an increased incidence of complete AV block.

TABLE 19–1. TYPES OF TRICUSPID ATRESIA

	Pulmonary Blood Flow	Frequency (%)
Type I: No Transposition of Great Arteries (TGA)		**70**
A. No VSD, with pulmonary atresia	↓	(10)
B. Small VSD, with pulmonary stenosis	↓	(50)
C. Large VSD, no pulmonary stenosis	⇆↑	(10)
Type II: D-TGA		**30**
A. VSD with pulmonary atresia	↓	(2)
B. VSD with pulmonary stenosis	⇆↓	(8)
C. VSD without pulmonary stenosis	↑↑	(20)
Type III: L-TGA		Very rare
A. Pulmonary/subpulmonary stenosis	↓	
B. Subaortic stenosis	↑	**100**

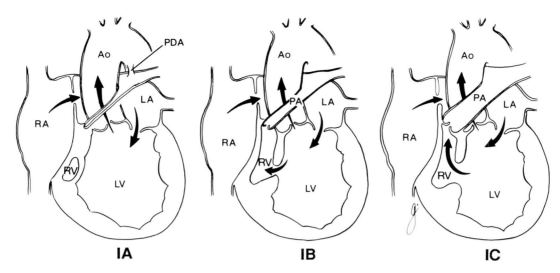

Figure 19–2. Type I: Tricuspid atresia without transposition of the great arteries. Type IA: Pulmonary blood flow depends on a patent ductus arteriosus or bronchial collaterals because of pulmonary atresia. Type IB: Restrictive pulmonary blood flow due to a small VSD, small right ventricular cavity, and infundibular pulmonary stenosis. Type IC: Normal or increased pulmonary blood flow due to a large VSD and an adequate pulmonary outflow tract.

Pathophysiology

Hypoxemia is always present because the entire systemic venous blood must pass from the right atrium to the left atrium where it mixes with the pulmonary venous blood. The degree of hypoxemia may be mild or severe depending on the ratio of systemic to pulmonary blood flow and the absolute pulmonary blood flow. Complete mixing is usually achieved at the left atrial level, so that the left ventricular, right ventricular, pulmonary arterial, and systemic arterial saturations are equal.

Over 70% of patients with TA have decreased pulmonary blood flow and present with cyanosis (types IA, IB, IIA, IIB, and IIIA). They do not exhibit signs of heart failure unless a restrictive ASD is present. Most of these infants have type IB with normally related great arteries, a small VSD, and right ventricular outflow obstruction. Their cyanosis is severe and progressive, sometimes associated with hypoxic spells similar to those experienced by infants with tetralogy of Fallot. Increasing cyanosis and cyanotic spells may be due to sponta-

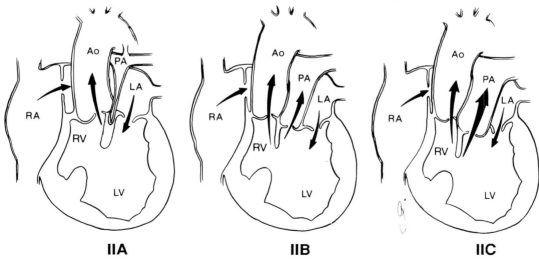

Figure 19–3. Type II: Tricuspid atresia with transposition of the great arteries. Type IIA: Transposed great arteries with large VSD and pulmonary atresia. Pulmonary blood flow depends upon a patent ductus arteriosus or bronchial collaterals. Type IIB: Transposed great arteries with large VSD and pulmonary stenosis. Pulmonary blood flow tends to equal systemic blood flow. Type IIC: Transposed great arteries with a normal or enlarged pulmonary artery. Pulmonary blood flow is primarily determined by the pulmonary vascular resistance.

neous closure of the VSD, especially a muscular VSD, and progression of infundibular narrowing that further reduces pulmonary blood flow.

The remaining 30% of children with TA have increased pulmonary blood flow (types IC, IIC, and IIIB) and present with congestive heart failure. High pulmonary to systemic blood flow ratios account for inadequate systemic perfusion and a volume burden on the single ventricle. Ventricular end-diastolic volume and pressure increase, a result of excessive pulmonary blood flow and fluid retention associated with an activated renin-angiotensin-aldosterone mechanism. Most of these patients present in early infancy with severe failure and TGA, a large VSD, and no right ventricular or pulmonary artery obstruction (type IIC). Those who have type IC with normally related great arteries and a large VSD or PDA and those who have type IIIB with L-transposition have a more moderate increase in pulmonary blood flow and present later with mild congestive failure. The tendencies for muscular VSDs to get smaller and infundibular stenosis to progress actually benefit these children for months or years by producing a more balanced flow. However, any reduction in the size of the VSD in patients with TA and transposed great arteries whose left ventricle ejects directly and without obstruction into the pulmonary artery (type IIC) will result in excessive pulmonary blood flow and reduced systemic blood flow.[5]

When the ASD is small, the flow of blood from the right atrium to the left atrium is restricted and the right atrial and systemic venous pressures are increased. Left ventricular output is decreased, not only because of decreased filling but also owing to an increase in afterload as higher intraventricular pressures are needed to achieve adequate systemic perfusion pressures. These patients present in the neonatal period with significant cyanosis and inadequate systemic perfusion.

Natural History

Infants with either decreased pulmonary blood flow or severe congestive heart failure are unlikely to survive beyond infancy without surgery. Children who survive because of balanced systemic and pulmonary circulations generally exhibit adequate exercise tolerance and growth velocity until the second decade of life. After years of receiving combined pulmonary and systemic venous return, a cardiomyopathy develops secondary to chronic volume overload. Surgically untreated infants with decreased pulmonary blood flow have myocardial dysfunction with reduced ejection fractions and larger than normal end-diastolic volumes.[6,7] Although reduced ejection fractions may be related to hypoxemia, older patients who have survived because of palliative systemic to pulmonary arterial shunts have a progressive decrease in ejection fraction and a larger end-diastolic volume.[6] In some patients, dilatation of the mitral valve annulus causes mitral incompetence, arrhythmias, and pulmonary vascular obstructive disease.[8–11] After age 15, mortality increases predominately owing to heart failure and pulmonary vascular obstructive disease.[8–11]

Diagnostic Features

The clinical presentation and therapy depend upon the associated cardiac anomalies that are responsible for pulmonary blood flow being either decreased, normal, or increased. All children with TA are cyanotic because of mixing at the atrial level. However, those with decreased pulmonary blood flow (because of a small VSD, a small right ventricular chamber, right ventricular outflow tract

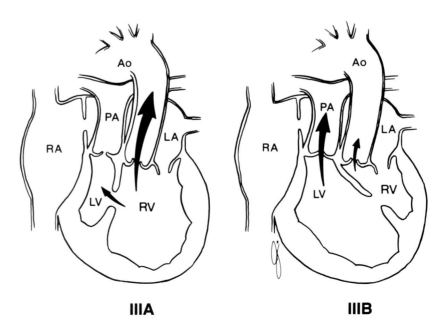

Figure 19–4. Type III: Tricuspid atresia with L-transposition of the great arteries. Type IIIA: Pulmonary or subpulmonary stenosis. Type IIIB: Subaortic stenosis. Ventricular inversion is illustrated.

IIIA

IIIB

obstruction, and/or pulmonary artery obstruction) are profoundly cyanotic. Those with excessive pulmonary blood flow (due to a large VSD or TGA without obstruction to pulmonary blood flow) present with congestive heart failure as the dominant clinical problem and a mild degree of cyanosis. Congestive heart failure accounts for tachypnea, tachycardia, hepatic enlargement, decreased oral intake, and decreased growth velocity.

The diagnosis of TA depends upon typical radiographic, echocardiographic, and catheterization findings. Radiographic findings are determined by the volume of pulmonary blood flow and size of the interventricular septal defect. A square cardiac silhouette is present with a large ASD that straightens the right atrial border and enlarges the left atrium. With a small septal defect, the right atrium is greatly enlarged, whereas the pulmonary artery segment is small owing to reduced flow. Left ventricular hypertrophy, P pulmonale due to right atrial enlargement, and left axis deviation are present on electrocardiograph (ECG). ECG is now the primary modality for the initial diagnosis. The combination of M-mode and two-dimensional echocardiography can define the size and location of cardiac chambers, great artery entrances, valves, and flow pathways. Doppler techniques can measure pressure gradients across stenotic orifices and estimate pulmonary artery pressures to determine the need for atrial septectomy. Magnetic resonance imaging can clarify the relationship of viscera to atria, great arteries to one another, size of the cardiac chambers, and possible distortion of the pulmonary arteries, particularly after palliative systemic to pulmonary artery shunts.[12,13] At cardiac catheterization, low oxygen saturation in the left atrium is noted. Angiography demonstrates a triangular filling defect due to an absent or diminutive right ventricle.

Anesthesia and Perioperative Management

Anesthetic Considerations for Palliative Procedures

Procedures to Increase Pulmonary Blood Flow. When cyanotic infants requiring procedures to increase pulmonary blood flow come to the operating room, it is crucial to avoid aggravation of preexisting hypoxemia. Hypoxemia is particularly likely to occur during (1) induction of anesthesia, (2) lung retraction, and (3) distal shunt anastomosis when the branch pulmonary artery is clamped, further reducing pulmonary blood flow. A cyanotic infant who is awake and capable of struggling is likely to become profoundly hypoxic during an awake intubation, which provokes breathholding and bradycardia, as well as the release of endogenous catecholamines that further increases PVR. Instead, by means of a mask induction with 50% oxygen, 50% nitrous oxide, and halothane or an intravenous induction with incremental doses of fentanyl, gradual control of the airway can be accomplished

in most patients without hypoventilation or noxious stimulation. At the moment effective ventilation by bag and mask is assured, a neuromuscular blocking drug is administered and endotracheal intubation performed.

After induction, nitrous oxide is discontinued and 100% oxygen is provided throughout the rest of the procedure. Pure oxygen will protect the patient from hypoxemia due to hypoventilation and intrapulmonary shunting. It also decreases PVR and the impact of any intravenous air emboli that may reach the systemic circulation, unlike nitrous oxide, which enlarges these gas-containing spaces. Cyanotic neonates are unable to experience Pa_{O_2} levels high enough to cause damage to the eyes, which eliminates even a theoretical risk of hyperoxia-related retinopathy prematurity.

Hypoxia due to hypoventilation, atelectasis, and perhaps a decrease in cardiac output when the lung is retracted must be offset by requiring that the dependent lung expand sufficiently to lift the mediastinum with each breath. Routine, intermittent reinflation of the retracted lung will help to minimize intrapulmonary shunting. At other times, pulse oximetry signals the need for the surgeon to interrupt surgery temporarily to allow reexpansion of the lung.

Immediately prior to clamping of the branch pulmonary artery, 50–100 U/kg of heparin are administered to reduce the likelihood of shunt thrombosis and 1 mEq/kg of sodium bicarbonate is given to offset the acidosis that develops as a result of the decreased pulmonary blood flow. In polycythemic patients, hemodilution to a hemoglobin of 14 or 15 g by controlled blood loss in exchange for isotonic crystalloid may be desirable to decrease blood viscosity and improve flow through the shunt. Blood loss at the time of unclamping of the systemic-pulmonary shunt may require prompt transfusion. A well-functioning shunt usually decreases diastolic blood pressure owing to increased pulmonary blood flow at the expense of the systemic flow. The blood pressure can usually be increased by the administration of isotonic fluid. Occasionally, inotropic agents are needed to maintain adequate blood pressure until the ductus arteriosus closes. After the clamps are released and the shunt is noted to be functioning, the prostaglandin infusion is discontinued. Most patients can be safely extubated in the operating room. Intercostal nerve blocks are relatively contraindicated because of the large collateral vessels in patients with decreased pulmonary blood flow.

Procedures to Decrease Pulmonary Blood Flow. Oxygen is a selective pulmonary vasodilator. It increases an already excessive blood flow and decreases systemic flow and systemic blood pressure. Therefore, the F_{IO_2} needs to be titrated between 21 and 100% to maintain the Sp_{O_2} between 80 and 90% unless an extra margin of safety is indicated as during intubation and lung retraction. When the pulmonary artery band is applied (a fixed resistor), the F_{IO_2} is increased to at least 50% to minimize the contribution of hypoxemia to pulmonary vasoconstriction (dynamic resistor).

Infants who require pulmonary artery banding to relieve severe congestive failure will tolerate little, if any, myocardial depression and often require inotropic support preoperatively or during the induction of anesthesia.[5] An air/oxygen mixture and incremental doses of fentanyl provide satisfactory anesthesia without myocardial depression in these cases. Other infants with mild failure tolerate a mask induction with halothane and perhaps extubation in the operating room at the end of the procedure. An intra-arterial catheter is useful to compare systemic pressures with those obtained by the surgeon in the distal pulmonary artery at the time the band is tightened. Central venous pressure (CVP), if it is measured, will decrease slightly as the pulmonary blood flow is reduced. An increase in CVP suggests excessive impedance to ejection of the pulmonary ventricle and the band should be loosened.[14] An excessively tight band will severely decrease systemic arterial oxygen saturation often heralded by bradycardia.

Procedures to Enlarge Interatrial Communications. Because of the risk of hemodynamic collapse, an intra-arterial catheter for continuous monitoring of systemic pressures and a central venous catheter for the delivery of vasoactive drugs are warranted. Resuscitation is necessary more often than in other closed-heart procedures. Immediately before the application of the vascular clamp, the retracted lung is temporarily released and the child is hyperventilated with 100% oxygen for 2 minutes. Atropine and sodium bicarbonate, 1 mEq/kg, are administered in anticipation of bradycardia and acidemia that are likely to result from decreased cardiac output while the clamp is in place. Warmed blood products are prepared for immediate transfusion to replace blood loss that will be intentional to some extent, for the purpose of flushing air out of the atria.

Anesthetic Considerations for Reparative Procedures

Premedication. Effective pharmacologic sedation is beneficial prior to a Fontan procedure. Children about to undergo a Fontan procedure are sophisticated enough to be terrified of the procedure or, at least, to be upset by their family's apprehension. The separation of a screaming child from the parent becomes a highly undesirable memory. In addition, it increases the risk of a stormy induction complicated by breathholding and laryngospasm that would aggravate preexisting hypoxemia. Although these children have preexisting cyanosis, premedication in children older than 12 months of age provides effective sedation with only transient or no exacerbation of hypoxemia. Diazepam, 0.3–0.5 mg/kg,

combined with hydroxyzine, 1–2 mg/kg, administered orally 1 hour before the separation of the child from the parents provides safe and effective sedation.

Anesthetic Induction. Anesthetic agents and techniques must be selected to preserve a margin of safety that is already compromised by preexisting hypoxemia and left ventricular dysfunction due to chronic volume overload. The patient's cardiac reserve is compromised either when the pulmonary blood flow is decreased and the child is profoundly cyanotic and polycythemic or when the pulmonary blood flow is excessive and there is a volume burden on the single ventricle.

It is reasonable to perform a mask induction with halothane in most children scheduled for a Fontan procedure, who tend to be between 1 and 4 years of age and arrive without an intravenous catheter. A mask induction is performed with 50% oxygen, 50% nitrous oxide, and halothane increased by 0.5% every three breaths up to 3%. Just before induction, or as consciousness is lost, the essential monitors are applied. During the induction, noninvasive blood pressures are obtained every 15–20 seconds. Ventilation is gently assisted, then controlled, usually by the time an IV catheter is inserted. Pancuronium and fentanyl are given, halothane and nitrous oxide discontinued, and 100% oxygen maintained throughout the rest of the anesthetic. The myocardial depressant effect of halothane is usually acceptable. Even when hypotension requires decreasing its concentration and converting to a narcotic-based technique, it is usually possible to gain gradual control of the airway and acquire intravenous access. Systemic perfusion pressure must be maintained to provide adequate pulmonary blood flow through a systemic to pulmonary shunt.

When myocardial reserve is marginal because of poorly compensated congestive heart failure or severe hypoxemia, an intravenous induction is carried out after the essential monitors are applied and the patient is preoxygenated. For example, a high-dose (50–100μg/kg) fentanyl technique is used, supplemented with additional doses of a benzodiazepine. Small incremental doses of fentanyl can be given without unacceptable cardiovascular depression or muscle rigidity.[16,17] Once the airway is controlled, or as a consequence of muscle rigidity induced by fentanyl, pancuronium is administered. A total dose of at least 20 μg of fentanyl is given prior to intubation. This is one of many techniques that offers gradual control of the airway and hemodynamic stability while eliminating the need for additional anesthetics during the rewarming phase of bypass and the early postbypass period.

Fluid Management. Cyanotic patients with hematocrits over 60% have hyperviscosity, increased systemic vascular resistance, decreased cardiac output, sludging, the potential for thrombosis, and a poorly defined coagulopathy. Once an IV catheter is inserted, the rapid infusion of about 5 mL/kg of Ringer's lactate solution helps to restore the preoperative fluid deficit and minimize the effects of positive-pressure ventilation and myocardial depressants that tend to decrease cardiac output and increase the likelihood of complications from hyperviscosity.

Patients undergoing a Fontan procedure receive two peripheral intravenous catheters and a double-lumen central venous catheter. There is an increased risk of bleeding from pericardial adhesions resulting from previous palliative surgery, and peripheral venous access is likely to be difficult to acquire postoperatively when the veins are obscured by edema. A double-lumen central venous catheter allows continuous measurement of CVP and delivery of vasoactive drugs to the central circulation.

Termination of Cardiopulmonary Bypass. Once the right ventricle has been eliminated from the circulation by the Fontan operation, pulmonary perfusion depends on a filling pressure in the right atrium that is higher than the pressure in the left atrium to overcome PVR. The left ventricle is required to overcome the systemic vascular resistance followed by the PVR in series. Measures to decrease PVR, including hyperventilation, increased FIO_2, and an alkalotic pH of 7.6 are helpful as bypass is discontinued. Eventually, spontaneous ventilation will enhance venous return, improve ventilation to perfusion matching, and increase cardiac output. Although hypoxemia due to intracardiac shunts will no longer compromise left ventricular performance, preoperative myocardial dysfunction due to chronic volume overload, aggravated by 80–100 minutes of hypothermic cardiopulmonary bypass, may result in left ventricular failure when bypass is terminated.

Before discontinuing cardiopulmonary bypass, it is important to establish normal sinus rhythm to maximize cardiac output. Left atrial contraction will augment ventricular filling. However, a normal sinus rhythm and contractile atria are not essential to obtain a satisfactory result.[18] Under the best of circumstances, it is necessary to maintain a CVP of at least 15–20 mm Hg and left atrial pressures under 10 mm Hg an interatrial gradient of 7–10 mm Hg. The higher the mean CVP that is required, the greater the immediate intraoperative and early postoperative mortality and morbidity.[19,20] A CVP of greater than 20 mm Hg correlates with a poor prognosis. Elevated left atrial pressure suggests ventricular or AV valve dysfunction. At these times, it is useful to decrease systemic and PVR with sodium nitroprusside, 1–2 μg/kg/min, and enhance contractility with either dopamine, 10 μg/kg/min, or isoproterenol, 0.1 μg/kg/min.[21,22]

If the right atrial pressure is elevated more than 10 mm Hg over the left atrial pressure, obstruction to pulmonary blood flow from the right atrium through the lungs is suggested. A higher PA pressure results from either small pulmonary arteries or an increased PVR. If the PA pressure is low, and the difference between it and the mean right atrial pressure is greater than 1–2 mm Hg, stenosis somewhere within the RA-PA pathway is likely, perhaps requiring revision of the pathway.[23]

Augmentation of Venous Return. Phasic external compression of the lower body can be used to augment systemic venous return. Anti-shock air pants over Webril (Jobst Institute, Inc, Toledo, OH) can be applied (from the ankles to the costal margins) after the induction of general anesthesia.[24] Just prior to discontinuing cardiopulmonary bypass and continuing for at least 24 hours, support of the systemic venous circulation occurs with 1-minute cycles of 30–50 mm Hg for 45 seconds followed by 15 seconds of decompression. Heck and Doty reported that by relocating peripherally sequestered fluid to the central circulation, right atrial pressure increased by a mean of 7 mm Hg (44%), systolic arterial pressures increased an average of 20 mm Hg (30%), left atrial pressure increased a mean of 7 mm Hg (93%), and none of the nine patients received inotropes or vasodilating agents.[24] Milliken et al found similar improvements in hemodynamic variables with the use of an inflatable abdominal binder (extra-large adult blood pressure cuff) attached to a Jobst extremity pump.[25] By augmenting venous return, right atrial pressure is increased without the necessity of large fluid volume infusions and without massive fluid sequestration in the lower body and intra-abdominal cavity as a consequence of inadequate right-sided hemodynamics.

Surgical Techniques

Palliative Procedures. Almost all patients with TA require palliative surgery within the first year of life. These procedures are intended to (1) increase pulmonary blood flow when it is diminished (small VSD, pulmonic stenosis) by means of a systemic-pulmonary artery anastomosis or a venous-pulmonary anastomosis; (2) decrease pulmonary blood flow when it is excessive (large VSD) by means of pulmonary artery banding; or (3) enlarge a restrictive atrial communication by means of an atrial septectomy. Rarely, when the VSD is restrictive, as in patients with D-transposition of the great arteries, enlargement of the VSD is necessary.

Operations to Increase Pulmonary Blood Flow. A systemic-pulmonary artery anastomosis is indicated in over 70% of patients with TA. Many have severe cyanosis at birth and depend on the patency of their ductus arteriosus until a surgically created systemic to pulmonary shunt, "an artificial ductus," is established. Until then, ductal patency can be maintained by the administration of prostaglandin E_1 at a rate of 0.05–0.1 µg/kg/min. Prostaglandin E_1 improves systemic arterial oxygenation and stabilizes the acid-base balance in neonatal patients.[26] Complications of prostaglandin infusion include accidental interruption of the infusion, apnea, fever, seizures, vasodilatation, and peripheral edema.[27] In addition to ductal dependency, indications for systemic-pulmonary shunts include significant or progressive hypoxemia and polycythemia due to decreased pulmonary blood flow.

Generally, the procedure of choice is a Blalock-Taussig shunt in which an end-to-side anastomosis is performed between the subclavian artery and the pulmonary artery on the side opposite the aortic arch. A modified Blalock-Taussig shunt using an interposed polytetrafluoroethylene (Gore-Tex) prosthetic graft can be performed on either side. These shunts are rarely large enough to cause heart failure and are preferred if a Fontan procedure is planned for the future because the success of a Fontan operation depends on the presence of a low PVR. These shunts can be easily ligated at the time of corrective surgery.

When this shunt cannot be established, a central shunt, connecting the ascending aorta to the main pulmonary artery using a prosthetic graft, may be accomplished. Both the Waterston shunt (side-to-side anastomosis of the ascending aorta to the right pulmonary artery) and the Potts shunt (side-to-side anastomosis of the descending thoracic aorta to the left pulmonary artery) are obsolete because of the inability to control the size of the shunt orifice. These shunts often led to excessive pulmonary blood flow, congestive heart failure, pulmonary hypertension, and eventually pulmonary vascular obstructive disease.

Glenn Procedure.

In 1958, Glenn succeeded in creating a more physiologic circulation for cyanotic patients with TA by performing a palliative operation that provided pulmonary blood flow without adding to the volume load of the systemic ventricle as occurred with systemic to pulmonary artery shunts.[28] The Glenn shunt is an end-to-side anastomosis of the distal end of the divided right pulmonary artery to the superior vena cava with division of the superior vena cava–right atrial junction and proximal right pulmonary artery (Fig 19–5). This procedure confirmed experimental evidence that systemic venous pressure provided adequate driving force for pulmonary blood flow.[28] However, long-term evaluation has shown deterioration to occur about 5 years after the initial palliation because of decreased flow through the shunt as PVR increases and collateral circulation through the inferior vena cava develops.[6] Deterioration is probably due to microthrombi in the pulmonary capillary bed. Today, a modified Glenn shunt is commonly used as an interim palliation for high-risk candidates for the Fontan procedure (see below).

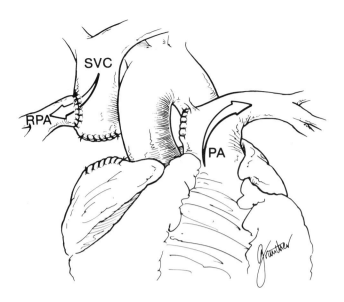

Figure 19–5. Glenn shunt, an end-to-side anastomosis of the superior vena cava to the distal end of the divided right pulmonary artery. The superior vena cava–right atrial junction and the proximal right pulmonary artery are divided.

Operations to Decrease Pulmonary Blood Flow.

Pulmonary artery banding is indicated in patients with TA when excessive pulmonary blood flow causes severe heart failure. Most of these patients have type IIC with TGA and no obstruction to pulmonary blood flow. Balanced pulmonary and systemic blood flow is expected when the pulmonary artery is sufficiently constricted by a band to decrease distal pulmonary artery pressure to one third to one half of systemic pressure. The systemic pressure increases as systemic blood flow increases. Pulmonary artery banding is rarely indicated in patients with type IC who have moderate increases in pulmonary blood flow because their VSD decreases in size.

Operations to Enlarge a Restrictive Interatrial Communication.

Enlargement of the ASD is indicated to obtain better mixing of blood and decompression of the right atrium. Between 4 and 33% of patients with TA have been reported to have a restrictive ASD.[29] A gradient between the right and left atria as little as 2–5 mm Hg may be clinically significant. In neonates, balloon atrial septostomy at the time of cardiac catheterization effectively ruptures the membrane of the fossa ovalis. When a balloon septostomy is inadequate, further enlargement of the ASD is usually accomplished by a Blalock-Hanlon operation. In older children with a thick interatrial septum, a thoracotomy can be avoided by blade atrial septostomy performed at the time of cardiac catheterization.[31]

ATRIAL SEPTECTOMY. The Blalock-Hanlon operation is performed via a right lateral thoracotomy. A portion of both the right and left atria with a portion of the interatrial septum is isolated from the circulation by application of a vascular clamp. Two parallel incisions are made, one into the right atrial wall and another into the left atrial wall with the interatrial septum trapped between these incisions. The septum is pulled into the operating field and excised. Systemic and pulmonary venous return may be significantly reduced during the few minutes of partial occlusion. Preexisting hypoxemia often worsens and cardiac output is reduced.

A less commonly used surgical septectomy is performed by the "inflow occlusion" technique. Because the cardiac output is equal to the cardiac input, there will be no cardiac output for about 60 seconds while snares are tightened around the venae cavae. The right atrium is opened and the septum is retracted and excised. The venae cavae snares are released to flush air out of the right atrium prior to its closure, necessitating the transfusion of at least 30–50 mL of blood. Resuscitative drugs for asystole are frequently required.

Reparative Surgical Procedures

Fontan Procedure. The original Fontan operation was successfully performed in 1968 by Fontan and Baudet.[32] They offered the first physiologic correction for TA by completely separating systemic and pulmonary circulations from one another. This procedure was based on the principle that right atrial pressure was adequate to drive blood through the lung provided that the PVR was normal, making a ventricle unnecessary. Right atrial connection to the pulmonary artery was subsequently found to be unnecessary for pulmonary blood flow.[33] In an experimental model, pulsation in a valveless chamber elevated pressure within the chamber and decreased forward flow. Maximal forward output was achieved by streamlining blood flow through a valveless right atrial tunnel of uniform caliber.

The original operation consisted of the insertion of an aortic homograft between the right atrium and the proximal end of the transected right pulmonary artery, ligation of the main pulmonary artery, closure of the ASD, and, two steps that have since been discarded, construction of a Glenn shunt and placement of a valve in the right atrial–inferior vena cava junction. Since 1968, many modifications of this operation have been proposed for the treatment of TA and other single-ventricle complexes.[34–36] Figure 19–6 illustrates some of the most popular modifications of the Fontan procedure currently used in patients with TA.

SELECTION CRITERIA. The success of a Fontan procedure depends upon proper patient selection so the single ventricle can perform the work imposed by both systemic

and pulmonary vascular resistances. This requires an unobstructed circulation and nearly normal systolic and diastolic ventricular function (Table 19–2).[37]

The Fontan procedure is absolutely contraindicated if PVR exceeds $4 U/m^2$, if severe hypoplasia of the pulmonary arteries is present, if the patient is an infant (because of high PVR), if the left ventricular end-diastolic pressure is greater than or equal to 25 mm Hg, and if the left ventricular ejection fraction is greater than or equal to 45%. Additionally, there are a number of relative contraindications. Patients who are between 1 and 2 years of age may safely undergo a Fontan operation only if all other anatomic criteria are met because young children do not tolerate high systemic venous pressures as well as older children. Although older patients (>15 years of age) are at no greater risk than children of 1–2 years, they are subject to decreased ventricular function, ventricular hypertrophy, and valvular dysfunction.[38,39]

If the PVR is $2–4 U/m^2$, a child over the age of 2 may undergo a Fontan operation. Mean pulmonary artery pressure of greater than 15 mm Hg is probably acceptable if the elevation is due to excessive pulmonary blood flow that will be reduced by a corrective operation. Central pulmonary hypoplasia must be repaired to ensure success. However, decreased pulmonary artery size is less predictive of outcome than originally thought.[40–42] Left ventricular end-diastolic pressure of greater than 15 mm Hg suggests left ventricular dysfunction and may contraindicate a Fontan operation. However, if associated with a large-volume burden, these high pressures may normalize after a corrective operation.[39] Severe left ventricular hypertrophy is a substantial risk factor for a Fontan operation whether it is associated with left ventricular volume overload, subaortic obstruction, or pulmonary artery banding.[38]

Mair and co-workers evaluated their experience with 176 patients with TA who had a Fontan procedure between 1973 and 1989.[19] They identified two risk factors that clearly influenced operative and late postoperative mortality: preoperative PVR and left ventricular diastolic function. They utilized a preoperative catheterization index (PCI) to select candidates for Fontan procedures.

$$PCI = PVR + \frac{LVEDP}{Qp + Qs}$$

A PCI less than 4 accurately predicted the postoperative right atrial pressure to be 20 mm Hg or less, a circumstance that was associated with a 95% early and 89% overall survival rate.[19]

PRE–FONTAN PHYSIOLOGY. Systemic to pulmonary shunting is universally present prior to the Fontan procedure with the exception of those patients who have undergone a Glenn procedure. The following are characteristics of "single"-ventricle physiology:[43]

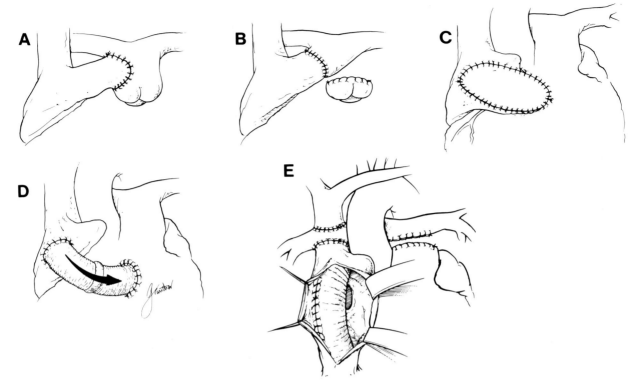

Figure 19–6. Modifications of the Fontan procedure. (*A*) Direct connection of the right atrial appendage to the side of the main pulmonary artery. (*B*) Direct connection of the right atrial appendage to the end of the pulmonary trunk (Kreutzer modification). (*C*) Right atrial–right ventricular connection with a pericardial patch as described by Bjork. (*D*) Right atrial–right ventricular connection with a valved conduit as described by Bowman. (*E*) Total cavopulmonary anastomosis with intra-atrial baffle.

1. The pulmonary circulation exists in parallel with the systemic circulation. Parallel shunting through the low-resistance circuit places a volume burden on the ventricle with progressive dependence on Starling compensatory mechanisms. The ventricle dilates increasing wall stress. Ventricular hypertrophy develops increasing myocardial substrate demands.[39]
2. Parallel shunting of blood into the pulmonary circuit decreases perfusion to the rest of the body. The body compensates for a smaller share of the total cardiac output by increasing sympathetic tone, which creates imbalances between myocardial substrate supply and demand.[43]
3. Parallel systemic and pulmonary circulations decrease oxygen saturation.

Recent Trends in Surgery. Preoperative evaluation of the lusitropic (relaxation) state in patients with borderline PVR helps to determine outcome. Both animal and human data suggest that a longer duration of volume burden leads to chronic cardiac dilatation and irreversible injury associated with myocardial fibrosis.[43] Endomyocardial biopsies obtained from Fontan candidates have shown that the degree of reversibility of injury correlates with myocardial elasticity and may predict reversibility of the dilatation injury.[43] In recognition of lusitropic dysfunction that develops in many Fontan candidates, some surgical teams recommend earlier surgery and use of a modified Glenn shunt to relieve the volume burden of a parallel circulation before irreversible changes occur in the myocardium.

The modified Glenn shunt is a superior vena cava to right pulmonary artery anastomosis with ligation of the superior vena cava to the right atrial junction. This pro-

TABLE 19–2. PATIENT SELECTION CRITERIA FOR THE FONTAN PROCEDURE

Absolute Contraindications
　Early infancy
　Pulmonary vascular resistance ≥ 4 U/m^2
　Severe hypoplasia of pulmonary arteries
　Ejection fraction $\leq 45\%$
　Ventricular end-diastolic pressure ≥ 25 mm Hg
Relative Contraindications
　Age <1–2 years
　Pulmonary vascular resistance 2–4 U/m^2
　Mean pulmonary artery pressure >15 mm Hg
　Previous pulmonary artery banding
　Severe left ventricular hypertrophy
　Stenotic or deformed pulmonary arteries
　Mitral insufficiency
　Subaortic obstruction

cedure leaves the pulmonary arteries in continuity as opposed to Glenn's original description of the shunt. The advantages of cavopulmonary anastomosis for palliation of TA include an increase in effective pulmonary blood flow, with a decrease in the total pulmonary blood flow, and elimination of the ventricular volume burden. Risks of pulmonary artery distortion and late pulmonary hypertension (associated with aortopulmonary shunt) are avoided. In addition, patients in whom pulmonary artery distortion is already present can undergo pulmonary artery reconstruction at the time of bidirectional cavopulmonary anastomosis. Bridges et al reported their experience with 38 patients who underwent bidirectional cavopulmonary anastomosis because they did not meet criteria for Fontan repair.[44] There were no deaths either early or late, median hospital stay was 8 days, and median arterial saturation increased from 79 to 84%. One of the patients with persistent cyanosis required a systemic to pulmonary artery shunt. These investigators found this operation to be successful in providing adequate relief of cyanosis and relief of ventricular volume overload.

Another surgical approach to the Fontan candidate with increased PVR is baffle fenestration with subsequent transcatheter closure. A fenestration in the vena cava to pulmonary artery baffle limits increases in right atrial pressure by allowing blood to shunt right to left. Although arterial saturation is decreased, cardiac output is maintained. Bridges et al reported the use of a baffle fenestration in 20 patients considered to be an increased risk for Fontan repair.[45] Nineteen of these 20 patients survived the operation with a mean arterial oxygen saturation of 86%, mean right atrial pressure of 15 mm Hg, and mean duration of pleural effusions of 6 days. Fifteen of 19 survivors tolerated test occlusion of the fenestration and subsequently underwent permanent transcatheter umbrella closure of the baffle fenestration. Complex intra-atrial baffles may also be required in patients with systemic or pulmonary venous anomalies.[46]

POSTOPERATIVE CARE

Circulation. After completion of the Fontan operation, the pulmonary and systemic circulations are in series resulting in the following improvements in cardiac physiology:[43]

1. Elimination of left-to-right shunting and the volume burden on the ventricle. The ventricular work to generate the same cardiac output decreases as do myocardial metabolic demands.
2. Elimination of shunting into the pulmonary circulation allows the total cardiac output to supply the systemic circulation. The increased inotropic state present in the pre–Fontan state is eliminated improving the myocardial supply/demand ratio.
3. The pulmonary circulation becomes a passive system with flow regulated by the pressure difference between the right and left atrial pressures. Pulmonary

blood flow is biphasic; initial flow occurs with atrial systole, whereas the second phase occurs during left atrial relaxation when blood from the central pulmonary arteries flows into the pulmonary veins.[47]
4. Placing the low-resistance pulmonary circulation in series with the systemic circulation decreases the radius and increases the length of the vascular bed. By the Poiseuille law, these changes increase the resistance of the circulation. This tends to increase ventricular afterload. However, afterload is also determined by ventricular size, so the decrease in ventricular size associated with the elimination of the volume burden may offset the effect of increased resistance.
5. Elimination of shunting with improvement in oxygen saturation.

Ventilation. From the time that cardiopulmonary bypass is discontinued, a pattern of ventilation that minimizes mean airway pressure is preferable to maximize pulmonary blood flow. This can be best achieved by delivering large tidal volumes, approximately 15 mL/kg, with a relatively short inspiratory time to allow for a prolonged exhalation. There should be no unnecessary positive end-expiratory pressure (PEEP) and the respiratory rate should be adjusted to maintain a normal P_{CO_2}. It is important to avoid other factors that may increase PVR such as a functional residual capacity that is either abnormally high or abnormally low, hypothermia, hypercarbia, or acidemia. In hemodynamically labile patients, it will be important to further decrease mean airway pressure by the use of muscle relaxants and sedatives. Conversion to spontaneous ventilation as early as possible enhances pulmonary blood flow. Extubation on the first postoperative day is achieved with safety in over 50% of patients.

Complications. Because thrombosis may occur along the right atrial suture line or within other parts of the Fontan pathway, some advocate the use of oral anticoagulants for 2–3 months postoperatively or until ventricular function and the velocity of flow have improved sufficiently as documented by serial echocardiography. Significant morbidity is related to elevated right atrial pressure. A large percentage of patients experience fluid retention for a period of weeks to months featuring hepatomegaly, ascites, pericardial effusions, peripheral edema, and pleural effusions, including chylothorax. Benign liver dysfunction, reflected by increased hepatic enzymes, results from chronic venous congestion. More serious is acute postoperative hepatic dysfunction resulting from decreased cardiac output, hypoperfusion, and hepatic hypoxia.[48] Some patients develop a protein-losing enteropathy owing to gastrointestinal congestion, reduced lymphatic drainage, and impaired intestinal absorption.[49]

Immediate and Long-term Outcome. Intermediate and long-term results after the Fontan procedure are very good as operative mortality has declined because of improved patient selection and modifications in surgical techniques. Valved conduits are no longer used because of their increased tendency to obstruction.[50] Various centers report an actuarial survival rate between 71 and 85%. Among survivors, 94–96% are in New York Heart Association functional class I or II.[19,51,52] There is an improvement in exercise tolerance, total work performed, and the ventilatory response to exercise. However, cardiac output, stroke volume, and heart rate response to graded exercise remain lower than normal. Additionally, mild hypoxemia persists after the Fontan operation, especially during exercise. This hypoxemia may result from persistent intrapulmonary right-to-left shunting or coronary sinus drainage to the left atrium.[53,54]

TRICUSPID STENOSIS

Congenital tricuspid stenosis is usually accompanied by an ASD and hypoplasia of the right ventricle, pulmonary valve, and pulmonary arteries. The narrowing is usually due to hypoplasia of the tricuspid annulus with relatively normal, although diminutive, valve leaflets. Stenosis caused by fusion of the commissures rarely occurs. The clinical manifestations of isolated congenital tricuspid stenosis are similar to those seen in TA.

In general, when the annulus is small, valvulotomy is not possible, and when it is severe, the treatment resembles that for TA. When stenosis is due to fusion of the leaflets, tricuspid valve commissurotomy may relieve the obstruction. Stenosis may be alleviated by plastic repair of the valve or valve replacement if the right heart is expected to handle the full cardiac output after closure of the interatrial communication. When there is severe hypoplasia of the tricuspid valve and the right ventricle, an atrioventricular or atriopulmonary conduit may be used. (See previous sections for diagnostic features, anesthesia and perioperative care, and surgical intervention.)

TRICUSPID INSUFFICIENCY

Congenital tricuspid valve insufficiency is usually associated with hypoplasia or atresia of the right ventricular outflow tract. In some cases, the insufficiency is functional. In other cases, the insufficiency is due to dysplastic valve cusps tethered to the right ventricular wall by abnormally short chordae tendineae and papillary muscles.

Clinical manifestations of significant tricuspid insufficiency include jugular venous distension, hepatic enlargement, edema, orthopnea, dyspnea, and a harsh pansystolic murmur. The chest radiograph reveals massive cardiomegaly with the pulmonary vascular pattern being diminished. The ECG demonstrates right axis deviation and a right bundle branch block (RBBB) pattern.

A transient form of tricuspid insufficiency due to papillary muscle dysfunction has been reported to occur in neonates with significant perinatal asphyxia and myocardial ischemia.[55] In older patients, a dilated annulus can be treated by annuloplasty or tricuspid valve replacement.

THE EBSTEIN ANOMALY

The Ebstein anomaly is the most common malformation responsible for congenital tricuspid insufficiency, occurring in about 0.5% of all children with congenital heart disease.[56] The basic pathologic anatomy consists of a spiraling downward displacement of the tricuspid annulus and leaflets into the body of the right ventricle associated with a variable degree of fusion of the leaflets to the wall of the ventricle (Fig 19–7). The functional consequences are (1) tricuspid regurgitation that may be insignificant to severe; (2) inadequate function of the distal pumping right ventricular chamber; (3) paradoxical motion of the aneurysmal "atrialized" proximal right ventricular chamber; (4) dilation of the right atrium; (5) right-to-left shunting through an ASD in most patients; and (6) tachyarrhythmias. There is a wide spectrum of deformity. Some patients are asymptomatic or have only mild cyanosis, whereas others have profound cyanosis with right ventricular failure and arrhythmias.[57]

Anatomy
Rather than originating from the annulus fibrosis, the medial (septal) leaflet of the tricuspid valve is attached to the ventricular septum in the Ebstein anomaly. These attachments take a spiraling, open, rather than

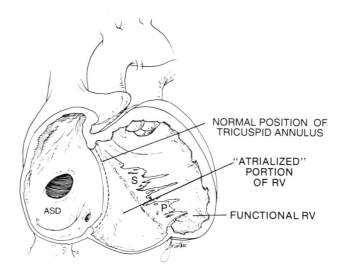

Figure 19–7. The Ebstein anomaly with spiraling displacement of the annulus and the leaflets of the tricuspid valve into the body of the right ventricle. This creates an ineffective atrialized proximal right ventricular chamber and a distal pumping right ventricular chamber.

closed, configuration, with the point of maximum displacement usually at the commissure between the septal and posterior leaflets. The anterior leaflet is enlarged and elongated, often described as sail-like, and is the least affected of the three leaflets. The septal and posterior leaflets vary considerably in size, with the septal leaflet being most dysplastic, sometimes vestigial, and the posterior leaflet being more often elongated than reduced in size. These leaflets usually have many, short chordae connected to multiple, small papillary muscles. The edge of the distal anterior leaflet is usually closely bound to the free wall of the ventricle, occasionally to the septum, and rarely to the medial and anterolateral papillary muscles, its normal attachment.

The function of the tricuspid valve in the Ebstein anomaly is primarily determined by the adherence of the anterior leaflet to the ventricular wall. Most valves are incompetent, although stenosis may occur to varying degrees. Stenosis results from partial adherence of the distal margin of one leaflet to another or obstruction of the right ventricular outflow tract by billowing of the anterior leaflet.[58]

The downward displacement of the valve divides the right ventricle into two parts. A proximal part is continuous with the right atrium and is referred to as the "atrialized" portion because it lies above the tricuspid valve and is functionally integrated with the right atrium. This atrialized chamber is often dilated. Occasionally, its wall is so thin that it moves paradoxically during ventricular systole and may even distend during atrial systole. The anatomic right atrium is consistently enlarged, sometimes massively. A dilated patent foramen ovale or an ostium secundum ASD is present in almost all cases.

The distal chamber is the functional right ventricle and, because it lies below the displaced valve, it is smaller than a normal ventricle. However, it is almost always dilated with a thinner wall than normal, containing fewer than the normal number of muscle fibers. This may be a feature of the developmental anomaly in addition to being a consequence of tricuspid insufficiency.[59]

Pathophysiology

Several mechanisms combine to produce the various manifestations of the Ebstein anomaly. Tricuspid incompetence is generally present, ranging from mild to severe. Infrequently, a variable degree of obstruction may exist between the two parts of the right ventricle, usually with incompetence. Right ventricular dysfunction occurs because of decreased myocardial thickness,[59] the small size of the functional right ventricular chamber, and/or the cardiomyopathy that develops from tricuspid valve dysfunction. Right-to-left shunting through an interatrial communication is often present, accounting for cyanosis and creating the potential for paradoxical emboli.

Paradoxical motion of the aneurysmal atrialized portion of the right ventricle may also contribute to right-sided dysfunction. During atrial systole, a portion of the blood in the right atrium is propelled into the atrialized ventricle, which dilates to accommodate this blood. During ventricular systole, the blood contained in the atrialized ventricle is forced back into the true atrium. This "ping-pong" effect leads to ineffective forward right ventricular output.

Cyanosis is a common sign of the Ebstein malformation. It occurs in more than half the patients and is severe in about a third.[60] Cyanosis is common in the newborn and may be severe when forward flow is restricted by high (neonatal) PVR, poor right ventricular contraction, and massive tricuspid incompetence.[61] The intense cyanosis due to shunting at the atrial level commonly resolves as PVR decreases, thus decreasing right atrial pressure. Cyanosis frequently recurs between the ages of 5 and 10 years as tricuspid insufficiency and right ventricular dysfunction lead to dilatation of right heart structures. As the tricuspid valve orifice dilates, a vicious cycle ensues. Increased insufficiency of the tricuspid valve leads to increased right atrial pressure causing a greater right to left shunt and worsening cyanosis. When episodes of recurrent cyanosis occur, paroxysmal tachycardia should be suspected because tachycardia enhances tricuspid insufficiency by reducing the duration of diastolic filling of the functional ventricle, thus increasing right atrial pressure.

Natural History

The extreme variability of the pathologic anatomy in the Ebstein anomaly accounts for the wide spectrum of functional abnormalities. Neonates may present with cyanosis, severe cardiomegaly, and congestive heart failure. Although one half of patients present during the first few months of life,[62] the onset of episodic cyanosis, dyspnea, fatigability, and palpitations may occur in infancy, childhood, or not until very late in life. Other patients may remain asymptomatic throughout a normal life-span with a mild deformity found only at autopsy.

Diagnostic Features

Although a normal sinus rhythm is usually present in the Ebstein anomaly, dilatation of the right atrium produces a wide variety of arrhythmias, mostly supraventricular. Paroxysmal atrial tachycardia occurs in more than 25% of patients and 5–20% of patients with the disorder have a Kent bundle associated with the Wolff-Parkinson-White syndrome.[63] Right bundle branch block is also common. Valve displacement can also be seen on echocardiography.

Cardiomegaly and decreased pulmonary vascular markings are commonly seen on chest radiograph. Right atrial dilatation and displacement of the right ventricular outflow track produce a funnel-shaped cardiac silhouette with severe forms of the Ebstein anomaly.

At cardiac catheterization, the right ventricle may be difficult to enter with a catheter. Alternatively entrance into the pulmonary outflow tract may require extensive manipulation due to its unusual position and dilatation. Simultaneous determination of electrocardiogram and intracardiac pressure demonstrate the characteristic finding of an atrial pressure waveform with a right ventricular electrogram in the atrialized right ventricle.

Anesthesia and Perioperative Management

The major anesthetic issues in children with the Ebstein anomaly are (1) decreased cardiac output, (2) right-to-left intracardiac shunting, and (3) the propensity for tachyarrhythmias. The success or failure to manage any one of these problems correlates with success or failure in the management of the others.

Forward flow through the residual functioning right ventricle is compromised by its reduced size and pumping capacity, as well as the inefficiency due to tricuspid incompetence. Forward flow is maximized and regurgitant fraction minimized by reducing PVR, maintaining a heart rate that is normal for age, optimizing right ventricular preload, and maintaining an adequate state of contractility.

A heart rate that is higher than normal may increase the regurgitant fraction, raise the right atrial pressure, and increase the right-to-left shunt producing more profound hypoxemia.[64] A baseline tachycardia may also increase the likelihood of tachyarrhythmias. Higher heart rates shorten diastole, which further impedes right ventricular filling and increases right atrial pressure.

Effective preoperative sedation and adequate depth of anesthesia decrease the likelihood of tachycardia. Patients with severe hemodynamic compromise benefit from the safety of an intravenous induction and maintenance of anesthesia with oxygen, fentanyl, and vecuronium. This is one of many combinations that avoid the myocardial depressant and arrhythmogenic effects of potent inhalation agents. When nonvagolytic drugs such as vecuronium, atracurium, and metocurine are given, narcotic-induced bradycardia is unopposed and may require treatment with atropine. Pancuronium is a useful neuromuscular blocking drug in these patients because it has modest vagolytic and sympathomimetic effects. Drugs that may precipitate tachycardia such as isoflurane, atropine, and gallamine should be avoided. The initial treatment of hypotension should depend upon intravenous fluids and/or phenylephrine rather than drugs with positive chronotropic effects.

Additional methods to avoid tachycardia and tachyarrhythmias include (1) continuing preoperative antiarrhythmic medications throughout the perioperative period; (2) avoiding pulmonary artery catheters and utilizing caution during placement of CVP monitors that might precipitate tachyarrhythmias[65]; and (3) minimizing mechanical stimulation of the irritable atria during dissection and cannulation. The risk of tachyarrhythmias may be so threatening as to warrant the use of femoral vessels to establish partial cardiopulmonary bypass. Because of its close proximity to the valve annulus, the AV node may be injured during tricuspid valve repair or replacement causing temporary or permanent conduction disturbances. Except for patients with the Wolff-Parkinson-White (WPW) syndrome who had division of accessory pathways, arrhythmias remain a significant problem in both the early and late postoperative period. Prolonged postoperative intensive care is indicated, followed by ambulatory monitoring, because ventricular tachycardia and ventricular fibrillation have been reported after uncomplicated intraoperative courses.[66]

Supraventricular arrythmias should be treated aggressively. If the arrhythmia is associated with significant hypotension, synchronized electrical cardioversion beginning with 0.5 J/kg should be performed. Adenosine, an endogenous purine nucleotide, depresses AV conduction and is effective for tachyarrhythmias that depend on a reentrant circuitry involved the AV node. Adenosine acts rapidly and has a short duration of action because its half-life is only a few seconds. If the initial dose of 50–100 µg/kg is ineffective, the dose may be doubled.[67–69] Adverse effects that subside within a few minutes include dyspnea, facial flushing, chest pain, and complete AV block. When SVT recurs or persists despite adenosine, longer-acting medications such as propranolol or procainamide are options to slow the heart rate. Digoxin slows AV nodal conduction but should be avoided in patients with the WPW syndrome because they become more susceptible to ventricular fibrillation with digoxin therapy. Verapamil should be avoided in all infants because it is rarely effective and it has been associated with significant, unpredictable hypotension and/or complete AV block.

Immediate and Long-term Outlook

Because of the high incidence of postoperative ventricular arrhythmias, a 20–40 µg/kg/min lidocaine infusion is started at the termination of cardiopulmonary bypass and maintained for at least 48 hours. Telemetry monitoring is maintained throughout the hospitalization. Long-term antiarrhythmic therapy may be necessary. Because of the variability of the pathologic anatomy, long-term outcome without therapy is unclear. With valve repair or replacement, additional valvular procedures may subsequently be required for progressive regurgitation, stenosis, or prosthetic failure.

Surgical Techniques

Surgical intervention is indicated for severe cyanosis, congestive heart failure, and/or severe arrhythmias. Patch closure of the ASD may be all that is necessary when the tricuspid valve and the distal right ventricular chamber function adequately. Most often, tricuspid insufficiency secondary to an Ebstein malformation is treated by closure of the ASD and plastic repair of the valve. In selected cases when the atrialized right ventricle is large, thin-walled, and moves paradoxically,[70] the repair advocated by Danielson (Fig 19–8) is performed. This repair excludes the ineffective aneurysmal atrial portion with plication by the use of pledgeted mattress sutures to bring the displaced line of insertion of the anterior and posterior leaflets back to the normal annulus.[66] If the valve remains incompetent, the diameter of the annulus can be further reduced by a posterior annuloplasty (Fig 19–9).

The indications for tricuspid valve replacement are controversial because the success of the Danielson repair has significantly reduced the need for replacement. Only 19% of Danielson's own patients received a valve replacement.[66] A low-profile prosthetic valve inserted at the true annulus or in a supra-annular position above the coronary sinus and conduction tissues (Fig 19–10) is used when valve replacement is necessary. Plication of the atrialized chamber is also done if it is aneurysmal.[67]

When the Wolff-Parkinson-White syndrome is present and there is a history of life-threatening paroxysmal tachyarrhythmias, electrophysiologic mapping permits obliteration of the accessory conduction pathway.[68] At the time of operation, the ASD is closed and valve defects are treated if necessary. Other arrhythmias are not indications for surgery because their incidence is not affected by correction of the defective valve.

Surgical management of neonates with palliative surgical procedures such as a systemic to pulmonary arterial shunt carries a high mortality.[63] Starns et al recently reported successful palliation of five neonates with

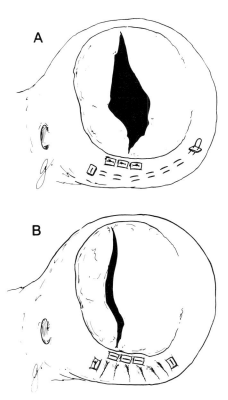

Figure 19–9. Danielson repair for the Ebstein anomaly. If the tricuspid valve remains incompetent following plication of the atrialized chamber (*A*), the diameter of the annulus can be further reduced by a posterior annuloplasty (*B*).

the Ebstein anomaly and ductus-dependent pulmonary blood flow.[70] They closed the tricuspid valve with autologous pericardium and created an aorta to pulmonary shunt with 4-mm polytetrafluoroethylene tubing. No operative or late deaths occurred and pulmonary blood flow is expected to support growth and development until an eventual Fontan procedure is performed.

CONGENITAL MALFORMATIONS OF THE MITRAL VALVE

The normal mitral valve apparatus consists of four primary components: (1) the fibrous annulus, (2) anterior (aortic) and posterior (mural) leaflets, (3) chordae tendineae, and (4) two papillary muscles. Realizing its complexity and central location, it is not surprising that congenital malformations of the mitral valve rarely involve just one of these primary components. Most often the entire valve is affected, and in three fourths of the patients, other congenital heart lesions coexist, usually involving the left-sided chambers and the aorta. Malformations of one or more of the components may produce stenosis, insufficiency, or combined stenosis and insufficiency.

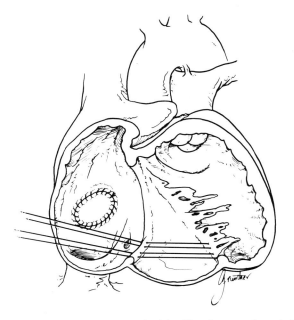

Figure 19–8. The Danielson repair of the Ebstein anomaly excludes the ineffective aneurysmal atrialized portion. The displaced lines of insertion of the anterior and posterior leaflets are plicated to the normal annulus.

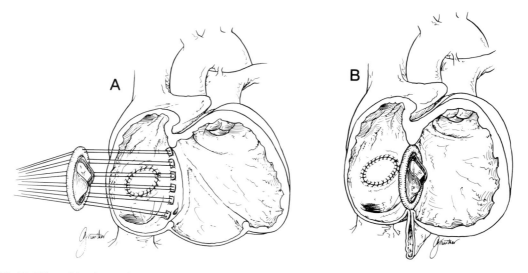

Figure 19–10. Tricuspid valve replacement with plication of the atrialized ventricle. (*A*) A low-profile prosthetic valve may be inserted either at the true annulus or, as illustrated, in a supra-annular position above the coronary sinus and the conduction tissue. (*B*) Plication of the atrialized chamber is done if it is aneurysmal.

Anatomy

Most congenital mitral stenosis, other than that within the hypoplastic left heart syndrome, occurs with a functionally adequate left ventricle. A relatively frequent cause is isolated fusion of the leaflets. Both papillary muscles are implanted directly onto the commissures, restricting the motion of the leaflets and reducing the orifice area.[71] Other causes of restricted leaflet motion include chordae that are shortened, thickened, fused, and/or abnormally attached. Leaflet motion may also be restricted by papillary muscles that are thickened and fused or even absent. The "parachute" mitral valve is another relatively frequent cause of mitral stenosis in which normal leaflets are attached to shortened chordae that converge on a single, large papillary muscle.[66] Stenosis results from obliteration of the interchordal spaces and the inability of the free edges of the mitral leaflets to open during diastole.

A supravalvular ring of thickened endocardium located just on the left atrial side of the mitral annulus is capable of producing variable degrees of obstruction above the mitral orifice. Although this abnormality of the left atrium may occur as an isolated defect, it is usually part of the Shone complex of four obstructive lesions in series: (1) a supravalvular ring, (2) a "parachute" mitral valve, (3) subaortic stenosis, and (4) coarctation of the aorta.[72] The "hammock" valve describes obstruction due to a combination of intermixed chordae and many short, abnormal papillary muscles implanted on the ventricle just underneath the posterior leaflet.[73] Hypoplasia of the annulus may be an isolated finding responsible for stenosis of the valve associated with a left ventricle of adequate size. Mitral stenosis occurring in association

with hypoplastic left heart syndrome is discussed in Chapter 16.

Congenital mitral insufficiency occurs from dilatation of the mitral annulus that prevents the leaflets from coming together during systole. Primary annular dilatation is a rare isolated finding in neonates, being associated with an ASD in 50% of cases.[74] Secondary annular dilatation results from left ventricular enlargement or other causes of mitral regurgitation. The most common leaflet anomaly is a cleft anterior leaflet. This occurs as either a true cleft that separates the anterior leaflet into two hemi-leaflets with abnormal chordae often attached to the free edges of the cleft, or a "tri-leaflet" mitral valve identical to that seen in partial endocardial cushion defects. In the rare case of an isolated posterior leaflet anomaly, perforations or localized agenesis is responsible for regurgitant flow.

Mitral valve prolapse is a common, almost always benign cause of mild regurgitation rarely requiring surgical intervention. Systolic billowing primarily involving the posterior leaflet is permitted by myxomatous degeneration of the leaflets, elongated thin chordae, and dilatation of the annulus. It is usually an isolated condition but may be associated with a variety of other diseases.[75]

Insufficiency associated with stenosis may be due to restriction of leaflet motion from commissure fusion, short thickened chordae and/or papillary muscles, or an Ebstein-type mitral valve. This is a rare malformation in which the attachment of the posterior leaflet is displaced downward into the left ventricle creating a proximal "atrialized" chamber and an effective, distal chamber.[76] Although a parachute valve[73] and a hammock valve usually produce only stenosis, both may also allow regurgitation as does any lesion that restricts leaflet mobility. Severe insufficiency (and sometimes stenosis) occurs with anomalous mitral arcade in which the anterior leaflet is immobilized by chordae that are so short and fused that the leaflet appears to connect directly to abnormal papillary muscles.[77]

Pathophysiology

Mitral Stenosis. Isolated mitral stenosis reduces filling of the left ventricle, which may be normal or small in size. Obstruction to left atrial emptying increases left atrial pressure, which in turn increases pulmonary venous pressure, mean pulmonary artery pressure, and PVR. In mild cases, the increase in left atrial pressure maintains a pressure gradient only during the rapid filling phase of diastole, whereas with more severe stenosis, a pressure gradient remains throughout diastole. Left atrial contraction contributes to left ventricular filling, although its effect is significantly reduced as the left atrium enlarges, which makes the duration of diastole more important. Left atrial contraction is rarely eliminated altogether because atrial fibrillation is unusual in children.

Increased pulmonary venous pressure causes perivascular edema and vascular engorgement, reduces lung compliance, and increases airway resistance by compression of adjacent small airways. In severe cases, the pulmonary arterial hypertension causes right ventricular failure and tricuspid regurgitation. The addition of other left-sided lesions such as aortic stenosis or coarctation may cause left ventricular failure, further increasing pulmonary venous pressure.

Mitral Regurgitation. The volume burden of chronic systolic regurgitation through the mitral valve causes the ventricle to dilate and hypertropy. Initially, end-diastolic volume increases, and the forward ejection fraction is maintained. The left atrium also dilates and becomes more compliant, accommodating the regurgitant volume. Because of the increased compliance of the left atrium, pressure changes do not reflect the volume of regurgitation. In contrast, acute mitral regurgitation produces a marked rise in left atrial pressure with giant V waves representing the regurgitant jet of blood ejected into a relatively normal-sized, noncompliant left atrium.

Natural History

Congenital mitral valve disease usually presents early in life with signs of pulmonary venous hypertension, particularly when other cardiac anomalies coexist. Overall, the onset of symptoms occurs within the first month of life in one third of cases and within the first year in three fourths of cases.[78] The most symptomatic infants are those who have low cardiac output, most often due to a combination of mitral stenosis and left ventricular outflow obstruction. By 4 years of age, surgery is performed

in 86% of patients with congenital mitral stenosis and left ventricular outflow obstruction, in 62% with mitral stenosis, and in 39% with mitral insufficiency.[79] Isolated congenital mitral insufficiency produces signs and symptoms of left atrial hypertension. However, mitral regurgitation is usually better tolerated than stenosis. In patients with mitral regurgitation, left heart failure usually develops gradually over a period of years as the regurgitant fraction exceeds 60%.[80] Most importantly, left ventricular dysfunction often becomes unpredictably irreversible. Although isolated congenital mitral insufficiency can produce pulmonary edema in infancy, associated lesions causing left ventricular outflow tract obstruction are usually responsible for early symptoms of left heart failure.[81]

Diagnostic Features

Early symptoms of congenital mitral stenosis or regurgitation include dyspnea, feeding difficulties, failure to thrive, coughing, and recurrent pulmonary infections.

Anesthesia and Perioperative Management

Mitral Stenosis. The most crucial anesthetic consideration is the need to control heart rate. A low-normal to normal heart rate will optimize left ventricular filling by prolonging diastolic filling time. On the other hand, moderate bradycardia may severely reduce cardiac output despite adequate filling time. This is particularly true in patients incapable of increases in stroke volume such as neonates or patients with small left ventricles. Loss of sinus rhythm and atrial contraction further reduces left ventricular filling.[82]

Control of the heart rate begins with effective psychologic preparation and pharmacologic sedation leading to a tranquil induction. The ventricular response to atrial fibrillation is controlled by continuing digoxin throughout the perioperative period in the rare child with this arrhythmia. Depth of anesthesia must be adequate at the time of intubation and other noxious stimuli. Other techniques to control heart rate include avoidance of prophylactic anticholinergics, positive chronotropes, and neuromuscular blocking agents with potent vagolytic effects. There should be minimal mechanical stimulation of the atria internally with catheters and guidewires and externally with surgical dissection and cannulation.

A normal to high-normal preload should be maintained. Excessive preoperative diuresis, perhaps evident only during induction, may require rapid restoration of intravascular volume with isotonic crystalloid. The CVP will have limited value in the presence of mitral stenosis, although trends will be useful in assessing preload and right ventricular function. Pulmonary artery catheters are used only in selected patients because insertion is more difficult in children, tachycardia is likely to be precipitated, and rupture of a pulmonary artery is more likely with pulmonary hypertension. Perioperative management with a central venous catheter initially and a left atrial catheter prior to discontinuing cardiopulmonary bypass are satisfactory alternatives to pulmonary artery catheterization in children.

Pulmonary Hypertension. Preexisting pulmonary hypertension will be aggravated by hypoxia, hypercarbia, acidemia, high mean airway pressures, sympathetic stimulation, hypothermia, and hypervolemia. Nitrous oxide may also increase PVR in children. Studies in adults have consistently documented that nitrous oxide increases PVR causing small increases in patients with normal PVR and large increases in patients with pulmonary hypertension.[83,84]

However, these findings in adults have not been corroborated by a comparable study in infants.[85] In 12 infants with recently repaired congenital heart disease with or without increased PVR, exposure to 50% nitrous oxide produced no significant change in pulmonary artery pressure or PVR. Indirect support for these results came from a study of infants and small children with cyanotic congenital heart disease and right-to-left shunting breathing 70% nitrous oxide and halothane during the induction of anesthesia.[86] As there was no decrease in arterial oxygen saturation on induction, this study suggested that there was no substantial increase in PVR due to 70% nitrous oxide. Nitrous oxide is often avoided because pure oxygen, a selective pulmonary vasodilator, protects the patient from hypoxemia due to hypoventilation and intrapulmonary shunting and minimizes the size of obvious or occult air emboli.

Most patients tolerate the myocardial depression that results from both halothane and nitrous oxide during an inhalation induction with 50% oxygen, 50% nitrous oxide, and halothane. After an intravenous catheter is established, a neuromuscular blocking agent is administered, nitrous oxide is discontinued, and anesthesia is maintained with isoflurane and fentanyl or a benzodiazepine and fentanyl. Even in patients with limited myocardial reserve, it is often possible to at least gain control of the airway using halothane. In patients with severe congestive heart failure, it may be safer to carry out an intravenous induction with incremental doses of fentanyl or sufentanil, perhaps adding incremental doses of a benzodiazepine.[87–89]

The use of ketamine in patients with increased PVR has been limited. Although ketamine might increase PVR, several studies in children with congenital heart disease have documented no significant change in PVR with intravenous ketamine, 2 mg/kg.[90,91] Although ketamine is a myocardial depressant, ejection fraction and cardiac output are preserved after ketamine induction in children with congenital heart disease, probably from the release of catecholamines by ketamine.[90,92]

Mitral Regurgitation. The anesthetic management of patients with mitral insufficiency is designed to improve forward flow. Afterload reduction with arterial vasodilators is the most effective maneuver to improve cardiac output, reduce the regurgitant fraction, and decrease pulmonary hypertension. As with mitral stenosis, preoperative management, with a central venous catheter initially and left atrial catheter prior to discontinuing cardiopulmonary bypass, is a satisfactory alternative to pulmonary artery catheterization. Arterial vasodilators such as nitroprusside are more effective than venodilators such as nitroglycerin[93] because they decrease impedance to left ventricular ejection in addition to decreasing the heart size.[94,95] A decrease in left ventricular size reduces the amount of mitral regurgitation by decreasing the orifice area as the components of the mitral apparatus become better aligned.[96] Inotropic drugs also are useful in reducing heart size and the regurgitant fraction associated with ventricular enlargement.[97]

Optimizing preload remains challenging even after the establishment of invasive monitors. Chronic mitral regurgitation leads to left ventricular dilatation and eccentric hypertrophy that increases ventricular compliance. Left ventricular volume may increase substantially with only a minimal increase in distending pressure. Even smaller pressure changes may not be reflected proximally because of the dilated, extremely compliant left atrium.

A normal to slightly increased heart rate is desirable. With an increased heart rate, the shortened systolic time interval decreases the regurgitant fraction. Bradycardia increases ventricular volume, further increasing the regurgitant fraction.

Anesthetic Induction and Maintenance. The fundamental goals of the anesthetic are to avoid increases in afterload and significant myocardial depression. These goals can be accomplished by many different anesthetic techniques and agents. Except for severe regurgitation with congestive heart failure, a mask induction with 50% oxygen, 50% nitrous oxide, and halothane can be consistently and safely titrated until the airway is controlled and intravenous access established. Narcotic-oxygen anesthesia, supplemented with a benzodiazepine or low concentrations of isoflurane, is often selected for patients with significant myocardial dysfunction.

Termination of Cardiopulmonary Bypass. Problems that complicate weaning from cardiopulmonary bypass after mitral valvuloplasty or replacement are (1) pump failure (particularly in patients who had severe heart failure preoperatively), (2) coronary air or clot embolization after manipulation of the left atrium, and (3) an inability to overcome the increased afterload following the elimination of the left atrium as a low pressure vent. Some causes specifically related to valve replacement include paravalvular leak, injury to the AV node or circumflex artery when the valve is sutured to the annulus, and malfunction of the valve because it is too big, its orientation is wrong, or there is interference by suture, the papillary muscle, or the left atrial catheter. Combinations of an inotrope (isoproterenol, amrinone, or dopamine) and an arterial vasodilator (nitroprusside) are often necessary for discontinuation of cardiopulmonary bypass. An occasional patient requires afterload reduction provided by an intra-aortic balloon pump to separate from cardiopulmonary bypass.

Surgical Technique for Congenital Mitral Valve Disease

Severe symptoms and signs of pulmonary venous hypertension, congestive failure refractory to medical management, and failure to thrive are indications for surgical reconstruction or replacement of the mitral valve. Early repair of associated extracardiac lesions, such as a PDA or coarctation of the aorta, may significantly improve cardiac function.[98] Because there are many disadvantages of prosthetic valves, delaying surgery in marginal cases may lead to a better result with valve repair or, if replacement is necessary, permit insertion of an adult-sized prosthesis once the child has grown.

Mitral Valve Repair. Although a "commissurotomy" was performed successfully for mitral stenosis as a closed procedure as early as 1952,[99] the best functional results with valve repair are currently achieved using total cardiopulmonary bypass. Some reconstructive techniques of the mitral valve include the following.[100,101]

Excision of a supravalvular left atrial ring.

Plication of a dilated annulus (perhaps with the insertion of a Carpentier mitral ring) (Fig 19–11). The use of this prosthetic device before the age of 10 years may create stenosis as the child grows).

Suturing of clefts (Fig 19–12) and perforations.

Separation of fused structures.

Plication of excess leaflet tissue.

Shortening of elongated chordae and/or papillary muscles.

Excision of obstructive tissue.

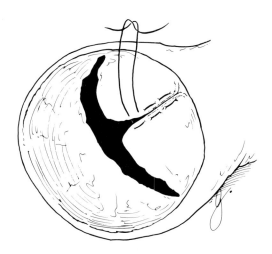

Figure 19–12. Suture closure of a cleft anterior mitral leaflet.

Mitral Valve Replacement. Valve replacement is necessary in 10–15% of patients requiring surgery for congenital mitral valve disease. The decision may be made by surgical inspection. When a patient has difficulty weaning from cardiopulmonary bypass following a valve repair, reestablishment of cardiopulmonary bypass and valve replacement may be necessary. Residual valvular incompetence, suspected by the presence of a thrill within the left atrium associated with an increased left atrial pressure, can be verified by epicardial or transesophageal echocardiography. The surgeon inserts the largest mitral valve prosthesis that will fit within the annulus (and still function properly) so reoperation for outgrowth will be delayed or unnecessary. A mechanical valve is usually chosen despite its risk of rapid failure and tendency to cause thromboembolism requiring long-term anticoagulation.[102] It is necessary to use a low-profile mechanical valve, such as the St. Jude bileaflet valve or the Bjork-Shiley tilting disc valve, whenever the left ventricular chamber is small, as in patients with mitral stenosis. A high-profile mechanical valve such as the Starr-

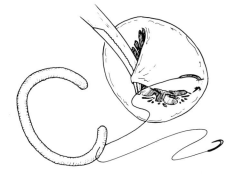

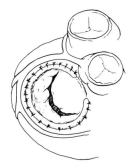

Figure 19–11. Plication of a dilated mitral annulus with insertion of a Carpentier ring.

Edwards ball valve will not only impinge on the left ventricular wall but also restrict ball excursion within the cage. Occasionally, it may produce significant left ventricular outflow tract obstruction.

Postoperative Care. After valve repair, PVR usually decreases, although inotropic support and afterload reduction may still be required. A combination of isoproterenol and nitroprusside is advantageous. Isoproterenol has a potent inotropic effect without unacceptable tachycardia in most situations and will decrease PVR. Despite a reduction in left atrial pressure with surgical repair, mobilization of excessive pulmonary extravascular water occurs over days, requiring gradual withdrawal of mechanical ventilation.

Immediate and Long-term Outcome. Valvular repair rather than replacement is practiced whenever possible even with a less optimal hemodynamic result. Most patients with either congenital mitral stenosis or insufficiency will have at least some incompetence after valve repair, and most patients with mitral stenosis will have a residual diastolic pressure gradient. However, the hemodynamic improvement usually permits the child to grow and be reasonably active. About 20% of patients will need reoperation on the valve up to 10 years postoperatively.[71]

Porcine heterograft and aortic homograft valves are rarely used in infants, children, and young adults because of early failure due to calcification and degeneration leading to stenosis and insufficiency.

REFERENCES

1. Edwards JE, Burchell HB: Congenital tricuspid atresia: A classification. *Med Clin North Am* 33:1177, 1949
2. Vlad P: Tricuspid atresia. In Keith JD, Rowe RD, Vlad P (eds): *Heart Disease in Infancy and Childhood*, 3rd ed. New York: Macmillan, 1978, pp 518–541
3. Michler RE, Rose EA, Malm JR: Tricuspid atresia. In Arciniegas EA (ed): *Pediatric Cardiac Surgery*. Chicago: Year Book Medical, 1985, pp 297–313
4. Bharati S, McAllister HA, Tatooles CJ, et al: Anatomic variations in underdeveloped right ventricle related to tricuspid atresia and stenosis. *J Thorac Cardiovasc Surg* 72: 383–400, 1976
5. Tingelstad JB, Lower RR, Owell TR, et al: Pulmonary artery banding in tricuspid atresia with transposed great arteries. *Am J Dis Child* 121:434–437, 1971
6. Laks H, Mudd JF, Standeven JW, et al: Long term effect of the superior vena cava pulmonary artery anastomosis on pulmonary blood flow. *J Thorac Cardiovasc Surg* 74:253–260, 1977
7. Nishioka K, Kamiya T, Ueda T, et al: Left ventricular volume characteristics in children with tricuspid atresia before and after surgery. *Am J Cardiol* 47:1105–1110, 1981
8. Rosenthal A, MacDonald D II: Tricuspid atresia. In Adams FH, Emmanouilides GC, Riemenschneider TA, (eds): *Moss' Heart Disease in Infants, Children and Adolescents*, 4th ed. Baltimore: Williams & Wilkins, 1989, pp 348–361
9. Nishioka K, Kamiya T, Ueda T, et al: Left ventricular volume characteristics in children with tricuspid atresia before and after surgery. *Am J Cardiol* 47:1105–1110, 1981
10. Moodie DS, Ritter DG, Tajik AJ, et al: Long-term follow-up in the unoperated univentricular heart. *Am J Cardiol* 53:1124–1128, 1984
11. Moodie DS, Ritter DG, Tajik AJ, et al: Long-term follow-up after palliative operation for univentricular heart. *Am J Cardiol* 53:1648–1651, 1984
12. Julsrud PR, Ehman RL, Hagler DJ, Ilstrup DM: Extracardiac vasculature in candidates for Fontan surgery: MR imaging. *Radiology* 173:503–506, 1989
13. Didier D, Higgins CB, Fisher MR, et al: Congenital heart disease: Gated MR imaging in 72 patients. *Radiology* 158: 227–235, 1986
14. Doty DB: Pulmonary artery banding. In Glenn WWL, (ed): *Thoracic and Cardiovascular Surgery*. New York: Appleton-Century-Crofts, 1983, pp 681–687
15. Stow RT, Burrows FA, Lerman J, Roy WL: Arterial oxygen saturation following premedication in children with cyanotic congenital heart disease. *Can J Anaesth* 35:63–66, 1988
16. Reves JG, Kissin I, Fournier SE, Smith LR: Additive negative inotropic effect of a combination of diazepam and fentanyl. *Anesth Analg* 63:97–100, 1984
17. Tomichek RC, Rosow CE, Philbin DM, et al: Diazepam-fentanyl interaction—Hemodynamic and hormonal effects in coronary artery surgery. *Anesth Analg* 62:881–884, 1983
18. Behrendt DM, Rosenthal A: Cardiovascular status after repair by Fontan procedure. *Ann Thorac Surg* 29:322–330, 1980
19. Mair DD, Hagler DJ, Puga FJ, et al: Fontan operation in 176 patients with tricuspid atresia. *Circulation* 82(suppl IV):IV-164–IV-169, 1990
20. Sanders SP, Wright GB, Keane JF, et al: Clinical and hemodynamic results of the Fontan operation for tricuspid atresia. *Am J Cardiol* 49:1733–1740, 1982
21. Fyman PN, Goodman K, Casthely PA, et al: Anesthetic management of patients undergoing Fontan procedure. *Anesth Analg* 65:516–519, 1986
22. Williams DB, Kiernan PD, Schaff HV, et al: The hemodynamic response to dopamine and nitroprusside following right atrium-pulmonary artery bypass. *Ann Thorac Surg* 34: 51–57, 1982
23. Kirklin JW, Barratt-Boyes BG: Tricuspid atresia. In Kirklin JW, Barratt-Boyes BG (eds): *Cardiac Surgery*. New York: John Wiley & Sons, 1986, pp 857–888
24. Heck HA, Doty DB: Assisted circulation by phasic external lower body compression. *Circulation* 64:(suppl II)118–122, 1981
25. Milliken JC, Laks H, George B: Use of a venous assist device after repair of complex lesions of the right heart. *J Am Coll Cardiol* 8:922–929, 1986
26. Freed MD, Heymann MA, Lewis AB, et al: Prostaglandin E$_1$ in infants with ductus arteriosus-dependent congenital heart disease. *Circulation* 64:889–905, 1981

27. Lewis A, Freed M, Heymann M, et al: Side effects of therapy with prostaglandin E₁ in infants with critical congenital heart disease. *Circulation* **64**:893–898, 1981

28. Glenn WWL: Circulatory bypass of the right side of the heart: II. Shunt between superior vena cava and distal right pulmonary artery. Report of a clinical application. *N Engl J Med* **259**:117–120, 1958

29. Dick M, Gyler DC, Nadas AS: Tricuspid atresia. Clinical course in 101 patients. *Am J Cardiol* **36**:327–337, 1975

30. Deverall PB, Lincoln JCR, Aberdeen E, et al: Surgical management of tricuspid atresia. *Thorax* **24**:239–245, 1969

31. Park SC, Neches WH, Mullins CE, et al: Blade atrial septostomy. A collaborative study. *Circulation* **66**: 258–266, 1982

32. Fontan F, Baudet E: Surgical repair of tricuspid atresia. *Thorax* **26**:240–248, 1971

33. Deleval MR, Kilner P, Gewillig M, Bull C: Total cavopulmonary connection: A logical alternative to atriopulmonary connection for complex Fontan operations. *J Thorac Cardiovasc Surg* **96**:682–695, 1988

34. Bjork VO, Olin CL, Bjarke BB, et al: Right atrial right ventricular anastomosis for correction of tricuspid atresia. *J Thorac Cardiovasc Surg* **77**:452–458, 1979

35. Bowman FO, Malm JR, Hayes CJ, et al: Physiological approach to surgery for tricuspid atresia. *Circulation* **58**(suppl I):I-83–I-86, 1978

36. Kreutzer G, Galindex E, Bono H, et al: An operation for the correction of tricuspid atresia. *J Thorac Cardiovasc Surg* **66**:613–621, 1973

37. Haas GS, Laks H, Pearl JP: Modified Fontan procedure. *Adv Cardiac Surg* **1**:111–154, 1990

38. Kirklin JK, Blackstone EH, Kirklin JW, et al: The Fontan operation. Ventricular hypertrophy, age, and date of operation as risk factors. *J Thorac Cardiovasc Surg* **92**:1049–1064, 1986

39. Mayer JE, Hegalson H, Jonas RA, et al: Extending the limits for modified Fontan procedures. *J Thorac Cardiovasc Surg* **92**:1021–1028, 1986

40. Girod D, Rice M, Mair D, et al: Relationship of pulmonary artery size to mortality in patients undergoing the Fontan operation. *Circulation* **72**(suppl II):II-93–II-96, 1985

41. Fontan F, Fernandez G, Costa F, et al: The size of the pulmonary arteries and the results of the Fontan operation. *J Thorac Cardiovasc Surg* **98**:771–724, 1989

42. Nakata S, Imai Y, Takanashi Y, et al: A new method for the quantitative standardization of cross-sectional areas of the pulmonary arteries in congenital heart diseases with decreased pulmonary blood flow. *J Thorac Cardiovasc Surg* **88**:610–619, 1984

43. Pasque MK: Fontan hemodynamics. *J Cardiac Surg* **3**:45–52, 1988

44. Bridges ND, Jonas RA, Mayer JE, et al: Bidirectional cavopulmonary anastomosis as interim palliation for high-risk Fontan candidates. Early results. *Circulation* **82**(suppl IV): IV-170–IV-176, 1990

45. Bridges ND, Lock JE, Castaneda AR: Baffle fenestration with subsequent transcatheter closure. Modification of the Fontan operation for patients at increased risk. *Circulation* **82**:1681–1689, 1990

46. Vargas FJ, Mayer JE, Jonas RA, Castaneda AR: Anomalous systemic and pulmonary venous return connections in conjunction with atriopulmonary anastomosis (Fontan-Kreutzer). *J Thorac Cardiovasc Surg* **93**:523–532, 1987

47. Nakazawa AM, Nojima K, Okuda H, et al: Flow dynamics in the main pulmonary artery after the Fontan procedure in patients with tricuspid atresia or single ventricle. *Circulation* **75**:1117–1123, 1987

48. Matsuda H, Covino E, Hirose H, et al: Acute liver dysfunction after modified Fontan operations for complex cardiac lesions: Analysis of the contributing factors and its relation to the early prognosis. *Thorac Cardiovasc Surgery* **96**:219–226, 1988

49. Hess J, Kruizinga K, Bijleveld CMA, et al: Protein-losing enteropathy after Fontan operation. *J Thorac Cardiovasc Surg* **88**:606–609, 1984

50. Fernandez G, Costa F, Fontan F, et al: Prevalence of reoperation for pathway obstruction after Fontan operation. *Ann Thorac Surg* **48**:654–659, 1989

51. Annecchino FP, Brunelli F, Borhi A, et al: Fontan repair for tricuspid atresia: Experience with 50 consecutive patients. *Ann Thorac Surg* **45**:430–436, 1988

52. Stefanelli G, Kirklin JW, Naftel DC, et al: Early and intermediate-term (10 year) results of surgery for univentricular atrioventricular connection ("single ventricle"). *Am J Cardiol* **54**:811–821, 1984

53. Rhodes J, Garofano RP, Bowman FR Jr, et al: Effect of right ventricular anatomy on the cardiopulmonary response to exercise: Implications for the Fontan procedure. *Circulation* **81**:1811–1817, 1990

54. Zellers T, Driscoll D, Mottram C, et al: Exercise tolerance and cardiorespiratory response to exercise before and after the Fontan operation. *Mayo Clin Proc* **64**:1489–1497, 1989

55. Bueciarelli RL, Nelson EM, Egan EA, et al: Transient tricuspid insufficiency of the newborn. A form of myocardial dysfunction in stressed newborns. *Pediatrics* **59**:330–337, 1977

56. Rowe RD, Freedom RM, Mehrizi A: *The Neonate with Congenital Heart Disease.* Philadelphia: WB Saunders, 1981, pp 515–528

57. Anderson KR, Zuberbuhler JR, Anderson RH, et al: Morphologic spectrum of Ebstein's anomaly of the heart. A review. *Mayo Clin Proc* **54**:174–180, 1979

58. Sealy WC: The cause of the hemodynamic disturbances in Ebstein's anomaly based on observations at operation. *Ann Thorac Surg* **27**:536–546, 1979

59. Anderson KR, Lie JT: The right ventricle myocardium in Ebstein's anomaly: A morphometric histopathologic study. *Mayo Clin Proc* **54**:181–184, 1979

60. Kumar AJ, Fyler DC, Miettinen OS, Nadas AS: Ebstein's anomaly: Clinical profile and natural history. *Am J Cardiol* **28**:84–95, 1971

61. Newfield EA, Cole RB, Paul MH: Ebstein's malformation of the tricuspid valve in the neonate. Functional and anatomic pulmonary outflow tract obstruction. *Am J Cardiol* **19**:727–731, 1969

62. Schiebler GL, Adams P, Anderson RC, et al: Clinical study of twenty-three cases of Ebstein's anomaly of the tricuspid valve. *Circulation* **19**:165–187, 1959

63. Van Mierop LHS, Kutsche LM, Victorica BE: Ebstein anomaly. In Adams FH, Emmanouilides GC (eds): *Moss' Heart Disease in Infants and Adolescents.* 4th ed. Baltimore: Williams & Wilkins, 1989, pp 361–371

64. Blount SG, McCord MC, Gelb IJ: Ebstein's anomaly. *Circulation* **15**:210–224, 1957

65. Linter SPK, Clarke K: Caesarean section under extradural analgesia in a patient with Ebstein's anomaly. *Br J Anaesth* **56**:203–205, 1984

66. Danielson GK, Fuster V: Surgical repair of Ebstein's anomaly: *Ann Surg* **196**:499–504, 1982

67. Arciniegas E: Surgical treatment of Ebstein's anomaly. In Tucker BL, Lindesemith GG, Takahashi M (eds): *Second Clinical Conference on Congenital Heart Disease.* New York: Grune & Stratton, 1982, pp 293–318

68. Sealy WC, Gallaher JJ, Pritchett ELC, Wallace AG: Surgical treatment of tachyarrhythmias in patients with both an Ebstein's anomaly and a Kent bundle. *J Thorac Cardiovasc Surg* **75**:847–853, 1978

69. Overholt ED, Rheuban KS, Gutgesell HP, et al: Usefulness of adenosine for arrhythmias in infants and children. *Am J Cardiol* **61**:336–340, 1989

70. Starnes VA, Pitlick PT, Bernstein D, et al: Ebstein's anomaly appearing in the neonate. A new surgical approach. *J Thorac Cardiovasc Surg* **101**:1082–1087, 1991

71. Shone JD, Sellers RD, Anderson RC, et al: The developmental complex of "parachute mitral valve," supravalvular ring of left atrium, subaortic stenosis and coarctation of the aorta. *Am J Cardiol* **11**:714–725, 1963

72. Roberts WC, Cohen LS: Left ventricular papillary muscles. *Circulation* **46**:138–154, 1972

73. Glancy DL, Chang MY, Dorney ER, Roberts WC: Parachute mitral valve. Further observations and associated lesions. *Am J Cardiol* **27**:309–313, 1971

74. Carpentier A, Branchini B, Cour JC, et al: Congenital malformations of the mitral valve in children: Pathology and surgical treatment. *J Thorac Cardiovasc Surg* **72**:854–866, 1976

75. Gingell RL, Vlad P: Mitral valve prolapse. In Keith JD, Rowe RD, Vlad P (eds): *Heart Disease in Infancy and Childhood.* New York: Macmillan, 1978, p 810

76. Ruschhaupt DG, Bharati S, Lev M: Mitral valve malformation of Ebstein type in absence of corrected transposition. *Am J Cardiol* **38**:109–112, 1976

77. Layan TE, Edwards JE: Anomalous mitral arcade: A type of congenital mitral insufficiency. *Circulation* **35**:389–395, 1967

78. Van der Horst RL, Hastreiter AR: Congenital mitral stenosis. *Am J Cardiol* **20**: 773–783, 1967

79. Kirklin JW, Barratt-Boyes BG: Congenital mitral valve disease. In Kirklin JW, Barratt-Boyes BG (eds): *Cardiac Surgery.* New York: John Wiley & Sons, 1986, p 1098

80. Lake CL: Valvular heart disease. In *Cardiovascular Anesthesia.* New York: Springer-Verlag, 1985, p 150

81. Freed MD, Keane JF, Van Praagh R, et al: Coarctation of the aorta with congenital mitral regurgitation. *Circulation* **49**:1175–1184, 1974

82. Scott KD, Marpole DGF, Bristow JD, et al: The role of left atrial transport in aortic and mitral stenosis. *Circulation* **41**:1031–1041, 1970

83. Schulte-Sasse U, Hess W, Tarnow J: Pulmonary vascular responses to nitrous oxide in patients with normal and high pulmonary vascular resistance. *Anesthesiology* **57**:9–13, 1982

84. Hilgenberg JC, McCammon RL, Stoelting RK: Pulmonary and systemic vascular resistance responses to nitrous oxide in patients with mitral stenosis and pulmonary hypertension. *Anesth Analg* **59**:323–326, 1980

85. Hickey PR, Hansen DD, Strafford M, et al: Pulmonary and systemic hemodynamic effects of nitrous oxide in infants with normal and elevated pulmonary vascular resistance. *Anesthesiology* **65**:374–378, 1986

86. Hensley FA, Larach DR, Stauffer RA, Waldhausen JA: The effect of halothane/nitrous oxide/oxygen mask induction on arterial hemoglobin saturation in cyanotic heart disease. *J Cardiothorac Anesth* **1**:289–296, 1987

87. Hickey P, Hansen DD: Fentanyl- and sufentanil-oxygen-pancuronium anesthesia for cardiac surgery in infants. *Anesth Analg* **63**:117–124, 1984

88. Moore RA, Yang SS, McNicholas KW: Hemodynamic and anesthetic effects of sufentanil as the sole anesthetic for pediatric cardiac surgery. *Anesthesiology* **62**:725–731, 1985

89. Hansen DD, Hickey PR: Anesthesia for hypoplastic left heart syndrome: Use of high-dose fentanyl in 30 neonates. *Anesth Analg* **65**:127–132, 1986

90. Hickey PR, Hansen DD, Cramolini GM, et al: Pulmonary and systemic hemodynamic responses to ketamine in infants with normal and elevated pulmonary vascular resistance. *Anesthesiology* **62**:287–293, 1985

91. Morray JP, Lynn AM, Stamm SJ, et al: Hemodynamic effects of ketamine in children with congenital heart disease. *Anesth Analg* **63**:895–899, 1984

92. Bini M, Reves JG, Berry D, et al: Ejection fraction during ketamine anesthesia in congenital heart disease patients. *Anesth Analg* **63**:186, 1984 (abstr)

93. Pierpoint GL, Talley RC: Pathophysiology of valvar heart disease. *Arch Intern Med* **142**:998–1001, 1984 (abstr)

94. Goodman DJ, Rossen RM, Holloway EL, et al: Effect of nitroprusside on left ventricular dynamics in mitral regurgitation. *Circulation* **50**:1025–1032, 1974

95. Harshaw CW, Grossman W, Munro AB, McLaurin LP: Reduced systemic vascular resistance as therapy for severe mitral regurgitation of valvular origin. *Ann Intern Med* **83**:312–316, 1975

96. Perloff JW, Roberts WC: The mitral apparatus. Functional anatomy of mitral regurgitation. *Circulation* **46**:227–239, 1972

97. Thomas SJ, Lowenstein E: Anesthetic management of the patient with valvular heart disease. *Int Anesth Clin* **17**:67–96, 1979

98. Collins-Nakai RL, Rosenthal A, Castaneda AR, et al: Congenital mitral stenosis: A review of 20 years experience. *Circulation* **56**:1039–1047, 1977

99. Bower BD, Gerrard JW, D'Abreu AL, Parsons CG: Two cases of congenital mitral stenosis treated by valvotomy. *Arch Dis Child* **28**:91–97, 1953

100. Carpentier A: Congenital malfunction of the mitral valve. In Stark J, deLeval M (eds): *Surgery for Congenital Heart Defects.* New York: Grune & Stratton, 1983, pp 453–466

101. Edmunds LH, Wagner HR: Congenital anomalies of the mitral valve. In Arciniegas EA (ed): *Pediatric Cardiac Surgery.* Chicago: Year Book Medical, 1985, pp 325–336

102. Dunn JM: Prosthetic cardiac valves in children. In Morse D, Steiner RM, Fernadez J (eds): *Guide to Prosthetic Cardiac Valves.* New York: Springer-Verlag, 1985, pp 191–208

Chapter 20 | Anomalies of the Aortic Arch and Valve

David A. Rosen and Kathleen R. Rosen

Children with anomalies of the aortic arch and valve are frequently asymptomatic. The presentation is often a murmur or a slight decrease in activity. Infants and neonates with these anomalies are more likely to present with congestive heart failure than older children. Table 20–1 is a schematic presentation of congestive heart failure associated with these lesions. Cyanosis rarely appears with these aortic lesions but can be associated with them if they have progressed to advanced stages when pulmonary hypertension and pulmonary edema become a problem. The association of these lesions with abnormalities in the coronary arteries brings ischemic changes to the arena of congenital heart disease.

Although this chapter discusses anomalies of the aortic arch and valve individually, they frequently occur in combination with other aortic and with nonaortic lesions. It is up to the cardiac team to determine which lesion predominates and to care for patients according to their primary and secondary congenital malformations.

CONGENITAL AORTIC STENOSIS

Aortic stenosis (AS), one of the five most common congenital heart lesions, accounts for approximately 5–10% of all congenital heart defects. Obstruction to left ventricular outflow can occur at valvar (85%), subvalvar (8–10%), or supravalvar levels (Fig 20–1). Isolated supravalvar AS is often a cardiac manifestation of the Williams syndrome. The incidence of congenital AS may be significantly underestimated. Bicuspid aortic valves are frequent precursors of valvar AS and may occur in up to 1% of the general population.[1] Additional cardiovascular anomalies, especially ventricular septal defect (VSD), patent ductus arteriosus (PDA), and coarctation of the aorta, are noted in 20% of patients with valvar AS and over 50% of patients with subvalvar AS. Valvar and subvalvar AS occur two to four times more frequently in boys than in girls. Acquired bicuspidlike valves occur by fusion of the tricuspid aortic valves and are usually the result of rheumatic heart disease.[2]

Anatomy

The normal aortic valve has three cusps and an area of 2 cm^2 per square meter of body surface area (BSA). Valvar AS can be classified as mild, moderate, or severe according to the size of the valve orifice[3]; Table 20–2). The structural abnormality in valvar AS may be limited to either the valve annulus or cusps or it may involve both structures.[4] Valve cusps may be abnormal in form (fused, thickened, dysplastic) or number (bicuspid or unicuspid). In the congenital bicuspid aortic valve, the raphe between the hemicusps is below the edges of the valve cusps. This feature differentiates it from a fused tricuspid aortic valve, in which there is fusion at one valve commissure. The fusion of the two hemicusps produces a raphe that is at the same height as the free edges of the cusps.[2] Poststenotic dilatation of the ascending aorta accompanies valvar AS.

Subvalvar AS or left ventricular outflow tract narrowing is rarely present at birth but develops later during childhood.[5,6] Development of subaortic stenosis may be related to the presence of other congenital heart defects.[7]

Narrowing of the left ventricular outflow tract (LVOT) presents in three different forms: (1) A discrete fibrous membrane located within 1 cm of the aortic valve (seen in three quarters of patients); (2) A thicker muscular ridge or collar (seen in 10%); (3) diffuse, "tunnel-like" muscular narrowing of the entire LVOT (seen in 10–15%).

Narrowing of the ascending aorta, beginning above the sinuses of Valsalva, also occurs in three forms: (1) An hourglass-shaped internal constriction seen in the majority of patients; (2) diffuse narrowing of the entire as-

TABLE 20–1. PRESENTATION OF AORTIC ARCH AND VALVE ANOMALIES

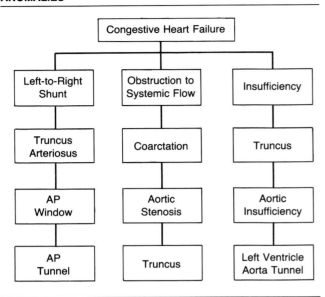

cending aorta described in 25%; and (3) a discrete supravalvar membrane.[8] Involvement of the origins of the brachiocephalic vessels secondary to the Coanda effect is manifested in more than 80% of patients by in-

creased right arm blood pressure.[9] The coronary arteries are exposed to the high LV-generated pressure necessary to achieve flow through the stenotic aorta. Patients with supravalvar AS exhibit dilated and tortuous coronaries and are at increased risk for coronary artery disease. The coronary arteries are also at risk for obstruction from adhesion of the valve leaflets to the obstructing ridge of aortic tissue or from obliteration of the coronary ostia.[10]

Pathophysiology

Although a large variety of anatomic locations and shapes exists in AS, the pathophysiology is similar. Age, however, does influence the physiologic expression of disease. Critical aortic stenosis is seen in newborn infants either shortly after birth or coincidentally with closure of the ductus arteriosus. The transitional circulation results in circulatory failure when the neonatal LV is unable to generate adequate flow through the obstructed LVOT. Right-to-left flow through the ductus arteriosus in the presence of a VSD decompresses the LV and provides perfusion to the lower body. Alternatively, the RV may perfuse the entire body via the duct.

In older children, the LV becomes hypertrophied and classically shows supernormal performance rather than heart failure. Decreased wall stress (afterload) and elevated ejection fraction are seen in congenital, but not acquired, AS and persist into adulthood.[11] LV function

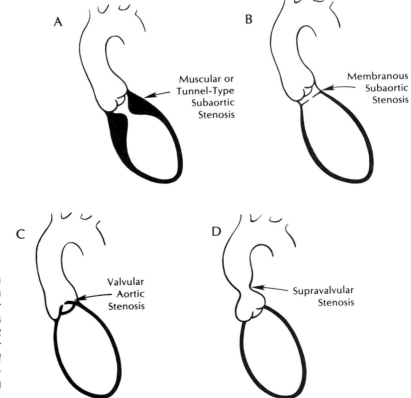

Figure 20–1. Types of congenital aortic stenosis. (A) Fibromuscular or tunnel-type subaortic stenosis with obstruction to left ventricular emptying by muscular overgrowth of the entire outflow tract. (B) Membranous subaortic stenosis in which a membrane is present 1–2 cm below the aortic valve orifice obstructing ventricular outflow. (C) The thickened, domed, fused leaflets of congenital valvular stenosis. (D) The hourglass-shaped narrowing of the supravalvular aorta producing supravalvular stenosis.

TABLE 20–2. CLASSIFICATION AND MANAGEMENT OF AORTIC STENOSIS

Classification	PSEG (mm Hg)	VALVE AREA (m²/m² BSA)	FOLLOW-UP (yr)	Activity Restrictions	Surgery
Trivial	<25	>0.7	2	None	No
Mild	25–50	>0.7	1–2	None if treadmill normal	No
Moderate	50–75	0.5–0.7	1	Light exercise only	Yes, only if symptomatic or + treadmill
Severe	>75	<0.5	Treat	Light recreation only	Yes

PSEG, peak systolic ejection gradient.

and thickness decrease to normal after relief of the obstruction.[12] These patients are at risk for the development of unfavorable myocardial oxygenation supply/demand ratios secondary to ventricular hypertrophy. Myocardial oxygen balance is quantified by the ratio of diastolic to systolic pressure time index. The subendocardial region is at greatest risk for inadequate coronary blood flow.[13] Subendocardial fibroelastosis is a frequent autopsy finding in infants with congenital AS.[14,15] Exercise increases the systolic ejection gradient and therefore increases LV workload, whereas the accompanying tachycardia further impedes coronary flow.[16,17]

In addition to left ventricular hypertrophy and increased work, the physiology of subvalvar and supravalvar AS is frequently complicated by the development of aortic insufficiency (AI). In supravalvar stenosis, the valve shows thickening and abnormal attachment of the leaflets.[18] Valve thickening is acquired in subvalvar stenosis as the normal valve is subject to the high-velocity jet flow.[19]

Natural History

Many older reports emphasized the dire prognosis associated with the severe neonatal form of aortic stenosis. Mortality rates greater than 50% were observed.[20] Many of these infants also had a small LV chamber, a diminutive aortic or mitral valve annulus, or abnormal papillary muscles, and may have fulfilled the diagnostic criteria of hypoplastic left heart syndrome. When these infants are excluded, early and late surgical mortality rates for isolated valvar AS in infancy are 0–15% and 18–24%, respectively[14,21,23] (Table 20–3).

Congenital valvar AS that presents after the first year of life has a much better prognosis. The mean age of death without treatment is 35 years. Early surgical mortality is 2–4% and late surgical deaths occur in 14–20%.[24,25] The incidence of late mortality increases 1.5% per year after the first 5 years. Significant residual stenosis or insufficiency after surgery increases the risk for late cardiac death. Reoperation rates are also quite high and may approach 40%.[24,26] Although only 2% will require additional surgery within the first 10 years, the rate of reoperation increases 3.3% each year thereafter.[24]

Surgical mortality for subvalvar and supravalvar

stenosis is a function of the specific type of lesion. Discrete limited areas of narrowing are relatively easy to repair with low surgical morbidity and mortality rates.[18,27] Tunnel-type subaortic stenosis and diffuse narrowing of the ascending aorta are difficult to treat and are associated with significant morbidity and mortality.[28–30]

Sudden cardiac death is associated with all types of AS and is frequently precipitated by strenuous exercise. Sudden death may occur in as many as 7.5% of patients with AS.[31] The proposed mechanism of sudden death is believed to be dysrhythmia secondary to ischemia or fibrotic involvement of the conduction system.[32] Myocardial infarction, congestive heart failure, and bacterial endocarditis are other causes of late cardiac death. The turbulent flow produced by the high-velocity systolic jets in AS increases the potential for development of endocarditis. This risk does not decrease following repair because of the inherent residual abnormalities of the aortic valve or LVOT.

Diagnostic Features and Methods of Diagnosis

Newborn infants with AS present with signs of circulatory collapse, cyanosis, or congestive heart failure. Hypotension, tachycardia, respiratory distress, poor peripheral prefusion, and irritability are nonspecific signs of physiologic distress in the neonate. Murmur is usually absent. Further studies are necessary to differentiate between the causes of shock in the newborn.

Congestive heart failure is the typical presentation

TABLE 20–3. RECENT SURVIVAL STATISTICS OF SOME AORTIC VALVE AND ARCH ANOMALIES

University of Michigan Congenital Heart Survival Statistics 1986–1991		
Lesion	No. of Cases	Deaths
Truncus Arteriosus	34	4
Interrupted Arch, VSD	22	1
Subaortic Stenosis (Konno) (mean age 5.9 yr)	21	3
Critical Aortic Stenosis (Neonatal)	17	1

in older infants. Difficulty in feeding, poor weight gain, and decreased growth indicate exercise intolerance in infants. Respiratory distress, hepatomegaly, peripheral edema, and diminished peripheral pulses are common signs of congestive failure. A hyperactive precordium and gallop rhythm may also be noted. In infants, the classic murmur of AS is infrequent.

The great majority of older children with all types of AS are completely asymptomatic at the time of diagnosis. A systolic ejection murmur is noted on routine examination. The typical AS murmur is loud, harsh, high-pitched, and crescendo-decrescendo in form. It is best heard at the base of the heart and radiates to the jugular notch. An aortic ejection click associated with valvar AS can be heard at the apex but is uncommon with other forms of AS. The presence of an early low-pitched diastolic murmur suggests the occurrence of aortic insufficiency. Physical examination may reveal a left ventricular lift, and when the left ventricular/aortic ejection gradient is >25 mm Hg, a thrill is usually palpable.[31] The most common complaint of the child with AS is easy fatigability. Other more serious symptoms include dyspnea on exertion, angina, and syncope. Epistaxis, abdominal pain, and profuse sweating are unusual symptoms of AS.

Supravalvar AS is associated in up to 50% of cases of the Williams syndrome.[18,28] The main manifestations of this syndrome are narrowing of pulmonary and systemic arteries, mental retardation, auditory hyperacusis, abnormalities of the teeth, decreased mobility of the cervical spine, husky voice, characteristic elfin facies, and a friendly, "cocktail party" personality. A prominent high forehead and epicanthal folds, small mandible, and underdeveloped nasal bridge make up the elfin facial features. Familial and sporadic forms of AS are also described.

The electrocardiogram in congenital AS can be entirely normal or have signs of increased ventricular work. Infants less than 1 month old typically demonstrate right ventricular hypertrophy. Older infants and children may show signs of left ventricular hypertrophy (LVH) and LV strain patterns. An R wave in lead V_6 or an S wave in lead V_1 indicates LVH. A flattened, biphasic, or inverted T wave or ST depression in V_6 is related to severe stenosis in children.[33] These electrocardiographic (ECG) changes are not specific to AS.

The chest radiograph shows cardiomegaly and pulmonary congestion in neonates or older patients with congestive heart failure or significant aortic insufficiency. In the absence of failure, cardiac size is normal. A rounding of the LV apex accompanies LVH. Left atrial enlargement suggests severe stenosis. Poststenotic dilation of the ascending aorta may be seen in older children.

Visualization of the anatomy of AS is easily accomplished with echocardiography, which has eliminated the need for invasive angiography in many cases. Noninvasive diagnosis is especially useful in the critically ill neonate and for routine serial examinations in older children. The LVOT and subaortic narrowing are better delineated by two-dimensional echocardiography than by angiography. Systolic ejection gradient, aortic insufficiency, and LVH can be estimated by Doppler echocardiography.[34] Prenatal diagnosis of AS can be made with echocardiography. Anticipation of delivery of an infant with AS may affect the outcome favorably by minimizing delays in instituting supportive and palliative therapies.[35]

Cardiac catheterization is reserved for those patients who are surgical candidates. The peak systolic ejection gradient is used to classify the severity of the stenosis and indications for surgery (see Table 20–2).[36] If cardiac output is reduced or a shunt is present, the pressure gradient measured at angiography will not be accurate. Patients with obvious mild or severe valvar AS by echocardiography do not require angiography prior to surgery. Combined right heart and left heart catheterization is recommended for supravalvar and subvalvar AS because of the high incidence of associated cardiac lesions.

Anesthetic and Perioperative Management

Children with supravalvar AS may present with unusual facies or the "elfin facies" of the Williams syndrome and frequently are mentally handicapped. They are occasionally difficult to intubate. Most children presenting for repair of AS, regardless of type, are usually not New York Heart Association class 4 and therefore can tolerate options other than a high-dose narcotic technique. It is important that they not be hypovolemic; therefore, NPO (nothing by mouth) times should be optimized or an intravenous infusion started. Children over 1 year of age are usually premedicated so that they can come to the operating room sedated. The standard monitors are used. In addition, a thermodilution cardiac output pulmonary artery catheter, though not of great value in most repairs of congenital heart disorders, may provide very useful information in anesthesia for AS surgery.

Unless LVEDP is markedly elevated (>16 mm Hg), an inhalation induction is tolerated, and once intravenous access is obtained, the technique may be changed to a narcotic-based technique if the myocardial performance is questionable. The key to anesthesia for AS lesions is maintenance of the heart rate at normal, avoidance of tachycardia, avoidance of a decrease in SVR, and avoidance of myocardial depressants. Heart rate maintenance should be of paramount importance in choosing all the medications given before repair. Not only tachycardia but bradycardia as well should be avoided because bradycardia decreases cardiac output and enhances congestive heart failure if already present (Table 20–4).

Surgical Therapy

Valvulotomy is imperative in the neonate with critical AS. Traditionally, open valvulotomy with exposure of

TABLE 20–4. MANAGEMENT OF AORTIC LESIONS

Lesion	HR Concerns	Anesthetic Goals: PVR-SVR balance	Other Concerns
Aortic stenosis	Avoid increase		Avoid postoperative hypertension Watch for signs of myocardial ischemia
Aortic insufficiency	Avoid decrease		Avoid postoperative hypertension PVCs are an ominous sign
Coarctation	Avoid increase		Keep mean distal aortic pressure >45 during cross-clamp HTN postoperatively
Truncus arteriosus type 1	Avoid increase		Patient at risk for pulmonary hypertensive crisis
Truncus arteriosus types 2 and 3	Avoid increase		Patient at risk for pulmonary hypertensive crisis
Truncus arteriosus type 4	Avoid increase		Variant of tetralogy of Fallot
Patent ductus arteriosus (PDA)			Diastolic pressure will rise
Interrupted arch	Avoid increase		Patient at risk for pulmonary hypertensive crisis
Aortopulmonary window			Similar in physiology to PDA

Symbols: Δ, pulmonary vascular resistance; □, coronary blood flow; ○, systemic vascular resistance.

the valve has been performed, with either cardiopulmonary bypass or in-flow occlusion.[21,37] Experience with alternative methods is increasing.[21,38] Closed valvulotomy, by which Hegar dilators or balloons are progressively inserted into the LV and through the aortic valve, has several advantages. Surgical approach through the left chest allows simultaneous repair of coarctation and is associated with minimal formation of adhesions, thus facilitating the inevitable reoperation.[38] Reduced medical cost is a secondary benefit of the closed procedure.

Sharp incision of the fused commissures with cardiopulmonary bypass is the standard primary surgical approach in older children.[24,26] Ultimately reoperation and valve replacement is expected (see section on surgery for aortic insufficiency below). Prosthetic valve placement is delayed as long as possible in children because of continued growth and difficulties inherent in anticoagulant therapy. The use of bioprosthetic valves avoids the need for anticoagulation in children but is associated with a very high incidence of valve calcification.[39] Early experience with homograft and autograft valves is encouraging; calcification of these valves is delayed and there is no need for anticoagulant therapy.[40,41] With autograft valves, the child's own pulmonary valve is in the aortic position; the valve may grow with the child, so that the need for reoperation on the systemic valve may be minimized.[42,43]

Balloon dilatation is a promising method of treatment for either primary or recurrent valvar or discrete subvalvar AS.[44,45] This technique can be used either as a primary method or for relief of recurrent stenosis after surgical valvuloplasty. Short-term and intermediate results are comparable with those of surgical treatment; long-term follow up is unavailable. In balloon dilatation, a balloon catheter is placed retrograde across the aortic valve and inflated several times at several atmospheres of pressure to open the valve orifice along the fused commissures. The recommended ratio of balloon to annulus diameters is 90–100%[46,47] Ventricular ectopy, hypotension, or bradycardia may occur during balloon inflation. Interventional angiography frequently requires general anesthesia to maintain optimal operative conditions during placement of the catheter. Vascular complications related to the bulk of current angioplasty equipment are frequent, as described later.

Surgery is recommended for subvalvar gradients greater than or equal to 30 mm Hg or if there is a possibility of very rapid progression and secondary valve dysfunction (aortic regurgitation).[48,49] Treatment of discrete fibrous or muscular subvalvar stenosis involves excision of the extra tissue during bypass. During repair, the ventricular septum, the conduction system, septal coronary artery, and left-sided valves are at risk. Tunnel-type stenosis is much more difficult to repair. It is not easy to visualize the site of stenosis, and the mitral valve may be involved. Aortoventriculoplasty or septoplasty

(Konno procedure) may be necessary, with widening of the outflow tract and annulus with a Dacron patch graft and replacement of the aortic valve or valved conduit bypass graft. A conduit from the left ventricle to the descending aorta leaves the native outflow tract unaltered and creates a "double-outlet left ventricle," which provides some retrograde flow to the ascending aorta.[50]

Repair of discrete hourglass-type supravalvar stenosis is similarly straightforward. Resection of the discrete obstruction is performed via a lateral aortotomy with patch closure into the single noncoronary cusp or an extended bisinus approach.[51] Like subaortic lesions, diffuse supravalvar stenosis is difficult to relieve surgically. The brachiocephalic and coronary circulations may be compromised during the repair and residual gradients are frequent. Approaches to the surgical treatment of the lesion include a long-segment aortoplasty, LV to descending aorta conduits, and replacement of the entire aortic root with a valve.

Postoperative Care

After the relief of the aortic obstruction, the hypertrophied myocardium may result in systemic hypertension. Hypertension should be controlled with β-blockers or vasodilators. β-Blockers are particularly useful if there has been a dynamic component to the obstruction. Otherwise, sodium nitroprusside is often used for precise control of the blood pressure. Nitroglycerin may be used if manipulation of the coronaries during repairs causes changes suggestive of myocardial ischemia. Early extubation, another means of controlling blood pressure, is a possibility, particularly in those lesions in which ventriculotomy has not been performed. Extubation may be delayed for 24–48 hours in cases of tunnel-like subvalvar AS that require extensive myocardial resection. Because subvalvar AS repairs are so close to the conduction system, a temporary pacemaker must be present. Slow heart rates after discontinuation of bypass pump should be treated with a pacemaker rather than with chronotropic agents, which may exacerbate any residual obstruction.

Immediate and Long-term Results

Surgical attempts to reduce the pressure gradient of valvular AS are successful in the majority of cases if the lesion is isolated and discrete. Significant residual gradients are more likely with diffuse lesions and occur in up to 25% of patients. These operations are usually palliative rather than curative. Aortic insufficiency (AI) is seen in approximately 15% of patients postoperatively but gradually develops in 90% of patients over the next 20 years.[24] Both residual AS and AI increase the risk of late sudden death.[24] However, moderate residual stenosis is better tolerated than insufficiency.[37] Reoperation will probably be necessary in all patients within 40 years of the original procedure for either stenosis or insufficiency.[24] If the primary procedure was performed in infancy then a second valvulotomy may be tried in lieu of valve replacement. Subvalvar lesions can also recur.

After repair of supravalvar AS, there may be problems with myocardial blood flow resulting from decreased flow to the hypertrophied left ventricle, a secondary effect of the sudden decrease in coronary driving pressure that occurs after the obstruction has been relieved.[52] Other potential complications affecting long-term morbidity and mortality are arrhythmias, congestive heart failure, coronary insufficiency, embolism, and bacterial endocarditis.

Postoperative Results of Balloon Angioplasty. Balloon dilatation valvuloplasty fails to relieve the obstruction adequately in 5–30% of children.[43,44,53–55] Aortic insufficiency is induced or worsened in 33–60% of patients.[43,54,55] Mild to moderate insufficiency is most common. Severe AI is associated with unicommissural valves or injury to the valve during angiography.[46] Major life-threatening complications are reported in 5% of patients, including LV perforation with tamponade, avulsion, or perforation of the aortic or mitral valve cusps, femoral artery avulsion or rupture, dislodgement of the balloon with embolization, exsanguination requiring transfusion, and death during the procedure.[47] Serious complications are more frequent in infants under 1 year of age.[47] Injury to the femoral artery from the large angioplasty catheters occurs in up to 45% of patients.[56] Simple iliofemoral thrombosis is the most common complication; thrombolytic drugs can restore the pulse in the majority of cases. Complete or partial disruption of the artery may require surgical repair of the vessel or volume resuscitation. Cardiac conduction abnormalities are also a potential problem after balloon aortic valvulotomy. Transient His-Purkinje abnormalities have been reported in up to 38% of patients.[57] Fortunately, complete heart block or AV node dysfunction appears to be very rare (<1.5% of cases).[57]

AORTIC VALVE INSUFFICIENCY

Anatomy

Unlike congenital aortic valvular stenosis, aortic valve insufficiency (AI) is an acquired lesion. It is frequently the result of the repair of aortic stenosis (whether surgically or by balloon dilatation) and is due to fibrosis, thickening, and contracture of the aortic valve leaflets.

Both AI and aortic stenosis may occur after rheumatic heart disease, although stenosis takes longer to develop. Insufficiency is also the primary complication seen with juvenile rheumatoid arthritis, in which it progresses more rapidly than it does in rheumatic fever. Other less common etiologies of AI in the child include bacterial endocarditis and the Marfan syndrome. The Marfan syndrome that is present at birth causes dilation

of the aortic sinus of Valsalva; in older children with the Marfan syndrome, incompetency of the aortic valve is more commonly associated with progressive dilation of the aortic root, which causes separation of the valve commissures and impaired coaptation of the valve leaflets.[58]

In doubly committed subarterial or infundibular VSDs, aortic insufficiency is caused by inadequate support of the right coronary cusp and the Venturi effect of the VSD. The association of aortic insufficiency and VSD is more common in East Asia (20–30%) than in the United States (3%).[59]

Pathophysiology

Aortic valve insufficiency occurs when the valve leaflets cannot close the aortic orifice during diastole. Insufficiency is an important finding because a regurgitant area as small as 20% of the valve can double the workload of the left ventricle. Over time, the left ventricle dilates. Initially the increased left ventricular volume does not increase end-diastolic pressure because of an increase in left ventricular compliance. This process functions in conjunction with reflex peripheral dilation to reduce the afterload and improve forward flow. Another compensatory mechanism, left ventricular hypertrophy, has the effect of normalizing left ventricular wall pressure.[60] The insufficiency increases preload, which increases left ventricular stroke volume. As a consequence of the compensatory mechanisms, systolic pressure increases but the diastolic pressure decreases widening the pulse pressure.

Aortic insufficiency steadily increases myocardial oxygen consumption. Myocardial blood flow occurs in diastole, and because the aortic valve is insufficient, the blood flow through the coronaries is reduced. Subsequently, the myocardial oxygen supply decreases, yet the demand steadily increases leading to ischemia, failure of the compensatory mechanisms, and left ventricular failure. A normal ejection fraction is a particularly ominous sign with this lesion. If AI has existed for some time in the presence of rheumatic heart disease, aortic stenosis is usually present as well. This restriction to forward flow interferes with the ventricle's ability to deal with the regurgitant flow and causes the compensatory mechanisms to fail more quickly.

Natural History

The progression of the natural history of aortic insufficiency is presented in Table 20–5. AI is initially asymptomatic but eventually leads to pulmonary edema, heart failure, and angina pectoris. Ventricular arrhythmias are present in unoperated patients with AI. Multiple PVCs are commonly associated with advanced disease and are related to reduced ejection fraction rather than the degree of aortic regurgitation.[61] Five percent of cases of sudden death in the pediatric cardiac population are due to aortic regurgitation.[62] The presence of ventricular arrhythmias in this lesion is so ominous that it is consid-

TABLE 20–5. NATURAL HISTORY OF AORTIC VALVE INSUFFICIENCY

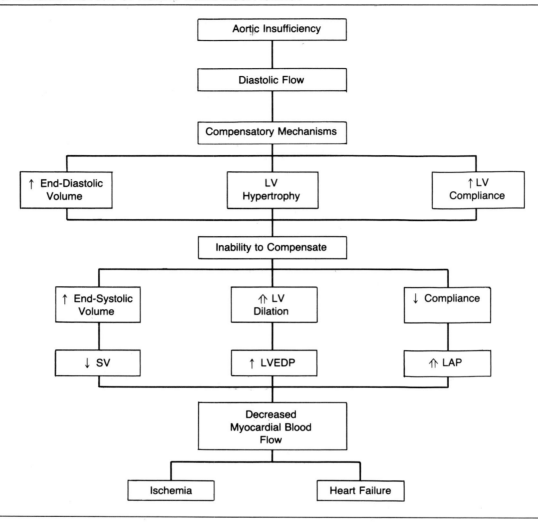

ered as an indication for surgical replacement of the valve.

Diagnostic Features

A number of physical findings are associated with AI. There is an increased left ventricular impulse with a wide pulse pressure and a bounding pulse. On auscultation, a diastolic thrill is often heard at the left third intercostal space. The S_1 is decreased, whereas the S_2 is normal or single. The severity of the regurgitation can be gauged by listening for a high-pitched decrescendo diastolic murmur at the third or fourth left intercostal space. As the severity increases, the murmur generally becomes louder and longer. When heart failure becomes severe and the regurgitation increases, the murmur of aortic regurgitation may decrease or even disappear.

Auscultation of the heart may also reveal a mid-diastolic or presystolic rumble at the apex of the heart. This sound, called the Austin Flint murmur, results from a flutter motion in the mitral valve produced by the aortic regurgitant flow and left atrial filling. It is associated with moderate to severe aortic insufficiency. Austin Flint murmurs occur after left ventricular hypertrophy has developed and the diastolic pressure has fallen below 60 mm Hg.

The electrocardiogram initially shows a normal appearance with subsequent left ventricular hypertrophy and ST and T wave changes indicative of strain. Enlargement of the left atrium is a sign of progressive disease.

The chest radiograph demonstrates cardiomegaly, with the left ventricle dilating inferiorly and leftward. The ascending aortic arch is often dilated, with a prominent aortic knob. Findings of pulmonary venous congestion are seen in more advanced disease. The cardiothoracic ratio appears to be important: The postoperative mortality rate is 30% in patients with cardiothoracic ratios above 0.64 and 7% in those with cardiothoracic ratios below 0.64.[63]

Echocardiography is extremely helpful in diagnosis. The lesion can be detected even with M-mode echocardiography. For example, the M-mode finding of fluttering of the mitral valve is noted from the regurgitant aortic flow and is seen in the majority of isolated lesions. In cases of at least moderate aortic regurgitation, two-dimensional echocardiography demonstrates doming of the mitral valve. Echocardiography is especially useful in assessing left ventricular function, particularly in patients with asymptomatic disease. When the shortening fraction falls below 25% in these patients, left ventricular failure is likely to occur.[64] Although Doppler evaluation of the aortic valve is highly diagnostic, with a sensitivity of at least 90%,[65] it still falls short in determining severity of disease. In this respect, color-flow Doppler appears to be the only real echocardiographic tool for directly assessing the quantity of regurgitant flow.

Aortography is also used to quantitate aortic regurgitation. It uses a 4-point scale: 1 + represents a small wisp of contrast going into the ventricle, and when the rating reaches 4 +, the entire ventricle fills and does not clear for several systoles. Exercise testing may also be a useful tool in evaluating aortic insufficiency because it identifies signs of early left ventricular dysfunction.

Anesthetic and Perioperative Management

The goal of anesthetic management in AI is the encouragement of forward flow (see Table 20–4). Calm relaxed patients have a lower systemic vascular resistance and more forward flow. With older children, therefore, premedication is indicated. Patients should also receive any chronic vasodilator therapy, digitalis, or diuretics preoperatively. It is important that electrolytes be normal and that the volume status be appropriate for the patient.

Children with preserved ventricular function may desire to be anesthetized via inhalation induction. With inhalation induction, however, regurgitant flow tends to produce a higher concentration of agent in the myocardium than in the brain. Isoflurane, which reduces systemic vascular resistance and increases heart rate, is a good choice in these cases. Intravenous induction with a benzodiazepine and a narcotic is chosen in those patients with severely compromised ventricular function. Anesthetic inductions will be slowed by the lack of net forward flow from the left ventricle.

Surgical Technique

Valve replacement is the usual surgical approach to aortic insufficiency because valve repair usually does not eliminate the hemodynamic problems necessitating surgery. Prosthetic valves are commonly used in children, but homografts may also be used. Replacement generally incurs a small amount of stenosis but also results in a well-functioning valve.

The choice of valve frequently depends on the sizes available and the child's activity level. Normally active children, who get cut and bruised, will experience difficulty and danger with mechanical valves that require constant anticoagulation. Moreover, chronic anticoagulation would be a severe problem in a patient who became pregnant.

Bioprosthetic valves are sometimes preferred over mechanical valves because they have a lower incidence of thrombosis and do not require the same degree of anticoagulation; aspirin may be sufficient. With tissue valves in children, there is a higher incidence of calcification, which may result in a much earlier need for replacement than with a mechanical valve. The increased calcification is felt to be secondary to an immunologic response to the presence of a calcium-binding amino acid or possibly secondary to the relatively large calcium uptake in the pediatric patient.[66,67]

Homografts inserted in the aortic position require no anticoagulation and have superior hemodynamics with lower transvalvar gradients than do small-sized mechanical or bioprosthetic valves. Even the smallest mechanical or bioprosthetic valves (19 mm) requires supporting structures and a subaortic resection (konno) to fit into the aortic root of a small child. On the other hand, when a homograft is used in children, particularly larger children with larger roots, the valve may be inserted "freehand," without supporting structures. The experience with homografts is limited, but a recent report examining 15 years of experience with homograft valves in the aortic position appears encouraging.[67] A human valve, being a tissue valve, offers the clear advantage of not requiring anticoagulation and does not undergo premature degeneration.[67] Homografts, or at least the leaflets, may also remain "viable," thus decreasing formation of Ca^{2+}.

Another option is to place the patient's pulmonary valve in the aortic position (by autograft) and use a homograft for the pulmonary valve. The valve may grow as the child does, and it may have significant advantages over an aortic valve homograft.[67]

The choice of valve depends on a great number of factors: the child, the child's family, social situations, the cardiologist's approach to anticoagulation in the small child, the surgeon, and availability of materials.

Postoperative Care

Postoperatively the dilated left ventricle will no longer be receiving the large regurgitant volume; the potential for some degree of stenosis, particularly when mechanical valves are used, may necessitate inotropic support for a few days. Although extubation is usually not immediate, prolonged intubation is usually not required. Vasodilators are used after surgery to lower the afterload and prevent hypertension. Amrinone, frequently chosen for its inotropic effect and vasodilation, seems to be particularly suited to these patients' needs.

Immediate and Long-term Results

When replacement of the aortic valve is appropriately timed, mortality is low. Mortality, however, may be as high as 20% in the failing heart.[68] Valve replacement in children usually reduces cardiac size and improves left ventricular function. Placement of a prosthetic valve in the aortic position is associated with thromboembolism, which generally requires some form of anticoagulation therapy specific to the valve used. Hemolysis may also occur, particularly if there is a paravalvular leak.

As was previously mentioned, calcification occurs when porcine valves are used in children. Aortic stenosis that develops from patient growth or calcification requires serial echocardiogram studies at least yearly. Furthermore, the mechanical valves must also be followed for failure, as pannus overgrowth around the valve annulus can cause them to become stenotic or regurgitant. In a very small percentage of cases (0.1%), the valve will fail for structural reasons. All types of valve replacements are at risk for the development of endocarditis, particularly because a primary indication for valve replacement is endocarditis-induced AI. An aortic homograft appears to offer some advantage in this situation if a tissue valve has been used.[67] Children must therefore receive prophylaxis for subacute bacterial endocarditis (SBE) whenever they undergo a procedure that places them at risk (see Chapter 26).

Common to most of the lesions in this section is turbulent flow. Consequently, they all show increased risk for SBE before operation and many will have an even greater risk after they have been repaired. The risk of death from endocarditis is significantly increased if the patient has undergone an open-heart surgical procedure. For example, a simple ventricular septal defect has an infective risk of endocarditis of 2.4 per 1000 patient-years. The addition of aortic insufficiency increases the risk. After surgery on the aortic valve, the risk increases to 3.8%. On the other hand, if the patient has isolated aortic stenosis that is untreated, the risk for bacterial endocarditis is only 1.8 per 1000 patient-years. If a patient has had endocarditis once, the risk of repeat infection increases geometrically. Following an open-heart procedure for congenital heart disease, the overall mortality for infective endocarditis is 50%.[69] Thus, there is definite need for SBE prophylaxis in these patients.

ANOMALIES OF THE AORTIC ARCH

Coarctation of the Aorta

Anatomy. Coarctation of the aorta results from a ridge-like thickening originating from the aortic media and protruding from the lateral and posterior walls of the aorta. The medial thickening is typical of coarctations that occur at any age, but with the growth of the child, the aortic lumen is further compromised. Preductal coarctations usually present in infancy, whereas juxta-ductal-postductal coarctations, which are more common, present later in life.

Coarctation of the aorta is often not an isolated lesion or localized disease. The process responsible for the coarctation appears to result in other changes, such as the formation of aneurysms in many of the body arteries. The fact that 32% of the aneurysms are proximal to the coarctation site suggests that hypertension is not the sole cause.[70] Coarctation of the aorta is often associated with bicuspid aortic valve. In this setting, cystic medial necrosis also is noted in the aorta, where it causes an intrinsic weakness that may be responsible for the aortic rupture that is not uncommonly seen in these patients in later life even after successful repairs of their coarctation.[71]

The area of narrowing may extend beyond a limited segment. An important issue in repairing coarctations in the neonate, when the coarctation is not small and discrete, is when to repair the aortic arch as well. Preoperative pressure assessment of the associated hypoplasia is not valuable because the coarctation provides back pressure that distorts the pressure gradients that may exist in the hypoplastic aortic arch. Qu et al have identified the minimum outside aortic diameter as 3.9 mm.[72] They have also urged that if the aortic arch index (distal aortic arch diameter to normal aortic ring diameter—the Rowlatt formula)[73] is less than 0.63, both the coarctation and the complete aortic arch should be repaired.

Pathophysiology. The major physiologic effect of coarctation of the aorta is the increased afterload on the systemic ventricle. When the systemic ventricle pumps against a fixed obstruction, the tension in the ventricle is increased and leads to ventricular hypertrophy. Systolic hypertension above the coarctation and systemic hypotension below the coarctation are common. In this condition, the aortic lumen is reduced by 45–55%. The hypertension is felt to be due not only to the obstruction but also to the change in arterial stiffness and capacity of the vascular system proximal to the aorta.[74] The arterial tracing shows a delayed slow upstroke, a rounded peak, and a smooth decline during diastole. Collaterals develop from the subclavian artery to bypass the coarctation site later in childhood. Intercostal arteries collateralize to anastomose below the coarctation site and are responsible for the "rib notching" seen on radiographs. There is a progressive widening of the pulse pressure above the coarctation and a progressive decrease of the pulse pressure below it.

Natural History. Coarctation of the aorta is a relatively common congenital heart malformation occurring in 1 in 1200 live births. The natural history of the disease, if left uncorrected, is death by the fourth decade. The most common identifiable mechanism of death in the uncorrected lesion is cardiac failure (25.5%), followed by aortic rupture (21%), endocarditis (18%), cerebrovascular hemorrhage (11.5%), and other unknown mechanisms.[75]

Diagnostic Features. Coarctation of the aorta is frequently identified on routine physical examination by the absence of femoral pulses. Coarctation is also associated with differential blood pressures in the arms and legs. Other presentations of this lesion in the neonate are tachypnea, poor feeding, and even cardiovascular collapse. In the neonate, the presence of a patent ductus arteriosus may obscure the diagnosis of coarctation; many children will also develop significant collaterals to further obscure the diagnosis. In children over 3 years old, a chest radiograph often discloses rib notching, which is due to erosion of the rib by dilated collateral vessels. Invasive diagnostic procedures in the small child may be associated with significant risk. Therefore, noninvasive evaluation methods, such as echocardiography, are preferred. Conventional two-dimensional echocardiography may fall short in predicting the angiographic severity of the lesion, whereas color Doppler correlates well with angiographic evaluation. Gradients should be measured in both systole and diastole.[76] The area of interest is the acceleration zone in the proximal descending aorta; the distal/proximal acceleration zone ratio is predictive of angiographic severity. The color flow Doppler determination of the width of the accelerating stream immediately proximal to the coarctation site also correlates reasonably well with the angiographic findings. Patients with severe coarctation will demonstrate continued acceleration toward the narrowing. The presence simply of acceleration in the aorta is not pathognomonic of coarctation because normal patients may demonstrate acceleration for a short distance in the proximal part of the descending aorta.[77] Spectral-pulsed and continuous-wave Doppler methods are also useful but must be interpreted cautiously because their results are affected by collaterals or a patent ductus arteriosus.

In utero echocardiographic interpretation has advanced to the point that coarctation can be determined as early as 18 weeks. This is usually not by visualization of a discrete coarctation but rather by noting relative sizes of the ventricles, diminished aortic flow, and a greater than 2:1 flow across the tricuspid and mitral valves. Coarctations diagnosed in this manner usually have a high degree of isthmal hypoplasia.[78] Congenital diaphragmatic hernia may present with similar findings.

Cine magnetic resonance imaging (MRI), like echocardiography, is noninvasive and allows accurate assessment of the degree of coarctation. It has the added advantage of providing definitive anatomy as well as dynamic spatial and temporal visualization of the flow both distal and proximal to the coarctation. Unlike echocardiography, which may be confused by the presence of a ductus, cine MRI is able to analyze ductal and coarctation flows separately.[79] With this technique, however, the patient must lie perfectly still during the examination and data are not obtained in real-time fashion, as with echocardiography. Realistically, only in those situations in which echocardiography is unreliable (eg, patients with lung disease or chest deformities) should MRI be used as the first line of noninvasive diagnostic procedures.

Anesthetic and Perioperative Management. Placement of monitors is critical in the anesthetic management of children with coarctation. The blood pressure above and below the coarctation should be closely monitored to prevent organ damage from hypertension or hypotension. The left arm should not be used for blood pressure monitoring because the subclavian artery may be used in the aortic repair or may be involved in the coarctation itself. An arterial catheter is particularly beneficial to assess and treat acidosis and to control alterations of blood pressure associated with the repair. In children with a well-developed collateral system, there are usually only minimal hemodynamic alterations when the aorta is clamped and unclamped and an arterial catheter may be omitted. Inotropic medications are rarely used after the repair if they were not required before the repair. Because vasodilators or other antihypertensive therapies are commonly used, peripheral intravenous access will frequently suffice and a CVP may not be necessary if the patient has not been on an inotropic support before surgery. Although the coarctation is usually approached via a left thoracotomy, the midline approach may be used in neonates if the coarctation is associated with hypoplasia of the aortic arch. A vascular shunt is rarely required for straightforward coarctations with good collaterals. Shunts may be used for lower body perfusion during aortic cross-clamping, however, and are more commonly used when there is significant upper body hypertension with low descending aortic pressures. A study by Watterson et al identified the critical level for arterial pressure in the descending aorta,[80] suggesting that the arterial pressure in the lower extremity should be maintained at greater than 45 mm Hg in children over 1 year of age. Furthermore, if the blood pressure in the descending aorta is less than 45 mm Hg, the position of the proximal clamp should be adjusted so that the subclavian artery is open and thus allows for collateral flow. Optionally, the distal clamp could be adjusted to allow maximal intercostal artery collaterals. The final step is reducing or stopping agents that might have an effect on blood pressure. If these techniques fail, lower body blood pressure should be supported by a shunt or left heart bypass. The anesthetic technique employed should allow for control of the blood pressure during aortic clamping and unclamping. The P_{CO_2} should also be maintained in the normal range because hyperventilation could decrease central nervous system blood flow. Hyperthermia must be avoided; the child should be allowed to cool down to 35°C. These procedures will allow the spinal cord to remain without blood flow for a longer time during the aortic occlusion. Nevertheless, the incidence of paraplegia, complicating coarctation repair, is reported to be in the range of 1 in 250.[80] Proposed mechanisms of paraplegia are interruption of the blood supply to the anterior spinal artery, inadequate distal flow during cross-clamping, or increased cerebral spinal fluid pressure.[80]

Anticoagulation of these patients during cross-clamping of the aorta is frequently used. With infants in their first year who present with congestive heart failure, heparin, 1 mg/kg, is given before clamping the aorta because of the resulting low-flow state. Infants not in failure or older children with well-developed collaterals probably do not benefit from systemic anticoagulation.

General anesthesia is used by most anesthesiologists for this procedure. When an inhalation agent is chosen, isoflurane is preferred, which controls blood pressure as well as helping to control the afterload if a left-to-right shunt is functional (see Table 20–4). Use of a light general anesthetic with an epidural catheter placed to the thoracic region remains controversial as neurologic injury is possible from the surgery itself when the cord blood flow is decreased. Total intravenous anesthesia can also be used; a high-dose narcotic technique is used in very sick neonates. Ketamine is usually not indicated because of preexisting hypertension.

Surgical Treatment. The approach to coarctation of the aorta depends on the size, length, and associated lesions. Surgical mortality is usually reported as low (<10%).[81] It is important that all the ductal tissue be excised at the time of surgery to prevent recoarctation. In neonates, a technique called subclavian flap angioplasty (SFA) is often used to repair the coarctation. This technique can have long-term effects on the hemodynamics of the left arm, namely, decreased growth, reduced blood flow, or even brachial plexus injury.[82] The best surgical technique, SFA, end-to-end repair, or prosthetic graft, is unclear. Balloon dilatation can be performed in neonates with good early results; however, early restenosis is very common. In the presence of isthmal hypoplasia balloon dilation is dangerous because it may lead to aortic dissection. On the other hand, balloon dilatation may still have a place in infants with other severe associated anomalies.[83] Balloon dilatation is the preferred treatment for recoarctation of the aorta after surgical repair.

There are many controversies in management of children with coarctation if they have other associated heart anomalies, such as ventricular septal defect. One study proposed banding of the pulmonary artery when there is aortic arch obstruction with a large VSD and peak ascending aortic velocity of less than 1 m/s.[84] Others recommend repairing the coarctation and then banding the pulmonary artery.[85] A third approach is repair of both the VSD and coarctation from a median sternotomy.

Postoperative Care. If the child was relatively asymptomatic before surgery, early extubation should be considered, but it is essential that adequate analgesia be provided. Inadequate pain control can contribute to hypertension. Hypertension, both systolic and diastolic, is a common problem after repair and must be carefully controlled. Two types of hypertension are observed after coarctation repair. The first type occurs during the first 24 hours and is related to the carotid baroreceptors. If sodium nitroprusside is used for hypertension, high doses are required. Nitroglycerin is usually not effective in controlling the hypertension, but β-blockers or angiotensin-converting enzyme inhibitors are often chosen. Even though the operation does not involve the abdomen, it is essential that a nasogastric tube be placed. This is necessary because many children have abdominal pain and ileus in the postrepair period. Gastrointestinal bleeding occurs infrequently and is usually attributed to mesenteric arteritis and occurs 1–5 days after repair. Delay in postoperative feeding seems to help minimize this problem, as does pretreatment with propranolol before the repair.

The second form of hypertension is associated with the arteritis seen below the level of the coarctation and is seen in about 50% of the patients who develop hypertension in the first 24 hours. There is increased secretion of norepinephrine for several days and angiotensin levels are elevated for 3–4 days. This hypertension responds well to β-blockers, arterial smooth muscle dilators, and angiotensin-converting enzyme inhibitors. If the child has undergone balloon angioplasty for dilatation of the coarctation, the systolic pressure falls while the diastolic pressure remains the same. Because renin activity and plasma catecholamines also remain unchanged, hypertension is not a problem.[86]

Because of the location of the surgery, injuries to the recurrent laryngeal nerve or phrenic nerve are also possibilities. Paraplegia is a relatively rare complication of coarctation repair occurring in 0.14–0.4% of cases.[87,88]

Immediate and Long-term Results. Except for a need for prophylactic antibiotics to prevent endocarditis, children after successful resection of a coarctation require no special restrictions. However, even after successful coarctation repair, the child must be followed for hypertension, which is reported in 17–50% of patients.[89] The higher incidence appears to be associated with repairs at later ages. Interestingly, hypertension seen after exercise is confined to the upper body and may be associated with early restenosis.[86] This exercise-induced hypertension tends to be associated with accelerated cardiovascular disease and early mortality despite a good repair. β-Blockade, and specifically cardioselective β-blockade, has been examined in an attempt to prevent the accelerated cardiovascular disease.[90] The cause of this exercise-induced differential upper body hypertension is thought to be secondary to the increased stiffness seen in the aorta above the coarctation site as well as the altered baroreceptor function.

Restenosis, another important complication, occurs in nearly 20% of patients. The surgical technique employed and the age at repair both appear to affect the rate of restenosis.[81] In many situations, it appears to be surgically related (ie, not completely removing all ductal tissue or coarctation tissue). There is also a significant incidence of aneurysmal dilatation after repair probably due to associated cystic medial necrosis of the aorta.[91] After patch angioplasty repairs of coarctation, children should be followed with repeated echocardiograms, computed tomography, and chest radiography for formation of aortic aneurysms. The incidence of aneurysms in patients with patch angioplasty repair may be up to 30%; there is a much lower incidence with end-to-end repair.[92]

Interrupted Aortic Arch

Anatomy. Interrupted aortic arch is a rare abnormality accounting for about 1% of congenital heart defects. There are three types of interrupted aortic arch, as depicted in Fig 20–2. Type A, which occurs in 43% of cases, places the interruption between the left subclavian artery and the aortic isthmus. Type B is the most common, occurring in 53% of cases, with the interruption between the left carotid and left subclavian arteries. Type C interruption (4% of cases) occurs when there is lack of continuity between the right and left carotid arteries. A ventricular septal defect is present in more than 80% of the type B and 50% of the type A cases. The ventricular septal defect seen with type B is usually a

defect in the infundibular (outlet) septum, which provides a substrate for subaortic stenosis when closed because of its malalignment. Naturally, a patent ductus arteriosus is seen in almost all cases (98%), but isolated interrupted aortic arch has been reported.[93]

The DiGeorge syndrome is associated with interrupted arch and significantly increases mortality. The syndrome consists of thymic hypoplasia associated with hypoparathyroidism and hypocalcemia. Facial anomalies and immunodeficiency are also common in the DiGeorge syndrome. Truncus arteriosus is seen in 33% of children with interrupted arch and the DiGeorge syndrome. Double-outlet right ventricle is also associated with interrupted arch.[94] Less frequent associations are with aortopulmonary window, single ventricles, endocardial cushion defects, bicuspid aortic valve, and other left-sided obstructive lesions. Obviously, a patent ductus arteriosus or some other aberrant connection must almost always be present for the child to survive.

Pathophysiology. The blood flow to the descending aorta of patients with interrupted aortic arch depends upon patency of the ductus arteriosus. When the ductus starts to close, the lower body is hypoperfused, metabolic acidosis develops, and renal insufficiency occurs. Most of the cardiac output is directed into the pulmonary circulation by the ductal closure and decreasing pulmonary vascular resistance. Associated pathophysiologic problems include shunting through ventricular septal defects or aortopulmonary windows and left ventricular outflow obstruction caused by a malaligned interventricular system or mitral valve attachments.

Natural History. Patients with interrupted aortic arch usually die early in infancy, typically when the ductus closes. Blood flow in the ductus is usually reversed and deterioration, which starts early in the newborn period, is usually rapid. As the ductus closes, more blood flow is forced into the lungs and less blood is sent to the de-

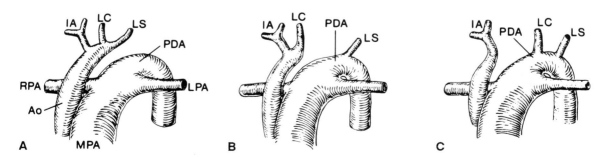

Figure 20–2. Types of aortic arch interruption. (*A*) In type A, the defect is distal to the left subclavian artery. (*B*) Type B has the interruption between the left subclavian (LS) and left carotid (LC) arteries. (*C*) Type C has the discontinuity between the innominate (IA) and left carotid arteries. Ao, aorta; MPA, main pulmonary artery; RPA, right pulmonary artery; LPA, left pulmonary artery; PDA, patent ductus arteriosus. (*From Arciniegas E (ed): Pediatric Cardiac Surgery. Chicago, Year Book Medical, 1985, p 109, with permission.*)

scending aorta. A mortality rate of 90% in untreated patients is expected within the first year of life.

Diagnostic Features. In infants, the presenting symptoms of interrupted aortic arch are similar to those of coarctation but with more severe symptoms. Acidosis is often a problem because of limited perfusion. The chest radiograph demonstrates cardiomegaly with increased pulmonary vascular markings.

Neonates with interrupted aortic arch, like those with coarctation of the aorta, may be subjected to significant risk by invasive diagnostic procedures. In most cases, two-dimensional echocardiography can be used effectively to evaluate neonates with congenital arch obstruction. Two factors that may make echocardiography difficult are the presence of a widely patent ductus (in infants receiving prostaglandin E [PGE] therapy) and the absence of a thymus, which hampers visualization.[84] It is important to scan in the high parasternal and suprasternal notch areas to exclude an aortopulmonary window or the origin of the left subclavian artery distal to the coarctation. The left sidedness or right sidedness of the aortic arch should be determined. If the therapy is going to be based on the echocardiogram, it is also necessary to exclude ventricular septal defect, left ventricle outflow obstruction, and mitral valve abnormalities.

Surgical Therapy. Treatment of interrupted aortic arch is heavily influenced by associated anomalies. Patients are maintained on PGE_1 therapy to maintain the patency of the ductus arteriosus. The lesion is repaired in either one or two stages. In the one-stage repair, the ventral septal defect is closed and the aorta is repaired as well. The one-stage repair is almost always done with bypass and often requires profound hypothermia and circulatory arrest. If the resources and anatomy to do the one-stage repair are available, this procedure appears to have a lower mortality than the two-stage repair (42% versus 72%) (see Table 20–3).[74,95] The two-stage repair consists of pulmonary artery banding and restoration of the integrity of the aorta. Patients with a univentricular heart will require a staged procedure.

Anesthesia and Perioperative Management. A high-dose narcotic such as fentanyl is used because of the complexity of the surgery in repair of interrupted aortic arch and the condition of the infant. When circulatory arrest is planned during the operation, fentanyl concentrations above 20 ng/mL may be maintained throughout the procedure by an initial loading dose of 35 μg/kg of fentanyl followed by a continuous infusion at 0.3 μg/kg/min. Membrane oxygenators such as the SciMed, which bind fentanyl, can be primed with 130 ng of fentanyl per cm square centimeter of membrane surface area so that precipitous decreases in fentanyl con-

centration or massive increases in glucose (preventing high glucose concentrations appears to be important in improving neurologic outcome after circulatory arrest) are avoided at initiation of bypass.

Monitors should be placed to evaluate the blood pressure above and below the aortic interruption. A central venous catheter is needed because these infants usually require inotropic support. Multiple sites are used to monitor temperature to assure that no residual heat sinks are present during cooling and rewarming from circulatory arrest.

After the period of circulatory arrest and reinstitution of blood flow, urine output may be absent. Mannitol is used to increase the renal plasma flow that has been inhibited by the vasopressin release associated with cardiopulmonary bypass. Furosemide and ethacrynic acid may also be employed but are not administered until the patient has warmed. These children are followed closely for adequate urine output after bypass. Institution of peritoneal dialysis is begun early if renal failure is apparent.

Postoperative Care. Children who have undergone repair of interrupted aortic arch are not candidates for early extubation and may be returned to the intensive care unit on continuous narcotic infusions. Initially they are at risk for pulmonary hypertensive crisis. Long-term hospitalization, up to 6 months, is not uncommon with this lesion.

Immediate and Long-term Results. Modern surgical techniques allow children with interrupted aortic arch to survive to mid-childhood. They must be followed closely for the development of left ventricular outflow tract obstruction, the relief of which may play a significant role in their survival.[95] The obstruction may be at the level of the aortic arch, but subaortic stenosis is also associated with this lesion.[96] Residual or recurrent gradients at the anastomosis may be relieved by surgery or angioplasty. Accordingly, a child with interrupted aortic arch should have SBE prophylaxis throughout life (see Chapter 26).

Truncus Arteriosus

Truncus arteriosus is a rare congenital heart lesion representing fewer than 1% of all cases of congenital heart disease.

Anatomy. Crucial to the understanding of truncus arteriosus is the septation that occurs over a 5-day period about 4 weeks after conception (see Chapter 3).[94] There are two classification systems for the anatomy of the defect. The older system, still in use, was proposed by Collett and Edwards in 1949.[98] Their classification (Table 20–6) is based on where the arrest in embryologic development occurred when the pulmonary arteries were

TABLE 20–6. CLASSIFICATION OF TRUNCUS ARTERIOSUS

Type	Anatomic Finding	Pulmonary Blood Flow
I	The MPA arises from the truncus and divides into the left and right pulmonary arteries	Increased
II	The pulmonary arteries arise from the posterior aspect of the truncus	Increased-normal
III	The pulmonary arteries arise from the lateral aspects of the truncus	Increased-normal
IV Not a truncus; grouped with TOF and PA	No pulmonary arteries; lungs supplied by bronchial arteries from the descending aorta	Decreased

being differentiated from the sixth aortic arches. Type 1 truncus arteriosus places the defect very low in the ascending aorta, whereas type 4 has the pulmonary arteries originating in the aorta below the arch vessels. Type 1 is the most common (48–68% of cases) and type 2 is the second most common (29–48%). Types 3 and 4 each represent fewer than 10% of truncus cases. Type 4 does not represent a true truncus, but is an extreme form of tetralogy of Fallot with pulmonary atresia; it is often referred to as pseudotruncus.

Van Praagh and van Praagh made Collett and Edwards' classification system more accurate and complete, first by dividing each of Collett and Edwards' four groups into A (with ventricular septal defect) and B (without ventricular septal defect). In addition, their classification system better describes the location of the pulmonary arteries. Lesions of the B type are very uncommon because the persistence of the truncus arteriosus is almost always associated with a VSD. Most of the time, the truncus will straddle the ventricular septum, but in 40% of cases, it is oriented to either the left or right ventricle.[99] The VSD is large because of a deficiency in the infundibular septum.

The truncal valve, which is critical to the diagnosis, contains a single semilunar valve. The presence of this valve differentiates this lesion from aortic and pulmonary valve atresia. Unfortunately, the truncal valve is frequently abnormal, typically being described as thick, fleshy, polypoid, or soft. The number of leaflets also typically varies from one to five; most truncal valves (69%) have three, but 2% will have five or more leaflets.[100] As could be expected, regurgitation is commonly observed (in 50% of patients).[94]

Because stenosis in the pulmonary arteries is rare, the child must undergo the repair early on or else receive a pulmonary artery band to protect the pulmonary vasculature. One of the pulmonary arteries is absent in about 16% of truncus cases, with the absent pulmonary artery being on the same side as the aortic arch. Truncus, unlike other truncoconal abnormalities, exhibits normal distal (but not proximal) coronary arteries.[101] Anomalies of the coronary artery ostial origin are common, occurring in

37–45% of patients.[102] The types and incidence of associated anomalies are in Table 20–7.

The cardiac conduction system in truncus has a correctly positioned sinus and atrioventricular node. However, the conduction system is remote from the ventricular septal defect. Unlike most VSDs, the VSD in truncus is infundibular, not perimembranous.

Pathophysiology. There is obligatory mixing of systemic and pulmonary blood in truncus arteriosus because of the absence of a separation between the systemic and pulmonary circulations. Fortunately, streaming and the increased pulmonary resistance of the neonate direct flow toward the systemic circulation. As the pulmonary vascular resistance decreases in the young infant, streaming still accounts for some differential flow. Pulmonary artery saturation is usually 10% less than the systemic saturation, but pulmonary overload rapidly occurs and the child develops congestive heart failure. If the condition is uncorrected, the child's pulmonary vascular resistance increases and irreversible vascular disease ensues at a very young age.

Natural History. Truncus arteriosus is a relatively rare congenital heart defect but mortality is high: 50% of patients die by 2.5 months and 80% by 1 year of age, with the most common cause being heart failure.[94]

TABLE 20–7. INCIDENCE OF ANOMALIES ASSOCIATED WITH TRUNCUS ARTERIOSUS

Associated Anomaly	Incidence (%)
Abnormal coronary ostia	37–49
ASD	9–20
Aberrant subclavian artery	4–10
Persistent left superior vena cava	4–9
Tricuspid stenosis	6
Extracardiac anomalies	21–30
Single coronary artery	13
Single pulmonary artery	16
Partial anomalous pulmonary venous return	1

Diagnostic Features. The child with truncus usually presents with severe congestive heart failure (CHF) caused by the increased pulmonary:systemic blood flow ratio and, frequently, by truncal valve regurgitation. Like other children with lesions causing increased pulmonary flow, these patients have tachypnea, difficulty in feeding, and irritability. On auscultation, a loud murmur and a single second heart sound are heard. A wide pulse pressure is found. The ECG is nonspecific, typically showing biventricular hypertrophy with an axis of +90 to +150. First- or second-degree heart block is found in 10% of patients. The chest radiograph shows a wide mediastinum from the superior pulmonary arteries and a large heart with increased pulmonary markings. The aorta is to the right in 30–35% of cases. The position of the aorta and increased vascular markings are pathognomonic of truncus arteriosus.

Echocardiographic diagnosis of truncus arteriosus identifies the origin of the pulmonary arteries from the common trunk and the presence of the semilunar valve (truncal valve). Doppler and color flow studies are usually effective in evaluating the competency of the valve and can determine stenosis in it. Some echocardiographers suggest that it may be difficult to distinguish truncus from tetralogy of Fallot or from pulmonary atresia plus a ventricular septal defect by echocardiography alone. In such cases, angiograms would be necessary to define the pulmonary artery anatomy clearly and to plan for separation of the pulmonary and systemic flow. A single truncal injection may be all that is needed, but a large dose of contrast dye will be needed because of the large run-off. When older children are catheterized, it is extremely important to attempt to determine pulmonary vascular resistance. A study from the Mayo Clinic found an increased incidence of mortality in children with two pulmonary arteries who had pulmonary vascular resistance greater than 8 Wood units/m^2.[103] When pulmonary vascular resistance cannot be estimated, pressures in the pulmonary artery of half the systemic pressure or less indicate a good surgical candidate. When pulmonary artery pressure is systemic, systemic saturation of 85% or more suggests that the PVR is in the acceptable range. Cine MRI would also be helpful and might obviate the need for an arteriogram.

Anesthetic and Perioperative Management. Anesthesia is managed as previously described for critically ill neonates with complete mixing lesions. These children will typically not require preoperative sedative medications. Very sick infants in severe failure may be receiving positive inotropic drugs. The monitors required are arterial and central venous pressure catheters. Umbilical arterial and venous catheters can be used if they are in good position. A good position for the umbilical venous catheter is in the atrium or inferior vena cava (IVC), having passed through the ductus venosus in the liver. Frequently, the surgeon will place intracardiac catheters,

such as a left atrial line, at the time of surgery. Intubation is occasionally a problem because of an association of facial dysmorphism with truncus.[104] Because of the association of the DiGeorge syndrome in truncus (26%), calcium levels must be closely monitored.[94]

The anesthetic technique must be adjusted for the type of truncus (see Table 20–4). If the type is 1 or 2 and the pulmonary blood flow is increased, a technique that will not increase systemic vascular resistance should be used. For this reason, ketamine is not recommended in these cases. A high-dose narcotic technique is most often used. Pulmonary blood flow, which is usually excessive, should be limited. Pulmonary vascular resistance (PVR) is not likely to increase with safe ventilatory management, but hyperventilation can reduce PVR, worsening the situation. Using positive end-expiratory pressure (PEEP), avoiding 100% oxygen, and maintaining normal Pco_2 will maintain pulmonary vascular resistance.

In type 1 truncus, the systemic blood flow must be very carefully controlled. Decreasing systemic vascular resistance increases systemic flow but also decreases coronary artery perfusion. The balance may be so precarious that simply opening the chest could disrupt the relative flows and cause the heart to fail, particularly if the truncal valve is regurgitant. If effective system flow ceases before bypass, the surgeon may be able to improve flow by restricting flow to the pulmonary arteries.

The size of the infant and the location of the pulmonary arteries typically determine whether the operation is performed using circulatory arrest. After cardiopulmonary bypass, it is important to realize that the ventricle has a smaller preload and a higher resistance. Agents that decrease the pulmonary artery pressure while maintaining left ventricular output are frequently chosen for inotropic support. Because pulmonary vascular crisis can have severe consequences in these infants, they are often maintained on narcotic infusions for the first few days after surgery. Injury to the conduction system surrounding the ventricular septal defect closure is usually not a problem because the conduction system is remote. However, patients may require pacing for a short period after discontinuation of bypass.

Surgical Technique. Timing of the repair is considered crucial; the optimum time is the first month after birth. There used to be a belief that repair of the child with truncus should not be attempted until the child's pulmonary vascular resistance decreased and heart failure developed. This approach has become rare. Some institutions still place children with truncus on digitalis and diuretics and, if the failure is well controlled, allow the child to grow for 4–6 months before repair. The upper age limit with this approach is imposed by the need to perform the repair before fixed pulmonary hypertension begins. Unfortunately, approximately 25% of these patients will develop pulmonary vascular disease by three months.

Pulmonary artery banding is rarely done in this operation because the band may severely distort the pulmonary arteries and hinder a good repair at a later date; furthermore, an effective band is very difficult to achieve. If the pulmonary arteries are to be banded and two are present, banding both arteries is preferable to banding only one according to some evidence. In one study, placing a single band was associated with a higher incidence of pulmonary obstructive disease and the band typically produced severe obstruction in the right pulmonary artery.[105]

Surgical repair now consists of removing the pulmonary arteries from the truncal artery. If the truncal valve is not competent, it must be replaced. Replacement in this case is often done by inserting a valved homograft in the aortic position because it is difficult to find an artificial valve that can be sutured into the aortic position in a small neonate. The ventricular septal defect is closed. The distal end of a second valved homograft is then connected to the pulmonary arteries and the proximal end is sutured to the right ventricular outflow tract.[106] Surgical mortality as reported by Ebert and Bove is low (10%).[107,108] Truncus repair must be considered a staged procedure because the conduit will need to be replaced as the child grows.

Because of the limitations of the homograft, a new technique for type 1 and type 2 truncus has been developed that does not require a conduit. The pulmonary arteries are removed from the common truncus arteriosus and the ventricular septal defect is closed through a ventriculotomy. The pulmonary arteries are then connected directly to the right ventricle, with the anterior wall of the pulmonary arteries being reconstructed with a patch.[109,110] It is not yet apparent whether the valveless technique has any long-term advantages over the use of conduits, although when a valve has to be replaced, cryopreserved homografts and conduits appear to be much superior to mechanical and other tissue valves. The ability to repair this lesion without the need for long-term anticoagulation is a real advantage in children.

Postoperative Care. Complete atrioventricular block has been reported and must be rapidly corrected to prevent myocardial ischemia. There also is almost always some degree of left ventricular dysfunction, which is readily managed with inotropic support.[111] Episodes of pulmonary hypertension can also occur, but these are minimized by narcotic infusions for the first 48 hours postoperatively. These patients remain intubated for several days after repair of truncus to minimize pulmonary hypertensive crises.

Immediate and Long-term Results. The outcome is excellent after uncomplicated truncus repair without valve stenosis or regurgitation (see Table 20–3). Truncal valve regurgitation, particularly if it is associated with stenosis, necessitates frequent and careful follow-up.[108]

If a conduit is used, the patient should be followed yearly with echocardiography to determine the onset of conduit stenosis and resultant ventricular changes. In the long term, some of these patients have immunologic deficits because of reduced total T-cell percentages and T helper cells.[112] They are, therefore, thought to belong to the spectrum of the DiGeorge syndrome.[101] Naturally, these children are at high risk for bacterial endocarditis and must receive regular prophylaxis as high-risk patients.

Patent Ductus Arteriosus

The ductus arteriosus is an integral structure in fetal circulation. The complex cascade of events that occurs during the transition from fetal to neonatal circulation (see Chapter 4) normally results in the functional closure of the ductus arteriosus from approximately 15 hours to 4 days after birth, a closure sequence seen even in preterm infants born at 20 weeks of gestation.[113] This stage is caused by the medial smooth muscles in the ductus wall. Although the vessel remains anatomically patent, flow through it is remarkably diminished. Anatomic obliteration of the ductus arteriosus is complete by approximately 1 month after birth,[114] owing to infolding of the endothelium, disruption of the subintimal layers, and small hemorrhages and necroses in the subintimal region. During this interval, the ductus is susceptible to various physiologic and pharmacologic influences that promote ductal patency, such as hypoxia and prostaglandins.

The incidence of isolated patent ductus arteriosus (PDA) is 1 in 2500 live full-term births, accounting for approximately 10% of all congenital heart defects. Girls are affected almost twice as often as boys. Prenatal exposure to rubella virus, especially during the first trimester, significantly increases the risk of PDA. Isolated PDA is seen in 50% of these patients; it is part of more complex congenital heart disease in up to 85%.[115]

The observation of PDA in preterm infants is related to birth weight rather than the presence of respiratory distress syndrome.[113] Forty-two percent of infants weighing less than 1000 g or 20% of infants at less than 1750 g have a PDA.[116] The ductus arteriosus in premature infants is quite large in relation to the aorta and pulmonary artery and is structurally immature.

Anatomy. The isolated PDA typically arises from the anterior surface of the main pulmonary artery near its junction with the left pulmonary artery and joins the posterior descending aorta soon after the origin of the left subclavian artery. The ductus arteriosus develops from the left sixth aortic arch, providing a conduit between the aorta and the pulmonary artery during intrauterine life. If there is a right aortic arch, the ductus may be on the right, joining the right pulmonary artery and the right aortic arch just distal to the right subclavian artery. It is possible for the ductus to be bilateral.

The ductus arteriosus is structurally different from

the true vascular tissue of the aorta and pulmonary artery. The internal media is not composed of elastic fibers; smooth muscle in both longitudinal and circumferential arrangements is seen instead.[117] It constricts when exposed to elevations in Pa_{O_2}. This response becomes more dramatic as the fetus matures (Fig. 20–3). In preterm infants, the muscular layer is thin and poorly contractile. Premature infants are at risk for pulmonary disease (hyaline membrane disease, pneumonia, meconium aspiration) accompanied by hypoxemia. The premature lung may also be less efficient in the metabolism of prostaglandins that promote patency. These facts may explain the increased incidence of PDA in premature infants.

Pathophysiology. In the fetus, flow from the right ventricle is diverted from the high-resistance pulmonary bed via the ductus arteriosus to the descending aorta. It has been shown in lambs that 90% of the right ventricular of 59% or the combined ventricular output flows through the ductus arteriosus.[118] Diversion of the blood away from the quiescent lung parenchyma allows adequate perfusion of the fetus at a reduced cardiac output.

The hemodynamics of PDA are similar to those of a VSD, in which the left-to-right shunt is governed by relative resistance. When the ductus is small, left-to-right flow is determined by the capacity of the ductus to impede flow from the aorta to the pulmonary artery. Alternatively, when the ductus is large, the shunted blood flow is determined by the ratio of pulmonary vascular resistance to systemic vascular resistance.

Natural History After birth and the fall in pulmonary vascular resistance, the natural history of patent ductus arteriosus is similar to that of other lesions with predominant left-to-right shunt flow (Table 20–8). The increased size of the left atrium may open the foramen ovale and thus increase left-to-right shunting at the atrial level. This condition combines with the development of pulmonary edema to increase the work load on the right side of the heart in later stages.

Several compensatory mechanisms operate in the patent ductus for maintenance of myocardial performance (Frank-Starling mechanism, sympathetic system, and myocardial hypertrophy). Stimulation of the sympathetic system, in turn, stimulates the myocardium and causes the release of norepinephrine as well as catecholamine release from the adrenal glands. This release causes the increased heart rate and sweating seen in children with PDA. Premature infants, however, lack complete development of these compensatory mechanisms and are less tolerant of a PDA than older children or even infants born at term.

When these compensatory mechanisms are absent or underdeveloped, heart failure results. The reduced diastolic pressure also adds to the problem of reduced myocardial blood flow, which in the presence of anemia can place the myocardium at risk for inadequate oxygen supply. The risk of subacute bacterial endocarditis with PDA, even in the presence of minimal shunt blood flow from a small patent ductus, generally mandates closure of the ductus.

Diagnostic Features. The signs of isolated PDA in the child can include tachypnea, diaphoresis, decreased exercise tolerance, failure to thrive, recurrent respiratory infections, lobar emphysema or collapse, cardiac failure, cardiac enlargement, bacterial endocarditis, and irreversible pulmonary vascular disease. Most often, however, PDA presents with a murmur diagnosed on routine physical examination. The murmur is described as a continuous machine murmur, which gets louder throughout systole with a peak at the second heart sound and then gets softer throughout diastole. The murmur is loudest

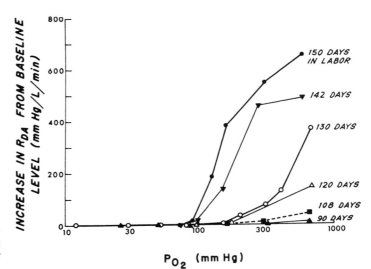

Figure 20–3. The increased responsiveness of the ductus arteriosus to oxygen increases with length of gestation. R_{DA} is the control ductus arteriosus resistance. (*From McMurphy DM, et al; 1972, pp 232–238, with permission.*)

TABLE 20–8. NATURAL HISTORY OF PATENT DUCTUS ARTERIOSUS

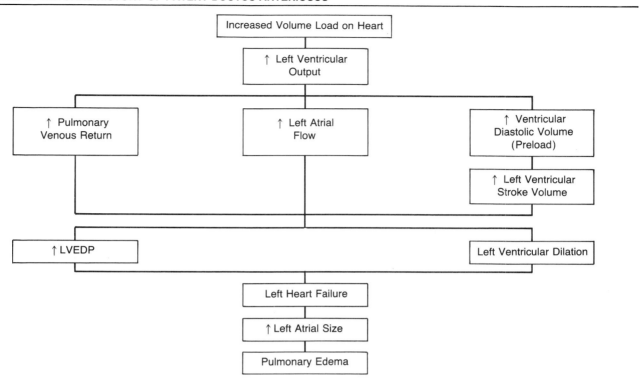

at the first or second intercostal space at the left sternal border. The pulse pressure is wide, often with prominent or bounding pulses.

The ECG is usually normal. In cases with large left-to-right flow, there may be left ventricular hypertrophy or left atrial enlargement. Right ventricular hypertrophy is present if the PDA has caused pulmonary occlusive disease.

The chest radiographic findings are also dependent on ductal flow. In small PDAs with limited left-to-right shunt, the chest radiograph is normal. As the shunt increases, the pulmonary artery becomes more prominent, with a prominent aortic knob. As the shunt flow continues to increase, there will be left heart enlargement and an increase in pulmonary vascular markings.

Echocardiography is the main diagnostic procedure for PDA in many institutions. Two-dimensional echocardiography can reliably identify the aortic end of the ductus. Continuous-wave Doppler can detect abnormal flow in the pulmonary artery. Color flow Doppler can visualize the jet of abnormal flow and determine more information about the size and shape of the ductus.

Ductal closure should not be done without ascertaining whether it will benefit the patient. In isolated PDA, a challenge with vasodilators or 100% oxygen is used to show that the pulmonary vasculature is still reactive. Fixed pulmonary hypertension from an isolated ductus is rare at the present time but would result in decreased cardiac output and rapid deterioration when the ductus is closed.

Anesthetic and Perioperative Management. A child presenting for closure of a PDA is usually given antibiotic prophylaxis, whether the ductus is closed in the catheterization laboratory or in the surgical suite.[116] Preoperative medications are usually given when the procedure is done in the catheterization laboratory but are not necessary. When done surgically, closure of PDA should be considered as a limited thoracotomy. Usually, it is very short in duration and the blood loss is minimal, although blood loss may become significant if the ductus is torn during ligation. Secure intravenous access is necessary, but an arterial catheter is not essential. A functioning pulse oximeter and end-tidal CO_2 monitoring will give almost all the monitoring information needed. Placement of monitors, which is very critical with this lesion, should make it possible for the anesthesiologist to assess whether the correct structure has been ligated. The surgeon may test-occlude to confirm the correct structure. Having a pulse oximeter on a lower extremity and placing the blood pressure cuff on the right arm are reasonable choices; this placement allows determination of whether the descending aorta or the ascending aorta is compromised. If the pulmonary artery is occluded, there is a decrease in saturation and end-tidal CO_2. Ligation of a hemodynamically significant ductus increases the diastolic pressure. There may be an initial increase in systolic pressure as well but this is usually transient (see Table 20–4).

The anesthetic technique for surgical repair is variable, but in severely ill preterm neonates, adequate anesthesia and analgesia are important to prevent further stress. Techniques involving high doses of narcotics (50 μg/kg fentanyl) are often used, but some researchers have documented the effective use of high spinals or epidural anesthesia. In older children, the choice of technique should permit extubation at the end of the case. As in the younger child, a technique that will provide good postoperative analgesia is important to enhance deep breathing and minimize pulmonary complications. Standard techniques of intravenous narcotic given around the clock or, in older children, by patient-controlled analgesia are effective. Intercostal nerve blocks are also effective in controlling the pain and can be done by the surgeon under direct vision or by the anesthesiologist with standard techniques. Other mechanisms of pain relief that have been employed include intrapleural local anesthetics and epidural narcotics.

When the PDA is closed in the catheterization laboratory, sedation is needed, and many cardiologists insist that the child be absolutely still at the time of occluder placement. Because nonsurgical closure is usually presented to the family as a way to avoid general anesthesia, a deep sedation technique is often used. A continuous midazolam infusion (0.25 mg/kg bolus followed by infusion at 0.4–4.0 μg/kg/min) with a bolus of ketamine (0.1–0.5 mg/kg) at the time of occluder placement can provide optimum conditions for the cardiologists, ie, a sedated spontaneously breathing patient.

Surgical Technique. The approach to PDA is usually through a left posterolateral thoracotomy (fourth to fifth intercostal space), but it can be approached through a median sternotomy, which is often done in children who have a PDA and other cardiac malformations. In children with ductus-dependent lesions, the ductus is usually isolated before bypass and then ligated once on bypass. Unrecognized PDA can cause significant problems during bypass for other lesions, as the blood will tend to go from the aortic cannula to the ductus and flood the lungs. This condition usually manifests itself by low systemic blood pressure and high mixed venous oxygen saturation during bypass. The treatment is to isolate and ligate the ductus. If isolation and ligation are difficult, the heart should be allowed to eject until it is isolated in order to promote flow to the lower part of the body. Phenylephrine should not be used in this situation to increase blood pressure because it will only aggravate the problem and further limit blood flow to the lower part of the body.

Because the ductus may resemble the descending aorta and the main pulmonary artery in size, care must be taken to ligate the correct vessel at the time of surgery. Test occlusion may be done. The ductus may be ligated with suture or clipped and may or may not be transected. There is a tendency to avoid clips because they interfere with subsequent MRI. Postoperatively, the child requires a chest tube for 24 hours and must stay in the hospital 3–5 days. Another 2–4 weeks must pass before the child returns to unrestricted activity.

Nonsurgical closure of the ductus is a possibility in selected patients. A noninterventional approach with indomethacin may be tried in preterm infants; however, this drug is not effective in term infants or older children. Catheter closure of PDA has been performed since 1977, and the equipment and technique have improved significantly since then.[119] It can now be done in children weighing as little as 7 kg and as young as 3 months and has an overall success rate of 84–98%.[120,121] The first devices were foam-disk hooked devices. The Rashkind PDA occluder, a hookless double-disk system, was then developed. The disks are inserted via the femoral artery into the aorta, across the ductus, and into the pulmonary artery. They can also be inserted via the venous system into the PDA. This nonsurgical approach to closure, when successful, eliminates the need for a thoracotomy and an extended hospitalization and can be done at the time of the angiogram. Though general anesthesia is not specifically indicated, the patient needs to lie still during placement of the catheter. The deep sedation often approximates general anesthesia. Morphine preoperatively followed by ketamine, 1.5–5.0 mg/kg IV, for a 95-minute procedure has been reported.[122]

The delivery system for this closure device requires that the patient weigh more than 7 kg, and the catheter must traverse a tight bend to be positioned correctly. After successful application of the occlusion device, patients have been discharged home.

Embolization can occur with this form of closure, although incidence of embolization has decreased from 16 to 3.6%.[120] Incomplete closure of the ductus is also possible if the size of the ductus or if the device is incorrectly placed. Embolization or incomplete closure may require an operative procedure. When the ductus is approached surgically after failure of an occlusion device, however, there is usually an increased operative risk from anemia as a result of blood loss from the catheterization.

The consensus from centers that perform catheter closure of a PDA is that if it is possible to manage the patient medically to a body weight of 8 kg, the PDA should be closed in the catheterization laboratory with an occluding device. If the child cannot be medically managed or the device cannot be seated correctly, surgery is performed.

Immediate and Long-term Results. Mortality for surgical repair of PDA is low (<1%). Recannulation of the ductus has been reported to occur if the ductus is not divided. Other specific injuries associated with the surgery include injury to the recurrent laryngeal nerve, which on extubation may cause problems from unilateral vocal cord paralysis. The thoracic duct may also be injured, with chylothorax resulting.

Complications of PDA closure are rare, although closure can reveal other, previously undetected congenital anomalies that may result in death. For example, when the patient has previously undetected congenital anomalies of the coronary arteries, as when the coronary artery arises from the pulmonary artery, closure of the ductus results in considerably less oxygen in the blood supplied to these arteries; less oxygen is then delivered to the heart, and infarction or failure may result. Another possible complication is a postoperative ductal aneurysm.

Bacterial endocarditis is a primary indication for closure of an otherwise asymptomatic PDA. Endocarditis remains a risk for at least a year after the ductus has been complete closed.[123]

Aortopulmonary Window

Aortopulmonary (AP) window is a rare anomaly resulting from incomplete fusion of the conotruncal ridge. Three types are found: type 1 is in the proximal portion of the ascending aorta on the medial wall just above the sinus of Valsalva; type 2 is more distal in the ascending aorta and opens into the origin of the right pulmonary artery; and in type 3 the right pulmonary artery originates from the posterior part of the ascending aorta and is separate from the main pulmonary artery. The presence of two semilunar valves (annuli) distinguishes type 3 from truncus arteriosus. Associated anomalies occur in about 50% of patients with AP window.[124]

Pathophysiology. The pathophysiology of AP window is similar to that of patent ductus arteriosus but is usually more severe. The increased left-to-right shunt produces early and severe symptoms of increased pulmonary blood flow. The direct connection between the pulmonary and systemic circuits resembles truncus and delay of surgical correction rapidly increases pulmonary vascular resistance. Endocarditis and pulmonary rupture are also potential complications.

Natural History. Although the pathophysiology and clinical picture are similar to those of patent ductus arteriosus, patients with AP window usually die in early childhood (<2 years of age) from heart failure, pulmonary vascular obstructive disease, or endarteritis if they do not receive surgical correction.

Patients rarely survive past 20 years of age without correction unless the defect is very small (<10 mm).

Diagnostic Features. Patients with AP window typically present like other children in cardiac failure, with tachypnea, difficulty in feeding, and poor weight gain. The chest radiograph shows cardiomegaly with increased vascular markings. The ECG demonstrates left ventricular hypertrophy or biventricular hypertrophy. The diagnosis is made by echocardiography or angiography. There are some reports that the echocardiogram may be superior because it is better able to define associated anomalies and interpretation is not complicated by overlapping structures.[125] It is important that the diagnostic technique chosen evaluate pulmonary vascular resistance because the child with elevated pulmonary vascular resistance will do poorly following repair.

Anesthetic and Perioperative Management. There are conflicting reports in the literature as to whether AP window is part of the spectrum of malformations seen with the DiGeorge syndrome.[104,124] Anomalies of the VATER (vertebral defects, tracheoesophageal fistula, radial and renal dysplasia) association are seen with this lesion.[124] The anesthesia plan depends on the surgical approach. If an extracardiac approach is planned, the anesthetic is similar to that for ligation of a patent ductus arteriosus. However, if bypass is used, the anesthetic management and concerns are similar to those with truncus arteriosus. It is unlikely that circulatory arrest would be needed to repair AP window. If circulatory arrest is used, there seems to be a disproportionate amount of blood shunted away from the vital organs with this lesion, with a significant increase in Qp/Qs during surface cooling[126] (see Table 20–4).

Surgical Technique. Repair of AP window depends on location. Because the lesion is extracardiac, simple dissection and ligation, as with a patent ductus arteriosus, may be possible if the lesion is small. Unfortunately, most patients will require cardiopulmonary bypass, with a patch placed in the aorta to divide the two circulations. Abnormal coronary arteries or pulmonary arteries, lesions commonly associated with AP window, may complicate discontinuation of cardiopulmonary bypass.

Postoperative Care. The postoperative management of AP window is similar to that of children after surgical closure of patent ductus arteriosus. Patients should be closely monitored postoperatively for pulmonary hypertensive crisis.[127]

Immediate and Long-term Results. Survival after closure of uncomplicated AP windows (without associated cardiac defects) approaches 80–90%.[128] Long-term outcome of uncomplicated defects corrected in infancy is excellent. However, outcome is affected by method of repair (recurrence or residual defect), pulmonary vascular obstructive disease, and other cardiac anomalies.

Aortic Left Ventricular Tunnel

Aortic left ventricular tunnel is a rare congenital abnormality in which an endothelial track forms between the aorta and the left ventricle. The presentation of this lesion is very similar to that of aortic regurgitation. The tunnel originates above the right coronary artery and enters the left ventricle just below the right and left aortic cusps. The aortic regurgitation is apparent at birth. The primary diagnostic tool has been angiography, but echocardiography may be able to show the intracardiac portion of the tunnel better, and color flow Doppler may be able to distinguish valve regurgitation from tunnel regurgitation (a distinction particularly difficult with angiography). Anesthetic management is similar to that of a patient with severe aortic insufficiency. Immediate results from surgical closure of the tunnel are usually good, but long-term aortic regurgitation may be severe. There is some evidence that early repair of the tunnel, even in the absence of symptoms, may minimize the long-term aortic regurgitation.[129]

Vascular Rings

The term *vascular rings* denotes a group of anomalies of the great vessels and their branches that cause respiratory or feeding problems in infants. The incidence of vascular rings is small but probably is underestimated. A great number of these lesions are probably asymptomatic. Associated congenital heart disease, primarily tetralogy of Fallot and transposition of the great vessels, is seen in up to 20% of patients.[130]

Anatomy. Vascular rings are persistent embryonic structures present during the fetal development of the aortic arch. They are described by their anatomic features. Rings are more commonly associated with right-sided arches than with left-sided arches. The most common type of complete rings is a double aortic arch with both arches remaining patent. The next most common form of complete ring occurs when there is a right aortic arch and the right subclavian artery is retropharyngeal with a left-sided ductus arteriosus (Fig 20–4). Association of congenital heart disease with this lesion is uncommon. The third most common presentation is a right aortic arch with mirror-image branching and a left ligamentum arteriosum. Cyanotic congenital heart disease is very highly associated with this abnormality (98%). The most frequent finding in a complete ring is a left aortic arch with a right descending aorta and a right ligamentum arteriosum. This lesion also has a high incidence of associated congenital heart disease. A left aortic arch with an anomalous right subclavian artery is probably the most common aortic arch anomaly, occurring in 0.5% of the population, but is rarely symptomatic.[131]

The most common incomplete rings are a retropha-

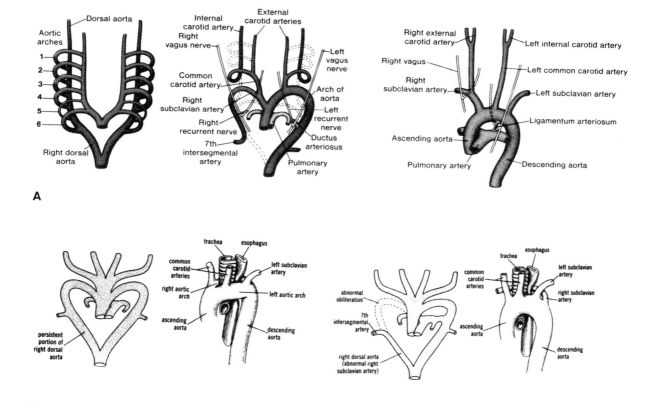

Figure 20–4. Development of double aortic arch and abnormal right subclavian artery, two common forms of vascular ring that result in varying degrees of tracheoesophageal compression (*B*), contrasted with the normal development of the aortic arch (*A*). (*From Sadler TW: Langman's Medical Embryology, 5th ed. Baltimore: Williams & Wilkins, 1985, p 202, with permission.*)

ryngeal right subclavian artery, innominate artery compression, and a pulmonary artery sling. Associated congenital abnormalities are very common (50–80%) in children with anomalous pulmonary arteries resulting in pulmonary artery slings.

Pathophysiology. Vascular rings produce symptoms by the compression of the trachea or esophagus or both. *Complete* rings totally surround and compress the structure; *incomplete* rings only compress it.

Natural History. Children with symptomatic vascular rings may show symptoms of respiratory distress, dysphagia, wheezing, or cyanosis as early as the day after birth and are usually symptomatic by 3 months of age. However, symptoms have been noted to develop after 1 year of age (Table 20–9). With tracheal obstruction, hyperinflation of the lungs progressively develops. Failure to thrive, poor growth, and feeding difficulties are chronic problems with vascular rings obstructing the esophagus.

Diagnostic Features. The symptoms of vascular rings include a harsh cry, inspiratory stridor, dysphagia, chronic cough, bronchopneumonia, and difficulty in feeding. Symptoms are milder and of later onset and dysphagia is less prominent in patients with a right aortic arch and retroesophageal component than in patients with a double aortic arch.[131]

The ECG is normal, as is the cardiac examination. Echocardiographic evaluation can be helpful in identifying double aortic arch. Other modalities that are particularly beneficial in defining the anatomy are digital subtraction angiography, computed tomographic (CT) scanning with contrast, and MRI. CT and MRI appear to be particularly useful investigational tools in pulmonary artery slings.

The chest radiograph with the barium swallow may be the simplest approach to evaluation. The lateral chest radiograph may show the compression of the trachea. In patients with pulmonary artery slings, bronchus suis should be considered if the chest radiograph shows differential atelectasis in the various lobes. Bronchus suis is the independent origin of the right upper bronchus from the trachea. The barium swallow esophagram shows typical changes of most of the malformations except when the problem arises from an anomalous innominate artery. A bronchogram may demonstrate the defect but similar information can be gained without the risk. When an anomalous innomiante artery is the problem, the child presents with stridor. After the barium study shows no abnormality, bronchoscopy is performed, and a pulsatile mass is seen in the trachea. It may be difficult or impossible to wean a child with a vascular ring from mechanical ventilation until surgical repair is completed.

Anesthetic and Perioperative Management. The choice of anesthesia depends upon the type of vascular ring. With a double aortic arch, adequate ventilation may be ascertained by end-tidal CO_2 monitoring and pulse oximetry alone. Arterial and central venous catheters are frequently employed with anomalous pulmonary arteries, which are more complex. Secure intravenous access is important because all of these conditions may have a period of uncontrolled bleeding. Because endotracheal tube placement may be critical, it is advisable to have a variety of sizes available. Just as with an anterior mediastinal mass, rings may cause tracheal compression; the child may deteriorate on induction and may totally decompensate when neuromuscular blocking agents are given. In such a case, an inhalation induction with the child spontaneously breathing is recommended, with neuromuscular blocking agents used only when control of the airway has been fully assessed. Tube placement may be especially difficult with anomalous pulmonary arteries, particularly if a bronchus suis is present. Because double-lumen tubes are generally not available for the smaller infants, two small endotracheal tubes may be

TABLE 20–9. PRESENTATION OF COMPLETE AND INCOMPLETE VASCULAR RINGS

Finding	Symptoms	Postoperative Course
Left aortic arch with right descending aorta and right ductus	Dysphagia	Short
Double aortic arch	Severe symptoms: Stridor, dyspnea, cough	Short-term postoperative tracheal obstruction
Right aortic arch with mirror image branching	Congenital heart disease predominates	Depends upon repair of CHD
Right aortic arch with anomalous left subclavian	Usually asymptomatic	Short
Left arch and right retroesophageal right subclavian	Usually asymptomatic	Short
Anomalous innominate artery	Tracheal compression	Patient may have tracheomalacia
Pulmonary artery sling	Obstructive emphysema or right lung atelectasis	May be prolonged

placed into the trachea, positioning one to ventilate the bronchi proximal to the obstruction and passing the second, longer tube distal to the obstruction.

Once the airway has been secured, maintenance of anesthesia can proceed. If tracheomalacia or stenosis will not be a problem postoperatively, a technique that will allow extubation at the end of the case is employed. Thoracic epidural catheters placed via the caudal canal plus light general anesthesia to provide good intraoperative and postoperative analgesia may be used. Many of the children with vascular rings will present with a history of respiratory disease; consequently, good postoperative analgesia is important to minimize postoperative pulmonary complications.

Surgical Technique. The surgical approach to a vascular ring depends on which anomaly is actually present. Surgical repair is indicated when the symptoms are severe or complications of the lesion appear (such as aspiration or repeated pneumonia). Surgery is approached in most of the complete vascular rings by a left posterolateral thoracotomy. Identification and division of the ring usually correct the problem. A right thoracotomy is used when the patient has a left-sided aortic arch and a right-sided ligamentum arteriosum.

The anomalous innominate artery is approached via an anterior thoracotomy or a sternotomy. The artery is sutured to the underside of the sternum.

Correction of the incomplete ring caused by a pulmonary artery sling is a more challenging problem. Usually the pulmonary artery has to be divided and then reanastomosed to the main pulmonary artery. The compression of the trachea or bronchus may require reconstruction as well. The approach must be individualized but a median sternotomy with bypass may be necessary, particularly when tracheal reconstruction is needed in a young child. The repair has a perioperative mortality of 40–50%.[130]

Postoperative Care. Symptomatic children requiring preoperative mechanical ventilation are returned to the intensive care unit postoperatively. They may require ventilatory support for weeks to months in spite of a successful surgical repair. Those with the most difficult course have complete cartilaginous tracheal rings that demonstrate tracheobronchial stenosis. Those with tracheomalacia may have a prolonged ventilatory course postoperatively. Children with minimal pulmonary disease at the time of surgery may be extubated at the end of surgery. Because many of these children also have a history of respiratory disease, good postoperative analgesia is important to minimize postoperative pulmonary complications.

Immediate and Long-term Results. In one large series on vascular rings, early mortality was 4.9%, whereas late mortality was 3.4%. Most of the children who died were younger than 6 months of age.[132] Another problem associated with repair of the pulmonary artery is postoperative obstruction or stenosis. The result of pulmonary artery repairs is assessed with ventilation perfusion scans. These patients will also frequently present for bronchoscopy and tracheostomy. In double aortic arch, if the two vessels do not separate well after division, aortopexy may become necessary.[132] Injuries to the recurrent laryngeal nerve, phrenic nerve, or thoracic duct are common after repair of vascular rings or slings. Fortunately, for the most common complete vascular ring, long-term results are excellent owing to the simplicity of the surgical repair.

REFERENCES

1. Roberts WC: The congenitally bicuspid aortic valve: A study of 85 autopsy cases. *Am J Cardiol* **26**:72–83, 1970
2. Cardella JF, Kanjuh VI, Edwards JE: Association of the acquired bicuspid aortic valve with rheumatic disease of the atrioventricular valves. *Am J Cardiol* **63**:876–877, 1989
3. Latson LA: Aortic stenosis: Valvar, supravalvar, and fibromuscular subvalvar. In Garson A, Bricker JT, McNamara DG (eds): *The Science and Practice of Pediatric Cardiology.* Philadelphia: Lea & Febiger, 1990, pp 1334–1352
4. Anderson RH: Editorial note: The anatomy of aortic valvar stenosis. *Int J Cardiol* **26**:355–359, 1990
5. Freedom RM, Fowler RS, Duncan WJ: Rapid evolution from "normal" left ventricular outflow tract to fatal subaortic stenosis in infancy. *Br Heart J* **45**:605–609, 1981
6. Freedom RM, Dische MR, Rowe RD: Pathologic anatomy of subaortic stenosis and atresia in the first year of life. *Am J Cardiol* **39**:1035–1044, 1977
7. Cassidy SC, Van Hare GF, Silverman NH: The probability of detecting a subaortic ridge in children with ventricular septal defect or coarctation of the aorta. *Am J Cardiol* **66**: 505–508, 1990
8. O'Connor WN, Davis JB Jr, Geissler R, et al: Supravalvular aortic stenosis: Clinical and pathologic observations in 6 patients. *Arch Pathol Lab Med* **109**:179–185, 1985
9. French JW, Guntheroth WG: An explanation of asymmetric upper extremity blood pressures in supravalvular aortic stenosis: The Coanda effect. *Circulation* **52**:31–36, 1970
10. Martin MM, Lemmer JH Jr, Shaffer E, et al: Obstruction to the left coronary ostium in supravalvar aortic stenosis. *Ann Thoracic Surg* **45**:16–20, 1988
11. Assey ME, Wisenbaugh T, Spann JF, et al: Unexpected persistence into adulthood of low wall stress in patients with congenital aortic stenosis: Is there a fundamental difference in the hypertrophic response to a pressure overload present from birth? *Circulation* **75**:973–979, 1987
12. Dorn GW, Donner R, Assey ME, et al: Alterations in left ventricular geometry, wall stress, and ejection performance after correction of congenital aortic stenosis. *Circulation* **78**: 1358–1365, 1988
13. Krovetz LJ, Kurlinski JP: Subendocardial blood flow in children with congenital aortic stenosis. *Circulation* **54**:961–965, 1976

14. Leung MP, McKay R, Smith A, et al: Critical aortic stenosis in early infancy: Anatomic and echocardiographic substrates of successful open valvulotomy. *J Thorac Cardiovasc Surg* **101**:526–535, 1991

15. Sandor GGS, Ollet PM, Trusler GA, et al: Long-term follow-up of patients after valvulotomy for congenital valvular aortic stenosis in children. *J Thorac Cardiovasc Surg* **80**:171–176, 1980

16. Lewis AB, Heymann MA, Stranger P, et al: Evaluation of subendocardial ischemia in valvar aortic stenosis in children. *Circulation* **49**:978–984, 1974

17. Cueto L, Moller JH: Haemodynamics of exercise in children with isolated aortic valvular disease. *Br Heart J* **35**:93–98, 1973

18. Flaker G, Teske D, Kilman J, et al: Supravalvular aortic stenosis: A 20 year clinical perspective and experience with patch aortoplasty. *Am J Cardiol* **51**:256–260, 1983

19. Roberts WC: Valvular, subvalvular and supravalvular aortic stenosis: Morphologic features. *Cardiovasc Clin* **5**:97–126, 1973

20. Pelech AN, Dyck JD, Trusler GA, et al: Critical aortic stenosis. *J Thorac Cardiovasc Surg* **94**:510–517, 1987

21. Turley K, Bove EL, Amato JJ, et al: Neonatal aortic stenosis. *J Thorac Cardiovasc Surg* **99**:679–684, 1990

22. Karl TR, Sano S, Brawn WJ, Mee RBB: Critical aortic stenosis in the first month of life: Surgical results in 26 infants. *Ann Thorac Surg* **50**:105–109, 1990

23. Balaji S, Keeton BR, Sutherland GR, et al: Aortic valvulotomy for critical aortic stenosis in neonates and infants aged less than one year. *Br Heart J* **61**:358–360, 1989

24. DeBoer DA, Robbins RC, Maron BJ, et al: Late results of aortic valvulotomy for congenital valvar stenosis. *Ann Thorac Surg* **50**:69–73, 1990

25. Hseih K, Keane JF, Nadas AS, et al: Long-term follow-up of valvulotomy before 1968 for congenital aortic stenosis. *Am J Cardiol* **58**:338–341, 1986

26. Wheller JJ, Hosier DM, Teske DW, et al: Results of operation for aortic valve stenosis in infants, children, and adolescents. *J Thorac Cardiovasc Surg* **96**:474–477, 1988

27. Hardesty RL, Griffith BP, Matthews RA, et al: Discrete subvalvular aortic stenosis: An evaluation of operative therapy. *J Thorac Cardiovasc Surg* **74**:352–361, 1977

28. Keane JF, Fellows KE, LaFarge CG, et al: The surgical management of discrete and diffuse supravalvar aortic stenosis. *Circulation* **54**:112–117, 1976

29. Weisz D, Hartmann AF Jr, Weldon CS: Results of surgery for congenital supravalvar aortic stenosis. *Am J Cardiol* **37**:73–77, 1976

30. Reis RL, Peterson LM, Mason DT, et al: Congenital fixed subvalvular aortic stenosis. An anatomical classification and correlations with operative results. *Circulation* **43**(suppl 1: 44):1–11, 1971

31. Friedman WF, Pappelbaum SJ: Indications for hemodynamic evaluation and surgery in congenital aortic stenosis. *Pediatr Clin North Am* **18**:1207–1225, 1971

32. James TN, Jordan JD, Riddick L, Bargeron LM: Subaortic stenosis and sudden death. *J Thorac Cardiovasc Surg* **95**:247–254, 1988

33. Wagner HR, Weidman WH, Ellison RC, Miettinen OS: Indirect assessment of severity in aortic stenosis. *Circulation* **56**(suppl 1):1–20, 1977

34. Bengur AR, Snider R, Serwer GA, et al: Usefulness of the Doppler mean gradient in evaluation of children with aortic valve stenosis and comparison to gradient at catheterization. *Am J Cardiol* **64**:756–761, 1989

35. Huhta JC, Carpenter RJ, Moise KJ, et al: Prenatal diagnosis and postnatal management of critical aortic stenosis. *Circulation* **75**:573–576, 1987

36. Gutgesell HP and the Committee on Congenital Cardiac Defects of the Council on Cardiovascular Disease in the Young: Recreational and occupational recommendations for young patients with heart disease: A statement for physicians. *Circulation* **74**:1195A–1198A, 1986

37. Burch M, Redington N, Carvalho JS, et al: Open valvotomy for critical aortic stenosis in infancy. *Br Heart J* **63**:37–40, 1990

38. Duncan A, Sullivan I, Robinson P, et al: Transventricular aortic valvotomy for critical aortic stenosis in infants. *J Thorac Cardiovasc Surg* **93**:546–550, 1987

39. Milano A, Vouhe PR, Baillot-Vernant F, et al: Late results after left-sided cardiac valve replacement in children. *J Thorac Cardiovasc Surg* **92**:218–225, 1986

40. Barratt-Boyes BG, Roche AHG, Whitlock RML: Six year review of the results of free-hand aortic valve replacement using an antibiotic sterilized homograft valve. *Circulation* **55**:353–362, 1977

41. Gerosa G, McKay R, Ross DN: Replacement of the aortic valve or root with a pulmonary autograft in children. *Ann Thorac Surg* **51**:424–429, 1991

42. Santangelo KL, Elkins RC, Stelzer P, et al: Normal left ventricular function following pulmonary autograft replacement of the aortic valve in children. Fifth International Symposium on Cardiac Bioprostheses, Avignon, France, May 25, 1991 (abstr)

43. Gerosa G, McKay R, Davies J, Ross DN: Comparison of the aortic homograft and the pulmonary autograft for aortic valve or root replacement in children. *J Thorac Cardiovasc Surg* **102**:51–61, 1991

44. Rao PS: Balloon aortic valvuloplasty. *Clin Cardiol* **13**:458–466, 1990

45. Lababidi Z, Weinhaus L, Stoeckle H, Walls JT: Transluminal balloon dilatation for discrete subaortic stenosis. *Am J Cardiol* **59**:423–425, 1987

46. Sholler GF, Perry SB, Sanders SP, Lock JE: Balloon dilation of congenital aortic valve stenosis: Results and influence of technical and morphologic features on outcome. *Circulation* **78**:351–360, 1988

47. Rocchini AP, Beekman RH, Shachar GB, et al: Balloon aortic valvuloplasty: Results of the valvuloplasty and angioplasty of congenital anomalies registry. *Am J Cardiol* **65**:784–789, 1990

48. Shem-Tov A, Schneeweiss A, Motro M, Neufield HN: Clinical presentation and natural history of mild discrete subaortic stenosis: Follow-up of 1–17 years. *Circulation* **66**:509–512, 1982

49. Douville EC, Sade RM, Crawford FA, Wiles HB: Subvalvar aortic stenosis: Timing of operation. *Ann Thorac Surg* **50**:29–34, 1990

50. Reder RF, Dimich I, Steinfeld L, Litwak RS: Left ventricle to aorta valved conduit for relief of diffuse left ventricular outflow obstruction. *Am J Cardiol* **39**:1068–1071, 1977

51. Braunstein PW, Sade RM, Crawford FA, Oslizlok PC: Repair of supravalvar aortic stenosis: Cardiovascular, morphometric and hemodynamic results. *Ann Thorac Surg* **50**:700–707, 1990

52. Sharma BK, Fujiwara H, Hallman GL, et al: Supravalvar aortic stenosis: A 29-year review of surgical experience. *Ann Thorac Surg* **51**:1031–1039, 1991

53. Rao PS, Thapar MK, Wilson AD, et al: Intermediate-term follow-up results of balloon aortic valvuloplasty in infants and children with special reference to causes of restenosis. *Am J Cardiol* **64**:1356–1360, 1989

54. Sullivan ID, Wren C, Bain H, et al: Balloon dilatation of the aortic valve for congenital aortic stenosis in childhood. *Br Heart J* **61**:186–191, 1989

55. Vogel M, Benson LN, Burrows P, et al: Balloon dilatation of congenital aortic valve stenosis in infants and children: Short term and intermediate results. *Br Heart J* **62**:148–153, 1989

56. Burrows PE, Benson LN, Williams WG, et al: Iliofemoral arterial complications of balloon angioplasty for systemic obstructions in infants and children. *Circulation* **82**:1697–1704, 1990

57. Carlson MD, Palacios I, Thomas JD, et al: Cardiac conduction abnormalities during percutaneous balloon mitral or aortic valvulotomy. *Circulation* **79**:1197–1203, 1979

58. Geva T, Sanders SP, Diogenes MS, et al: Two-dimensional and Doppler echocardiographic and pathologic characteristics of the infantile Marfan syndrome. *Am J Cardiol* **65**:1230–1237, 1990

59. Gumbiner CH, Takao A: Ventricular septal defects. In Garson A, Bricker JT, McNamara DG (eds): *Science and Practice of Pediatric Cardiology*. Philadelphia: Lea & Febiger, 1990, p 1005

60. El Said GM, El Refaee MM: Rheumatic heart disease. In Garson A, Bricker JT, McNamara DG (eds): *Science and Practice of Pediatric Cardiology*. Philadelphia: Lea & Febiger, 1990, pp 1512–1520

61. Garson A: Ventricular arrhythmias. In Garson A, Bricker JT, McNamara DG (eds): *Science and Practice of Pediatric Cardiology*. Philadelphia: Lea & Febiger, 1990, p 1891

62. Garson A, McNamara D: Sudden death in a pediatric cardiac population. *J Am Coll Cardiol* **5**:134B–137, 1985

63. Braun LO, Kincaid OW, McGoon DC: Prognosis of aortic valve replacement in relation to the preoperative heart size. *J Thorac Cardiovasc Surg* **63**:381, 1973

64. Henry WL, Robert OB, Rosing DR: Observation on the optimum time for operative intervention for aortic regurgitation: Serial echocardiographic evaluation of asymptomatic patients. *Circulation* **62**:484–492, 1980

65. Veyrat C, Abitbol G, Bas S, et al: Quantitative assessment of valvular regurgitations using the pulsed doppler technique. *Ultrasound Med Biol* **10**:201–213, 1984

66. Rocchini AP, Weesner KM, Heidelberger K, et al: Porcine xenograft valve failure in children: An immunologic response. *Circulation* **64**:II162–II171, 1983

67. Gerosa G, McKay R, Davies J, Ross DN: Comparison of the aortic homograft and the pulmonary autograft for aortic valve or root replacement in children. *J Thorac Cardiovasc Surg* **102**:51–61, 1991

68. Park MK: Acquired heart disease. In Park MK (ed): *Pediatric Cardiology for Practitioners*. Chicago: Year Book Medical, 1984, pp 217–218

69. Karl T, Wensley D, Stark J, et al: Infective endocarditis in children with congenital heart disease: Comparison of selected features in patients with surgical correction or palliation and those without. *Br Heart J* **58**:57–65, 1987

70. Skandalakis JE, Edward BF, Gray SW, et al: Coarctation of the aorta with aneurysm. *Surg Gynecol Obstet* **111**:307–326, 1960

71. Lindsay J: Coarctation of the aorta, bicuspid aortic valve and abnormal ascending aortic wall. *Am J Cardiol* **61**:184–185, 1988

72. Qu R, Yokota M, Kitano M, et al: Surgical indication for aortic arch hypoplasia in infants. *J Cardiovasc Surg* **31**:796–800, 1990

73. Rowlatt UF, Rimoldi HJA, Lev M: The quantitative anatomy of the normal child's heart. *Pediatr Clin North Am* **10**:499–587, 1963

74. Morriss MJH, McNamara DG: Coarctation of the aorta and interrupted aortic arch. In Garson A, Bricker JT, McNamara DG (eds): *Science and Practice of Pediatric Cardiology*. Philadelphia: Lea & Febiger, 1990, pp 1353–1381

75. Mitchell IM, Pollock JCS: Coarctation of the aorta and poststenotic aneurysm formation. *Br Heart J* **64**:332–333, 1990

76. Carvalho JS, Redington AN, Shinebourne EA, et al: Continuous wave Doppler echocardiography and coarctation of the aorta: Gradients and flow patterns in the assessment of severity. *Br Heart J* **64**:133–137, 1990

77. Simpson IA, Soho DJ, Valdez-Cruz LM, et al: Color Doppler flow mapping in patients with coarctation of the aorta: New observations and improved evaluation with color flow diameter and proximal acceleration as predictors of severity. *Circulation* **77**:736–744, 1988

78. Allan LD, Chita SK, Handerson RH, et al: Coarctation of the aorta in prenatal life: An echocardiographic, anatomical and functional study. *Br Heart J* **59**:356–360, 1988

79. Simpson IA, Chung HJ, Glass RF, et al: Cine magnetic resonance imaging for evaluation of anatomy and flow relations in infants and children with coarctation of the aorta. *Circulation* **78**:142–148, 1988

80. Watterson KG, Dhasmana JP, O'Higgins JW, Wisheart JD: Distal aortic pressure during coarctation operation. *Ann Thorac Surg* **49**:978–990, 1990

81. Sciolaro C, Copeland J, Cork R, et al: Long-term follow-up comparing subclavian flap angioplasty to resection with modified oblique end to end anastomosis. *J Thorac Cardiovasc Surg* **101**:1–13, 1991

82. Van Son JAM, van Asten WNJC, van Lier HJJ, et al: A comparison of coarctation resection and subclavian flap angioplasty using ultrasonography: Monitored postductal reactive hyperemia. *J Thorac Cardiovasc Surg* **100**:817–829, 1990

83. Redington AN, Booth P, Shore DF, Rigby ML: Primary balloon dilatation of coarctation of the aorta in neonates. *Br Heart J* **64**:277–281, 1990

84. Glassow PF, Huhta JC, Yoon GG, et al: Surgery without angiography for neonates without aortic arch obstruction. *Int J Cardiol* **18**:417–425, 1988

85. Yamaguchi M, Tachibana H, Hosokawa Y, et al: Early and

late results of surgical treatment of coarctation of the aorta in the first three months of life. *J Cardiovasc Surg* **30**:169–172, 1989

86. Choy M, Rocchini AP, Beekman RH, et al: Paradoxical hypertension after repair of coarctation of the aorta in children: Balloon angioplasty versus surgical repair. *Circulation* **75**:1186–1191, 1987

87. Brewer LA, Fosburg RG, Mulder GA, Berska JJ: Spinal cord complications following surgery for coarctation of the aorta: A study of 66 cases. *J Thorac Cardiovasc Surg* **64**:368–378, 1972

88. Crawford FA, Sade RM: Spinal cord injury associated with hyperthermia during aortic coarctation repair. *J Thorac Cardiovasc Surg* **87**:616–618, 1984

89. Malan JE, Benatar A, Levin SE: Long-term follow-up of coarctation of the aorta repaired by patch angioplasty. *Int J Cardiol* **30**:23–32, 1991

90. Karey REW, Carton JL, Blackman MS: Atenalol therapy for exercise-induced hypertension after aortic coarctation repair. *Am J Cardiol* **66**:1233–1236, 1990

91. Isner JM, Donaldson RF, Fulton D, et al: Cystic medial necrosis in the coarctation of the aorta: A potential factor contributing to adverse consequences observed after percutaneous balloon angioplasty of coarctation sites. *Circulation* **75**:686–695, 1987

92. Bromberg B, Beekman RT, Rocchini AP, et al: Aortic aneurysm after patch aortoplasty repair of coarctation: A prospective analysis of prevalence, screening tests and risks. *J Am Coll Cardiol* **14**:734–741, 1989

93. Matsumoto M, Okamoto Y, Konishi Y, et al: Isolated interruption of the aortic arch. *J Cardiovasc Surg* **29**:574–576, 1988

94. Williams RL, Sommerville RJ: Truncus arteriosus. In Garson A, Bricker JT, McNamara DG (eds): *The Science and Practice of Pediatric Cardiology*. Philadelphia: Lea & Febiger, 1990, pp 1127–1133

95. Scott WA, Rocchini AP, Bove EL, et al: Repair of interrupted aortic arch in infancy. *J Thorac Cardiovasc Surg* **96**:564–568, 1988

96. Monro JL, Bunton RW, Sutherland GR, Keeton BR: Correction of interrupted aortic arch. *J Thorac Cardiovasc Surg* **98**:421–427, 1989

97. Orts-Llorca F, Puerta Fonolla J, Sobrado J: The formation, septation and fate of the truncus arteriosus in man. *J Anat* **134**(Part 1):41–56, 1982

98. Collett RW, Edwards JE: Persistent truncus arteriosus: A classification according to anatomic types. *Surg Clin North Am* **29**:1245–1270, 1949

99. Ceballos R, Soto B, Kirklin JW, Bargeron LM Jr: Truncus arteriosus: An anatomical-angiographic study. *Br Heart J* **49**:589–599, 1983

100. Fuglestad SJ, Puga FJ, Danielson GK, Edwards WD: Surgical pathology of the truncal valve: A study of 12 cases. *Am J Cardiovasc Pathol* **2**:39–47, 1988

101. De la Cruz MV, Cayre R, Angelini P, et al: Coronary arteries in truncus arteriosus. *Am J Cardiol* **66**:1482–1486, 1990

102. Mair DD, Edwards WD, Julsrud PR, et al: Truncus arteriosus. In Adams FH, Emmanouilides GC, Riemenschneider TA (eds): *Heart Disease in Infants and Children*, 4th ed. Baltimore: Williams & Wilkins, 1989, pp 504–515

103. Marcelletti C, McGoon DC, Danielson GK, et al: Early and late results of repair of truncus arteriosus. *Circulation* **55**:636–641, 1977

104. Radford DJ, Perkins L, Lachman R, Thong YH: Spectrum of DiGeorge syndrome in patients with truncus arteriosus: Expanded DiGeorge syndrome. *Pediatr Cardiol* **9**:95–101, 1988

105. McFaul RC, Mair DD, Feldt RH, et al: Truncus arteriosus and previous pulmonary arterial banding: Clinical and hemodynamic assessment. *Am J Cardiol* **38**:626–632, 1976

106. Elkins RC, Steinberg JB, Razook JD, et al: Correction of truncus arteriosus with truncal valvular stenosis or insufficiency using two homografts. *Ann Thorac Surg* **50**:728–733, 1990

107. Ebert PA, Turley K, Stanger P, et al: Surgical treatment of truncus arteriosus in the first 6 months of life. *Ann Surg* **200**:451–456, 1984

108. Bove EL, Beekman RH, Snider AR: Repair of truncus arteriosus in the neonate and young infant. *Ann Thorac Surg* **47**:499–506, 1989

109. Barbero-Marcial M, Riso A, Atik E, Jatene A: A technique for correction of truncus arteriosus types I and II without extracardiac conduits. *J Thorac Cardiovasc Surg* **99**:364–369, 1990

110. Sharma BK, Pilato M, Ott DA: Surgical repair of type II truncus arteriosus without a conduit. *Ann Thorac Surg* **50**:479–481, 1990

111. Zannini L, Galli R, Curien N, et al: Surgery of truncus arteriosus in the first 2 years of life: Analysis of a consecutive series of 22 patients. *G Ital Cardiol* **12**:723–728, 1982

112. Radford DJ, Lachman R, Thong YH: The immunocompetence of children with congenital heart disease. *Int Arch Allergy Appl Immunol* **81**:331–336, 1986

113. Reller MD, Colasurdo MA, Rice MJ, McDonald RW: The timing of spontaneous closure of the ductus arteriosus in infants with respiratory distress syndrome. *Am J Cardiol* **66**:75–78, 1990

114. Heymann MA, Rudolph AM: Control of the ductus arteriosus. *Physiol Rev* **55**:62–78, 1975

115. Gittenberger-DeGroot AC, Moulaert AJ, Hitchcock JF: Histology of the persistent ductus arteriosus in cases of congenital rubella. *Circulation* **62**:183–186, 1980

116. Ellison RC, Peckham GJ, Lang P, et al: Evaluation of the preterm infant for patent ductus arteriosus. *Pediatrics* **71**:364–372, 1983

117. Gittenberger-DeGroot AC, van Ertbruggen I, Moulaert AJ, Honnek E: The ductus arteriosus in the preterm infant: Histologic and clinical observations. *J Pediatr* **96**:88–93, 1980

118. Rudolph AM, Heymann MA: Medical treatment of the ductus arteriosus. *Hosp Pract* **12**:57–65, 1977

119. Dyck ID, Benson LN, Smallhorn JF, et al: Catheter occlusion of the persistently patent ductus arteriosus. *Am J Cardiol* **62**:1089–1092, 1988

120. Rashkind WJ, Mullins CE, Hellenbrand WE, Tait MA: Nonsurgical closure of patent ductus: Clinical application

of the Rashkind PDA Occluder. *Circulation* **75**:583–592, 1987

121. Ali Khan MA, Mullins CE, Nihill MR, et al: Percutaneous catheter closure of the ductus arteriosus in children and young adults. *Am J Cardiol* **64**:218–221, 1989
122. Wessel DL, Keane JF, Parness I, Lock JE: Outpatient closure of the patent ductus arteriosus. *Circulation* **77**:1068–1071, 1988
123. Mullins CE: Patent ductus arteriosus. In Garson A, Bricker JT, McNamara DG (eds): *Science and Practice of Pediatric Cardiology*. Philadelphia: Lea & Febiger, 1990, pp 1055–1069
124. Kutsche LM, Van Mierop LHS: Anatomy and pathogenesis of aortopulmonary septal defect. *Am J Cardiol* **59**:443–447, 1987
125. Sreeram N, Walsh K: Aortopulmonary window with aortic origin of the right pulmonary artery. *Int J Cardiol* **31**:249–251, 1991
126. Mavroudis C, Gott JP, Katzmark S: The effect of surface cooling on blood flow distribution in infant pigs with mature left to right shunts. *Cryobiology* **22**:243–250, 1985
127. Ravikumar S, Wright CM, Hawker RE, et al: The surgical management of aortopulmonary window using the anterior sandwich patch closure technique. *J Cardiovasc Surg* **29**:629–632, 1988
128. Doty DB, Richardson JV, Falkousky GE, et al: Aortopulmonary septal defect: Hemodynamics, angiography, and operation. *Ann Thorac Surg* **32**:244–250, 1981
129. Sreeram N, Franks R, Walsh K: Aortic-ventricular tunnel in a neonate: Diagnosis and management based on cross sectional and colour Doppler ultrasonography. *Br Heart J* **65**:161–162, 1991
130. Morrow RW: Aortic arch and pulmonary artery abnormalities. In Oski FA, DeAngelis CD, Feigin RD, Warshaw JB (eds): *Principles and Practice of Pediatrics*. Philadelphia: JB Lippincott, 1990, pp 1450–1456
131. Arciniegas E, Hakimi M, Hertzler JH, et al: Surgical management of congenital vascular rings. *J Thorac Cardiovasc Surg* **77**:721–727, 1979
132. Becker CI, Ilbawi MN, Idriss FS, DeLeon SY: Vascular anomalies causing tracheoesophageal compression. *J Thorac Cardiovasc Surg* **97**:725–731, 1989

Chapter 21 | Myocardial and Coronary Anomalies

Howard P. Gutgesell

CARDIOMYOPATHY

Cardiomyopathies are commonly divided into dilated (congestive) and hypertrophic types. Other forms of cardiomyopathy are seen in infants of diabetic mothers and in patients with glycogen storage disease.

Dilated Cardiomyopathy

The term *dilated cardiomyopathy* (also called *congestive cardiomyopathy*) is applied to the large group of primary and secondary myocardial diseases characterized by cardiac dilatation and decreased myocardial contractility. It is apparent that dilated cardiomyopathy is not a single disease but an end result of myocardial injury from a wide variety of metabolic, infectious, nutritional, or toxic conditions (Table 21–1). Although it is common practice to attempt to establish a precise etiology by means of cultures, serologic tests, and metabolic studies, the precise underlying cause is undetermined in the majority of patients presenting with clinical and laboratory features of dilated cardiomyopathy.

Endocardial Fibroelastosis. Primary endocardial fibroelastosis (EFE) is characterized by a diffuse, "milky" thickening of the endocardium, especially that of the left ventricle.[1] The heart is enlarged, with a dilated left ventricular cavity. Although the etiology is unknown, it is believed that EFE is a sequel to a viral interstitial myocarditis.[2] A *secondary* form of EFE is seen in a heterogeneous group of congenital cardiac lesions characterized by increased left ventricular wall stress. Aortic atresia and severe aortic stenosis are the most common.

Primary EFE is typically manifested by the development of congestive heart failure in a previously healthy infant. Symptoms similar to those of patients with dilated cardiomyopathy described below occur in the first year of life in 80% of patients. Definitive diagnosis can be made only by myocardial biopsy or autopsy.

Anthracycline-induced Heart Disease. Two anthracyclines are used extensively in the treatment of leukemia and solid tumors: doxorubicin (Adriamycin) and daunorubicin. Their clinical effectiveness is limited by their cardiotoxicity, which results in a dilated cardiomyopathy that is often irreversible. The most important risk factor for the development of congestive heart failure is the total cumulative dose: Less than 1% of patients receiving under 500 mg/m^2 of doxorubicin develop heart failure, whereas over 30% of those receiving more than 600 mg/m^2 develop cardiotoxicity.[3] Mediasternal irradiation appears to enhance the cardiotoxic effects of doxorubicin.[4]

Patients receiving anthracycline therapy generally have frequent evaluation of cardiac function by echocardiography, radionuclide angiography, or even myocardial biopsy.[5,6] Therapy is discontinued in the presence of decreased left ventricular function. However, recent studies have demonstrated abnormal ventricular function in long-term survivors even when ventricular function was thought to be normal during chemotherapy.[7]

Carnitine Deficiency. Carnitine, a quaternary ammonium compound, is an essential cofactor for transport of long-chain fatty acids into mitrochondria for oxidation. Several carnitine deficiency syndromes have been described and are classified as systemic (low plasma and tissue carnitine concentrations) or myopathic (normal plasma concentration but low skeletal muscle concentration). Cardiac enlargement with congestive heart failure occurs in occasional patients with both forms of carnitine deficiency and responds to treatment with L-carnitine.[8]

Tripp et al[9] described a family in which a dilated cardiomyopathy developed in four of five children, three

TABLE 21–1. CAUSES OF DILATED CARDIOMYOPATHY

Infection
    Viral (especially Coxsackie and other enteroviruses)
    Bacterial
    Mycoplasma
    Rickettsial (Rocky Mountain spotted fever)
    Protozoal (visceral larva migrans)
Metabolic/Nutritional
    Hypocalcemia
    Hypokalemia
    Hypomagnesemia
    Thiamine deficiency (beriberi)
    Carnitine deficiency
Toxins
    Anthracyclines
    Alcohol
    Cobalt, other heavy metals
Miscellaneous
    Ischemic (anomalous left coronary artery)
    Hereditary
    Neuromuscular disease
    Postpartum cardiomyopathy

of whom died suddenly and were found to have EFE at autopsy. The surviving child had severe plasma and tissue carnitine deficiency; left ventricular function was markedly improved following oral L-carnitine therapy. The case is of importance because it illustrates that endocardial fibroelastosis is a nonspecific pattern of injury of the immature myocardium, and that at least one form of dilated cardiomyopathy is amenable to specific therapy. All patients with dilated cardiomyopathy should be investigated for carnitine deficiency.

Natural History. In a review of 161 patients and children with primary myocardial disease seen at the Boston Children's Hospital 1945 through 1974, Greenwood et al[10] reported that one third of the patients died, one third recovered, and one third survived with residual cardiac disease. More recent studies have demonstrated 1-year survival rates of 63–83% and 5-year survival rates of 34–77%.[11–14] Older age at presentation, very poor ventricular function, and rhythm abnormalities seem to indicate poor prognosis. Improved medical therapy with potent diuretics, afterload reduction, and better antiarrhythmic drugs will probably reduce the early mortality rate, but improvement in long-term outcome will require better understanding of the underlying disease process and specific therapy.

Diagnostic Features. The most common modes of presentation of infants and children with dilated cardiomyopathy are (1) tachypnea and exercise intolerance secondary to congestive heart failure; (2) arrhythmia; and (3) cardiomegaly detected at the time of chest radiograph obtained as part of the evaluation of another med-

ical condition. Although many patients ultimately develop severe cardiac failure with pulmonary edema and low cardiac output, others are surprisingly asymptomatic despite radiographic or echocardiographic evidence of cardiomegaly and decreased left ventricular performance. The physical examination typically demonstrates a quiet precordium with normal or decreased first and second heart sounds and a third heart sound or summation gallop. A soft, blowing apical murmur of mitral insufficiency is present in approximately a third of patients. Hepatomegaly is frequently present, and ascites and peripheral edema may occur in cases of severe biventricular failure.

The chest radiograph reveals cardiomegaly with pulmonary venous congestion. The electrocardiogram (ECG) is variable. The most common pattern, especially in patients with chronic cardiomyopathy, is one of left ventricular hypertrophy. Generalized low voltage with T wave flattening or inversion suggests an acute inflammatory process or pericardial effusion. In EFE, the ECG is notable for marked ventricular hypertrophy.[15] Echocardiography is the most useful noninvasive diagnostic test and reveals a dilated left ventricle with reduced indices of systolic function.[16] The left atrium and occasionally the right ventricle are enlarged. With the widespread use of echocardiography, cardiac catheterization and angiography are infrequently performed in children suspected of having dilated cardiomyopathy. Exceptions are patients undergoing aortography to exclude a coronary artery anomaly, those undergoing myocardial biopsy to exclude myocarditis, and those considered for cardiac transplantation.

Anesthesia and Perioperative Management. Dilated cardiomyopathy itself is not amenable to surgical therapy other than heart transplantation. Thus, in most cases, anesthesia will be administered for surgical treatment of noncardiac conditions. The following aspects of the hemodynamics of dilated cardiomyopathy should be considered in planning anesthetic management: (1) Cardiac output is usually normal or slightly diminished. (2) The decreased myocardial contractility is partially balanced by increased left ventricular end-diastolic (and thus pulmonary venous) pressure. Thus, volume replacement must be sufficient to maintain an adequate cardiac output but not so vigorous as to produce pulmonary edema. These principles are no different than for patients with normal hearts, but the room for error is less in patients with cardiomyopathy. (3) Because decreased ventricular function is virtually the sine qua non of dilated cardiomyopathy, it seems prudent to avoid potent inhalation anesthetic agents, such as halothane, that directly depress myocardial contractility.[17] Intraoperative and postoperative monitoring of intravascular volume and ventricular function by echocardiography or intravascular catheters may be advantageous.

Hypertrophic Cardiomyopathy

The term *hypertrophic cardiomyopathy* has become the most widely used name for the cardiac disorder characterized by myocardial hypertrophy, especially of the ventricular septum, small- or normal-sized ventricular cavities, dilated atria, and histologic evidence of myocardial fiber disarray.[18] The disorder was initially called idiopathic hypertrophic subaortic stenosis (IHSS) in the United States, muscular subaortic stenosis (MSS) in Canada, and hypertrophic obstructive cardiomyopathy (HOCM) in England.

Pathophysiology. Hypertrophic cardiomyopathy is characterized by abnormal *diastolic* function. The hypertrophied ventricular walls are stiff, with abnormal patterns of relaxation. This results in elevated left ventricular end-diastolic pressure and, consequently, elevated left atrial, pulmonary venous, and pulmonary capillary pressures. Indices of left ventricular *systolic* function are generally normal or even above normal. Thus, hypertrophic cardiomyopathy is one of the small number of cardiac disorders in which the patient may have symptoms of congestive heart failure (eg, pulmonary edema) in the presence of a hypercontractile left ventricle.

Hemodynamic studies demonstrate a dynamic pressure gradient in the subaortic region of the left ventricle in many patients with hypertrophic cardiomyopathy. Some patients have an outflow gradient at rest, whereas in others, the gradient is manifest only after provocative measures such as the administration of isoproterenol or amyl nitrite.[19] The gradient is the result of an already narrowed outflow tract (secondary to septal hypertrophy) further narrowed by systolic anterior motion (SAM) of the mitral valve and its chordae against the septum. The gradient is increased by conditions that either increase myocardial contractility (digitalis, sympathomimetics), decrease afterload (vasodilators, exercise), or decrease ventricular volume (tachycardia, hypovolemia). Likewise, the gradient can be diminished or abolished by conditions that decrease contractility (β-adrenergic blockade) or increase afterload (squatting, α-adrenergic stimulation).

The presence or absence of an outflow gradient seems to have less clinical importance than was initially believed, and there is disagreement as to whether the presence of a pressure *gradient* actually represents outflow *obstruction*.[20] Outflow gradients may also be present on the right side of the heart, especially in severe cases presenting in early childhood. Several of the early descriptions of this condition in children noted right and left ventricular outflow gradients.[21]

Natural History. Many children with hypertrophic cardiomyopathy have a stable clinical course with few symptoms during childhood.[22] Paradoxically, the risk of sudden death seems to be greatest in young patients,

including those with no functional limitations and little or no outflow gradient.[23] Sudden death is particularly apt to occur during or immediately after exercise and competitive sports are contraindicated in patients with hypertrophic cardiomyopathy. Cardiac arrhythmias, particularly atrial fibrillation, are common. Patients with hypertrophic cardiomyopathy are at risk of developing endocarditis, usually on the thickened mitral valve that contacts the septum in systole. Progression of hypertrophic cardiomyopathy with an outflow gradient to a dilated cardiomyopathy with depressed ventricular function is a serious, but uncommon, outcome.[24]

Diagnostic Features. Hypertrophic cardiomyopathy is inherited as an autosomal dominant condition with a high degree of penetrance.[25] Although symptoms most commonly become apparent in late adolescence or young adulthood, the condition has been observed at autopsy, in stillborns,[26] and in octogenarians.[27] In one elderly woman, hypertrophic cardiomyopathy was diagnosed during anesthesia.[28] Dyspnea is the most common symptom, followed by chest pain, fatigue, and syncope. Many patients with laboratory features of the disease may have no symptoms, and the first manifestation of the disease may be sudden death.[29]

Common physical findings include the presence of an exaggerated and sometimes bifid apical impulse, a prominent S_3 or S_4, and a variable systolic murmur. The murmur is typically heard best midway between the left sternal border and the apex and is due to subaortic "obstruction," mitral insufficiency, or both. The peripheral pulses are brisk, in distinction to the damped pulses of fixed forms of left ventricular outflow obstruction such as aortic valve stenosis.

The diagnosis of hypertrophic cardiomyopathy can be established by noninvasive techniques. The ECG is usually abnormal, the most common findings being ST segment and T wave abnormalities, left ventricular hypertrophy, and prominent Q waves in the inferior and lateral leads. The chest radiograph may reveal cardiomegaly, especially with left ventricular hypertrophy. Echocardiography has largely replaced cardiac catheterization and angiography as the definitive diagnostic test in this condition. The echocardiographic features of hypertrophic cardiomyopathy include asymmetric septal hypertrophy (with a septal/left ventricular wall ratio of ≥1.3), normal or supranormal indices of systolic function, systolic anterior motion of the mitral valve, and systolic vibration of the aortic valve leaflets.

Anesthesia and Perioperative Management. Most surgical procedures in children with hypertrophic cardiomyopathy will be noncardiac procedures for coexistent medical conditions. Halothane and similar negative inotropic agents are well tolerated, especially if volume expansion and vasoconstrictors are used to counteract vasodilation.[30] Halothane was thought actually to improve hemodynamics in one case.[31] Because of their effects on systemic vascular resistance, enflurane and isoflurane are less advantageous, although they have been used successfully in a small number of reported cases.[30,32,33] Spinal or epidural anesthesia, which decrease systemic vascular resistance, should be used cautiously if at all.[30,32,34] Isoproterenol, epinephrine, and other positive inotropic agents may likewise have deleterious effects.

Fluid administration and replacement of blood losses must also be judicious to avoid hypotension or pulmonary edema. In older children undergoing extensive procedures with large losses of blood, preoperative insertion of a Swan-Ganz catheter for monitoring pulmonary arterial wedge pressure is desirable. Antibiotic prophylaxis against bacterial endocarditis should be given to all patients with hypertrophic cardiomyopathy prior to and after surgery.

A recent survey of 35 patients with hypertrophic obstructive cardiomyopathy undergoing major noncardiac surgery revealed no significant ventricular dysrhythmias or intraoperative deaths. However, there was one patient with perioperative myocardial infarction, eight patients with atrial arrhythmias or premature ventricular contractions, and five patients with significant perioperative hypotension requiring vasopressors.[30] However, the ventriculoaortic gradient is always labile in patients with hypertrophic cardiomyopathy. It can be increased by decreased preload or afterload and increased myocardial contractility.

Surgical and Medical Therapy. The mainstay of medical therapy for hypertrophic cardiomyopathy has been β-adrenergic blockade, recently with the longer-acting β-blockers. β-Blockade is more effective for relieving angina than in relieving dyspnea or preventing arrhythmias or sudden death.

The calcium channel blocking agents, primarily verapamil and nifedipine, are widely used as alternatives to β-adrenergic blockade in the management of hypertrophic cardiomyopathy.[35] Verapamil decreases contractility and enhances myocardial relaxation,[36–38] thus decreasing the systolic outflow gradient and enhancing diastolic filling. Amiodarone has been shown to improve survival in the subset of patients with ventricular tachycardia.[39] Automatic implantable defibrillators have also been used successfully in patients with life-threatening ventricular tachyarrhythmias.[40]

A variety of surgical procedures aimed at reducing the left ventricular outflow gradient have been proposed.[41] They are typically reserved for symptomatic patients with substantial outflow gradients and lack of response to medical therapy. A transaortic approach with resection of a large wedge of tissue from the left ventricular side of the septum is the most widely used procedure (so-called septal myotomy-myectomy).

Cardiomyopathy of Infants of Diabetic Mothers

A unique form of cardiomyopathy is present in a small percentage of infants of diabetic mothers. The hearts of these infants are large, with thick walls (especially the interventricular septum) and small or normal-sized ventricular cavities.[42–43] Systolic indices of ventricular function are usually normal, although some observers have reported a dilated form of cardiomyopathy.[44] The pathologic and hemodynamic features of the cardiomyopathy of infants of diabetic mothers are very similar to those of hypertrophic obstructive cardiomyopathy. The major difference is the transient nature of the cardiomyopathy; by 6–12 months of age, wall thickness and cavity dimensions have returned to normal.[42]

The etiology of the cardiomyopathy of infants of diabetic mothers is unknown, although the presence of a similar cardiomyopathy in infants with nesidioblastosis suggests that elevated insulin levels in utero may be a causative factor. Because the cardiomyopathy is transient, specific therapy is rarely necessary.

The preoperative evaluation of infants of diabetic mothers should include echocardiography to determine if cardiomyopathy is present and whether it is of the obstructive or dilated form. Subsequent management should then follow the principles outlined previously for these forms of cardiomyopathy.

Glycogen Storage Disease

Glycogen storage disease is produced by deficiency of enzymes involved in the degradation of glycogen. In type II (Pompe disease), caused by deficiency of alpha-1,4-glucosidase, there is accumulation of excessive amounts of glycogen in the cardiac muscle cells. This results in marked cardiomegaly, with hypertrophy of the ventricular septum and free walls,[45,46] often with features of ventricular outflow obstruction. Patients with glycogen storage disease develop heart failure at an early age and few survive beyond 6 months of life.

CONGENITAL CORONARY ARTERY ANOMALIES

Anomalous Origin of the Coronary Arteries from the Pulmonary Artery

Anatomy. Anomalous origin of the left coronary artery from the pulmonary artery (ALCA) is a rare cardiovascular anomaly with a high infant mortality rate.[47,48] Anomalous origin of the left anterior descending coronary, the right coronary artery, and both coronary arteries from the pulmonary artery have also been described, but these conditions are extremely rare and will not be included in the present discussion. When the left coronary artery arises from the pulmonary trunk, myocardial perfusion must be provided directly from the pulmonary artery or from collaterals from the right coronary artery (which arises in a normal manner from the aortic root).

Pathophysiology. Myocardial perfusion is typically adequate in the early neonatal period when pulmonary pressure is high but generally becomes insufficient as pulmonary pressure and resistance regress by 1–2 months of age.[49] Myocardial ischemia or infarction with left ventricular dysfunction frequently become apparent between 1 and 6 months of age. During this phase, depending upon the extent of the coronary collaterals, there may be actual left-to-right shunting of oxygenated blood from the right coronary artery through collaterals to the left coronary artery and into the main pulmonary artery creating a so-called "myocardial steal."

Natural History. It has been estimated that 90% of untreated patients with ALCA die in the first year of life.[47] However, occasional patients are asymptomatic in early childhood and the lesion is discovered at the time of evaluation of a heart murmur or chest pain later in childhood or adulthood.

Diagnostic Features. The most common presentation of ALCA is one of congestive heart failure (tachypnea, cardiomegaly) in an infant with either no murmur or the murmur of mitral insufficiency. ECG typically reveals evidence of anterolateral myocardial infarction. Thallium scintigraphy[50] as well as two-dimensional and Doppler echocardiography[51,52] generally allow distinction of this condition from other causes of dilated cardiomyopathy. Aortic angiography (Fig 21–1) provides a precise diagnosis and allows assessment of the collateral vessels.

Anesthesia and Perioperative Management. Symptomatic infants undergoing surgery for ALCA have pulmonary venous congestion, marginal cardiac output, decreased myocardial contractility due to myocardial ischemia or infarction, and a high likelihood of developing ventricular arrhythmias. Although experience is limited because of the rarity of the condition, the principles used for adults with severe coronary insufficiency seem applicable.[53,54] Fluid administration must be very judicious in order to assure adequate cardiac output without pulmonary edema. Catecholamines (dopamine, dobutamine) may be useful to augment cardiac output, but their potential to increase myocardial oxygen consumption and produce arrhythmias warrants caution.

Surgical and Medical Therapy. The initial treatment of symptomatic infants with ALCA is essentially the application of the principles of the modern coronary care unit to the infant: cardiac monitoring, antiarrhythmia therapy, diuretics, and afterload-reducing agents are typically employed. Ultimately, surgical intervention is considered, but there is disagreement as to whether this should be performed in early infancy[55,56] or later in child-

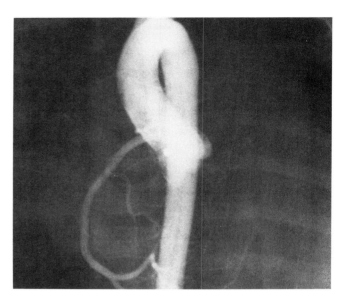

Figure 21–1. Ascending aorta angiogram in a 5-month-old infant with anomalous origin of the left coronary artery. Only the large right coronary artery is visualized arising from the aorta; the left coronary artery was subsequently opacified in a retrograde manner by collateral vessels from the right coronary artery.

hood[57] and as to whether the optimal procedure is simply to ligate the left coronary artery near its origin,[49,58] perform a saphenous vein graft,[59] reimplant the left coronary into the aorta,[55,60] create an intrapulmonary artery neocoronary artery,[61,62] or perform an internal mammary or subclavian artery to left coronary anastomosis.[63,64]

Of the surgical techniques mentioned above, only the creation of a transpulmonary tunnel[61,62] between the aorta and left coronary definitely requires cardiopulmonary bypass. Ligation of the left coronary at its origin and subclavian-coronary anastomosis are performed without bypass, whereas saphenous vein grafts and direct aortic reimplantation are often performed with bypass standby.

Anomalous Origin of the Anterior Descending Coronary Artery from the Right Coronary Artery in Tetralogy of Fallot

In approximately 8% of patients with tetralogy of Fallot, the anterior descending coronary artery arises from the right coronary artery and crosses the right ventricular overflow tract as it descends toward the apex.[65–67] This condition, which should be identified by preoperative angiography, is of importance at the time of intracardiac repair because the artery can be injured or severed if a conventional right ventriculotomy is performed (see Chapter 14).

Aberrant Coronary Artery Origin from the Aorta. Either the left or right coronary artery may have an abnormal origin from the aorta itself, a condition not to be confused with anomalous origin of the coronary artery from the pulmonary trunk (described earlier). Origin of the left coronary artery from the anterior (right) sinus of Valsalva, or from the right coronary artery itself, with a subsequent course between the aorta and the right ventricular infundibulum, has been associated with sudden death in children and young adults, especially during exercise.[68,69] Aberrant origin of the right coronary artery from the left sinus of Valsalva is thought to have a benign clinical course.[69]

Surgical experience with these conditions has been very limited, but coronary bypass would be advised for symptomatic patients with origin of the left coronary artery from the right sinus of Valsalva. The general principles of anesthetic management of coronary disease would seem applicable.

Congenital Coronary Arteriovenous Fistula

Anatomy. Either or both of the coronary arteries may have a fistulous connection to the cardiac chambers or the pulmonary artery. The right ventricle is the most common site of termination of the fistula. The involved coronary artery is typically dilated and tortuous and the heart itself mildly to moderately enlarged.

Natural History. The majority of patients diagnosed before 20 years of age are asymptomatic. In an analysis of 13 new and 174 previously reported cases, Liberthson et al[70] found a history of preoperative symptoms or complications related to the fistula in only 19% (including congestive heart failure in 6%, bacterial endocarditis in 3%, and death in one patient). In contrast, 63% of patients over 20 years at the time of diagnosis had symptoms or complications that included congestive heart failure in 19%, endocarditis in 4%, myocardial infarction in 9%, death in 4%, and fistula rupture in one patient.

Diagnostic Features. The most common clinical finding is a continuous murmur heard best at the mid left sternal border. The ECG is usually normal. The chest radiograph is likewise usually normal, although in patients with a large shunt, the heart size and pulmonary vascular markings may be increased.

The differential diagnosis includes other lesions that produce continuous murmurs. These include patent ductus arteriosus, anomalous coronary artery from the pulmonary artery, ventricular septal defect with aortic insufficiency, aortopulmonary window, and ruptured sinus of Valsalva. The correct diagnosis may be made by echocardiography, which often demonstrates the marked dilatation of the involved coronary artery. Contrast echocardiography, with injection into the aortic root, demonstrates the site of termination of the fistula. Coronary arteriography is generally performed prior to surgical repair.

Surgical and Medical Therapy. Although most pediatric patients are asymptomatic, surgical repair of coronary arteriovenous fistula is usually recommended because of the high incidence of complications late in life.[71] Surgical technique has consisted of either distal ligation (especially if the coronary artery terminates at the fistula) or the use of interlocking mattress sutures under the coronary artery to close the fistula while maintaining patency of the vessel.[72,73] Although most fistulas can be closed without bypass, it is generally advisable to have a pump-oxygenator on standby. The anesthetic management is determined by the type and presence of symptoms or complications.

KAWASAKI SYNDROME

The Kawasaki syndrome (also called the mucocutaneous lymph node syndrome) is an acute febrile exanthem of children. It was first described by Kawasaki[74,75] in Japan in 1967 and has subsequently been recognized in children from all continents and all racial groups.

Pathophysiology

The acute syndrome consists of fever, conjunctival injection, oral erythema with crusting of the lips, induration of the hands and feet followed by erythema and desquamation of the soles and palms, a diffuse erythematous rash, and lymphadenopathy. Current guidelines help establish the diagnosis,[76] although atypical cases are common.[77,78] Cardiac involvement, which occurs in about 20% of cases of the Kawasaki syndrome, consists of pancarditis during the first week or two of the illness and the development of coronary artery aneurysms (Fig 21–2) between the second and sixth week of illness.[79,80]

Natural History

The pancarditis of the early phase of the illness may produce pericardial effusion, decreased ventricular function with congestive heart failure, mitral insufficiency, and cardiac arrhythmias (premature ventricular contractions, paroxysmal atrial tachycardia, or heart block). The pathologic changes associated with these findings include perivasculitis of the coronary arteries and aorta, inflammation of the pericardium, myocardium, and endocardium, and inflammation of the cardiac conduction system.[81]

Coronary angiography demonstrates coronary aneurysms in 17–20% of patients studied in the fourth week of the disease. Coronary artery aneurysms are the most striking and most widely studied aspect of cardiovascular involvement in the Kawasaki syndrome and either directly or indirectly contribute to the mortality rate of about 1%. Potential sequelae include rupture of the aneurysm with hemorrhage into the pericardial space and aneurysm thrombosis with myocardial infarction. Serial

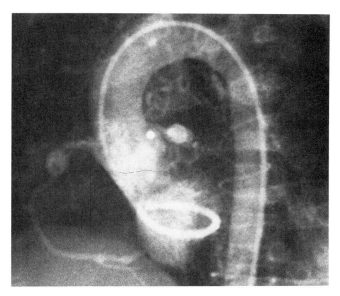

Figure 21–2. Aortic root injection in a 9-month-old infant 2 months after the onset of the Kawasaki syndrome. Note the pea-sized aneurysms on the proximal portions of the left and right coronary arteries.

angiographic studies have demonstrated apparent resolution of coronary aneurysms in a substantial number of patients. Recent data suggest that the normal appearing arteriogram may be produced by intimal thickening and smooth muscle proliferation.[82]

Diagnostic Features

The majority of the coronary aneurysms involve the proximal portions of the left and right coronary artery (see Fig 21–2), areas that can be generally visualized by two-dimensional echocardiography. In experienced hands, echocardiography is over 90% accurate in the detection of coronary aneurysms and is the most widely used method for studying patients with this condition.[83,84]

Anesthesia and Perioperative Management

Certainly the administration of anesthesia would be unusual in the acute stage of the Kawasaki syndrome (pancarditis stage) unless necessary for treatment of a concurrent illness. The abdominal pain present in about one fourth of patients might be confused with appendicitis or other surgical conditions.[85] Anesthetic management should emphasize judicious fluid administration, the use of anesthetic agents that minimize myocardial depression, and preparedness to deal with tachy- or bradyarrhythmias. Although experience is very limited and anesthetic problems have not been documented,[86–89] anesthetic management should be comparable to that used for adults with coronary artery disease with special efforts to minimize myocardial oxygen consumption and systemic hypotension.

Surgical Therapy

A small number of patients with coronary insufficiency secondary to coronary thrombosis or stenosis may be candidates for coronary bypass surgery, especially those with giant aneurysms.[88–91] Internal mammary grafts to the involved coronary artery appear preferable to saphenous vein grafts because of the high incidence of graft thrombosis.[92,93]

REFERENCES

1. Fishbein MC, Ferrans VJ, Roberts WC: Histologic and ultrastructural features of primary and secondary endocardial fibroelastosis. *Arch Pathol Lab Med* **101**:49–54, 1977
2. Hutchins GM, Vie SA: The progression of interstitial myocarditis to idiopathic endocardial fibroelastosis. *Am J Pathol* **66**:483–496, 1972
3. Lenaz L, Page JA: Cardiotoxicity of Adriamycin and related anthracyclines. *Cancer Treat Rev* **3**:111–120, 1976
4. Minow RA, Benjamin RS, Lee ET, Gottlieb JA: Adriamycin cardiomyopathy: Risk factors. *Cancer* **39**:1397–1402, 1977
5. Alexander J, Dainiak N, Berger HJ, et al: Serial assessment of doxorubicin cardiotoxicity with quantitative radionuclide angiography. *N Engl J Med* **300**:278–283, 1979
6. Bristow MR, Mason JW, Billingham ME, Daniels JR: Doxorubicin cardiomyopathy: Evaluation by phonocardiography, endomyocardial biopsy, and cardiac catheterization. *Ann Intern Med* **88**:168–175, 1978
7. Lipshultz SE, Colan SD, Gelber RD, et al: Late cardiac effects of doxorubicin therapy for acute lymphoblastic leukemia in childhood. *N Engl J Med* **324**:808–815, 1991
8. Chapoy PR, Angelini C, Brown WJ, et al: Systemic carnitine deficiency—A treatable inherited lipid-storage disease presenting as Reye's syndrome. *N Engl J Med* **303**:1389–1394, 1978
9. Tripp ME, Katcher ML, Peters HA, et al: Systemic carnitine deficiency presenting as familiar endocardial fibroelastosis: A treatable cardiomyopathy. *N Engl J Med* **30**:385–390, 1981
10. Greenwood RD, Nadas AS, Fyler DC: The clinical course of primary myocardial disease in infants and children. *Am Heart J* **92**:549–560, 1976
11. Taliercio CP, Seward JB, Driscoll DJ, et al: Idiopathic dilated cardiomyopathy in the young: Clinical profile and national history. *J Am Coll Cardiol* **6**:1126–1131, 1985
12. Toshihiro I, Benson LN, Freedom RM, Rowe RD: Natural history and prognostic risk factors in endocardial fibroelastosis. *Am J Cardiol* **62**:431–434, 1988
13. Chen SC, Nouri S, Balfour I, et al: Clinical profile of congestive cardiomyopathy in children. *J Am Coll Cardiol* **15**:189–193, 1990
14. Griffin ML, Hernadex A, Martin TC, et al: Dilated cardiomyopathy in infants and children. *J Am Coll Cardiol* **11**:139–144, 1988
15. Sellers FJ, Keith JD, Manning JA: The diagnosis of primary endocardial fibroelastosis. *Circulation* **29**:49–59, 1964
16. Ghafour AS, Gutgesell HP: Echocardiographic evaluation of left ventricular function in children with congestive cardiomyopathy. *Am J Cardiol* **44**:1332–1338, 1979

17. Bowers JR: Anesthesia and cardiomyopathies: Report of two cases. *Anesth Analg* **50**:1013–1316, 1971

18. Roberts WC, Ferrans VJ: Pathologic anatomy of the cardiomyopathies: Idiopathic dilated and hypertrophic types, infiltrative types and endomyocardial disease with and without eosinophilia. *Hum Pathol* **6**:287–342, 1975

19. Braunwald E, Lambrew CT, Rockoff SD, et al: Idiopathic hypertrophic subaortic stenosis. *Circulation* **30**(suppl IV): IV–1–IV–213, 1964

20. Murgo JP, Alter BR, Dorethy JF, et al: Dynamics of left ventricular ejection in obstructive and nonobstructive hypertrophic cardiomyopathy. *J Clin Invest* **66**:1369–1382, 1980

21. Neufield HN, Ongley PA, Edwards JE: Combined congenital subaortic stenosis and infundibular pulmonary stenosis. *Br Heart J* **22**:686–690, 1960

22. Maron BJ, Tajik AJ, Ruttenberg HD, et al: Hypertrophic cardiomyopathy in infants: Clinical features and natural history. *Circulation* **65**:7–17, 1982

23. Maron BJ, Roberts WC, Epstein SE: Sudden death in hypertrophic cardiomyopathy: A profile of 78 patients. *Circulation* **65**:1388–1394, 1982

24. Beder SD, Gutgesell HP, Mullins CE, McNamara DG: Progression from hypertrophic obstructive cardiomyopathy to congestive cardiomyopathy in a child. *Am Heart J* **104**: 155–156, 1982

25. Clark CE, Henry WL, Epstein SE: Familial prevalence and genetic transmission of idiopathic hypertrophic subaortic stenosis. *N Engl J Med* **289**:709–714, 1973

26. Maron BJ, Edwards JE, Henry WL, et al: Asymmetric septal hypertrophy (ASH) in infancy. *Circulation* **50**:809–820, 1974

27. Hamby RI, Aintablian A: Hypertrophic subaortic stenosis is not rare in the eighth decade. *Geriatrics* **31**:71–74, 1976

28. Lanier W, Prough DS: Intraoperative diagnosis of hypertrophic obstructive cardiomyopathy. *Anesthesiology* **60**:61–63, 1984

29. Maron BJ, Roberts WC, Edwards JE, et al: Sudden death in patients with hypertrophic cardiomyopathy: Characterization of 26 patients without functional limitation. *Am J Cardiol* **41**:803–806, 1978

30. Thompson RC, Liberthson RR, Lowenstein E: Perioperative anesthetic risk of noncardiac surgery in hypertrophic obstructive cardiomyopathy. *JAMA* **254**:2419–2421, 1985

31. Reitan JA, Wright RG: The use of halothane in a patient with asymmetrical septal hypertrophy: A case report. *Can Anaesth Soc J* **29**:154–156, 1982

32. Boccio RV, Chung JH, Harrison DM: Anesthetic management of Caesarian section in a patient with idiopathic hypertrophic subaortic stenosis. *Anesthesiology* **65**:663–665, 1986

33. Freilich JD, Jacobs BR: Anesthetic management of cerebral aneurysm resection in a patient with idiopathic hypertrophic subaortic stenosis. *Anesth Analg* **71**:558–560, 1990

34. Loubser P, Suh K, Cohen S: Adverse effects of spinal anesthesia in a patient with idiopathic hypertrophic subaortic stenosis. *Anesthesiology* **60**:228–230, 1984

35. Rosing DR, Kent KM, Maron BJ, Epstein SE: Verapamil therapy: A new approach to the pharmacologic treatment of hypertrophic cardiomyopathy. II. Effects on exercise capacity and symptomatic status. *Circulation* **60**:1208–1213, 1979

36. Spicer RL, Rocchini AP, Crowley DC, et al: Hemodynamic effects of verapamil in children and adolescents with hypertrophic cardiomyopathy. *Circulation* **67**:413–420, 1983

37. Hanrath P, Mathey DG, Kremer P, et al: Effect of verapamil on left ventricular filling in hypertrophic cardiomyopathy. *Am J Cardiol* **45**:1258–1264, 1980

38. Rosing DR, Condit JR, Maron BJ, et al: Verapamil therapy: A new approach to the pharmacologic treatment of hypertrophic cardiomyopathy. III. Effects of long-term administration. *Am J Cardiol* **48**:545–553, 1981

39. McKenna WJ, Oakley CM, Krikler DM, Goodwin JF: Improved survival with amiodarone in patients with hypertrophic cardiomyopathy and ventricular tachycardia. *Br Heart J* **53**:412–416, 1985

40. Kron J, Oliver RP, Norsted S, Silka MJ: The automatic implantable cardioverter-defibrillator in young patients. *J Am Coll Cardiol* **16**:896–902, 1990

41. Mohr R, Schaff HV, Danielson GK, et al: The outcome of surgical treatment of hypertrophic obstructive cardiomyopathy. *J Thorac Cardiovasc Surg* **97**:666–674, 1989

42. Gutgesell HP, Speer ME, Rosenberg HS: Characterization of the cardiomyopathy in infants of diabetic mothers. *Circulation* **61**:441–450, 1980

43. Gutgesell HP, Mullins CE, Gillette PC, et al: Transient hypertrophic subaortic stenosis in infants of diabetic mothers. *J Pediatr* **89**:120–125, 1976

44. Poland RL, Walter LJ, Chang C: Hypertrophic cardiomyopathy in infants of diabetic mothers. *Pediatr Res* **9**:269, 1975 (abstr)

45. Ehlers KH, Hagstrom JWC, Lukas DS, et al: Glycogen storage disease of the myocardium with obstruction to left ventricular outflow. *Circulation* **25**:96–109, 1962

46. Rees A, Elbl F, Minhas K, Solinger R: Echocardiographic evidence of outflow tract obstruction in Pompe's disease (glycogen storage disease of the heart). *Am J Cardiol* **37**: 1102–1106, 1976

47. Wesselhoeft H, Fawcett JS, Johnson AL: Anomalous origin of the left coronary artery from the pulmonary trunk: Its clinical spectrum, pathology, and pathophysiology, based on a review of 140 cases with seven further cases. *Circulation* **38**:403–425, 1968

48. Askenazi J, Nadas AS: Anomalous left coronary artery originating from the pulmonary artery: Report on 15 cases. *Circulation* **51**:976–987, 1975

49. Case RB, Morrow AG, Stainsby W, Nestor JO: Anomalous origin of the left coronary artery. The physiologic defect and suggested surgical treatment. *Circulation* **17**:1062–1068, 1958

50. Gutgesell HP, Pinsky WW, DePuey EG: Thallium–201 myocardial perfusion imaging in infants and children: Value in distinguishing anomalous left coronary artery from congestive cardiomyopathy. *Circulation* **61**:596–599, 1980

51. Fisher EA, Sepehri B, Lendrum B, et al: Two dimensional echocardiographic visualization of the left coronary artery in anomalous origin of the left coronary artery from the pulmonary artery: Pre- and postoperative studies. *Circulation* **63**:698–704, 1981

52. King DH, Danford DA, Huhta JC, Gutgesell HP: Nonin-

vasive detection of anomalous origin of the left main coronary artery from the pulmonary trunk by pulsed Doppler echocardiography. *Am J Cardiol* **55**:608–609, 1985

53. DiNardo JA: *Anesthesia for Cardiac Surgery.* East Norwalk, CT: Appleton & Lange, 1990, pp 59–84

54. Tarhan S: *Cardiovascular Anesthesia and Postoperative Care,* 2nd ed. Chicago: Year Book Medical, 1989, pp 261–284

55. Arciniegas E, Farooki ZQ, Hakimi M, Green EW: Management of anomalous left coronary artery from the pulmonary artery. *Circulation* **62**(suppl I):I–180–I–189, 1980

56. Neches WH, Mathews RA, Park SC, et al: Anomalous origin of the left coronary artery from the pulmonary artery: A new method of surgical repair. *Circulation* **50**:582–587, 1974

57. Driscoll DJ, Nihill MR, Mullins CE, et al: Management of symptomatic infants with anomalous origin of the left coronary artery from the pulmonary artery. *Am J Cardiol* **47**: 642–648, 1981

58. Nadas AS, Gamboa R, Hugenholtz PG: Anomalous left coronary originating from the pulmonary artery: Report of 2 surgically treated cases with a proposal of hemodynamic and therapeutic classification. *Circulation* **29**:167–175, 1964

59. El-Said GM, Ruzyllo W, Williams RL, et al: Early and late results of saphenous vein graft for anomalous origin of the left coronary artery from pulmonary artery. *Circulation* **48**(suppl III):III–2–III–6, 1973

60. Cooley DA, Hallman GL, Bloodwell RD: Definitive surgical treatment of anomalous origin of the left coronary artery from the pulmonary artery: Indications and results. *J Thorac Cardiovasc Surg* **52**:798–808, 1966

61. Takeuchi S, Imamura H, Katsumoto K, et al: New surgical method for repair of anomalous left coronary artery from pulmonary artery. *J Thorac Surg* **78**:7–11, 1979

62. Midgley FM, Watson DC, Scott LP, et al: Repair of anomalous origin of the left coronary artery in the infant and small child. *J Am Coll Cardiol* **6**:1231–1234, 1984

63. Meyer BW, Stefanik G, Stiles QR, et al: A method of definitive surgical treatment of anomalous origin of left coronary artery: A case report. *J Thorac Cardiovasc Surg* **56**:104–107, 1968

64. Pinsky WW, Fagan LR, Kraeger RR, et al: Anomalous left coronary artery: Report of two cases. *J Thorac Cardiovasc Surg* **65**:810–814, 1973

65. Longenecker CG, Reemstma K, Creech O Jr: Anomalous coronary artery distribution associated with tetralogy of Fallot: A hazard in open cardiac repair. *J Thorac Cardiovasc Surg* **42**:258–262, 1961

66. Dabizzi RP, Caprioli G, Aizaai L, et al: Distribution and anomalies of coronary arteries in tetralogy of Fallot. *Circulation* **61**:95–102, 1980

67. Fellows KE, Freed MD, Keane JR, et al: Results of routine preoperative coronary angiography in tetralogy of Fallot. *Circulation* **51**:561–566, 1975

68. Cheitlin MD, DeCastro CM, McAllister HA: Sudden death as a complication of anomalous left coronary origin from the anterior sinus of Valsalva: A not-so-minor congenital anomaly. *Circulation* **50**:780–787, 1974

69. Liberthson RR, Dinssmore RE, Fallon JT: Aberrant coronary artery origin from the aorta: Report of 18 patients, review of literature and delineation of natural history and management. *Circulation* **59**:748–754, 1979

70. Liberthson RR, Sagar K, Berkoben JP, et al: Congenital coronary arteriovenous fistula: Report of 13 patients, review of the literature and delineation of management. *Circulation* **59**:849–854, 1979

71. Daniel TM, Graham TP, Sabiston DC Jr: Coronary artery-right ventricular fistula with congestive heart failure: Surgical correction in the neonatal period. *Surgery* **67**:985–994, 1970

72. Hallman GL, Cooley DA, Singer DB: Congenital anomalies of the coronary arteries: Anatomy, pathology and surgical treatment. *Surgery* **59**:133–144, 1966

73. Cooley DA, Ellis PR: Surgical consideration of coronary arterial fistula. *Am J Cardiol* **10**:467–474, 1962

74. Kawasaki T: Acute febrile mucocutaneous syndrome with lymphoid involvement with specific desquamation of the fingers and toes. *Jpn J Allergy* **16**:178–222, 1967

75. Kawasaki T, Kosaki F, Okawa S, et al: A new infantile acute febrile mucocutaneous lymph node syndrome (MCLS) prevailing in Japan. *Pediatrics* **54**:271–276, 1974

76. American Heart Association Committee on Rheumatic Fever, Endocarditis, and Kawasaki Disease: Diagnostic guidelines for Kawasaki disease. *Am J Dis Child* **144**:1218–1219, 1990

77. Avner JP, Shaw KN, Chin AJ: Atypical presentation of Kawasaki disease with early development of giant coronary artery aneurysms. *J Pediatr* **114**: 605–606, 1989

78. Rowley AJ, Gonzales-Crussi F, Gidding SS, et al: Incomplete Kawasaki disease with coronary artery involvement. *J Pediatr* **110**:409–413, 1987

79. Kata H, Koeke S, Yammamoto M, et al: Coronary aneurysms in infants and young children with acute febrile mucocutaneous lymph node syndrome. *J Pediatr* **86**:892–898, 1975

80. Kato H, Koike S, Tanaka C: Coronary heart disease in children with Kawasaki disease. *Jpn Circulation J* **43**:469–476, 1979

81. Fujiwara H, Hamashima Y: Pathology of the heart in Kawasaki disease. *Pediatrics* **61**:100–107, 1978

82. Sasaguri Y, Kato H: Regression of aneurymsm in Kawasaki disease: A pathological study. *J Pediatr* **100**:225–231, 1982

83. Satomi G, Nakamura K, Narai S, Takao A: Systematic visualization of coronary arteries by two-dimensional echocardiography in children and infants: Evaluation in Kawasaki's disease and coronary arteriovenous fistula. *Am Heart J* **107**:497–505, 1984

84. Capannari TE, Daniels SR, Meyer RA, et al: Sensitivity, specificity and predictive value of two-dimensional echocardiography in detecting coronary artery aneurysms in patients with Kawasaki disease. *J Am Coll Cardiol* **7**:355–360, 1976

85. Wheeler RA, Najmaldin AS, Soubra M, et al: Surgical presentation of Kawasaki disease (mucocutaneous lymph node syndrome). *Br J Surg* **77**:1273–1274, 1990

86. Kitamura S, Kawachi K, Oyama C, et al: Severe Kawasaki heart disease treated with an internal mammary artery graft in pediatric patients. *J Thorac Cardiovasc Surg* **89**:860–866, 1985

87. Kitamura S, Seki T, Kawachi K, et al: Excellent patency

and growth potential of internal mammary artery grafts in pediatric coronary artery bypass surgery. New evidence for a "live" conduit. *Circulation* **78**:1129–1139, 1988

88. Suma K, Takeuchi Y, Shiroma K, et al: Cardiac surgery of eight children with Kawasaki disease (mucocutaneous lymph node syndrome). *Jpn Heart J* **22**:605–616, 1981

89. Takeuchi Y, Suma K, Asai T, Kusakawa S: Surgical experience with coronary arterial sequelae of Kawasaki disease in children. *J Cardiovasc Surg* **22**:231–238, 1981

90. Tartara K, Kusakawa S: Long-term prognosis of giant coronary aneurysm in Kawasaki disease: An angiographic study. *J Pediatr* **111**:705–710, 1987

91. Kitamura S, Kawashima Y, Fujita T, et al: Aortocoronary bypass grafting in a child with coronary artery obstruction due to mucocutaneous lymph node syndrome: Report of a case. *Circulation* **53**:1035–1040, 1976

92. Kitamura S, Kawachi K, Harima R: Surgery for coronary heart disease due to mucocutaneous lymph node syndrome (Kawasaki disease): Report of 6 patients. *Am J Cardiol* **51**:444–448, 1983

93. Sandiford FM, Vargo TA, Shih J, et al: Successful triple coronary artery bypass in a child with multiple coronary aneurysms due to Kawasaki's disease. *J Thorac Cardiovasc Surg* **79**:283–287, 1980

Chapter 22 | Heart and Lung Transplantation in Children

James M. Steven and C. Dean Kurth

HISTORY OF HEART TRANSPLANTATION

The first laboratory experiments with heart transplantation are credited to Carrell and Guthrie[1] at the University of Chicago, who performed heterotopic heart transplants in 1905, a technique in which the donor heart remains in the normal or orthotopic position by anastomosing the graft to the carotid artery and jugular vein of a puppy. They demonstrated that contractile function returned even after 75 minutes of graft ischemia. In a series of experiments conducted in the Soviet Union from 1940 to 1956, Demikhov achieved graft viability for 32 days using a canine intrathoracic heterotopic model.[2] He also demonstrated functional viability of the graft by excluding the recipient heart from the circulation for periods extending to 15 hours. In 1957, Webb and Howard extended the survival of the graft for ischemic periods of 8 hours by 4°C crystalloid cardioplegic arrest and topical cooling.[3] Orthotopic heart replacement, which necessitated preservation of the recipients' other vital organs during the procedure as well as the need for the graft to assume immediately all the circulatory work, posed other technical and physiologic challenges. Working on dogs at the University of Maryland in 1958, Goldberg achieved brief survival of recipients after orthotopic heart transplantation using cardiopulmonary bypass and anastomosis of the graft to a left atrial cuff to avoid individual pulmonary vein anastomoses.[4] This technique was modified by Cass and Brock in the following year to include an analogous right atrial cuff obviating the need for individual caval anastomoses.[5] These investigators formed the foundation of a technique that Shumway and Lower consolidated and refined at Stanford University to the classic description of orthotopic heart transplantation in 1960.[6]

They also found that the canine recipients survived 6–21 days, and that survival was limited by immunologic problems rather than the technical aspects of the operation. This view was elegantly confirmed by canine autotransplants in demonstrating nearly normal long-term function at rest and during exercise.[7]

Although the technical aspects of the procedure had been detailed by the early 1960s, the ability to modulate rejection of the grafted heart was several years away. Mann observed delayed graft failure in his canine heterotopic heart transplants in 1933.[8] In 1959, Schwartz discovered the immunosuppressive properties of 6-mercaptopurine.[9] A related compound, azathioprine, was subsequently shown to be more effective in treating kidney graft rejection.[2] Because corticosteroids were also effective in the treatment of kidney rejection, Lower and Shumway incorporated both azathioprine and high-dose steroids into a regimen for treating acute graft rejection and obtained long-term survival of dogs after orthotopic heart transplantation.[10]

Much to the surprise of those who had spent years laying the foundation for heart transplantation, the first human transplant was performed by the South African surgeon Christian Barnard in 1967.[11] At that time, death was defined in terms of cardiorespiratory activity rather than cessation of brain function, so close proximity of a suitable recipient as well as the timely death of a donor were needed. Barnard, inspired by his brief observation of Lower in Virginia, placed a donor on cardiopulmonary bypass 5 minutes after the cessation of cardiac and respiratory function, cooled the heart, and removed it for transplantation. Because of fears of rejection, an aggressive immunosuppression regimen, including high-dose prednisone, hydrocortisone, azathioprine, antinomycin C, and local irradiation, was used. Unfortunately, the patient died from *Pseudomonas* pneumonia on the eighteenth postoperative day. Despite the outcome, this operation captured the fancy of many cardiac surgeons, leading to 101 transplants performed by 64 surgical teams in 24 countries over the next year. After dismal results, most centers abandoned the procedure, whereas clinical activity continued in the few centers with long-standing research programs in heart transplantation.

Further improvement in outcome came with better methods to monitor and treat graft rejection. In 1972, the Stanford group developed a program of myocardial surveillance for rejection that employed transcatheter biopsy forceps designed by Caves[12] and a reproducible histologic grading system developed by Billingham.[13] The next year, Oyer added rabbit antithymocyte globulin (ATG) to the therapy of acute rejection.[14] Although these improvements had brought the 1-year survival at Stanford from 20% in 1968 to nearly 70% by 1976, the greatest single improvement in immunotherapy resulted from the addition of cyclosporine A to the maintenance regimen in 1980. This drug, initially described by Calne[15] in 1977, not only increased 1-year survival to 80% but it dramatically sped rehabilitation and shortened the time to discharge of these patients.[16] The introduction of cyclosporine is generally recognized as the milestone marking the modern era of renewed interest in human heart transplantation.

Parallel developments in organ procurement became necessary to meet the growing demand for heart transplantation. Early among these included the incorporation of criteria to establish irreversible cessation of neurologic function state statutes defining death. The Harvard ad hoc committee to define brain death released a report in 1968 that served as a template upon which many states expanded their statutory definition of death to include irreversible cessation of neurologic function.[17] Most states adopted some variant of these criteria in the early 1970s, dramatically improving flexibility in organ procurement and avoiding the period of warm ischemia that was impossible to avoid under earlier statutes. In 1977, the Stanford program further increased the number of organs available for transplantation by initiating a program whereby organs could be transported from great distances.[18] Using cold cardioplegia and topical cooling to 4°C, donor hearts tolerated ischemic periods of 4 hours without discernible injury to graft histology or function.

The clinical evolution of pediatric heart transplantation stretches back nearly as far as the initial adult experiment by Barnard. In 1967, Kantrowitz, working at Maimonides/Downstate Medical Center in New York, transplanted the heart of an anencephalic neonate into an 18-day-old infant with tricuspid atresia.[19] The following year, Cooley performed a heart-lung transplant in a 2-month-old infant with complete common atrioventricular canal defect.[20] Despite the technical success, both infants survived only a few hours. Over the next 12 years, only 11 pediatric heart transplants were performed worldwide. In the early 1980s, heart transplantation was performed in a number of adolescents as an extension of adult programs. By 1984, heart transplants were again

offered to infants, and from 1984 to 1988, over 200 transplants were performed in children under 10, 65 of whom were less than 1 year of age. At Loma Linda University in 1985, Bailey began advocating heart transplantation for neonates with certain congenital heart malformations, such as hypoplastic left heart syndrome.[21] He suggested that transplantation during the neonatal period in which immunologic tolerance exists would reduce the morbidity and mortality that accompanied rejection and immunotherapy in children. Since that time, heart transplantation in infants has become increasingly common. However, given normal life expectancy, the life-long need for immunosuppression, and the actuarial rate of complications following the transplant, pediatric heart transplantation carries considerable uncertainty. Nevertheless, heart transplantation represents a rewarding component of any multifaceted approach to pediatric heart disease.

HEART TRANSPLANTATION

Patient Demographics and Selection

Heart transplantation is offered to alter the natural history of cardiac disease. Thus, the risk of morbidity and mortality related to conventional medical and surgical management must exceed that associated with heart transplantation. Early mortality results from graft failure, rejection, and opportunistic infection, whereas late mortality usually results from rejection, graft atherosclerosis, or lymphoproliferative disease. Morbidity can result from any of these complications as well as the effect of immunosuppressive therapy on the growth and development of the child. Data collected by the International Registry since 1985 reveal a 2-year survival after heart transplantation of 72% in children from 1 to 18 years of age, 62% for children under 1 year of age, and 77% in adults[22] (Fig 22–1).

The number of heart transplants worldwide increased 19% in the years 1987–1990, whereas pediatric (<18 years) heart transplantation grew 73%.[22] This figure results from the increase in transplants in children under 5 years of age (Fig 22–2). From Cooley's report until 1983, all recipients were older than 4 years of age, whereas in 1990, children under 5 years of age accounted for about half of all pediatric heart transplants, over 70% of which were performed in infants (<1 year old).[23] This age category represents the most rapidly growing population subset during the past 5 years. As of 1989, 169 recipients under 1 year of age, 65% of whom were less than 2 months old, have received heart transplants at 29 centers worldwide.[23]

The indications for heart transplantation in children have also changed in the last few years. Although among all pediatric heart transplants performed to date myocardial disease still represents the most common indication,

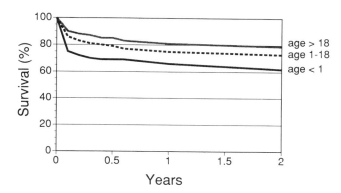

Figure 22–1. Actuarial survival in three age groups. Differences in 2 year survival can be entirely related to operative mortality. Beyond the first month postoperatively, mortality is comparable in the three age groups. (*Data from the Registry of the International Society for Heart and Lung Transplantation.[22]*)

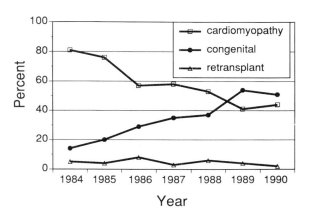

Figure 22–3. Distribution of pediatric heart transplants by indication, presented as a percentage of the transplants performed in each year. Since 1989, congenital heart malformations represent the most common indication. (*Data from the Registry of the International Society for Heart and Lung Transplantation[22] and J.M. Kreitt, personal communications.*)

congenital malformations represent a growing fraction (Fig 22–3).[22] In fact, 1989 was the first year in which pediatric transplants performed for congenital malformations exceeded those for cardiomyopathy.[23] Cardiomyopathy in pediatric patients is usually idiopathic or the result of viral myocarditis and, less commonly, the product of familial, metabolic, or hypertrophic conditions or cancer therapy with radiation and anthracycline drugs. Rarely, anomalous origin of the left coronary artery from the pulmonary artery may result in infarction and ischemic cardiomyopathy. Examples of congenital malformations that merit consideration for heart transplantation include children with transposition of the great arteries who, after a Mustard or Senning procedure, develop right ventricular failure; children who have a single ventricle

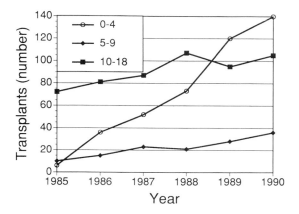

Figure 22–2. Distribution of pediatric heart transplants by age, presented as the number of transplants performed in each year. The number of transplants has increased in each of these pediatric age groups, but the greatest increase has occurred in children under 5 years. (*Data from the Registry of the International Society for Heart and Lung Transplantation[22] and J.M Kreitt, personal communications.*)

and develop ventricular failure or elevated pulmonary vascular resistance that precludes a Fontan operation; children who have truncus arteriosus with severe truncal valve insufficiency; and children with hypoplastic left heart syndrome (HLHS). Although Bailey has shown a 3-year survival of 84% following primary heart transplantation for HLHS,[24] the estimated 1000 children born each year with this lesion presently exceeds the current donor pool. Despite estimates that over 3000 neonates born each year in the United States would be treated optimally with heart or heart-lung transplants,[25,26] in fact, only 67 donors under 1 year of age were accepted in 1990 (United Network for Organ Sharing, unpublished data). Rare indications for heart transplantation include intramyocardial tumors that result in either obstruction or malignant arrhythmias that are otherwise unmanageable. Graft failure necessitates transplantation in approximately 4%.[23]

As with adults, the most important hemodynamic information in the evaluation of a child for transplantation is the determination of pulmonary vascular resistance (PVR). Most adult transplant programs will not offer orthotopic heart transplant when PVR exceeds 6 Wood units/m^2 [27–31] because regression analysis suggests that this doubles postoperative mortality.[28] An absolute value for PVR contraindicating transplantation has not been defined in children. Addonizio et al confirmed that right ventricular failure does not develop after transplant in children with preoperative PVR less than 6 Wood unit.[32,33] However, they did not find an increased mortality owing to greater values for PVR unless accompanied by the need for preoperative inotropic support.[33] Fricker et al suggest that heart transplantation is contraindicated when PVR exceeds 10 Wood units/m^2 in children.[34] However, neonates exhibit PVR that approaches systemic vascular resistance (SVR), which usually exceeds 10 Wood units/m². Although PVR typically decreases during the first few days of life, it may be increased in lesions such as HLHS and truncus arteriosus. In this case, consideration must be given to the source of the donor. Neonatal donor hearts may better tolerate the additional right ventricular pressure work associated with increased PVR.

Several strategies have been developed to manage children with high PVR. Usually, the etiology of elevated PVR is attributable to pulmonary vascular disease from prolonged high pressure and flow due to systemic to pulmonary communications or pulmonary venous hypertension from ventricular failure. Some groups place prognostic importance on the response of PVR to vasodilators such as nitroprusside or prostaglandin E₁ to distinguish a dynamic increases in pulmonary vascular tone from fixed pulmonary vascular disease.[29–32,34] In theory, dynamic processes will resolve rapidly on correction of the underlying hemodynamic abnormality with transplantation. The Stanford protocol accepts children with PVR of 7–8 Wood units/m² if PVR decreases with vasodilators.[30,31] In our experience, in two of three transplant candidates who had PVR over 10 Wood units who received amrinone infusions for approximately 2 weeks, PVR decreased to less than 6 Wood units/m². However, all three had good early postoperative hemodynamics after orthotopic heart transplantation.

Other strategies for managing the child with increased PVR include increasing the donor heart size (body weight 125–210% that of the recipient)[33] and minimizing the ischemic time. For this reason, some programs have advocated intact donor transport to the transplant center.[21,36] Alternate solutions include heart-lung[32,33] and heterotopic heart transplant.[32,33] In the latter, the recipient heart remains to assist in right ventricular pressure work, thus preserving pulmonary blood flow.[38,39] Both approaches carry increased mortality.[22,23,39] Heterotopic heart transplantation offers a 5-year survival of only 54%; both operative and late mortality are increased[23] (Fig 22–4). The outcome following heart-lung transplantation is slightly worse than heterotopic heart transplantation.[22]

Other contraindications to heart transplantation include recent pulmonary infarction; severe central nervous system, hepatic, or renal dysfunction; certain infections (eg, hepatitis, human immunodeficiency virus [HIV], cytomegalovirus [CMV], tuberculosis, varicella); or neoplasms that might be exacerbated by immunosuppression.[29,35,37] Pulmonary abscesses develop in about 50% of those with recent pulmonary infarction after immunosuppression commences.[40,41] A stable social situation is of vital importance because these children will require years of close follow-up along with life-long immunosuppressive therapy.

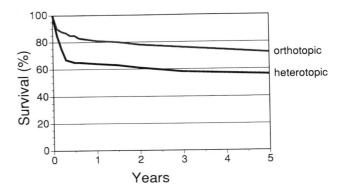

Figure 22–4. Comparison of orthotopic and heterotopic heart transplantation by actuarial survival. Heterotopic transplantation carries higher operative and late mortality. (*Data from the Registry of the International Society for Heart and Lung Transplantation.*[22])

Recipient Preparation

Upon selection for transplantation, the candidate's blood is ABO typed and screened for antibodies against sera of random blood donors. Unless the recipient reacts to more than 10% of the sera in the antibody screen, donor matching is based solely on ABO type.[42] Children who exhibit greater than 10% reaction undergo serum cross match with the donor once identified. Histocompatibility matching by HLA type is not routinely performed given the limited donor pool. The benefit of HLA matching remains controversial.[27,28,43–45] Because the administration of homologous blood products may serve to stimulate antibody responses, pretransplant transfusions should be avoided whenever possible. If a transfusion becomes necessary, blood showing evidence of infection by hepatitis viruses, HIV, and CMV should be avoided. The average wait on the transplant list in most centers is 3–4 weeks.[24,31,34]

Donor Selection

Selection Process. Once a prospective donor meets the criteria for brain death and parental consent is obtained, the child's weight and blood type are entered into the United Network for Organ Sharing (UNOS) system. Donor weight and blood type determine the basis of a match. In general, the donor should be within 80–160% of the recipient's weight, although the upper limit may be increased to over 200% under certain circumstances, such as an elevated PVR in the recipient.[33,46] A period of cardiac arrest is common among potential pediatric donors. If cardiovascular function has been restored to the normal range with minimal or no inotropic support, a history of cardiac arrest does not contraindicate donation. Guidelines from Loma Linda University are purportedly more liberal in this respect as they only require a shortening fraction of 28% or more irrespective of inotropic support.[24] Echocardiographic evaluation of the donor heart is performed to determine structural or functional abnormalities.

Although graft ischemic times less than 4 hours have high success,[18] it may become necessary to extend this time under exceptional circumstances, such as the procurement of neonatal hearts.[46] At Stanford University, over half (58%) the pediatric procurements take place outside the immediate vicinity of the transplant center, whereas 29% occur in the same hospital and 22% in a nearby hospital.[37] Although more common in the early experience with pediatric transplants, the transport of intact donors effectively limits ischemic time.[21,36]

A history of laboratory findings that suggest systemic disease (eg, extracranial malignancy) or infection in the donor preclude consideration. Subclinical infection or carrier status, however, rarely does. Despite the morbidity and mortality associated with CMV infection in the early postoperative period of immunosuppression,[41,47] the limited donor pool renders it impractical to exclude a donor on the basis of a positive CMV antibody titer.[47] Recent experience indicates that CMV infection in the donor may not increase mortality in the recipient.

Heart Procurement. Because anesthesiologists rarely travel with the procurement team, anesthetic management of brain dead organ donors is provided by anesthesiologists at the institution where the procurement will take place. Although this aspect of care is often viewed as undesirable, anesthetic management is vital to the performance of the graft.

The initial step in a multiple organ procurement is median sternotomy to enable the direct inspection of the heart by the cardiac transplant team. The team ready to procure the abdominal viscera then commences the process of freeing the vascular and visceral connections of these organs to the point at which their preservative solutions can be administered, whereupon inflow occlusion is accomplished with caval tourniquets, the aorta is cross-clamped, and cold (4°C) crystalloid cardioplegia infused into the coronaries from the aortic root. The donor heart excision follows, removing the right atrium at the caval insertions, the left atrium at the pulmonary vein insertions, the aorta at the level of the innominate, and the pulmonary artery at the proximal right and left branches. When the recipient has a congenital malformation or subsequent surgery that has left the child with significant abnormalities of the great arteries or veins, longer segments of donor vessels should be obtained.

Multiple factors render the donor an anesthetic challenge. The management of the multiple-organ donor is the subject of recent reviews.[48,49] Despite meeting criteria for transplantation, the heart often has been injured by cardiac arrest, hypotension or catecholamine admin-

istration, and the lack of normal neuroendocrine stimulation.[50] If the donor has had a head injury, management often includes fluid restriction, dehydration, and inotropic support to maintain cerebral perfusion pressure. That strategy should be completely abandoned once the diagnosis of brain death is made and the child becomes a candidate for organ donation. Fluids should be administered as necessary to restore and maintain normal intravascular volume. Diabetes insipidus, resulting in polyuria, hypovolemia, and hypernatremia, commonly complicates management,[48–51] and may be treated with crystalloid replacement and vasopressin. Substantial blood loss can occur in the operating suite during preparations for the procurement of abdominal organs. Blood products should be administered as necessary to preserve satisfactory hemodynamics.

The hemodynamic response to surgery is oftentimes difficult to predict. Hypertension and tachycardia may follow surgical stimulation as a result of spinal reflexes akin to the mass reflex or as a result of persistent brain stem reflexes.[49,52] Conversely, donors may become hypotensive and bradycardic as they lack compensatory sympathetic reflexes to preserve hemodynamics under conditions of hypovolemia or myocardial dysfunction.[48–51] In addition, inotropic support may become necessary if arterial blood pressure remains more than 20% below normal for age despite adequate intravascular volume. Dopamine is often used for this purpose because of its effect on splanchnic circulation. If the hypertensive response to surgical stimuli is of sufficient magnitude to pose a risk of myocardial injury or to substantially contribute to blood losses, vasodilators such as nitroprusside or trimethaphan should be employed.[48,49,52] β-Adrenergic blockers should not be used to treat the hypertension because they decrease posttransplant myocardial function.

Recipient Management

Perioperative Considerations. The hemodynamic principles that govern anesthetic care for heart transplantation are similar, although perhaps more extreme, than those for reparative or palliative cardiac surgery. Management is described for the two largest groups of patients presenting for transplantation, ie, patients with dilated cardiomyopathy and congenital malformations.

Dilated cardiomyopathy represents an exaggerated adaptive mechanism whereby the heart dilates in response to changes in the composition of the myocardium in an attempt to preserve cardiac output. The Laplace law, which relates pressure directly to wall tension and inversely to the radius of the ventricle, predicts that dilation places the heart at a mechanical disadvantage because wall tension must increase in order to maintain ventricular and systemic pressure. A dysfunctional, dilated heart is exquisitely sensitive to changes in preload, afterload, and contractility. Once these children reach the early phase of the plateau in the Starling curve, where increasing preload does not increase cardiac output, a decrease in preload typically reduces output.[54] Contractility is already maximal; hence, stroke volume decreases when exposed to negative inotropic drugs or increased afterload (Fig. 22–5).[54] The inability to increase stroke volume renders these children unable to maintain cardiac output when bradycardia occurs.[54]

Increased PVR commonly accompanies both cardiomyopathies[56] and congenital heart malformations[56–60] of sufficient severity to merit transplantation. Further increases in PVR usually promote hypoxemia, which is caused by increased right-to-left shunting of blood, or exacerbate right ventricular failure, which is caused by right ventricular pressure demands that exceed compensatory capacity. Cardiac output decreases[60] causing precipitous deterioration in the child's well-being. In general, a dilated ventricle failing on account of volume overload or cardiomyopathy is very sensitive to anesthetic agents. A heart adequately compensated for the pressure work of increased PVR, however, tolerates and

merits doses of anesthetic agents, such as narcotics, capable of blunting the sympathetic response that may further increase PVR following airway and surgical stimuli.[61] Airway management assumes paramount importance because oxygenation and ventilation regulate PVR.[62,63]

The detailed anesthetic management of congenital heart malformations afflicting individual heart transplant recipients is described in previous chapters. The lesions are classified physiologically into four types: shunts, admixture of pulmonary and systemic venous return, valvular regurgitation, or obstruction to blood flow. An anesthetic should be designed to minimize the cardiac work of these physiologic abnormalities while maximizing oxygen delivery to the tissues. In children with anomalies that result in left-to-right shunts, the left ventricle labors under the increased volume work necessary to meet systemic flow demands while some output is lost to the shunt. Anesthetic management should strive for minimal alteration in PVR because decreasing PVR and increasing pulmonary flow compared with systemic flow (Qp:Qs) increases the volume burden on the left ventricle. Conversely, increased PVR or decreased SVR worsen hypoxemia in right-to-left shunting. Lesions, such as the single ventricle, in which there is complete mixing of pulmonary and systemic venous return display dramatic fluctuations of Qp:Qs. Optimal management strikes a delicate balance between the excessive volume work of a large Qp:Qs and the extreme hypoxemia of reduced Qp:Qs.

The principles used in managing children with valvar regurgitation or flow obstruction are similar to those used in adults. Valvular regurgitation, a common finding in the atrioventricular valves of children with end-stage dilated cardiomyopathies, imposes a volume load on the respective ventricle. It responds well to decreasing resistance distal to the valve and keeping heart rate normal to slightly elevated in order to limit the time during the cardiac cycle for regurgitation to occur. Obstructive lesions produce a pressure burden that is reduced by lowering the resistance distal to the obstruction and decreasing heart rate to maximize the outflow time. An exception is left ventricular outflow obstruction in which decreased systemic resistance jeopardizes coronary flow to the hypertrophic myocardium.

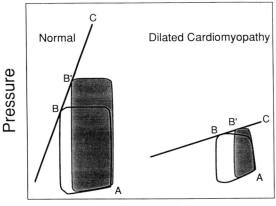

Figure 22–5. Ventricular pressure-volume curves illustrating response to increased afterload. Open circles represent baseline relationship in a normal ventricle and one with dilated cardiomyopathy (DCM). The area within the loop represents stroke volume (SV). Points A represent the end of ventricular filling and the beginning of isovolumic contraction. Points B occur as the ventricular pressure falls below aortic pressure, the aortic valve closes, and ejection ceases. The slope of lines C reflect ventricular contractility. Initially, the heart with myocardial disease dilates to maintain contractility (Frank-Starling mechanism) but ultimately this compensation fails and contractility diminishes. With an increase in afterload, the aortic valve closes at B' resulting in SV represented by the shaded loops. A normal ventricle maintains SV despite a substantial change in afterload, whereas the DCM ventricle suffers a dramatic reduction in SV with a small change in afterload. (*Adapted from Clark NJ, Martin RD: Anesthetic considerations for patients undergoing cardiac transplantation. J Cardiothorac Anesth 2:519–542, 1988, with permission.*)

Preinduction. The preanesthetic evaluation should focus on cardiovascular and pulmonary function. An anesthetic plan is devised by integrating cardiac anatomy, indication for transplantation, and the optimal hemodynamics as outlined above.

Although heart transplants are rarely scheduled, the time necessary to procure the donor heart usually provides time for patient preparation. The recipient should be made NPO (nothing by mouth) as soon as a donor organ has been identified. Children who critically depend on preload to maintain cardiac output (ie, dilated cardiomyopathy or failing, volume overloaded ventricle) should have a maintenance intravenous infusion begun. Most transplant programs administer a pretransplant dose of cyclosporine, either intravenously or orally.[25,35,37,43] Although many centers omit sedative premedication for heart transplant recipients,[55,64] an individualized approach based upon the hemodynamic state of the child and the plan for induction should be used. Sedative premedication in infants under 6 months old and all children with dilated cardiomyopathy or other causes of severe ventricular dysfunction is usually avoided. However, sedative premedication is desirable in children with congenital heart malformations with moderate or no ventricular failure in whom an inhalation induction is planned, particularly if their anatomy limits pulmonary blood flow.

Although monitoring practices vary widely between institutions, all subscribe to the minimum standards defined by the American Society of Anesthesiologists. Invasive monitors in awake children are seldom placed prior to induction. An intra-arterial catheter, usually placed after induction, is the only invasive monitor routinely employed in the prebypass period. Central venous pressure is monitored only when required for preoperative management. If central venous access is needed, the right internal jugular, which is a potential route of catheterization for myocardial biopsy, is avoided whenever possible.[64] The placement of pulmonary artery catheters in infants and small children is difficult and not without risk.[65] Most centers performing large numbers of pediatric heart transplants consider the value of the information gained does not warrant the additional risk of pulmonary artery catheterization.[64,66,67]

Induction and Maintenance of Anesthesia. The selection of anesthetic agents for the induction of anesthesia depends largely upon the desired or tolerable effects each agent might have on the hemodynamics as well as whether the recipient is at high risk of pulmonary aspiration (Table 22–1). The unscheduled nature of the surgery that abridges the customary period of withholding food coupled with the preoperative oral dose of cyclosporine generates concern about gastric fluid volume. A classic rapid-sequence induction may destabilize hemodynamic function. On the other hand, pulmonary aspiration in a child with elevated PVR about to undergo transplantation and immunosuppression is equally devastating. A coordinated transplant team usually can arrange a period of 4–6 hours without oral intake when the recipient is notified at the time of initial donor referral. Gastric fluid volume and pH may also be altered by administration of a histamine$_2$ blocking agent[68,69] or nonparticulate antacid.[70] This combination should reduce the risk of pulmonary aspiration sufficiently to permit a gradual rather than a rapid-sequence induction of anesthesia. However, if pulmonary aspiration represents the overriding concern, rapid-sequence induction techniques using a variety of anesthetic agents (eg, fentanyl, sufentanil, etomidate, or ketamine along with muscle relaxants) have been described.[55,66,71–74]

The uptake and distribution of both inhalational and intravenous agents may appear unusual in these children. The uptake of volatile agents in children with congenital heart malformations is influenced by pulmonary blood flow and the solubility characteristics of the agent. Uptake in the presence of left-to-right shunts is influenced by the opposing effects of increased pulmonary blood flow, which slows the increase in alveolar concentration, against the increased pulmonary artery anesthetic concentration because the shunted blood has already passed through the lungs. A normal rate of induction usually results.[75] Uptake of anesthetic in malformations with reduced pulmonary blood flow depends on the solubility of the anesthetic agent. Although reduced pulmonary blood flow limits the amount of anesthetic that can be taken up, this effect is offset by the more rapid

TABLE 22–1. TYPICAL ANESTHETIC TECHNIQUES USED FOR HEART TRANSPLANTATION

	Dilated Cardiomyopathy		Congenital Malformation (Mild Ventricular Dysfunction)		
Premedication	None		Atropine Pentobarbital (≥6 mo; 4 mg/kg PO) Meperidine (≥12 mo; 3 mg/kg PO)		
Induction					
Rapid	Ketamine Succinyl choline		Ketamine Succinyl choline	or	Thiopental Succinyl choline
Gradual	Fentanyl Scopolamine Pancuronium		Fentanyl Scopolamine Pancuronium	or	Halothane Nitrous oxide Pancuronium
Maintenance	Fentanyl Scopolamine Pancuronium		Fentanyl Scopolamine Pancuronium		

rise in alveolar concentration that occurs, particularly with soluble anesthetics.[76,77] Despite a 50% right-to-left shunt, the arterial concentration of anesthetic is relatively unaffected when using a soluble agent such as methoxyflurane, whereas arterial concentration is markedly reduced with insoluble drugs (eg, N_2O).[77] When cardiac output is low, dramatic increases in alveolar concentration ensue[76] and cardiac output may plummet. The change in uptake and distribution of intravenous agents is most notable in children with dilated cardiomyopathy. A delay in the peak effect suggests either increased volume of distribution (V_D) or slow delivery of the drug.[55,78–81] Fentanyl pharmacokinetics in adults with poor left ventricular function reveal normal V_D, thus suggesting the absence of hemodynamic responses to stimuli after lower fentanyl doses related more to diminished myocardial reserve than the depth of anesthesia.[82] These characteristics necessitate a slow induction in order to avoid anesthetic overdose.

In the 25 years since Ozinsky described the initial anesthetic for heart transplantation in which he used thiopental, succinylcholine, and halothane,[83] virtually every anesthetic agent has been used in these patients. Each technique has desirable and detrimental effects. Large surveys indicate that narcotic-based anesthetics remain the most popular because of negligible direct effects on contractility.[64,66,84,85] Although the reduction in endogenous catecholamine responses, heart rate, and systemic vascular resistance that may accompany large doses of these agents may destabilize some children, moderate doses (10–30 μg/kg fentanyl, 2–5 μg/kg sufentanil) preserve satisfactory hemodynamics in most patients despite significant ventricular dysfunction.[55,61,73,74,82]

Ketamine provides analgesia while ensuring superior amnesia to that offered by narcotics alone.[86] This arylcycloalkylamine indirectly releases catecholamines that support the circulation.[86,87] The increased systemic vascular resistance that accompanies catecholamine release will reduce stroke volume in dilated, cardiomyopathic ventricles that are unable to increase contractility.[73] In a child with dilated cardiomyopathy, elevated basal serum catecholamine levels, depleted myocardial norepinephrine stores, and downregulation of myocardial β receptors,[55,88] ketamine directly depresses the myocardium.[86,87,89] The influence of ketamine on PVR remains a subject of debate.[73,90–92]

Benzodiazepines, which have mild hemodynamic effects alone, cause systemic hypotension owing to synergistic myocardial depression[93] or reduction in SVR[94] when given with narcotics. Etomidate offers inconsequential hemodynamic changes at the customary induction doses.[71,72,74] This drug causes short-term suppression of hormonal stress response, an effect unlikely to be of clinical importance in the recipient receiving large doses of immunosuppressive steroids postoperative-

ly.[72,95] The direct myocardial depression and variable effects on SVR produced by induction doses of barbiturates have limited their use to children who have fair hemodynamic reserve.[96]

Inhaled agents are less commonly used for induction as they cause hypotension.[64] The hemodynamic properties of each volatile agent on heart rate, contractility, and vascular resistance should be considered in the context of the desirable cardiovascular effects. Despite an increased incidence of hypotension, they offer the advantage of a slow induction and the ability to titrate the drug to effect. Nitrous oxide produces myocardial effects ranging from mild depression[97–99] to cardiovascular collapse.[100] The effect of nitrous oxide on PVR remains controversial.[97–99]

The selection of neuromuscular blocking drugs merits consideration of their individual effects on heart rate, histamine release, and ganglionic blockade both alone and in combination with the other anesthetic agents employed. Vecuronium, for example, exerts minimal effect on heart rate or the sympathetic ganglion and causes imperceptible histamine release,[101] yet it may cause profound bradycardia in combination with synthetic narcotics such as sufantanil.[102]

A satisfactory induction technique incorporates incremental doses of fentanyl (total dose 5–50 μg/kg) and pancuronium because the vagotonic effects of this narcotic are offset by the vagolytic effects of pancuronium. Sedation and amnesia with scopolamine (7–10 μg/kg) are given to children over 1 year of age. In the hemodynamically unstable recipient, induction with ketamine (0.5–4.0 mg/kg) preserves hemodynamic function somewhat better than fentanyl. Fentanyl (20–50 μg/kg) and sufentanil blunt changes in PVR and circulating catecholamines providing the most stable hemodynamic profile during cardiopulmonary bypass and in the postbypass and early postoperative period.

In conjunction with drug selection and administration, skillful airway management assumes vital importance in these children. Many children have limited tissue oxygen delivery owing to reduced arterial oxygen content or cardiac output, which is particularly sensitive to changes in ventilation.

Irrespective of the elegance with which an anesthetic plan is constructed and executed, hemodynamic collapse may result. A few children are sufficiently compromised that muscle relaxants alone precipitate cardiovascular collapse. Initial resuscitative efforts should include bolus infusions of fluids and inotropic agents, but rapidly established CPB is preferable to large doses of vasoconstrictors that may prevent uniform cooling.

Surgical Technique. The replacement of a heart with the typical arrangement of great arteries and veins generally follows the original technique of Lower and Shumway.[6] Bicaval cannulation and hypothermic cardiopulmonary bypass provide satisfactory operating conditions in selected children, whereas deep hypothermic circulatory arrest may be preferred in neonates, infants, and children requiring extensive vascular reconstruction as a component of heart transplantation.[35-37,46] The surgeon excises the recipient's heart leaving a posterior cuff of left and right atrial tissue to which the graft is sewn[6] (Fig 22–6). This technique avoids the potential for bleeding and obstruction at individual pulmonary vein and vena cava anastomoses and shortens the operative time. Great arterial anastomoses are performed at the ascending aorta and main pulmonary artery.

The anatomic complexities of many cardiovascular malformations and the operations used to treat them demand some creativity on the part of the transplant surgeon.[103] For example, in transplantation of neonates with hypoplastic left heart syndrome, the diminutive ascending aorta and arch must be reconstructed[46,104] (Fig 22–7). Children with transposition of the great arteries after intra-atrial baffle procedures (eg, Mustard or Sen-

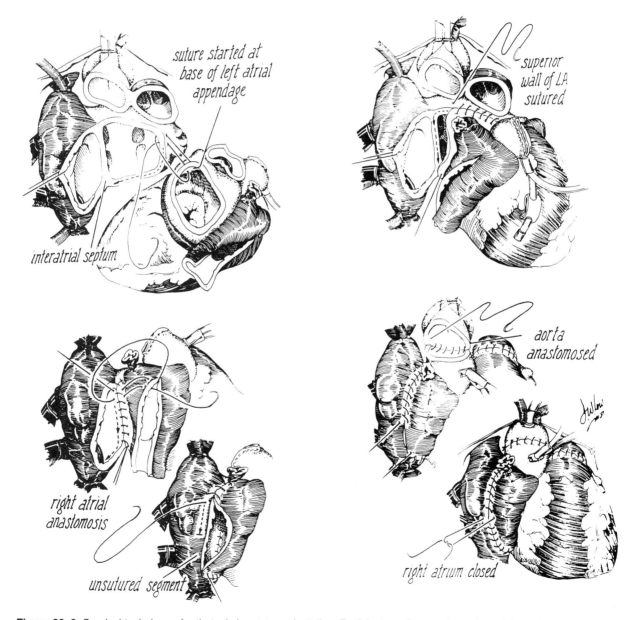

Figure 22–6. Surgical technique of orthotopic heart transplantation. Recipient cardiectomy is performed in such a manner as to leave a cuff of right and left atrial tissue. The posterior wall of the graft LA is excised and the remaining LA wall sutured to the recipient LA cuff. A longitudinal incision in the donor RA is subsequently anastomosed to the RA cuff. Main pulmonary artery and ascending aorta anastomoses complete the procedure. (*Adapted from Edmunds LH, Norwood WI, Low DW: Atlas of Cardiothoracic Surgery. Philadelphia: Lea & Febiger, 1990, p 73, with permission.*)

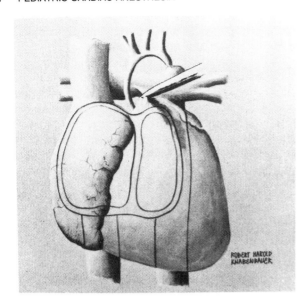
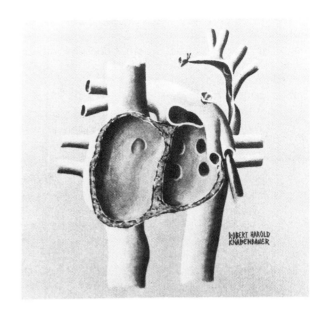
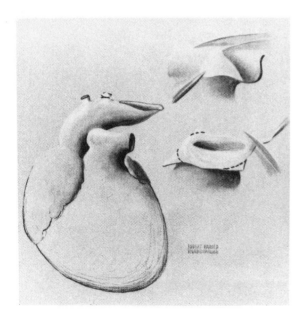
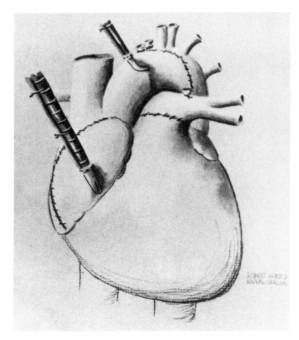

Figure 22–7. Surgical technique of orthotopic heart transplantation in infants with hypoplastic left heart syndrome. Atrial anastomoses are carried in a manner analogous to typical heart transplants. Donor cardiectomy is modified to include a long segment of ascending aorta and aortic arch. Donor aorta is incised longitudinally to enable reconstruction of the hypoplastic native aortic arch. The pulmonary artery anastomosis may require modification to accommodate the enlarged main PA usually present in these recipients. (*Adapted from Bailey[46,104] with permission.*)

ning) represent another example as redirection of the great arteries comprises a part of their transplant. Extensive pulmonary artery reconstruction is common in such lesions as truncus arteriosus and tetralogy of Fallot with pulmonary atresia. Superior vena caval reconstruction complicates transplantation in children after a Glenn or Fontan procedure. Perhaps the most challenging are the heterotaxy syndromes in which virtually every case is unique. The risks of obstruction to blood flow–prolonged ischemia, postoperative bleeding, and the increased PVR that accompanies many of these lesions makes the operative mortality quite high.[22,31]

Heterotopic heart transplantation is employed when the recipient's PVR exceeds the level at which orthotopic transplant seems safe[33,35,38,39] or when the only available donor for an unstable recipient is too small.[38,39] The anastomoses allow both hearts to contribute to the circulation simultaneously, enabling, for example, the hypertrophied, native right ventricle of a child with high PVR to continue to do most of the pulmonary pressure work. The technical complexities of this operation and the high-risk population on whom it is performed result in higher operative and late mortality compared with orthotopic transplantation.[22,39] Alternate strategies for both of these treatment groups exist, such as heart-lung transplantation or a mechanical heart, but these carry increased risk as well.[22,105–106]

Separation from Cardiopulmonary Bypass After Transplantation.

Mild tachycardia augments cardiac output in the newly implanted graft as diminished compliance[107,108] and sympathetic denervation limit the ability of the ventricle to change stroke volume.[108,109] A heart rate between 100 and 110 in adults and 130 and 150 in neonates accomplishes this goal.[29,55,67] Although β_1 sympathomimetic drugs such as isoproterenol and, to a lesser extent, dopamine, exhibit greater efficacy at increasing cardiac output with this tachycardia,[109,110] a pacemaker (atrial, ventricular, or AV sequential) should be employed in the event that these drugs are unable to increase heart rate or are arrhythmogenic.

Techniques to minimize PVR are vital in the management of children during separation from CPB after heart transplant. Management of ventilation is the most specific and powerful way to alter PVR.[62,63,111,112] Prior to termination of CPB, the lungs should be well inflated using the Valsalva maneuver to eliminate atelectatic areas and then ventilated at normal tidal volumes to achieve moderate to extreme hypocapnia (ie, Pa_{CO_2} 20–30 mm Hg). Ventilation should be near functional residual capacity (FRC) as the pulmonary vasculature becomes distorted and PVR rises when lung volume increases or decreases significantly with respect to this point[113] (Fig 22–8). When lung volume is higher or lower than FRC, pulmonary vessel diameter decreases owing to unfavorable geometry.[113] Lung volumes below FRC distort the extra-acinar vessels, whereas lung volumes above FRC compress alveolar capillaries. Cassin demonstrated the effect of lung expansion, CO_2 elimination, and hypoxia on fetal PVR (Fig 22–9).[62] Acidosis increases baseline PVR and shifts the hypoxic pulmonary vasoconstriction curve to the right such that the critical Po_2 at which the PVR begins to rise increases as the pH falls (Fig 22–10).[63] Large tidal volumes (V_T) (20–25 mL/kg) at a frequency (f) of 20–30/min reliably accomplish these objectives. This method of ventilation also optimizes inspiratory and expiratory time and prevents the development of inadvertent positive end-expiratory pressure (PEEP). Because PEEP might augment FRC and thereby increase PVR, it is reserved for severe pulmonary abnormalities, most commonly pulmonary edema, that limit lung compliance (C_L) and the ability to maintain normal FRC and arterial oxygenation.

When ventilatory measures are inadequate to reduce PVR to ensure satisfactory right ventricular function and cardiac output, pharmacologic therapy is initiated. Virtu-

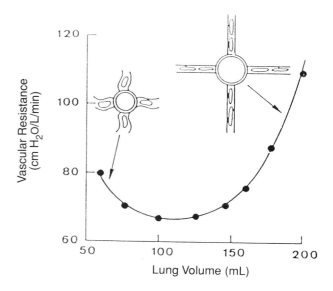

Figure 22–8. Effect of lung volume on pulmonary vascular resistance. At low lung volumes, resistance is high because extra alveolar vessels become tortuous. At high volumes, the capillaries are stretched and their caliber is reduced. (*From West JB: Respiratory Physiology—The Essentials. Baltimore: Williams & Wilkins, 1974, with permission.*)

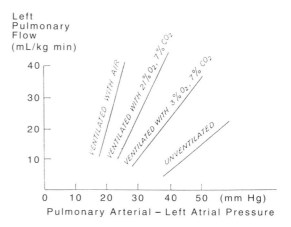

Figure 22–9. Effect of lung inflation, ventilation, and oxygenation on PVR. On the x-axis is pulmonary perfusion pressure and on the y-axis is pulmonary blood flow. Slope of the lines represents PVR. (*Modified from Cassin S, et al: The vascular resistance of the foetal and newly ventilated lung of the lamb. J Physiol 171:61–79, 1964, with permission.*)

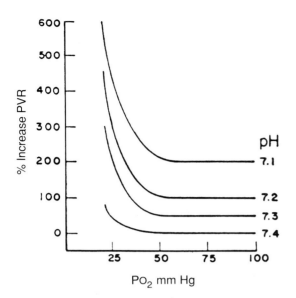

Figure 22–10. Influence of changing arterial oxygen tension (Po₂) and pH on PVR. Systemic acidosis increases PVR independently while accentuating hypoxic pulmonary vasoconstriction. Acidosis and hypoxia increase PVR and interact synergistically. (*From Rudolph AM, Yuan S: Response of the pulmonary vasculature to hypoxia and H⁺ ion concentration changes. J Clin Invest 45:399–411, 1966, with permission.*)

ally all drugs exert similar effects on systemic and pulmonary vascular resistance beds. β₂-Adrenergic agonists (isoproterenol),[114,116] vasodilators (nitroglycerin, nitroprusside), α-adrenergic antagonists (tolazoline),[112,117] and calcium channel blockers[115,116,118] have all been used with some success under certain circumstances. More promising recently are the eicosanoids (PGE₁ and prostacyclin) and their analogues (iloprost).[115–117,119] Experimental studies suggest that adenosine triphosphate (ATP), through its stimulation of endothelium-derived relaxing factor (EDRF), may be a selective pulmonary vasodilator because of extensive first-pass clearance from the lung.[120] Nitric oxide, a free radical postulated to be EDRF, exhibits selective pulmonary vasodilation when administered by inhalation in both animal and human experiments.[121–123] Hemoglobin scavenging clears nitric oxide in the lung before it can produce systemic vasodilation.[121,122] If these pharmacologic therapies fail to provide satisfactory hemodynamics, mechanical right ventricular assist (RVAD) is employed. However, evidence that RVAD improves survival is lacking.

Once heart rate, contractility, and PVR are satisfactory, CPB is terminated. Intravascular volume, guided by CVP or direct atrial pressure determinations, should be maintained at slightly increased levels (8–15 mm Hg) because the denervated heart adjusts output on the basis of the Frank-Starling relationship rather than neurally mediated changes in heart rate and contractility.[29,55,80,107,124]

When cardiac function appears sufficient, protamine is administered to antagonize the heparin effect. Protamine administration carries both dose-related and idiosyncratic risks of hemodynamic compromise.[125,127] The dose-related reduction in SVR and mild negative inotropy attributed to histamine release rarely appears in neonates and young children. Rare, but potentially devastating, complement C5a-mediated increases in PVR may occur after protamine administration in allergic individuals.[125,126] Recent investigation has shown complement activation commonly occurs without hemodynamic consequences in humans after heparin reversal with protamine, whereas increases in thromboxane B₂ are reproducibly linked to pulmonary vasoconstriction.[127] Postoperative hemorrhage is best managed with infusion of whole blood less than 48 hours old.[128] This therapy promotes coagulation more effectively than component replacement, avoids large fluctuations in hematocrit, and reduces the incidence of hypotension resulting from vasoactive substances in components such as enriched platelet concentrates. Azathioprine, 5 mg/kg, and methyl prednisolone, 10 mg/kg, also are administered after terminating CPB in most centers.

Postoperative Management. Critical problems facing the recipient include graft failure, arrhythmias, hemorrhage, and rejection. Denervation and ischemic injury largely determine the level of cardiac function after transplantation. The ischemic injury results in a spectrum of cardiac function abnormalities, beginning with reduced ventricular compliance[107] and, in severe instances, systolic performance as well.[109] These functional abnormalities should resolve over a period of hours to days if satisfactory hemodynamics can be maintained using supportive measures as long as complicating features, such as elevated PVR or acute rejection, do not delay or preclude the resolution of ischemic injury.[107,109]

Postoperative ventilatory manipulations reduce PVR by both mechanical and chemical mechanisms. Thus, the objectives of postoperative mechanical ventilation are maintenance of normal FRC, moderate to marked hypocapnia (Paco₂ 20–28 mm Hg) achieved with minimal mean airway pressure. A volume-limited ventilator whose tubing compliance is 1.7 mL/cm H₂O, V_T 20–30 mL/kg, f 20–25/minutes, inspiratory time 0.5–0.6 second (I:E 1.0:3.5) is used. PEEP is not used except in children with poor lung compliance. The pharmacologic therapy for elevated PVR is not as reliable. Isoproterenol,[114–116] PGE₁, and prostacyclin[115–117,119] occasionally lower PVR without adversely lowering SVR. Vasodilators are rarely effective. The pulmonary hypertension ensuing from left ventricular failure generally resolves within months of transplantation.[129]

CARDIAC DENERVATION. The management of the denervated heart must take into account its abnormal responses to both changing bodily demands and pharmacologic agents. A normal autonomically mediated increase in heart rate and contractility occur in response to increased O_2 demand with the result that left ventricular end-diastolic volume (LVEDV) remains constant or diminishes slightly. The denervated heart, however, relies upon increased venous return to augment LVEDV and increase cardiac output (the Frank-Starling mechanism).[109,124,130] Heart rate and contractility increase only under the direct stimulation of the circulating catecholamines that are released several minutes later.[109,130,131] The salutary effect of pharmacologic or pacemaker management that results in mild tachycardia after heart transplantation exists because cardiac output increases while reducing LVEDV and therefore wall tension.[109,110] Maximal heart rate and cardiac output are lower in the denervated heart, thus AV oxygen extraction increases and lactate production becomes significant at lower demand levels.[109,132]

The response of the transplanted heart to cardiovascular drugs depends upon their mechanism of action (Table 22–2). Agents acting directly on myocardial receptors retain normal potency. Experimental evidence suggests an increased adrenergic responsiveness to directly acting drugs following denervation,[133–137] but the importance of this finding in the clinical setting is unclear.[55,138,139] Drugs affecting the heart indirectly via the autonomic nervous system are ineffective.[138,140]

The need to support a failing heart in the early postoperative period reflects either ischemic injury,

acute rejection, or unsuitable recipient physiology, most commonly due to elevated PVR. In the absence of these conditions, sufficient preload should produce acceptable cardiac output. Inotropic agents are generally quite effective, with the caveat that only the direct-acting component of their hemodynamic profile will be evident in the denervated heart.[55,138] Isoproterenol is usually administered until moderate tachycardia or a rhythm disturbance ensues and dopamine added if further inotropy seems warranted. The advantages of isoproterenol include an increase in cardiac output surpassing that of pacing alone,[109,110] a reduction in LVEDV, and thus wall tension, that accompanies moderate tachycardia in the denervated heart,[108] as well as a salutary effect on PVR.[114,116] Dopamine uniquely benefits renal function[141] and may offset the kidney injury resulting from hypoperfusion or cyclosporine.

Mechanical support of the circulation after transplant is reserved for desperate situations in which other measures fail to achieve adequate organ perfusion.[142] Although these techniques can be quite effective, the additional risk they impart to the immunocompromised patient limits their reasonable application to children who have suffered a self-limited myocardial injury or as a bridge to retransplantation.[105,106,142] Support may take the form of intra-aortic balloon counterpulsation, selective right and left ventricular assist devices,[106,142] or the total artificial heart.[105]

Evaluation and management of cardiac rhythm represents an important as well as unique challenge in the denervated heart. Sinus tachycardia is usually observed during early reperfusion.[110,124] Careful investigation may reveal two atrial pacemakers, one each from recipient and donor, if the implanting technique included anastomosis of the graft to a right atrial cuff.[140] Slowing of the intrinsic rate often occurs in the early postoperative period,[64,78] during which reduced ventricular compliance limits stroke volume[107,109,110] and, in the absence of autonomic reflex response to increase rate or contractility, cardiac output decreases. Chronotropic drugs or pacemaker therapy may become necessary several hours postoperatively;[29,55,64,67,80,84] thus pacemaker wires are placed on most cardiac allografts.

A variety of arrhythmias occur after transplantation, particularly in the first 6 months.[143] Atrial arrhythmias are most common with premature atrial contractions (PACs) noted in 67% of the recipients.[143] At least 40% of transplant recipients exhibit atrial arrhythmias or heart block during acute graft rejection.[143] Ventricular arrhythmias, usually premature ventricular contractions, occur in 30–40% of the recipients.[143] Malignant ventricular arrhythmias, such as ventricular tachycardia and ventricular fibrillation, are rare but may accompany severe rejection or coronary insufficiency.[38,143]

The response to antiarrhythmic drugs coincides with the degree to which they act directly on the heart (see

TABLE 22–2. ELECTROPHYSIOLOGIC ACTIONS OF VARIOUS DRUGS UPON THE DENERVATED HEART

Drug	Sinus Rate	Atrioventricular Conduction
Cardiovascular Drugs		
Atropine	–	–
Calcium channel blockers	↓	↓
Digoxin		
Initial	–	–
Chronic	–	↓
Epinephrine	↑	↑
Isoproterenol	↑	↑
Norepinephrine	↑ *	↑ *
Nitroprusside	–	–
Phenylephrine	–	–
Procainamide	↓ *	↓ *
Propranolol	↓	↓
Anesthetic Agents		
Edrophonium	–	–
Neostigmine	–	–
Narcotics	–	–
Pancuronium	–	–

* Opposite from response of innervated hearts.
(Adapted from: Fowles RE, Reitz BA, Ream AK: Drug interactions in a transplanted or artificial heart. In Kaplan JA (ed): Cardiac Anesthesia, Vol 2. Cardiovascular Pharmacology. Orlando, FL: Grune & Stratton, 1983, p 650.)

Table 22–2). Atropine ordinarily blocks the effect of acetylcholine released from the vagus; in the denervated heart, it has no effect.[140] Class IA antiarrhythmics, such as procainamide, normally act via a combination of indirect, atropinelike properties and direct suppression of Purkinje system automaticity.[144] Although these agents are useful in the treatment of supraventricular tachycardias or atrial flutter, the absence of associated tachycardia unmasks their negative inotropy after heart transplantation.[145] Class IB drugs, such as lidocaine or phenytoin, suppress ventricular automaticity independently of the autonomic nervous system and are effective in the denervated heart.[145] β-Adrenergic blocking drugs, class II, retain their usual activity.[78,133] Bretylium, a class III agent, also exhibits mixed direct and indirect effects through the autonomic system. The net effect on the denervated heart remains poorly understood,[144] thus limiting its use to refractory ventricular tachycardia or fibrillation. The calcium channel blockers, which constitute class IV, directly suppress the sinus and AV nodes[146] and thus retain their usual efficacy after heart transplantation.[145] These drugs, however, possess potent negative inotropic actions as well.[118] Class V, comprising other agents (eg, digoxin and adenosine), must be considered individually. Digoxin acts in a biphasic manner. The early reduction in AV conduction is largely vagally mediated.[147] Later in the course of digoxin therapy, its direct action influences AV conduction in the transplant recipient.[147] Although adenosine retains its efficacy in terminating supraventricular tachycardias via direct sinus node depression and slowing of atrial-His conduction,[148] reports suggesting increased sensitivity after heart transplantation warrant reduction in the initial dose.[149]

Persistent bradycardia occasionally merits the implantation of a permanent pacemaker. In the Stanford University experience, VVI pacemakers were placed in the 8% of pediatric heart recipients who exhibited episodes of bradycardia to rates below 40 or symptomatic bradycardia irrespective of rate.[31]

POSTOPERATIVE HEMORRHAGE. Hemorrhage is an early postoperative problem associated with considerable morbidity and mortality.[23,84] Postbypass coagulopathy complicates postoperative management most commonly in children with congenital heart malformations.[23] These children often require more extensive reconstructions in association with heart transplantation, including long suture lines on the aorta or pulmonary arteries. Previous palliative or reparative cardiac surgery usually entails more rough dissection leading to raw surfaces that tend to bleed. Furthermore, cyanotic heart disease is commonly associated with a preoperative coagulopathy arising from abnormal platelet number[150] or function,[151] factor levels,[152] and fibrinolysis. Preoperative coagulopathies may also occur in children who were receiving coumadin or heparin or have secondary hepatic disease.

In the vast majority, postoperative hemorrhage can be controlled with the administration of whole blood less than 48 hours old.[128] Component therapy with fresh frozen plasma and platelets is reserved for the treatment of prolonged prothrombin time, partial thromboplastin time, or thrombocytopenia unresponsive to fresh whole blood. Early enthusiasm for desmopressin,[153] which increases factor VIII and the von Willebrand factor, has waned since subsequent studies showed no reduction in blood loss.[154] Only one study in acyanotic children evaluated desmopressin in pediatric heart surgery and found no effect.[155] In a recent randomized prospective controlled study, there was no benefit in either cyanotic or acyanotic children undergoing cardiac surgery (L. M. Reynolds, personal communications). Aprotinin is a new drug that appears to reduce hemorrhage after open-heart surgery[156–158] primarily through inhibition of fibrinolysis,[158,159] although some have suggested a platelet protective effect during CPB.[160] Aprotinin is limited to investigational use in the United States.

IMMUNOSUPPRESSION. The incidence of rejection is highest in the first 6 months after transplant.[24,31,34,64] The higher doses of immunosuppressive therapy necessary during this early period convey the greatest associated risk of oportunistic infection as well.[31,41] Diffuse radiodensity in the lung, an indication of congestive heart failure, is an early indicator of rejection.[28,145] Diagnostic evaluation of radiographic density in the lung should simultaneously consider the lung as an initial avenue for opportunistic infection.[31,41,145] Disseminated infection may impair pulmonary function and ultimately give rise to the acute respiratory distress syndrome.[145]

Outcome after heart transplantation improved with progress in immunosuppression regimens.[16,37] Nonspecific drugs, such as glucocorticoids, that impose numerous side effects and global immunosuppression, have been replaced by specific T-cell inhibitors such as cyclosporine. Cyclosporine[15,16,161] selectively activates T suppressor cells while inhibiting B-cell and cytotoxic T-cell proliferation.[162] Serum levels determined by radioimmunoassay range from 100 to 300 ng/mL.[31,37] Because cyclosporine is 80% bound to red blood cells,[163] whole blood radioimmunoassay (RIA) values are higher, 200–1000 ng/mL.[34] High-pressure liquid chromatography provides the most accurate levels,[163] but the assay is too complex to be practical for most laboratories.

Cyclosporine causes renal,[16,161,164] hepatic,[161,165] and neurologic toxicity.[161,166] These toxicities are largely dose related and are reduced by monitoring blood levels[167] or minimizing the dose through the use of multiple-drug immunosuppression regimens.[166,168] Hepatic toxicity consists of asymptomatic mild, reversible elevations in bilirubin and, occasionally, transaminases suggesting cholestasis.[165] As many as half the patients receiving cyclosporine will have tremors and a few develop seizures.[31,161,166,169] Cosmetic side effects like hypertrichosis and gingival hyperplasia also occur.[37] Renal toxicity, usually dose related[166,167,170] and reversible,[168] is the most frequent and important injury. Tubulointerstitial injury progresses ultimately to focal glomerular sclerosis.[164] Most centers observe an improvement by dose reduction or elimination of the drug altogether if a reduction in glomerular filtration rate or a serum creatinine over 2 mg/dL occurs.[31,34,166–168,170] Hypertension afflicts virtually all pediatric heart transplant recipients[31,171] as a result of decreased renal sodium excretion and expanded plasma volume.[172,173] Although commonly attributed to cyclosporine,[172] these changes are exacerbated by steroids because hypertension has not been observed in patients from the Loma Linda program where steroids are not included in routine maintenance immunosuppression.[24]

Azathioprine, combined with a corticosteroid, most commonly prednisone, effects a dramatic reduction in the proliferation of all nonspecific host immune cells.[162] A purine antagonist, azathioprine, inhibits both DNA and RNA synthesis, and thus all immune functions requiring cell proliferation.[162] Corticosteroids exert nonspecific anti-inflammatory effects.[162] In sufficient doses, these drugs produce global immunosuppression[10,31] and impair growth.[31,174]

The dosage and scheduling of immunosuppression vary among institutions (Table 22–3), but most use cyclosporine, azathioprine, and prednisone for maintenance.[22,31,34] The greatest variation appears in the dosage of cyclosporine, which is determined by one of several blood assays.[163] Given the wide variability in therapeutic and toxic effects in infants and small children, cyclosporine, 10 mg/kg/day, is often administered, increasing the dose until a small change in serum creatinine or other toxicity becomes evident, resulting in a dose range of 8–45 mg/kg/day. Azathioprine receives more uniform treatment; most centers administer approximately 2 mg/kg/day to maintain the white blood cell count between 4000 and 5000/mm³.[24,31,34] At Loma Linda, infants transplanted under 6 months of age are tapered off azathioprine after the first year.[24] In response

TABLE 22–3. IMMUNOSUPPRESSION PROTOCOLS AT FOUR PEDIATRIC TRANSPLANT CENTERS

Drug	Stanford	Pittsburgh	Loma Linda	Childrens Hospital of Philadelphia
Cyclosporine				
Induction				
Dose	10 mg/kg/d	5 mg/kg/d	4–8 mg/kg/d	6–10 mg/kg/d
Target	200–300 ng/mL serum	700–1000 ng/mL blood	400–800 ng/mL blood	Mild ↑ creatinine
Maintenance				
Date	After 30 d	After 90 d	After 180 d	Same
Target	100–200 ng/mL	500 ng/mL blood	200–400 ng/mL blood	
Azathioprine				
First year				
Dose	2 mg/kg/d	1–2 mg/kg/d	2–3 mg/kg/d	2–3 mg/kg/d
Target	WBC 4000–5000		WBC >3500	WBC >4000
Second year	Same	Same	<6 mo—none >6 mo—1–2 mg/kg/d	Same
Corticosteroids				
Induction				
Drug	Prednisone	Prednisone	Methyl prednisolone	Prednisone
Dose	0.6 mg/kg/d	3 mg/kg/d	25 mg/kg bid × 4	2 mg/kg/d
Maintenance				
Date	By 6 weeks	By day 10		By 6 weeks
Drug	Prednisone	Prednisone	None	Prednisone
Dose	0.2 mg/kg/d	0.2 mg/kg/d		0.3 mg/kg/d
Subsequent				
Date	By 6 months			After 6 weeks
Dose	0.2 mg/kg/qod	Same	None	Passive taper: not ↑ with weight
ATG				
Induction days		Days 1–5		
Dose		1–2 mg/kg, maximum 100 mg		
OKT3 monoclonal				
Induction days	Days 1–14			Replace cyclosporine
Dose	0.1 mg/kg, maximum 5 mg			0.1 mg/kg, maximum 5 mg

to the deleterious effects of corticosteroids on growth, most centers limit the dose of these drugs in children. After 6 months, the Stanford group reduces steroid administration frequency to every other day in an attempt to discontinue them altogether if possible.[37] In fact, the Loma Linda program has eliminated corticosteroids altogether from the maintenance regimen of neonatal recipients.[24,25] Another approach is to set the dose of prednisone at 0.3 mg/kg/day 6 months after transplant and refrain from increasing the dose as the child grows, thereby accomplishing a "passive" taper.

Currently employed primarily to treat acute rejection, the latest immunotherapeutic drugs are specific antibodies acting against T cells. Polyclonal antithymocyte globulins (ATG), described in 1972 as adjuncts to immunosuppression induction and acute rejection therapy following heart transplantation,[175] opsonize T cells enabling their elimination by the reticuloendothelial system.[176] The murine monoclonal antibody OKT3, initially reported in 1983[176] and administered to cardiac allograft recipients in 1987,[177,178] interferes with antigen recognition by binding to CD3 T-cell surface antigen.[176-178] Among numerous minor side effects that accompany the administration of OKT3, life-threatening pulmonary edema afflicts 2–10% of treated patients.[178,179] Total lymphoid irradiation[180,181] has been successfully employed to treat refractory rejection in a limited number of children.[31]

These drugs have been added to the induction regimens at several large centers. ATG was added to the induction therapy, postoperative days 1–5, at both Pittsburgh University[34] and Stanford University.[175] Since then, Stanford has shifted to OKT3 for 10–14 days based upon a lower rate of early rejection.[163,182] Incidentally, the Pittsburgh group reports a dramatic reduction in accelerated coronary atherosclerosis in children who received ATG during induction.[183] Despite these reports, the International Registry has failed to detect appreciable improvement in survival in patients receiving OKT3 in conjunction with traditional triple-drug therapy.[22,23] The Children's Hospital of Philadelphia group currently reserves OKT3 (0.1–0.2 mg/kg/day) to replace cyclosporine for children who demonstrate significant reversible renal dysfunction at the time of transplant.

Prior to the ubiquitous use of cyclosporine, monitoring for rejection relied on noninvasive signs. Evidence of congestive heart failure accompanied by low-voltage ECG, new arrhythmias, S_3 gallop, and increased LV thickness on echocardiogram virtually sealed the diagnosis of rejection.[37] However, signs of rejection are more subtle on cyclosporine therapy[16] necessitating a more objective and sensitive system. To this end, endomyocardial biopsy was developed by Cave and Billingham (Table 22–4).[12,13] In the Stanford experience, 50% of those exhibiting grade 2 changes on biopsy resolve without acceleration in therapy.[37] Thus, "pulse" therapy for acute rejection follows biopsies exhibiting myocyte ne-

TABLE 22–4. THE BILLINGHAM CRITERIA FOR HISTOLOGIC GRADING OF ACUTE CARDIAC REJECTION

Grade	Histology	Usual Therapy
I	None	Maintenance immunosuppression
II (mild)	Mononuclear cell infiltrate	Maintenance immunosuppression Increased frequency of surveillance
III (moderate)	Cellular infiltrate Patchy myocyte necrosis	Pulse steroids (IV in first year); antithymocyte therapy (ATG, OKT3) if hemodynamically unstable
IV (severe)	Mononuclear cellular infiltrate Neutrophil infiltrate Diffuse myocyte necrosis Intramural hemorrhage	Pulse steroids Antithymocyte therapy

crosis (grade 3 or 4). Typical adult transplant protocols call for as many as 15 routine biopsies in the first year and gradually diminishing to 2–4 in successive years.[163] Technical problems posed by neonates and small infants cause most pediatric programs to modify these protocols, with many avoiding biopsy altogether in neonates.[24,35,36]

In recipients in whom endomyocardial biopsy is not possible, noninvasive signs of rejection assume a screening role. Infants with rejection typically develop congestive heart failure, arrhythmias, or interstitial pulmonary radiodensities. Some programs would treat presumptively with "pulse" immunosuppression, whereas others might seek confirmatory laboratory evidence, the value of which is controversial.[24,36,46] Laboratory studies include echocardiography,[184-186] magnetic resonance imaging (MRI),[187] radionuclide scans,[188,189] and T-cell assays.[36,190] Diastolic dysfunction indices represent early echocardiographic evidence of rejection.[184,185] Systolic function abnormalities characterize advanced rejection. A preponderance of isolated reports citing exotic tests purport to provide noninvasive evidence of rejection. They include dynamic function analysis, such as LV torsional deformation[191]; or MRI of T_2 relaxation time (spin-spin relaxation time, a parameter characterizing tissue water) and cardiac tissue intensity[187]; alterations in end-diastolic or stroke volumes using technetium 99[188]; evidence of myocardial necrosis by myocardial uptake of indium 111_{Tn}–labeled monoclonal antibodies against cardiac myosin[189]; or changes in the general immune state deduced by an increase in all T-cell subsets (T3, T4, and T8) without the changes in the T4:T8 ratio that characterize viral infection.[190] To date, none has gained widespread acceptance as definitive noninvasive evidence for rejection.

Outcome Following Heart Transplantation

Survival. Survival after pediatric heart transplantation is slightly lower than that in adults, which is entirely related to the higher operative mortality (see Fig 22–2).[22] Heart transplantation for congenital heart disease carried a twofold increase in operative risk related to the increased likelihood of technical difficulties with the anastomoses, hemorrhage, and right heart failure from elevated PVR.[22] Infants under 1 year old have an operative mortality of 24%,[22] perhaps related to the larger proportion of patients with congenital heart disease in this age group. Any rigorous comparison of outcome following transplantation with any other therapy should consider mortality in those awaiting transplant. Although this figure probably varies widely with the specific indication for transplantation and the condition of the child, the Stanford group reported seven deaths among 60 children listed (12%), 6 of whom died within 30 days.[31]

The causes of death and their relative frequency following heart transplantation are similar in adults and children except that graft failure is more common in the latter (Fig 22–11). Graft failure may result from obstructed blood flow, hemorrhage, ineffective myocardial preservation or increased PVR, and accounts for 40% of the pediatric mortality as opposed to 25% of the adult deaths.[22] Between 70 and 80% of the mortality after pediatric heart transplant occurs in the first 6 months.[22,31] By the end of the first postoperative month, infection becomes the most common cause of death, replaced after 6 months by rejection, including accelerated coronary atherosclerosis (Fig 22–12).[22]

Infection. International Registry statistics place infection as the third most common cause of death after pediatric heart transplant, accounting for 20% of deaths,[22] although there is variability from center to center depending on the potency of the immunosuppressive regimen employed. Thus, the Stanford pediatric heart transplant program reports very low mortality from rejection (16% of all deaths); however, 62% of their deaths resulted from infection.[31] Alternatively, the Pittsburgh heart transplant program reports a much higher incidence of rejection episodes (all children surviving 2 weeks suffer at least one episode in the first 2 months),[34] but only 18% of their deaths resulted from infection.[41] Similarly, the period of highest infection risk is the early postoperative period when immunosuppression is greatest.[22] All of the lethal infections in the Pittsburgh series[41] and 80% of those in the Stanford patients were evident within 3 months of transplant or retransplant.[31] Worldwide experience suggests that infection is the most common cause of death from 1–6 months post-transplant.[22]

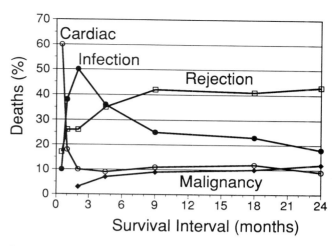

Figure 22–12. Prevalence of lethal complications as a function of time after heart transplant expressed as a percentage of deaths at each interval. This pattern is reproducible for heart and heart-lung recipients whether children or adults. "Cardiac" deaths include operative/technical difficulties, uncontrolled hemorrhage, and graft failure as might occur with increased PVR. (*Data from the Registry of the International Society for Heart and Lung Transplantation.*[22])

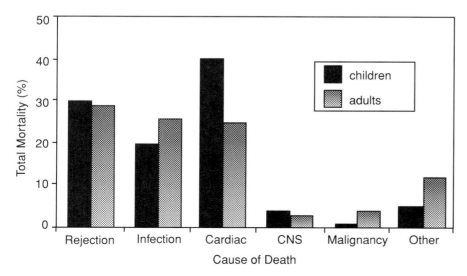

Figure 22–11. Causes of death, expressed as a fraction of all mortality, after orthotopic heart transplantation in children and adults. The most notable difference occurs in "cardiac" deaths, which include operative/technical difficulties, uncontrolled hemorrhage, and graft failure. (*Modified from data of the Registry of the International Society for Heart and Lung Transplantation.*[22])

The distribution of infectious agents in pediatric[31,41] and adult patients[192] is comparable; for example, at Stanford, 48% of pediatric infections were bacterial, 37% viral, 12% fungal, and 3% protozoal.[31] Viral and fungal organisms play a role in 90% of the lethal infections.[31] Bacterial infection usually presents in the first 2 weeks after transplant. Thirty percent of the bacterial infections resulted in bacteremia, all of which were associated with gram-negative pulmonary infections.[41] One patient had developed a pulmonary infarct prior to transplant that evolved into a pulmonary abscess 30 days postoperatively, a complication reported to affect 50% of adults with recent pretransplant pulmonary infarction.[40]

Viral infection tends to occur later in the postoperative course.[41] CMV represented the most prevalent (70%) and serious (14% mortality) of the viral infections in the Pittsburgh program.[41] At least 86% of the clinical CMV infections occurred in previously seronegative children.[41] CMV infection exhibited a mean onset 33 days post-transplant.[41] CMV pneumonia was associated with both cases of bacterial lung abscess diagnosed in this series. Although CMV screening of donors and matching CMV status of donor and host remains impractical owing to the limited donor pool, this series was reported at a time when blood products were not screened either. During the initial hospitalization, 43% of the previously seronegative children converted.[41] In adults, seroconversion and reactivation both occur in approximately 50%, but all lethal CMV infections occurred in previously seronegative recipients.[47] In many centers, all blood products are screened prior to administration to transplant recipients and listed transplant candidates to avoid administration of CMV antibody–positive blood products to CMV seronegative recipients whenever feasible. Therapy for CMV includes antiviral agents such as ganciclovir[193–195] and a reduction in immunosuppressive drugs.[193] However, the latter is controversial because CMV infection has also been associated with increased risk of rejection and graft atherosclerosis.[196] Prophylactic administration of acyclovir[197,198] and CMV immune globulin[198,199] both represent promising therapies that have proven effective in reducing the incidence of serious CMV infections in seronegative recipients. Recent evidence that non-A, non-B hepatitis afflicts 48% of the recipients of organs from hepatitis C seropositive donors has led some programs to restrict the use of these organs to life-saving circumstances.[200] Despite the potential gravity of any viral infection in transplant patients, the minor childhood respiratory and gastrointestinal viruses seem well tolerated.

Fungal and protozoal infections are always serious, although fortunately they represent only 7 and 4%, respectively, of the infections.[41] In the Stanford series, 50% of the children with fungal infections died,[31] whereas all children with fungal infection died in the Pittsburgh series.[41] Protozoal infection, usually *Pneumo-cystsis* pneumonia, typically follows aggressive immunotherapy for recalcitrant rejection.[41]

Rejection. Episodes of rejection afflict virtually all pediatric heart recipients. In the Stanford series, 70% of the children had at least one episode of rejection in the first 3 months, 85% by 6 months, and all by 5 years.[31] After the first 6 months, the incidence of rejection fell to 0.2 episodes/100 patient-days.[31] Between 1974 and 1989, 11% of the Stanford pediatric heart recipients lost their graft to rejection, although this rate has progressively declined with improvements in immunotherapy.[31] For instance, the addition of cyclosporine reduced the proportion of children losing their graft from 33 to 7%, and none has lost a graft from rejection since the addition of OKT3 and total lymphoid irradiation in 1986.[31] The International Registry, however, reports rejection as the second leading cause of death in pediatric heart recipients, resulting in 30% of the overall mortality.[31] In contrast to the Stanford report, the International Registry includes deaths related to accelerated coronary atherosclerosis as rejection complications.

The initial therapy of acute rejection consists of "pulse" corticosteroids.[24,31,34,35] In the early postoperative period, intravenous methyl prednisolone serves as the most common therapeutic modality. After the first year post-transplant, oral prednisone is generally regarded as sufficient.[31,34] If evidence of rejection persists or hemodynamic deterioration occurs, the therapy is intensified to include specific T-cell immunosuppressive agents such as ATG or OKT3.[24,31,34,35] OKT3 is more effective,[177,178,182] albeit more toxic, than ATG.[178,179] Repeated exposure to OKT3 may stimulate the development of an anti-idiotypic antibody that diminishes its effectiveness over time.[182] Total lymphoid irradiation has been successful in the Stanford series when employed in children whose rejection remains unresponsive to other therapy.[37] Retransplantation remains the ultimate recourse for uncontrolled rejection, but the operative mortality is 34%.[22]

Coronary atherosclerosis is a serious source of late morbidity and mortality affecting as many as 50% of adults surviving 5 years after heart transplant.[201–204] The incidence is less certain in pediatrics varying between 0 and 28% in children followed from 6 months to 6 years after transplant.[24,31,183] The Stanford pediatric transplant program reports a 15% incidence overall, with a 21% prevalence among recipients surviving more than 2 years.[31] Although the pathologic changes of advanced coronary disease become evident as soon as 25 days post-transplant, angiographic abnormalities are rarely visualized before 2 years.[31] In the Pittsburgh series, all of the children who died from recurrent, unremitting rejection between 6 and 11 months postoperatively had histologic evidence of diffuse coronary arteritis, lymphocyte infiltration, and myocyte necrosis.[183] In the children diagnosed with coronary disease after the first year, 50–100% will die or require retransplantation.[31,183] Coronary atherosclerosis may manifest clinically as congestive heart failure, sudden death,[183] or, rarely, angina[205] because ischemia usually remains silent in the denervated heart.[31,206]

Numerous observations, for example, the appearance of a lymphocyte infiltration around the coronaries,[183] indicate an immunologic mechanism for coronary atherosclerosis after heart transplantation.[203,207] A strong association exists between the frequency of rejection episodes and coronary disease in children who die in the first year.[183] Late development of coronary disease is temporally related to recurrent mild focal rejection noted on endomyocardial biopsy.[183] Although some studies show an increased likelihood of coronary disease with HLA A2 or A3 mismatches[14] or anti-HLA antibody production in the recipient,[208] others fail to demonstrate an association.[183,209] The side effects of immunosuppressive therapy (eg, prednisone and hyperlipidemia, cyclosporine and hypertension) may also play a role in accelerated coronary atherosclerosis.[202,209] However, animal models demonstrate that coronary disease occurs irrespective of the use of immunosuppressive drugs.[207,210] In fact, Pahl suggests that improvements in immunotherapy, specifically the addition of ATG to the induction sequence, may have reduced the incidence of coronary disease in the Pittsburgh series.[183]

Epidemiologic studies indicate that other risk factors contribute to accelerated coronary atherosclerosis.[31,196,209,211] None of the children in the Stanford series who received their transplant before age 14 exhibited coronary disease.[31] Between 14 and 18 years, the changes were only evident pathologically.[31] In this series, atherosclerosis was evident on angiography only in children after age 18.[31] Hypercholesterolemia and hypertriglyceridemia occurred in over 50% of children after 6 months of immunotherapy with prednisone.[183] Institutions that have omitted prednisone from routine maintenance immunosuppression purportedly have lower risk of coronary disease.[24,212,213] Alternatively, dietary therapy, such as ω–3 fish oil supplementation,[214] may reduce the risk. An association between seroconversion for CMV and accelerated coronary disease in recipients has also been noted.[196]

The therapeutic options after the development of accelerated coronary atherosclerosis remain limited. The diffuse, distal nature of the coronary involvement often precludes percutaneous transluminal angioplasty or even coronary artery bypass grafting. Retransplantation remains the most common therapy[31,202] despite the higher risk of operative mortality[22,202] and recurrent coronary disease.[202]

Malignancy accounts for 5% of the overall mortality after adult heart transplantation and 12% of the mortality among those who survive longer than 2 years.[22] The postulated mechanism is a reduction in host defenses related to immunosuppression that enables tumor proliferation.[215] Lymphomas account for more than half these malignancies,[31,216] most commonly associated with positive Epstein-Barr virus (EBV) titers.[215,217] Reductions in immunosuppressive therapy successfully treat many of these lymphomas,[215,217] occasionally with the addition of acyclovir,[31,217] lending support to this "host-permissive" mechanism. The more benign nature of this process has led to the term *lymphoproliferative disorder* (LPD) rather than lymphoma.

In children, malignancies account for only 1–2% of the mortality after heart transplantation.[22] Among children transplanted at Stanford University, 11% developed malignancies, 83% of whom had lymphoproliferative disease.[31] Half of the malignancies were discovered incidentally at autopsy, suggesting a higher incidence of subclinical disease.[31] One child with generalized lymphoproliferative disease responded to reduction in immunosuppression and acyclovir, whereas another with central nervous system (CNS) LPD achieved remission with radiation therapy.[31] Of the six children with malignancies, only one child (17%) succumbed to unremitting LPD.[31] In the same series, neither of the two children transplanted for doxorubicin cardiomyopathy relapsed as a result of immunosuppression.[31]

Neurologic dysfunction immediately following heart transplantation most commonly arises from ischemia suffered either prior to transplant or perioperatively.[169] Alternate mechanisms of injury include CNS infection,[41,169] usually opportunistic, toxicity of immunosuppressive drugs,[161,166,169] or, rarely, CNS lymphoma.[169,217]

Cardiovascular rehabilitation occurs rapidly with 90–100% of the survivors discharged New York Heart Association class I.[31,34,46] Children who received heart transplants at Stanford spent an average of 6.8 days per year in the hospital during the first year, which diminished to 0.9 days per year in the fifth year.[31] In fact, 27% required no further hospitalizations.[31] Follow-up cardiac catheterization confirms normal growth of the pulmonary artery and aortic anastomoses.[30,218] In the absence of acute rejection, hemodynamic studies generally reveal normal cardiac output with high-normal end-diastolic pressures and atrial pressures.[30,109,171,218,219] Heart rate typically remains slightly elevated.[109,219] Intrinsic cardiac function,[124] including impulse formation,[140] conduction,[140] length-tension relationships,[84,124,130] and coronary autoregulation[64,84,124] remain intact following transplant. In patients with cardiomyopathy, PVR generally normalizes over the first month postoperatively[129]; the time course for resolution of elevated PVR associated with congenital heart disease has not been reported.

As noted previously, the denervated heart increases cardiac output in response to exercise by initially relying upon the Frank-Starling mechanism and subsequently circulating catecholamines.[109,130] This limits maximal heart rate and cardiac output during exercise resulting in increased oxygen extraction and earlier lactate production when compared with controls.[109,132] For heart transplant recipients, maximal increases in oxygen consumption achieved during exercise are limited to 70% of controls.[132] However, heart recipients rarely perceive limitations in their daily activities.

Although development is normal in children after heart transplant, growth impairment is reported in 79% of the children transplanted before age 14 at Stanford.[31,174] Disturbance in linear growth is highly correlated to corticosteroid dose, and is thus directly related to the frequency of cardiac rejection episodes.[174] Linear growth improves if steroid therapy can be tapered to an alternate-day dosing. At Loma Linda, where steroids are administered only to treat rejection, normal growth has been observed in transplant recipients.[46]

HEART-LUNG AND LUNG TRANSPLANTATION

Heart-lung and lung transplants are becoming more established in pediatric practice. The major indications include the Eisenmenger syndrome and other congenital cardiovascular malformations associated with pulmonary vascular disease, primary pulmonary hypertension, cystic fibrosis, and pulmonary fibrosis (Fig 22–13).[22] Primary pulmonary or pulmonary vascular disease without end-stage heart failure is increasingly treated with lung transplant alone. Thus, 23% of the patients receiving single lung transplants in 1990 had primary pulmonary hypertension of the Eisenmenger syndrome.[22] The risks of uncontrollable postoperative hemorrhage in patients who had previous thoracotomies render transplants in these patients relatively contraindicated in some programs.[213,220]

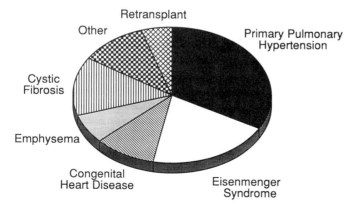

Figure 22–13. Indications for heart-lung transplantation from 1981–1990. (*Data from the Registry of the International Society for Heart and Lung Transplantation.*[22])

Donor Management

Donor identification and management for lung or heart-lung transplantation is more selective than heart transplantation because only 10% of potential donors meet the criteria.[220] The screening process is designed to eliminate the prospect of significant acquired lung disease, aspiration, or pulmonary edema. Thoracic capacity should be no greater than that of the recipient because larger lungs are at risk for postoperative atelectasis and subsequent infection.[220] Upon diagnosis of brain death, intravascular volume should be restored to a maximal CVP of 8–10 mm Hg. If diabetes insipidus occurs, desmopressin helps prevent the accumulation of excess lung water that may follow excessive crystalloid replacement.[220] If arterial blood P_{O_2} is over 100 mm Hg and a peak inflating pressure is under 30 cm H_2O at a ventilator tidal volume of 15 mL/kg, PEEP 5 cm H_2O, F_{IO_2} 0.4 pulmonary function is adequate for transplantation.[220] Specific antimicrobial therapy should address tracheal secretions that reveal a predominant organism.[220]

Intraoperatively, the donor receives 30 mg/kg methyl prednisolone and a prostaglandin E_1 (PGE_1) infusion beginning at 25 ng/kg/min and doubled every 2 minutes until systemic arterial pressure decreases 10–20%.[220] This dose is typically 100 ng/kg/min, which causes maximal pulmonary vasodilation for uniform cooling during infusion of pulmoplegic solution.[220] Pulmoplegic solution with modified Euro Collins solution (per liter: K^+ 108 mEq, Mg^{+2} 60 mEq, HCO_3 9.3 mEq, HPO_4^- 85 mEq, $H_2PO_4^-$ 15 mEq, 2.5% dextrose)[78,220] is infused into the pulmonary artery after cardioplegia has been infused into the aortic root.[220] The lungs are inflated and the trachea stapled to retain lung volume in that position. Division of the venae cavae, aorta, and trachea permits the removal of the heart and lungs en bloc, whereupon the organs are transported at 4°C.[220]

Recipient Management

The anesthetic management of children undergoing heart-lung or lung transplantation centers around manipulation of PVR. Anesthetic or ventilatory techniques that increase PVR can result in acute right ventricular failure and reduced cardiac output in children without intracardiac communications or severe hypoxemia in those with the Eisenmenger syndrome or congenital heart malformations with a right-to-left shunt. Moderate to extreme hyperventilation in conjunction with anesthetic agents that have a salutary or neutral effect on PVR and effectively blunt the pulmonary vascular response to tracheal intubation and surgery are used. Despite evidence that ketamine increases PVR under some circumstances,[92] it preserves systemic vascular tone,[86,91,92] making it the agent of choice in the child with a severe Eisenmenger syndrome. In children with the Eisenmenger syndrome, a slight decrease in SVR due to drugs such as fentanyl might dramatically increase the right-to-left shunt. In our experience, if PVR exceeds the SVR to the extent that substantial right-to-left shunting occurs continuously, ketamine has a negligible effect on the ratio of PVR:SVR. Alternatively, SVR can be maintained by the administration of an α-adrenergic agonist while using other anesthetic techniques. Nitrous oxide carries the disadvantages of negative inotropy and possibly pulmonary vasoconstriction[97-100] that, coupled with its propensity to expand small gas bubbles in the pulmonary vasculature after implantation,[78] make it undesirable in heart-lung transplants.

Several considerations assume importance in the selection and placement of a tracheal tube. The tube should be large enough to seal the airway and enable adequate ventilation if lung compliance decreases or airway resistance increases. Tracheal tubes larger than 4.5 mm inside diameter generally permit bronchoscopic removal of clots at the tracheal anastomosis.[221] Too large a tube risks compression necrosis of the tracheal anastomosis. Because the tube will invade the surgical field, sterile technique is recommended for tracheal intubation.[78] The distal orifice of the tube should reside just below the vocal cords in order to remain above the anastomosis.

The surgical technique requires excision of the lungs and heart individually, taking care to identify and preserve the phrenic, vagus, and recurrent laryngeal nerves.[220,222] The heart is excised in a fashion analogous to any heart recipient unless the organ is to be employed in a "domino" transplant, in which case, division of the venae cavae follows the technique of donor procurements.[220] A button of left pulmonary artery at the ligamentum arteriosum is left to preserve the integrity of the recurrent laryngeal nerve. Meticulous hemostasis, particularly in the posterior mediastinum, precedes implantation because this area will later be inaccessible.[220] Implantation occurs en bloc with the tracheal anastomosis first so the lungs can be gently reinflated with air (F_{IO_2} 0.21).[78,221] Aortic and right atrial (or caval) anastomoses complete the procedure.[220]

In order to limit oxidative injury in the postischemic lung,[223] ventilation is adjusted after separation from CPB to give the lowest F_{IO_2} that results in a Pa_{O_2} over 70 mm Hg in conjunction with a level of PEEP that minimizes F_{IO_2} without compromising hemodynamics.[221] If hypoxemia persists, common etiologies are excessive lung water and left ventricular dysfunction causing elevated pulmonary venous pressures. Both problems occur in the context of severed lymphatic connections precluding interstitial fluid elimination.[224] The hypoxemia usually responds to measures designed for increasing LV function, for diuretics, and for PEEP. The evidence suggests that lymphatic channels reform after a few weeks.[225]

Hemorrhage is particularly troublesome after heart-lung transplantation. Extensive systemic to pulmonary collaterals, coagulopathy due to hepatic dysfunction from passive congestion, and pleural scars from previous thoracotomies all contribute to the bleeding. Uncontrollable bleeding related to previous thoracotomy accounts for as much as half the operative mortality in the children undergoing heart-lung transplantation.[213]

Outcome Following Heart-Lung Transplantation

Although heart-lung and lung transplants have been performed in infants as young as 2 months of age, only 50 transplants in children under 10 years of age have been reported to the International Registry since 1981.[22] From available data, outcome is not related to age. In fact, outcome among the three lung transplant options (heart-lung, single, and double lung) is similar.[22] Operative mortality is 16–19%, usually related to hemorrhage or graft failure.[22] These deaths account for one third of the total mortality (Fig 22–14).[22] As with heart transplants, infection becomes the most important cause of death between 1 and 6 months postoperatively, but the proportion of deaths due to infection is higher—25–35%.[22] Rejection follows as the most important cause of death beyond 6 months, being responsible for 20% of the overall mortality.[22] Outcome following heart-lung or lung transplant is significantly worse than that after heart transplant alone (Fig 22–15).[22] One-year survival worldwide is approximately 60% and five-year survival approaches 40%,[22] although the Stanford program reports improving results.[220]

In addition to the complications described for heart transplantation, these children also experience lung graft disease. A diffuse pulmonary vascular process that histologically resembles accelerated atherosclerosis occurs.[226,227] An obliterative bronchiolitis may appear[220,224,228] that contributes significantly to morbidity and mortality. The mechanism for this process is probably the repair of recurrent episodes of rejection or infection. Among the hospital survivors of heart-lung transplantation performed at Stanford University between 1981 and 1986, 63% developed obliterative bronchiolitis and 42% of those died from the process.[220] Although the addition of azathioprine to the immunosuppression protocol reduced the incidence of obliterative bronchiolitis to 20%, 40% of these patients still succumbed to obliterative bronchiolitis with superimposed pneumonia.[220]

In lung transplant recipients, fever, cyanosis, and a lung infiltrate represent the most challenging common condition confronting the clinician. The differential diagnosis includes myocardial dysfunction due to ischemia or rejection, pulmonary infection or rejection, or increased interstitial fluid due to severed lymphatic channels. Transbronchial biopsy provides accurate diagnosis. The ability to monitor perivascular and perialveolar cellular infiltrates in the lung assumes tremendous importance because over 60% of pulmonary rejection episodes

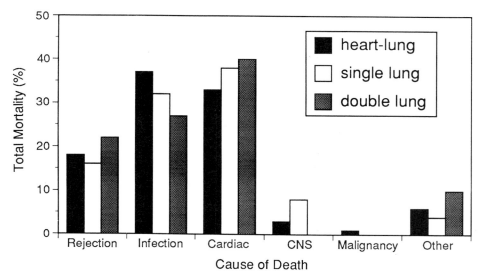

Figure 22–14. Causes of death, expressed as a fraction of total mortality, following heart-lung and lung transplantation. "Cardiac" deaths include operative/technical difficulties, uncontrolled hemorrhage, and graft failure as might occur with increased PVR. (*Data from the Registry of the International Society for Heart and Lung Transplantation.*[22])

may occur without cardiac rejection.[220,227] This technique, however, presents severe logistical problems in small children. Another sensitive indicator of pulmonary rejection is flow-related pulmonary function. A reduction of more than 20% in the FEF_{25-75} or the FEV_1 necessitates a transbronchial biopsy by the Stanford protocol.[220] Although pulmonary rejection reduces FEV_1 and PaO_2, the FEF_{25-75} provides the most sensitive index of pulmonary rejection (Fig 22–16).[220] Whether these noninvasive studies provide sufficient sensitivity and specificity in the diagnosis of pulmonary rejection in children too small for endobronchial biopsy remains unclear.

After lung or heart-lung transplantation, dramatic symptomatic relief often ensues, although pulmonary function is not normal.[224,229] Denervation of the lung results in reduced bronchomotor tone at rest and eliminates the cough reflex to airway stimuli distal to the anastomosis.[221] Early follow-up studies conducted in the mid–1980s revealed nearly normal pulmonary function[229]

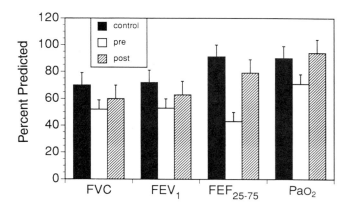

Figure 22–16. Pulmonary function changes during rejection episodes that follow lung transplantation. FVC, forced vital capacity; FEV_1, forced expired volume in 1 second; FEF_{25-75}, forced expired flow from 25–75% of FVC; PaO_2, arterial oxygen tension. Control studies are conducted after transplantation when free of rejection. Pre- and post- changes were measured during histologic lung rejection before (pre-) and after (post-) rejection therapy was instituted. Changes in FEF_{25-75} consistently provided the most sensitive measure of lung rejection. Effective therapy restored pulmonary function. (*Data from Starnes VA: Heart-lung transplantation: An overview. Cardiol Clin 8:159–168, 1990.*)

Figure 22–15. Actuarial 2-year survival following heart-lung and single lung transplantation compared with that after orthotopic heart transplantation. (*Data from the Registry of the International Society for Heart and Lung Transplantation.*[22])

and pulmonary artery pressure[230] in the early postoperative period. Initially, a substantial proportion of survivors developed a gradual reduction in flow-related pulmonary function over time.[228] More recent methods of immunosuppression and monitoring reveal that many of the pulmonary function abnormalities noted during rejection are reversible if promptly treated.[220] Heart-lung and lung transplantation are still evolving therapies.

Anesthetic Management of Children After Heart Transplantation

Over 3000 heart and lung transplants are performed each year, a total exceeding 17,000 since 1982.[22] As a result, anesthesiologists practicing outside the centers performing these procedures are increasingly likely to encounter such patients. The estimated incidence of noncardiac procedures for heart transplant recipients ranges from 10 to 28%.[139,231–236] The incidence of general surgical problems after heart transplant is 10 times that following other cardiac operations.[138] The mortality after these general surgical procedures may reach 31%.[233]

Common Surgical Interventions Following Heart Transplantation

There are no published series of pediatric heart transplant recipients undergoing other surgical procedures. However, in adults, surgical interventions involve virtually all surgical subspecialties, although exploratory laparotomy for an acute abdomen is among the most common.[138,139,231] Because the immunocompromised state of transplant recipients warrants an aggressive approach, the findings at laparotomy frequently are not remediable by surgery. Typical intra-abdominal diseases, some of which may be related to corticosteroid therapy, include cholecystitis, peptic ulcer disease, pancreatitis, and perforated bowel.[138,139,235] Pancreatitis, which often follows procedures requiring CPB and may be related to infection and drug therapy as well, represents a particularly frequent cause of acute abdomen after heart transplantation.[138,232,234,235] The tissue diagnosis of a neoplastic process necessitates surgery.[216,217] Infectious complications may prompt diagnostic or therapeutic procedures such as open lung biopsy or the evaluation of a CNS process.[41]

Preoperative Evaluation. Preoperative evaluation and intraoperative management require an understanding of the physiology of the denervated heart. After the early postoperative period, hemodynamic function should be near normal unless rejection is present.[30,109,171,218,219] The compensatory responses of the denervated heart to increased metabolic demand are the Frank-Starling mechanism to increase cardiac output early and circulating catecholamines to increase heart rate and contractility subsequently.[109,130] In the face of rejection, symptoms of congestive heart failure are abnormalities in

diastolic and ultimately systolic function.[107,110,186,191] Arrhythmias also frequently complicate the first 6 months after transplant and become particularly prominent during acute rejection.[143] Silent coronary disease may afflict up to 25–44% of those who have survived 3 years.[201,203,204] Finally, side effects commonly accompany immunosuppressive therapy, such as the hypertension[31,171] and renal insufficiency[166–168,170] associated with cyclosporine therapy.

Preoperative Management. Depending upon the overall condition of the child, the anesthetic plan may range from a complicated integration of a variety of critical considerations to one in which the past history of heart transplantation becomes virtually incidental. The extent to which preanesthetic medication becomes safe, even necessary, defies any simple generalization and remains a matter of judgment based largely upon the hemodynamic and emotional state of the child as well as the anticipated actions that such drugs might have. Most children have received steroid therapy sufficiently recently to have a suppressed hypothalamic-pituitary axis, thus meriting stress steroid replacement by any of the accepted protocols. All children should benefit from the basic cardiovascular and respiratory monitoring afforded by ECG, noninvasive blood pressure, stethoscope, pulse oximetry, and respiratory gas analysis. In children transplanted more than 2 years previously, particularly adolescents, the possibility of myocardial ischemia should be entertained. The benefits of invasive monitoring in measuring the status and abnormal response of the cardiovascular system must be weighed against the risks of the usual complications and the more serious consequences of iatrogenic infection.

Intraoperative Management. The selection of anesthetic agents requires a judgment as to the basic hemodynamic state in light of other conditions bearing upon management, such as elevated intracranial pressure or an overriding risk of reflux and aspiration of stomach contents. Because the cardiac output relies upon venous return during conditions of normal and increased demand, the preservation of intravascular volume deserves particular attention. Similarly, anesthetic agents that possess significant negative inotropy may limit the heart's ability to respond to changes in EDV and should thus be avoided. Others have noted interactions between azathioprine, cyclosporine, and various anesthetic drugs. Azathioprine acts as a cholinesterase inhibitor that antagonizes competitive relaxants and prolongs the effects of depolarizing agents,[237] whereas cyclosporine potentiates the effects of barbiturates, fentanyl,[238] and muscle relaxants.[239]

The implications of cardiac denervation deserve consideration in drug selection. As noted previously, stimuli that exert cardiac actions via the autonomic nervous system exert no effect in the denervated heart whether the stimulus is pharmacologic, mechanical (eg, oropharyngeal vagal reflexes), or an autoregulatory reflex (eg, baroreceptor responses to blood pressure changes).[64,78,138] Anesthetic agents also exert indirect cardiac effects. The vagolytic effects of pancuronium and the vagotonic effects of narcotics are not evident in transplanted hearts.[64,138] Nitrous oxide, which acts as a sympathetic stimulant as well as a direct myocardial depressant, normally benefits from the offsetting nature of these actions. In the absence of sympathetic innervation, the myocardial depression becomes increasingly evident.[138] Similarly, tachycardia indicating sympathetic discharge due to light anesthesia or hypovolemia is delayed until circulating catecholamines influence cardiac β receptors directly.[138]

The same potential hazards apply to regional techniques employed in heart transplant recipients. The rapid changes in preload and systemic vascular resistance that accompany spinal or epidural anesthesia represent a significant threat to the heart devoid of sympathetic reflex compensation.[64] Given sufficient augmentation of circulating volume,[236] a block with more gradual, controllable onset (eg, epidural versus spinal)[138] and prompt recognition and treatment of hemodynamic disturbances with direct-acting sympathomimetic agents would seemingly provide the greatest safety. Nevertheless, both spinal and epidural techniques have been safely used.[236]

REFERENCES

1. Carrel A, Guthrie CC: The transplantation of veins and organs. *Am Med* **10**:1101, 1905
2. McGregor CC: Evolution of heart transplantation. *Cardiol Clin* **8**:3–10, 1990
3. Webb WR, Howard HS: Restoration of function of the refrigerated heart. *Surg Forum* **8**:302–306, 1957
4. Goldberg M, Berman EF, Akman LC: Homologous transplantation of the canine heart. *J Int Coll Surg* **30**:575–586, 1958
5. Cass MH, Brock R: Heart excision and replacement. *Guy's Hosp Rep* **108**:285–290, 1959
6. Lower RR, Shumway NE: Studies on orthotopic homotransplantation of the canine heart. *Surg Forum* **11**:18–19, 1960
7. Dong E, Hurley EJ, Lower RR, Shumway NE: Performance of the heart two years after autotransplantation. *Surgery* **56**:270–273, 1964
8. Mann FC, Priestley JT, Markowitz J, Yater WM: Transplantation of the intact mammalian heart. *Arch Surg* **26**:219–224, 1933
9. Schwartz R, Eisner A, Dameshek W: The effect of 6-mercaptopurine on primary and secondary immune responses. *J Clin Invest* **38**:1394–1402, 1959
10. Lower RR, Dong E, Shumway NE: Long-term survival of cardiac homografts. *Surgery* **58**:110–119, 1965
11. Barnard CN: A human cardiac transplant: An interim report of a successful operation performed at Groote Schuur Hospital. *S Afr Med J* **41**:1271–1274, 1967
12. Caves PK, Billingham ME, Schulz WP, et al: Transvenous biopsy from canine orthotopic heart allografts. *Am Heart J* **85**:525–530, 1973
13. Caves PK, Stinson EB, Billingham ME, Shumway NE: Serial transvenous biopsy of the transplanted human heart. Improved management of acute rejection episodes. *Lancet* **1**:821–826, 1974
14. Bieber CP, Hunt SA, Schwinn DA, et al: Complications in long-term survivors of cardiac transplantation. *Transplant Proc* **13**:207–211, 1981
15. Calne RY, White DJG, Rolles K, et al: Prolonged survival of pig orthotopic heart grafts treated with cyclosporin A. *Lancet* **1**:1183–1185, 1978
16. Oyer PE, Stinson EB, Jamieson SW, et al: Cyclosporine in cardiac transplantation. A 2 1/2 year follow-up. *Transplant Proc* **15**:2546–2552, 1983
17. Beecher HK, Adams RD, Barger AC, et al: A definition of irreversible coma: Report of the Ad Hoc Committee of the Harvard Medical School to examine the definition of brain death. *JAMA* **205**:85–88, 1968
18. Watson DC, Reitz BA, Baumgartner WA, et al: Distant heart procurement for transplantation. *Surgery* **86**:56–59, 1979
19. Kantrowitz A, Haller SD, Joos H, et al: Transplantation of the heart in an infant and an adult. *Am J Cardiol* **22**:782–790, 1968
20. Cooley DA, Bloodwell RD, Hallman GL, et al: Organ transplantation for advanced cardiopulmonary disease. *Ann Thorac Surg* **8**:30–42, 1969
21. Bailey LL, Nehlsen-Cannarella SL, Dorshow RW, et al: Cardiac allotransplantation in newborns as therapy for hypoplastic left heart syndrome. *N Engl J Med* **315**:949–951, 1986
22. Kreitt JM, Kaye MP: The Registry of the International Society for Heart and Lung Transplantation: Eighth Official Report—1991. *J Heart Lung Transplant* **10**:491–498, 1991
23. Kreitt JM, Kaye MP: The Registry of the International Society for Heart Transplantation: Seventh Official Report—1990. *J Heart Transplant* **9**:323–330, 1990
24. Boucek MM, Kanakriyeh MS, Mathis CM, et al: Cardiac transplantation in infancy: Donors and recipients. *J Pediatr* **116**:171–176, 1990
25. Bailey LL, Assaad AN, Trimm F, et al: Orthotopic transplantation during early infancy as therapy for incurable congenital heart disease. *Ann Surg* **208**:279–285, 1988
26. Penkoske PA, Rowe RC, Freedom RM, et al: The future of heart and heart-lung transplantation in children. *Heart Transplant* **3**:233–238, 1984
27. Griepp RB, Stinson EB, Dong E, et al: Determinants of operative risk in human heart transplantation. *Am J Surg* **122**:192–196, 1971
28. Kirklin JK, Naftel DC, McGiffin DC, et al: Analysis of morbid events and risk factors for death after cardiac transplantation. *J Am Coll Cardiol* **11**:917–924, 1988
29. Renlund DG, Bristow MR, Lee HR, O'Connell JB: Medical aspects of cardiac transplantation. *J Cardiothorac Anesth* **2**:500–512, 1988

30. Starnes VA, Bernstein D, Oyer PE, et al: Heart transplantation in children. *J Heart Transplant* 8:20–26, 1989

31. Baum D, Bernstein D, Starnes VA, et al: Pediatric heart transplantation at Stanford: Results of a 15-year experience. *Pediatrics* 88:203–214, 1991

32. Addonizio LJ, Gersony WM, Robbins RC, et al: Elevated pulmonary vascular resistance and cardiac transplantation. *Circulation* 76(suppl V):V-52–V-55, 1987

33. Addonizio LJ, Hsu DT, Fuzesi L, et al: Optimal timing of pediatric heart transplantation. *Circulation* 80(suppl III): III-84–III-89, 1989

34. Fricker FJ, Griffith BP, Hardesty RL, et al: Experience with heart transplantation in children. *Pediatrics* 79:138–146, 1987

35. Jacobs JL, Sands BB, Norwood WI: Cardiac transplantation. In Holbrook PR (ed): *Textbook of Pediatric Critical Care*. Philadelphia: WB Saunders, 1993 pp 332–338

36. Mavroudis C, Harrison H, Klein JB, et al: Infant orthotopic cardiac transplantation. *J Thorac Cardiovasc Surg* 96: 912–924, 1988

37. Bernstein D, Starnes VA, Baum D: Pediatric heart transplantation. *Adv Pediatr* 37:413–439, 1990

38. Barnard CN, Wolpowitz A: Heterotopic versus orthotopic heart transplantation. *Transplant Proc* 11:309–312, 1979

39. Barnard CN, Barnard MS, Cooper DKC, et al: The present status of heterotopic cardiac transplantation. *J Thorac Cardiovasc Surg* 81:433–439, 1981

40. Young JN, Yazbeck J, Esposito G, et al: The influence of acute preoperative pulmonary infarction on the results of heart transplantation. *J Heart Transplant* 5:20–22, 1986

41. Green M, Wald ER, Fricker FJ, et al: Infections in pediatric orthotopic heart transplant recipients. *Pediatr Infect Dis J* 8:87–93, 1989

42. Jacobs JL, Williams JF: Pediatric heart transplantation. *Cardiol Clin* 8:149–157, 1990

43. Addonizio LJ, Rose EA: Cardiac transplantation in children and adolescents. *J Pediatr* 111:1034–1038, 1987

44. Yacoub M, Festenstein H, Doyle P, et al: The influence of HLA matching in cardiac allograft recipients receiving cyclosporine and azathioprine. *Transplant Proc* 19:2487–2489, 1987

45. Opelz G: Collaborative Heart Transplant Study; Effect of HLA matching in heart transplantation. *Transplant Proc* 21:794–796, 1989

46. Bailey LL, Wood M, Razzouk A, et al: Heart transplantation during the first 12 years of life. *Arch Surg* 124:1221–1226, 1989

47. Wreghitt TG, Hakim M, Gray JJ, et al: Cytomegalovirus infection in heart and heart and lung transplant recipients. *J Clin Pathol* 41:660–667, 1988

48. Gelb AW, Robertson KM: Anaesthetic management of the brain dead for organ donation. *Can J Anaesth* 37:806–812, 1990

49. Ghosh S. Bethune DW, Hardy I, et al: Management of donors for heart and heart-lung transplantation. *Anaesthesia* 45:672–675, 1990

50. Griepp RB, Stinson EB, Clark DA, et al: The cardiac donor. *Surg Gynecol Obstet* 133:792–798, 1971

51. Randell T, Orko R, Hockerstedt K: Peroperative fluid management of the brain-dead multiorgan donor. *Acta Anaesthesiol Scand* 34:592–595, 1990

52. Wetzel RC, Setzer N, Stiff JL, Rogers MC: Hemodynamic responses in brain dead organ donor patients. *Anesth Analg* 64:125–128, 1985

53. Weber KT, Janicki JS: The heart as a muscle-pump system and the concept of heart failure. *Am Heart J* 98:371–384, 1979

54. Parmley WW: Pathophysiology of congestive heart failure. *Am J Cardiol* 56:7A–11A, 1985

55. Clark NJ, Martin RD: Anesthetic considerations for patients undergoing cardiac transplantation. *J Cardiothorac Anesth* 2:519–542, 1988

56. Rabinovitch M: Pulmonary hypertension. In Adams FH, Emmanouilides GC, Riemenschneider TA (eds): *Heart Disease in Infants, Children, and Adolescents*, 4th ed. Baltimore: Williams & Wilkins, 1989, pp 856–880

57. Heath D, Edwards JE: The pathology of hypertensive pulmonary vascular disease. *Circulation* 28:533–547, 1958

58. Meyrick B, Reid L: Pulmonary hypertension. Anatomic and physiologic correlates. *Clin Chest Med* 4:199–217, 1983

59. Burrows FA, Rabinovitch M: The pulmonary circulation in children with congenital heart disease: Morphologic and morphometric considerations. *Can Anaesth Soc J* 32:364–373, 1985

60. Burrows FA, Klinck JR, Rabinovitch M, Bohn DJ: Pulmonary hypertension in children: Perioperative management. *Can Anaesth Soc J* 33:606–628, 1986

61. Hickey PR, Hansen DD, Wessel DL, et al: Blunting of stress responses in the pulmonary circulation of infants by fentanyl. *Anesth Analg* 64:1137–1142, 1985

62. Cassin S, Dawes GS, Mott JC, et al: The vascular resistance of the foetal and newly ventilated lung of the lamb. *J Physiol (Lond)* 171:61–79, 1964

63. Rudolph AM, Yuan S: Response of the pulmonary vasculature to hypoxia and H^+ ion concentration changes. *J Clin Invest* 45:399–411, 1966

64. Demas K, Wyner J, Mihm FG, Samuels S: Anaesthesia for heart transplantation: A retrospective study and review. *Br J Anaesth* 58:1357–1364, 1986

65. Nicolson SC, Steven JM, Betts EK: Monitoring the pediatric patient. In Blitt CD (ed): *Monitoring in Anesthesia and Critical Care Medicine*. New York: Churchill Livingstone, 1990, pp 739–786

66. Borland LM: Anesthesia for organ transplantation in children. *Int Anesthesiol Clin* 23:173–199, 1985

67. Martin RD, Parisi F, Robinson TW, Bailey L: Anesthetic management of neonatal cardiac transplantation. *J Cardiothorac Anesth* 3:465–469, 1989

68. Manchikanti L, Colliver JA, Marrero T, et al: Ranitidine and metoclopramide for prophylaxis of aspiration pneumonitis in elective surgery. *Anesth Analg* 63:903–910, 1984

69. Godsouzian N, Coté CJ, Liu LMP, Dedrick DF: The dose-response effects of oral cimetidine on gastric pH and volume in children. *Anesthesiology* 55:533–536, 1981

70. Gibbs CP, Banner TC: Effectiveness of Bicitra as a preoperative antacid. *Anesthesiology* 61:97–99, 1984

71. Kates RA, Stack RS, Hill RF, et al: General anesthesia for patients undergoing percutaneous transluminal coronary angioplasty during acute myocardial infarction. *Anesth Analg* 65:815–818, 1986

72. Cooper SC, Lell WA: Hormonal effects of an induction dose of etomidate for patients undergoing urgent myocar-

dial revascularization. *J Cardiothorac Anesth* 2:171–176, 1988

73. Gutzke GE, Shah KB, Glisson SN, et al: Cardiac transplantation: A prospective comparison of ketamine and sufentanil for anesthetic induction. *J Cardiothorac Anesth* 3:389–395, 1989

74. Waterman PM, Bjerke R: Rapid-sequence induction in patients with severe ventricular dysfunction. *J Cardiothorac Anesth* 5:602–606, 1988

75. Tanner GE, Angers DG, Barash PG, et al: Effect of left-to-right, mixed left-to-right and right-to-left shunts on inhalational anesthetic induction in children. A computer model. *Anesth Analg* 64:101–107, 1985

76. Eger EI: Ventilation, circulation, and uptake. In Eger EI (ed): *Anesthetic Uptake and Action.* Baltimore: Williams & Wilkins, 1974, pp 122–145

77. Stoelting RK, Longnecker DE: Effect of right-to-left shunt on the rate of increase in arterial anesthetic concentration. *Anesthesiology* 36:352–356, 1972

78. Ream AK, Fowles RE, Jamieson S: Cardiac transplantation. In Kaplan JA (ed): *Cardiac Anesthesia,* 2nd ed. Orlando, FL: Grune & Stratton, 1987, pp 881–891

79. Reitz BA, Fowles RE, Ream AK: Cardiac transplantation. In Ream AK, Fogdall RP (eds): *Acute Cardiovascular Management: Anesthesia and Intensive Care.* Philadelphia: JB Lippincott, 1982, pp 549–567

80. Fernando NA, Keenan RL, Boyan CP: Anesthetic experience with cardiac transplantation. *J Thorac Cardiovasc Surg* 75:531–535, 1978

81. Benowitz NL, Meister W: Pharmacokinetics in patients with cardiac failure. *Clin Pharmacokinet* 1:389–405, 1976

82. Wynands JE, Wong P, Whalley DG, et al: Oxygen-fentanyl anesthesia in patients with poor left ventricular function: Hemodynamics and plasma fentanyl concentrations. *Anesth Analg* 62:476–482, 1983

83. Ozinsky J: Cardiac transplantation—The anaesthetist's view: A case report. *S Afr Med J* 41:1268–1270, 1967

84. Grebenik CR, Robinson PN: Cardiac transplantation at Harefield. A review from the anaesthetist's standpoint. *Anaesthesia* 40:131–140, 1985

85. Hensley VA, Martin DE, Larach DR, et al: Anesthetic management for cardiac transplantation in North America–1986 survey. *J Cardiothorac Anesth* 1:427–429, 1987

86. White PF, Way WL, Trevor AJ: Ketamine—Its pharmacology and therapeutic uses. *Anesthesiology* 56:119–136, 1982

87. Traber DL, Wilson RD, Priano LL: Differentiation of the cardiovascular effects of CI–581. *Anesth Analg* 47:769–777, 1968

88. Braunwald E: Heart failure: Pathophysiology and treatment. *Am Heart J* 102:486–490, 1981

89. Schwartz DA, Horowitz LD: Effects of ketamine on left ventricular performance. *J Pharmacol Exp Ther* 194:410–414, 1975

90. Morray JP, Lynn AM, Stamm SJ, et al: Hemodynamic effects of ketamine in children with congenital heart disease. *Anesth Analg* 63:895–899, 1984

91. Hickey PR, Hansen DD, Cramolini GM, et al: Pulmonary and systemic hemodynamic responses to ketamine in infants and children with normal and elevated pulmonary vascular resistance. *Anesthesiology* 62:287–293, 1985

92. Wolfe RR, Loehr JP, Schaffer MS, Wiggins JW: Hemodynamic effects of ketamine, hypoxia and hyperoxia in children with surgically treated congenital heart disease residing ≥ 1,200 meters above sea level. *Am J Cardiol* 67:84–87, 1991

93. Stanley TH, Webster LR: Anesthetic requirements and cardiovascular effects of fentanyl-oxygen and fentanyl-diazepam-oxygen anesthesia in man. *Anesth Analg* 57:411–416, 1978

94. Tomicheck RC, Rosow CE, Philbin DM, et al: Diazepam-fentanyl interaction—Hemodynamic and hormonal effects in coronary artery surgery. *Anesth Analg* 62:881–884, 1983

95. Fragen RJ, Shanks CA, Molteni A, Avram MJ: Effects of etomidate on hormonal responses to surgical stress. *Anesthesiology* 61:652–656, 1984

96. Conway CM, Ellis DB: The haemodynamic effects of short-acting barbiturates. *Br J Anaesth* 41:534–542, 1969

97. Lappas DG, Buckley MJ, Laver MB, et al: Left ventricular performance and pulmonary circulation following addition of nitrous oxide to morphine during coronary-artery surgery. *Anesthesiology* 43:61–69, 1975

98. Schulte-Sasse U, Hess W, Tarnow J: Pulmonary vascular responses to nitrous oxide in patients with normal and high pulmonary vascular resistance. *Anesthesiology* 57:9–13, 1982

99. Hickey PR, Hansen DD, Stafford M, et al: Pulmonary and systemic hemodynamic effects of nitrous oxide in infants with normal and elevated pulmonary vascular resistance. *Anesthesiology* 65:374–378, 1986

100. Davidson JR, Chinyanga HM: Cardiovascular collapse associated with nitrous oxide anaesthetic: A case report. *Can Anaesth Soc J* 29:484–488, 1982

101. Morris RB, Cahalan MK, Miller RD, et al: The cardiovascular effects of vecuronium (ORG NC45) and pancuronium in patients undergoing coronary artery bypass grafting. *Anesthesiology* 58:438–440, 1983

102. Starr NJ, Sethna DH, Estafanous FG: Bradycardia and asystole following the rapid administration of sufentanil with vecuronium. *Anesthesiology* 64:521–523, 1986

103. Chartrand C, Guerin R, Kanagh M, Stanley P: Pediatric heart transplantation: Surgical considerations for congenital heart diseases. *J Heart Transplant* 9:608–617, 1990

104. Bailey LL, Concepcion W, Shattuck H, Huang L: Method of heart transplantation for the treatment of hypoplastic left heart syndrome. *J Thorac Cardiovasc Surg* 92:1–5, 1986

105. Griffith BP, Hardesty RL, Kormos RL, et al: Temporary use of the Jarvik-7 total artificial heart before transplantation. *N Engl J Med* 316:130–134, 1987

106. Farrar DJ, Hill D, Gray LA, et al: Heterotopic prosthetic ventricles as a bridge to cardiac transplantation: A multicenter study in 29 patients. *N Engl J Med* 318:333–340, 1988

107. Davies RA, Koshal A, Walley V, et al: Temporary diastolic noncompliance with preserved systolic function after heart transplantation. *Transplant Proc* 19:3444–3447, 1987

108. Ingels NB, Ricci DR, Daughters GT, et al: Effects of heart rate augmentation on left ventricular volumes and cardiac output of the transplanted human heart. *Circulation* 56(suppl II):II-32–II-37, 1977

109. Schroeder JS: Hemodynamic performance of the human transplanted heart. *Transplant Proc* **1**:304–308, 1979

110. Stinson EB, Caves PK, Griepp RB, et al: Hemodynamic observations in the early period after human heart transplantation. *J Thorac Cardiovasc Surg* **69**:264–270, 1975

111. Peckham GJ, Fox WW: Physiologic factors affecting pulmonary artery pressure in infants with persistent pulmonary hypertension. *J Pediatr* **93**:1005–1010, 1978

112. Drummond WH, Gregory GA, Hyman MA, Phibbs RA: The independent effects of hyperventilation, tolazoline and dopamine on infants with persistent pulmonary hypertension. *J Pediatr* **98**:603–611, 1981

113. West JB: *Respiratory Physiology—The Essentials.* Baltimore: Williams & Wilkins, 1974

114. Daoud FS, Reeves JT, Kelly DB: Isoproterenol as a potential pulmonary vasodilator in primary pulmonary hypertension. *Am J Cardiol* **42**:817–822, 1978

115. Prielipp RC, Rosenthal MH, Pearl RG: Hemodynamic profiles of prostaglandin E_1, isoproterenol, prostacyclin, and nifedipine in vasoconstrictor pulmonary hypertension in sheep. *Anesth Analg* **67**:722–729, 1988

116. Prielipp RC, McLean R, Rosenthal MH, Pearl RG: Hemodynamic profiles of prostaglandin E_1, isopoterenol, prostacyclin, and nifedipine in experimental porcine pulmonary hypertension. *Crit Care Med* **19**:60–67, 1991

117. Bush A, Busst CM, Knight WB, Shinebourne EA: Comparison of the haemodynamic effects of epoprostenol (prostacycline) and tolazoline. *Br Heart J* **60**:141–148, 1988

118. Stone PH, Antman EM, Muller JE, Braunwald E: Calcium channel blocking agents in the treatment of cardiovascular disorders. Part II: Hemodynamic effects and clinical applications. *Ann Intern Med* **93**:886–904, 1980

119. Bush A, Busst C, Booth K, et al: Does prostacycline enhance the selective pulmonary vasodilator effect of oxygen in children with congenital heart disease? *Circulation* **74**:135–144, 1986

120. Fineman JR, Crowley MR, Soifer SJ: Selective pulmonary vasodilation with ATP-$MgCl_2$ during pulmonary hypertension in lambs. *J Appl Physiol* **69**:1836–1842, 1990

121. Frostell C, Fratacci MD, Wain JC, et al: Inhaled nitric oxide—A selective pulmonary vasodilator reversing hypoxic pulmonary vasoconstriction. *Circulation* **83**:2038–2047, 1991

122. Pepke-Zaba J, Higenbottam TW, Dihn-Xuan AT, et al: Inhaled nitric oxide as a cause of selective pulmonary vasodilation in pulmonary hypertension. *Lancet* **338**:1173–1174, 1991

123. Zellers TM, Vanhoutte PM: Endothelium-dependent relaxations of piglet pulmonary arteries augment with maturation. *Pediatr Res* **30**:176–180, 1991

124. Kent KM, Cooper T: The denervated heart—A model for studying autonomic control of the heart. *N Engl J Med* **291**:1017–1021, 1974

125. Lowenstein E, Johnston WE, Lappas DG, et al: Catastrophic pulmonary vasoconstriction associated with protamine reversal of heparin. *Anesthesiology* **59**:470–473, 1983

126. Morel DR, Zapol WM, Thomas SJ, et al: C5a and thromboxane generation associated with pulmonary vaso- and broncho-constriction during protamine reversal of heparin. *Anesthesiology* **66**:597–604, 1987

127. Hobbhahn J, Conzen PF, Habazettl H, et al: Heparin reversal by protamine in humans—Complement, prostaglandins, blood cells and hemodynamics. *J Appl Physiol* **71**:1415–1421, 1991

128. Manno CS, Hedberg KW, Kim HC, et al: Comparison of the hemostatic effects of fresh whole blood, stored whole blood and components after open heart surgery in children. *Blood* **77**:930–936, 1991

129. Bhatia SJS, Kirshenbaum JM, Shemin RJ, et al: Time course of resolution of pulmonary hypertension and right ventricular remodeling after orthotopic cardiac transplantation. *Circulation* **76**:819–826, 1987

130. Pope SE, Stinson EB, Daughters GT, et al: Exercise response of the denervated heart in long-term cardiac transplant recipients. *Am J Cardiol* **46**:213–218, 1980

131. McLaughlin PR, Kleiman JH, Martin RP, et al: The effect of exercise and atrial pacing on left ventricular volume and contractility in patients with innervated and denervated hearts. *Circulation* **58**:476–483, 1978

132. Savin WM, Haskell WL, Shroeder JS, Stinson EB: Cardiorespiratory responses of cardiac transplant patients to graded, symptom-limited exercise. *Circulation* **62**:55–60, 1980

133. Cannom DS, Rider AK, Stinson EB, Harrison DC: Electrophysiologic studies in the denervated transplanted human heart: II. Response to norepinephrine, isoproterenol and propranolol. *Am J Cardiol* **36**:859–866, 1975

134. Borrow KM, Neumann A, Arensman FW, Yacoub MH: Left ventricular contractility and contractile reserve in humans after cardiac transplantation. *Circulation* **71**:866–872, 1985

135. Vatner DE, Lavallee M, Amano J, et al: Mechanisms of supersensitivity to sympathomimetic amines in the chronically denervated heart of the conscious dog. *Circ Res* **57**:55–64, 1985

136. Yusuf S, Theodoropoulos S, Mathias CJ, et al: Increased sensitivity of the denervated transplanted human heart to isoprenaline both before and after β-adrenergic blockade. *Circulation* **75**:696–704, 1987

137. Gilbert EM, Eiswirth CC, Mealey PC, et al: β-Adrenergic supersensitivity of the transplanted human heart is presynaptic in origin. *Circulation* **79**:344–349, 1989

138. Bailey PL, Stanley TH: Anesthesia for patients with a prior cardiac transplant. *J Cardiothorac Anesth* **4**:38–47, 1990

139. Kanter SF, Samuels SI: Anesthesia for major operations on patients who have transplanted hearts. A review of 29 cases. *Anesthesiology* **46**:65–68, 1977

140. Cannom DS, Graham AF, Harrison DC: Electrophysiological studies in the denervated transplanted human heart: Response to atrial pacing and atropine. *Circ Res* **32**:268–278, 1973

141. Hilberman M, Maseda J, Stinson EB, et al: The diuretic properties of dopamine in patients after open-heart surgery. *Anesthesiology* **61**:489–494, 1984

142. Zumbro GL, Kitchens WR, Shearer G, et al: Mechanical assistance for cardiogenic shock following cardiac surgery, myocardial infarction, and cardiac transplantation. *Ann Thorac Surg* **44**:11–13, 1987

143. Schroeder JS, Berke DK, Graham AF, et al: Arrhythmias after cardiac transplantation. *Am J Cardiol* **33**:604–607. 1974

144. Mason JW, Winkle RA, Rider AK, et al: The electrophysiologic effects of quinidine in the transplanted human heart. *J Clin Invest* **59**:481–489, 1977

145. Stein KL, Darby JM, Grenvik A: Intensive care of the cardiac transplant recipient. *J Cardiothorac Anesth* **2**:543–553, 1988

146. Antman EM, Stone PH, Muller JE, Braunwald E: Calcium channel blocking agents in the treatment of cardiovascular disorders. Part I: Basic and clinical electrophysiologic effects. *Ann Intern Med* **93**: 875–885, 1980

147. Ricci DR, Orlick AE, Reitz BA, et al: Depressant effect of digoxin on atrioventricular conduction in man. *Circulation* **57**:898–903, 1978

148. Camm AJ, Garratt CJ: Adenosine and supraventricular tachycardia. *N Engl J Med* **325**:1621–1629, 1991

149. Ellenbogen KA, Thames MD, DiMarco JP, et al: Electrophysiological effects of adenosine in the transplanted human heart: Evidence of supersensitivity. *Circulation* **81**:822–828, 1990

150. Gross MA, Keefer V, Liebman J: The platelets in cyanotic heart disease. *Pediatrics* **42**:651–658, 1968

151. Maurer HM, McCue CM, Robertson LW, Higgins JC: Correction of platelet dysfunction and bleeding in cyanotic congenital heart disease by simple red cell volume reduction. *Am J Cardiol* **35**:831–835, 1975

152. Ekert H, Gilcrist GS, Stanton R, Hammond D: Hemostasis in cyanotic heart disease. *J Pediatr* **76**:221–230, 1970

153. Salzman EW, Weinstein MJ, Weintraub RM, et al: Treatment with desmopressin acetate to reduce blood loss after cardiac surgery. A double-blind randomized trial. *N Engl J Med* **314**:1402–1406, 1986

154. Hackmann T, Naiman SC: Con: Desmopressin is not of value in the treatment of post-cardiopulmonary bypass bleeding. *J Cardiothorac Vasc Anesth* **5**:290–293, 1991

155. Seear MD, Wadsworth LD, Rogers PC, et al: The effect of desmopressin acetate (DDAVP) on postoperative blood loss after cardiac operations in children. *J Thorac Cardiovasc Surg* **98**:217–219, 1989

156. Blauhut B, Gross C, Necek S, et al: Effects of high-dose aprotinin on blood loss, platelet function, fibrinolysis, complement, and renal function after cardiopulmonary bypass. *J Thorac Cardiovasc Surg* **101**:958–967, 1991

157. Harder MP, Eijsman L, Roozendaal KJ, et al: Aprotonin reduces intraoperative and postoperative blood loss in membrane oxygenator cardiopulmonary bypass. *Ann Thorac Surg* **51**:936–941, 1991

158. Havel M, Teufelsbauer H, Knöbl P, et al: Effect of intraoperative aprotonin administration on postoperative bleeding in patients undergoing cardiopulmonary bypass operation. *J Thorac Cardiovasc Surg* **101**:968–972, 1991

159. Marx G, Pokar H, Reuter H, et al: The effects of aprotinin on hemostatic function during cardiac surgery. *J Cardiothorac Vasc Anesth* **5**:467–474, 1991

160. van Oeveren W, Jansen NJG, Bidstrup BP, et al: Effects of aprotinin on hemostatic mechanisms during cardiopulmonary bypass. *Ann Thorac Surg* **44**:640–645, 1987

161. Calne RY, Rolles K, White DJG, et al: Cyclosporin A initially as the only immunosuppressant in 34 recipients of cadaveric organs; 32 kidneys, 2 pancreases, and 2 livers. *Lancet* **2**:1033–1036, 1979

162. Woodley SL, Renlund DG, O'Connell JB, Bristow MR: Immunosuppression following cardiac transplantation. *Cardiol Clin* **8**:83–96, 1990

163. Valantine HA: Long-term management and results in heart transplant recipients. *Cardiol Clin* **8**:141–148, 1990

164. Myers BD, Ross J, Newton L, et al: Cyclosporine-associated chronic nephropathy. *N Engl J Med* **311**:699–705, 1984

165. Schade RR, Guglielmi A, Van Thiel DH, et al: Cholestasis in heart transplant recipients treated with cyclosporine. *Transplant Proc* **15**:2757–2760, 1983

166. Schüler S, Warnecke H, Hetzer R: Prevention of toxic side effects of cyclosporine in heart transplantation. *Transplant Proc* **19**:2518–2521, 1987

167. Moyer TP, Post GR, Sterioff S, Anderson CF: Cyclosporine nephrotoxicity is minimized by adjusting dosage on the basis of drug concentration in blood. *Mayo Clin Proc* **63**:241–247, 1988

168. Hunt SA, Stinson EB, Oyer PE, et al: Results of "immunoconversion" from cyclosporine to azathioprine in heart transplant recipients with progressive nephrotoxicity. *Transplant Proc* **19**:2522–2524, 1987

169. Hotson JR, Enzmann DR: Neurologic complications of cardiac transplantation. *Neurol Clin* **6**:349–365, 1988

170. Trento A, Griffith BP, Hardesty RL, et al: Cardiac transplantation: Improved quality of survival with a modified immunosuppressive protocol. *Circulation* **76**(suppl V):V48-V51, 1987

171. Pahl E, Fricker FJ, Trento A, et al: Late follow-up of children after heart transplantation. *Transplant Proc* **20**: 743–746, 1988

172. Curtis JJ, Luke RG, Jones P, Diethelm AG: Hypertension in cyclosporine-treated renal transplant recipients is sodium-dependent. *Am J Med* **85**:134–138, 1988

173. Thompson ME, Shapiro AP, Johnsen AM, et al: New onset of hypertension following cardiac transplantation: A preliminary report and analysis. *Transplant Proc* **15**:2573–2577, 1983

174. Uzark K, Crowley D, Callow L, Bove E: Linear growth after pediatric heart transplantation. *Circulation* **78**(suppl II):II–492, 1988 (abstr)

175. Bieber CP, Griepp RB, Oyer PE, et al: Use of rabbit antithymocyte globulin in cardiac transplantation—Relationship of serum clearance rates to clinical outcome. *Transplantation* **22**:478–488, 1976

176. Cosimi AB: The clinical usefulness of anti-lymphocyte antibodies. *Transplant Proc* **15**:583–589, 1983

177. Costanzo-Nordin MR, Silver MA, O'Connell JB, et al: Successful reversal of acute cardiac allograft rejection with OKT3 monoclonal antibody. *Circulation* **76**(suppl V):V-71–V-80, 1987

178. Bristow MR, Gilbert EM, Renlund DG, et al: Use of OKT3 monoclonal antibody in heart transplantation: Review of the initial experience. *J Heart Transplant* **7**:1–11, 1988

179. Ortho Multicenter Transplant Study Group: A randomized trial of OKT3 monoclonal antibody for acute rejection of renal transplants. *N Engl J Med* **313**:337–342, 1985

180. Kahn DR, Hong R, Greenberg AJ, et al: Total lymphatic

irradiation and bone marrow in human heart transplantation. *Ann Thorac Surg* 38:169–171, 1984

181. Strober S, Dhillon M, Schubert M, et al: Acquired immune tolerance to cadaveric renal allografts—A study of three patients treated with total lymphoid irradiation. *N Engl J Med* 321:28–33, 1989

182. Starnes VA, Oyer PE, Stinson EB, et al: Prophylactic OKT3 used as induction therapy for heart transplantation. *Circulation* 80(suppl III):III–79–III–83, 1989

183. Pahl E, Fricker FJ, Armitage J, et al: Coronary arteriosclerosis in pediatric heart transplant survivors: Limitation of long-term survival. *J Pediatr* 116:177–183, 1990

184. Dawkins KD, Oldershaw PJ, Billingham ME, et al: Noninvasive assessment of cardiac allograft rejection. *Transplant Proc* 17: 215–217, 1985

185. Valantine HA, Fowler MB, Hunt SA, et al: Changes in Doppler echocardiographic indexes of left ventricular function as potential markers of acute cardiac rejection. *Circulation* 76(suppl V):V–86–V–92, 1987

186. Johnson DE, Gollub SB, Wilson DB, et al: Systolic anterior motion of the mitral valve as a manifestation of heart transplantation rejection. *J Heart Transplant* 7:289–291, 1988

187. Kurland RJ, West J, Kelley S, et al: Magnetic resonance imaging to detect heart transplant rejection: Sensitivity and specificity. *Transplant Proc* 21:2537–2543, 1989

188. Novitsky D, Cooper DKC, Boniaszcuk J, et al: Prediction of acute cardiac rejection using radionuclide scanning to detect left ventricular volume changes. *Transplant Proc* 17:218–220, 1985

189. First W, Yasuda T, Segall G, et al: Noninvasive detection of human cardiac transplant rejection with indium–111 antimyosin (Fab) imaging. *Circulation* 76(suppl V):V–81–V–85, 1987

190. Ertel W, Reichenspurner H, Lersch C, et al: Cytoimmunological monitoring in acute rejection and viral, bacterial or fungal infection following transplantation. *Heart Transplant* 4:390–394, 1985

191. Hansen DE, Daughters GRT, Alderman EL, et al: Effect of acute human cardiac allograft rejection on left ventricular systolic torsion and diastolic recoil measured by intramyocardial markers. *Circulation* 76:998–1008, 1987

192. Hofflin JM, Potasman I, Baldwin JC, et al: Infectious complications in heart transplant recipients receiving cyclosporine and corticosteroids. *Ann Intern Med* 106:209–216, 1987

193. Harmon WE: Opportunistic infections in children following renal transplantation. *Pediatr Nephrol* 5:118–125, 1991

194. Goodrich JM, Mori M, Gleaves CA, et al: Early treatment with ganciclovir to prevent cytomegalovirus disease after allogeneic bone marrow transplantation. *N Engl J Med* 325:1601–1607, 1991

195. Mai M, Nery J, Sutker W, et al: DHPG (ganciclovir) improves survival in CMV pneumonia. *Transplant Proc* 21:2263–2265, 1989

196. Grattan MT, Moreno-Cabral CE, Starnes VA, et al: Cytomegalovirus infection is associated with cardiac allograft rejection and atherosclerosis. *JAMA* 261:3561–3566, 1989

197. Hibberd PL, Rubin RH: Prevention of cytomegalovirus infection in the pediatric renal transplant patient. *Pediatr Nephrol* 5:112–117, 1991

198. Balfour HH, Chance BA, Stapleton JT, et al: A randomized, placebo-controlled trial of oral acyclovir for the prevention of cytomegalovirus disease in recipients of renal allografts. *N Engl J Med* 320:1381–1387, 1989

199. Snydman DR, Werner BG, Heinz-Lacey B, et al: Use of cytomegalovirus immune globulin to prevent cytomegalovirus disease in renal-transplant recipients. *N Engl J Med* 317:1049–1054, 1987

200. Pereiera BJG, Milford EL, Kirkman RL, Levey AS: Transmission of hepatitis C virus by organ transplantation. *N Engl J Med* 325:454–460, 1991

201. Pascoe EA, Barnhart GR, Carter VH, et al: The prevalence of cardiac allograft arteriosclerosis. *Transplantation* 44:838–839, 1987

202. Gao SZ, Schroeder JS, Hunt S, Stinson EB: Retransplantation for severe accelerated coronary artery disease in heart transplant recipients. *Am J Cardiol* 62:876–881, 1988

203. Uretsky BF, Murali S, Reddy PS, et al: Development of coronary artery disease in cardiac transplant patients receiving immunosuppressive therapy with cyclosporine and prednisone. *Circulation* 76:827–834, 1987

204. Gao SZ, Schroeder JS, Alderman EL, et al: Prevalence of accelerated coronary artery disease in heart transplant survivors. Comparison of cyclosporine and azathioprine regimens. *Circulation* 80(suppl III):III–100–III–105, 1989

205. Stark RP, McGinn AL, Wilson RF: Chest pain in cardiactransplant recipients: Evidence of sensory reinnervation after cardiac transplantation *N Engl J Med* 324:1791–1794, 1991

206. Rowan RA, Billingham ME: Myocardial innervation in long-term heart transplant survivors: A quantitative ultrastructural survey. *J Heart Transplant* 7:448–452, 1988

207. Lurie KG, Billingham ME, Jamieson SW, et al: Pathogenesis and prevention of graft arteriosclerosis in an experimental heart transplant model. *Transplantation* 31:41–47, 1981

208. Petrossian GA, Nichols AB, Marboe CC, et al: Relation between survival and development of coronary artery disease and anti-HLA antibodies after cardiac transplantation. *Circulation* 80(suppl III):III–122–III–125, 1989

209. Gao SZ, Schroeder JS, Alderman EL, et al: Clinical and laboratory correlates of accelerated coronary artery disease in the cardiac transplant patient. *Circulation* 76(suppl V): V–56–V–61, 1987

210. Cramer DV, Qian S, Harnaha J, et al: Cardiac transplantation in the rat. I. The effect of histocompatibility differences on graft atherosclerosis. *Transplantation* 47:414–419, 1989

211. Thompson J, Eich D, Ko D, et al: Hyperchoslesterolemia as a marker of early coronary artery disease post cardiac transplantation. *Circulation* 76(suppl IV):IV–167, 1987 (abstr)

212. Yacoub M, Alivizatos P, Khaghani A, Mitchell A: The use of cyclosporine, azathioprine, and antithymocyte globulin with or without low-dose steroids for immunosuppression of cardiac transplant patients. *Transplant Proc* 17:221–222, 1985

213. Radley-Smith R, Yacoub MH: Heart and heart-lung transplantation in children. *Circulation* 76(suppl IV):IV24, 1987 (abstr)

214. Starris GE, Mitchell RS, Billingham ME, et al: Inhibition of accelerated cardiac allograft arteriosclerosis by fish oil. *J Thorac Cardiovasc Surg* 97:841–855, 1989

215. Nalesnik MA, Makowka L, Starzl TE: The diagnosis and treatment of posttransplant lymphoproliferative disorders. *Curr Probl Surg* 25:365–472, 1988

216. Kirkorian JG, Anderson JL, Bieber CP, et al: Malignant neoplasms following cardiac transplantation. *JAMA* 240:639–643, 1978

217. Starzl TE, Nalesnik MA, Porter KA, et al: Reversibility of lymphomas and lymphoproliferative lesions developing under cyclosporine-steroid therapy. *Lancet* 1:583–587, 1984

218. Kanakriyeh MS, Mullins CE, Parisi F, et al: Late hemodynamic results after orthotopic heart transplantation in early infancy. *Circulation* 78(suppl II):II294, 1988 (abstr)

219. Greenberg ML, Uretsky BF, Reddy S, et al: Long-term hemodynamic follow-up of cardiac transplant patients treated with cyclosporine and prednisone. *Circulation* 71:487–494, 1985

220. Starnes VA: Heart-lung transplantation: An overview. *Cardiol Clin* 8:159–168, 1990

221. Robertson KM, Borland LM: Anesthesia for organ transplantation. In Motoyama EK, Davis PJ (eds): *Smith's Anesthesia for Infants and Children*, 5th ed. St Louis: CV Mosby, 1990, pp 689–722

222. Jamieson SW, Stinson EB, Oyer PE, et al: Operative technique for heart-lung transplantation. *J Thorac Cardiovasc Surg* 87:930–935, 1984

223. Deneke SM, Fanburg BL: Oxygen toxicity of the lung: An update. *Br J Anaesth* 54:737–749, 1982

224. Ettinger NA, Trulock EP: Pulmonary considerations of organ transplantation. Part 3. *Am Rev Respir Dis* 144:433–451, 1991

225. Jamieson SW: Recent developments in heart and heart-lung transplantation. *Transplant Proc* 17:199–203, 1985

226. Higenbottam T, Stewart S, Wallwork J: Transbronchial lung biopsy to diagnose lung rejection and infection of heart-lung transplants. *Transplant Proc* 20:767–769, 1988

227. Starnes VA, Theodore J, Oyer PE, et al: Evaluation of heart-lung recipients with prospective serial transbronchial biopsies and pulmonary function studies. *J Thorac Cardiovasc Surg* 98:683–690, 1989

228. Burke CM, Dawkins KD, Blank N, et al: Post-transplant obliterative bronchiolitis and other late sequelae in human heart-lung transplantation. *Chest* 86:824–829, 1984

229. Theodore J, Jamieson SW, Burke CM, et al: Physiologic aspects of human heart-lung transplantation. Pulmonary function status of the post-transplanted lung. *Chest* 86:349–357, 1984

230. Dawkins KD, Jamieson SW, Hunt SA, et al: Long-term results, hemodynamics, and complications after combined heart and lung transplantation. *Circulation* 71:919–926, 1985

231. Steed DL, Brown B, Reilly JJ, et al: General surgical complications in heart and heart-lung transplantation. *Surgery* 98:739–744, 1985

232. Colon R, Frazier OH, Kahan BD, et al: Complications in cardiac transplant patients requiring general surgery. *Surgery* 103:32–38, 1988

233. Jones MT, Menkis AH, Kostuk WJ, McKenzie FN: Management of general surgical problems after cardiac transplantation. *Can J Surg* 31:259–262, 1988

234. DiSesa VJ, Kirkman RL, Tilney NL, et al: Management of general surgical complications following cardiac transplantation. *Arch Surg* 124:539–541, 1989

235. Merrell SW, Ames SA, Nelson EW, et al: Major abdominal complications following cardiac transplantation. *Arch Surg* 124:889–893, 1989

236. Melendez JA, Delphin E, Lamb J, Rose E: Noncardiac surgery in heart transplant recipients in the cyclosporine era. *J Cardiothorac Vasc Anesth* 5:218–220, 1991

237. Dretchen KL, Mortenroth VH, Standaert FG, Walts LF: Azathioprine: Effects of neuromuscular transmission. *Anesthesiology* 45:604–609, 1976

238. Cirella VN, Pantuck CB, Lee YJ, Pantuck EJ: Effects of cyclosporine on anesthetic action. *Anesth Analg* 66:703–706, 1987

239. Gramstad L, Gjerløw JA, Hysing ES, Rugstad HE: Interaction of cyclosporin and its solvent, Cremophor, with atracurium and vecuronium. *Br J Anaesth* 58:1149–1155, 1986.

Chapter 23 | Pediatric Cardiac Intensive Care

Edward E. Lowe

Advances in diagnostic modalities, pharmacology, anesthesia, and surgical techniques and greater understanding of pathophysiologic processes have led to an improved prognosis for patients with congenital heart disease. Despite this, major cardiovascular complications continue to be encountered in the postoperative period.

LOW CARDIAC OUTPUT

Etiologies for low cardiac output postoperatively may be multiple in nature. All essentially affect the determinants of cardiac performance: contractility, preload, afterload, and heart rate (Fig. 23–1).

Contractility

Myocardial Injury Secondary to Surgical Trauma. Myocardial contractility may be reduced by surgical trauma.[1–5] Incisions in the myocardium disrupt continuity of muscle fibers as well as possibly injuring conductive pathways. Tissue manipulation may promote edema formation, swelling, or bleeding. These phenomena, in turn, may adversely affect function by decreasing compliance and causing ischemia.

Myocardial Dysfunction Secondary to Chronic Volume and Pressure Overload. Certain congenital heart defects expose the myocardium to chronic volume and pressure overload. The end result may be either secondary cardiomyopathies or myocardial ischemia.[5–11] Ventricular mass increases early when there are sustained increases in volume or pressure.[5–6] The hypertrophy occurring after volume overload is hypothesized to be secondary to increased diastolic pressures in the chamber leading subsequently to eccentric hypertrophy.[6] Muscular hypertrophy secondary to pressure overload is hy-

pothesized to result from increased systolic pressure within that chamber subsequently leading to concentric hypertrophy. Eccentric hypertrophy is defined as an increase in ventricular mass associated with dilatation or increase in ventricle volume, whereas concentric hypertrophy is defined as an increase in ventricular mass or wall thickness associated with a normal-sized ventricle. Initially, these are normal adaptive changes permitting normal myocardial function. However, if volume and/or pressure overload become extreme or are prolonged, damage of muscle fibers and even changes at the cellular level may occur leading to impaired myocardial contractility.

Congenital cardiac lesions that may be associated with chronic left or right ventricular volume overload are atrial septal defect, ventricular septal defect, aortopulmonary window, large patent ductus, atrioventricular (AV) canal, and tricuspid atresia. Pressure overload affecting the left ventricle can be seen in outflow tract obstruction such as subaortic, aortic valvular, or aortic supravalvular stenosis and coarctation of the aorta. Pressure overload of the right ventricle can be present in tetralogy of Fallot, pulmonary stenosis, and pulmonary hypertension.

Ischemic Changes. Chronic volume and pressure overload may also cause ischemic changes in the myocardium leading to myocardial failure. Boucek and coworkers[11] studied total creatine kinase (CK) and myocardial isoenzyme (CKMB) activity prospectively in 282 children with congenital heart disease. Significant elevations in percent CKMB and CKMB activity were found in the symptomatic infants and children with large left-to-right shunts secondary to ventricular septal defect (VSD) or AV canal, aortic coarctation or stenosis, and cyanotic congenital heart defects such as transposition of the great vessels and right ventricular outflow tract ob-

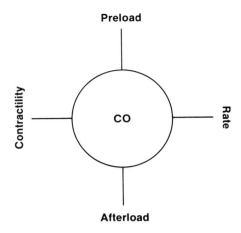

Figure 23–1. Determinants of cardiac output.

struction. They concluded that volume or pressure overload and arterial oxygen saturation possibly cause myocardial cell injury.

One major factor contributing to the ischemic changes is the development of an imbalance between oxygen supply and demand. For example, in aortic stenosis with elevated left ventricular pressure, myocardial perfusion may be compromised in times of stress. In cyanotic heart disease, the oxygen supply might be limited by a decreased oxygen content or an increased coronary artery resistance secondary to polycythemia. Increased myocardial muscle mass requires a greater oxygen supply, and supply is easily compromised in lesions causing ventricular hypertrophy.

Coronary Artery Injury. During surgical repair of congenital heart lesions, there is an ever-present possibility of coronary artery air embolism or injury. Coronary artery injury is difficult to avoid when coronary anatomy is abnormal, as in tetralogy of Fallot where the anterior descending coronary artery passes over the anterior right ventricular wall in the area of the ventriculotomy.[3,8]

Residual Effects of Myocardial Preservation. Because many cardiac operations performed with cardiopulmonary bypass require cross-clamping of the aorta at some time during repair, there is always the potential for global myocardial ischemia.[5,12] Cross-clamping of the aorta interferes with coronary blood flow because the arterial input from the pump oxygenator enters the aorta distal to the clamp. Aortic cross-clamping is associated with temporary functional depression ("stunning") without permanent structural or biochemical changes even with modern methods of myocardial protection.[13]

Interstitial and cellular myocardial edema are associated with aortic cross-clamping.[5] Cellular edema and swelling result from depletion of energy stores, abnormalities in transport of ions across cell membranes, and

formation of osmotically active intracellular molecules in the face of ischemia.[14,15] Myocardial edema, in turn, reduces ventricular compliance and leads to decreased cardiac output.

Before the extensive use of cardioplegia in cardiac surgery, global myocardial ischemia leading to cell death and myocardial necrosis was frequent in patients undergoing cardiopulmonary bypass.[12,16,17] The etiology of this condition was reperfusion of a heart severely damaged by ischemia. A sustained contracture occurred, which was referred to as "stone heart"[18,19] (see Chapter 11).

Metabolic Derangements. Myocardial insufficiency in the postoperative period leading to decreased cardiac output may be secondary to a number of metabolic derangements. These derangements include hypoxemia, electrolyte abnormalities, hypercarbia, acidosis, and hypoglycemia. Hypoglycemia is especially likely in infants who are receiving small amounts of fluids without enough glucose to meet metabolic demands. Failure to recognize and promptly correct these derangements perpetuates the problem.

Hypoxemia. Hypoxemia depresses myocardial contractility. Certain patients with congenital heart disease, especially those with increased pulmonary blood flow or congestive heart failure preoperatively, continue to have pulmonary dysfunction postoperatively. Phrenic nerve injury leading to lung volume diminution has been reported in 1.9% of open and 1.3% of closed pediatric cardiac surgical procedures.[20] Patients with pulmonary dysfunction postoperatively often have increased airway secretions that promote atelectasis and plugging of endotracheal tubes. Each of the above situations promotes ventilation:perfusion mismatching and pulmonary shunting and decreases oxygenation. Hypoxemia stimulates anaerobic metabolism that can cause metabolic acidosis. In turn, this depresses the myocardium causing further decreases in cardiac output, compromised tissue perfusion, and worsened metabolic acidosis.

Electrolyte Abnormalities. Normal levels of sodium, potassium, calcium, and magnesium are essential for excitable membrane function and muscular contraction. Serum and whole-body concentrations of each of these electrolytes can be altered postoperatively.

Alterations in serum sodium, unless extreme, seldom have significant direct effects on the myocardium. Most of the cardiovascular effects of sodium are secondary to its association with hyper- or hypovolemia. Abnormalities in potassium, calcium, magnesium, or phosphate may significantly alter myocardial and peripheral vascular function.[21]

HYPOKALEMIA. In the postoperative cardiac patient, hypokalemia is usually secondary to inadequate potassium replacement of losses caused by diuretic therapy. Hypokalemia has its most significant effects on electrophysiologic events in the heart producing conduction and rhythm disturbances. Arrhythmias associated with digitalis toxicity are enhanced in the presence of hypokalemia. Electrocardiographic (ECG) changes seen with, but not necessarily limited to, hypokalemia are prolongation of the PR and QT intervals, ST segment depression, flattened T waves, and U waves. Automaticity is increased and ventricular ectopic beats, tachycardia, and fibrillation are common in extreme hypokalemia.

HYPERKALEMIA. With the use of potassium cardioplegia, residual hyperkalemia may occur in the immediate post-bypass period. Hyperkalemia may also occur with inadvertent rapid administration of fluids containing potassium as well as when renal failure occurs secondary to low cardiac output states. Elevated potassium decreases automaticity, conductivity, and contractility of the heart.[21] Typical ECG changes associated with hyperkalemia are elevated T waves, prolonged PR interval, loss of P waves, widened QRS complexes, fibrillation, and cardiac standstill. Standstill usually occurs in diastole. ECG abnormalities depend not only upon the degree of hyperkalemia but also upon the rate at which it occurs.

The initial goal in treatment of hyperkalemia is to antagonize the effects of potassium on the heart and shift the elevated extracellular potassium into the intracellular space. Calcium antagonizes the cardiac effects of potassium. Potassium is shifted to the intracellular space by producing an alkalotic state with hyperventilation or sodium bicarbonate or by glucose and insulin. Excess serum potassium can be removed from the body with ion exchange resins such as sodium polystyrene sulfonate (Kayexalate) or by dialysis.

CALCIUM. Hypocalcemia is a potential problem in the postoperative period. A decrease in ionized calcium levels has been demonstrated after CPB.[22] Hypocalcemia is more important in infants and small children because they lack the reserve stores to maintain normal ionized calcium levels. Calcium stores increase with age and muscle mass, but adult calcium stores levels are not present until adolescence.[23]

The importance of calcium in the electrophysiologic contractile process has been reviewed extensively.[24–26] Basically, in cardiac cells, multiple ionic transmembrane fluxes are responsible for the action potential (Fig 23–2). Five phases are recognized:

Phase 0: Rapid depolarization generated by sodium influx through fast channels
Phases 1 and 2: Beginning repolarization and combined calcium and sodium influx through slow channels

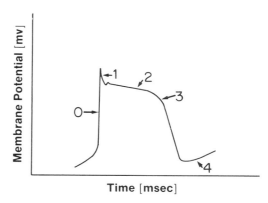

Figure 23–2. A diagrammatic representation of the five phases of action potential in ventricular muscle.

Phase 3: Repolarization resulting from potassium flux from the interior to the exterior of the cell
Phase 4: Resting membrane potential generated by active pumping of sodium out of the cell

Intracellular calcium also regulates activity between contractile proteins in all forms of muscle. In cardiac and skeletal muscles, the inhibition of the troponin-tropomyosin complex on the cross bridges between actin and myosin is released by calcium. Calcium also is required for activation of adenosine triphosphatase (ATPase) that provides the energy for contraction by catalyzing ATP hydrolysis. Calcium is stored in the sarcoplasmic reticulum but, unlike skeletal muscle that can regulate calcium, both cardiac and vascular smooth muscles need the influx of extracellular calcium to function. Therefore, hypocalcemia, especially decreased ionized calcium, decreases myocardial contractility and vascular smooth muscle tone.

MAGNESIUM. Extracorporeal hemodilution and intense diuresis can cause hypomagnesemia in the postoperative period.[27] This electrolyte is essential for many metabolic pathways and function of enzyme systems at the cellular level. Similar to calcium, magnesium is important for neurochemical transmission and muscle contraction. Cardiovascular effects of hypomagnesemia include depressed myocardial contractility, coronary artery spasm, arrythmias and increased sensitivity to digitalis.[27]

Acid-Base Abnormalities. Acidotic states, whether metabolic or respiratory, have significant effects on the cardiovascular system. These effects are complex because in the intact preparation, there is an interaction between direct and indirect effects (Table 23–1).[28] The direct effect of hydrogen ions and CO_2 on the myocardium is depression of function. Indirect effects are secondary to increased stimulation of the sympathetic nervous system by increased hydrogen ions and CO_2 levels that may

TABLE 23–1. DIRECT AND INDIRECT EFFECTS OF ACUTE ACIDOSIS AND HYPERCARBIA

	Acidosis		Hypercarbia	
	Direct	*Indirect*	*Direct*	*Indirect*
Myocardial Contractility	Depression	Stimulation	Depression	Stimulation
Coronary Arteries	D	?	D	?
Pulmonary Vascular	O–C	C	O–C	C
Systemic Vascular	D	C	D	C
Renal Vasculature	D	C	D	C
Cerebral Vasculature	O	?	D	?

Abbreviations: D, dilation; C, constriction; O, no minimal effect.
(Data from Pavlin EG, Hornbein TF: Effects of acid-base imbalance on organ function. Refresher Courses in Anesthesiology 9:120, 1981.)

overcome the direct depressant effects. Respiratory acid-base changes may be more pronounced than metabolic changes because biologic membranes are more permeable to carbon dioxide. Acidotic states also decrease the cardiovascular response to catecholamines.[29]

The effects of alkalosis on the myocardium are not as clear as the effects of acidosis. Alkalosis, however, has been shown to depress cardiac output.[30] It also has a significant effect on ion fluxes, especially potassium and calcium, which may lead to cardiac arrhythmias. The arrhythmias, in turn, compromise myocardial function.

Residual Drug Effects. Despite reports that β-adrenergic antagonists and calcium antagonists taken by adult patients for angina, arrhythmias, and hypertension interact with anesthetic agents to decrease myocardial contractility, it is well accepted that control of the medical problem probably outweighs the danger of possible interactions with anesthetic agents.[31–37] In the pediatric patient with hypertrophic subaortic stenosis and infundibular pulmonary stenosis, β-adrenergic antagonists are important adjuncts in treatment and should not be discontinued preoperatively in these lesions. There is a theoretical possibility of these drugs causing residual problems with myocardial contractility in the postoperative period. Plachetka showed significant propranolol concentrations after bypass in patients who received propranolol up to 2–4 hours before cardiac surgery possibly secondary to redistribution or altered metabolism.[38]

DECREASED PRELOAD

Classically, preload is related to end-diastolic fiber length.[39,40] Clinically, preload is usually assessed by measuring end-diastolic pressure (pulmonary capillary wedge pressure or left atrial pressure for the left ventricle and central venous pressure for the right ventricle) or end-diastolic volumes (by echocardiography). Measurement of end-diastolic volume is reported to be a more reliable indicator of preload than end-diastolic pressure[39,41] Figure 23–3 illustrates the relationships between preload and stroke volume in normal and compromised myocardium. Figure 23–4 shows the relationship between end-diastolic volume and pressure, which illustrates the importance of compliance in assessing preload. Because pressures can be measured continuously, they are used clinically to assess preload. Multiple factors, such as hypovolemia, cardiac tamponade, pulmonary effects, residual anatomic defects, and arrhythmias, contribute to decreased preload and lead to low cardiac output.

Hypovolemia

Decreased intravascular volume may result from inadequate surgical hemostasis. It has been suggested that the use of positive end-expiratory pressure (PEEP) may decrease mediastinal bleeding.[42] This finding has not been confirmed.[43,44] Meticulous control of bleeding before closure of the chest is essential.

Inadequate heparin neutralization as a cause of continued bleeding can be assessed by appropriate clotting studies. The activated clotting time is abnormal in the presence of heparin excess but is also prolonged in primary fibrinolysis, deficiencies in factors of the intrinsic coagulation system, and disseminated intravascular coagulation (DIC). It does not specifically detect abnormal clotting secondary to platelet dysfunction, thrombocytopenia, or deficiencies in factors of the extrinsic coagulation system.[45]

Bleeding secondary to thrombocytopenia or platelet dysfunction can be secondary to the effects of cardiopulmonary bypass on platelets,[46] central catheters,[47] or

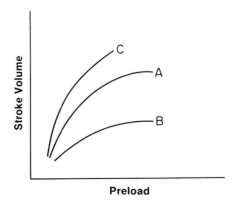

Figure 23–3. Relationship between preload and stroke volume in normal (A), depressed (B), and stimulated (C) myocardium.

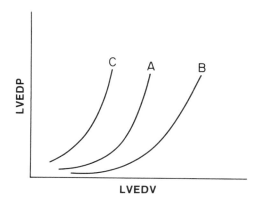

Figure 23–4. Left ventricular end-diastolic volume and pressure relationship (compliance). Curve A, normal; B, increased compliance; C, decreased compliance. LVEDV, left ventricular end-diastolic volume; LVEDP, left ventricular end-diastolic pressure. (*Modified from Sill JC, White RD: Chapter 7. In Tarhan S (ed): Cardiovascular Anesthesia and Postoperative Care. Chicago: Year Book Medical, 1982, p 186, with permission.*)

medications such as sodium nitroprusside.[48] Heparin may also cause thrombocytopenia.[49] Therefore, platelet transfusions may be required after cardiopulmonary bypass and in the postoperative period to control hemorrhage.

Patients with cyanotic heart disease and significant polycythemia have decreased clotting factors. A relationship between the degree of polycythemia and thrombocytopenia[50] and impairment of platelet aggregation[51] has been shown. Cyanotic heart disease is also often accompanied by a decrease in factors II, V, VII, VIII, and IX and fibrinogen.[52] All of these factors may increase bleeding. Despite the deficiency of many clotting factors in cyanotic heart disease, DIC occurs infrequently.[53]

Translocation of fluid from the intravascular space may also contribute to hypovolemia. This is a frequent phenomenon associated with major surgical procedures and trauma. In patients who have undergone cardiopulmonary bypass, decreased intravascular colloid osmotic pressure secondary to hemodilution and destruction of serum proteins may occur promoting loss of intravascular fluid to the extravascular tissues.[5]

A second etiology of increased fluid translocation leading to possible hypovolemia is increased permeability associated with cardiopulmonary bypass and deep hypothermia. Complement activation leading to a total-body inflammatory response occurs during cardiopulmonary bypass.[54–57] Vascular permeability increases and leukocytes aggregate resulting in pulmonary sequestration and contributing to pulmonary dysfunction.[58] This phenomenon has been referred to as the "postpump syndrome."

Recent reports also have indicated a possible link

between increased capillary permeability leading to loss of intravascular fluid and leukotrienes.[64] Leukotrienes are mediators of hypersensitivity and inflammation. An increased level of leukotrienes has been identified in patients undergoing pulmonary bypass.[59]

A number of studies on the effect of desmopressin acetate (DDAVP) on postoperative cardiac surgery blood loss have been reported. Although there are reports of decreased blood loss after DDAVP, other studies show no beneficial effect.[60–63] Aprotinin, tranexamic acid, and ε-aminocaproic acid decrease surgical blood loss in adults but have not been studied extensively in children.

Cardiac Tamponade

Cardiac tamponade is an ever-present possibility in the postoperative cardiac surgery patient. It compromises diastolic filling and, therefore, cardiac output. Most frequently, cardiac tamponade is secondary to continued bleeding, but when it occurs late in the postoperative course, it may also be associated with the postcardiotomy syndrome.

The traditional "Beck triad" of low blood pressure, jugular venous distention that corresponds to elevated right atrial pressure, and muffled heart sounds[64] is present in less than 50% of cases.[65] Specific physical signs depend upon intravascular volume, rate of pericardial fluid accumulation, and intrapericardial tension.[66] Other findings that may be helpful in diagnosing cardiac tamponade are widening of the mediastinum on the chest radiograph, significant pericardial fluid by echocardiography, and sudden cessation of chest tube bleeding, with increased filling pressures and hypotension. A decrease in surface ECG electrode voltage and pulsus paradoxus may also be present. If one can compare intrapericardial pressure with atrial pressure, tamponade is unlikely if intrapericardial pressure is equal to or less than atrial pressure. If it is higher than atrial pressure, tamponade or chest tube clotting has occurred.[67]

When tamponade compromises cardiovascular stability, drainage is mandatory. Until this can be accomplished, however, certain therapeutic interventions should be undertaken to support the patient. Ventricular filling pressures, heart rate, and ejection fraction must be maintained. Maintenance of adequate preload with volume loading, therefore, is important. The use of β agonists to maintain heart rate and contractility may be helpful. Extreme tachycardia must be avoided, however, because it may compromise the time for diastolic filling and systolic ejection. α Agonists may be harmful because of the depressant effects of increased afterload on myocardial contractility in this condition.

Another etiology of cardiac tamponade, the postpericardiotomy syndrome, is well recognized.[68,69,71] The postpericardiotomy syndrome occurs after opening the pericardium even when cardiopulmonary bypass is not used. Characteristically, it occurs from a few days to 1–2 weeks after pericardiotomy.[68] Fever, chest pain, pericardial friction rubs, pericardial effusions, and pleural effusions may be present. The white blood cell count may be normal or elevated. Antiheart antibodies as well as viral titers are increased.[72] In most patients, the syndrome responds quickly to treatment with anti-inflammatory agents and corticosteroids. Occasionally, however, patients may develop all of the signs and symptoms of cardiac tamponade and require pericardial drainage.

Pulmonary Effects on Preload

The effects of positive-pressure ventilation and PEEP upon the cardiovascular system can be complex. Cardiac output may be compromised because positive airway pressure decreases preload, alters resistances in the pulmonary and systemic circuits, and actually causes ventricular dysfunction[73] (see Chapter 24).

Preload may be compromised by the transmission of positive airway pressure to the intrapleural space. Positive intrapleural pressure is then transmitted to both the great veins and right atrium impeding venous return and, therefore, diastolic volume and filling pressure.[74–76,77] Volume augmentation and the use of intermittent mandatory ventilation offset these effects.[73,75,76,78]

Cardiovascular performance may be compromised by pleural collections of air. A tension pneumothorax decreases venous return and right heart filling. If severe, it will compromise ventilation leading to hypercarbia and hypoxemia, which may further compromise myocardial function. Examination usually reveals decreased or distant breath sounds and a hyperresonant percussion note on the affected side. Heart sounds and the trachea may be shifted toward the opposite side. Neck vein distention secondary to obstruction of venous return may also be present. If there is time to obtain a chest radiograph, this is the most reliable method of establishing the diagnosis. It will usually show collapse of the lung and possibly depression of the hemidiaphragm on the affected side. Shift of the heart and mediastinum toward the opposite side is common. If the patient is rapidly deteriorating, a large-bore needle attached to a syringe and stopcock is used to evacuate the air immediately. Relief of tension is followed by insertion of a chest tube, placing it to water seal, and applying 10–20 cm H_2O negative pressure.

INCREASED AFTERLOAD

Afterload is related to ventricular wall tension during systole.[40] Impedance to systolic ejection increases as afterload increases. Resistances across the pulmonary and systemic circulatory beds and obstructive valvular and subvalvular lesions may all contribute to this phenomenon. In the compromised heart, end-systolic volumes increase and stroke volume or cardiac output decreases (Fig 23–5). As Figure 23–5 illustrates, a severely compromised myocardium is more greatly affected by increased afterload.

Pulmonary Etiologies

The importance of right ventricular function to overall cardiac performance has recently been reemphasized.[79–81] Therefore, changes that increase the afterload of the right ventricle must be considered when assessing myocardial dysfunction and low cardiac output in the postoperative cardiac patient.

Any number of factors may increase pulmonary vascular resistance, which, in turn, increases right ventricular afterload (Table 23–2). Many congenital heart defects may be associated with pulmonary vascular changes and increased pulmonary resistance.[81–83] Both increased pulmonary blood flow and chronic hypoxemia associated with congenital heart lesions are associated with vascular changes and pulmonary hypertension (see Chapter 18).

Afterload may also be altered by positive airway pressures and contribute to impairment of right ventricular function. Increasing lung volumes secondary to positive pressure may compress pulmonary vessels impeding pulmonary blood flow. Thus, right ventricular afterload increases.[73–75] Normally, under these circumstances, right ventricular contractility increases to maintain stroke volume. If the myocardium is unable to increase its contractility, assuming preload is optimal, right ventricular failure will occur.

Increases in pulmonary vascular resistance severe enough to compromise right ventricular function occur secondary to hypoxemia, hypercarbia, and metabolic acidosis.[84,85] These conditions perpetuate decreased cardiac output because the longer they exist, the more severe each becomes.

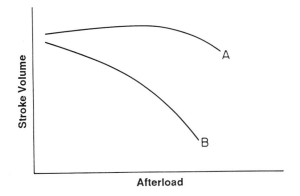

Figure 23–5. A diagrammatic representation of relationship between increasing afterload and stroke volume in normal and depressed myocardium. Curve A, normal myocardium; B, depressed myocardium.

TABLE 23–2. FACTORS ALTERING PULMONARY VASCULAR RESISTANCE

Increase	Decrease
Hypoxia	Oxygen
Hypercarbia	Hypocarbia
Acidosis	Alkalosis
Sympathetic stimulation	Tolazoline
Increased pulmonary blood flow*	Nitroprusside
Elevated airway pressure	Nitroglycerin
Pulmonary emboli	Prostaglandin E₁
Hypothermia	Isoproterenol
	Dobutamine

* Effect greater over time due to alteration in vascular wall.

Pulmonary vascular obstruction secondary to embolic phenomena may also occur in the postoperative cardiac patient. Several pathophysiologic processes contribute to increases in pulmonary vascular resistance after pulmonary embolization. Hemodynamically, emboli reduce the size of the pulmonary vascular bed. Ventilation-perfusion mismatch leads to hypoxemia. Vasoconstriction secondary to arteriolar reflexes or release of serotonin from platelet or other vasoactive substances occurs.[86] Stresses such as pain and airway irritation that stimulate the sympathetic nervous system also can increase right ventricular afterload because both pulmonary vascular resistance and pulmonary artery pressure are increased.

Left ventricular function can also be compromised by positive airway pressure and increased pulmonary vascular resistances.[73,77,87] Increased right ventricular afterload increases right ventricular volume and pressure shifting the interventricular septum toward the left ventricle. Left ventricular pressure increases and volume decreases leading to a decreased left ventricular output demonstrating ventricular interdependence.[73,77,87]

A second mechanism, mechanical interference occurring with positive-pressure ventilation, decreases ventricular output.[73,87] With increasing lung volumes, the pericardium may be stretched and the heart compressed. This decreases ventricular compliance, which increases end-diastolic pressures within the heart at decreased end-diastolic volumes. Under such circumstances of decreased compliance, elevated end-diastolic pressure associated with decreased output would give the impression of a failing myocardium. In actuality, the problem is end-diastolic tamponade.[87] Treatment under these circumstances is volume augmentation and possibly decreasing mean airway pressure rather than inotropic support.

Increased Systemic Resistance

Multiple factors in the postoperative cardiac patient increase systemic vascular resistance and, in turn, left ventricular afterload. Low cardiac output, acidosis, stress,

hypothermia, and inotropic agents are examples. In the normal heart, increases in afterload result in a compensatory increase in contractility to maintain stroke volume. In the diseased or compromised heart, compensation is limited and stroke volume tends to decrease (see Fig 23–5).[88]

Increased viscosity of blood increases afterload. Polycythemia can persist into the postoperative period, particularly after palliative procedures for cyanotic heart disease such as the creation of systemic to pulmonary shunts.

Residual Obstructive Lesions

A residual defect after repair of a congenital heart lesion is a possible factor contributing to low cardiac output. Residual outflow tract obstruction or ventricular septal defect may occur after tetralogy of Fallot repair. Valve abnormalities in aortic stenosis, pulmonic stenosis, and mitral stenosis are additional examples.[89–91] Baffle obstruction of the superior vena cava or pulmonary veins has been observed after a Mustard repair for transposition of the great vessels as well.[92]

Diagnosis of Low Cardiac Output Syndrome

The development of sophisticated monitoring modalities to assess cardiovascular function has contributed to increased success in the care of the patient with congenital heart disease. Both invasive and noninvasive modalities are used to assess the status of postoperative cardiac patients.

Physical and Clinical Indicators. In the array of sophisticated monitoring, the information that may be obtained by simple observation is often relegated to a minor role today. This is unfortunate because physical examination is quite helpful in evaluating cardiac output.

A conscious patient with poor perfusion appears restless and confused. If uncorrected, the level of consciousness decreases. Peripheral vasoconstriction develops secondary to a compensatory increase in systemic vascular resistance resulting in a mottled appearance of the skin and delayed capillary refill. Peripheral pulse volume is diminished. If skin temperature is monitored, it will be decreased. The temperature gradient between the skin and environment has been used to assess perfusion adequacy.[93–95] Usually great toe skin temperature is halfway between body core and environmental temperatures. With significant decreases in peripheral perfusion, the toe to environmental temperature gradient is less than 2°C. When this gradient approaches 0.5°C, shock can be life threatening.[94] Hennings and co-workers report that great toe temperature is a more reliable predictor of survival or mortality in shock states than either blood pressure or cardiac output in the adult patient.[93] Meskhishvili and associates showed that in infants and small babies after open-heart surgery, cardiac index and the temperature of the big toe correlated well.[95] In their studies, Hennings and co-workers concluded that the cardiac index and normalization of skin temperature in the first 6 hours postoperatively are significant variables for postoperative hemodynamic recovery.[96] Despite favorable reports of core-peripheral temperature gradients being a useful indicator of cardiovascular stability, Woods and co-workers could not demonstrate a consistent correlation between such gradients and the cardiac index or systemic vascular resistance in patients in shock.[96]

Although pulse rate and blood pressure are important in assessing cardiovascular stability, they may be misleading in low cardiac output states. If the cardiovascular system is responsive, the pulse often increases in response to a low cardiac output. However, this is not the case if low cardiac output is secondary to sinus bradycardia resulting from sinoatrial (SA) node dysfunction or AV block. Blood pressure alone may or may not reflect adequacy of myocardial function. Because blood pressure is the product of cardiac output and systemic vascular resistance, both must be assessed to make a definite decision concerning the relationship of blood pressure to adequacy of perfusion. An elevated or normal pressure does not ensure adequate perfusion.

Under normal circumstances, urinary output reflects the adequacy of volume status and perfusion. In children, 1 mL/kg/h of urine is acceptable. Urine volume may be used to monitor perfusion only when high-output renal failure, the diuretic phase of acute tubular necrosis, and osmotic diuresis have been ruled out. Therefore, not only urine volume but urinary content must be considered as indicators of adequate perfusion.

Metabolic Indicators. Low cardiac output states, like other forms of shock, inadequately supply vital substrates to tissues leading to anaerobic metabolism and increasing metabolic acidosis. Measurement of arterial blood gases reveals increasing base deficits and decreasing serum bicarbonate levels. The pH may be low or normal depending upon the degree of respiratory compensation.

Measuring lactate concentration is also useful in low perfusion states.[97,98] Michael and Weil reported that an increase in arterial lactate from 2 to 8 mm/L, remaining near 8 mm/L for more than 2 hours, decreased survival rates from 90 to 10% in patients with acute perfusion failure.[97] They also reported that pulmonary artery and central venous lactate levels correlated well with arterial levels under conditions of shock in critically ill patients. Vincent and colleagues also reported poor survival in patients in shock who had sustained elevations of arterial lactate levels after volume resuscitation, and they recommended that other forms of therapy be instituted if lactate levels do not decrease by 10% or more within 1 hour after treatment has begun.[98]

Mixed Venous Oxygen Tensions and Saturations. In low perfusion states, mixed venous oxygen tensions and saturations are reduced because of greater oxygen extraction from blood at the tissue level. Controversy exists in the literature concerning their usefulness as indicators of adequate cardiac function. Several investigators suggest that mixed venous oxygen saturations reflect either changes in cardiac output[99] or early signs of hemodynamic instability.[100–102] Others have found inconsistent or no correlation between mixed venous oxygen saturation and cardiac output.[101,102] In pediatric cardiac patients postoperatively, Parr and colleagues[103] reported cardiac death was associated with low mixed venous oxygen tensions but that death was better predicted by the combination of cardiac index and mixed venous oxygen tension. Mixed venous oxygen tensions greater than 30 mm Hg and a cardiac index over 2 L/m^2/min in postoperative pediatric cardiac patients are recommended.

Although venous oxygen tensions and saturations can be used as trend monitors for hemodynamic instability in postoperative cardiac patients, they cannot replace direct measurements of cardiac output.[104] When oxygen utilization at the tissue level is impaired, as in cyanide toxicity and septic shock, mixed venous oxygen tensions and saturations cannot be used as indicators of perfusion.

Central Venous and Pulmonary Artery Catheters. Central venous pressure (CVP) measurements are estimates of right ventricular filling pressure.[105] To be accurate, the catheter must be located in the right atrium. In patients with normal cardiac and pulmonary function, CVP correlates with pulmonary capillary wedge (PWP) pressures. Mangano[106] found good correlation between the CVP and PWP, with the CVP predicting normality or abnormality in the pulmonary capillary wedge pressure 96% of the time in adult patients with ejection fractions of 0.5 or greater and no dyssynergy of the left ventricle. In patients with ejection fractions less than 0.4 or in those with ventricular dyssynergy, CVP measurements did not predict changes in left ventricular function. It must be also noted that CVP values do not necessarily correspond to left ventricular filling pressure numerically even in the patient with a normal heart.[107] In pediatric cardiac patients postoperatively, CVP measurements may be used to estimate left-sided filling pressures as well as to guide volume therapy when significant disparity in function of the right and left ventricles is absent.

Pulmonary artery catheters are used to measure pulmonary artery pressures and pulmonary capillary wedge pressures, to determine cardiac output by thermodilution, to help derive values for pulmonary or systemic vascular resistance, oxygen consumption, and shunting, and for cardiac pacing in selected patients with congenital heart disease.

Normally, the PWP at end expiration is a measurement of left ventricular end-diastolic pressure (LVEDP) in the absence of mitral valve dysfunction.[108] The terms *pulmonary diastolic pressure* (PAD) and *PWP* are often used interchangeably, but if the pulmonary artery diastolic pressure is 5 mm Hg or more greater than PWP, as in pulmonary hypertension, they should not be used synonymously.[109] Table 23–3 is a useful guide for interpretation of values obtained from the pulmonary artery catheter.

Cardiac Output and Derived Values. Cardiac output measurement is a useful clinical monitor of cardiovascular function. It may be obtained by either thermodilution or dye dilution techniques at the bedside. Other indices of cardiovascular function may be obtained from the cardiac output values (see Chapter 8).

Echocardiography. Echocardiography, as discussed in Chapter 6, can be used to assess structure and function of the heart as well as to follow the results of therapeutic intervention at the patient's bedside postoperatively.[110,111] Doppler echocardiography can be used to determine cardiac output in a noninvasive or semi-invasive manner (see Chapter 8).

Management of Low Cardiac Output

As demonstrated in Fig 23–1, cardiac output is determined by the interaction of heart rate, preload, afterload, and contractility. Manipulation of these variables by volume addition, pharmacologic interventions, and electromechanical supportive devices to optimize cardiovascular function is often necessary in the postoperative patient.

Heart Rate Manipulation. Significant changes in heart rate may compromise cardiac performance. Bradycardia requires treatment only if it significantly affects hemodynamics, leading to hypotension and low cardiac output, or if accompanied by electrical instability (such as ectopic ventricular depolarization, which might lead to more dangerous ventricular arrhythmias).

Atropine, 10–20 μg/kg, may be used to treat brady-

cardia. If atropine is ineffective, isoproterenol, 0.05–0.1 μg/kg/min, is usually effective. A potential hazard of increasing heart rate excessively is the increase in myocardial oxygen demands that could lead to myocardial ischemia.[112–114] Excessive increases in heart rate may also be detrimental to diastolic filling, which may be arrhythmogenic, especially in an environment of hypoxemia, hypercarbia, or acidosis associated with low cardiac output.

Preload Manipulation. Cardiac output cannot be maximal without adequate preload. Optimal preload can be estimated by monitoring filling pressures and cardiac output or blood pressure during volume expansion. Left atrial pressure, pulmonary capillary wedge pressure, or, under certain circumstances, pulmonary artery diastolic pressures or right atrial pressures (CVP) may be used to determine preload. With volume expansion, if filling pressures increase with no improvement or decrease in blood pressure and/or cardiac output, preload augmentation is probably optimal (see Fig 23–3). When this occurs, another treatment modality such as inotropic support, afterload reduction, or mechanical support with balloon augmentation is indicated. Optimal preload varies from patient to patient because of differences in myocardial compliance.

Several different fluids may be used to provide adequate preload. If the patient is hypovolemic secondary to blood loss with decreased hemoglobin or hematocrit, blood replacement is a logical choice. If preload is reduced and hemoglobin or hematocrit are at acceptable levels, then other fluids such as colloids (fresh frozen plasma, albumin, or hydroxyethyl starch) or crystalloids (balanced salt solutions) or combinations of the two are appropriate. Each fluid has its advocates and detractors.

Those favoring colloid or combination therapy point out the importance of maintaining colloidal osmotic pressure in maintaining adequate plasma volume, maintenance of satisfactory cardiac function indices with small volumes of fluid, and minimizing fluid in extravascular spaces after resuscitation.[115–119] One disadvantage of colloid or combination therapy occurs in patients with increased permeability of pulmonary-capillary membranes. In this situation, the membrane leak may be intensified by colloid therapy leading to deterioration of pulmonary function.[119,120]

The advantages of using balanced salt solutions in low output or hypovolemic states after trauma, surgery, or hemorrhage also have their advocates.[121–124] Some report the importance of replenishing both intravascular and interstitial fluid space losses.[121–124] Balanced salt solutions have a composition similar to these losses. In acute hemorrhagic shock, decreases in extracellular fluid volume can be significant and balanced salt solutions of value when given with blood.[124]

TABLE 23–3. PRESSURE ALTERATIONS IN CARDIOPULMONARY DYSFUNCTION

Defect	RAP	PAP	PADP	PAOP
Pulmonary vascular resistance increase	I	I	I	N–D
Right ventricular failure	I	N–D	N–D	N–D
Cardiogenic shock	I	I	I	I
Hypovolemic shock	D	D	D	D
Cardiac tamponade	I	I	I	I

Abbreviations: RAP, right atrial pressure; PAP, mean pulmonary artery pressure; PADP, pulmonary diastolic pressure; PAOP, pulmonary artery occlusion pressure (wedge pressure); I, increased; D, decreased; N, no change.

The rational selection of fluid for augmentation of preload can only be made after evaluation of the physiologic processes occurring in each patient, what fluids have been lost, and the expected effects of the fluid administration on the physiologic compensatory mechanisms of the patient.

Manipulation of Contractility. When preload is optimal and cardiac output, perfusion, or blood pressure remain suboptimal, additional cardiovascular support such as inotropic agents, mechanical support, afterload reduction, or a combination of these modalities will be required.

Pharmacologic Manipulation of Contractility

Dopamine. A naturally occurring endogenous catecholamine, dopamine has both dopaminergic effects, which may augment renal function, and β-adrenergic effects, which increase contractility with less chronotropic or arrhythmogenic side effects than isoproterenol or epinephrine. The cardiovascular effects vary according to the dosage. At low dosages ($\leq 5\mu$g/kg/min) dopamine stimulates dopaminergic receptors, causing vasodilation in splanchnic, renal, coronary, and cerebral vascular beds.[125] This is suggested as the explanation for increased renal blood flow, glomerular filtration rate, and sodium excretion at low doses of dopamine.[126] This effect is not antagonized by either α or β antagonists but is attenuated by haloperidol and phenothiazines.[125] The inotropic effects of dopamine are due to β_1 receptor–agonist action, which is both direct and indirect at doses of 5–10 μg/kg/min. Indirect activity results from stimulation of catecholamine release in the myocardium.[125] In dosages between 10 and 20 μg/kg/min, a mixture of β and α effects are present, and almost complete α effects are present with dosages greater than 20 μg/kg/min.[125,127] These α effects lead to widespread vasoconstriction and increases in systemic vascular resistance. In cyanotic lambs with chronic hypoxemia due to intracardiac right-to-left shunt, the hemodynamic effects of dopamine (5–20 μg/kg/min) were similar to acyanotic animals.[128] Usual doses are 2–20 μg/kg/min.

However, differences in the effects of dopamine in infants and children have been reported.[130–134] Guller and co-workers[129] showed an increased incidence of arrhythmias in children aged 2–15 years at dopamine dosages greater than 10 μg/kg/min. Although not all patients developed arrhythmias at higher dosages, dopamine should be used with caution at dosages between 10 and 20 μg/kg/min in children. Miall-Allen[130] demonstrated inadequate response of mean arterial pressure in hypotensive preterm neonates to 5 μg/kg/min compared with 10 μg/kg/min of dopamine, and they recommended starting at 10 μg/kg/min in these patients. Dopamine

may be a less effective inotrope if stress has depleted endogenous catecholamine stores in the pediatric patient.

Several animal studies noted less response to exogenous catecholamines, decreased catecholamine levels, β receptor affinity, and density in the myocardium of fetal and neonatal animals.[131,132,133,134] Voelkel and co-workers[135] demonstrated decreased density of β receptors, decreased adenylate cyclase activity in myocardium, and a decreased response to isoproterenol after chronic hypoxemia in an animal model. The importance of these observations in animal models to human neonates and pediatric patients is incompletely known. In postoperative cardiac patients under 2 years of age with low cardiac output, higher doses of dopamine than needed in adults were required to increase cardiac output.[136]

One possible adverse effect of dopamine in the pediatric cardiac patients is the tendency to increase pulmonary vascular resistance.[137,138] This could increase afterload on the right ventricle contributing to decreased contractility and cardiac output. Other investigators noted decreased pulmonary vascular resistance with dopamine.[139]

Dobutamine. Dobutamine is a synthetic catecholamine with a structure similar to isoproterenol. Its direct β_1-adrenergic agonist effect on the myocardium increases myocardial contractility with minimal peripheral vascular effects.[140] Dobutamine has less chronotropic effect than isoproterenol, does not stimulate the release of endogenous catecholamines, and has no dopaminergic effects.[140,141] Multiple reports suggest a superiority of dobutamine over dopamine for treatment of myocardial failure, increasing cardiac output or index with less effect upon heart rate, systemic vascular resistance, and pulmonary vascular resistance.[139,141–143] Dobutamine decreases pulmonary vascular resistance in low cardiac output states and attenuates hypoxic pulmonary vasoconstriction.[127,129,138–141] Dobutamine augments coronary artery blood flow.[144]

In pediatric patients with cardiac failure, dobutamine augments cardiac output and decreases wedge pressure and systemic resistance.[145,146] Heart rate increases in pediatric cardiac patients.[146] The usual dose of dobutamine is 1–10 μg/kg/min.

Epinephrine. Epinephrine is a naturally occurring catecholamine with both α- and β-adrenergic effects. It stimulates both β_1 and β_2 receptors. The β_1 effects increase myocardial contractility, accelerate the sinoatrial node, and increase conductivity through atrioventricular node and Purkinje system.[127] Epinephrine decreases the ventricular muscle refractory period.[127] These effects increase cardiac output, heart rate, and dysrhythmias. Although epinephrine dilates the coronary arteries, oxygen demand, which is increased both by increased rate and augmentation of contractility, may outstrip supply. The β_2 effects on peripheral vasculature promote vasodilation, especially in muscle vasculature.[147] At low dosages (<0.02 μg/kg/min), the β_2 effects decrease systemic vascular resistance and blood pressure despite increased myocardial contractility. The β_2 receptor stimulation also promotes relaxation of bronchial smooth muscle and inhibits mast cell degranulation and release of histamine.[148] The β_2 activity stimulates renin release in the kidney.[149]

The α effects of epinephrine on the peripheral vasculature predominate at all but minimal dosages.[127,147] Both systemic vascular resistance and venous resistance increase. The increased blood pressure increases left ventricular afterload and may actually decrease peripheral perfusion. Renal perfusion decreases because of renal vascular constriction decreasing the excretion of sodium and chloride.[150] Increased venous resistance decreases venous capacitance and promotes venous return to the heart.

Epinephrine has significant metabolic effects. These include stimulation of lipolysis, glycogenolysis, gluconeogenesis, and ketone production. Combined with inhibition of insulin release, these effects increase plasma levels of glucose, free fatty acids, lactate, and β-hydroxybutyrate.[151]

The effects of epinephrine are complex. When used as an inotropic agent at low dosages, it will increase myocardial contractility and decrease systemic vascular resistance through its β_1 and β_2 effects. Heart rate and systolic pressure increase and diastolic pressure decreases with epinephrine infusions, thereby widening pulse pressures at dosages of 0.02 μg/kg/min or less. As dosage increases, diastolic pressures also increase. At higher dosages, it continues to stimulate the myocardium but the α-adrenergic effects predominate in the peripheral vasculature increasing systemic vascular resistance. As systemic vascular resistance increases, afterload increases, and this effect may require blocking with a vasodilator.[152] Epinephrine, therefore, has both beneficial and harmful effects in low cardiac output syndrome. The usual dosage range for continuous infusion of epinephrine is 0.05–1.0 μg/kg/min.

Norepinephrine. Like epinephrine, norepinephrine is a naturally occurring catecholamine. Though mainly regarded for its α-adrenergic effects on peripheral vasculature, norepinephrine also has β_1-adrenergic effects in the heart.[127] Infusion of norepinephrine increases systemic vascular resistance and systolic, diastolic, and mean arterial pressures. Heart rate usually decreases secondary to baroreceptor stimulation, and cardiac output is unchanged or decreased.[127] Norepinephrine constricts the venous side of the circulation like epinephrine, decreasing venous capacitance and increasing venous return or preload. With increased preload, contractility, and afterload, myocardial work and oxygen demand increase.

Norepinephrine significantly constricts renal and splanchnic vascular beds decreasing renal, hepatic and intestinal blood flow, which may compromise function of these organs.[147] Pulmonary vasoconstriction is also reported to occur with norepinephrine, which increases pulmonary vascular resistance and right ventricular afterload. Thus, norepinephrine is relatively contraindicated in patients with pulmonary hypertension or decreased right ventricular function.

Several investigators have reported improved cardiovascular performance using norepinephrine in combination with vasodilator agents such as phentolamine or nitroprusside in patients with low cardiac output.[153,154] The vasodilators appear to attenuate the α-adrenergic effects of norepinephrine. Increases in pulmonary vascular resistances secondary to norepinephrine also were attenuated by phentolamine.[155] An increased heart rate with the combination of norepinephrine and vasodilators could be detrimental in patients with ischemic heart disease.[153]

Usual infusions of norepinephrine are 0.05–1.0 μg/kg/min. When used in combination with phentolamine, a 1.0:2.5 ratio of norepinephrine to phentolamine is effective in low cardiac output.

Isoproterenol. Isoproterenol is a synthetic catecholamine with β_1- and β_2-adrenergic effects. When administered by infusion in doses of 0.05–0.5 μg/kg/min, it increases myocardial contractility, heart rate, and cardiac output if preload is adequate.[127] The β_2-adrenergic effect on the peripheral vasculature decreases systemic vascular resistance, so blood pressure may not increase. Although it may cause dysrhythmias, isoproterenol stimulates intrinsic pacemakers in bradydysrhythmias or complete heart block.

Two effects of isoproterenol may alter the myocardial oxygen demand and supply relationship: (1) increased heart rate and contractility increase oxygen demand, and (2) peripheral dilatation decreases diastolic pressure, which may compromise coronary blood flow.[156] Isoproterenol, therefore, is not ideal in patients with ischemic heart disease. It might be of benefit, however, in patients without ischemic heart disease (eg, congenital heart disease) because it decreases afterload in both the systemic and pulmonary circulations. Isoproterenol not only relaxes bronchial smooth muscle, a β_2-adrenergic effect, but causes pulmonary artery vasodilation.[138] In patients with pulmonary disease, it attenuates hypoxic pulmonary vasoconstriction and increases intrapulmonary shunting.[127]

Calcium. Calcium is essential for the normal function of electrophysiologic and contractile processes of the heart.

In the plasma, calcium exists in three forms: (1) bound to plasma protein, (2) freely soluble but un-ionized, and (3) ionized and unbound. It is the ionized form that is the most biologically active.[157]

Calcium has significant inotropic effects, but the concentration of serum ionized calcium prior to administration of calcium influences the magnitude of its inotropic effects. Drop and Scheidegger demonstrated a greater inotropic response when correcting hypocalcemia to normocalcemia than when changing normocalcemia to hypercalcemia.[158] Calcium infusion acutely increasing ionized calcium may promote bradycardia or progress to significant ventricular arrhythmias.[159] Calcium also enhances the effects of cardiac glycosides. Therefore, calcium should be administered cautiously to a digitalized patient.[157] An acute increase in ionized calcium causes vasoconstriction in the coronary, systemic, and cerebral vasculature.[160] The increased resistance in coronary and systemic vascular beds may decrease the oxygen supply to the myocardium and increase left ventricular afterload.

When used as an inotropic agent, calcium in the ionized form is the most effective. Calcium chloride consistently increases plasma ionized calcium concentrations.[161] Many investigators, therefore, advocate that the chloride salt of calcium be used when treating low cardiac output states. The usual recommended dose of calcium chloride in low cardiac output in infants and children is 10–20 mg/kg slowly into a central vein. Comparing calcium chloride and gluconate, Coté et al demonstrated that equivalent doses of elemental calcium resulted in equivalent changes in ionized calcium levels and hemodynamic effects.[162] The dose of calcium gluconate is three times the chloride dose on a weight basis, but it can be administered via peripheral veins.

Amrinone. Although not specifically approved for use in children, amrinone may prove beneficial in postoperative pediatric patients. It is a nonadrenergic, nonglycoside drug with both positive inotropic and peripheral vasodilating effects. It is thought to exert its pharmacologic actions by phosphodiesterase inhibition leading to an increase in cyclic adenosine monophosphate (AMP).[163] Amrinone compares favorably with dobutamine and dopamine in the treatment of adult patients with congestive heart failure.[164]

Amrinone has proven effective in treating low cardiac output after cardiac surgery.[165] Concern regarding its use in infants has occurred secondary to findings of negative inotropic effects on neonatal animal myocardium.[166] After studying amrinone pharmacokinetics in neonates and infants after postcardiac surgery, Lawless et al concluded that higher initial bolus doses were required on a body weight basis in these patients compared with adults.[167] They demonstrated a significant difference in half-life (longer in neonates) and clearance (lower in neonates) between neonates and infants. There was no difference in the volume of distribution. Thrombocytopenia has occurred with amrinone therapy.[168] The recommended amrinone dose schedule is an initial bolus of 0.5–0.75 mg/kg followed by an infusion of 5–10 μg/kg/min and not to exceed 10 mg/kg in 24 hours.

Mechanical Manipulation of Contractility. There is a subgroup of patients in whom cardiac output from left ventricular dysfunction persists despite optimum therapy with preload augmentation, inotropic agents, and afterload manipulation. These patients often benefit from a transplant, or they can be supported until transplantation, for example, with mechanical assist devices.

Intra-aortic Balloon Counterpulsation (IABC). This was one of the first mechanical devices other than cardiopulmonary bypass used to assist the failing myocardium.[169] This device decreases myocardial oxygen requirements, reduces left ventricular work, and increases coronary blood flow[169,170] (see Chapter 10).

The balloon is usually placed via the femoral artery and positioned with the tip just distal to the left subclavian artery. By timing balloon inflation and deflation correctly, diastolic coronary filling and reduction of impedance to systolic ejection are obtained. Balloon inflation is timed to occur immediately after closure of the aortic valve. Closure of the aortic valve is represented by the dicrotic notch of the arterial pressure waveform. If a radial arterial pulse wave is being monitored, inflation is set to occur just prior to the dicrotic notch. This timing is required because there is a delay of approximately 50 milliseconds in adults between aortic valve closure centrally and the dicrotic notch on a peripheral arterial waveform. Correct timing of inflation occurs when the diastolic augmentation peak is maximal.[171]

Timing of balloon deflation must be correct to allow unobstructed ventricular ejection. Correct timing of deflation occurs when the end-diastolic dip is 10–15 mm Hg below the level of the unaugmented diastolic pressure and the systolic peak following an augmented beat, compared with the systolic pressure of an unaugmented beat, is maximally reduced.

Though balloon augmentation in adults is common, its use in pediatric patients has been somewhat limited because of technical problems.[172] Among these are size restraints. In infants and small children, even the deflated balloon occupies too much of the aortic lumen and fails to decrease aortic impedance to systolic ejection. At very rapid spontaneous heart rates, at times it is difficult to set timing intervals for inflation and deflation of the intra-aortic balloon. When the ratio of augmentation to nonaugmentation is lengthened (eg, going from 1:1 to 1:2) in an attempt to correct this problem, augmentation is insufficient to be of benefit. The successful use of IABC has been reported in children 5 years of age or older using balloons of 4 and 12 mL on nos. 7 and 9 French catheter.[173] Veasy et al, using 2.5- or 5.0-mL balloons on a no. 5 French catheter, obtained cardiovascular improvement in four of five infants with postoperatively low cardiac output.[174] (see also Chapter 10).

Weaning from IABC begins when left ventricular function improves and the need for inotropic support decreases.[169,171] Assistance is gradually reduced by increasing the ratio of augmentation to nonaugmentation. When the patient maintains adequate cardiovascular parameters for 6–12 hours at a ratio of 1:8, the device is removed.[169,171]

Multiple complications have been reported with the use of IABC.[169,171,175] These include ischemia in extremities distal to the site of balloon insertion, vessel perforation, thrombosis, emboli formation, thrombocytopenia, and wound infection at the insertion site.

Extracorporeal Membrane Oxygenation (ECMO).

Since Baffles et al[176] reported the use of ECMO for support in congenital heart disease in 1970, ECMO and ventricular assist devices have been used for pediatric cardiovascular failure.[177–182] The goals of ECMO in low cardiac output states are to (1) maintain adequate tissue perfusion, (2) minimize myocardial energy expenditure, (3) maximize potential functional cardiac recovery, and, in some cases (4) act as a bridge to transplantation. Success rates of this mode of therapy have varied among different institutions, but most agree that ECMO improves survival rates in pediatric patients with low cardiac output syndromes and severe pulmonary hypertension[176–182] (see Chapter 10).

Afterload Manipulation.

Low cardiac output states compromising perfusion cause compensatory increases in sympathetic activity and vasoconstriction that increase afterload. The increased afterload and vasoconstriction secondary to myocardial failure is controlled by vasodilating agents.

In the acute setting, agents used for afterload reduction ideally should have a rapid onset of action, a short duration of action, and be easily controlled. Four agents meeting these criteria are nitroprusside, phentolamine, trimethaphan, and nitroglycerin. Other agents with longer durations of action that are unsuitable for intravenous administration may be used for chronic afterload reduction.

The predominant site of action of vasodilators may be arterial, venous, or both.[183] The effect of decrease in arterial resistance on afterload is quite obvious. It may not be appreciated that dilatation of the venous side of the circulation that decreases preload can influence afterload as well. Afterload (ie, myocardial systolic wall tension) is a function of both intraventricular pressure and volume. An agent that promotes venous dilatation and, therefore, decreases preload may lower ventricular

volume, which diminishes afterload without affecting systemic vascular resistance.[183] In hypotensive patients, vasodilator therapy should be used with the utmost caution and complete hemodynamic monitoring. Often a combination of a positive inotropic drugs and vasodilator is optimum.[153,154,183]

Sodium Nitroprusside.

Sodium nitroprusside dilates both arterial resistance and venous capacitance vessels.[184] The onset of action is rapid (within seconds) and the duration of effect is short (1–3 minutes).[184] When administered by continuous infusion in doses of 0.5–1.0 μg/kg/min, precise control of its hemodynamic effects is possible.

Cardiovascular effects of nitroprusside are the combined result of venous pooling (decreased preload) and arteriolar vasodilation (decreased afterload). Left ventricular function influences which of the vascular effects predominates.[185] With normal or near-normal left ventricular function, the effect of decreased venous capacitance appears to be more important than impedance reduction. Decreased preload under these circumstances causes either little change or a decrease in cardiac output, which may require volume augmentation. When left ventricular impairment is present, afterload reduction predominates, improving myocardial function and cardiac output.[185]

Nitroprusside favorably influences oxygen demand in the failing heart by both preload and afterload reduction. Ventricular volume, filling pressure, and wall tension are reduced. Because of improvement in function[184] and possibly alteration in baroreceptor activity,[186] increases in heart rate occur less frequently when nitroprusside is administered in heart failure compared with the normal heart.[184,185] Concern in regard to nitroprusside's effects upon myocardial blood supply has been raised. Nitroprusside may divert blood away from ischemic areas of the myocardium in coronary artery insufficiency.[187] Other investigators failed to show this effect in studies of regional myocardial perfusion.[188] Because coronary insufficiency is unlikely in the pediatric population, these concerns are unimportant in the patient with most congenital heart defects. Nitroprusside may have both beneficial and adverse effects on the pulmonary circulation. Because of its pulmonary vascular dilating effects, it reduces the afterload of the right ventricle when pulmonary hypertension is present. Like most vasodilators, however, it can attenuate hypoxic pulmonary vasoconstriction and increase intrapulmonary shunt.

In addition to inadvertent hypotension, one of the potentially most harmful side effects of nitroprusside is cyanide toxicity. Normally, cyanide from nitroprusside metabolism combines with oxyhemoglobin to form methemoglobin. Methemoglobin follows one of two pathways: (1) combination with methemoglobin to form cyanmethemoglobin, or (2) detoxification by rhodanase, an enzyme found in the liver and kidney.[189] In the presence of thiosulfate and hydroxocobalamin (vitamin B_{12}), it is converted to thiocyanate, which is excreted by the kidney. If the above pathways are unable to handle the amount of cyanide produced, cyanide toxicity occurs. Under these circumstances, cyanide accumulates in the tissues, combines with cytochrome oxidase, interferes with oxidative phosphorylation, and leads to histotoxic anoxia at the tissue level.

Early signs of cyanide toxicity include metabolic acidosis and increased mixed venous oxygen tensions. Patients may also develop neurologic dysfunction and cardiovascular collapse. Treatment consists of discontinuation of the nitroprusside infusion and administration of thiosulfate (150 mg/kg) and nitrates (sodium or amyl nitrate) to create methemoglobin, which combines with cyanide ions to form cyanmethemoglobin.[189]

The formation of cyanide ions appears to be rate limited during nitroprusside infusion. The usual recommended maximum dose of nitroprusside is 8 μg/kg/min or 0.5 mg/kg/h. Tinker and Michenfelder showed that cyanide toxicity did not occur in patients receiving this dose for up to 48 hours.[189] Thiocyanate may accumulate in patients with compromised renal function, so dosage should be reduced.[190]

Nitroglycerin. Nitroglycerin, a direct acting vasodilator, has its predominant effect on venous capacitance but also causes some arterial vasodilation.[183–185] Therefore, it can be expected to alter preload more than afterload. Usual doses of nitroglycerin are 0.25–5.0 μg/kg/min intravenously. Administration of nitroglycerin to patients with mild heart failure causes little change in cardiac output, but in severe heart failure, greater augmentation of cardiac output occurs.[191] Nitroglycerin is advantageous for ischemic myocardium because it dilates coronary arteries, improves endocardial blood supply, and reverses myocardial ischemia.[187,188,191]

Pulmonary vascular resistance is also decreased by nitroglycerin. It is beneficial in patients with pulmonary hypertension. When pulmonary congestion is a prime problem in the failing heart, nitroglycerin may be of benefit because of its predominant effect on preload and pulmonary vasculature. In this situation, nitroglycerin decreases both ventricular filling pressure and pulmonary artery pressure.[183]

Side effects of nitroglycerin include hypotension, particularly in hypovolemic patients or with large doses, which increases the degree of arterial vasodilation and methemoglobinemia.[192]

Trimethaphan. Trimethaphan is a ganglionic blocking agent dilating both arteriolar resistance and venous capacitance vessels. These effects are mediated by ganglionic blockade, direct action, and histamine release. Trimethaphan is metabolized partially by pseudocholinesterase.

Ganglionic blockade, which decreases both sympathetic and parasympathetic discharges, causes variable chronotropic effects. If tachycardia does occur, it can be attenuated by β-adrenergic blockade. Parasympathetic blockade with trimethaphan causes pupillary dilation, which may last for several hours after the drug is stopped. This can be disturbing, especially if the neurologic status of the patient is in question. Patients may also develop tachyphylaxis to the vasodilating effects of this drug. The usual dose is 2.5–30.0 μg/kg/min by continuous intravenous infusion.

Phentolamine. Phentolamine is an β-adrenergic blocking drug with a primary effect on arteriolar resistance. It reduces systemic vascular resistance and the afterload of the left ventricle, but reflex tachycardia can be a problem.[153,185] Tachycardia associated with this drug can be attenuated with β-adrenergic blocking drugs. The dose for continuous intravenous infusion is 1–2 μg/kg/min.

Hydralazine. Hydralazine is a direct-acting vasodilator with a predominant effect on arterial vascular beds. This is manifested by vasodilation in both systemic and pulmonary circulation. Hydralazine appears to have a beneficial effect on afterload in patients with decreased left ventricular function and mitral regurgitation, in whom combination preload-afterload reduction causes hypotension and the need for repeated preload augmentation.

Diastolic hypotension can be a problem with hydralazine and, coupled with reflex tachycardia, can be harmful in patients with ischemic heart disease. Rebound hypertension may occur after bolus administration of the drug. After chronic administration of hydralazine, salt and water retention may become a problem requiring the use of diuretics.[185] Tolerance unresponsive to increased dose or intravenous administration occurs in 30% of adult patients.[193] A lupuslike syndrome may also occur with chronic use of the drug.[185] Doses for continuous intravenous infusion are 0.25–1.5 μg/kg/min.[194,195]

ARRHYTHMIAS

Postoperative arrhythmias result from myocardial injury, metabolic disturbances, and autonomic imbalance. Arrhythmias contributing to hemodynamic instability must be promptly recognized and treated.

Mechanisms

The mechanisms of arrhythmia formation are secondary either to disturbances in impulse formation (automaticity), conduction, or both. Alterations that disturb phase 0 or phase 4 depolarization may affect automaticity (see Fig 23–2).[196] Factors that reduce automaticity (eg, parasympathetic stimulation, digitalis, and anesthetic agents) in higher pacemaker sites favor the occurrence of pacemaker activity in lower areas of the cardiac conductive system. When automaticity is enhanced in areas other than the sinoatrial node, ectopic pacemaker activity can occur. Factors such as sympathetic stimulation, hypoxemia, and hypercarbia may contribute to enhanced automaticity.

Conduction disturbance may lead to prolongation or actual block of the passage of impulses between different areas of the heart's conductive system. They probably also account for the mechanism of reentry, which is thought to be the cause of many cardiac arrhythmias. Electrophysiologic studies of reentry reveal a phenomenon where an impulse from a common pathway divides into two separate pathways. A unidirectional block is encountered in one area. The impulse in the unblocked pathway proceeds, and meanwhile the excitability of the blocked pathway recovers and becomes stimulated by retrograde stimulation from the unblocked impulse. When reentrant phenomena become sustained, arrhythmias such as premature atrial contractions, atrial fibrillation, ventricular premature beats, and other tachyrhythmias occur.[197]

Supraventricular Arrhythmias

By definition, any arrhythmias whose impulse formation or reentry site occurs above the bundle of His bifurcation are considered supraventricular.[198]

Sinus Bradycardia. Secondary to a decreased rate of depolarization of sinus pacemaker cells, sinus bradycardia may significantly impair cardiac output because stroke volume cannot always compensate for the slower rate. ECG findings are normal configuration of P waves, QRS complexes, and T waves. PR intervals are normal and rhythm is regular. Treatment is required only if hemodynamic instability is present. Assuming primary etiologies (eg, hypoxemia, parasympathetic reflexes) have been removed, chronotropic enhancement by atropine (parasympatholytic, promoting sympathetic predominance), isoproterenol (β_1 receptor stimulation), or pacing (atrial pacing as long as AV block is absent) may correct the problem.

Sinus Tachycardia. Sinus tachycardia is significant when it compromises cardiac filling or emptying. Etiologic factors are hypoxia, hypercarbia, hypovolemia, excess sympathetic stimulation, or any factor that increases the metabolic rate. ECG findings are rapid rate with normal rhythm, normal P waves, QRS complexes, and T waves but PR and QT intervals may be shortened because both are rate dependent. Treatment of the underlying cause will usually correct the problem.

Atrial Flutter. Atrial flutter is the result of an ectopic focus in the atrium usually firing at a rate between 250 and 350.[199] P waves are identical, usually regular, and have a saw-tooth appearance on the ECG and are referred to as flutter waves. Usually only an occasional P

wave is conducted through the AV node creating different degrees of AV block (2:1, 4:1, and so on). Preceded by a number of flutter waves, QRS complexes appear normal but may be irregular. Treatment modes available are overdrive atrial pacing, cardioversion, or increasing AV block and slowing ventricular rate with digoxin, β-adrenergic blocking agents, or calcium channel blockers.

Atrial Fibrillation. When multiple ectopic foci in the atrium fire continuously, atrial fibrillation (AF) occurs.[199] Atrial rates of 300–500 are present. P waves are not discernible and the base line wanders. QRS complexes will usually be normal but irregular secondary to irregular stimulation and conduction through the AV node of atrial impulses. Treatment modalities include cardioversion, which will often restore normal sinus rhythm, particularly in recent-onset AF. The ventricular response can be controlled by the use of β-adrenergic blocking agents, calcium channel blockers, or digoxin.

Atrioventricular Junctional Rhythm. When a junctional pacemaker controls both atrial and ventricular rates, an atrioventricular junctional rhythm is present. Three forms are recognized: (1) junctional escape rhythm with a rate of 30–60/min, which occurs when diminished sinus node pacemaker activity is present; (2) accelerated junctional rhythm, which is secondary to increased automaticity producing a rate of 60–100; and (3) junctional tachycardia, producing rates greater than 100. ECG findings include P waves that precede, follow, or are hidden within the QRS complex. The QRS-T wave pattern is usually normal. Treatment is required only if bradycardia is accompanied by hemodynamic instability.

Paroxysmal Supraventricular Tachycardias. Paroxysmal supraventricular tachycardias (SVT) may be either atrial or junctional in nature. They may compromise hemodynamic stability because of interference with cardiac filling or emptying. The rate is usually between 150 and 250. P waves, if present, are abnormal but are usually lost within the preceding T wave. QRS complexes are regular. ST and T wave changes often occur. Treatment modalities include (1) maneuvers to increase vagal tone (Valsalva maneuver or carotid sinus massage); (2) a calcium channel blocker (verapamil), which may cause significant negative inotropic and chronotropic effects, however, in patients taking β-adrenergic blockers, and in children; (3) cardioversion, which will often convert this dysrhythmia; and (4) adenosine, which acts by decreasing conduction through the AV node (has not been studied in children).

Atrioventricular Heart Blocks. Delayed or complete absence of conduction of sinus node impulses to the ventricles define AV heart blocks. They are commonly classified as first-degree AV block, second-degree AV block, and complete heart block.

First-Degree AV block. First-degree AV block is present when the PR interval is prolonged but all of the sinus node impulses are conducted to the ventricle. PR intervals of greater than 0.2 seconds define first-degree heart blocks in adults. In infants and children, however, normal maximal PR intervals vary with heart rate (see Table 5–2). The ECG has normal P waves, prolonged PR interval, and normal QRS complexes. Treatment is usually not required.

Second-Degree AV Block. Second-degree AV block is characterized by an atrial rate that is faster than the ventricular rate. A certain number of the impulses from the SA node are conducted to the ventricle at regular intervals, however, at ratios of 2:1 and 3:1. This form of AV block is divided into two major types. In Mobitz I (Wenckebach) rhythm, the ECG reveals gradual lengthening of the PR interval and decreasing RR interval to the point of nonconduction of an atrial impulse to the ventricle. P waves and QRS complexes are usually normal, but ventricular rhythm will be irregular. With Mobitz II rhythm, atrial beats are conducted consecutively with constant PR intervals before a dropped beat occurs. There may also be multiple P waves per QRS complex in more advanced forms of block. P waves are usually normal, with regular atrial rhythm, but regular or irregular ventricular rhythm can occur. PR interval length may vary but will be constant. The width of the QRS complex will be determined by the location of the block. It is normal with blocks at the level of bundle of His, but widened when at bundle branch level.

Mobitz I block rarely requires treatment except with bradycardia, for which pacing may be indicated. Mobitz II blocks are more significant, for they may progress to complete heart block. Ventricular pacing is usually indicated.

Complete Heart Block. Complete heart block (CHB) is present when all atrial impulses fail to be conducted to the ventricles. ECG findings are a slow ventricular rate in the range of 30–40/min. P waves are normal, QRS complexes are widened, and no relationship between P waves and QRS complexes is present. CHB requires ventricular pacing, but the rate may be enhanced by isoproterenol until pacing can be established.

Ventricular Arrhythmias

Ventricular premature contractions (PVCs) arise from ectopic foci within the ventricular myocardium. They may be initiated by autonomic imbalance, ischemic injury, electrolyte imbalance, especially potassium depletion, and digitalis toxicity. ECG findings include absent P waves, wide QRS complexes, and ST segment direction usually opposite the QRS complex. A compensatory pause often occurs after the PVC and before the next sinus impulse (P wave). When a PVC is coupled with one normal beat, the result is bigeminy, two normal beats, trigeminy, and so on. These beats may be isolated or recur repeatedly. When PVCs should be treated is controversial. It would appear that if they are frequent (> 6/min), multifocal, occur in such a manner that the R on T phenomenon occurs, or are significantly interfering with cardiovascular function, treatment should be instituted. Treatment consists of correction of underlying causes if possible. If a specific cause is not apparent or has been corrected but PVCs are still present, lidocaine, β-adrenergic blocking agents, or other antiarrhythmic agents usually correct the problem.

Ventricular tachycardia is defined as more than three premature ventricular contractions in a row at a rate between 100 and 250. P waves are usually absent but occasionally may occur and be conducted in a retrograde manner. QRS complexes are wide and regular. Cardiac output is decreased because filling, emptying, and contractility are compromised. Treatment modalities include lidocaine, procainamide, bretylium, or β-adrenergic blocking agents. If drug therapy is unsuccessful or cardiac output is reduced, DC countershock should be used.

Impulse discharge is chaotic and no QRS complex is discernible on the ECG in ventricular fibrillation. Cardiac output is compromised because myocardial contractility is essentially nonexistent. Treatment is external cardiac massage and defibrillation with DC countershock. After defibrillation, lidocaine, procainamide, or bretylium may be used to maintain normal rhythm.

Arrhythmias Associated with Specific Anomalies

Life-threatening cardiac arrhythmias are associated with several congenital cardiac defects, including tetralogy of Fallot, transposition of the great arteries, and AV septal defects.[200]

After repair of tetralogy of Fallot, the incidence of right bundle branch block is 59%[201] and that of complete heart block is 1%.[202] An increased incidence of ventricular arrhythmias also occurs.[203,204] Sudden death has been reported in 2–3% of patients after repair of tetralogy.[202,205] The cause of sudden death may be either secondary to heart block, tachyarrhythmias, or both.[200] These conduction disturbances are thought to be secondary to injury of the conduction pathways at surgery. Other arrhythmias reported after tetralogy of Fallot repair include SA node dysfunction, AV node conduction defects, and supraventricular arrhythmias (see Chapter 14[200]).

After Mustard repairs of transposition of the great arteries, supraventricular dysrhythmias and AV conduction defects inducing complete heart block often occur.[200,206] Hypotheses offered to explain the origin of arrhythmias after Mustard repair include (1) sinus node or sinus node artery damage, [207] (2) internodal pathway interruption, [208] and (3) AV node conductive tissue damage. [206] An incidence of sudden death of 2–8% has been reported after repair of transposition of the great vessels (see Chapter 15). [209,210]

Preoperative arrhythmias are more common in children with sinus venosus atrial septal defects (ASDs) and ASDs of the secundum type. [200] Junctional and low atrial rhythms are common in sinus venosus defect. [211] Secundum defects in older patients are associated with atrial flutter or fibrillation. Increased shunting and pulmonary hypertension are coincident with preoperative arrhythmias in patients with ASDs. [212,213] Postoperatively, junctional rhythms, AV dissociation, and ectopic atrial rhythms are common, but usually self-limited, in children. [213,214]

Arrhythmias after closure of ventricular septal defects (VSDs) are similar to those associated with repair of tetralogy of Fallot. [200] Right bundle branch block is the most common but occurs less frequently if the defect is repaired via atriotomy. [215,216] Complete heart block may occur after repair of VSD. Ventricular arrhythmias occur after a ventriculotomy has been performed for VSD repair (see Chapter 13). [217]

Conduction disturbances are the most common arrhythmias after AV canal repairs. Studies of the conduction system in this defect have revealed abnormalities in placement of left bundle branches, hypoplasia of bundle fibers, and abnormal origin of left bundle fibers from the common bundle. [218] Prolongation of the PR interval on the ECG is common secondary to delayed intra-atrial activation. [219] A 29–33% incidence of complete heart block, either transient or permanent, has been reported postoperatively. [220] Intraoperative mapping of the conduction system decreases this complication (see Chapter 13).

Therapy

Antiarrhythmic Drugs. Antiarrhythmic medications have been classified according to pharmacologic effects on electrophysiologic cardiac events. [221] Class I drugs decrease depolarization rates, functioning like local anesthetics to block fast inward sodium channels. Subclasses are identified by their effects on action potential duration (APD) and effective refractory period (ERP). [222] APD is defined as the total time between depolarization and return to normal negative resting potentials. ERP is defined as the period during depolarization when a cell will not depolarize if stimulated again. Class IA drugs prolong APD and ERP. Class IB drugs shorten both APD and ERP. Class IC drugs have little effect on APD and shorten ERP. Class II drugs have β-adrenergic blocking action, class III drugs markedly prolong APD and ERP, and class IV drugs antagonize slow inward calcium cur-

rents. Some antiarrhythmic medications have mixed actions.

Class I Drugs. Procainamide is a class IA drug that prolongs APD and ERP while slowing conduction. [222] Effective for treating both ventricular and supraventricular arrhythmias, procainamide increases AV block accompanying arrhythmias secondary to digitalis toxicity. Significant hypotension secondary to vasodilation or myocardial depression can occur. If either the PR or QRS interval is prolonged 0.02 seconds or greater, intravenous administration of procainamide should be discontinued [223]; therefore, it should be administered slowly intravenously. For emergency treatment, an intravenous loading dose of 3–5 mg/kg followed by infusion of 20–80 μg/kg/min may be used. Procainamide may also be administered intramuscularly or orally. The intramuscular dose is 20–30 mg/kg/24 h and the oral dose is 15–50 mg/kg/24 h. Maximum recommended dosage for both intramuscular and oral routes per 24 hours is 4 g. Two grams is the intravenous maximum recommended dose per 24 hours. Patients on chronic procainamide therapy may develop a lupuslike syndrome.

Quinidine is a class IA antiarrhythmic medication that has actions similar to procainamide. It may be useful in the treatment of atrial and ventricular premature contractions. Because it may enhance AV nodal conduction, quinidine should be administered only after digitalization in patients with atrial flutter or fibrillation because 1:1 AV conduction may occur. It may be administered intravenously, intramuscularly, or orally. Intravenous dosage is 2–10 mg/kg every 3–6 hours, administered slowly and with ECG monitoring. Administration intravenously is no longer recommended in pediatric patients. [223] The oral dose is 30 mg/kg/24 h.

Lidocaine is a class IB drug that shortens both APD and ERP. It may decrease ERP of AV node resulting in an accelerated response of the ventricle in atrial flutter or fibrillation. [222] Lidocaine is most useful in the treatment of ventricular arrhythmias. The dosage schedule is 1 mg/kg bolus followed by an infusion of 20–50 μg/kg/ min.

Tocainide and mexiletine are two newer class IB drugs with actions similar to lidocaine used for a long-term ventricular arrhythmia therapy. Tocainide is associated with blood dyscrasias (agranulocytosis, bone marrow depression, thrombocytopenia, aplastic anemia) and pulmonary fibrosis. [222] These side effects are not common with mexiletine. Neither drug is commonly used in pediatrics. Oral doses in children are mexiletine, 4–15 mg/kg/d in three doses, and tocainide, 20–40 mg/ kg/d in three doses. [224]

Flecainide and encainide are newer class IC drugs used to treat ventricular arrhythmias. [222] Flecainide has more myocardial depressant effect than encainide, which limits its use. Dose-dependent arrhythmia enhancement has occurred with class IC drugs. They are not commonly used in pediatrics. Doses for children are encainide, 2–5 mg/kg/d orally, and flecainide, 1–2 mg/kg/day intravenously in four doses.[224]

Class II Drugs. Propranolol and other β-adrenergic antagonists are class II antiarrhythmics. Their major antiarrhythmic effects are secondary to β-adrenergic blockade. Propranolol is effective in the treatment of both supraventricular and ventricular arrhythmias. It can decrease the ventricular response to atrial fibrillation, a response more pronounced in digitalized patients. The recommended intravenous dosage is 0.01–0.1 mg/kg. The drug should be administered slowly with ECG and blood pressure monitoring. Propranolol may cause significant hypotension and bradycardia. Recommended oral doses are 0.5–4.0 mg/kg/24 h to a maximum of 60 mg/24 h in children.

Esmolol is a new short-acting β₁-adrenergic antagonist effective for the treatment of supraventricular tachycardias and ventricular arrhythmias. Esmolol is also used to treat hypertension. The intravenous dosage is an initial dose of 0.5–1.0 mg/kg as a bolus, followed by an infusion of 50–300 μg/kg/min. Side effects are similar to those of propranolol.

Class III Drugs. Bretylium is a class III antiarrhythmic drug that significantly prolongs APD but initially stimulates catecholamine release and prevents reuptake of norepinephrine. It has been useful in the treatment of ventricular tachycardia and fibrillation refractory to other modes of therapy. The acute intravenous dose for ventricular fibrillation is 5 mg/kg, which may be followed by 10 mg/kg every 15–30 minutes to a total dose of 30 mg/kg.[223] The maintenance dose is 5–10 mg/kg every 6 hours. Hypotension may occur with administration of bretylium.

Amiodarone is a unique class III drug with multiple pharmacodynamic actions (antagonizes cardiac sodium and calcium currents, prolongs cardiac repolarization, a noncompetitive β-blocker).[222] Amiodarone has been shown to be effective treatment for a variety of arrhythmias (supraventricular, ventricular) but major side effects limit its use (pulmonary fibrosis, abnormal liver function tests, corneal opacities, thyroid dysfunction, peripheral neuropathy, bradycardia). The pediatric dose schedule is 5–10 mg/kg/d for 10 days and then reduced to 3–5 mg/kg/d.[224]

Class IV Drugs. Verapamil is a class IV antiarrhythmic useful in the treatment of supraventricular arrhythmias in the pediatric population. Its antiarrhythmic action is secondary to blockade of slow calcium channels. AV nodal conduction is also slowed. Verapamil causes significant myocardial depression as well as peripheral vasodilation resulting in hypotension. It should be used with caution, if at all, in patients receiving β-adrenergic antagonists because AV block may be enhanced to the point of complete AV block or standstill. The recommended intravenous dosage in the pediatric population for arrhythmia control varies according to age: 0–1 year, both initial and repeat doses of 0.1–0.2 mg/kg (maximum single dose range 0.75–2.0 mg); 1–15 years, initial dose of 0.1–0.3 mg/kg (total dose 2–5 mg) and repeat dose of 0.1–0.2 mg/kg (total dose 2–5 mg).[225] The initial dose should be administered slowly over at least 1 minute, and repeat doses, if required, should be administered 30 minutes after the first dose. Continuous ECG and blood pressure monitoring is mandatory during intravenous administration of verapamil for arrhythmias.

Class V Drugs

ADENOSINE. A class V antiarrhythmic, adenosine is useful for conversion to sinus rhythm of paroxysmal supraventricular tachycardia (PSVT) when other maneuvers have failed. It appears to slow AV nodal conduction and interrupt AV nodal reentry mechanisms. Adenosine is not effective in the treatment of atrial flutter or fibrillation. The dosage in adults is 6–12 mg and in pediatric patients 50–200 μg/kg intravenously. Possible side effects are hypotension, bradycardia, and sinus arrest, but these are usually transient because of the short half-life of adenosine.

Although there are many other antiarrhythmic drugs, they are either not used in the acute situations or doses for pediatric patients are not firmly established. For these reasons, they are not discussed here.

Cardioversion and Defibrillation. Cardioversion and defibrillation are important modalities in the treatment of cardiac tachyarrhythmias. Cardioversion utilizes DC countershock synchronized to prevent administration during the "vulnerable" period of the ventricle. Defibrillation utilizes an unsynchronized DC countershock to terminate arrhythmias, and it is usually reserved for ventricular tachycardia and fibrillation. Cardioversion is often successful in the treatment of atrial fibrillation, flutter, and supraventricular tachycardia unresponsive to medication or vagal maneuvers.

When defibrillation is used in infants and children, the initial energy level recommended is 2 W-s/kg.[226] If unsuccessful, this dose can be doubled. If repeated attempts at defibrillation are unsuccessful, conditions such as hypoxia, acidosis, or electrolyte imbalance should be sought and corrected before higher energies are given.[227]

Cardiac Pacemakers. Postoperative pediatric cardiac patients may require either temporary or permanent pacemaker implantation. Damage to conductive pathways may occur at the time of surgery, as discussed previously.

At the time of open-heart procedures in pediatric patients, many cardiothoracic surgeons place epicardial leads in the right atrial and ventricular myocardium for initiating temporary pacing if the need arises in the post-operative period. Some institutions also use transvenous pacing leads and electrodes. If cardiac impulse generation difficulties (eg, sick sinus syndrome) or conduction defects that compromise cardiovascular stability persist, a permanent pacemaker system is used. Williams and Hesslein recommend permanent pacemaker implantation in symptomatic complete AV block if the condition persists up to 2 weeks.[228] Other indications for permanent pacing are recommended by Dreifus and co-workers.[229] Another indication for pacing in the postoperative period is the use of overdrive pacing at rapid rates to convert certain tachyarrhythmias (atrial fibrillation and supraventricular tachycardia).

Components of Pacemakers. Pacemaker systems consist of a pulse generator or power source, pacemaker leads, and electrodes. The pulse generator in most modern pacemakers contains a lithium battery and consists of three circuits: (1) timing circuit (controls pacing intervals); (2) output circuit (controls charging and discharging of the impulse); and (3) sensing circuit (senses intracardiac electrical signal). The rates, output, and modes of the pacemaker generators can be programmed. Mechanisms incorporated in the circuitry allow sensing circuits to discriminate between true and false cardiac electrical signals. Other modifications permit a refractory period for the pulse generator when nonsensing occurs for a fixed time interval following depolarization of cardiac muscle. This prevents sensing at inappropriate times in the cardiac cycle.

When temporary pacing is required, an external pulse generator is used. Many models of these generators are available. Ideal characteristics include (1) a method to control output and amplitude, enabling the defining of the threshold for capture and alteration of output if changes in threshold occur; (2) a method to alter mode of pacing (fixed or demand mode); (3) a provision for either atrial or ventricular or AV sequential pacing; (4) a method to alter pacing rate in all modes; and (5) indicators to show impulse generation and sensing.

Pacemaker leads and electrodes deliver pulse generator signals to the heart and, in those pacemakers with a sensing circuit, convey electrical potentials from the heart to the pulse generator. Two types of pacemaker lead systems are available: unipolar and bipolar. When two leads and a pair of electrodes are used, the system is designated as bipolar. A single lead and electrodes connecting the pulse generator to the heart constitutes a unipolar lead system. In this system, the second electrode is either attached to a metal plate on the pulse generator or is the case of the generator. In both systems,

current flows from the cathode to the myocardium and returns to the anode from the myocardium. With the unipolar system, the body tissue must conduct the return impulses to complete the circuit.

Advantages and disadvantages have been reported for both systems. Bipolar leads provide lower-amplitude signals to the generator than do unipolar lead systems, which may compromise sensing in some situations. Unipolar systems, however, are more affected by external signals such as skeletal muscle potentials or electromagnetic interference. Pacer spikes on the ECG are clearer when unipolar leads are utilized. Bipolar systems can be converted to unipolar systems by disconnecting the anode lead from the pacemaker and attaching a lead from the chest wall to the anode of the pulse generator.

Pacemaker Classification. A useful classification of modes of cardiac pacing has been organized by the Inter-Society Commission for Heart Disease Resources (ICHD).[230] Using a five-letter code, the first letter indicates the chamber paced, second letter indicates the chamber sensed, third letter, the response to the sensed signal, fourth letter the programmable function, and fifth letter special tachyarrhythmic functions. The letters used are V, ventricle; A, atrium; D, double or dual (also triggering and inhibition); I, inhibited; T, triggered; O, not applicable or nonprogrammable; P, programmable; R, reverse (generator-activated by rapid rather than slow heart rates); S, scanning; B, bursts; and E, external. The following examples indicate common pacing modes using this system. In fixed mode (VOO), the ventricle is paced but does not sense or respond to external signals. The pacemaker emits a signal at a fixed rate regardless of cardiac electrical activity. This can lead to competition between the pacemaker and cardiac electrical events and promote arrhythmias. *Asynchronous* is another term used to describe this mode of pacing. In ventricular inhibited (VVI) mode, the ventricle is stimulated, the R wave sensed, and the pacemaker is inhibited when depolarization occurs (demand pacemaker). The rate of the pacemaker is programmed, and if ventricular depolarization occurs normally at a rate greater than the pacemaker rate, it senses the R wave and its timing circuit is reset to zero. When an R wave is sensed within a preset time interval, however, the pacemaker will stimulate the ventricle at the set rate. This is the most widely used pacemaker today.

Two other modes of pacing temporarily, atrial and AV sequential pacing, are occasionally used in postoperative cardiac patients. Both modes enhance the atrial contribution to cardiac output by providing an "atrial kick." For atrial pacing to be effective, AV conduction must be normal. If AV sequential pacing is used, it is done in either the asynchronous or synchronous (demand) mode. In both, the pacemaker rate is set at a specific AV time interval. A danger inherent in using the asynchronous mode is precipitation of arrhythmias. When the synchronous, or demand, mode is used, both the atrium and ventricle are stimulated, but the ventricular R wave is sensed. The classification of these two modes are DOO (asychronous AV sequential pacing) and DVI (synchronous AV sequential pacing). Other more complicated pacemakers, including those with tachyarrhythmic functions or automatic implantable defibrillators, may occasionally be used in the pediatric population.

Cardiopulmonary Resuscitation (CPR).

Precipitating factors leading to cardiac arrest in pediatric patients include hypoxia secondary to airway obstruction and pulmonary parenchymal disease, hypotension associated with sepsis, metabolic disorders, loss of circulatory blood volume, and parasympathetic reflexes. Cardiac arrhythmias are a less frequent cause compared with adults and asystole is found more frequently. Despite differences in the frequency of precipitating events of cardiac arrest in infants and children compared with adults, prompt recognition and initiation of therapy are essential for successful outcome. Initial priorities of quickly establishing an unobstructed airway, adequate ventilation, and circulatory support are the same.

Airway and Ventilation.

Establishing an unobstructed airway is the first priority. Removing foreign material from the mouth and pharynx (eg, vomitus) may be accomplished by suctioning if available. One of three maneuvers may be used to maintain the airway without artificial aids when resuscitation is initiated:

1. Head tilt and chin lift. Head is placed in sniffing position and chin is brought forward by lifting upward on mentum of the mandible.
2. Jaw thrust. Mandible is brought forward by lifting at its angles.
3. Combination of 1 and 2.

Ventilation must be initiated if the patient is not breathing spontaneously after initial airway-clearing maneuvers have been performed. In the older child and adolescent, mouth-to-mouth ventilation can be used with the nose pinched closed or sealed by the rescuer's cheek. Ventilation of the infant may be performed by covering the mouth and nose simultaneously with the resuscitator's mouth. Adequacy of ventilation may be assessed by observing expansion of the victim's chest. One must be careful not to apply too large a tidal volume, especially in the infant. This can promote gastric distention, which could be followed by compromised lung expansion, gastric rupture, or regurgitation with aspiration. If gastric distention occurs, decompression can be accomplished by inserting an orogastric tube temporarily. Decompression should not be accomplished by applying pressure to the abdomen.

On many occasions, especially in the hospital setting, airway maintenance after initial CPR includes insertion of artificial airways (oropharyngeal airways and endotracheal tubes) and ventilation with self-inflating bags, nonrebreathing or partial rebreathing devices. These devices should allow the administration of 100% oxygen. Several things must be considered before placement of an artificial airway. Most patients can be adequately ventilated without their use. Establishment of an airway and initiation of ventilation must not be prolonged by attempting to place an artificial airway. Patients with pharyngeal reflexes intact may not tolerate an oropharyngeal airway. Placement of a nasopharyngeal airway may cause epistaxis secondary to nasal mucosal or adenoid trauma. Parasympathetic reflexes may occur with the placement of airways or laryngoscopy in pediatric patients.

Selecting the correct size airway, mask, or endotracheal tube is important. If a mask of the incorrect size is used, it may be difficult to obtain a tight seal and much of the ventilation will be wasted. An oropharyngeal airway that is too short will push the base of the tongue against the posterior pharyngeal wall. If too long, it impinges upon the epiglottis, obstructing the laryngeal opening. An estimation of the correct size oropharyngeal airway can be made by placing the airway beside the cheek and noting the distance from the lips to the angle of the mandible. An airway of the correct length extends just beyond the mandibular angle.

ENDOTRACHEAL TUBE SIZES. Estimation of the correct internal diameter of the endotracheal tube can be made from the following:

Premature infant: 2.5–3.0 mm
Normal newborn to 3 months of age: 3.0–3.5 mm
3 months to 1 year: 3.5–4.0 mm
1–2 years: 4.0–4.5 mm
After 2 years of age, the following formula has proven to be useful: internal diameter (ID) in mm = (age + 16)/4.

To prevent undue pressure on the tracheal mucosa leading to edema or tissue changes in the cricoid region, an audible leak should be present between 10 and 20 cm H_2O inflating pressure, especially if the tube is required for long periods of time.[231] If cuffed endotracheal tubes are used in children, a tube approximately 1 mm smaller than predicted usually needs to be placed. Cuffed tubes are usually not placed in children younger than 10–12 years of age.

ENDOTRACHEAL INTUBATION. When anticipating laryngoscopy for endotracheal tube placement, several differences between the pediatric airway compared with the adult airway should be considered:

1. The tongue is relatively larger in relation to the oral cavity.

2. The glottis is more cephalad with the vocal cords slanting upward and backward.
3. The epiglottis is Ω shaped and narrower.
4. The cricoid ring, not the glottic opening, is the narrowest portion of the airway.

Because the tongue is relatively larger, it may be difficult to displace with the laryngoscope blade. The larynx appears more anterior and extending the head may make it difficult to visualize. Placing the head on a pillow and depressing the shoulders and larynx often overcomes this problem. It is often difficult to lift the short, narrow, Ω-shaped epiglottis with the laryngoscope blade. Finally, an endotracheal tube that passes easily between the vocal cords may exert undue pressure at the cricoid level.

During intubation of any patient in cardiac arrest, it is probably wise to assume that there is a danger of passive regurgitation or vomiting. Application of cricoid pressure (Sellick maneuver) at the time of laryngoscopy is a reasonable precaution.

Circulatory Support. Recommendations for CPR in the infant and small child consider anatomic and physiologic differences. In evaluating the presence of a pulse, the carotid artery is palpated in the older child and adult, but the brachial or femoral pulse is more accessible in infants. If a pulse is not present, chest compressions should be instituted immediately. The patient should be supine on a firm surface that supports the back and spine. When a firm surface is unavailable for an infant, the rescuer may encircle the chest with both hands and support the back with the fingers. Sternal compressions may then be performed by the thumbs. Alternatively, the palm of the hand may be utilized for support. Chest compressions are applied to the lower third of the sternum approximately 2 fingerbreadths below the intermammary line in the infant. The sternum is compressed up to 2.5 cm at a rate of 100 times per minute, using two or three fingers.[225] In the child, chest compressions are applied with the heel of one hand on the sternum approximately 2 fingerbreadths above the xiphisternal junction. The fingers should not make contact with the chest wall to prevent injury to the ribs and lungs. A compression rate of 80–100 per minute is used, depressing the sternum 2.5–4.0 cm.

These compression rates take into consideration the small stroke volumes and the requirement for increased heart rate to provide adequate cardiac output in infants and young children. It should be noted that precordial thumps are not recommended in infants and small children. In the adolescent, the heel of the hand is placed on the sternum approximately 1 fingerbreadth above the xiphisternal junction, with a compression rate of 60–80 per minute. Adequacy of cardiac compression is assessed by palpation of carotid, brachial, or femoral pulses de-

pending upon the patient's age. Pupillary size may also be beneficial in assessing adequacy of ventilation and chest compression. Normally the pupils will be small if central nervous system (CNS) perfusion and oxygenation are adequate. One limiting factor, however, is the effect of parasympatholytic or sympathomimetic medications used during resuscitative efforts, which cause pupillary dilation.

The current recommendations for coordination of ventilation and external cardiac massage is one breath per five compressions in all age groups.[225] Several investigators, secondary to research in animal models and humans, suggest that simultaneous ventilation with elevated inflation pressures and chest compressions improves carotid blood flow.[232,233] This is termed "new CPR" or SCV-CPR (simultaneous compression ventilation) and is based upon the hypothesis that forward blood flow in external cardiac massage is secondary to a gradient between intrathoracic and extrathoracic pressure in the arterial system and extrathoracic arterial-venous pressure differences rather than compression of the heart between the sternum and spinal column. Other investigators reported that despite the increased carotid flow with this method, cerebral perfusion pressure (CPP) was compromised secondary to an increase in intracranial pressure owing to raised intrathoracic pressure and venous obstruction.[232,234] However, this complication has also been reported for standard CPR.[235] New CPR requires endotracheal intubation and may, because of high inflation pressures, increase the risk of pulmonary barotrauma. At this time, its use is not recommended in pediatric patients.[225]

As in adults, ECG monitoring to elucidate cardiac rhythm should be established as soon as feasible during resuscitation. The ECG rhythm influences further treatment. Intravenous access should also be established for drug and possibly fluid administration, but ventilation and chest compression must not be interrupted while vascular access is obtained. The instillation of epinephrine, atropine, or lidocaine into the tracheobronchial tree via an endotracheal tube has proven effective in cardiopulmonary resuscitation when intravenous access cannot be quickly established. Rapid absorption of drugs can occur from the bone marrow making the intraosseous space (placement of a needle into marrow space of the tibia) a possible alternative route for access to the circulation during CPR.

Pharmacologic Support of CPR. Specific medications have been used traditionally during CPR for several major reasons: (1) correction of metabolic acidosis secondary to inadequate oxygen availability at the tissue level; (2) enhancement of myocardial contractility and alteration of peripheral resistance; (3) treatment of bradycardia; and (4) aid in the management of arrhythmias. The first-line drugs in CPR are epinephrine and bicarbonate with other inotropic and vasoactive drugs added as required.

The mixed α-β agonist, epinephrine, is used to increase myocardial contractility, heart rate, and systemic vascular resistance. This latter function improves coronary blood flow. It also may make ventricular fibrillation more amenable to electrical defibrillation. Indications for its use are asystole, bradycardia unresponsive to atropine, electromechanical dissociation, and fine ventricular fibrillation.[225] Epinephrine and other catecholamines appear to be less effective in an acidotic environment.[29] The dosage in pediatric patients during CPR is 0.01 mg/kg (10 μg/kg) of a 1:10,000 solution intravenously or endotracheally. This dose may be repeated every 5 minutes as required. Once spontaneous circulation is restored, persistent hypotension or poor perfusion may be treated with an epinephrine infusion if other inotropes are ineffective. The current recommended dose, preferably through a central catheter, is 0.1–1.0 μg/kg/min.[225]

Bicarbonate has been recommended for correction of metabolic acidosis in cardiopulmonary arrest for many years. It remains the drug of choice, but more cautious use of this medication in CPR has been advocated.[225,236,237] Acidemia associated with cardiopulmonary arrest is usually a combined respiratory-metabolic acidosis. If the major precipitating event has been respiratory in nature, acidosis will often be quickly corrected by initiating adequate ventilation and oxygenation, with a short period of cardiac massage to restore the circulation. Under these circumstances, the development of a significant metabolic acidosis is unlikely and bicarbonate administration would lead to alkalemia. The importance of adequate ventilation is emphasized. Carbon dioxide tension in the blood will increase if ventilation is inadequate after bicarbonate administration.[238]

Current recommendations are to use bicarbonate only after adequate ventilation, correction of hypoxemia, administration of epinephrine, and chest compressions have failed to reestablish adequate cardiovascular function or if a known metabolic acidosis is present.[225] The initial dosage can be 1 mEq/kg, with additional doses based on arterial blood pH. If blood gases are unobtainable, repeat doses of bicarbonate, 1 mEq/kg every 10 minutes, if arrest is uncorrected, may be given. Full-strength bicarbonate may be used in children, but it should be diluted to half strength in infants to prevent a sudden increase in serum osmolarity. Adverse effects of sodium bicarbonate administration include alkalemia that shifts potassium intracellularly, reduction of ionized calcium, hypernatremia, hyperosmolarity, and decreased availability of oxygen at the tissue level.

Atropine, a parasympatholytic agent, is indicated when sinus bradycardia is present. The dose is 0.01–0.02 mg/kg intravenously. It may also be instilled into the tracheobronchial tree. Atropine dilates the pupils, transiently interfering with neurologic assessment.

Other inotropic agents may be of benefit in maintaining cardiovascular function after the initial resuscitation period. Dopamine may improve blood pressure, perfusion, and coronary output. Dosages of 2–30 μg/kg/min have been used in pediatric patients. Dobutamine, which has primarily an inotropic effect on the myocardium, may be indicated in dosages of 5–20 μg/kg/min when myocardial function is less than optimal. Because it is mainly a β agonist, dobutamine may cause a degree of peripheral dilation. Isoproterenol, 0.01–1.0 μg/kg/min, is indicated for either sinus bradycardia or complete heart block. All of these drugs are given by intravenous infusion, preferably by a calibrated pump through a central venous catheter.

Calcium has been routinely used to increase myocardial contractility in the past. Because of recent findings of alterations in calcium homeostasis in ischemia and cell death,[239,240] and the question of its effectiveness in electromechanical dissociation or asystole,[241,242] current recommendations from the American Heart Association suggest its use only with documented hypocalcemia, hyperkalemia, hypermagnesemia, or calcium channel blocker overdose. Doses of calcium chloride, 20 mg/kg, are given slowly intravenously into a central venous catheter.

Lidocaine is the principal antiarrhythmic drug in pediatric patients with ventricular dysrhythmias. An initial dose of 1 mg/kg is administered as a bolus, followed by an intravenous infusion of 20–50 μg/kg/min. Other medications used for arrhythmias if lidocaine is ineffective are bretylium and procainamide.

REFERENCES

1. Oka Y, Lin T: Postoperative management: Complications. *Int Anesth Clin* **18**:217–231, 1980.
2. Winfield JM, Fox CL, Mersheimer WL: Etiological factors in postoperative salt retention and its prevention. *Ann Surg* **134**:626–640, 1951
3. Bharati S, Lev M: Sequelae of atriotomy and ventriculotomy on the endocardial conduction system and coronary arteries. *Am J Cardiol* **50**:580–587, 1982
4. Najafi H, Henson D, Dye WS, et al: Left ventricular hemorrhagic necrosis. *Ann Thorac Surg* **7**:550–580, 1969
5. Kirklin JW, Blackstone EH, Kirklin JK: General principles of cardiac surgery. In Braunwald E (ed): *Heart Disease: Textbook of Cardiovascular Medicine*, 2nd ed. Philadelphia: WB Saunders, 1984, pp 1797–1814
6. Panidis IP, Kotler MN, Fan Ren J, et al: Development and regression of left ventricular hypertrophy. *J Am Coll Cardiol* **3**:1309–1320, 1984
7. Graham TP Jr, Atwood GF, Boerth RC, et al: Right and left heart size and function in infants with symptomatic coarctation. *Circulation* **56**:641–647, 1977
8. Graham TP Jr: Ventricular performance in adults after operation for congenital heart disease. *Am J Cardiol* **50**:612–620, 1982

9. Liberthson RR, Boucher CA, Strauss HW, et al: Right ventricular function in adult atrial septal defect. *Am J Cardiol* **47**:56–60, 1981

10. Pearlman AS, Boer JS, Clark CE, et al: Abnormal right ventricular size and ventricular septal motion after atrial septal defect closure. *Am J Cardiol* **41**:295–301, 1978

11. Boucek RJ Jr, Kasselberg AG, Boerth RC, et al: Myocardial injury in infants with congenital heart disease, evaluation by creatine kinase MB isoenzyme analysis. *Am J Cardiol* **50**:129–135, 1982

12. Hultgren HN, Miyagawa M, Buch W, Angell WW: Ischemic myocardial injury during cardiopulmonary bypass surgery. *Am Heart J* **85**:167–176, 1973

13. Lucas SK, Elmer EB, Flaherty JT, et al: Effects of multiple dose potassium cardioplegia on myocardial ischemia, return of ventricular function and ultrastructural preservation. *J Thorac Cardiovasc Surg* **80**:102–110, 1980.

14. Leaf A: Maintenance of concentration gradients and regulation of cell volume. *Ann NY Acad Sci* **72**:396–404, 1959

15. Tranum-Jensen J, Janse MJ, Fiolet JWT, et al: Tissue osmolarity, cell swelling and reperfusion in acute regional myocardial ischemia in the isolated porcine heart. *Circ Res* **49**:364–381, 1981

16. Roberts WC, Bulkley BH, Morrow AH: Pathologic anatomy of cardiac valve replacement: A study of 224 necropsy patients. *Prog Cardiovasc Dis* **15**:539–587, 1973

17. Sapsford RN, Blackstone EH, Kirklin JW, et al: Coronary perfusion versus cold ischemic arrest during aortic valve surgery. *Circulation* **49**:1190–1199, 1974

18. Cooley DA, Reul GJ, Wukasch DC: Ischemic contracture of the heart—"Stone heart." *Am J Cardiol* **29**:575–577, 1972

19. Katz AM, Tuda M: The "stone heart" and other challenges to the biochemist. *Am J Cardiol* **39**:1073–1077, 1977

20. Watanabe T, Trusler GA, Williams WG, et al: Phrenic nerve paralysis after pediatric cardiac surgery. *J Thorac Cardiovasc Surg* **94**:383–388, 1987

21. Dubois GD, Arieff AI: Clinical manifestations of fluid and electrolyte disorders. In Arieff AI, Defronzo RA (eds): *Fluid, Electrolyte and Acid-Base Disorders.* New York: Churchill Livingstone, 1985, pp 1087–1144

22. Heining MPD, Linton RAF, Band DM: Plasma ionized calcium during open heart surgery. *Anaesthesia* **40**:237–241, 1985

23. Hall K, Enberg G, Ritzen M, et al: Somatomedin A levels in serum from healthy children and from children with growth hormone deficiency or delayed puberty. *Acta Endocrinol* **94**:155–165, 1980

24. Fleckenstein A: Specific pharmacology of calcium in myocardium, cardiac pacemaker and vascular smooth muscle. *Ann Rev Pharmacol Toxicol* **17**:149–166, 1977

25. Rasmussen H: The calcium messenger system, part 1. *N Engl J Med* **314**:1094–1100, 1986

26. Rasmussen H: The calcium messenger system, part 2. *N Engl J Med* **314**:1164–1169, 1986

27. Harris MN, Crowther A, Jupp RA, Aps C: Magnesium and coronary artery revascularization. *Br J Anaesth* **60**:779–783, 1988

28. Narins RG, Jones ER, Townsend R, et al: Metabolic acid-base disorders: Pathophysiology, classification, and treatment. In Arieff AI, Defronzo RA (eds): *Fluid, Electrolyte, and Acid-base Disorders.* New York: Churchill Livingstone, 1985, pp 269–384

29. Weil MH, Houle DB, Brown DB, et al: Vasopressor agents: Influence of acidosis on cardiac and vascular responsiveness. *Calif Med* **88**:437–440, 1958

30. Morgan BC, Crawford EW, Hornbein TF, et al: Hemodynamic effects of changes in arterial carbon dioxide tension during intermittent positive pressure ventilation. *Anesthesiology* **28**:866–873, 1967

31. Foex P, Prys-Roberts C: Anesthesia and the hypertensive patient. *Br J Anaesth* **46**:575–588, 1974

32. Alderman EL, Coltart J, Wettach GE, Harrison DC: Coronary artery syndrome after sudden propranolol withdrawal. *Ann Intern Med* **81**:625–627, 1974

33. Miller RR, Olson HG, Amsterdam EA, Mason DT: Exacerbation of coronary events after abrupt cessation of antianginal therapy. *N Engl J Med* **293**:416–418, 1975

34. Stanley TH, deLange S, Boscoe MJ, Bruijn N, et al: The influence of chronic preoperative propranolol therapy on cardiovascular dynamics and narcotic requirements during operation in patients with coronary artery disease. *Can Anaesth Soc J* **29**:319–324, 1982

35. Ponten J, Haggendol J, Milocco I, et al: Long term metoprolol therapy and neurolept-anesthesia in coronary artery surgery: Withdrawal versus maintenance of beta, adrenoreceptor blockade. *Anesth Analg* **62**:380–390, 1983

36. Casson WR, Jones RM, Parsons RS: Nifedipine and cardiopulmonary bypass. *Anaesthesia* **39**:1197–1201, 1984

37. Engelman RM, Hadji-Rousou I, Breyer RH, et al: Rebound vasospasm after coronary revascularization in association with calcium antagonist withdrawal. *Ann Thorac Surg* **37**:469–472, 1984

38. Plachetka JR, Solomon NW, Copeland JG: Plasma propranolol before, during and after cardiopulmonary bypass. *Clin Pharmacol Ther* **30**:745–751, 1981

39. Sibbald WJ, Calvin J, Driedger AA: Right and left ventricular preload and diastolic ventricular compliance: Implications for therapy in critically ill patients. *Crit Care State of the Art* **3**:3F, 1982

40. Perkin RM, Levin DL: Shock in the pediatric patient. Part I. *J Pediatr* **101**:163–169, 1982

41. Calvin JE, Driedger AA, Sibbald EJ: Does the pulmonary capillary wedge pressure predict left ventricular preload in critically ill patients? *Crit Care Med* **9**:437–443, 1981

42. Hoffman WS, Tomasello DN, MacVaugh H: Control of postcardiotomy bleeding with PEEP. *Ann Thorac Surg* **34**:71–73, 1982

43. Zurick AM, Urzua J, Ghattas M, et al: Failure of positive end expiratory pressure to decrease bleeding after cardiac surgery. *Ann Thorac Surg* **34**:608–611, 1982

44. Murphy DA, Finlayson DC, Craver JM, et al: Effect of positive end expiratory pressure on excessive mediastinal bleeding after cardiac operations: Controlled study. *J Thorac Cardiovasc Surg* **85**:864–869, 1983

45. Beynen FM, Tarhan S: Anesthesia for surgical repair of congenital heart defects in children. In Tarhan S (ed): *Cardiovascular Anesthesia and Postoperative Care,* 2nd ed. Chicago: Year Book Medical, 1989, pp 105–212

46. Peterson KA, Dewanjee MK, Kaye MP: Fate of indium[111]-labeled platelets during cardiopulmonary bypass per-

formed with membrane and bubble oxygenators. *J Thorac Cardiovasc Surg* 84:39–43, 1982

47. Kim YL, Richman K, Marshall B: Thrombocytopenia associated with Swan-Ganz catheterization in patients. *Anesthesiology* 53:261–262, 1980

48. Snow N, Lucas A, Gray LA Jr: Effect of sodium nitroprusside on postoperative blood loss in the cardiac surgical patient. *Crit Care Med* 9:827–828, 1981

49. King DJ, Kelton JG: Heparin associated thrombocytopenia. *Ann Intern Med* 100:535–540, 1984

50. Gross MA, Keefer V, Liebman J: The platelets in cyanotic heart disease. *Pediatrics* 42:651–658, 1968

51. Maurer HM, McCue CM, Robertson LW, Haggins JC: Correction of platelet dysfunction and bleeding in cyanotic congenital heart disease by simple red cell volume reduction. *Am J Cardiol* 35:831–835, 1975

52. Ekert H, Gilchrist GS, Stanton R, Hammond D: Hemostasis in cyanotic heart disease. *J Pediatr* 76:221–230, 1970

53. Hastreiter AR, Vanderhorst RL: Hemodynamics of neonatal cyanotic heart disease. *Crit Care Med* 5:23–28, 1977

54. Chenoweth DE, Cooper SW, Hugli TE, et al: Complement activation during cardiopulmonary bypass: Evidence for generation of C3a and C5a anaphylatoxins. *N Engl J Med* 304:497–503, 1981

55. Cavarocchi NC: Complement activation during cardiopulmonary bypass. *J Thorac Cardiovasc Surg* 91:252–258, 1986

56. Best N, Sinosich MJ, Teisner B, et al: Complement activation during cardiopulmonary bypass by heparin-protamine interaction. *Br J Anaesth* 56:339–343, 1984

57. Jones HM, Matthews N, Vaughan RS, Stark JM: Cardiopulmonary bypass and complement activation: Involvement of classic and alternate pathways. *Anaesthesia* 37:629–633, 1982

58. Craddock PR, Fehr J, Bridham KL, et al: Complement and leukocyte-mediated pulmonary dysfunction in hemodialysis. *N Engl J Med* 296:769–773, 1977

59. Swerdlow BN, Mihm FG, Goetzl EJ, Matthay MA: Leukotrienes in pulmonary edema fluid after cardiopulmonary bypass. *Anesth Analg* 65:306–308, 1986

60. Salzman EW, Weinstein MJ, Weintraub RM, et al: Treatment with desmopressin acetate to reduce blood loss after cardiac surgery: A double-blind randomized trial. *N Engl J Med* 314:1402–1406, 1986

61. Czer LSC, Bateman TM, Gray RJ, et al: Treatment of severe platelet dysfunction and hemorrhage after cardiopulmonary bypass: Reduction in blood product usage with desmopressin. *J Am Coll Cardiol* 9:1139–1147, 1987

62. Hackman T, Gascoyne RD, Naiman SC, et al: A trial of desmopressin (1-desamino–8-d-arginine vasopressin) to reduce blood loss in uncomplicated cardiac surgery. *N Engl J Med* 321:1437–1443, 1989

63. Seear MD, Wadsworth LD, Rogers PC, et al: The effect of desmopressin acetate (DDAVP) on postoperative blood loss after cardiac operations in children. *J Thorac Cardiovasc Surg* 98:217–219, 1989

64. Beck GS: Two cardiac compression triads. *JAMA* 104:715–716, 1935

65. Trinkle JK, Marcos J, Grover FL, Cuello LM: Management of the wounded heart. *Ann Thorac Surg* 17:230–236, 1974

66. Guberman B, Fowler NO, Engel PJ, et al: Cardiac tamponade in medical patients. *Circulation* 64:633–640, 1981

67. Levin DL, Perkin RM: Postoperative care of the pediatric patient with congenital heart disease. In Shoemaker WC, Thompson WL, Holbrook PR (eds): *Textbook of Critical Care*. Philadelphia: WB Saunders, 1984, pp 399–400

68. Moffet HL: Cardiovascular syndromes. In Moffet HL (ed): *Pediatric Infectious Disease*. Philadelphia: JB Lippincott, 1981, pp 411–429

69. Shabetai R: Diseases of the pericardium. In Hurst JW, et al (eds): *The Heart*, 7th ed. New York: McGraw-Hill, 1990, pp 1348–1374

70. Benzing G III, Kaplan S: Late complications of cardiac surgery. *Pediatr Clin North Am* 18:1225–1242, 1971

71. Drusin LM, Engle MA, Hagstrom JW, Schwartz MS: The postpericardiotomy syndrome: A six year epidemiologic study. *N Engl J Med* 272:597–602, 1965

72. Engle MA, Zobriskie JB, Senterfit LB, et al: Viral illness and the postpericardiotomy syndrome. A prospective study in children. *Circulation* 62:1151–1158, 1980

73. Perkin RM, Levin DL: Adverse effects of positive pressure ventilation in children. In Gregory GA: *Respiratory Failure in the Child. Clinics in Critical Care Medicine*. New York: Churchill Livingstone, 1981, pp 163–167

74. Morgan BC, Martin WE, Hornbein TF, et al: Hemodynamic effects of intermittent positive pressure respiration. *Anesthesiology* 27:584–590, 1966

75. Downs JB, Douglass ME, Sanfelippo PM, et al: Ventilatory pattern, intrapleural pressure and cardiac output. *Anesth Analg* 56:88–94, 1977

76. Downs JB, Douglas ME: Assessment of cardiac filling pressure during continuous positive pressure ventilation. *Crit Care Med* 8:285–289, 1980

77. Viquerat CE, Righetti A, Suter PM: Biventricular volumes and functions in patients with adult respiratory distress syndromes ventilated with PEEP. *Chest* 83:509–514, 1983

78. Walkinshaw M, Shoemaker WC: Use of volume loading to obtain preferred levels of PEEP. *Crit Care Med* 8:81–86, 1980

79. Weber KT, Janicki JS, Shroff SG, et al: The right ventricle: Physiologic and pathophysiologic considerations. *Crit Care Med* 11:323–328, 1983

80. Polak JF, Holman BL, Wynne J, Colucci WS: Right ventricular ejection fraction: An indicator of increased mortality in patients with congestive heart failure associated with coronary artery disease. *J Am Coll Cardiol* 2:217–224, 1983

81. Heath D, Edwards JE: The pathology of hypertensive pulmonary vascular disease. A description of six grades of structural changes in the pulmonary arteries with special reference to congenital cardiac septal defects. *Circulation* 18:533–547, 1958

82. Rabinovitch M, Haworth SG, Castaneda AR, et al: Lung biopsy in congenital heart disease: A morphometric approach to pulmonary vascular disease. *Circulation* 58:1107–1122, 1978

83. Rudolph AM: *Congenital Diseases of the Heart*. Chicago: Year Book Medical, 1974, pp 29–48

84. Rudolph AM, Yuan S: Response of the pulmonary vasculature to hypoxia and H$^+$ ion concentration changes. *J Clin Invest* 45:399–411, 1968

85. Comroe JH: *Physiology of Respiration*. Chicago: Year Book Medical, 1974, pp 155–156

86. Kuida H: Primary and secondary pulmonary hypertension: Pathophysiology, recognition and treatment. In Hurst JW, et al (eds): *The Heart*, 7th ed., New York: McGraw-Hill, 1990, pp 1191–1204

87. Laver MB, Strauss HW, Pohost GM: Right and left ventricular geometry: Adjustments during acute respiratory failure. *Crit Care Med* **7**:509–519, 1979

88. Ross J Jr, Braunwald E: The study of left ventricular function in man by increasing resistance to ventricular ejection with angiotensin. *Circulation* **29**:739–749, 1964

89. Ruzyllo W, Nihill MR, Mullin CE: Hemodynamic evaluation of 221 patients after intracardiac repair of tetralogy of Fallot. *Am J Cardiol* **34**:565–576, 1974

90. Moss AJ: What every primary physician should know about the postoperative cardiac patient. *Pediatrics* **63**:320–330, 1979

91. Nugent EW, Freedom RM, Nora JJ: Clinical course in pulmonary stenosis.*Circulation* **56**(suppl 1):38–47, 1977

92. Clarkson PM, Neutze JM, Barratt-Boyes BG, Brandt PWT: Late postoperative hemodynamic results and cineangiographic findings after Mustard atrial baffle repair of transposition of the great arteries. *Circulation* **53**:525–532, 1976

93. Hennings RO, Weiner F, Weil MH: Measurement of toe temperature for assessing the severity of acute circulatory failure. *Surg Gynecol Obstet* **149**:1–7, 1979

94. Joly HR, Weil MH: Temperature of great toe as an indication of the severity of shock. *Circulation* **39**:131–138, 1969

95. Alexi-Meskhishvilli V, Popov SA, Nikoljuk AP: Evaluation of hemodynamics in infants and small babies after open heart surgery. *Thorac Cardiovasc Surg* **32**:4–9, 1984

96. Woods I, Wilkins RG, Edwards JD, et al: Danger of using core/peripheral temperature gradient as a guide to therapy in shock. *Crit Care Med* **15**:850–852, 1987.

97. Michaels S, Weil MH: Measurement of blood lactate levels on central venous and pulmonary artery blood for estimating severity and prognosis. *Crit Care Med* **8**:263, 1980 (abstr)

98. Vincent J-L, Dufaye P, Berre J, et al: Serial lactate determinations during circulatory shock. *Crit Care Med* **11**:449–451, 1983

99. Martin WE, Cheung PW, Johnson CC, Wong KC: Continuous monitoring of mixed venous oxygen saturation in man. *Anesth Analg* **52**:784–793, 1973

100. Waller JL, Kaplan JA, Bauman DI, Craver JM: Clinical evaluation of a new fiberoptic catheter oximeter during cardiac surgery. *Anesth Analg* **61**:676–679, 1982

101. Baele PL, McMichan JC, Marsh HM, et al: Continuous monitoring of mixed venous oxygen saturation in critically ill patients. *Anesth Analg* **61**:513–517, 1982

102. Jamieson WRE, Turnbull KW, Larrieu AJ, et al: Continuous monitoring of mixed venous oxygen saturation in cardiac surgery. *Can J Surg* **25**:538–543, 1982

103. Parr GVS, Blackstone EH, Kirklin JW: Cardiac performance and mortality early after intracardiac surgery in infants and young children. *Circulation* **51**:867–874, 1975

104. Kohanna FH, Cunningham JN Jr, Catinella FP, et al: Cardiac output determination after cardiac operation: Lack of correlation between direct and indirect estimates. *J Thorac Cardiovasc Surg* **82**:904–908, 1981

105. Civetta JM: Invasive catheterization. In Shoemaker WC, Thompson WL (eds): *Critical Care State of the Art 1*. Fullerton, CA: Society of Critical Care Medicine, 1980, p 5

106. Mangano DT: Monitoring pulmonary arterial pressure in coronary artery disease. *Anesthesiology* **53**:364–370, 1980

107. Lowenstein E, Teplick R: To (PA) catheterize or not to (PA) catheterize—That is the question. *Anesthesiology* **53**:361–363, 1980

108. Sprung CL, Rackow EC, Civetta JM: Direct measurements and derived calculations using the pulmonary artery catheter. In Sprung CL (ed): *The Pulmonary Artery Catheter*. Baltimore: University Park Press, 1983, pp 105–140

109. Weil MH: Patient evaluation "vital signs" and initial care. In Shoemaker WC, Thompson WL (eds): *Critical Care State of the Art 1*: Fullerton, CA: Society of Critical Care Medicine, 1980, p 18

110. Ritter SB: Transesophageal real-time echocardiography in infants and children with CHD. *J Am Coll Cardiol* **18**:569–580, 1991

111. Muhuideen IA, Roberson DA, Silverman NH, et al: Intraoperative evaluation of CHD in infants and children. *Anesthesiology* **76**:165–171, 1992

112. Knoebel SB, McHenry PL, Phillips JF, Widlansky S: Atropine induced cardioacceleration and myocardial blood flow in subjects with and without coronary artery disease. *Am J Cardiol* **33**:327–332, 1974

113. Kurland G, Williams J, Lewiston NJ: Fatal myocardial toxicity during continuous infusion of intravenous isoproterenol therapy of asthma. *J Allergy Clin Immunol* **63**:407–411, 1979

114. Winsor T, Wright RW, Berger HJ: Isoproterenol toxicity. *Am Heart J* **89**:814–817, 1975

115. Brinkmeyer S, Saraf P, Motoyama E, Stezoski W: Superiority of colloid over electrolyte solution for fluid resuscitation (severe normovolemic hemodilution). *Crit Care Med* **9**:369–370, 1981

116. Shoemaker WC: Comparison of the relative effectiveness of whole blood transfusions and various types of fluid therapy in resuscitation. *Crit Care Med* **4**:71–78, 1976

117. Boutros A, Reuss R, Olson L, et al: Comparison of hemodynamic, pulmonary and renal effects of use of three types of fluids after major surgical procedures on the abdominal aorta. *Crit Care Med* **7**:9–13, 1979

118. Haupt M, Rackow EC: Colloid osmotic pressure and fluid resuscitation with hetastarch, albumin and saline solutions. *Crit Care Med* **10**:159–162, 1982

119. Shoemaker WC, Hauser CL: Critique of crystalloid versus colloid therapy in shock and shock lung. *Crit Care Med* **7**:117–124, 1979

120. Weil MH, Henning RJ, Puri VK: Colloid oncotic pressure: Clinical significance. *Crit Care Med* **7**:113–116, 1979

121. Shires GT, Williams J, Brown F: Acute changes in extracellular fluids associated with major surgical procedures. *Ann Surg* **154**:803–810, 1961

122. Virgilio RW, Smith DE, Zorins CK: Balanced electrolyte solutions: Experimental and clinical studies. *Crit Care Med* **7**:98–106, 1979

123. Shires GT, Carrico CT, Cohn D: The role of extracellular fluid in shock. *Int Anesth Clin* **2**:435–454, 1964

124. Shires GT: Role of sodium containing solutions in treatment of oligemic shock. *Surg Clin North Am* **45**:365–376, 1965

125. Goldberg LI: Dopamine: Clinical uses of endogenous catecholamine. *N Engl J Med* **291**:707–710, 1974

126. Parker S, Carlon GC, Isaacs M, et al: Dopamine administration in oliguria and oliguric renal failure. *Crit Care Med* **9**:630–632, 1981

127. Zaritsky A, Chernow B: Catecholamines in critical care medicine. *Crit Care Q* **6**:39–47, 1983

128. Bernstein D, Crane C: Comparative circulatory effects of isoproterenol and dopamine in lambs with experimental cyanotic heart disease. *Pediatr Res* **29**:323–328, 1991

129. Guller B, Fields AF, Coleman MG, Holbrook PR: Changes in cardiac rhythm in children treated with dopamine. *Crit Care Med* **6**:151–154, 1978

130. Miall-Allen V, Whitelaw AGL: Response to dopamine and dobutamine in the preterm infant less than 30 weeks gestation. *Crit Care Med* **17**:1166–1169, 1989

131. Driscoll DJ, Gillette PC, Lewis RM, et al: Comparative hemodynamic effects of isoproterenol, dopamine and dobutamine in the newborn dog. *Pediatr Res* **13**:1006–1009, 1979

132. Buckley NM, Gootman PM, Yellin EL, Brazeou P: Age related cardiovascular effects of catecholamines in anesthetized piglets. *Circ Res* **45**:282–292, 1979

133. Manders WT, Pagani M, Vatner SF: Depressed responsiveness to vasoconstrictor and dilator agents and baroreflex sensitivity in conscious, newborn lambs. *Circulation* **60**:945–955, 1979

134. Schumacher W, Mirkin BL, Shappard JR: Biological maturation and beta adrenergic effectors: Development of beta adrenergic receptors in rabbit heart. *Mol Cell Biochem* **58**:173–181, 1984

135. Voelkel NF, Hegstrand L, Reeves JT, et al: Effects of hypoxia on density of beta adrenergic receptors. *J Appl Physiol* **50**:363–366, 1981

136. Lang P, Williams RG, Norwood WI, Castaneda AR: The hemodynamic effects of dopamine in infants after corrective cardiac surgery. *J Pediatr* **96**:630–634, 1980

137. Mentzer RM, Alegre CA, Nolan SP: The effects of dopamine and isoproterenol on the pulmonary circulation. *J Thorac Cardiovasc Surg* **71**:807–814, 1976

138. Furman WR, Summer WR, Kennedy TP, Sylvester JT: Comparison of the effects of dobutamine, dopamine and isoproterenol on hypoxic pulmonary vasoconstriction in the pig. *Crit Care Med* **10**:371–374, 1982

139. Gray R, Shah PK, Singh B, et al: Low cardiac output states after open heart surgery: Comparative hemodynamic effects of dobutamine, dopamine and norepinephrine plus phentolamine. *Chest* **80**:16–21, 1981

140. Tuttle RR, Mills J: Development of a new catecholamine to selectively increase cardiac contractility. *Circ Res* **36**:185–196, 1975

141. Carlier J, El Allaf D: Old and new inotropic drugs. *Resuscitation* **11**:217–231, 1984

142. Leier CV, Hebon PT, Huss P, et al: Comparative systemic and regional hemodynamic effects of dopamine and dobutamine in patients with cardiomyopathic heart failure. *Circulation* **58**:466–475, 1978

143. Solomon NW, Plachetka JR, Copeland JG: Comparison of dopamine and dobutamine following coronary bypass grafting. *Ann Thorac Surg* **33**:48–54, 1982

144. Fowler MB, Alderman EL, Oesterle SN, et al: Dobutamine and dopamine after cardiac surgery: Greater augmentation of myocardial blood flow with dobutamine. *Circulation* **70**(suppl 1):105–111, 1984

145. Perkin RM, Levin DL, Webb R, et al: Dobutamine: A hemodynamic evaluation in children in shock. *J Pediatr* **100**:977–983, 1982

146. Bohn DJ, Poirier CS, Edmonds JF, Baker GA: Hemodynamic effects of dobutamine after cardiopulmonary bypass in children. *Crit Care Med* **8**:367–371, 1980

147. Hoffman BB, Lefkowitz RJ: Catecholamines and sympathomimetic drugs. In Gilman AG, Rall TW, Nies AS, Taylor P (eds): *Goodman and Gilman's The Pharmacological Basis of Therapeutics*, 8th ed. New York: Pergamon Press, 1990, pp 187–220

148. Assem EK, Schild HD: Inhibition by sympathomimetic amines of histamine release induced by antigen in passively sensitized human lung. *Nature* **224**:1028–1029, 1969

149. Vander AJ: Effect of catecholamines and the renal nerves on renin secretion in anesthetized dogs. *Am J Physiol* **209**:659–662, 1965

150. Gambos EA, Hulet WH, Bopp P, et al: Reactivity of renal systemic circulation to vasoconstrictor agents in normotensive and hypertensive subjects. *J Clin Invest* **41**:203–217, 1962

151. Clutter WE, Bier DM, Shah SD, Cryer PE: Epinephrine plasma metabolic clearance rates and physiologic thresholds for metabolic and hemodynamic actions in man. *J Clin Invest* **66**:94–101, 1980

152. Chernow B, Rainey TG, Lake CR: Endogenous and exogenous catecholamines in critical care medicine. *Crit Care Med* **10**:409–416, 1982

153. Kirsh MM, Bove E, Metmer M, et al: The use of levarterenol and phentolamine in patients with low cardiac output following open heart surgery. *Ann Thorac Surg* **29**:26–31, 1980

154. Wilson RF, Sukhnanden R, Thal AP: Combined use of norepinephrine and dibenzyline in clinical shock. *Surg Forum* **15**:30–31, 1964

155. Rhodes EL, O'Rourke PT, Lee R, et al: The effect of levarterenol and phentolamine on the hypertensive pulmonary vasculature. *Ann Thorac Surg* **16**:375–379, 1973

156. Mueller H, Ayres SM, Gregory JJ, et al: Hemodynamics, coronary blood flow, and myocardial metabolism in coronary shock: Response to L-norepinephrine and isoproterenol. *J Clin Invest* **49**:1885–1902, 1970

157. Mudge GH, Weiner IM: Agents affecting volume and composition of body fluids. In Gilman AG, Rall TW, Nies AS, Taylor P (eds): *Goodman and Gilman's The Pharmacological Basis of Therapeutics*, 8th ed. New York: Pergamon Press, 1990, pp 682–707

158. Drop LJ, Scheidegger D: Plasma ionized calcium concentration. *J Thorac Cardiovasc Surg* **79**:425–431, 1980

159. Bronsky D, Dubin A, Waldstein SS: Calcium and the electrocardiogram: The electrocardiographic manifestations of hyperparathyroidism and marked hypercalcemia from various etiologies. *Am J Cardiol* **7**:823–832, 1961

160. Drop LJ: Ionized calcium, the heart and hemodynamic function. *Anesth Analg* **64**:432–451, 1985

161. White RD, Goldsmith RS, Rodriguez R, et al: Plasma ionic calcium levels following injection of chloride, gluconate and gluceptate salts of calcium. *J Thorac Cardiovasc Surg* **71**:609–613, 1976

162. Coté CJ, Drop LJ, Daniels AL, Hoaglan DC: Calcium chloride versus calcium gluconate: Comparison of ionization and cardiovascular effects in children and dogs. *Anesthesiology* **66**:465–470, 1987

163. Mancini D, LeJemtel T, Sonnenblick E: Intravenous use of amrinone for the treatment of the failing heart. *Am J Cardiol* **56**:8B–15B, 1985

164. Benotti JR, McCue JE, Alpert JS: Comparative vasoactive therapy for heart failure. *Am J Cardiol* **56**:19B–24B, 1985

165. Goenen M, Pedemonte O, Baele P, et al: Amrinone in the management of low cardiac output after open heart surgery. *Am J Cardiol* **56**:33B–38B, 1985.

166. Ross-Ascuitto N, Ascuitto R, Chen V, Downing SE: Negative inotropic effects of amrinone in the neonatal piglet heart. *Circ Res* **61**:847–852, 1987.

167. Lawless S, Burckart G, Diven W, et al: Amrinone in neonates and infants after cardiac surgery. *Crit Care Med* **17**:751–754, 1989.

168. Ansell J, Tiarks C, McCue J, et al: Amrinone induced thrombocytopenia. *Arch Intern Med* **144**:949–952, 1984

169. Silvay G, Litwak R, Griepp RB: Circulatory assist devices. In Kaplan J.A. (ed): *Cardiac Anesthesia*, 2nd ed. Philadelphia: WB Saunders, 1987, pp 1021–1038.

170. Housman LB, Bernstein NEF, Braunwald NS, Dilley RB: Counter-pulsation for intraoperative cardiogenic shock: Successful use of intra-aortic balloon. *JAMA* **224**:1131–1133, 1973

171. Craver JM, Hatcher CR: The percutaneous intra-aortic balloon pump. In Hurst JW, et al (eds): *The Heart*, 7th ed. New York: McGraw-Hill, 1990, pp 2189–2193

172. Benzing G III: Department of Pediatric Cardiology, Cincinnati Children's Hospital Medical Center. Personal communication

173. Pollock JC, Charlton MC, Williams WG, et al: Intraaortic balloon pumping in children. *Ann Thorac Surg* **29**:522–528, 1980

174. Veasy LG, Blalock BA, Orth JL, et al: Intra-aortic balloon pumping in infants and children. *Circulation* **68**:1095–1100, 1983

175. Harvey JC, Goldstein JE, McCabe JC, et al: Complications of percutaneous intra-aortic balloon pumping. *Circulation* **64**(suppl 2):114–117, 1981

176. Baffles TG, Fridman JL, Bicoff JP, Whitehall JL: Extracorporeal circulation for support of palliative cardiac surgery in infants. *Ann Thorac Surg* **10**:354–363, 1970

177. Kanter KR, Pennington DG, Weber TR, et al: Extracorporeal membrane oxygenation for postoperative cardiac support in children. *J Thorac Cardiovasc Surg* **93**:27–35, 1987

178. Redmond CR, Graves ED, Falterman KW, et al: Extracorporeal membrane oxygenation for respiratory and cardiac failure in infants and children. *J Thorac Cardiovasc Surg* **93**:199–204, 1987

179. Rogers AJ, Trento A, Siewers RD, et al: Extracorporeal membrane oxygenation for postcardiotomy cardiogenic shock in children. *Ann Thorac Surg* **47**:903–906, 1989

180. Weinhous L, Canter C, Noetzel M, et al: Extracorporeal membrane oxygenation for circulatory support after congenital heart defects. *Ann Thorac Surg* **48**:206–212, 1989

181. Anderson HL, Attorri RJ, Custer JR, et al: Extracorporeal membrane oxygenation for pediatric cardiopulmonary failure. *J Cardiovasc Surg* **99**:1011–1021, 1990

182. Klein M, Shaheen KW, Whittlesey GC, et al: Extracorporeal membrane oxygenation for circulatory support of children after repair of congenital heart disease. *J Thorac Cardiovasc Surg* **100**:498–505, 1990

183. Braunwald E: Vasodilator therapy—A physiologic approach to treatment of heart failure. *N Engl J Med* **297**:331–333, 1977

184. Wood AJJ: Hypotensive and vasodilator drugs. In Wood AJJ and Wood M (eds): *Drugs and Anesthesia: Pharmacology for Anesthesiologists*, 2nd ed. Baltimore: Williams & Wilkins, 1990, pp 447–454

185. Cohn JN, Franciosa JA: Drug therapy: Vasodilator therapy of cardiac failure (part I). *N Engl J Med* **297**:27–31, 1979

186. Higgins CB, Vatner SF, Eckberg D: Alterations in the baroreceptor reflex in conscious dogs with heart failure. *J Clin Invest* **51**:715–724, 1972

187. Chiariello M, Gold HK, Leinbach RC, et al: Comparison between the effects of nitroprusside and nitro-glycerin on ischemic injury during acute myocardial infarction. *Circulation* **54**:766–773, 1976

188. Kerber RE, Martins JB, Marcus ML: Effect of acute ischemia, nitroglycerin and nitroprusside on regional myocardial thickening, stress and perfusion. *Circulation* **60**:121–129, 1979

189. Tinker JH, Michenfelder JD: Sodium nitroprusside: Pharmacology, toxicity and therapeutics. *Anesthesiology* **45**:340–354, 1976

190. Vesey CJ, Cole PV, Simpson PJ: Cyanide and thiocyanate concentrations following sodium nitroprusside infusion in man. *Br J Anaesth* **48**:651–660, 1976

191. Flaherty JT, Reid PR, Kelly DT: Intravenous nitroglycerin in acute myocardial infarction. *Circulation* **51**:132–139, 1975

192. Saxon SA, Silverman ME: Effects of continuous infusion of intravenous nitroglycerin on methemoglobin levels. *Am J Cardiol* **56**:461–464, 1985

193. Packer M: Vasodilator and inotropic therapy for severe chronic heart failure. *J Am Coll Cardiol* **2**:841–852, 1983

194. Marco JD, Standeven JW, Barner HB: Afterload reduction with hydralazine following valve replacement. *J Thorac Cardiovasc Surg* **80**:50–53, 1980

195. Swartz MT, Kaiser GC, Willman VL, et al: Continuous hydralazine infusion for afterload reduction. *Ann Thorac Surg* **32**:188–192, 1981

196. Cranefield PF, Wit AL, Hoffman BF: Genesis of cardiac arrhythmias. *Circulation* **47**:190–204, 1973

197. Smith WM: Mechanisms of cardiac arrhythmias and conduction disturbances. In Hurst JW, et al (eds): *The Heart*, 7th ed. New York: McGraw-Hill, 1990, pp 473–488

198. Marriott HJL, Myerburg RJ: Recognition of cardiac arrhythmias and conduction disturbances. In Hurst JW, et

al (eds). *The Heart*, 7th ed. New York: McGraw-Hill, 1990, pp 489–534

199. Dubin D: *Rapid Interpretation of EKGs*, 4th ed. Tampa, FL: Cover Publishing Co., 1990

200. Vetter VL, Horowitz LN: Electrophysiologic residual and sequelae of surgery for congenital heart defects. *Am J Cardiol* 50:588–604, 1982

201. Gelband H, Waldo AL, Kaiser GA, et al: Etiology of right bundle branch block in patients undergoing total correction of tetralogy of Fallot. *Circulation* 44:1022–1033, 1971

202. Wolff GS, Rowland TW, Ellison RC: Surgically induced right bundle branch block with left anterior hemiblock. *Circulation* 46:587–594, 1972

203. James FW, Kaplan S, Chou T: Unexpected cardiac arrest in patient after surgical correction of tetralogy of Fallot. *Circulation* 52:691–695, 1975

204. Gillete PC, Yeoman MA, Mullins CE, McNamara DG: Sudden death after repair of tetralogy of Fallot. *Circulation* 56:566–571, 1977

205. Quattlebaum TG, Varghese PJ, Neil CA, Donahoo JS: Sudden death among postoperative patients with tetralogy of Fallot. *Circulation* 54:289–293, 1976

206. Mari DD, Danielson GK, Wallace RB, McGoon DC: Long term follow-up of Mustard operation survivors. *Circulation* 49(suppl 2):46–53, 1974

207. Mustard WT, Keith JD, Trusler GA, et al: The surgical management of transposition of the great vessels. *J Thorac Cardiovasc Surg* 48:953–958, 1964

208. Isaacson R, Titus JL, Merideth J, et al: Apparent interruption of atrial conduction pathways after surgical repair of transposition of the great arteries. *Am J Cardiol* 30:533–535, 1972

209. Saalouke MG, Rios J, Perry LW, et al: Electrophysiologic studies after Mustard's operation for d-transposition of the great vessels. *Am J Cardiol* 41:1104–1109, 1978

210. Champsauer GL, Sokol DM, Trusler GA, Mustard WT: Repair of transposition of the great arteries in 123 pediatric patients. *Circulation* 47:1032–1041, 1973

211. Kyger ER, Frazier OH, Cooley DA: Sinus venosus atrial septal defect: Early and late results following closure in 109 patients. *Ann Thorac Surg* 25:44–50, 1978

212. Sealy WC, Farmer JC, Young WG, Brown IW: Atrial dysrhythmias and atrial secundum defects. *J Thorac Cardiovasc Surg* 57:245–250, 1969

213. Popper RW, Knott JMS, Selzer A, Gerbode F: Arrhythmias after cardiac surgery. 1. Uncomplicated atrial septal defect. *Am Heart J* 64:455–461, 1962

214. Chen SC, Arcilla RA, Moulder PV, Cassels DE: Postoperative conduction disturbances in atrial septal defect. *Am J Cardiol* 22:636–644, 1968

215. Rein JG, Freed MD, Norwood WI, Castaneda AR: Early and late results of closure of ventricular septal defect in infancy. *Ann Thorac Surg* 24:19–27, 1977

216. Hobbins SM, Izukawa T, Radford DJ, et al: Conduction disturbances after surgical correction of ventricular septal defect by the atrial approach. *Br Heart J* 41:289–293, 1979

217. Kulbertus HE, Coyne JJ, Hallidie-Smith KA: Conduction disturbance before and after surgical closure of ventricularseptal defect. *Am Heart J* 77:123–130, 1969

218. Feldt RH, DuShane JW, Titus JL: The atrioventricular conduction system in persistent common atrioventricular canal defect: Correlations with electrocardiogram. *Circulation* 42:437–444, 1970

219. Waldo AL, Kaiser GA, Bowman FO, Malm JR: Etiology of prolongation of the PR interval in patients with an endocardial cushion defect. *Circulation* 48:19–26, 1973

220. Levy MJ, Cuello L, Tuna N, Lillehei CW: Atrioventricularis communis. *Am J Cardiol* 14:587–598, 1964

221. Vaughan Williams EM: Classification of anti-dysrhythmic drugs reassessed after a decade of new drugs. *J Clin Pharmacol* 24:129–147, 1984

222. Roden DM, Woosley RL: Antiarrhythmic drugs. In Wood AJJ and Wood M (eds): *Drugs and Anesthesia: Pharmacology for Anesthesiologists*, 2nd ed. Baltimore: Williams & Wilkins, 1990, pp 461–462

223. Benitz WE, Tatro DS: *Pediatric Drug Hand Book*. 2nd ed. Chicago: Year Book Medical, 1988

224. Park MK: *The Pediatric Cardiology Handbook*. St Louis: Mosby–Year Book, 1991

225. Chameides L (ed): *Textbook of Pediatric Advanced Life Support*. Dallas: American Heart Association, 1988, pp 49–60

226. Gutgesell HP, Tacker WA, Geddes LA, et al: Energy dose for defibrillation in children. *Pediatrics* 58:898–901, 1976

227. Lake CL, Sellers TD, Nolan SP, et al: Energy dose and other variables possibly affecting ventricular defibrillation during cardiac surgery. *Anesth Analg* 63:743–751, 1984

228. Williams WG, Hesslein PS: Cardiac rhythm disturbances. In Arciniegas E (ed): *Pediatric Cardiac Surgery*. Chicago: Year Book Medical, 1985, pp 419–432.

229. Dreifuss LS, Fisch C, Griffen JC, et al: ACC/AHA guidelines for implantation of cardiac pacemakers and antiarrhythmia devices. *Circulation* 84:455–467, 1991

230. Kugler JD, Danford DA: Pacemakers in children: An update. *Am Heart J* 117:665–679, 1989

231. Finholt DA, Audenert SM, Stirt JA, et al: Endotracheal tube leak pressure and tracheal lumen size in swine. *Anesth Analg* 65:667–672, 1986

232. Criley JM, Niemann JT, Rosborough JP, et al: The heart is a conduit in CPR. *Crit Care Med* 9:373–374, 1981

233. Chandra N, Tsitlik J, Weisfeldt ML: Optimization of carotid flow during CPR in arrested dogs. *Crit Care Med* 9:379–381, 1981

234. Bircher N, Safar P: Comparison of standard and "new" closed-chest CPR and open chest CPR in dogs. *Crit Care Med* 9:384–385, 1981

235. Rogers ML, Nugent SK, Stidham GL: Effects of closed chest cardiac massage on intracranial pressure. *Crit Care Med* 7:454–456, 1979

236. Weil MH, Ruiz CE, Michaels S, Rackow EC: Acid-base determination of survival after cardiopulmonary resuscitation. *Crit Care Med* 13:888–892, 1985

237. Bishop RL, Weisfeldt ML: Sodium bicarbonate administration during cardiac arrest. *JAMA* 235:506–509, 1976

238. Ostrea EM, Odell CG: The influence of bicarbonate administration on blood pH in a "closed system." Clinical implications. *J Pediatr* 80:671–680, 1972

239. Katz A, Reuter M: Cellular calcium and cardiac cell death. *Am J Cardiol* 44:188–190, 1979

240. Clark RE, Christlieb IY, Ferguson TB, et al: Laboratory and initial clinical studies of nifedipine, a calcium antagonist for improved myocardial preservation. *Ann Surg* **193**: 719–732, 1981

241. Steuven HA, Thompson B, Aprahamian C, et al: The effectiveness of calcium chloride in refractory electromechanical dissociation. *Ann Emerg Med* **4**:626–629, 1985

242. Steuven HA, Thompson B, Aprahamian C, et al: Lack of effectiveness of calcium chloride in refractory asystole. *Ann Emerg Med* **4**:630–632, 1985

Chapter 24 | Postoperative Respiratory Function and Its Management

Douglas F. Willson

Because cardiac and pulmonary functions are interdependent, pulmonary complications after cardiac surgery in children are common and vexing problems. Multiple factors conspire to increase the likelihood of pulmonary injury perioperatively. The lung may have preoperative abnormalities secondary to congenital circulatory anomalies. Retraction during the surgical procedure and cardiopulmonary bypass may injure the lung mechanically and physiologically. Finally, anesthesia impairs pulmonary function. Any and all of these factors place the respiratory system at risk and necessitate meticulous postoperative respiratory care.

RESPIRATORY FUNCTION IN CHILDREN

Pulmonary function in children differs from adults both quantitatively and qualitatively. For a complete discussion, the reader is referred to standard texts.[1,2] Table 24–1 lists the most important differences and their clinical implications. These differences are more pronounced in infants and small children.

Probably the most notable difference clinically is metabolic rate. Oxygen consumption and carbon dioxide production may be as much as two to three times greater on a weight basis in the small infant relative to an adult.[3] Coupled with a lower functional residual capacity (FRC),[4] infants and children consequently have less respiratory reserve. Airway obstruction rapidly leads to cyanosis.

Lower lung compliance, along with increased chest wall compliance, manifests itself in a greater resting shunt fraction[5] in children (thus the lower Pa_{O_2} in small infants). Infants, particularly, breathe at tidal volumes overlapping closing volumes and are consequently prone to areas of low ventilation to perfusion ratios (V/Q). Normally, however, infants are quite active and are constantly reestablishing lung volumes with crying and movement. Sedation, lingering neuromuscular blockade, or residual anesthetic effects may exacerbate the tendency toward loss of lung volume postoperatively leading to cyanosis and respiratory distress.

A further reason for lack of respiratory reserve involves differences in muscular bulk and efficiency. Small children have little intercostal muscle and rely nearly exclusively on diaphragmatic contraction for normal tidal breathing. They are thus limited in their ability to increase their tidal volume and, in general, increase their minute ventilation primarily by increasing respiratory rate. Additionally, their diaphragmatic musculature has fewer type I slow fibers making them prone to fatigue with extremes of respiratory work.[6]

Finally, there is the obvious difference of size. Size, however, presents more subtle difficulties than just the technical problems of putting small tubes in small airways. For example, with 1 mm of subglottic tracheal edema, the normal infant subglottic tracheal diameter (6 mm) has a 33% reduction in diameter, a 55% reduction in cross-sectional area, and at least an 80% decrease in airflow at constant pressure.[7] The consequences of even a small amount of subglottic edema or injury—such as produced by a traumatic intubation or from a viral respiratory infection—may include croup, wheezing, and an increased frequency of atelectasis. In contrast, such minor trauma or infection in an adult or older child would pose little problem.

The final result of these and other differences in children's respiratory function is an increased likelihood

TABLE 24–1. DIFFERENCES IN RESPIRATORY PHYSIOLOGY IN CHILDREN

Higher carbon dioxide production and oxygen consumption
    Rapid onset of cyanosis when obstructed
Lower lung compliance/higher chest wall compliance
    Lower functional residual capacity
    Closure of small airways during tidal breathing
    Higher resting shunt
Less respiratory muscle bulk and efficiency
    Prone to fatigue and respiratory failure
Small airway size
    Prone to airway obstruction

of complications. The pulmonary system is clearly the most vulnerable organ system in children and it is no surprise that many of the difficulties seen in children after cardiac surgery revolve around this system either directly or indirectly.

PERIOPERATIVE CONCERNS

Many, if not most, postoperative respiratory difficulties can be anticipated because of preoperative or intraoperative events or circumstances. Surgery itself is unlikely to produce immediate improvement and, in fact, may further compromise respiration.

Preoperative Problems

Airway Concerns. Congenital heart disease (CHD) is frequently a component of chromosomal abnormalities or other complex congenital malformations (24–45% of children with CHD have extracardiac malformations).[8] The airway may thus be affected, such as in the choanal atresia/stenosis seen with the CHARGE association (coloboma, heart anomalies, atresia of choanae, mental and growth retardation, genitourinary anomalies, ear anomalies), the tracheoesophageal fistula with VATER (vertebral segmentation, tracheoesophageal fistula, congenital scoliosis, imperforate anus, renal abnormalities, absent radius) association, or the complex of abnormalities seen in trisomy 21. In addition to cardiac disease, children with the Down syndrome have compromised airways because of a flattened nasal bridge, small nose, large tongue, short neck, and generalized hypotonia. These features increase airway resistance, the risk of atelectasis/lung volume loss, and postintubation croup postoperatively. Similar inferences could be made about children with other syndromes associated with CHD.

Lung Disease. Normally, major thoracic surgery is delayed in the presence of respiratory infection or other lung disease. Unfortunately, this is not always possible, as in the premature infant with resolving respiratory distress syndrome requiring ligation of the ductus arteriosus. Similarly, children with large left-to-right shunts and consequent high pulmonary blood flow and pressure may have pulmonary dysfunction from increased interstitial lung water that may impair lung function postoperatively. In both of these examples, surgery must proceed before lung function can be greatly improved.

More problematic is the issue of preoperative respiratory infection. If the average child contracts 5–6 viral respiratory infections in the first year of life and the associated pulmonary dysfunction lasts 4–6 weeks,[9,10] the "window of opportunity" to perform corrective surgery in the first year of life is limited. Most anesthesiologists and surgeons would delay surgery in the presence of known viral respiratory infection. Unfortunately, the fact that the child is incubating a virus preoperatively is not always known. The influence on morbidity and mortality after cardiac surgery is speculative, at best, but the experience of Hall et al[11] of nearly 50% mortality in children with respiratory syncytial virus (RSV) and congenital heart disease is sobering. Those children with lesions involving pulmonary hypertension and right ventricular dysfunction would be at greatest risk.

Owing to the vulnerability of the young child's respiratory system, preoperative pulmonary problems cause great concern. The judgment of when to delay or proceed with surgery is a clinical one, but every attempt must be made to optimize pulmonary function preoperatively. Respiratory reserve is marginal even in normal infants and cardiac surgery alone may overstress this system.

Influence of the Cardiac Lesion. Chronic pulmonary hyperperfusion and hypertension cause pulmonary vascular changes. First described by Dammann and Ferencz,[12] these changes range from mild medial muscular hypertrophy to obliteration and occlusion of much of the pulmonary arterial tree. Types of congenital heart disease associated most often with pulmonary vascular disease are those in which both increased flow and pressure have existed since birth (eg, ventricular septal defect, patent ductus arteriosus, transposition of the great vessels). Such pulmonary vascular changes rarely occur in the first few years of life[13] and usually are asymptomatic. However, as these changes become more prominent (generally in the second decade), disturbances in V:Q matching and right ventricular failure develop (Eisenmenger complex). The more common situation is that infants with large left-to-right shunts have persistence of the fetal pattern of musculature in their pulmonary vascular bed.[14] In either case, pulmonary hypertension does not subside immediately postoperatively and right ventricular afterload may contribute to right ventricular failure.

Children who require ventilatory support preoperatively present a greater challenge. Most of these are children with pulmonary congestion and consequent poor lung compliance who require only a moderate amount of positive pressure to maintain adequate oxygenation and ventilation. These children usually are rapidly "weanable" after their cardiac problem has been corrected. Children with high pulmonary venous pressures (particularly seen with left-sided obstructive lesions) may suffer from air trapping (Fig 24–1) and be difficult to ventilate. Frequently, the respiratory failure is precipitated by viral respiratory infection and begins a cycle of respiratory failure requiring significant ventilator support—placing the child at risk for recurrent pneumonias, barotrauma, and declining nutrition. Surgery is prompted by the fact that the cardiac component is the only correctable aspect.

Nutrition. Nutrition is a major preoperative concern that is often underestimated. Greater than 25% of children with CHD are below the third percentile for weight and height.[15] Failure to thrive is a common problem. More disturbing is the starvation some children undergo in the hospital because they cannot tolerate the stress of feeding or the necessary volumes of fluid required to supply calories adequate for growth. As surgical correction is often delayed arbitrarily "until the child is bigger," at times the children are starved for months and correction of their cardiac lesion is attempted when all else fails. Malnutrition has subtle effects on every organ system in the body. The effects on three systems—immune, cardiac, and respiratory—are most pertinent to the postoperative course.

Multiple studies have demonstrated the association of malnutrition and depression of immune function ranging from impaired cell-mediated immunity[16] to decreased levels of complement and immunoglobulins.[17] Clearly, malnutrition increases the risk of postoperative infection.

The effects on the respiratory system have been recently reviewed by Askanazi and colleagues.[18] Respiratory drive,[19] muscular bulk and endurance,[20] and incidence of pneumonia[21] are all adversely affected by starvation.

Cardiac function may also be impaired. With severe protein-energy malnutrition, the heart is small, myocardial mass is diminished, and the myocardial fibrils show vacuolization and atrophy.[22,23] Depression of cardiac output, frequently with overt failure when refeeding is instituted, is common.[24]

Although all of these effects are seen in children with extreme malnutrition, the effects on most children with CHD are undoubtedly more subtle. However, the implications for the postoperative period are clear. Rapid restoration of positive nitrogen balance is the only solution. Often this means institution of parenteral nutrition immediately postoperatively rather than waiting for enteral feedings to be tolerated.

Intraoperative Problems

As with preoperative issues, intraoperative events or problems may have significant implications for the postoperative course. Some events, such as the effects of cardiopulmonary bypass on the lung, are unavoidable. Less subtle problems, such as cardiac arrest on induction or difficulties with coming off cardiopulmonary bypass, have important effects that are difficult to predict.

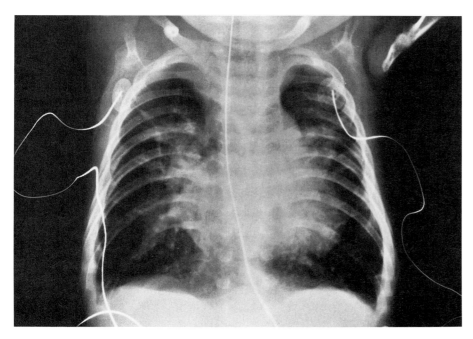

Figure 24–1. Chest radiograph of patient with air trapping secondary to pulmonary overperfusion and hypertension.

Prebypass Events. Induction of anesthesia with achievement of a secure airway is the first step in a sequence that leads to control of both cardiac and respiratory systems via cardiopulmonary bypass (CPB). They are "routine," yet there is an endless variety of things that can—and occasionally do—go wrong. Most of them have significant implications for postoperative respiratory care.

Significant issues in the prebypass period are the obvious concern to prevent hypotension and/or hypoxia. Aspiration of gastric contents, inadvertent main stem intubation, and airway trauma are others. Placement of intravascular catheters is another potential risk. Pneumothorax, bleeding, arrhythmias, and right atrial perforation produce ominous complications that have serious postoperative implications. The importance of each of these events to postoperative pulmonary and cardiac function is clear and should be reviewed on receiving the patient in the postoperative care unit.

Cardiopulmonary Bypass. Multiple studies have documented the deleterious effects of cardiopulmonary bypass (CPB) on pulmonary structure and function.[25,30] Although extracorporeal membrane oxygenation (ECMO) is used to treat respiratory failure,[31] Ratliff and colleagues[26] demonstrated a sequence of changes similar to those seen in shock or traumatic lung injury. The extent of these changes correlated directly to the duration of CPB, with significant morbidity associated with CPB longer than 120–150 minutes.[27]

Whether or not the lung is ventilated during bypass may affect postoperative pulmonary function,[32,33] but most anesthesiologists maintain the lungs on 2–5 cm of positive end-expiratory pressure (PEEP) during CPB. The use of a few large tidal volume breaths when ventilation is resumed should minimize the residual effects of static inflation.

Hypothermic arrest, which allows the surgeon to repair cardiac lesions in small infants in a quiet, bloodless field and without the limitations of venous and arterial cannulas, does not increase postoperative pulmonary complications.[34] In one uncontrolled series, pulmonary function was markedly improved because of a decrease in time on CPB.[35]

Postbypass Events. Weaning from bypass is fraught with additional potential disasters. Reestablishing ventilation means ascertaining that the tube remains well positioned—generally easily determined by observing the lungs directly. More subtle is the possible gradual obstruction of the endotracheal tube with blood and secretions. This usually manifests itself on the way to, or soon after arrival, in the postoperative unit. It is probably a good practice to suction the child prior to moving to the intensive care unit (ICU), as it may be delayed in the ICU by other pressing demands.

Reestablishing circulation is generally a cooperative effort with the surgeon and involves manipulation of volume, inotropes, and cardiac rate and rhythm. The degree of support needed and ease of separation from CPB have significant implications. Poor cardiac function and the need for high filling pressures to sustain cardiac output may necessitate positive pressure ventilation despite normal instrinsic pulmonary function.

Establishing a dry surgical field and achieving adequate chest tube drainage is within the surgical purview but should be noted by the anesthesiologist. Profuse bleeding after chest closure or obstruction of chest tube drainage are surgical problems that may impact upon cardiac and pulmonary function. Arterial blood gases should be obtained before transfer to the postoperative care unit.

Postoperative Concerns

There are a variety of postoperative pulmonary changes that are consequences of anesthesia and surgery and should be expected regardless of the specific procedures. Physical findings, chest radiographs, and ventilator settings should be reviewed early in the postoperative period.

Pain. Pain is one of the first consequences of surgery. Thoracotomy is said to be the most painful procedure,[36] probably because the incision moves and is stretched by respiration and coughing. The natural response is to splint and refrain from deep breathing and coughing to minimize pain. Atelectasis, pooling of secretions, and pneumonia may result. Control of pain is not only humane but is good medicine as it improves respiratory function.[37] Pain control is accomplished with systemically administered narcotics, epidural narcotics,[38] intercostal blocks,[39] intrapleural blocks,[40] lumbar epidural analgesia,[41] and cryoanalgesia,[42] as well as other techniques. A continuous infusion of morphine, 10–30 μg/kg/h, provides satisfactory relief of pain in most children.[43,44] Good pain control by any of these methods facilitates deep breathing, coughing, and early ambulation, all of which may prevent postoperative respiratory complications. A good illustration of this phenomenon is the frequent improvement in weaning or pulmonary function that occurs once the surgeon removes the chest tubes on postoperative day 2 or 3.

Anesthetic Effects. Lingering effects of anesthesia may also have deleterious consequences on pulmonary function. Inhaled anesthetics depress tracheal ciliary activity[45] and thus slow mucus clearance.[46] Inhaled and most intravenous anesthetics alter the ventilatory response to carbon dioxide[47] as well as to hypoxia.[48,49] Incomplete reversal of neuromuscular blocking drugs may further impair respiratory muscle function. Residual sedation may contribute to upper airway obstruction. The decrease in FRC accompanying anesthesia decreases lung compliance and increases work of breathing.[50] All of these effects persist into the postoperative period.[51] The degree to which these effects persist depends upon the length and type of procedure, type of anesthesia, and the condition of the patient.

Miscellaneous Effects. Direct trauma to the lung by compression and retraction, particularly using a thoracotomy approach, may produce large areas of atelectasis in the affected lung. Blood and secretions may obstruct distal airways preventing reexpansion of the areas involved and producing a fertile ground for infection. Aggressive pulmonary toilet and, when possible, avoidance of neuromuscular blockade and oversedation in the postoperative period can facilitate mobilization of these plugs. Surgical positioning during the procedure may have similar untoward effects. Pain control, aggressive pulmonary care, and early mobilization help to minimize morbidity.

Excessive fluid administration either intraoperatively or postoperatively may increase interstitial lung water and have deleterious effects on lung compliance. This may be a recurrent issue as high filling pressures may be necessary in the presence of poor myocardial function to maintain reasonable cardiac output. This is a common reason for inability to wean from mechanical ventilation after cardiac surgery. Often weaning must await improvement in cardiac function and postoperative diuresis.

Reversal of hypoxic pulmonary vasoconstriction (HPV) by the variety of vasoactive drugs used to bolster cardiac function may impair oxygenation. Most of the commonly used inotropic agents[52,53] have deleterious effects on V:Q matching in the lung, although these effects may be counterbalanced by their salutary effects on cardiac output. However, HPV is rarely a reason to modify or change the vasoactive agent but should be noted when using these drugs.

CAUSES OF POSTOPERATIVE RESPIRATORY FAILURE

Except for the simple cardiac repairs (eg, patent ductus arteriosus [PDA] ligation, atrial septal defect [ASD] repair), most children require a period of ventilatory support in the immediate postoperative period. The changes in respiratory function after anesthesia and cardiopulmonary bypass demand a variable interval for recovery before ventilation can be discontinued and the endotracheal tube removed. Any number of factors alone or in combination may contribute to respiratory failure and a systematic approach is necessary.

Nosocomial Infection

Rates of infection in the pediatric intensive care unit (PICU) are higher than in other areas of the hospital.

Reported pediatric nosocomial infection rates are in the range of 3–14%.[54–56] Age, length of stay, and invasive procedures all adversely affect that risk. Although the infection may begin in the urinary tract or central venous catheter, not uncommonly dissemination occurs and respiratory failure may be one of several manifestation. The site, likely organism, and reasonable empiric therapy are given in Table 24–2. A high index of suspicion and a low threshold to begin therapy is the norm in PICUs, particularly in children who have had multiple invasive catheters placed or artificial materials utilized to correct heart defects. Specific details regarding pulmonary infections are discussed later.

Upper Airway Problems

Vascular Rings and Tracheal Problems. Occasionally unrecognized airway problems such as vascular rings or tracheal stenosis present in the postoperative period. Compression of the airway due to vascular rings, either alone or in association with complex congenital heart disease, can be a preoperative cause of respiratory failure requiring intubation and positive pressure ventilation. After appropriate operative correction is accomplished, these children[57] rarely have immediate relief of respiratory symptoms,[57] usually because the underlying trachea is poorly developed. Often their symptoms worsen in the first postoperative week.[58] Such infants may need prolonged respiratory support for stenting of their airway and tracheobronchial toilet (see Chapter 20).

Croup. The most common postoperative airway problem is traumatic croup. Risk factors include (1) age of 1–4 years; (2) traumatic intubation; (3) a tight-fitting endotracheal tube; (4) coughing while intubated; (5) changes in patient position while intubated; (6) operations on the neck; and (7) duration of intubation greater than 1 hour.[59] Because all of the risks cannot be obviated even by meticulous technique, croup occurs in about 1% of pediatric patients.[59] Once it occurs, treatment with racemic epinephrine (2% in a 1:8 dilution administered via a hand-held nebulizer) is helpful.[60] Steroids, although unproven, are often quite helpful.

Vocal Cord Paralysis. Postoperative vocal cord paralysis is a rare cause of upper airway obstruction.[61] It results from inadvertent trauma to the recurrent laryngeal nerve either in the neck or thorax. Unilateral nerve injury causes stridor and hoarseness with the affected cord in a midline position if the injury is complete.[62] Vocal cord paralysis, however, rarely causes severe compromise unless both cords are injured.

Endotracheal Tube Problems. Certainly the most common cause of upper airway obstruction postoperatively is obstruction or displacement of the endotracheal

TABLE 24–2. EMPIRIC* THERAPY OF NOSOCOMIAL INFECTIONS IN THE PICU

Site	Likely Organisms	Reasonable Empiric Therapy	Comments
Bloodstream	CONS,† *Staphylococcus aureus, Enterococcus,* enterics‡, *Pseudomonas, Acinetobacter, Candida*	Vancomycin *plus* aminoglycoside§ or aztreonam or ceftazidime or M/A/P‖	*Haemophilus influenzae* is possible early, less likely later. Catheter-related infections can usually be treated with the catheter in place except for *Candida,* which cannot be cured without catheter removal.
Lung	*Enterics, Pseudomonas, Acinetobacter* (*Enterococcus, Staphylococcus* less common), RSV, influenza, adenovirus	M/A/P or ceftazidime *plus* aminoglycoside	*H. influenzae* or *Pneumococcus* are possible early. True pneumonia requires at least 2 wk of therapy. Do *not* treat colonization as pneumonia. Do a Gram stain of sputum, if you still remember how, or (even better) have someone else do it.
Urinary tract	Enterics, *Pseudomonas, Enterococcus, Candida,* rarely staphylococci; adenovirus in immunocompromised hosts	M/A/P *plus* aminoglycoside	Remove the catheter if possible. Fluconazole, a newer antifungal, is not nephrotoxic and has good activity in the urine but is only active against *Candida albicans.* Amphotericin B is still the antifungal of choice for serious fungal infections.
GI tract	*Clostridium difficile,* rotavirus	Oral vancomycin or metronidazole	Toxin identification without symptoms does not demand therapy.
Otitis media/sinusitis	Enterics, *Pseudomonas,* anaerobes, staphylococci	Clindamycin *plus* aminoglycoside or ampicillin/sulbactam	Tap the ears or sinuses. The "usual flora" is always unusual.
Meningitis	CONS, streptococci, *Candida, Listeria,* enterics, *Pseudomonas; Citrobacter* is reported in neonates	Vancomycin *plus* ceftazidime or piperacillin	Choose final antibiotic based on sensitivities and pharmacokinetics to maximize cerebrospinal fluid drug levels.

* Once an organism is identified, more specific therapy should be chosen.
† CONS, coagulase-negative *Staphylococcus.*
‡ Enterics, *E. coli, Klebsiella, Enterobacter, Serratia, Proteus.*
§ Aminoglycoside, gentamicin, or tobramycin or amikacin.
‖ M/A/P, mezlocillin, or azlocillin, or piperacillin, which cover enterics and *Pseudomonas,* but they should be used in conjunction with an aminoglycoside for treatment of a true gram-negative pneumonia.
(*From Havens PL: Nosocomial infections in the pediatric critical care unit. Pediatric Critical Care Clinical Review Series Part 3:107, 1989, with permission.*)

tube. As obvious as it may seem, it must be stressed because it is a predictable and frequent occurrence in a busy PICU. Meticulous nursing care and provision of adequate humidification are mandatory to prevent obstruction of small tubes with secretions. Nasotracheal tubes provide more secure anchoring than do oral tubes. They are also more comfortable for the child. Daily chest radiographs for review of tube placement are routine and are repeated whenever there is a question of tube position. Despite every precaution, accidental extubation occurs. Appropriate equipment and personnel must be immediately available to reintubate the trachea.

Sedation and Residual Paralysis. Lingering sedation may impair respiratory drive or lead to obstructive symptoms once the tube is removed. Sedation sometimes frustrates attempts to extubate children early postoperatively, particularly if large doses of narcotics were given intraoperatively. Similarly, residual weakness from intraoperative neuromuscular blocking drugs is common. Standard tests for recovery of neuromuscular function (head or leg lift, train-of-four) are helpful in evaluating the child prior to extubation. Even if the child appears strong, however, some intensivists make it a general practice to reverse neuromuscular blockers before extubation (neostigmine 0.1 mg/kg with glycopyrrolate 0.02 mg/kg).

Pulmonary Causes

Pulmonary pathology is rarely a cause of postoperative respiratory failure in isolation. Generally, pulmonary pathology occurs in conjunction with, or as a direct consequence of, the detrimental effects of the cardiac lesion or its operative repair on lung function. Variable degrees of ventilation perfusion mismatch, atelectasis, and derangement in pulmonary mechanics predispose the lung to the development of infection, pneumonia, and, most seriously, the respiratory distress syndrome.

Atelectasis. Atelectasis is common and occurs to some extent in all children postoperatively. More widespread atelectasis leads to persistent shunting and a fertile area for infection. Atelectasis is difficult to distinguish from infection both clinically and radiographically—except in retrospect. For that reason, it usually provokes aggressive investigation and sometimes broad-spectrum antibiotic coverage (with its attendant costs and morbidity). Treatment and prevention of atelectasis include meticulous tracheobronchial toilet, airway suction, and chest physiotherapy.[3] Adequate pain control is important to prevent splinting and allow coughing. Occasionally, persistent, localized atelectasis may require bronchoscopy both for diagnosis and therapy. With the newer fiberoptic scopes bronchoscopy can be accomplished in the ICU without the need for general anesthesia.[7]

It should be noted that oversedation and narcosis may contribute to atelectasis and pulmonary dysfunction. There is often a fine line between adequate analgesia and oversedation/respiratory depression.

Infection

Viral Infection. Postoperative pulmonary infection is a dreaded complication. Viral upper and lower respiratory tract infections are common in all children, particularly in the first year or two of life, so it is not surprising that this is of major importance in postoperative care. Such infections can be devastating in children with congenital heart disease.[11] As much as possible, children should be isolated from others with viral infections both before and after surgery. Surgery should probably be delayed in the presence of a viral upper respiratory infection (URI).[64–66]

Diagnosis of viral illness is difficult in view of the nonspecificity of fever, leukocytosis, and pulmonary infiltrate that are the usual manifestations. Such diagnostic difficulties are distressing as new and more effective antiviral agents become available (eg, ribavirin in respiratory syncytial virus [RSV] infection).[67] There is significant mortality with viruses such as RSV in congenital heart disease.[11] As the attack rate on wards in pediatric hospitals is quite high,[68] it would be wise to consider limiting surgical procedures when possible during outbreaks of RSV.

Bacterial Infection. Bacterial infection is also a significant risk. Many of these children are cachetic, have an injured lung from surgery, and have a perfect portal of entry via the endotracheal tube and other indwelling equipment. The risk of nosocomial pneumonia is highest in children in the PICU.[69] The incidence may reach 60% depending on the length of stay in the ICU and the child's underlying disease.[70]

The pathogenesis of colonization and subsequent infection is clear (Fig 24–2). Colonization with pathogenic organisms occurs rapidly in the intubated patient and is the first step.[71] There is no precise division, however, between colonization and infection—that is to say, at what point the isolation of bacteria from the endotra-

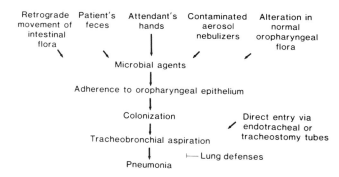

Figure 24–2. Important factors in the pathogenesis of nosocomial pneumonia. (*From Tobin MJ, Grenvik A: Nosocomial lung infection and its diagnosis. Crit Care Med 12:191–199, 1984, with permission.*)

cheal tube aspirate represents a true infection. Fever and leukocytosis are the rule rather than the exception early in the postoperative period and are thus nonspecific.[72] Blood cultures are helpful but are rarely positive even in the presence of infection.[73] More invasive techniques such as transthoracic needle biopsy or bronchoscopic alveolar lavage are more definitive means of diagnosis[74,75] but are rarely done in children because of technical difficulties and attendant morbidity. The usual approach is a clinical one: If one is suspicious of bacterial infection, culture the blood and trachea prior to treatment with broad-spectrum antibiotics. The length of treatment is frequently arbitrary and is dictated by clinical course and results of laboratory studies. The difficulty is that development of bacterial pneumonia in the ICU is associated with significant mortality (over 50% in one adult series).[76] In dealing with children with already compromised cardiopulmonary function and/or intracardiac prosthetic material, most prefer to be aggressive, perhaps overtreating rather than waiting for a nascent infection to become established.

Respiratory Distress Syndrome. The respiratory distress syndrome (RDS) is a spectrum of acute lung injury that can be induced by a variety of insults. The same pathologic process occurs in infants, children, and adults. It has also been termed "noncardiogenic pulmonary edema,"[77] referring to the initial manifestation of capillary leak from diffuse injury to the pulmonary vascular endothelium. The difficulty of establishing the diagnosis in the face of previous cardiac surgery is apparent and probably results in significant underrecognition.

Pathogenesis. Pathogenic mechanisms in RDS involve the lung's response to an initial injury. The activation of various endogenous systems would, at a local level, normally act to protect the lung and limit injury. However, widespread activation and amplification of this response results in diffuse injury.[78–80] Whatever the inciting event, the lung's response can be divided broadly into (1) primary response involving cellular and circulating mediators (eg, inflammatory cells, cytokines, complement, reactive oxygen species); (2) secondary results of the initial response (eg, surfactant deficiency, activation of the coagulation cascade; and (3) iatrogenic effects from supportive measures (oxygen toxicity, barotrauma). Once provoked, a cascade of mediators is loosed severely damaging pulmonary vascular endothelium. Diminished lung compliance, loss of lung volume with consequent ventilation, perfusion mismatch, destruction of pulmonary surfactant, and vascular thrombosis follow the capillary injury. Supportive care adds oxygen toxicity and barotrauma to the mix. The subsequent severe interstitial and intra-alveolar fibrosis is less well understood but appears to be a major cause of mortality.[81]

Etiology. Instigation of this pathophysiologic cascade is prompted by a variety of insults. Postoperatively, shock, infection, and aspiration all precipitate RDS. Recognition of RDS as distinguished from acute changes due to cardiac-related pulmonary edema may be difficult and often is only clear retrospectively.

Prognosis and Management. The clinical picture of RDS may involve only slowly worsening pulmonary status with diffuse alveolar infiltrates radiographically or these changes may occur suddenly and catastrophically. A method to avoid the progression of lung injury in RDS except to prevent the initial injury (eg, pneumonia, shock) is unknown, although several new lines of therapy are on the horizon.[82,83] Current management is directed at treating the underlying cause (eg, antibiotics for sepsis) and supportive care. Ventilatory assistance and improvement of cardiac function with inotropic drugs are routine but nonspecific therapy. The major focus is to support these patients with mechanical ventilation without further lung injury. The ventilatory therapeutic possibilities are discussed later in this chapter. Mortality in RDS is very high, ranging from 40–94%.[84,85]

Pneumothorax. Postoperative pneumothorax is most commonly due to obstruction of chest tube drainage from clot or from barotrauma related to mechanical ventilation. Another common scenario involves a partially obstructed endotracheal tube (particularly on first arrival in the ICU from the OR) where inspiration is not compromised but the expiratory phase is prolonged resulting in air trapping. "Breath-stacking" then leads to dangerous overdistention of the lung and sometimes to pneumomediastinum and pneumothorax. Finally, pneumothorax may also result from inadvertent pleural puncture during central venous catheter placement. Pneumothorax is poorly tolerated postoperatively and should be among the earliest considerations in the evaluation of cardiorespiratory failure.

The incidence of pneumothorax and pneumomediastinum related to positive-pressure ventilation in children was reported by Pollack at 5.6%.[86] Important etiologic factors are the level of positive pressure[87] and the underlying pulmonary problem. The incidence of pneumothorax from obstructed chest tubes is unknown. However, it is not infrequent. Careful attention to patency of chest tubes is important, as is a high level of suspicion for pneumothorax when a child on a ventilator abruptly deteriorates.

Pleural Effusions. Accumulation of fluid in the pleural space predictably diminishes lung compliance and may lead to loss of lung volume and respiratory failure. The most common causes in the early postoperative period include inadequate pleural drainage and/or fluid overload. Later, infection, chylothorax, and postpericardiotomy syndrome must also be considered. Because pericardial fluid accumulation may accompany pleural effusion, cardiac compression may occur as well.

Empyema. Empyema or effusion associated with infection is always a concern. The clinical findings include an exudative effusion with pneumonic infiltrates radiographically. It is most often related to an underlying necrotizing pneumonia caused by *Staphylococcus*, *Klebsiella*, *Pseudomonas*, or a variety of anaerobic bacteria.[88] Treatment is with adequate chest tube drainage and culture-specific antibiotics.

Postpericardiotomy Syndrome. Pleural effusion with the postpericardiotomy syndrome usually occurs days to weeks after surgery and is associated with other signs and symptoms, including fever, leukocytosis, and chest pain. Postpericardiotomy syndrome occurs in 27% of children undergoing procedures requiring pericardiotomy.[89] Pleural effusion rarely occurs in the absence of pericardial effusion and, along with other features, aids in differentiation from effusion due to infection. Occasionally, pericardiocentesis or thoracentesis is required for diagnosis and therapy. However, these children generally respond to medical management with aspirin or, failing that, corticosteroids.

Chylothorax. Chylothorax must always be considered in the differential diagnosis of pleural effusion. It occurs in approximately 1% of cardiac surgical procedures[90,91] and is common in extrapericardial procedures such as coarctectomy of the aorta or Blalock-Taussig shunts.[91] The onset of the effusion may be on the first postoperative day but is more common 2–3 days after surgery.[90,92] It is more commonly on the left but can occur bilaterally or on the right side.[93] The cause is surgical injury to the thoracic duct or its tributaries. The characteristics of chylous effusion are given in Table 24–3. Chylothorax generally responds to conservative therapy with chest tube drain-

TABLE 24–3. COMPOSITION AND CHARACTERISTICS OF CHYLE

Characteristics
  Milky appearance
    pH 7.4–7.8
    Specific gravity 1012–1025
    Sterile
    Fat globules staining with Sudan III
    Lymphocytes 400–6800/mm³
    Erythrocytes 50–600/mm³
Composition
  Total protein 21–59 g/L
    Albumin 12.0–41.6 g/L
    Globulin 11.0–30.8 g/L
    Fibrinogen 160–240 mg/L
  Total fat 6–40 g/L
    Triglycerides above plasma value
    Cholesterol plasma value or lower
  Sugar 2.7–11.1 mmol/L
  Urea 1.4–3.0 mmol/L
  Electrolytes similar to plasma values
  Pancreatic exocrine enzymes present
  Lipoprotein electrophoresis: Present chylomicron band
  Cholesterol/triglyceride ratio <1

(From Teba L, et al: Chylothorax review. Crit Care Med 13:49–52, 1985, with permission.)

age and provision of adequate caloric intake while reducing fat intake to reduce lymph flow.[91] In cases unresponsive to 1–2 weeks of medical management, surgical transthoracic duct ligation or pleuroperitoneal shunting is curative.[94]

Differential Diagnosis of Pleural Effusions. Differentiation among causes of pleural effusion is not always easy and necessarily requires analysis of pleural fluid. Transudative effusion, such as occurs in congestive heart failure, is characterized by a protein content of less than 3 g/100 mL, low lactate dehydrogenase (LDH), and a white blood cell count (WBC) less than 1000/mm³.[95] Exudative effusions have higher protein, LDH, and WBC values but beyond that may be difficult to differentiate. The reader is referred to two excellent reviews for more information on this subject.[96,97] Empyema is identifiable by the elevated WBC, whereas sympathetic effusions from underlying pneumonias are less dramatic. Chylous effusions are often initially serous in the absence of feeding. With feeding, however, they can be identified by their increased fat, cholesterol, and lymphocyte concentrations[95] (see Table 24–3). The effusion associated with postpericardiotomy syndrome is exudative and nonspecific.

Diaphragmatic Paralysis. Diaphragmatic paralysis secondary to direct operative injury[98] or prolonged topical hypothermia[90] of the phrenic nerve causes subtle but serious respiratory difficulties, particularly in small infants.[100,101] The incidence in Lynn's series from the Hospital for Sick Children in Toronto was 1.3%.[100] This injury does not present difficulties until the child is being weaned from the ventilator. One commonly finds a child with a relatively clear chest radiograph and good lung compliance who tolerates low-rate ventilation or continuous positive airway pressure (CPAP) quite well. On extubation, however, the child may develop respiratory distress and, on close inspection, demonstrate asymmetric chest movement. Although the diaphragm is stented with positive pressure, paradoxical movement of the paralyzed diaphragm is prevented. With removal of positive pressure, the affected diaphragm is free to ascend with negative pressure, thus compromising lung inflation with spontaneous breathing. Chest radiographs in the absence of positive pressure usually show elevation of the involved hemidiaphragm, but fluoroscopy or ultrasound may be needed to confirm the diagnosis. Older children and adults generally tolerate unilateral paralysis of the diaphragm, but owing to their compliant chest wall and lack of reserve, infants may not tolerate extubation. Treatment consists of reintubation and assisted ventilation or CPAP until function returns. If there is no return in 3–6 weeks, diaphragmatic plication may be necessary to allow successful weaning and extubation.[102,103]

Respiratory Failure of Cardiac Origin

The most common causes of respiratory failure postoperatively are cardiac in origin. These can be grouped into four categories in accordance with their predominant pathophysiology: (1) persistent (or created) left-to-right shunts; (2) left heart obstructive lesions; (3) hypoxemic lesions, bidirectional shunts; and (4) low cardiac output. Although the respiratory failure is in each case secondary to cardiac dysfunction, each manifests pulmonary signs and symptoms as determined by its specific pathophysiologic features. Additionally, these lesions may act synergistically with the previously discussed primarily pulmonary causes. It may be difficult at times to determine the relative contribution to the resultant respiratory failure.

Left-to-Right Shunts. Persistent or newly created left-to-right shunts may compromise respiratory function by the mechanisms illustrated in Fig 24–3. Increased pulmonary blood flow and/or pulmonary hypertension diminishes lung compliance[103,104] increasing work of breathing and contributing to the development of atelectasis. This is manifested clinically by rapid, relatively shallow respirations and signs of respiratory distress.

Large increases in pulmonary blood flow may cause enlargement of pulmonary arteries and left atrium such that major bronchi are compromised.[105] Lobar atelectasis is more frequent in small infants.[105] Such lung volume loss further diminishes compliance and potentially increases intrapulmonary shunt.

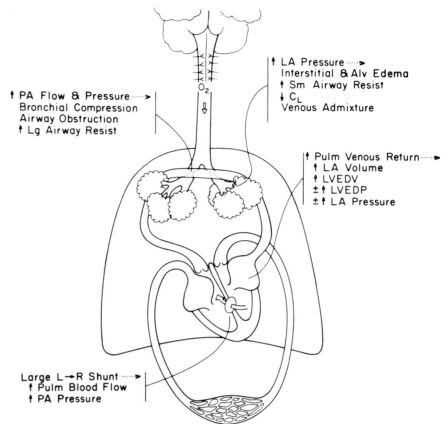

↑ PA Flow & Pressure ·····➤
Bronchial Compression
Airway Obstruction
↑ Lg Airway Resist

O₂
⇓

↑ LA Pressure ·····➤
Interstitial & Alv Edema
↑ Sm Airway Resist
↓ C_L
Venous Admixture

↑ Pulm Venous Return ·····➤
↑ LA Volume
↑ LVEDV
±↑ LVEDP
±↑ LA Pressure

Large L→R Shunt ·····➤
↑ Pulm Blood Flow
↑ PA Pressure

Figure 24–3. In patients with large left-to-right shunts, increased pulmonary blood flow and pressure can obstruct the bronchi. Increased pulmonary venous return and left atrial pressure may increase left ventricular end-diastolic volume (LVEDV) causing interstitial or alveolar pulmonary edema with resultant increased airway resistance and decreased lung compliance. (*From Lister G, Talner NS: Management of respiratory failure of cardiac origin. In Gregory GA (ed): Respiratory Failure in the Child. New York: Churchill Livingstone, 1981, pp 67–87, with permission.*)

A more subtle abnormality is the obstruction seen in the small airways resulting from increased pulmonary blood flow.[107] Because the small airways share the same interstitium with pulmonary vessels and lymphatics, dilatation or enlargement of these vessels may encroach on the lumen of poorly supported bronchioles. The obstruction is worse during exhalation (as the lung deflates and support for small airways decreases) and results in air trapping (see Fig 24–1). Clinically and radiographically, this may mimic air trapping due to asthma.

Pulmonary hypertension and increased blood flow has also been demonstrated to increase intrapulmonary shunting,[108] probably on the basis of atelectasis and pulmonary edema. Such right-to-left intrapulmonary shunting would potentially be improved by restoration of lung volume—as opposed to intracardiac causes of left-to-right shunt.

Common lesions with pulmonary overperfusion include palliative shunts (Blalock-Taussig, Waterston), pulmonary banding (where the band is too loose), or partial corrections (such as extracardiac correction of coarctation without closure of an associated ventricular septal defect). Medical therapy for these children postoperatively is broadly aimed at diminishing the intravascular volume while maintaining cardiac function and renal perfusion. Positive pressure ventilation may be

necessary to restore lung volumes and improve pulmonary compliance. Inotropic support may be helpful to maintain cardiac output at lower filling pressures and to encourage diuresis. Finally, afterload reduction has theoretical appeal as a means of improving forward flow but has been clinically disappointing,[109,110] probably because vasodilators dilate the pulmonary bed as much as the systemic vascular bed. If medical management is unsuccessful as manifested by an inability to wean from the ventilator or provide sufficient calories within fluid limitations, further surgical therapy is the only alternative.

Left Heart Obstructive Lesions. Left heart obstructive lesions are more common preoperatively but do occur postoperatively. Examples include mitral valve obstruction after repair of endocardial cushion defects, residual coarctation after coarctectomy, or obstructed pulmonary venous drainage after the Mustard procedure for repair of transposition of the great vessels. The physiology of respiratory failure is similar to that seen with pulmonary overcirculation but with the added element of low cardiac output. In general, although these patients may benefit from positive-pressure ventilation for their respiratory failure, their clinical course may be determined more by poor perfusion and oliguria than respiratory failure. They may develop respiratory acidosis and metabolic acidosis as well if cardiac output decreases. Medical treatment is limited. Diuresis and positive pressure ventilation may improve the pulmonary status but worsen cardiac output. Inotropic support is routine. Afterload reduction can be catastrophic because decreased arterial diastolic pressure impairs coronary flow and myocardial perfusion. Further surgical correction may be the only alternative.

Bidirectional Shunts. Intracardiac mixing or bidirectional shunting may persist after cardiac surgery or, in fact, may increase by design as with atrial septectomy, bidirectional Glenn procedures, and central shunts. The resultant physiology depends obviously on the initial physiology and its operative modification.

Patients in whom mixing of pulmonary and systemic blood has increased as a consequence of a palliative surgical procedure (eg, central shunts, atrial septectomy) may have increased pulmonary blood flow, decreased lung compliance, and increased intrapulmonary shunting—as do patients with left-to-right shunts. These patients may benefit from therapy to decrease pulmonary blood flow by diuresis and/or positive-pressure ventilation. However, as their arterial oxygen saturation depends directly on the relationship of the pulmonary to systemic blood flow[106] and their cardiac output, these measures may paradoxically improve lung function while having detrimental effects on cardiac function. Consequently, an empiric balance must be struck between their beneficial and harmful effects.

In these children, the relative contribution of cardiac and pulmonary systems to respiratory failure may be so intertwined that it is impossible to separate them, and one tends to amplify the other. Common ICU occurrences such as main stem intubation, obstructed endotracheal tubes, or loss of the airway through oversedation, or accidental extubation are poorly tolerated by these children. Obviously, particular care must be taken to avoid these incidents. Factors that improve oxygenation and respiratory function include (1) increased cardiac output, (2) decreased pulmonary vascular resistance (diminishing right-to-left shunting), and (3) increased pulmonary capillary oxygen content (Fig 24–4).

Low Cardiac Output. Low cardiac output, or true myocardial failure, is predictably the most common cause of postoperative death in children after cardiac surgery.[110–112] When the heart fails to keep up with circulatory demands, pulmonary congestion, hypoxemia, and hypercarbia result. Respiratory failure is secondary to cardiac failure, but therapy must be directed at both systems. Low cardiac output can occur after any cardiac repair but is more common after intracardiac procedures, procedures that require a ventriculotomy, and those with long bypass times. It should also be remembered that low cardiac output can result from mechanical problems

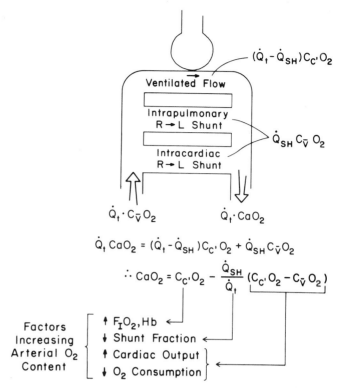

Figure 24–4. The factors that increase arterial oxygen content in patients with right-to-left shunts are (1) decreased difference between pulmonary capillary and mixed venous oxygen content (increased cardiac output and decreased oxygen consumption); (2) decreased shunt function; and (3) increased pulmonary capillary oxygen content (increased hemoglobin or fraction of inspired oxygen, F_{IO_2}). (*From Lister G, Talner NS: Management of respiratory failure of cardiac origin. In Gregory GA (ed): Respiratory Failure in the Child. New York: Churchill Livingstone, 1981, pp 67–87, with permission.*)

such as pericardial tamponade and tension pneumothorax.

The effect of low cardiac output on lung function is similar to that of pulmonary overcirculation. Simply put, increased filling pressures are required to maintain adequate cardiac output, thereby increasing lung water, diminishing compliance, escalating the work of breathing, worsening intrapulmonary shunt, and so on. Measures to treat low cardiac output are covered in Chapter 23 and include judicious use of inotropic and vasoactive drugs and optimization of preload. Positive-pressure ventilation improves heart failure by minimizing the oxygen cost of breathing and improving pulmonary dynamics. However, it also diminishes venous return and increases right ventricular afterload, both of which may have detrimental effects. Because no pulmonary maneuvers can correct the failing heart, the goal is to minimize intrapulmonary shunting and other pulmonary causes of hypoxia while attempting to improve cardiac function.

MECHANICAL VENTILATION

After major cardiac surgery children are generally supported with mechanical ventilation for a variable period of time. Although respiratory support may be life sustaining, it is clearly a two-edged sword. Deleterious effects, including impairment of cardiac performance, barotrauma, disturbed ventilation, perfusion in the lung, and infection, necessitate an awareness of potential hazards as well as benefits.

An exhaustive discussion of mechanical ventilation is beyond the scope of this chapter and the reader is referred to several excellent reviews on the mechanical ventilation in children.[113–116] The commonly varied ventilator parameters, modes of ventilation, and cardiorespiratory effects are reviewed here in practical terms.

Positive End-Expiratory Pressure

Positive end-expiratory pressure (PEEP) is commonly used with all forms of mechanical ventilation. Most children on ventilators are prone to gradual loss of lung volume either from sedation, inability to cough effectively, or the effects of their lung injury (diminished functional residual capacity, FRC). Decreased FRC is accompanied by increased pulmonary vascular resistance, lessened lung compliance, and increased shunt fraction. PEEP maintains lung volumes at end expiration and restores normal FRC. "Normal" FRC is a theoretical concept but has practical applications in achieving optimal or "best" PEEP. A "PEEP grid" can be empirically constructed for a given patient by gradually increasing PEEP to determine that PEEP at which static lung compliance is maximal and shunt is minimal. It should be noted that

above this ideal PEEP lung compliance, ventilation and cardiac output may decrease.[114] There is no reliable clinical method to determine optimal or best PEEP.

Continuous Positive Airway Pressure

Continuous positive airway pressure (CPAP) was first introduced by Gregory and colleagues[117] in their classic article on its use in infantile hyaline membrane disease. Theoretically, CPAP means that airway pressure is always positive. Practically speaking, CPAP generally refers to positive pressure used with spontaneous ventilation, whereas PEEP is used in conjunction with mechanical ventilation (note that it is quite possible to have a patient breathing spontaneously on PEEP and the term *CPAP* could be applied appropriately to most forms of positive-pressure ventilation). The advantages and disadvantages of CPAP are essentially those of PEEP except that allowing the patient to breathe spontaneously (as opposed to mechanical ventilation) lowers mean airway pressure, improves venous return, and improves distribution of ventilation relative to perfusion (Fig 24–5).

Intermittent Positive-Pressure Ventilation, Intermittent Mandatory Ventilation, and Synchronous Intermittent Mandatory Ventilation

Intermittent positive-pressure ventilation (IPPV), or intermittent mandatory ventilation (IMV), is a technique of mechanical ventilation that allows the patient to breathe and obtain fresh gas flow throughout the ventilator cycle. Although the merits of IMV or IPPV versus controlled mechanical ventilation (CMV) are controversial, in the author's opinion, there is no plausible advan-

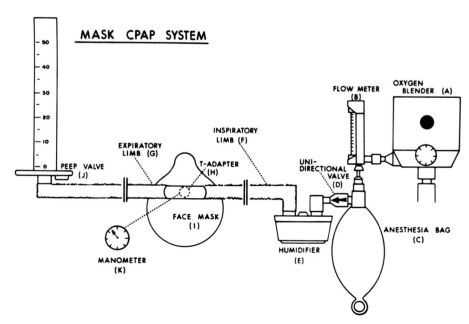

Figure 24–5. A diagram of a circuit to deliver CPAP.

tage to preventing the patient from obtaining fresh gas flow if the patient wishes to breathe above the ventilator rate (as with CMV). "Synchronous" IMV (SIMV), whereby the patient initiates the ventilator cycle within a given time frame (or the ventilator cycles itself), is a relatively new development. Theoretically, this improves patient tolerance by allowing the patient to "set the pace" and avoids the problem of the patient being out of synchrony with the machine. While it sounds attractive, there is no evidence that this is truly beneficial for children.

Peak Inspiratory Pressure

In a pressure-limited, time-cycled ventilator (Bournes BP200, Seacrest, most neonatal ventilators), pressure excursion (PIP-PEEP) and inspiratory time determine tidal volume. The advantage of pressure-limited ventilators is that they compensate for variable leaks around endotracheal tubes. On the down side, as lung compliance changes, tidal volumes change and ventilation may be too little or too much. Particularly as lung compliance improves, there is significant risk of overdistention and consequent barotrauma with pressure-limited ventilation.

PIP influences both ventilation (CO_2 removal) and oxygenation, as well as barotrauma,[118] just as tidal volume does with a volume ventilator mode. With volume ventilator modes, PIP reflects lung compliance (PEEP, inspiratory time, and flows being equal). The newer generations of ventilators can ventilate with either pressure or volume modes, as well as many others. Unfortunately, it is unclear whether the ventilator mode makes much difference (see later section on ventilator strategy).

Inspiratory to Expiratory Ratio

The inspiratory to expiratory ratio (I:E ratio) is another frequently manipulated variable. Prolonging inspiratory time increases mean airway pressure and, in general, improves oxygenation.[118,119] However, prolonged inspiratory time may also prevent adequate emptying of the lung. How rapidly a lung unit fills and empties is a function of its resistance (R) and compliance (C) (ie, time constant, $T = R \times C$). Lung units with long time constants (where compliance is high and/or resistance high), may have inadequate emptying time and develop "auto-PEEP."[118] A potential consequence of auto-PEEP is diminished tidal volumes, increased dead space ventilation, and hypercarbia. Inspiratory time cannot be prolonged indefinitely. Changes in the I:E ratio are not generally as effective as changes in tidal volume, PEEP, or PIP in improving oxygenation.[120]

Newer Modes of Mechanical Ventilation

Because no one mode of ventilation is superior to others, the number of modes of mechanical ventilation continues to proliferate. Among the newer modes are pressure

support ventilation (PSV), assist-control ventilation (ACV), airway pressure release ventilation (APRV), mandatory minute ventilation (MMV), and high-frequency ventilation (HFV).

Pressure Support Ventilation. This is a patient-triggered, pressure-limited mode of positive-pressure ventilation that delivers a preset positive pressure during the inspiratory phase (Fig 24–6). This approach has gained increasing acceptance because it allows the patient to control his or her own minute ventilation, is comfortable because the patient initiates every breath, and allows ventilatory assistance to be weaned progressively. There are several drawbacks, however. Because all breaths are initiated by the patient, diminished respiratory drive is not compensated. For small infants, the demand valves in most adult ventilators are too slow to keep up with their ventilatory rates (despite claims to the contrary by manufacturers). Finally, the small flows required by infants will cause the flow from the ventilator to cycle "off" rapidly once initiated because peak

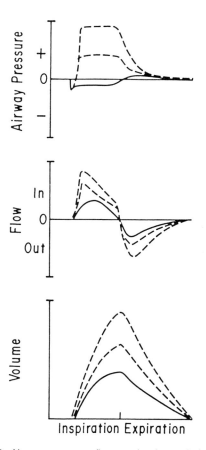

Figure 24–6. Airway pressure, flow, and volume during pressure support ventilation. Solid lines are unassisted breaths, whereas dashed lines indicate two different levels of pressure-assisted breaths. (*From MacIntyre NR: Respiratory function during pressure support ventilation. Chest 5:678, 1986, with permission.*)

pressure is reached nearly immediately. The result is very rapid, ineffective breaths. (In the Siemen's Servo 900 C, this can be remedied by turning down the working pressure of the ventilator. However, then the "SIMV + PSV" mode cannot be used.) Several new ventilators on the market are purported to have solved this problem.

Assist-Control Ventilation. This is a similar concept to PSV. Instead of assisting with pressure (or, actually, flow) when the patient initiates a breath, the ventilator delivers a given tidal volume with each triggering of the cycle. As with PSV, the patient can therefore "set" his or her own rate (and $PaCO_2$), but hypoventilation is not compensated. This differs from SIMV in that there is no set rate. One disadvantage over both PSV and SIMV is that it cannot easily be used during weaning.

Airway Pressure Release Ventilation.[122] This is a new approach that essentially cycles airway pressure (CPAP) between two different levels in the spontaneously breathing patient (Fig 24–7). "Releasing" airway pressure cyclically is purported to augment ventilation, while allowing the patient to breathe spontaneously throughout the ventilatory cycle. It avoids the high peak pressures, V:Q mismatch, and cardiac depression associated with positive-pressure ventilator breaths.

Mandatory Minute Ventilation. This is a "back-up" mode used with other modes that allows the patient to initiate his or her own ventilator breaths (eg, PSV, ACV). Simply stated, the MMV is set such that should minute volume fall the ventilator supplies the needed additional ventilation. MMV obviates the problem of apnea or hypoventilation with spontaneous breathing modes.

High-Frequency Ventilation. This uses rapid ventilator rates (usually > 100 breaths/min) and small tidal volumes to achieve ventilation and oxygenation.[123] Several types of high-frequency ventilators are available, including high-frequency jet ventilators (HFJV) and high-frequency oscillators (HFO). The advantages and theoretical aspects of HFV have been well covered by Drazen and co-workers.[124] Despite reams of literature and a number of commercially available machines, indications for the use of HFV are unclear.

Strategies of Mechanical Ventilation

Regardless of the underlying reason for respiratory support, adequate oxygenation and carbon dioxide elimination (ventilation) are the goals of therapy. Despite major technologic advances in the devices themselves, how a physician chooses to ventilate a patient to achieve these goals remains more of an art than a science—although volumes of "scientific" literature exist on this subject.

Many strategies to improve oxygenation have been studied. The only conclusions that can be reasonably supported are that mean airway pressure (MAP) and fraction of inspired oxygen (FIO_2) are the chief ventilator parameters that affect oxygenation—this appears to be true whether MAP is developed by use of PEEP, CPAP, IMV, HFV, or any other mode[118,123] (Fig 24–8). MAP relates closely to lung volume,[125] and recruitment of lung volume is likely the factor that improves oxygenation in all forms of mechanical ventilation. How best to develop MAP for a given type of lung disease to maximize benefit and minimize barotrauma is much debated.

Presuming that CO_2 production and cardiac output are relatively constant, carbon dioxide elimination is determined primarily by the alveolar ventilation supplied by the ventilator. Although, in the broad sense, alveolar ventilation is directly related to minute ventilation, simply changing the rate or tidal volume does not always improve CO_2 removal. Alveolar ventilation is minute ventilation minus dead space ventilation. Dead space ventilation is not a constant. The dead space to tidal volume ratio (V_D/V_T) is altered by PEEP changes in PIP, changes in rate and tidal volume, and so forth. In general, decreasing $PaCO_2$ is a direct function of increasing the rate or tidal volume. There are situations in which increasing the ventilator rate, for example, may actually decrease alveolar ventilation (such as with rapid rates in patients with asthma or bronchopulmonary dysplasia). Whether $PaCO_2$ should be normalized in situations in which high pressures and/or rates are required is unclear. Respiratory acidosis from mild hypercarbia is well tolerated.

Although the best mode of mechanical ventilation

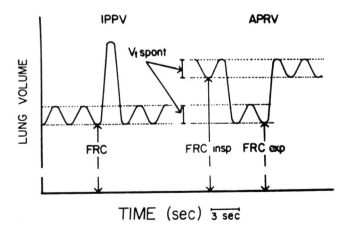

Figure 24–7. Theoretical changes in lung volume occurring during intermittent positive-pressure ventilation (IPPV) (left) as compared with airway pressure release ventilation (APRV). Functional residual capacity (FRC) is greater during APRV than during IPPV where FRC is similar to expiratory lung volume. (*From Stock MC, et al: Airway pressure release ventilation. Crit Care Med 15:462–466, 1987, with permission.*)

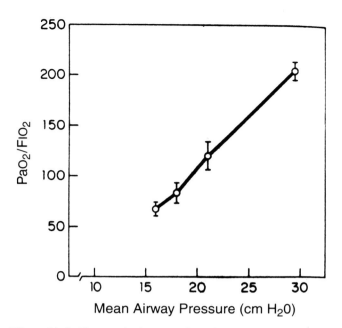

Figure 24–8. Changes in the mean Pao_2/Fio_2 ratio with increasing mean airway pressure (MAP) indicating improved arterial oxygenation. (*From Boros SJ: Variations in respiratory:expiratory ratio and airway pressure waveform during mechanical ventilation: The significance of mean airway pressures. J Pediatr 94:114–117, 1979, with permission.*)

for a given patient is unclear, some guidance can be gleaned from an understanding of the underlying pathophysiology. For example, the use of a rapid rate and small tidal volume is a reasonable approach in infantile hyaline membrane disease. These children have fast time constants (normal resistance, low compliance) and, at least initially, their lung disease is fairly homogeneous. Rapid rates and small volumes would not be appropriate for an asthmatic, however, as their time constants are long (high resistance, fairly normal compliance). Longer ventilatory cycles to allow distribution of tidal volume during inspiration and adequate emptying time during exhalation makes intuitive sense. More problematic is how best to support a patient with diffuse, inhomogeneous lung injury. The key issue is matching of ventilation with perfusion. In a homogeneous lung, convective flow generated by development of negative pressure gradient (spontaneous breathing) or positive pressure gradient (mechanical ventilation) distributes fairly evenly. With most forms of lung pathology, neither the lung nor the distribution of ventilation is homogeneous. Positive pressure does not solve the problem of maldistribution except to the extent that it can reexpand atelectatic areas (often at the expense of increasing dead space) and take over the oxygen cost of breathing. In this circumstance, experience, prejudices, and empiricism constitute the major influences on management.

Weaning and Extubation. Readiness for weaning is determined by a number of factors: (1) Did the child have any preoperative pulmonary problems? (2) What agents were used for anesthesia and has the child recovered? (3) What was the cardiac lesion? Is the child likely to have increased lung water or pulmonary hypertension? Is mixing an issue and, if so, what oxygen saturation should be expected? (4) What is the child's cardiac function now? What are the cardiac filling pressures and are these sufficient to maintain a reasonable cardiac output? Is the cardiac rhythm stable? (5) Were there any events during or after the surgery that are now compromising lung function? How long was cardiopulmonary bypass? (6) Does the child have any neurologic impairment in respiratory drive, muscle strength, or ability to protect the airway that would prevent extubation?

Attempts have been made to delineate rules, pulmonary functions, and other quantitative indicators to predict success in weaning and extubation. However, each child is different, and clinical judgment and observation are frankly more helpful than vital capacities, negative inspiratory forces, arterial blood gases, and the like. In general, if the child is awake and alert, has reasonable cardiac function without requiring high filling pressures, and has no pulmonary disease, weaning is unnecessary and mechanical ventilation can be terminated to evaluate breathing on a Mapleson D circuit (which is always available by the bedside). If the child appears comfortable, maintains his or her oxygen saturation, and moves air well on auscultation, extubation is accomplished. Extubation is done by an individual capable of performing immediate reintubation—and with ambu bag and mask, functioning laryngoscope, appropriate tubes, drugs, and suction at the bedside.

If a period of weaning is necessary, it begins when the patient requires an inspired oxygen concentration less than 50% and less than 10 cm PEEP to maintain adequate blood gases by gradually decreasing the rate of IMV. When the ventilator is at minimal settings, the child's contribution to ventilation is maximal, and spontaneous respiratory rate is less than 40 breaths per minute, a trial of CPAP can begin. During the CPAP trial, the pressure is gradually decreased to 2–3 cm H_2O If the arterial blood gases and clinical condition remain stable, the child's trachea is extubated as described previously.

In the absence of intrinsic pulmonary disease, success in weaning and extubation corresponds to diuresis with return of reasonable cardiac output at moderate to normal filling pressures. Furosemide and mannitol infusions postoperatively speed diuresis. Inotropic support is continued until the child is extubated. Those children whose filling pressures are increased remain on full ventilatory support. There is no wisdom in weaning or extubating a child whose cardiac function is marginal and for whom even a brief period of hypoxia could further impair cardiac function. Every attempt should be made to optimize inotropic support and give the child time to diurese and recover myocardial function. However, the present trend is toward early extubation to minimize the hazards of mechanical ventilation.[126,127]

Hazards of Mechanical Ventilation

The adverse effects of mechanical ventilation include the major problems in pulmonary and cardiac function listed in Table 24–4.

Cardiovascular Effects. Cardiovascular function can be significantly impaired by positive pressure. This depends to some degree on lung compliance,[128] but transmission of positive pressure to the intrapleural space diminishes venous return.[129] Additionally, increased mean airway pressure may increase pulmonary vascular resistance.[130] Right ventricular afterload increases, which is detrimental to right ventricular function. Major increases in mean airway pressure may increase right ven-

tricular afterload to the extent that stroke volume diminishes while end-diastolic pressures and volumes increase.[130] Increased end-diastolic volume affects left ventricular performance as well through encroachment on left ventricular filling by displacement of the interventricular septum (ventricular interdependence).[131,132] Each of these factors may lead to important decrements in cardiac output. In the postoperative period where cardiac performance is already compromised, this is a critical problem.

Pulmonary Effects. Mechanical ventilation has detrimental effects on the lungs. Problems include pulmonary infection and physiologic changes in distribution of ventilation and perfusion, lung compliance, and dead space ventilation. Parenchymal injury or barotrauma is the most disturbing issue. Alveolar rupture from overdistention is a common occurrence from positive pressure[86] and may lead to potentially disastrous pneumothorax, pneumomediastinum, or pneumopericardium. More chronic application of positive pressure has been associated with the development of chronic lung disease.[133]

Other Effects. Less critical are the effects of mechanical ventilation on renal function. Fluid and electrolyte retention are routine and may be related to changes in renal hemodynamics as well as ADH release.[134] Neurologic effects in children are limited to potential increases in intracranial pressure and diminished cerebral venous drainage. Other complications are listed in Table 24–4.

Airway problems are not specific to mechanical ventilation but result from the need for tracheal intubation to deliver positive pressure. These problems were reviewed by Blanc and Tremblay[135] and include a litany of complications ranging from oral mucosal injury to subglottic stenosis. The likelihood of these complications increases with the duration of intubation and mechanical ventilation.

TABLE 24–4. ADVERSE EFFECTS OF POSITIVE PRESSURE VENTILATION IN CHILDREN

Adverse physiologic responses
 Cardiovascular
  Decreased venous return
  Altered pulmonary and systemic vascular pressures and
   resistances
  Ventricular dysfunction
 Pulmonary
  Infection
  Altered ventilation/perfusion ratios
  Increased dead space
  Extravascular water accumulation
  Parenchymal damage
 Renal and fluid balance
  Inappropriate antidiuretic hormone secretion
  Altered renal and intrarenal hemodynamics
  Excessive fluid accumulation
 Neurologic
  Increased intracranial pressure
  Cerebral ischemia
 Gastrointestinal
 Acid-base balance
  Hypoventilation
  Hyperventilation
Airway problems
 Mucosal damage
 Pressure necrosis
 Malposition or extubation
 Partial or complete obstruction
Mechanical failure
 Power failure
 Malfunction

(From Perkin RM, Levin DL: Adverse effects of positive pressure ventilation. In Gregory GA (ed): Respiratory Failure in the Child. New York: Churchill Livingstone, 1981, pp 163–187, with permission.)

REFERENCES

1. Crone RK: The respiratory system. In Gregory GA (ed): *Pediatric Anesthesia.* New York: Churchill Livingstone 1983, pp 35–62.

2. Kendig EL, Cherniak V (eds): *Disorders of the Respiratory Tract in Children.* Philadelphia: WB Saunders, 1983, pp 177–187.

3. Lister G, Hoddman JIE, Rudolf AM: Oxygen uptake in infants and children. A simple method for measurement. *Pediatrics* **53**:656–662, 1974

4. Nelson NM: Neonatal pulmonary function. *Pediatr Clin North Am* **13**:769–799, 1966

5. Mansell A, Bryan C, Levison H: Airway closure in children. *J Appl Physiol* **33**:711–714, 1972

6. Keens, TG, Bryan AC, Levison H, Ianuzzo CD: Devel-

opmental pattern of muscle fiber types in human ventilatory muscles. *J Appl Physiol* **44**:909–912, 1978

7. Woods AM: Pediatric bronchoscopy, bronchography, and laryngoscopy. In Berry FA (ed): *Anesthetic Management of Difficult and Routine Pediatric Patients.* New York: Churchill Livingstone, 1986, pp 189–250

8. Noonan JA: Association of congenital heart disease with syndromes or other defects. *Pediatr Clin North Am* **25**:797–816, 1978

9. Collier AM, Pimmel RL, Hasselblad V, et al: Spirometric changes in normal children with upper respiratory infections. *Am Rev Respir Dis* **117**:47–53, 1978

10. McGill WA, Coveler LA, Epstein BS: Subacute upper respiratory infection in small children. *Anesth Analg* **58**:331–333, 1979

11. MacDonald NE, Hall CB, Suffin SC, et al: Respiratory syncytial virus infections in infants with congenital heart disease. *N Engl J Med* **307**:397–400, 1982

12. Dammann JF, Ferencz C: The significance of the pulmonary vascular bed in congenital hear disease: I. Normal lungs. II. Malformations of the heart in which there is pulmonary stenosis. III. Defects between the ventricles or great vessels in which both increased pressure and blood flow may act upon the lungs and in which there is a common ejectile force. *Am Heart J* **52**:7–17, 210–231, 1956

13. Nadas AS, Fyler DC: *Pediatric Cardiology.* Philadelphia: WB Saunders, 1972.

14. Hoffman JIE, Rudolf AM: Increasing pulmonary vascular resistance during infancy in association with ventricular septal defect. *Pediatrics* **38**:220–230, 1966

15. Mehrizi A, Drash A: Growth disturbance in congenital heart disease. *J Pediatr* **61**:418–429, 1962

16. Chandra RK: Rosette forming T-lymphocytes and cell mediated immunity in malnutrition. *Br Med J* **3**:608–609, 1974

17. Chandra RK: Serum complement and immunoconglutinin in malnutrition. *Arch Dis Child* **50**: 225–229, 1975

18. Askanazi J, Weissman C, Rosenbaum H, et al: Nutrition and the respiratory system. *Crit Care Med* **10**:163–172, 1982

19. Doekel RC, Zwillich CB, Scoggin CH, et al: Clinical semistarvation. Depression of hypoxic ventilatory response. *N Engl J Med* **295**:358–361, 1976

20. Arora NS, Rochester DF: Effect of general nutritional and muscular states on the human diaphragm. *Am Rev Respir Dis* **115**(suppl):84, 1977

21. James JW: Longitudinal study of the morbidity of diarrheal and respiratory infections in malnourished children. *Am J Clin Nutr* **25**:690–694, 1972

22. Smythe PM, Swanepoel A, Campbell JAH: The heart in kwashiorkor. *Br J Med* **1**:67–73, 1962

23. Piza J, Troper J, Cespedes R, et al: Myocardial lesions and heart failure in infantile malnutrition. *Am J Trop Med Hyg* **20**:343–355, 1971

24. Viart P: Hemodynamic findings during treatment of protein calories malnutrition. *Am J Clin Nutr* **31**:911–926, 1978

25. Jonmarker C, Larsson A, Werner O: Changes in lung volume and lung-thorax compliance during cardiac surgery in children 11 days to 4 years of age. *Anesthesiology* **65**:259–265, 1986

26. Ratliff NB, Young CNG, Hackel DB, et al: Pulmonary injury secondary to extracorporeal circulation. An ultra-structural study. *J Thorac Cardiovasc Surg* **65**:425–432, 1973

27. Asada S, Yamaguchi M: Fine structural change in the lung following cardiopulmonary bypass. *Chest* **59**:478–483, 1971

28. Turnbull KN, Miyagishima BA, Gerein AN: Pulmonary complications and cardiopulmonary bypass. A clinical study in adults. *Can Anaes Soc J* **21**:181–194, 1974

29. Rea HH, Harris EA, Seelye ER, et al: The effects of cardiopulmonary bypass upon pulmonary gas exchange. *J Thorac Cardiovasc Surg* **75**:104–120, 1978

30. Gale GD, Teasdale SKJ, Sanders DE: Pulmonary atelectasis and other respiratory complications after cardiopulmonary bypass and investigation of aetiological factors. *Can Anaesth Soc J* **26**:15–21, 1979

31. Bartlett RH, Ratliff DW, Cornell RG, et al: Extracorporeal circulation in neonatal respiratory failure: A prospective randomized study. *Pediatrics* **76**:479–487, 1985

32. Stanley TH, Liu WS, Gentry C: Effects of ventilatory techniques during cardiopulmonary bypass on post-bypass and post-operative pulmonary compliance and shunt. *Anesthesiology* **46**:391–395, 1977

33. Pennock JL, Pierce WS, Waldhausen JA: The management of the lungs during cardiopulmonary bypass. *Surg Gynecol Obstet* **145**:917–927, 1977

34. Bender HW, Fisher RD, Walker WE, Graham TP: Reparative cardiac surgery in infants and small children. Five years experience with profound hypothermia and circulatory arrest. *Ann Surg* **190**:437–443, 1979

35. Barash PG, Berman MA, Stansel HC, et al: Markedly improved pulmonary function after open heart surgery in infancy utilizing surface cooling, profound hypothermia, and circulatory arrest. *Am J Surg* **131**:499–503, 1976

36. Loan WB, Morrison JD: The incidence and severity of post-operative pain. *Br J Anaesth* **39**:695–698, 1967

37. Yaster M, Maxwell L: Pediatric regional anesthesia. *Anesthesiology* **70**:324–338, 1989

38. Shulman M, Sandler AN, Bradley JW, et al: Post-thoracotomy pain and pulmonary function following epidural and systemic morphine. *Anesthesiology* **61**:569–575, 1984

39. Faust RJ, Nauss LA: Post-thoracotomy intercostal block: Comparison of its effects on pulmonary function with those of intramuscular meperidine. *Anesth Analg* **55**:542–546, 1976

40. McIlvaine W, Knox R, Fennessey P, Goldstein M: Continuous infusion of bupivacaine via the intrapleural catheter for analgesia after thoracotomy in children. *Anesthesiology* **69**:261–264, 1988

41. Dalens B, Tanguy A, Haberer J: Lumbar epidural anesthesia for operative and postoperative pain relief in infants and young children. *Anesth Analg* **65**:1069–1073, 1986

42. Maiwand MO, Makey AR, Rees A: Cryoanalgesia after thoracotomy. Improvement of technique and review of 600 cases. *J Thorac Cardiovasc Surg* **92**:291–295, 1986

43. Koren G, Butt W, Chinyanga H, et al: Operative morphine infusion in newborn infants: Assessment of disposition characteristics and safety. *J Pediatr* **107**:963–967, 1985

44. Bray J: Postoperative analgesia provided by morphine infusion in children. *Anaesthesia* **38**:1075–1078, 1983

45. Forbes AR, Gamsu G: Mucociliary clearance in the canine lung during and after general anesthesia. *Anesthesiology* **50**:26–29, 1979

46. Lichtiger M, Landa JF, Hirsch JA: Velocity of tracheal mucus in anesthetized women undergoing gynecologic surgery. *Anesthesiology* **42**:753–756, 1975

47. Larson CP, Eger EI, Muallem M, et al: The effects of diethyl ether and methoxyflurane on ventilation. *Anesthesiology* **30**:174–184, 1969

48. Knill RL, Gelb AW: Ventilatory responses to hypoxia and hypercarbia during halothane sedation and anesthesia in man. *Anesthesiology* **49**:244–251, 1978

49. Hirshman CA, McCullough RE, Cohen PJ, Weil JV: Hypoxic ventilatory drive in dogs during thiopental, ketamine, or pentobarbital anesthesia. *Anesthesiology* **43**:628–634, 1975

50. Done HF, Rabson JG: The mechanics of the respiratory system during anesthesia. *Anesthesiology* **26**:168–178, 1965

51. Alexander JI, Spence AA, Parikh RK, Stuart B: The role of airway closure in post-operative hypoxemia. *Br J Anaesth* **45**:34–40, 1973

52. D'Oliveira M, Sykes MK, Chakrabart MK, et al: Depression of hypoxic pulmonary vasoconstriction by sodium nitroprusside and nitroglycerine. *Br J Anaesth* **53**:11–17, 1981

53. Furman WR, Summer WR, Kennedy TP, Sylvester JT: Comparison of the effects of dobutamine, dopamine, and isoproterenol on hypoxic pulmonary vasoconstriction in the pig. *Crit Care Med* **10**:371–374, 1982

54. Milliken J, Tait GA, Ford-Jones EL, et al: Nosocomial infections in a pediatric intensive care unit. *Crit Care Med* **16**:233–237, 1988

55. Pollock EMM, Ford-Jones, EL, Rebeyka I, et al: Early nosocomial infections in pediatric cardiovascular surgery patients. *Crit Care Med* **18**:378–384, 1990

56. Donowitz LG: High risk of nosocomial infection in the pediatric critical care patient. *Crit Care Med* **14**:26–28, 1986

57. Lincoln JCR, Deverall PB, Stark J, et al: Vascular rings compressing the esophagus and trachea. *Thorax* **24**:295–306, 1969

58. Kirklin JW, Barratt-Boyes BG: Vascular rings and slings. In Kirklin JW (ed): *Cardiac Surgery*. New York: John Wiley & Sons, 1993, pp 1365–1382

59. Koda BV, Jean IS, Andre JM, et al: Postintubation croup in children. *Anesth Analg* **56**:501–505, 1977

60. Westley CR, Cotton EK, Brooks TG: Nebulized racemic epinephrine by IPPB for the treatment of croup. *Am J Dis Child* **132**:484–487, 1978

61. Kirklin JW, Barratt-Boyes BG: *Cardiac Surgery*. New York, John Wiley & Sons, 1985, p 691

62. Parnell FW, Brandenburg TH: Vocal cord paralysis. A review of 100 cases. *Laryngoscope* **80**:1036–1045, 1970

63. MacKenzie CF, Shin B: Cardiorespiratory function before and after chest physiotherapy in mechanically ventilated patients with post-traumatic respiratory failure. *Crit Care Med* **13**:483–486, 1985

64. Jacoby DB, Hirshman CA: General anesthesia in patients with viral respiratory infections: An unsound sleep? *Anesthesiology* **74**:969–972, 1991

65. Dueck R, Prutow R, Richman D: Effect of parainfluenza infection on gas exchange and FRC response to anesthesia in sheep. *Anesthesiology* **74**:1044–1051, 1991

66. Tait AR, Knight PR: Intraoperative respiratory complications in patients with upper respiratory tract infections. *Can J Anaesth* **34**:300–303, 1987

67. Taber LH, Knight V, Gilbert BE, et al: Ribavirin aerosol treatment of bronchiolitis associated with respiratory syncytial virus infection in infants. *Pediatrics* **72**:613–618, 1983

68. Hall CB: Nosocomial viral respiratory infections: Perennial weeds on pediatric wards. *Am J Med* **70**:670–676, 1981

69. Sanford JP: Infection control in critical care units. *Crit Care Med* **2**:211–216, 1974

70. Tobin MJ, Grenvik A: Nosocomial lung infection and its diagnosis. *Crit Care Med* **12**:191–199, 1984

71. Freeman R, King B: Respiratory tract specimens from intensive care patients. Bacterial flora and cytological content. *Anaesthesia* **28**:529–530, 1973

72. Vilota ED, Barat G, Astorqui N, et al: Pyrexia following open heart surgery. The role of bacterial infection. *Anaesthesia* **29**: 529–536, 1974

73. Bartlett JG: Bacteriologic diagnosis of pulmonary infection. In Sacker MA (ed): *Diagnostic Techniques in Pulmonary Disease*, Part I. New York: Marcel Dekker, 1980

74. Zavala DC, Schoell JE: Ultrathin needle aspiration of the lung in infectious and malignant disease. *Am Rev Respir Dis* **123**:125–131, 1981

75. Higuchi JH, Coalson JJ, Johanson WG: Bacteriologic diagnosis of nosocomial pneumonia in primates: Usefulness of the protected specimen brush. *Am Rev Respir Dis* **125**: 53–57, 1982

76. Steven RM, Teres D, Skillman JT, Feingold DS: Pneumonia in an intensive care unit. *Arch Intern Med* **134**:106–111, 1974

77. Ashbaugh DG, Bigelow DB, Petty TL, Levine BE: Acute respiratory distress in adults. *Lancet* **2**:319–323, 1967

78. Kelly J: Cytokines of the lung. *Am Rev Respir Dis* **141**:765–788, 1990

79. Said SI, Foda HD: Pharmacologic modulation of lung injury. *Am Rev Respir Dis* **139**:1553–1564, 1989

80. Sibille YS, Reynolds HY: Macrophages and polymorphonuclear neutrophils in lung defense and injury. *Am Rev Respir Dis* **141**:471–501, 1990

81. Rinaldo JE, Rogers RM: Adult respiratory distress syndrome. Changing concepts of lung injury and repair. *N Engl J Med* **306**:900–909, 1982

82. Ziegler EJ, Fisher CJ, Sprung CL, et al: Treatment of gram-negative bacteremia and septic shock with HA–1A human monoclonal antibody against endotoxin. *N Engl J Med* **324**:429–436, 1991

83. Holm BA, Matalon S: Role of pulmonary surfactant in the development and treatment of adult respiratory distress syndrome. *Anesth Analg* **69**:805–818, 1989

84. Pfenniger J, Gerber A, Tschappeler H, Zimmeran A: Adult respiratory distress syndrome in children. *J Pediatr* **101**: 352–357, 1982

85. Holbrook PR, Taylor G, Pollack MM, Fields AI: Adult respiratory distress syndrome in children. *Pediatr Clin North Am* **27**:677–685, 1980

86. Pollack MM, Fields AI, Holbrook PR: Pneumothorax and pneumomediastinum during pediatric mechanical ventilation. *Crit Care Med* **7**:536–539, 1979

87. Glenski JA, Hall RT: Neonatal pneumopericardium: Analysis of ventilatory variables. *Crit Care Med* **12**:439–442, 1984

88. Finegold SM: Necrotizing pneumonias and lung abscess.

In Hoeprich PD (ed): *Infectious Diseases.* New York: Harper & Row, 1977, pp 309–317

89. Engle MA, Zabriskie JB, Senterfit LB, et al: Viral illness and the postpericardiotomy syndrome. A prospective study in children. *Circulation* **62**:1151–1158, 1980

90. Verunelli F, Giorgini V, Luisi VS, et al: Chylothorax following cardiac surgery in children. *J Cardiovasc Surg* **24**:227–230, 1983

91. McFarland JR, Holman CW: Chylothorax. *Am Rev Respir Dis* **105**:287–291, 1972

92. Kirklin JW, Barratt-Boyes BG: Postop care. In Kirklin JW, Barratt-Boyes BG (eds): *Cardiac Surgery*, 2nd ed. New York, John Wiley & Sons, 1993, pp 195–243

93. Teba L, Dedhia HV, Bowen R, Alexander JC: Chylothorax review. *Crit Care Med* **13**:49–52, 1985

94. Milsom JW, Kron IL, Rheuban KS, Rodgers BM: Chylothorax: An assessment of current surgical management. *J Thorac Cardiovasc Surg* **89**:221–227, 1985

95. Light RW: Pleural effusion. *Med Clin North Am* **61**:1339–1352, 1977

96. Sahn S: The pleura. State of the art. *Am Rev Respir Dis* **138**:184–234, 1988

97. Pistolesi M, Miniati M, Giuntini C: Pleural liquid and solute exchange. The state of the art. *Am Rev Respir Dis* **140**:825–847, 1989

98. Mickell JJ, Oh KS, Siewers RD, et al: Clinical implications of postoperative unilateral phrenic nerve paralysis. *J Thorac Cardiovasc Surg* **76**:297–304, 1978

99. Rousou JA, Parker T, Engelman RM, Breyer RH: Phrenic nerve paralysis associated with the use of iced slush and the cooling jacket for topical hypothermia. *J Thorac Cardiovasc Surg* **89**:921–925, 1985

100. Lynn AM, Jenkins JG, Edmonds JF, Burns JE: Diaphragmatic paralysis after pediatric cardiac surgery: A retrospective analysis of 34 cases. *Crit Care Med* **11**:280–282, 1982

101. Haller JA, Pickard LR, Tepas JJ, et al: Management of diaphragmatic paralysis in infants with special emphasis on selection of patients for operative plication. *J Pediatr Surg* **14**:779–785, 1979

102. Schwartz MZ, Filler RM: Plication of the diaphragm for symptomatic phrenic nerve paralysis. *J Pediatr Surg* **13**:259–263, 1978

103. Howlett G: Lung mechanics in normal infants and infants with congenital heart disease. *Arch Dis Child* **47**:707–715, 1972

104. Bancalari E, Jesse MJ, Gilband H, Garcia I: Lung mechanics in congenital heart disease with increased and decreased pulmonary blood flow. *Pediatrics* **90**:192–195, 1977

105. Stanger P, Lucase R, Edwards T: Anatomic factors causing respiratory distress in acyanotic congenital heart disease. Special reference to bronchial obstruction. *Pediatrics* **47**:760–769, 1969

106. Lister G, Talner NS: Management of respiratory failure of cardiac origin. In Gregory, GA (ed): *Respiratory Failure in the Child*. New York: Churchill Livingstone, 1981, pp 67–87

107. Motoyama EK, Laks H, Oh T, et al: Deflation flow-volume (DFV) curves in infants with congenital heart disease (CHD): Evidence for lower airway obstruction. *Circulation* **58**(suppl 2):107, 1978

108. Lees MH, Way C, Ross BB: Ventilation and respiratory gas transfer of infants with increased pulmonary blood flow. *Pediatrics* **40**:259–271, 1967

109. Linday LA, Levin AR, Klein AA, et al: Effect of vasodilators on left-to-right shunts in infants and children. *Pediatr Res* **14**:447, 1980 (abstr)

110. Kirklin JK, Blackstone EH, Kirklin JW, et al: Intracardiac surgery in infants under age three months: Predictors of postoperative in-hospital cardiac death. *Am J Cardiol* **48**:507–512, 1981

111. Parr GVS, Blackstone EH, Kirklin JW: Cardiac performance and mortality early after intracardiac surgery in infants and young children. *Circulation* **51**:867–874, 1975

112. Berdon WE, Baker DH: Vascular anomalies and the infant lung: Rings, slings, and other things. *Semin Radiol* **7**:39–64, 1972

113. Carlo WA, Martin RJ: Principles of neonatal assisted ventilation. *Pediatr Clin North Am* **33**:221–237, 1986

114. Tyler DC: Positive end-expiratory pressure. A review. *Crit Care Med* **11**:300–308, 1983

115. Sassoon CSH, Mahutto CK, Light RW: Ventilator modes: Old and new. *Crit Care Clin* **6**:605–634, 1990

116. Villar J, Winston B, Slutsky AS: Non-conventional techniques of ventilatory support. *Crit Care Clin* **6**:579–603, 1990

117. Gregory GA, Kitterman JA, Phibbs RH, Tooley WH: Treatment of the idiopathic respiratory distress syndrome with continuous positive airway pressure. *N Engl J Med* **284**:1333–1340, 1971

118. Boros SJ: Variations in inspiratory-expiratory ratio and airway pressure waveform during mechanical ventilation: The significance of mean airway pressure. *J Pediatr* **94**:114–117, 1979

119. Stewart AR, Finer NN, Peters KL: Effects of alterations of inspiratory and expiratory pressures, and expiratory/inspiratory ratios on mean airway pressure, blood gases, and intracranial pressure. *Pediatrics* **67**:474–481, 1981

120. Herman S, Reynolds EOR: Methods for improving oxygenation in infants mechanically ventilated for severe hyaline membrane disease. *Arch Dis Child* **48**:612–617, 1973

121. MacIntyre NR: Respiratory function during pressure support ventilation. *Chest* **89**:677–683, 1986

122. Stock MC, Downs JB, Frolicher DA: Airway pressure release ventilation. *Crit Care Med* **15**:462–466, 1987

123. Boros SH, Campbell K: A comparison of the effects of high-frequency high-tidal volume mechanical ventilation. *J Pediatr* **97**:108–112, 1980

124. Drazen JM, Kamm RD, Slutsky AS: High frequency ventilation. *Physiol Rev* **64**:505–543, 1984

125. Cartwright DW, Willis MM, Gregory GA: Functional residual capacity and lung mechanics at different levels of mechanical ventilation. *Crit Care Med* **12**:422–427, 1984

126. Heard GG, Lamberti JT, Park SM, et al: Extubation after surgical repair of congenital heart disease. *Crit Care Med* **13**:830–832, 1985

127. Schuller JL, Bovill JG, Nijveld A, et al: Extubation of the trachea after open heart surgery for congenital heart disease. *Br J Anaesth* **56**:1101–1108, 1984

128. Suter PM, Fairley HB, Isenberg MD: Optimal end-expiratory airway pressure in patients with acute pulmonary failure. *N Engl J Med* **292**:284–289, 1975

129. Qvist J, Pontoppidan H, Wilson RS, et al: Hemodynamic response to ventilation with PEEP: The effect of hypervolemia. *Anesthesiology* **42**:45–55, 1975

130. Cassidy SS, Eschenbacher WL, Robertson CH, et al: Cardiovascular effects of positive pressure ventilation in normal subjects. *J Appl Physiol* **47**:453–461, 1979

131. Brinker JA, Weiss JL, Lappe DL, et al: Leftward septal displacement during right ventricular loading in man. *Circulation* **61**:626–633, 1980

132. Rabotham JL, Lixfeld W, Holland L, et al: The effects of positive end-expiratory pressure on right and left ventricular performance. *Am Rev Respir Dis* **121**:677–683, 1980

133. Nash G, Blennerhasset JB, Pontoppidan H: Pulmonary lesions associated with oxygen therapy and artificial ventilation. *N Engl J Med* **276**:368–374, 1967

134. Baratz RA, Philbin DM, Patterson RW: Plasma antidiuretic hormone and urinary output during continuous positive pressure breathing in dogs. *Anesthesiology* **34**:510–513, 1971

135. Blanc FV, Tremblay NAG: The complications of tracheal intubation. A new classification with review of the literature. *Anesth Analg* **53**:202–213, 1974

Chapter 25 | Postoperative Complications

Carol L. Lake

The postoperative period is fraught with complications that may be responsible for both early and late mortality and morbidity. Conditions presenting preoperatively or developing intraoperatively are responsible for many postoperative complications, but some complications occur only postoperatively. Problems involving the cardiorespiratory systems are discussed in Chapters 23 and 24. Complications involving other or multiple systems are discussed here. These complications range in severity from occipital pressure ulcers[2] to brain death and include fluid and electrolyte imbalance, thermoregulatory abnormalities, pain, neuropsychologic dysfunction, hemostatic defects, hepatic failure, renal insufficiency, infection, and hormonal changes.

POSTOPERATIVE FLUID AND ELECTROLYTE REQUIREMENTS

Fluid Requirements

The postoperative fluid management must address the presence or absence of congestive heart failure, current intravascular volume status, the adequacy of blood and colloid replacement, the patient's ability to handle a fluid and sodium load, and the effect of cardiopulmonary bypass. Maintenance fluid requirements are based on preoperative body weight and reflect the need for less free water as the patient grows older. Simplified formulas derived from early work show that daily fluid requirements decrease from 100 mL/kg for the first 10 kg of body weight to 50 mL/kg for the next 10 kg and to 20 mL/kg for each kilogram over 20 kg.[3] Another method is to give 4 mL/h for 1–10 kg, an additional 2 mL/h for the next 10 kg, and 1 mL/kg for each kilogram over 20 kg. In addition, loss from nasogastric, rectal, ostomy, and chest

tubes must be added to these basic requirements. Infants on radiant warmers lose fluid through evaporation and these amounts must also be added. Humidified gases decrease the insensible losses as much as 10–15%.[4] Fever increases insensible loss by 10–12% for every degree increase in temperature above normal.

In the first 24 hours after cardiopulmonary bypass, only 50% of the maintenance fluid must be given. Over the subsequent 2–3 days, fluid allotments are increased toward full maintenance amounts. For those procedures not requiring bypass, immediate postoperative fluids are administered at 80–100% of maintenance. Adequate crystalloid or colloid therapy is important to decrease thrombotic events in cyanotic patients, although hemodilution also decreases blood viscosity and flow in acyanotic patients.[4–5]

Electrolyte Replacement

As infants and children have a greater proportion of free water loss to electrolyte loss, their electrolyte requirements are generally simple.

Sodium. It is usually adequate to administer 1–2 mEq/kg/d of sodium in the postoperative period. Many colloid preparations (5% albumin has 145 mEq/L) used for the maintenance of the vascular volume are high in sodium, and fluids for flushing pressure monitoring catheters usually contain sodium as normal saline. These sources of sodium should be considered when calculating daily sodium administration.

Potassium. Potassium administration must be carefully controlled in the postoperative period. Serum potassium concentrations should be monitored frequently in all postoperative cardiac patients. Both hyperkalemia and hypokalemia predispose a patient with an already irritable myocardium to dysrhythmias. Because of the risk of low cardiac output and resultant decreased renal blood

---

Portions of the text originally appeared in a chapter by Drs. James Bland and Jean Wright in the first edition of this book.[1]

flow in the postoperative period, potassium should not be added to postoperative intravenous fluids until cardiac output and renal perfusion are assured.

Respiratory alkalosis, prolonged cardiopulmonary bypass duration, and the use of diuretics all increase the likelihood of hypokalemia. Hypokalemia should be treated by adding 1–3 mEq/kg/d of potassium to the intravenous (IV) fluid. If severe hypokalemia is present and the clinical situation warrants urgent treatment, no more than 0.3 mEq/kg/h is given by continuous infusion through a central venous catheter over 1 hour. Serum potassium is then rechecked. Because of its sclerosing effect on veins and tissue damage if extravasation occurs, potassium bolus supplements should be given through central catheters.

Hyperkalemia is treated by temporizing or definitive measures. Temporizing measures include administration of calcium, bicarbonate, or glucose plus insulin. Potassium moves from the intravascular to the intracellular compartment by a change in blood pH with bicarbonate 1–2 mEq/kg IV. Glucose ($D_{50}W$, 1 mL/kg) and insulin (0.1 U/kg) augment the movement of potassium into the cell. Calcium chloride (10 mg/kg) or gluconate (7.5 mg/kg) opposes the effects of hyperkalemia on cardiac cell membranes. Rapid infusion of calcium should be avoided to prevent bradycardia or arrest.

Definitive treatment of hyperkalemia requires its removal from the patient by ion exchange resins that remove about 1 mEq of potassium per gram of resin given either orally or rectally. Rectal administration is used most frequently in the postoperative period because the greatest sodium/potassium exchange occurs in the colon. Sodium absorption, which accompanies the potassium loss, may result in congestive heart failure. In critical hyperkalemic states, potassium is most effectively removed by peritoneal or hemodialysis.

HYPOTHERMIA AND HYPERTHERMIA

Both hypothermia and hyperthermia are potentially harmful for the postoperative patient. Hypothermia results in peripheral vasoconstriction, increased systemic vascular resistance, sympathetic activation, and shivering. On admission to the intensive care unit, the central temperatures of most patients are in the range of 34–35°C. During the subsequent 8–12 hours, body temperature increases to normal (within 5–6 hours) and often to above normal temperatures of 38–40°C.[6] However, the shivering associated with hypothermia causes an imbalance between whole-body oxygen supply and demand reducing mixed venous oxygen saturation.[7] In addition to the depression of cardiorespiratory function by hypothermia, hepatic and renal function also are decreased. Radiant heat lamps, thermal blankets, and warm environments minimize heat loss and facilitate postoperative rewarming in infants and children.[8,9]

Hyperthermia increases metabolic demands and oxygen consumption, which are deleterious conditions in postoperative cardiac patients. Malignant hyperthermia must always be eliminated first as a cause. Casella and co-workers reported an association between postoperative fever, complications, and increased total creatine kinase activity in a series of children after cardiac surgery.[10]

Fevers should be treated with antipyretics such as acetaminophen while their etiology is determined. For patients unresponsive to conventional antipyretic therapy, cooling blankets, centrally acting drugs such as chlorpromazine, or the combination of vasodilators and a cooling fan may be used. However, care should be taken not to cause shivering, which increases metabolic oxygen demands and carbon dioxide production.

PAIN MANAGEMENT

A rapidly changing area is the management of postoperative pain in children after heart surgery. Pain may be deleterious by causing vasoconstriction, elevated catecholamines, hypercoagulability, immunosuppression, and decreased pulmonary volumes/coughing,[11] and it may even result in adverse outcomes after neonatal cardiac surgery.[12] Postoperative pain must be differentiated from agitation resulting from separation anxiety, hypoxia, air hunger, low cardiac output, or inadequate ventilation. In the absence of hypoventilation or hypoperfusion, agitation responds well to a combination of analgesics, anxiolytics, and supportive care from nursing staff and parents. When anxiety is the principal problem, droperidol, 0.05 mg/kg, diazepam, 0.02 mg/kg, midazolam, 0.07 mg/kg, or lorazepam, 0.01 mg/kg, are helpful. Other alternatives include ketamine (10–70 μg/kg/min) alone or in combination with midazolam (0.4–2.0 μg/kg/min).[13] Infusions of midazolam, 2–6 μg/kg/min, provided satisfactory sedation without drug accumulation in pediatric cardiac patients in Booker and Lloyd-Thomas' series.[14,15] Propofol is not recommended for prolonged infusion in pediatric patients.

Neuromuscular blockers should never be used as substitutes for analgesia. However, they may be useful to decrease oxygen consumption in the shivering patient and to augment ventilation in the patient breathing asynchronously with the ventilator. Each of the neuromuscular blockers has intrinsic cardiovascular properties that determine the proper choice for each clinical situation.

Techniques

The management of postoperative pain in children is in a state of evolution. Table 25–1 provides suggested dosages for the various techniques.

Intravenous Opioids. Intravenous analgesics may be administered by intravenous bolus, infusions, or a com-

TABLE 25–1. POSTOPERATIVE PAIN MANAGEMENT IN PEDIATRIC CARDIAC PATIENTS

Technique	Drug	Dose	Adverse Effects
Intravenous infusion (extubated patients)	Morphine	10 μg/kg/h	Respiratory depression
	Sufentanil	0.1–0.2 μg/kg/h	Respiratory depression
	Fentanyl	1–2 μg/kg/h	Respiratory depression
Intravenous infusion (intubated patients)	Morphine	20 μg/kg/h	Rapid development of tolerance
	Sufentanil	2 μg/kg/h	
	Fentanyl	8–10 μg/kg/h	
Intrapleural	Bupivacaine	Bolus 0.66 mg/kg Infusion 0.25–1.5 mg/kg/h	Seizures if plasma bupivacaine >2–4 μg/mL
	Lidocaine	0.5% solution at 0.3 mL/kg/h (not to exceed 0.5 mL/kg/h)	Seizures
Epidural	Morphine	Loading dose 0.05–0.07 mg/kg Infusion 10 μg/kg/h	Respiratory depression
	Fentanyl*	Loading dose 0.5–1.0 μg/kg Infusion 2–5 μg/kg/h	Respiratory depression
	Bupivacaine	0.1% at 0.3–0.5 mL/h	Seizures, cardiac toxicity

* A combination of a smaller dose of fentanyl with bupivacaine 0.1% at 0.3–0.5 mL/h decreases potential for toxicity

bination. Narcotic infusions have been the routine for several years. Morphine, 0.05–0.1 mg/kg, or fentanyl, 2 μg/kg, are useful in bolus doses. Infusions of either morphine or fentanyl are advantageous in children in whom hypertension or agitation would stress newly sutured anastomoses or increase postoperative bleeding. Safe and effective infusions of morphine are 10–30 μg/kg/h,[16] fentanyl, 0.3 μg/kg/h after a loading dose of 35 μg/kg, and sufentanil, 2 μg/kg/h. Because of the prolonged elimination half-life of morphine in newborns compared with older children, infusions over 10 μg/kg/h should be administered cautiously to this age group.[17]

Intravenous patient-controlled analgesia (PCA) can be effectively used in children at age 5 or younger if the child can differentiate painful stimuli and is coordinated enough to play video games. Bolus doses of morphine, 0.025 mg/kg, are given on demand with a lockout interval of 10 minutes between doses. An alternative is continuous infusion of a smaller dose (morphine, 0.015 mg/kg/h) with smaller demand boluses of 0.015 mg/kg.

Regional Blocks

Intercostal Nerve Blocks. For children undergoing thoracotomy, intercostal nerve blocks performed at the time of surgery or in the postoperative period provide significant analgesia. As in adults, plasma concentrations of the local anesthetic bupivacaine, 2–4 mg/kg, placed in the intercostal space of children indicate rapid absorption (peak concentrations in 5–15 minutes).[18] In addition, the volume of distribution of intercostal bupivacaine is larger and the clearance faster in children than in adults.[18]

Intrapleural Catheters. Intrapleural 20-gauge catheters placed via an 18-gauge Tuohy needle posteriorly through the intercostal space immediately below the thoracotomy

incision provide analgesia with either boluses or infusions of local anesthetics into the intrapleural cavity. Bolus doses of 0.66 mg/kg of 0.25% bupivacaine followed by 0.25–1.5 mg/kg/h infusions have been used successfully in children after repair of aortic coarctation.[19] These doses maintained arterial plasma bupivacaine concentrations at less than 2–4 μg/mL in most children, the reported range for central nervous system toxicity. Agarwal and co-workers reported a child who developed seizures at a bupivacaine level over 5 μg/mL during intrapleural infusion after thoracotomy for lung biopsy.[20]

Epidural Blocks. Because lumbar or thoracic epidural catheter placement is technically more challenging and associated with potential dural puncture or nerve injury, postoperative epidural analgesia in children less than 10 years of age is often provided via epidural catheters placed in the caudal canal and threaded cephalad to lumbar or thoracic regions.[21,22] Because spread of local anesthetic or analgesic can be assumed to be symmetric from the tip of the catheter, Gunter and co-workers calculated a loading dose of bupivacaine to be 0.05 × weight (kg) × number of segments to be blocked. An infusion of 0.175% bupivacaine with 1:200,000 epinephrine at 0.15 mL/kg/h provided satisfactory postoperative analgesia in children undergoing thoracic procedures, including ligation of patient ductus arteriosus.[21]

Bolus doses of 2.5 mg/kg and continuous infusions of 1.25–2.5 mg/kg bupivacaine are commonly used. These doses provide adequate analgesia without attaining toxic levels of 4 μg/mL.[23] However, the elimination half-life and volume of distribution of bupivacaine are greater in infants than in children owing to increased serum protein binding with aging.[24,25] Seizure activity in children during bupivacaine infusions at 1.25–2.5 mg/kg/h via a caudally placed epidural catheter were reported by Agarwal, McCloskey and colleagues.[20,26] Thus, McCloskey and colleagues suggest the use of lower doses for bupivacaine epidural infusions: 0.2–0.4 mg/kg/h in infants, and 0.2–0.75 mg/kg/h in children.[26] Because most of the studies of postoperative epidural analgesia are in children undergoing noncardiac surgery, the use of reduced doses of local anesthetics may be especially appropriate in children with congenital heart disease.

Morphine, in bolus doses of 0.07 mg/kg diluted to 3–10 mL, has been administered into the caudal canal to provide postoperative analgesia in thoracic and other surgical procedures.[27] Urinary retention was the most common complication (50% of children) of this technique in Valley and Bailey's series,[27] but vomiting was more common in Attia et al's series.[28] Pruritus[27,28] and excessive sedation also occurred. Attia and co-workers also reported a decreased slope in the ventilatory response to carbon dioxide in children given epidural morphine after noncardiac surgery.[28] However, minute ventilation, tidal volume, and rate were unaffected. In a dose-response study of children receiving 0.033, 0.067, and 0.10 mg/kg of caudal epidural morphine after lower abdominal procedures, Krane and co-workers noted a similar frequency and intensity of side effects with all doses but a longer duration of action with the 0.10 mg/kg dose.[29] Epidural sufentanil, 0.75 μg/kg, produces rapid-onset (3 minutes) but short-duration (∼ 3 hours) analgesia in children after noncardiac surgery.[30] The incidence and severity of side effects was similar to that seen with morphine in noncardiac pediatric patients, although drowsiness was the most common side effect.[28,30]

Rosen and co-workers described administration of caudal epidural morphine, 0.075 mg/kg, to children with normal hemostatic function after cardiac surgery by single injections, continuous infusions, or PCA.[31] No respiratory depression or pruritus occurred in their series. Only 4 of 16 patients had nausea. Urinary retention was not a problem owing to indwelling Foley catheters. However, pruritus was a common complaint after epidural morphine, which was reported in 88% of children in Dalen et al's series.[32]

MANAGEMENT OF COAGULATION ABNORMALITIES

Postoperative Bleeding

The approach to the child who has excessive postoperative bleeding includes knowledge of the classic pathways of hemostasis (Fig 25–1), points in the pathways that have been altered by the effects of the surgical procedure, the effect of cardiopulmonary bypass on coagulation proteins, and subsequent pharmacologic interventions. Bleeding may result from preexisting coagulopathies, particularly in cyanotic children with hematocrit values above 70%.[33–36] Inadequate reversal of

heparin and damage to or removal of clotting factors and platelets by the oxygenator and cardiotomy suction are part of the differential diagnosis. Use of blood from an autotransfusion system may cause dilutional thrombocytopenia and reduced clotting factors. The principal differential diagnosis is between hemostatic defects and inadequate surgical hemostasis.

Measurements of the activated clotting time (ACT), prothrombin time (PT), activated partial thromboplastin time (PTT), and platelet count are the initial step. If cardiopulmonary bypass was used and the patient was anticoagulated with heparin, the ACT should be returned to preoperative control levels. Titration of protamine to the remaining heparin activity decreases postoperative bleeding by 50%.[37] Neutralization of the heparin is documented by manual protamine titration or automated titration using the commercially available Hemochron (International Technidyne, Edison, NJ) or Hepcon (HemoTec, Englewood, CO) system. The ACT and heparin blood levels do not correlate well owing to the variability of antithrombin III levels.[38] However, ACT does correlate with heparin activity.

Protamine is a weaker anticoagulant than heparin and prolongs the PTT, although the thrombin time remains normal. Therefore, the thrombin time, in conjunction with the PTT, is useful to discriminate between inadequate protamine administration and protamine overdose. Other more specific tests, such as PT and platelet count, should be performed if bleeding persists after adequate heparin neutralization. Fibrinogen concentrations, clot retraction, fibrin degradation products, individual factor assays, and template bleeding time may be needed as the workup progresses. If the coagulation profile is normal but bleeding persists, particularly from only one chest drainage tube, surgical bleeding is the most likely cause.

Indications for Reoperation. Guidelines for mediastinal reexploration in pediatric patients are indicated in Table 25–2. Compulsory reoperation is indicated when the rate of bleeding is greater than 5% of the patient's blood volume per hour for more than 3 hours. Failure to reexplore in a timely fashion may risk cardiac tamponade or, at least, excessive and unnecessary administration of blood and blood products.

Blood Product Administration. The optimal blood product in the immediate postoperative period in children with congenital cardiac disease is unclear. After cardiopulmonary bypass, partial thromboplastin time and prothrombin time are commonly prolonged. Manno and co-workers compared transfusion with very fresh whole blood less than 6 hours old and stored at room temperature, whole blood 24–48 hours old, and reconstituted blood cells, platelets, and fresh frozen plasma in children undergoing open heart surgery with cardiopulmonary by-

INTRINSIC SYSTEM

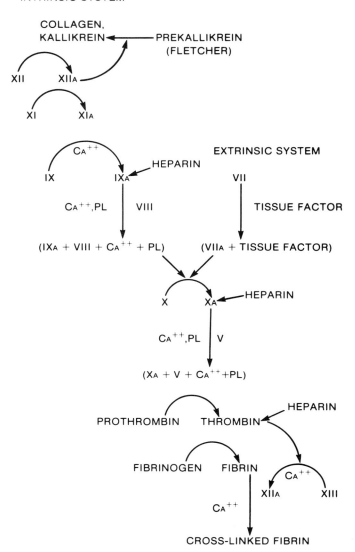

Figure 25–1. The extrinsic (tissue) and intrinsic pathways of hemostasis are a cascade of enzymatic reactions. The points at which heparin interferes with the clotting process are indicated. Roman numerals indicate clotting factors. PL, platelets; Ca^{++} (Ca^{2+}), calcium ion; A, activated. (*From Lake CL: Cardiovascular Anesthesia. New York: Springer-Verlag, 1985, p 367, with permission.*)

pass.[39] Postoperative blood loss was greatest in patients receiving reconstituted blood and least in those receiving 24- to 48-hour-old whole blood. Platelet aggregation responses were most reduced and prothrombin and activated partial thromboplastin times more prolonged in patients receiving reconstituted blood. In general, blood losses were comparable in patients receiving either very fresh whole blood or 24- to 48-hour-old whole blood. Thus, the use of completely screened (for infection), refrigerated 24- to 48-hour-old whole blood appears preferable for general postoperative transfusions. Component therapy, as described below, is indicated to replace erythrocytes or deficient factors.

Packed Cells. Blood components rather than whole blood are now used almost exclusively in transfusion therapy. Banked whole blood loses factor V, factor VIII,

2,3-diphosphoglycerate, and platelets during storage. The depletion is more severe when blood is preserved with citrate phosphate dextrose-adenine and stored for 35 days. Therefore, red cells are administered only to increase the oxygen-carrying capacity of the blood. Replacement of packed erythrocytes is usually performed in 10–20 mL/kg amounts in addition to milliliter-for-milliliter replacement of chest and mediastinal drainage with packed cells in the immediate postoperative period.

Prolonged hemolysis may occur in some patients after corrective cardiac surgery. This phenomenon occurs most frequently after the insertion of prosthetic valve grafts, and conduits.[40] Hemoglobin in serum or urine, decreased haptoglobin, and decreased red cell survival all suggest hemolytic anemia. Postoperative hemolytic anemia may be acute, chronic, or delayed

TABLE 25–2. GUIDELINES FOR REOPERATION FOR BLEEDING IN PEDIATRIC PATIENTS

	Blood Loss as % of Total Blood Volume	Weight (kg)	3	6	10	20	30	50
		Blood Volume (mL)	225	510	850	1600	2250	3750
Blood loss (mL) In any 1 hr	10		25	50	85	160	225	375
In any 2 consecutive hours	8		20	40	70	130	180	300
In any 3 consecutive hours	6		15	30	50	95	135	225
In any 4 consecutive hours	20		50	100	170	320	450	750

(*From Stark J: Postoperative care. In Stark J, De Laval M (eds): Surgery for Congenital Heart Defects. New York: Grune & Stratton, 1983, p 157, with permission.*)

(beginning long after discharge). Occasionally, the hemolysis may be so severe as to require removal of the synthetic material and replacement with pericardium or other natural materials.

Plasma. Fresh frozen plasma is administered to replenish depleted clotting factors. It contains all of the coagulation factors at levels of activity similar to those of normal plasma. Although it may be indicated in patients with multiple hemostatic defects, those with hepatic dysfunction who are bleeding, and massively transfused patients with factor deficiencies causing coagulopathy, prophylactic administration has not been demonstrated to decrease transfusion requirements in adult cardiac surgical patients.[41] When fresh frozen plasma is required, the initial therapeutic dose is 10–15 mL/kg.[42]

Platelets. Adequate numbers and function of platelets must be present to ensure hemostasis. Thrombocytopenia and platelet abnormalities occur for a variety of reasons after cardiopulmonary bypass. Patients who have had passive congestion of the liver and spleen from congestive heart failure or liver disease may sequester platelets in both organs. Non–blood-containing solutions used to prime the oxygenator may result in dilutional thrombocytopenia at the end of bypass. Dilutional thrombocytopenia is the most common cause of thrombocytopenia after multiple transfusions.[43] The presence of heparin prevents platelet aggregation and produces thrombocytopenia.[44] Even after platelet transfusions in patients who have undergone cardiopulmonary bypass, platelet aggregation and platelet plug formation may be significantly abnormal even if supposedly normal platelets are transfused.[45]

When indicated, platelets can be administered as individual units, or in "hyperpacked" units, which reduces the volume of fluid that must be given to infants or patients requiring fluid restriction. Hyperpacked platelet units concentrate 1 unit of platelets into 10 mL of volume. It is essential to restore both platelet function and numbers of platelets. Platelet transfusions are indicated for acute thrombocytopenia to less than 60,000/mm^3, but may be clinically indicated for higher platelet counts if platelet function is reduced. Platelet transfusion should be administered slowly as they may be associated with transfusion reactions. Patients who have had previous transfusion reactions and probably those who are hemodynamically unstable should be pretreated with H$_1$ and H$_2$ blockers and acetaminophen prior to platelet transfusion. Administration of 0.2 U/kg of regular platelet packs should increase the platelet count by 100,000/mm^3.

Autotransfused Blood (Direct and Chest Tube). Autologous blood transfusion systems reduce the patient's exposure to blood products but do have certain small, predictable complications. Red cell lysis, heparin anticoagulation, hemodilution, and removal of clotting factors or platelets occur during blood salvage and reinfusion. Techniques similar to those commonly employed in adults also are used in children, including preoperative autologous blood donations, acute normovolemic hemodilution, intraoperative salvage, and blood processing.[46] The volumes of blood collected preoperatively or salvaged perioperatively, however, are smaller in children and the present equipment is less efficient for pediatric use. A detailed discussion of the methods and equipment is beyond the scope of this chapter and the reader is referred to the review article by Stehling.[47] However, the use of the Haemonetics Cell Saver system has been shown actually to increase blood loss in adult patients during cardiac surgery, probably as a consequence of decreased platelet aggregation.[48]

METHODS TO REDUCE PERIOPERATIVE BLEEDING

Pharmacologic Therapy

Aprotinin. Aprotinin is an inhibitor of fibrinolysis, thrombin and fibrinogen receptors, and platelet aggregation and activation. It also improves the relations between platelets and the microvasculature. Although it is not currently approved for enhancing hemostasis in the United States, studies elsewhere suggest that it decreases blood loss and transfusion requirements in adult cardiac surgical patients.[49,50]

The activity of aprotinin is expressed as either kallikrein-inactivating units (KIU) or milligrams of protein where 1 mg equals 7143 KIU. Aprotinin therapy in children with body surface areas over 1.16 m^2 is usually initiated at adult doses of 2×10^6 KIU prior to cardiopulmonary bypass and continued with infusions of 0.5×10^6 KIU throughout surgery. An additional bolus of 1×10^6 KIU is added to the prime volume of the extracorporeal circuit in adult patients to compensate for the expected hemodilution. In children whose body surface areas are less than 1.16 m^2, a dose of 240 mg/m^2 is given as the loading dose and the dose added to the extracorporeal circuit with an infusion maintained at 56 mg/m^2/h throughout the perioperative period.[51] The desired plasma aprotinin concentration is 200 KIU/mL.[51] The use of hemofiltration systems during cardiopulmonary bypass decreases plasma aprotinin concentrations by adherence of aprotinin to the filters and actual filtrations of aprotinin.[51]

Despite the lack of adverse responses to aprotinin in adults,[52,55] there is one report of a severe anaphylactic reaction in a 3.5-year-old child receiving aprotinin prior to cardiac surgery.[53] However, the protein is of bovine origin. In addition, the artifactual increase in activated clotting time (ACT) necessitates maintenance of ACT at greater than 750 seconds to ensure adequate anticoagulation during cardiopulmonary bypass.[54] Although aprotinin is selectively absorbed by renal tissues, it does not have deleterious effects on renal function.[52,55]

Desmopressin. Desmopressin, 1-deamino–8-D-arginine vasopressin, is a synthetic vasopressin that increases factor VIII von Willebrand (VIIIvWF), factor VIII coagulant (VIIIc), and factor VIII–related antigen (VIIIr:Ag) activity by release from storage sites. Doses of 0.3 μg/kg are effective within 10 minutes of infusion and peak in 35 minutes in patients with type I von Willebrand's disease or mild factor VIII deficiency. The elimination half-life is 2.5–4.5 hours. Although initial studies suggested that desmopressin reduced blood loss in cardiac surgical patients,[56,57] subsequent studies failed to confirm these benefits.[58] Seear and co-workers found no differences in postoperative blood loss, bleeding time, or other coagulation tests in children given desmopressin after cardiac surgery.[59] These results were further confirmed by Sarraccino and co-workers.[60]

In children undergoing repair of atrial septal defects, ventricular septal defects, tricuspid atresia, or univentricular heart, Turner-Gomes and co-workers noted that both the antigenic (vWF:Ag) and biologic (vWF:rist) activity of von Willebrand factor increased and antithrombin III decreased after cardiopulmonary bypass.[61] These changes are likely to predispose to platelet aggregation and thrombus formation alone, suggesting that desmopressin might be detrimental in children with congenital heart disease. In addition, other risks of desmopressin include hypotension, decreased systemic vascular resistance,[62] and seizures secondary to hyponatremia.[63]

ε-Aminocaproic Acid. ε-Aminocaproic acid is an inhibitor of fibrinolysis by binding to plasmin and preventing breakdown of fibrinogen by plasmin. It is given in an intravenous loading dose of 100–150 mg/kg followed by an infusion of 10–15 mg/kg/h. These doses produce effective plasma concentrations of 13 mg/dL with an elimination half-life of 80 minutes. A nonrandomized and unblinded study by Sterns and colleagues demonstrated decreased chest tube blood loss with ε-aminocaproic acid given immediately after discontinuation of cardiopulmonary bypass and before protamine administration.[64] Although localized and generalized fibrinolysis may accompany cardiopulmonary bypass, McClure and co-workers were unable to demonstrate a reduction in blood loss in cyanotic children undergoing corrective cardiac surgery with cardiopulmonary bypass using a randomized, double-blind technique.[65] Studies in adults suggest that ε-aminocaproic acid therapy slightly decreases postoperative bleeding after cardiac surgery.[66]

Tranexaminic Acid. Tranexaminic acid, another inhibitor of fibrinolysis, provides more intense and sustained antifibrinolytic action than ε-aminocaproic acid. Horrow and co-workers demonstrated decreased blood loss and need for fresh-frozen plasma in adult cardiac surgical patients given 10 mg/kg of tranexaminic acid followed by an infusion of 1 mg/kg for 10 hours after cardiac surgery.[67] Although tranexaminic acid has been given to children undergoing other types of surgical procedures, its use in children undergoing cardiac surgery has not been reported.

Use of PEEP

Several studies have examined the use of positive endexpiratory pressure to decrease postoperative bleeding after cardiac surgery.[68,69] Hoffman and others felt that small amounts of PEEP (5 cm) applied prophylactically did not affect postoperative bleeding but that larger amounts were effective in controlling bleeding in those patients having massive postoperative hemorrhage.[69] Neither of these studies included children and, therefore, extrapolation of their data to children cannot be made.

HEPATIC DYSFUNCTION

Postoperative liver dysfunction, demonstrated by clinical jaundice, elevations of liver enzymes, and coagulation disturbances, occurs in as many as 23% of adult patients after cardiac surgery.[70] Several factors contribute to this complication. Long periods of cardiopulmonary bypass damage erythrocytes and add to the bilirubin load of the liver. Other important factors in the development of jaundice are the presence and severity of right heart failure, hypotension, hypoxemia, and the amount of blood transfused.

Similar factors are applicable to the pediatric cardiac surgical population. Jenkins et al reported a series of 11 children, 6 after Fontan procedures, who developed hepatic failure in association with low cardiac output and increased central venous pressures.[71] Matsuda and colleagues analyzed these and other factors in children undergoing Fontan procedures.[72] There was a positive correlation of low cardiac output, low urine output, and increased central venous pressure with a liver dysfunction score derived from abnormalities in total bilirubin, prothrombin time, and alanine aminotransferase.

Postoperative hepatic dysfunction is usually transient and self-limited. Transient elevation of serum bilirubin, alkaline phosphatase, and liver enzymes alanine aminotransferase (ALT, SGPT) or aspartate aminotransferase (AST, SGPT) occur within the first 3 days postoperatively and normalize by 1 week. Jaundice occurring later is associated with low cardiac output or congestive failure. Frequent analysis of liver enzymes, bilirubin, albumin, and alkaline phosphatase are necessary to monitor hepatic function in these patients. Careful attention to electrolytes, metabolism of drugs dependent on hepatic breakdown, avoidance of hypoglycemia, and maintenance of hemostatic function are essential to management of children with hepatic failure. In Jenkins' series, hepatic failure had a 45% mortality rate.[71]

RENAL DYSFUNCTION

Preexisting renal disease is unusual in the pediatric population. Most children develop acute renal failure (ARF) in the intensive care unit secondary to other disease processes or complications of major surgery. However, children with trisomy 21, trisomy 18, the VATER (vertebral segmentation, tracheoesophageal fistula, congenital scoliosis, imperforate anus, renal abnormalities, absent radius) syndrome, Turner syndrome, the Rubinstein-Taybi syndrome, and the fetal alcohol syndrome should be evaluated preoperatively for renal anomalies. A simple preoperative assessment by palpation of the kidneys on physical examination, urinalysis, renal ultrasound, and visualization of a nephrogram during catheterization detects renal abnormalities associated with these syndromes.

Furthermore, the preoperative presence of low cardiac output syndrome, congestive heart failure, long-term use of diuretics, cyanosis, hypotension, hypoxia, and the use of vasopressors all add to the risk of ARF in the patient undergoing cardiac surgery. Severe obstructive lesions of the left heart, coarctation of the aorta, and interrupted aortic arch may produce ARF before, during, or after repair.[73] Moreover, the hypertonic contrast media used in cardiac catheterization may cause medullary necrosis in infants.

The mortality rate in the general postoperative patient with renal failure is 25–65% and the underlying illness is the major determinant of mortality.[74,75] ARF occurs more frequently after pediatric cardiac surgery with an incidence of 8% as reported by Chesney and co-workers.[76] It also occurs more frequently after cardiovascular surgery than after other surgical procedures, which may be a consequence of factors occurring before, during, and after the operation.[73] Hyperuricemia is known to occur in cyanotic patients, and urate crystals may be deposited in the kidney contributing to postoperative renal failure. Despite this association, Ellis and colleagues did not find a high incidence of renal failure in these patients, although they recommended measurement of uric acid levels in cyanotic patients undergoing cardiac surgery.[77]

Preexisting Renal Disease

The pathogenesis of ARF in infants is multifactorial. In normal neonates, glomerular filtration rate and total renal blood flow based on surface area are less than in older children and adults. There is a preponderance of juxtamedullary blood flow in comparison to cortical blood flow.[78]

Glomerular enlargement has been described in many children with cyanotic congenital heart disease. It is unknown whether there is a decrease in the actual number of nephrons in children with cyanotic congenital heart disease (with compensatory hypertrophy of glomeruli) or if hypertrophy develops among a normal number of nephrons. The glomerular alterations in congenital heart disease occur in three stages. The first stage is that of ectasia of glomerular capillaries in children less than 5 years of age. During the next 10 years, glomerular enlargement and mesangial proliferation occur, with destructive changes in the capillary walls. Finally, glomerular sclerosis ensues in the second decade of life. Glomerular enlargement appears to occur as a result of hypoxia at an early age. This enlargement has also been associated with benign proteinuria. Other causes of proteinuria in this population include an increase in venous pressure and alterations in glomerular capillary basement membrane. All these causes of proteinuria contribute to the higher incidence of nephrotic syndrome seen in children with congenital heart disease.[79] These physiologic differences are increased by cardiac failure and by angiocardiography.

A few studies describe renal clearances in children with congenital heart disease. The glomerular filtration rate (GFR) in children with cyanotic congenital heart disease has been reported to be either normal or low in relation to body surface area. Renal plasma flow and renal blood flow, as obtained by *para*-aminohippurate clearance and xenon washout, are reduced in those with cyanotic and acyanotic lesions.[79] The most consistent abnormality in renal function in children with congenital heart disease is reduced renal plasma flow. This reduction in plasma flow must be primarily due to changes in outer cortical flow because studies involving extraction ratios indicate that it is not caused by a shift of blood flow from cortex to medulla. Successful surgical correction of congenital heart defects may not result in a return of renal plasma flow to normal and a reduced renal blood flow may therefore be permanent. Because of the decreased renal blood flow, a compensatory increase in GFR must occur by increasing the filtering surface area and the pressure gradient across the nephron.

Relation of Renal Problems to Low Cardiac Output State

Many of the structural and functional abnormalities observed in the kidneys of children with congenital heart disease are similar to those described in malnourished children. Gruskin noted that the majority of children with a reduction in outer cortical flow were physically small. Postnatal growth in children who have had heart failure may lag up to 2 years behind that of normal children; cell number, body potassium, and cell mass are affected.[79] Renin secretion is increased in congenital cardiovascular disease, decreasing blood flow to the outer renal cortex.

Acute renal failure occurs in both "closed" and "open" cardiac procedures. In addition to preoperative hypoxia, hypotension, and hypoperfusion effects on the kidneys, there may be intraoperative interference with, or interruption of, blood flow to the kidney, which may be an important factor in the development of ARF. Hypoventilation, hypotension, hypoxemia, dysrhythmias during the operative period, and possible direct toxic effects of anesthetic agents may also be important factors.[73] Bradyarrhythmias causing a decrease in cardiac output and hypotension appear to be the most consistent risk factors in the development of ARF.[76]

The adequacy of the technical repair and the type of intraoperative myocardial protection during induced ischemia are two major determinants of postoperative cardiac function and renal function. Aortic cross-clamp time also appears to be an important factor because of the risk of ischemia injury to an unprotected myocardium during that time.[73] These factors may produce a low cardiac output state and incipient renal failure. Furthermore, the treatment of the low cardiac output state with vasopressors, which constrict the renal vascular bed, tends to worsen the situation.

Diagnosis of Acute Renal Failure

The diagnosis of ARF in postoperative patients is usually clouded by the previously discussed factors. *Acute tubular necrosis* (ATN) is a histologic term that is not synonymous with ARF. True ATN, which is diagnosed by histologic criteria, occurs in only 60% of children with ARF.[76] The hallmark of ARF is reduced urine output. Oliguria in the older child is defined as less than 20 mL/h of urine output. In the preterm and term newborn, oliguria may be harder to define in that some newborns do not void until 24 hours of age. Accepted standards of adequate urine output are 2 mL/kg/h in infants and smaller children. Low-output failure is associated with less than 300 mL/m^2/d, whereas high-output failure is associated with urine volumes of more than 1000 mL/m^2/d.[73] This volume of urine production generally allows adequate handling of solute load. The urinary values and parameters used to diagnose ARF may be greatly altered in this population, particularly in the low birth weight infant.[80] Besides the routine serum and urinary electrolytes, osmolality, creatinine, and blood urea nitrogen, the fraction excretion of sodium (FE_{Na}) is the best test to discriminate between prerenal and renal causes of ARF. Accuracy of this single test has been reported as high as 90%.[81] The FE_{Na} in ARF is is usually greater than 1–2% in the absence of diuretics (Table 25–3). As renal failure progresses, the blood urea nitrogen increases 10 mg/100 mL/d and urinary sodium to 30 mEq/L or more.[73]

Management of Acute Renal Failure

Nephrotoxic Drugs. Aminoglycosides, diuretics, and angiographic contrast media may precipitate ARF in the postoperative period. Especially during the early postoperative period, when urine output is inconsistent, aminoglycoside usage should be strictly monitored. Peak and trough blood levels should be monitored. As urine out-

TABLE 25–3. DIAGNOSIS OF RENAL FAILURE IN CHILDREN

	ARF	Normal
Urine volume	<1 mL/kg/h	>2 mL/kg/h
Urine sodium	>60 mEq/L	20–40 mEq/L
U/P osmolarity	<1.1:1	>1.2:1
U/P urea	<3	3–8
FE_{Na}	>1	<1

put decreases, the ability to clear aminoglycosides falls and the risk of toxicity increases. The repeated administration of these drugs should be determined by the blood level and not by a predetermined schedule.

Engelman and co-workers[82] and Lawson and colleagues[83] in their animal studies showed that renal cortical ischemia associated with cardiopulmonary bypass could be reversed with diuretics. However, large doses of loop diuretics have been associated with the development of ARF. These drugs may accelerate the developing failure in the hypovolemic patient, especially in combination with aminoglycosides or in the situation of metabolic acidosis.

Diuretic Usage. Both mannitol and furosemide have been used to increased urine output in the patient with ARF, but there is not clear evidence that these drugs are effective in decreasing the morbidity or mortality associated with ARF in humans.[82] No amount of diuretic obviates the need for adequate restoration of blood volume, which should always be considered before diuretic therapy.[84] In the absence of congestive heart failure, mannitol (0.5 mL/kg of a 20% solution) followed by furosemide (1–5 mg/kg IV) may be given. An increase in urine output does not always indicate an improvement in renal function. Signs and symptoms of ARF should still be followed until the situation clears. If the child is going to respond to furosemide, it will usually be to a dose of 5 mg/kg or less. Increasing the dose beyond that range does not produce a higher success rate. Davis and colleagues reported the use of low-dose dopamine after cardiopulmonary bypass in adults to improve renal function.[85] This experience also appears to be applicable to the pediatric population.

Potassium-Calcium Balance. Acute renal failure invariably results in several metabolic derangements, not the least of which is hyperkalemia. With the loss of renal function, potassium accumulates in the body at a rate of 0.4–0.8 mEq/L/d (0.2–0.3 mEq/kg body weight/d).[86] The physiologic effects of potassium accumulation are worsened by infection, malnutrition, and acidosis. The most significant effect of hyperkalemia is the development of lethal arrhythmias, particularly asystole. Although electrocardiographic (ECG) signs of hyperkalemia may be masked in cardiac surgical patients, the sequence of ECG changes include tall, peaked T waves, decreased R wave amplitude, lengthening of PR and QRS intervals, and disappearance of P waves. If these dysrhythmias occur during a rather brief increase in serum potassium (as in hyperkalemia after succinylcholine), they are much more amenable to therapy than in the patient with a serum potassium of 7.5 mEq/L, anuria, and an already irritable myocardium. Hyperkalemia continues to be a problem until excreted or dialyzed.[5] All sources of potassium intake should be eliminated. The

therapy of hyperkalemia was discussed earlier in this chapter.

Hypocalcemia may also develop in the postoperative course during ARF or from citrate blood use. It is more common in newborns and small infants, particularly if they are septic or greatly stressed, on account of their poor calcium regulatory mechanisms. Whenever hypocalcemia is symptomatic (tetany, seizures, neuromuscular weakness), calcium should be given to counteract the effects of hyperkalemia on the myocardium. Calcium gluconate (0.5 mL or 10% solution) can be given at a rate of 4 mg/kg/h until symptoms subside. Maintenance calcium can then be given at 250 mg/kg/d in divided doses or as a continuous infusion in the hyperlimentation fluid.

Hypocalcemia, hypoglycemia, and hypomagnesemia may precipitate seizures in ARF.[87] When seizures occur, biochemical abnormalities should be investigated. Chesney reported hypoglycemia in 50% of infants with ARF after major cardiac surgery.[76] Hyponatremia is treated by fluid restriction or administration of sodium bicarbonate which also ameliorates acidosis. Nutritional support is vital to prevent negative protein and caloric balance in renal failure. Parenteral hyperalimentation should provide at least 1 g/kg of protein and 30–50 cal/kg/d.[73] Despite careful management of the problems previously described, reported mortality rates in pediatric patients with renal failure after heart surgery are high (65%) increasing to 85% in anuric patients.[73,76,77]

Dialysis and Functional Recovery. Slow continuous ultrafiltration or continuous arteriovenous hemofiltration are useful techniques in oliguric children.[88] In Zobel et al's series, achievement of normovolemia reduced vasopressor requirements, increased mean arterial pressure, and improved acidosis.[88] Dialysis, usually peritoneal because of the large peritoneal surface area in children, is initiated when there is intractable hyperkalemia, excessive hypervolemia resulting in hypertension and heart failure, acidosis unresponsive to bicarbonate, and uremic encephalopathy (eg, disorientation, seizures). Peritoneal dialysis can be performed continuously and without anticoagulation. However, it is less efficient, more time consuming, and associated with greater risk of infection. Recovery from low-output renal failure is indicated by increasing urine volume. Functional recovery may be delayed beyond recovery of urine output necessitating careful fluid and electrolyte balance during the recovery period.

NEUROLOGIC PROBLEMS

Acute neurologic morbidity has been reported to occur in 2–25% of children undergoing surgical repairs of congenital cardiac defects.[89] Neurologic symptoms include alterations of consciousness, seizures, hemiparesis, choreoathetoid syndromes, hypoxic-ischemic encephalopathy, subdural hematoma, or cerebral atrophy. Older surgical series report a somewhat lower incidence of neurologic defect ranging from 1–3%[90] to 4–5%.[91]

Cerebral and peripheral neurologic disorders following cardiac surgery occur in children despite meticulous attempts to prevent known causes, such as air and particulate emboli, and advances in surgical techniques or extracorporeal circulation. It is probably safe to assume that although catastrophic neurologic damage may be related to some untoward event in the perioperative period, such as massive air embolus or prolonged and refractory hypotension and hypoxia, less dramatic neurologic or neuropsychiatric changes may be multifactorial in origin. The pediatric patient, especially the small infant who requires cardiac surgery, may also be at risk because of factors associated with congenital heart disease such as prematurity, low birth weight, failure to thrive, other congenital anomalies, nutritional or metabolic imbalance, anemia, chronic cyanosis,[92] pulmonary insufficiency, and infection. Deep or profound hypothermia with circulatory arrest is commonly employed for the correction of the more complex defects in infants whose perioperative mortality rate ranges from 10–20% and in whom neurologic and other complications may be expected to increase.

Central Nervous System

Etiology and Prevention. Prevention of nervous system injury during congenital cardiac procedures is more important than treatment because present management is largely supportive and ineffective. Among the mechanisms alone or in combination that contribute to postoperative central nervous system dysfunction are hypoxia due to low blood flow or circulatory arrest, embolization of particulate matter or air, and metabolic abnormalities.

Hypoxia Due to Decreased Blood Flow or Circulatory Arrest. Inadequate cerebral perfusion during repair or palliation of congenital heart defects results in hypoxia at the cellular level and can cause transient or permanent neurologic sequelae. Multiple factors affect the delivery to, and utilization of, oxygen by the brain and can be manipulated to some extent to prevent ischemic episodes. Reduction in the cerebral blood flow or oxygen content of the blood or increases in cerebral metabolic activity when the normal compensatory mechanism to increase blood flow is blunted or absent may produce ischemia.

The level of arterial pressure necessary to prevent cerebral ischemia in infants and children undergoing cardiovascular surgical procedures is not clearly defined. It is probably safe to conclude that the compliant vascular system in young patients promotes better perfusion of vital organs at any reasonable pressure that would occur in older patients with arteriosclerotic vessels. Several authors indicate that mean arterial pressures of 30–50 mm Hg are acceptable on bypass provided no other signs of inadequate perfusion are present (metabolic acidosis, facial plethora, increased central venous pressure, P_{O_2} of venous return blood less than 40 mm Hg, uneven cooling, decreased urine output, continuing loss of pump volume, or difficulty maintaining physiologic flow rates).[93–95] Even in adults, lower mean perfusion pressures of 45–55 mm Hg do not increase neurologic dysfunction unless other risk factors are present, such as preexisting neurologic problems, prolonged duration of cardiopulmonary bypass, or degenerative valvular disease.[96] There appears to be an increased incidence of preexisting neurologic abnormalities in infants and children undergoing surgery for hypoplastic left heart syndrome.[97] Although profound hypothermia and circulatory arrest expedite surgical repair in neonates, the duration of perfusion and the duration of circulatory arrest clearly affect neurologic outcome (see Chapter 10). Neither the safe duration of circulatory arrest nor its efficacy compared with low-flow bypass have been documented experimentally.

Embolization

PARTICULATE EMBOLI. Particulate emboli may be formed by microaggregation of the patient's own platelets and leukocytes; cellular aggregation and generation of gaseous microemboli with oxygenators (particularly bubble oxygenators); the return of significant quantities of debris from the operative site, fat, and activated platelets via the cardiotomy suction apparatus; exogenous particles retained in the oxygenator during the manufacturing process; and material contained in transfused blood or intravenous solutions. These microemboli, generated by the extracorporeal circuit, may reduce cerebral blood flow causing focal or generalized changes including stroke, infarction, cerebral edema, and brain death.

Various methods have been devised to reduce damage to the nervous system by particulate emboli. Recirculation of the perfusate through a filter prior to institution of cardiopulmonary bypass, the use of filters on the cardiotomy return tubing and arterial inflow tubing of oxygenator,[98,99] and membrane oxygenation rather than bubble oxygenation[100] are the commonly used methods.

AIR EMBOLISM. Air emboli may enter the vascular system via intravenous infusion tubing and be transmitted to the systemic circulation in patients with right-to-left shunts such as tetralogy or transposition of the great arteries. Paradoxical air emboli, resulting when air enters the vascular system in patients with left-to-right shunts such as atrial or ventricular septal defects, occur when sudden increases in intrathoracic pressure (caused by coughing or extreme positive-pressure ventilatory maneuvers) change intracardiac dynamics. However, some paradoxical emboli occur in the absence of these events. Air emboli associated with cardiopulmonary bypass are prevented by careful circuit setup and placement of cannulas and rigorous removal of air from cardiac chambers and great vessels before discontinuation of bypass. If air embolism occurs, therapy with phenytoin (10 mg/kg IV slowly as a loading dose followed by 3 mg/kg three times a day), mannitol, 0.5 g/kg, methylprednisolone, 30 mg/kg, and barbiturates may be useful.

Postcardiotomy Delirium. Postoperative confusion, delirium, or frank psychosis are less prevalent in the pediatric population than in adults after cardiopulmonary bypass. The incidence ranges from 13 to 57% in adults.[101,102] In reviewing 550 intracardiac procedures using profound hypothermia and circulatory arrest for correction of congenital defects in infants and children between 1971 and 1979, Tharion and co-workers reported transient psychosis or hallucinations in 1.8%.[91] Kornfeld et al reported a 30% incidence of delirium in adults having repair of congenital heart defects but none in children.[103] In later work from the same institution, there was no delirium in patients less than 25 years of age with a 26% incidence in patients over age 45 versus 12% in patients less than 45 years of age.[104] In another study of 100 consecutive patients in which cardiopulmonary bypass was used, Sveinsson reported six patients with frank delirium, four with slight decreases in the ability to concentrate, and three with clouding of consciousness.[105] Eighty-seven percent were without any psychologic changes, including five children aged 6–12 years.

The clinical picture of postcardiotomy delirium or psychosis is quite characteristic. There is usually a lucid period of 2–5 days following surgery. The patient then may experience perceptual distortion of visual, tactile, proprioceptive, and auditory stimuli, which is associated with anxiety, restlessness, inability to concentrate, and mild confusion. These symptoms may progress to paranoid delusions, gross disorientation, illusions, and frank hallucination, usually of the visual type. Although the psychosis is usually relatively benign, it can cause significant management problems for the staff and deprive the patient of rest, sleep, and needed family support.

Preventive measures are important in postcardiotomy delirium. Because sleep deprivation may be an important precursor of the psychosis, sleep should be monitored during the early postoperative period, appropriate pain medication administered, and sleeping patients protected as much as possible from procedures or extraneous stimuli that might interrupt sleep. Careful and thorough preoperative orientation of patients and their families as to what to expect during the immediate postoperative period is very important. Information about the possibility of perceptual disturbances or confusion postoperatively should probably be included together with assurances that these problems are self-limited. Particularly anxious patients or families may benefit from pre- and postoperative psychiatric consultation. When psychosis or delirium is recognized (perceptual disturbance being the initial stage of delirium) and metabolic or cerebrovascular causes ruled out, medication with a butyrophenone, phenothiazine, or a minor tranquilizer may be indicated. Continued reassurance and reorientation by nursing staff and family and incorporation into the environment of familiar items such as toys, television, radio, and visits by siblings or other family members may be of great help.

Metabolic Causes of Postoperative Central Nervous System Abnormalities. Depression of the central nervous system or seizure activity may result from factors other than embolization or decreased perfusion. Hypoglycemia, hyponatremia, hypocalcemia, hypomagnesemia, hypernatremia, and uremia cause seizures and can be identified by laboratory analysis of blood. Drug-induced narcosis resulting from decreased metabolism of narcotics, barbiturates, or tranquilizers is likely in low cardiac output states.

Management of Neurologic Complications. Despite prophylactic measures and meticulous attention to perfusion and oxygenation, neurologic deficits occur. Supportive therapy should be applied to ensure arterial oxygenation and cerebral perfusion. Measures may include the use of increased inspired oxygen concentrations, ventilation with positive end-expiratory pressure if needed, and neuromuscular blocking drugs to ensure oxygenation, with positive inotropic drugs and/or vasodilators to enhance systemic perfusion. Fluid overload should be avoided and diuretics may be useful to prevent or treat cerebral edema. If seizure activity is present, anticonvulsant therapy should be initiated (Table 25–4).

Reversible causes of neurologic dysfunction during the postoperative period should be considered. Subdural hematoma is rare after cardiac surgery but has been reported in the pediatric population.[107,108] However, in McConnell's series, the subdural hematomas, which probably occurred during anticoagulation for extracorporeal circulation, were small and did not produce any mass effects.[106] Propranolol and hydralazine have been reported to result in changes in acute mental status, including depression, confusion, and hallucinations.[109,110]

Peripheral Nervous System Injuries

Peripheral nerves may be injured during pediatric cardiac surgical procedures by improper positioning of patients on the operating table, by direct surgical trauma during dissection and electrocautery, and by a combination of position and surgical events that results in ischemia to individual nerves or nerve groups, the sympa-

TABLE 25–4. MANAGEMENT OF POSTOPERATIVE NEUROLOGIC DYSFUNCTION

General Measures

Maintain adequate arterial perfusion pressure using volume expansion and catecholamine support if necessary.

Maintain adequate arterial oxygenation using controlled ventilation, positive end-expiratory pressure, and neuromuscular blockade if needed.

Avoid fluid overload. Monitor filling pressures and give diuretics as needed.

Seizures

Protect airway and ensure adequate ventilation using 100% oxygen, bag, mask at first, and endotracheal intubation and positive-pressure ventilation if seizure cannot be stopped quickly.

Rule out metabolic causes of seizures and treat accordingly:

Hypoxia: Administer 100% oxygen and ventilate

Hypoglycemia: Administer intravenous glucose, 0.5–1.0 g/kg

Hypocalcemia: Administer intraveous calcium gluconate, 100–200 mg/kg *SLOWLY*

Hyponatremia: Administer intravenous sodium chloride, 1–2 mL/kg of 3% solution; restrict intravenous free water administration

Hypernatremia: Must be corrected *SLOWLY* with diuretics and low- or no-sodium-containing solutions

Hyperpyrexia (fever): Active cooling using cooling mattress, fans, cold compresses, antipyretics aspirin or acetaminophen by mouth or rectal suppository in proper doses

Anticonvulsant Therapy

Phenobarbital: Load with 5–10 mg/kg given intravenously *SLOWLY;* maintain with 5 mg/kg/24 h

Diazepam: 0.1–0.2 mg/kg given intravenously q4h

Phenytoin: 1.5–3.0 mg/kg intravenously q8h

Consider CT scan to rule out subdural hematoma

Cerebral Edema

Hyperventilate to a Pco_2 of 25–30 mm Hg; maintain Po_2 above 100 mm Hg; consider neuromuscular blockers to prevent coughing and straining; avoid positive end-expiratory pressure if oxygenation is not a problem in order to prevent increases in intrathoracic pressure that may be transmitted to the head.

Elevate head 30°

Restrict fluids

Mannitol 1–2 g/kg initial dose; 250 mg/kg q4–6 h

Steroids (probably not effective for cerebral edema due to hypoxia but should probably be used empirically; methylprednisolone 5 mg/kg intravenously q12h; dexamethasone 0.25 mg/kg q6h

Consider intracranial pressure monitoring for severe cerebral edema

Postcardiotomy Delirium

Verbal reassurance by medical personnel and family

Reorientation of patient in quiet and unstimulating environment away from other critically ill patients; calendars, clocks, music, television may step up the reorientation

Ensure that the patient gets as much undisturbed sleep as possible to avoid sleep-deprivation syndrome

Butyrophenone therapy (haloperidol 0.05–0.15 mg/kg/d) for severe cases

Drug-induced Neurologic Dysfunction

Drugs known to cause neurologic dysfunction may be withdrawn or given in reduced doses:

Propranolol

Hydralazine

Droperidol

Phenothiazines

---

thetic chain, or the spinal cord.[110] Improper positioning of patients on the operating table results in stretching or compression of nerves that disrupts nerve fibers or causes neural ischemia. In the supine position for median sternotomy, one or both arms of the patient may be abducted to permit access to intravascular catheters. The angle of abduction should be 90 degrees or less at the shoulder to prevent excessive traction on the brachial plexus (especially if both arms are abducted). In the lateral decubitus position for thoracotomy, a small (rolled sheets) should be placed in the dependent axillary area and the head should be supported on pads to maintain alignment of the cervical and thoracic spine. Padding should also be placed between the slightly flexed legs and under the feet in the thoracotomy position.[111] In children with the Down syndrome, special support of the head and neck is essential to prevent cervical spinal cord injury in the 20% of these patients who have atlantoaxial subluxation.[112]

Phrenic Nerve Injury. Phrenic nerve injury is associated with birth trauma, surgical procedures in the neck and upper thorax such as hyperalimentation catheter insertion into the jugular system or repair of tracheoesophageal fistula or tracheostomy, and the surgical treatment

of congenital heart disease. In one series of over 1800 consecutive cardiac surgical procedures, there were 32 cases of unilateral phrenic nerve damage (an incidence of 1.7%).[113] In this report, there was a particularly high incidence in infants undergoing Blalock-Taussig shunts (7% incidence in Blalock-Taussig procedures, contributing 22% of the total number of phrenic nerve injuries). In a later series, the incidence of phrenic injury and diaphragmatic paralysis in 2700 patients after cardiac surgery was 1.3%.[114] An increased incidence associated with Blalock-Taussig shunts was unconfirmed in this report, but the number of such shunts in the series was quite small.[114] Another report of 26 children with diaphragmatic paralysis and eventration (congenital in 10, resulting from birth trauma in 4, and from operative phrenic nerve injury in 12) confirmed the increased association with Blalock-Taussig procedures as well as a high incidence of associated anomalies and prematurity.[115] Diagnosis is usually by clinical findings (paradoxical movement of the upper abdomen inward and upward on inspiration) or radiographic findings (elevated hemidiaphragm without descent on inspiration). Ross Russell and colleagues, however, report the measurement of phrenic nerve latency to direct phrenic nerve stimulation in a series of 37 children.[116] Using this technique, 10% of the children were noted to have decreased phrenic nerve conduction.

Therapy for phrenic nerve dysfunction includes prolonged ventilatory support or diaphragmatic plication. Plication of the affected diaphragm was performed in 21 of 26 patients in Smith and co-workers' series, with a mortality rate of 67% attributed to the associated anomalies and prematurity of the patients.[115] Stewart and colleagues reported recovery of diaphragmatic function with tracheostomy and prolonged mechanical ventilation.[117] A sequential approach to treatment has been proposed by Haller and co-workers in which treatment of associated parenchymal lung disease and cardiac dysfunction is performed over 2–6 weeks.[118] This approach balances the possibility of diaphragmatic recovery over time with iatrogenic complications from prolonged mechanical ventilatory support. Affatato and co-workers noted that phrenic nerve paralysis was well tolerated in children older than 1 year, but infants benefited from early diaphragmatic plication[119] (see Chapter 24).

Bilateral phrenic nerve injury after the Mustard repair of transposition of the great arteries was reported in four infants.[117] These patients were managed with tracheostomy and prolonged mechanical ventilation. Their recovery period ranged from 30 to 103 days and the outcome was satisfactory. The authors attributed the bilateral paralysis to electrocautery injury of the phrenic nerves during removal of a generous portion of pericardium for the repair to produce a large intracardiac baffle to avoid pulmonary or systemic venous obstruction with baffle contraction.

Another etiology for phrenic nerve dysfunction in adults is topical hypothermia (iced saline slush infused into the pericardium).[120] Special insulated topical cooling devices of various sizes have been devised for children to minimize phrenic nerve damage.[121]

Brachial and Cervical Plexus Injury. Brachial plexus injury occurs from several mechanisms. One mechanism is the position of the patient during median sternotomy and another is fracture of the first rib. In positioning a patient for median sternotomy, care must be taken to avoid abduction of the arms beyond a 90-degree angle from the chest wall in the supine position. It is also better to flex the elbows to 90 degrees and to elevate them several inches above the level of the table with towels or foam padding. If the arm is to be extended, limiting the abduction to 90 degrees and positioning the radial side of the hand anteriorly is the safest way to prevent stretching of the plexus.[122]

The damage to the brachial plexus caused by the median sternotomy itself was initially thought to result from stretching of the plexus with sternal retraction or arm position. However, van der Salm and co-workers found that brachial plexus injury associated with median sternotomy is probably due to fracture of the first rib with direct physical damage to the nerves.[123] It was related to the position of the sternal retractor and the width of the sternal opening. The position of the arms during the surgery did not seem to influence the presence or absence of brachial plexus damage, but arm position was either at the patient's side or not more abducted more than 90 degrees.

Van der Salm and associates also reported several cases of the Horner syndrome in conjunction with brachial plexus injuries, and at autopsy on one patient, they found that the cervical sympathetic chain on the ipsilateral side of the neurologic damage from the rib fracture was surrounded by hematoma.[124] The Horner syndrome has also been reported after internal jugular venous cannulation in children.[125] It may also occur after ligation of patent ductus arteriosus or the creation of systemic to pulmonary shunts.[126] Likewise, the recurrent laryngeal nerve may be injured during pediatric cardiovascular procedures resulting in vocal cord paralysis and hoarseness. Procedures during which the recurrent laryngeal nerve is at increase risk include repair of coarctation of the aorta, ligation of the ductus arteriosus, creation of pulmonary to systemic shunts, and tracheostomy.[111,126]

Intercostal Nerve Injury Damage to the intercostal nerves resulting in intercostal neuritis during intrathoracic operations is not an uncommon complication. It is probably the most frequently encountered problem in adults.[111] Intercostal nerve damage may occur from excessive stretching and tension on the nerve root during opening of the chest, from compression by a chest tube left in place for a prolonged period of time, or from damage by a needle during thoracentesis.[127,128] The infant or child who manifests undue pain or chest wall tenderness may be suspected of having intercostal neuritis. Such patients may benefit from therapeutic intercostal nerve block with 0.25% bupivacaine using a maximum dose of 1.5 mg/kg.

INFECTION

Although primary postoperative infection accounts for as few as 4% of the total number of postoperative deaths, it is an ever-present concern. Infection should always be considered a preventable form of morbidity and mortality. In the recent series by Pollock et al, wound infections comprised 28% and nonwound infections 72% of the postoperative infections.[129] Sepsis, mediastinitis, and pneumonia lead the list of postoperative infections. Sternal wound infections are increased with emergency or elective opening of the sternum on the ward rather than in the operating room. Sepsis in the newborn can be particularly difficult to diagnose as fever is rarely present. Instead, lethargy, feeding intolerance, hyperglycemia, and metabolic acidosis may be the only clues to sepsis.

Foreign materials, including central catheters, endotracheal tubes, Foley catheters, prosthetic valve, and graft materials all provide routes and hosts of infection. Because of the risk of bacteremia with nasal intubation,[130] some have recommended the avoidance of nasal endotracheal tubes in patients at high risk for endocarditis. Prolonged intubation may predispose to otitis, sinusitis, and tracheitis. Sternal wound infections are particularly difficult to treat, especially in cyanotic patients. On occasion, repeated debridement and musculocutaneous skin flaps are required to ensure healing.[131] Sepsis persisting despite antibiotics in the presence of prosthetic valves or materials may necessitate removal of these substances.

Prophylactic antibiotics are generally administered before and after surgery to children with congenital heart disease who may be hypoxic, in congestive heart failure, and have poor nutritional status. Antibiotic coverage is aimed at staphylococcal organisms in all patients and at gram-negative organisms in neonates and debilitated patients. Preoperative prophylaxis is indicated in Chapter 26, Appendix 1. Prophylactic coverage is continued for at least 48 hours postoperatively or longer when prosthetic valves and materials are present.

There is also a risk of infection from contaminated blood or blood products. All banked blood and blood products are screened for hepatitis, syphilis, and human immunodeficiency virus (HIV). Despite the screening process, some units pass the screen but contain low titers of viruses that may be transmitted to the recipient. Furthermore, the patients themselves may harbor the viruses and have previously undiagnosed diseases present in the postoperative period. Even malaria may occur in the postoperative period as undiagnosed fever in areas considered to be malaria free. Two children were reported with malaria within the first 3 postoperative days owing either to transfusion of infected blood or activation of a latent infestation by the stress of surgery.[132]

In patients with congenital heart disease associated with forms of asplenia, there is an increased frequency of fatal septicemia with encapsulated bacteria, particularly *Klebsiella* and *Escherichia coli* in children under 6 months of age. This particular group of patients needs continuous antibiotic prophylaxis with either amoxicillin or ampicillin.

At times, the postcardiotomy syndrome may be confused with postoperative sepsis (see Chapter 24). Persistent fever despite antibiotic coverage, leukocytosis, and elevated sedimentation rate all can mimic sepsis. The postpericardiotomy syndrome is generally benign unless pericardial effusion and tamponade develop.

Postoperative cardiac patients are still at risk for bacterial endocarditis long after hospital discharge. Palliative surgery does not decrease the incidence of endocarditis.[40] In fact, areas of turbulent flow, such as those surrounding shunt sites and deformities of valvular cusps, as in the bicuspid aortic valve associated with coarctation, are particularly at risk.

HORMONAL CHANGES

A stress response similar to that of adults occurs in older infants and children during cardiopulmonary bypass and postoperatively.[133] In smaller infants (under 10 kg in weight), the stress response is more limited. Milne and co-workers reported hyperglycemia during cardiopulmonary bypass that persisted for 7 days postoperatively. Serum insulin concentrations increased during bypass but returned to normal in the postbypass and postoperative periods. A similar response was noted with growth hormone. Cortisol increased transiently in the early postoperative period but rapidly returned to normal levels.[133] Mitchell and co-workers recently reported that triiodothyronine and thyroxine decrease with initiation of cardiopulmonary bypass.[134] Thyroid hormone levels partially recover by 3–6 hours after bypass but decrease again at 48 hours. By 5 days postoperatively, thyroid hormones were normal except in children with multisystem failure. These changes are clinically significant because of the recent findings of the inotropic effects of triiodothyronine.[134]

REFERENCES

1. Bland JW, Wright JA: General intensive care. In Lake CL (ed): *Pediatric Cardiac Anesthesia.* East Norwalk, CT: Appleton & Lange, 1988, pp 363–385
2. Neidig JR, Kleiber C, Oppliger RA: Risk factors associated with pressure ulcers in the pediatric patient following open-heart surgery. *Prog Cardiovasc Nurs* 4:99–106, 1989
3. Holliday MA, Segar WE: The maintenance need for water in parenteral fluid therapy. *Pediatrics* 19:823–832, 1957
4. Williams DR, Oh W: Effects of radiant warmers on insensible water loss in newborn infants. *Am J Dis Child* 128:511–514, 1984
5. Wood JH, Polyzoidis KS, Kee DB Jr, et al: Augmentation of cerebral blood flow induced by hemodilution in stroke patients after superficial temporal-middle cerebral arterial bypass operation. *Neurosurgery* 15:535–539, 1984
6. Sladen RN: Temperature and ventilation after hypothermia cardiopulmonary bypass. *Anesth Analg* 64:816–820, 1985
7. Ralley FE, Ramsay JG, Wynands JE, et al: Effect of heat humidified gases on temperature drop after cardiopulmonary bypass. *Anesth Analg* 63:1106–1110, 1984
8. Sharkey A, Lipton JM, Murphy MT, Giesecke AH: Inhibition of postanesthetic shivering with radiant heat. *Anesthesiology* 66:249–252, 1987
9. Goudsouzian NG, Morris RH, Ryan JF: The effects of warming blanket on maintenance of body temperature in anesthetized infants and children. *Anesthesiology* 39:351–353, 1973

10. Casella ES, Soule LM, Blanck TJJ: Creatine kinase activity and temperature in children after cardiac surgery. *J Cardiothorac Vasc Anesth* **2**:156–163, 1988

11. Tyler DC: Respiratory effects of pain in a child after thoracotomy. *Anesthesiology* **70**:873–874, 1989

12. Anand KJS, Hickey PR: Halothane-morphine compared with high-dose sufentanil for anesthesia and postoperative analgesia in neonatal cardiac surgery. *N Engl J Med* **326**:1–9, 1992

13. Rosen DA, Rosen KR: Pain and sedation in the pediatric patient: The 1990 approach to a very old problem. In Vincent JL (ed): *Update in Intensive Care and Emergency Medicine*. Update 1990. New York: Springer-Verlag, 1990, pp 758–769

14. Booker PD, Beechey A, Lloyd-Thomas AR: Sedation of children requiring artificial ventilation using an infusion of midazolam. *Br J Anaesth* **58**:1104–1108, 1986

15. Lloyd-Thomas AR, Booker PD: Infusion of midazolam in paediatric patients after cardiac surgery. *Br J Anaesth* **58**:1109–1115, 1986

16. Lynn AM, Opheim KE, Tyler DC: Morphine infusion after pediatric cardiac surgery. *Crit Care Med* **12**:836–866, 1984

17. Lynn AM, Slattery JT: Morphine pharmacokinetics in early infancy. *Anesthesiology* **66**:136–139, 1987

18. Rothstein P, Arthur GR, Feldman HS, et al: Bupivacaine for intercostal nerve blocks in children: Blood concentrations and pharmacokinetics. *Anesth Analg* **65**:625–632, 1986

19. McIlvaine WB, Knox RF, Fennessey PV, Goldstein M: Continuous infusion of bupivacaine via intrapleural catheter for analgesia after thoracotomy in children. *Anesthesiology* **69**:261–264, 1988

20. Agarwal R, Gutlove DP, Lockhaart CH: Seizures occurring in pediatric patients receiving continuous infusion of bupivacaine. *Anesth Analg* **75**:284–286, 1992

21. Gunter JB, Eng C: Thoracic epidural anesthesia via the caudal approach in children. *Anesthesiology* **76**:935–938, 1922.

22. Bosenberg AT, Bland BAR, Schulte-Steinberg O, Downing JW: Thoracic epidural anesthesia via caudal route in infants. *Anesthesiology* **69**:265–269, 1988

23. Jorfeldt L, Lofstrom B, Pernow B, et al: The effect of local anesthetics on central circulation and respiration in man and dog. *Acta Anaesthesiol Scand* **12**:153–168, 1968

24. Mazoit JX, Denson DD, Samii K: Pharmacokinetics of bupivacaine following caudal anesthesia in infants. *Anesthesiology* **68**:387–391, 1988

25. Ecoffey C, Desparmet J, Berdeaux A, et al: Bupivacaine in children: Pharmacokinetics following caudal anesthesia. *Anesthesiology* **63**:447–448, 1985

26. McCloskey JJ, Haun SE, Deshpande JK: Bupivacaine toxicity secondary to continuuous caudal epidural infusion in children. *Anesth Analg* **75**:287–290, 1992

27. Valley RD, Bailey AG: Caudal morphine for postoperative analgesia in infants and children: A report of 138 cases. *Anesth Analg* **72**:120–124, 1991

28. Attia J, Ecoffey C, Sandouk P, et al: Epidural morphine in children: Pharmacokinetics and CO$_2$ sensitivity. *Anesthesiology* **65**:590–594, 1986

29. Krane EJ, Tyler DC, Jacobson LE: The dose response of caudal morphine in children. *Anesthesiology* **71**:48–52, 1989

30. Benlabed M, Ecoffey C, Levron J-C, et al: Analgesia and ventilatory response to CO$_2$ following epidural sufentanil in children. *Anesthesiology* **67**:948–951, 1987

31. Rosen KR, Rosen DA: Caudal epidural morphine for control of pain following open heart surgery in children. *Anesthesiology* **70**:418–421, 1989

32. Dalen B, Tanguy A, Haberer J-P: Lumbar epidural anesthesia for operative and postoperative pain relief in infants and young children. *Anesth Analg* **65**:1069–1073, 1986

33. Leggett PL, Doyle D, Smith WB, et al: Elective cardiac operation in a patient with severe hemophilia and acquired factor VIII antibodies. *J Thorac Cardiovasc Surg* **87**:556–560, 1984

34. Roskos RR, Gilchrist GS, Kazmier FJ, et al: Management of hemophilia A and B during surgical correction of transposition of the great arteries. *Mayo Clin Proc* **58**:182–186, 1983

35. Wilson CJ, Frankville D, Robinson B, et al: Perioperative management of coronary artery bypass surgery in a patient with factor IX deficiency. *J Thorac Cardiovasc Anesth* **5**:160–161, 1991

36. Milam JD, Austin SF, Nihill MR, et al: Uses of sufficient hemodilution to prevent coagulopathies following surgical correction of cyanotic heart disease. *J Thorac Cardiovasc Surg* **89**:623–629, 1985

37. Guffin AV, Dunbar RW, Kaplan JA, Bland JW: Successful use of a reduce dose of protamine after cardiopulmonary bypass. *Anesth Analg* **55**:110–113, 1976

38. Jobes DR, Schwartz AJ, Ellison N, et al: Monitoring heparin anticoagulation and its neutralization. *Ann Thorac Surg* **31**:161–166, 1981

39. Manno CS, Hedberg KW, Kim HC, et al: Comparison of hemostatic effects of fresh whole blood, stored whole blood, and components after open heart surgery in children. *Blood* **77**:930–936, 1991

40. Gersony WM, Krongrad E: Evaluation and management of patients after surgical repair of congenital heart diseases. *Prog Cardiovasc Dis* **18**:39–56, 1975

41. Roy RC, Stafford MA, Hudspeth AS, Meredith JW: Failure of prophylaxis with fresh frozen plasma after cardiopulmonary bypass. *Anesthesiology* **69**:254–257, 1988

42. ASA Committee of Transfusion Medicine: *Questions and Answers About Transfusion Practices*. 2nd ed. Park Ridge, IL: American Society of Anesthesiologists, 1992, p 29

43. Miller RD, Robbins TO, Toping MJ, Barton SL: Coagulation defects associated with massive blood transfusions. *Ann Surg* **174**:794–801, 1971

44. Cines DB, Kaywin P, Bina M, et al: Heparin-associated thrombocytopenia. *N Engl J Med* **303**:788–795, 1980

45. Harker LA, Malpass TW, Branson HE, et al: Mechanisms of abnormal bleeding in patients undergoing cardiopulmonary bypass: Acquired transient platelet dysfunction associated with selective granule release. *Blood* **56**:824–834, 1980

46. DePalma L, Luban NL: Autologous blood transfusion in pediatrics. *Pediatrics* **85**:125–128, 1990

47. Stehling L: Autologous transfusion. *Int Anesthesiol Clin* **28**:190–196, 1990

48. Boldt J, Zickman B, Czeke A, et al: Blood conservation techniques and platelet function in cardiac surgery. *Anesthesiology* **75**:426–432, 1991

49. Royston D, Bidstrup BP, Taylor KM, Sapsford RN: Effects

of aprotinin on need for blood transfusion after repeat open-heart surgery. *Lancet* **2**: 1289–1291, 1987

50. Van Oeveren W, Jansen NJG, Bidstrup BP, et al: Effects of aprotinin on hemostatic mechanisms during cardiopulmonary bypass. *Ann Thorac Surg* **44**:640–645, 1987

51. Elliot MJ, Allen A: Aprotinin in paediatric cardiac surgery. *Perfusion* **5**(suppl):73–76, 1990

52. Blauhut B, Gross C, Necek S, et al: Effects of high-dose aprotinin on blood loss, platelet function, fibrinolysis, complement, and renal function after cardiopulmonary bypass. *J Thorac Cardiovasc Surg* **101**:958–967, 1991

53. Bohrer H, Bach A, Fleisher F, Lang J: Adverse haemodynamic effects of high-dose aprotinin in a paediatric cardiac surgical patient. *Anaesthesia* **45**:853–854, 1990

54. Royston DL: A prolonged activated clotting time is an unreliable indicator of thrombus formation during aprotinin therapy. *J Thorac Cardiovasc Surg* 1993 (in press.)

55. Royston D: High-dose aprotinin therapy: A review of the first five years' experience. *J Cardiothorac Vasc Anesth* **6**: 76–100, 1992

56. Czer LSC, Bateman TM, Gray RJ, et al: Treatment of severe platelet dysfunction and hemorrhage after cardiopulmonary bypass: Reduction in blood product usage with desmopressin. *J Am Cell Cardiol* **9**:1139–1147, 1987

57. Salzman EW, Weinstein MJ, Weintraub RM, et al: Treatment with desmopressin acetate to reduce blood loss after cardiac surgery. *N Engl J Med* **314**:1402–1406, 1986

58. Rocha E, Llorens R, Paramo JA, et al: Does desmopressin acetate reduce blood loss after surgery in patients on cardiopulmonary bypass? *Circulation* **77**:1319–1323, 1987

59. Seear MD, Wadsworth LD, Rogers PC, et al: The effect of desmopressin acetate (DDAVP) on postoperative blood loss after cardiac operation in children. *J Thorac Cardiovasc Surg* **98**:217–219, 1989

60. Sarraccino S, Adler E, Gibbons PA, et al: DDAVP does not decrease post bypass bleeding in acyanotic children. *Anesthesiology* **70**:A1057, 1989

61. Turner-Gomes SO, Andrew M, Coles J, et al: Abnormalities in von Willebrand factor and antithrombin III after cardiopulmonary bypass operations for congenital heart disease. *J Thorac Cardiovasc Surg* **103**:387–397, 1992

62. Frankville DD, Harper GB, Lake CL, Johns RA: Hemodynamic consequences of desmopressin administration after cardiopulmonary bypass. *Anesthesiology* **74**:988–996, 1991

63. Shepherd LL, Hutchinson RJ, Worden EK, et al: Hyponatremia and seizures after intravenous administration of desmopressin acetate for surgical hemostasis. *J Pediatr* **114**:470–471, 1989

64. Sterns LP, Lillehei CW: Effect of epsilon aminocaproic acid to reduce bleeding during cardiac bypass in children with congenital heart disease. *Can J Surg* **10**:304–307, 1967

65. McClure PD, Izsak J: The uses of epsilon aminocaproic acid to reduce bleeding during cardiac bypass in children with congenital heart disease. *Anesthesiology* **40**:604–608, 1974

66. Van der Salm TJ, Ansell JE, Okike ON, et al: The role of epsilon-aminocaproic acid in reducing bleeding after cardiac operation: A double-blind, randomized study. *J Thorac Cardiovasc Surg* **95**:538–540, 1988

67. Horrow JC, Hlavacek J, Strong MD, et al: Prophylactic tranexaminic acid decreases bleeding after cardiac operations. *J Thorac Cardiovasc Surg* **99**:70–74, 1990

68. Zurick AM, Urzua J, Ghattas M, et al: Failure of positive end-expiratory pressure to decrease postoperative bleeding after cardiac surgery. *Ann Thorac Surg* **34**:608–611, 1982

69. Hoffman WS, Tomasello DN, Mc Vaugh H: Control of postcardiotomy bleeding with PEEP. *Ann Thorac Surg* **34**: 71–73, 1982

70. Chu CM, Chang CH, Liaw YF, Hsieh MJ: Jaundice after open heart surgery: A prospective study. *Thorax* **39**:52–56, 1984

71. Jenkins JG, Lynn AM, Wood AE, et al: Acute liver failure following cardiac operations in children. *J Thorac Cardiovasc Surg* **84**:865–871, 1982

72. Matsuda H, Covino E, Hirose H, et al: Acute liver dysfunction after modified Fontan operation for complex cardiac lesions. *J Thorac Cardiovasc Surg* **96**:219–226, 1988

73. John EG, Levitsky S, Hastreiter AR: Management of acute renal failure complicating cardiac surgery in infants and children. *Crit Care Med* **8**:562–569, 1980

74. Ellis D, Gartner JC, Galvis AG: Acute renal failure in infants and children: Diagnosis, complications, and treatment. *Crit Care Med* **9**:607–617, 1981

75. Rigden S, Barratt TM, Dillon MJ, et al: Acute renal failure complicating cardiopulmonary bypass in children. *Arch Dis Child* **57**:425–530, 1981

76. Chesney RW, Kaplan BS, Freedman RM, et al: Acute renal failure: An important complication of cardiac surgery in infants. *J Pediatr* **87**:381–388, 1975

77. Ellis EN, Brouhard BH, Conti VR: Renal function in children undergoing cardiac operations. *Ann Thorac Surg* **36**: 167–172, 1983

78. Spitzer A: Renal physiology. *Pediatr Clin North Am* **18**:377–393, 1971

79. Gruskin AB: The kidney in congenital heart disease—An overview. *Adv Pediatr* **24**:133–189, 1977

80. Arant BS: Development patterns of renal functional maturation compared in the human neonate. *J Pediatr* **92**:705–712, 1978

81. Mathew OP, Jones AJ, James E, et al: Neonatal renal failure: Usefulness of diagnostic indices. *Pediatrics* **65**:57–60, 1980

82. Engelman RM, Gouge TH, Smith SJ, et al: The effect of diuretics and renal hemodynamics during cardiopulmonary bypass. *J Surg Res* **16**:268–276, 1974

83. Lawson DH, Macadam RF, Singh H, et al: Effect of furosemide and antibiotic induced renal damage in rats. *J Infect Dis* **126**:593–600, 1972

84. Abel RM, Buckley MJ, Austen WG, et al: Etiology, incidence and prognosis or renal failure following cardiac operations: Results of a prospective analysis of 500 consecutive patients. *J Thorac Cardiovasc Surg* **71**:323–333, 1976

85. Davis RF, Lappas DG, Kirklin JK, et al: Acute oliguria after cardiopulmonary bypass: Renal functional improvement with low dose dopamine infusion. *Crit Care Med* **10**: 852–856, 1982

86. Williams GS, Klenk EL, Winters RW: Acute renal failure in pediatrics. In Winters RW (ed): *The Body Fluid in Pediatrics*. Boston: Little, Brown, 1973, p 523

87. Reese GN, Appel SH: Neurologic complications of renal failure. *Semin Nephrol* **1**:137–150, 1981

88. Zobel G, Stein JI, Kuttnig M, et al: Continuous extra-corporeal fluid removal in children with low cardiac output after cardiac operations. *J Thorac Cardiovasc Surg* **101**: 593–597, 1991

89. Ferry PC: Neurologic sequelae of open-heart surgery in children. *Am J Dis Child* **144**:369–373, 1990

90. Mohri H, Dillard DH, Merendino KA: Hypothermia: Halothane anesthesia and the safe period of total circulatory arrest. *Surgery* **72**:345–351, 1972

91. Tharion HJ, Johnson DC, Celermajer JM, et al: Profound hypothermia with circulatory arrest. *J Thorac Cardiovasc Surg* **84**:66–72, 1979

92. Newburger JW, Silbert AR, Buckley LP, et al: Cognitive function and age at repair of transposition of the great arteries in children. *N Engl J Med* **310**:1495–1499, 1984

93. Beynen FM, Tarhan S: Anesthesia for surgical repair of congenital heart defects in children. In Tarhan S (ed): *Cardiovascular Anesthesia and Postoperative Care*, 2nd ed. Chicago: Year Book Medical, 1989, p 144

94. Lake CL: *Cardiovascular Anesthesia*. New York: Springer-Verlag, 1985, p 1986

95. Hickey PR, Wessel DL: Anesthesia for treatment of congenital heart disease. In Kaplan JA (ed): *Cardiac Anesthesia*, 2nd ed. Orlando, FL: Grune & Stratton, 1987, p 676

96. Kollka R, Hilberman M: Neurologic dysfunction following cardiac operation with low flow, low pressure CPB. *J Thorac Cardiovasc Surg* **79**:432–437, 1980

97. Glauser TA, Rorke LB, Weinberg PM, Clancy RR: Congenital brain anomalies associated with the hypoplastic left heart syndrome. *Pediatrics* **85**:984–990, 1990

98. Aris A, Solanes H, Camera ML, et al: Arterial line filtration during cardiopulmonary bypass. *J Thorac Cardiovasc Surg* **91**:526–533, 1986

99. Reed CC, Clark DK: *Cardiopulmonary Perfusion*. Houston: Texas Medical Press, 1975, pp 258–270

100. Solis RT, Kennedy PS, Beall AC, et al: Cardiopulmonary bypass microembolization and platelet aggregation. *Circulation* **52**:103–108, 1975

101. Kornfeld DS, Heller SS, Frank KA, et al: Delirium after coronary artery bypass surgery. *J Thorac Cardiovasc Surg* **76**:93–98, 1978

102. Dubin WR, Field HL, Gastfriend DR: Postcardiotomy delirium: A critical review. *J Thorac Cardiovasc Surg* **77**: 586–594, 1979

103. Kornfeld DS, Zimberg S, Malm JR: Psychiatric complications of open heart surgery. *N Engl J Med* **273**:287–292, 1965

104. Heller SS, Frank KA, Malm JR: Psychiatric complications of open-heart surgery: A reexamination. *N Engl J Med* **283**:1015–1020, 1970

105. Sveinsson JS: Postoperative psychosis after heart surgery. *J Thorac Cardiovasc Surg* **70**:717–726, 1975

106. McConnell JR, Fleming WH, Chu W-K, et al: Magnetic resonance imaging of the brain in infants and children before and after cardiac surgery. *Am J Dis Child* **144**:374–378, 1990

107. Krous HF, Tenckhoff L, Gould NS, et al: Subdural hematoma following open heart operations. *Ann Thorac Surg* **19**:269–276, 1975

108. Peters NL, Anderson KC, Reid PR, et al: Acute mental status changes caused by propranol. *Johns Hopkins Med J* **143**:163–164, 1978

109. Shopsin B, Hirsch J, Gershon S: Visual hallucinations and propranolol. *Biol Psychiatry* **10**:105–107, 1975

110. Nicholson MJ, McAlpine FS: Neural injuries associated with surgical positions and operations. In Martin JT (ed): *Positioning in Anesthesia and Surgery*. Philadelphia: WB Saunders, 1978, pp 193–224

111. Hatcher CR, Miller JI: Operative injuries to nerves during intrathoracic procedures. In Cordell RA, Ellison RG (eds): *Complications of Intrathoracic Surgery*. Boston: Little, Brown, 1979, pp 363–365

112. Moore RA, McNicholas KW, Warran SP: Atlantoaxial subluxation with symptomatic spinal cord compression in a child with Down's syndrome. *Anesth Analg* **66**:85–88, 1987

113. Mickell JJ, Oh KS, Siewers RD, et al: Clinical implications of postoperative unilateral phrenic nerve paralysis. *J Thorac Cardiovasc Surg* **76**:297–304, 1978

114. Lynn AM, Jenkins JG, Edmons JF, Burns JE: Diaphragmatic paralysis after pediatric cardiac surgery: A retrospective analysis of 34 cases. *Crit Care Med* **11**:280–292, 1983

115. Smith CD, Sade RM, Crawford EA, Othersen HB: Diaphragmatic paralysis and eventration in infants. *J Thorac Cardiovasc Surg* **91**:490–497, 1986

116. Ross Russell RI, Mulvey D, Laroche C, et al: Bedside assessment of phrenic nerve function in infants and children. *J Thorac Cardiovasc Surg* **101**:143–147, 1991

117. Stewart S, Alexson C, Manning J: Bilateral phrenic nerve paralysis after the Mustard procedure. *J Thorac Cardiovasc Surg* **92**:138–141, 1986

118. Haller JA, Pickard LR, Tepas JJ, et al: Management of diaphragmatic paralysis in infants with special emphasis on selection of patients with operative plication. *J Pediatr Surg* **14**:779–785, 1979

119. Affatato A, Villagra F, DeLeon JP, et al: Phrenic nerve paralysis following pediatric cardiac surgery. Role of diaphragmatic plication. *J Cardiovasc Surg* **29**:606–609, 1988

120. Chandler KW, Rozas CJ, Kory RC, Goldman AL: Bilateral diaphragmatic paralysis complicating local cardiac hypothermia during open-heart surgery. *Am J Med* **77**:243–249, 1984

121. Villamater J, Charlton G, Spector ML, et al: A topical myocardial cooling device for paediatrics. *Perfusion* **1**:289–292, 1986

122. Prince SR, Laurence RL, Hackel AJ: Percutaneous catheterization of the internal jugular vein in infants and children. *Anesthesiology* **44**:170–174, 1976

123. Van der Salm TJ, Cerada J-M, Cutler BS: Brachial plexus injury following median sternotomy. *J Thorac Cardiovasc Surg* **80**:447–452, 1980

124. Van der Salm TJ, Cutler BS, Okike ON: Brachial plexus injury following median sternotomy. II. *J Thorac Cardiovasc Surg* **83**:914–917, 1982

125. Forestner JE: Ipsilateral mydriasis following carotid artery puncture during attempted cannulation of the internal jugular vein. *Anesthesiology* **52**:438–439, 1980

126. Loomis JC: Care of the pediatric patient following cardiovascular surgery. In Ream AM, Fodgall R: *Acute Car-*

diovascular Management—Anesthesia and Intensive Care. Philadelphia: JB Lippincott, 1982, p 674

127. Jackson L, Keats AS: Mechanism of brachial plexus palsy following anesthesia. *Anesthesiology* **26**:190–194, 1965

128. Tolmie JD, Comer PB, Pauca AL, Parkin CE: Anesthetic complications of intrathoracic surgery. In Cordell RA, Ellison RG (eds): *Complications of Intrathoracic Surgery.* Boston: Little, Brown, 1979, pp 3–23

129. Pollock EM, Ford-Jones EL, Rebeyka I, et al: Early nosocomial infections in pediatric cardiovascular surgery patients. *Crit Care Med* **18**:378–384, 1992

130. Berry FA, Blankenbaker WL, Ball CG: Comparison of bacteremia occurring with nasotracheal and orotracheal intubation. *Anesth Analg* **52**:873–877, 1973

131. Jurkiewicz MJ, Bostwick J, Hester T, et al: Infected median sternotomy wound: Successful treatment by muscle flaps. *Ann Surg* **191**:738–744, 1980

132. Mok CK, Cheung KL, Wai KH, Ong GB: Malaria complicating open heart surgery. *Thorax* **35**:389–391, 1980

133. Milne EMG, Elliott MJ, Pearson DT, Holden MP: The effect on intermediary metabolism of open-heart surgery with deep hypothermia and circulatory arrest in infants of less than 10 kilograms body weight. A preliminary study. *Perfusion* **1**:29–40, 1986

134. Mitchell IM, Pollock JCS, Jamieson PG, et al: The effects of cardiopulmonary bypass on thyroid function in infants weighing less than five kilograms. *J Thorac Cardiovasc Surg* **103**:800–805, 1992

Chapter 26 | Anesthesia for Noncardiac Surgery in Children and Adults with Congenital Heart Disease

David D. Frankville

As a result of remarkable progress in diagnosis and management, the life expectancy of patients with congenital heart disease is steadily increasing. Consequently, more children will grow to become adults and more will undergo noncardiac surgery. These patients are a special challenge to the anesthesiologist for three reasons. First, the diversity of anatomy and physiology defies easy categorization, so that it is difficult to apply general principles of management. Second, cardiovascular and pulmonary capacity can be severely limited. Third, there is little objective data upon which to formulate an anesthetic plan.

Even a relatively simple anatomic lesion such as a ventricular septal defect can result in a wide spectrum of physiologic impairments, all resulting from the same basic physiology of a left-to-right shunt. A patient's condition can change dramatically with time or compensatory mechanisms. These compensatory mechanisms may be inadequate or even contribute to further physiologic impairment. Some children who undergo surgical palliation demonstrate residual physiologic limitations, whereas others appear to be quite normal. Because of the diversity of disease that can result from a single cardiac defect, a knowledge of the natural history of both corrected and uncorrected congenital heart defects is required in addition to an understanding of the basic anatomy and physiology.

The two factors that most influence the choice of anesthesia and monitoring for noncardiac surgery are (1) the magnitude of the surgical procedure, and (2) the degree of cardiovascular and pulmonary impairment caused by the congenital heart defect. Unlike the multitude of anatomic defects responsible for congenital heart disease, cardiovascular impairment can generally be traced to one of four distinct etiologies: hypoxemia, pulmonary disease, cardiac failure, or dysrhythmias (Fig 26–1). These physiologic abnormalities can occur alone or in combination.

HYPOXEMIA (CYANOSIS)

The term *cyanosis* is defined as a blue coloration of the skin and mucous membranes due to the presence of reduced hemoglobin. Recently, utilization of the oximeter has minimized the importance of discussing the "minimum" amount of reduced hemoglobin necessary to produce cyanosis. The use of the term *hypoxemia* rather than cyanosis is helpful in avoiding this confusion. Clinical detection of hypoxemia is not always reliable, especially in the infant, and noninvasive measurement of oxygen saturation should be performed. Hypoxemia is often associated with congenital heart defects resulting in decreased pulmonary blood flow and right-to-left shunting; however, patients with increased pulmonary blood flow can also suffer from hypoxemia (Table 26–1). Chronic hypoxemia is a systemic disorder that disrupts all the major organ systems.

Several issues should be considered about the long-term complications of chronic hypoxemia. First, the pathophysiology associated with chronic hypoxemia must not be confused with the physiologic adjustments to

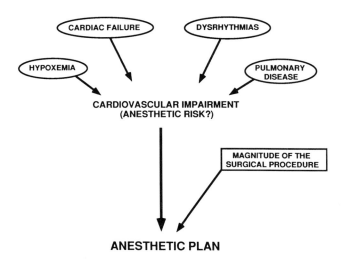

FIGURE 26–1. Factors influencing anesthetic management of the patient with congenital heart disease. The physiologic consequences of a congenital heart defect ultimately impair cardiovascular function. The presence and severity of these derangements, along with the magnitude of the surgical procedure, greatly influence the choice of anesthetic technique and monitoring for noncardiac surgery.

acute hypoxia. Second, data from experiments using adult humans or animals may not apply to the neonate or infant. Third, the physiologic responses to hypoxemia secondary to congenital heart disease may be quite different from those resulting from a low inspired oxygen content. Lastly, there is often concurrent pressure or volume overloading of the heart, and the ventricular dys-

function associated with hemodynamic stress can be superimposed upon that caused by chronic hypoxemia.

Cardiovascular System

Acute hypoxemia initiates both local vascular and centrally mediated responses. The result is a complex but coordinated cardiovascular, respiratory, and neurohumoral response that maintains oxygen delivery to vital organs. In response to acute hypoxemia, there is an immediate increase in ventilation, heart rate, and cardiac output. Blood flow is directed away from the musculature and abdominal organs toward the brain and heart. Systemic blood pressure remains relatively stable. Oxygen consumption and mixed venous oxygen saturation are both reduced. The net result of these changes is to preserve oxygen delivery to the brain and heart at the expense of other organ systems.[1–3]

As time progresses, the heart rate remains slightly elevated, but cardiac output returns to normal. The chemoreceptor response to hypoxia is decreased and ventilation is reduced.[4] However, a mild respiratory alkalosis persists. The most significant compensatory mechanism is the development of polycythemia, which allows adequate oxygen delivery to tissues without a persistent increase in cardiac output. Cerebral and myocardial oxygenation return to normal, whereas visceral and musculoskeletal oxygen delivery remain low despite the increased hematocrit.[5,6]

The consequences of chronic hypoxemia are different for the infant than the adult. In the normal infant, up to 36% of metabolism may be devoted to growth. Although hypoxemic children have normal total oxygen

TABLE 26–1. PHYSIOLOGIC ABNORMALITIES ASSOCIATED WITH SEVERAL CONGENITAL HEART DEFECTS

Cardiac Defect	Hypoxemia	Pulmonary Blood Flow	Cardiac Load	Dysrhythmias*
Anomalous pulmonary venous connection	+	↑	V	
Aortic stenosis			P	
Atrial septal defect†		↑	V	SVT
Atrioventricular canal	+	↑	V	CHB, SVT
Coarctation of the aorta			P	
Corrected transposition	±	↑ OR ↓	P / V	CHB
Ebstein anomaly	+	↓	V	SVT, VENT
Patent ductus arteriosus†		↑	V	
Pulmonary atresia with VSD	+	↓	V	
Pulmonary stenosis			P	
Single ventricle	+	↑ OR ↓	V	
Tetralogy of Fallot	+	↓	V	VENT
Transposition of the great vessels	±	↑ OR ↓	P / V	SVT, CHB
Tricuspid atresia	+	↓	V	SVT
Truncus arteriosus†	+	↑	V	
Ventricular septal defect†		↑	V	CHB

Abbreviations: V, volume load; P, pressure load; SVT, supraventricular tachycardia; VENT, ventricular tachycardia or ventricular fibrillation; CHB, complete heart block.

* Including late postoperative dysrhythmias.

† Hypoxemia and decreased pulmonary blood flow when the pulmonary vascular resistance is greater than systemic vascular resistance.

consumption and what appears to be adequate oxygen delivery to tissues, the metabolic activity of many organs remains low and growth is usually retarded. This indicates that chronically hypoxemic children expend more metabolic activity on nongrowth functions.[5,6] It has been postulated that anabolic metabolism is inhibited because of reduced stores of adenosine triphosphate (ATP) and decreased replication of deoxyribonucleic acid (DNA).

Heart. At rest, chronic hypoxemia does not appear to be associated with impaired left ventricular function, and in the presence of polycythemia, myocardial oxygen delivery appears to be normal. However, the ability to increase cardiac output in response to exercise or pharmacologically induced tachycardia is reduced.[7,8] This reduction of maximal exercise capability is thought to be secondary to myocardial dysfunction caused by chronic hypoxemia. Several mechanisms for myocardial dysfunction have been postulated, including recurrent episodes of severe hypoxemia, decreased coronary perfusion pressure secondary to systemic to pulmonary artery shunting, and increased blood viscosity leading to microvascular occlusion. All of these mechanisms result in myocardial ischemia and fibrosis, a common postmortem finding, even in the hypoxemic infant. Ultimately, ventricular diastolic compliance is reduced, and a greater ventricular end-diastolic volume is required to maintain stroke volume. Thus, cardiac reserve is reduced or ventricular failure occurs.

Children undergoing surgery to correct hypoxemia (eg, "total repair" of tetralogy of Fallot) before the age of 2 years can have normal left ventricular function postoperatively. However, those undergoing surgery after 2 years of age have normal left ventricular function only at rest. The reduced ability to increase cardiac output[9–11] in response to exercise suggests that chronic hypoxemia is associated with irreversible myocardial damage if allowed to persist.

Acute hypoxemia stimulates myocardial hypertrophy and has been demonstrated in adults with ischemic heart disease and in experimental studies of newborn rats.[3,12] Although it is likely that hypoxemia alone stimulates ventricular hypertrophy in the newborn human, most congenital cardiac defects also place additional volume or pressure workload on the heart, making it impossible to distinguish the predominant etiologic factor. Chronic hypoxemia also leads to several myocardial abnormalities that are similar to those that occur in response to hemodynamic stress. Bernstein[13] has demonstrated a 45% reduction of β receptor density in left ventricles exposed to hypoxemia but protected from additional cardiac workload. Adenylate cyclase activity was also decreased 39%, and circulating epinephrine was greatly increased. These data indicate that increased sympathetic tone persists during chronic hypoxemia leading to downregulation of β receptors. The reduction

of β receptors may contribute to the decreased myocardial function that occurs with chronic hypoxemia. Although decreased receptor sensitivity to epinephrine and depletion of myocardial norepinephrine was not demonstrated, this pathology is strikingly similar to that found in the failing adult ventricle.[14]

Hematology. Chronic hypoxemia is associated with two hematologic alterations that are of concern to the anesthesiologist: the development of polycythemia and abnormal hemostasis.

Polycythemia

Polycythemia is the major adaptive response to chronic hypoxemia. Tissue hypoxia increases both cardiac output and the oxygen-carrying capacity of the blood that allows normal systemic oxygen delivery without a large sustained increase of cardiac output. Hypoxia triggers release of erythropoietin from specialized cells in the kidney, which then stimulates bone marrow production of red blood cells and an increase of the circulating blood volume. Erythrocyte mass may be as great as three times normal, and blood volume may be over 100 mL/kg.[15]

As the hematocrit increases, blood viscosity increases dramatically (Fig 26–2). Although the hematocrit appears to be the major determinant of viscosity in larger vessels, other variables attain importance in the smaller vessels. These include the protein content, blood flow velocity, and red blood cell distensibility. Alignment of red cells within small blood vessels (Fahraeus-Lindqvist effect) reduces viscosity. In children with cyanotic heart disease, hyperviscosity is associated with thromboses of intracranial veins and sinuses, sometimes resulting in stroke. Children under the age of 5 years are at highest risk, particularly when there is concurrent iron deficiency, fever, or dehydration.[16] Adults with cyanotic congenital heart disease appear to be at decreased risk for thrombotic intracranial accidents, even with hematocrits of greater than 65%, but instead suffer from a propensity toward intracranial bleeding.[17] The etiology of this age-related difference is unknown.

In some patients with cyanotic heart disease, the elevated hematocrit ultimately limits pulmonary and systemic blood flow. This excessive erythroid response has been termed "decompensated erythrocytosis."[15] These patients exhibit fluctuating hematocrits and suffer symptoms of increased blood viscosity that include fatigue, faintness, headache, visual disturbances, depressed mentation, myalgias, and paresthesias of the toes and fingers (Table 26–2). There appears to be no relationship between the type of cardiac defect or degree of hypoxemia and the development of decompensated erythrocytosis.

The microcytic red cells seen with iron deficiency are extremely rigid resulting in significant increases in blood viscosity. Those with "decompensated erythrocy-

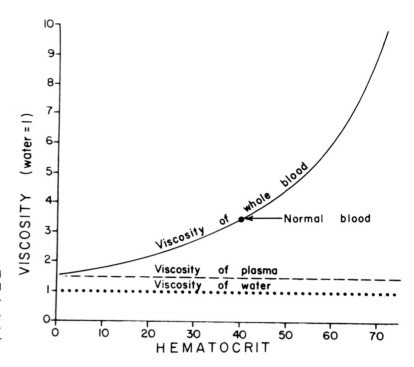

Figure 26–2. Relationship between blood viscosity and hematocrit. Hematocrit is the primary determinant of blood viscosity. Increasing the hematocrit will increase both systemic and pulmonary vascular resistance. (*From Guyton, AC (ed): Textbook of Medical Physiology, 7th ed. Philadelphia: WB Saunders, 1986, p 207, with permission.*)

tosis" often exhibit microcytosis secondary to depleted iron stores.[18] Inappropriate phlebotomies can further reduce iron stores and significantly impair tissue oxygen delivery by a combination of decreased hemoglobin content and increased numbers of microcytic cells. Iron deficiency should always be suspected when symptoms of hyperviscosity are present and the hematocrit is less than 65%.

Preoperative phlebotomy is indicated for those patients with significant symptomatic hyperviscosity and hematocrits greater than 65%.[17] Dehydration must first be corrected before a decision to remove blood is made. The objective is to reduce the hematocrit to a level at which symptoms of hyperviscosity are relieved. Ideally, a reduction of hematocrit will increase the stroke volume, increase systemic blood flow, and enhance systemic oxygen delivery. Quantitative intravascular fluid replacement of phlebotomized blood is essential in achieving these goals.

Patients with compensated erythrocytosis have stable hematocrits and symptoms of hyperviscosity are often absent even when hematocrits reach 70%. Microcytosis is uncommon in this population and therapeutic phlebotomies are seldom necessary.[17]

Hemostasis

As many as one out of five patients with congenital heart disease (both cyanotic and acyanotic) have laboratory evidence of abnormal hemostasis.[19] Abnormal hemostasis appears to correlate with the degree of hypoxemia and erythrocytosis; however, the etiology remains unclear. Reported hemostatic abnormalities include thrombocytopenia, platelet dysfunction, hypofibrinogenemia, accelerated fibrinolysis, and factor deficiencies.[17,20] Deficiency of von Willebrand factor has been reported in patients with acyanotic heart disease,[21] but there are no reports suggesting this occurs in cyanotic patients. Prolongation of the prothrombin time or the partial thromboplastin time is the most common laboratory abnormality. Patients may exhibit easy bruising, epistaxis, heavy menses, and hemoptysis. Drugs such as aspirin, heparin, nonsteroidal anti-inflammatory agents, and other anticoagulants may exacerbate the already abnormal hemostasis. Significant spontaneous hemorrhage is rare, but the risk of excessive perioperative bleeding is real even when tests of coagulation are normal. Reduction of red blood cell mass has been reported to correct

TABLE 26–2. SYMPTOMS OF HYPERVISCOSITY SYNDROME

Central Nervous System
  Headache
  Faintness
  Dizziness
  Blurred vision
  Amaurosis fugax
  Depressed mentation
General
  Fatigue
  Lassitude
  Muscle weakness
  Myalgias
  Paresthesias of the fingers, toes, and lips

the hemostatic defects in some polycythemic patients.[17] Enough blood is removed to reduce the hematocrit to less than 65%. The partial thromboplastin time can be used to assess the response to preoperative phlebotomy. Blood removed from the patient should be saved for possible autologous transfusion during or after the operation.

Other hematologic changes associated with cyanotic congenital heart disease include an increase in 2,3-diphosphoglycerate and urate levels. Although 2,3-diphosphoglycerate levels are usually elevated, the correlation with the degree of hypoxia or erythrocyte mass is poor. The oxygen-hemoglobin dissociation curve is generally normal or only slightly shifted to the right. In addition, uric acid levels may be elevated secondary to decreased excretion by the kidney. However, urate nephropathy and urolithiasis only rarely occur. Arthralgias are common in adults with cyanotic congenital heart disease but attacks of gout are uncommon.

Central Nervous System

Congenital heart defects that result in chronic hypoxemia also are associated with impairment of neurologic development. The cognitive, sensory, and motor systems are all affected. Children with chronic hypoxemia appear to be at greater risk of neurologic damage than children with acyanotic congenital heart disease.

Brain abscess can occur in any child with congenital heart disease; however, it is most frequently seen in patients with a right-to-left shunt, particularly older children with tetralogy of Fallot.[22] Although relatively rare, the consequences are grave, and the diagnosis can easily be missed. Symptoms include headache, vomiting, lethargy, personality changes, convulsions, and focal neurologic signs. Blood cultures are often negative and patients may not exhibit fever. The mortality is high, and rapid surgical drainage combined with antibiotics is justified. The incidence of cerebrovascular thrombosis and hemorrhage appears to be decreasing in recent years. This is probably related to earlier and more satisfactory palliation of most congenital heart defects.

As a group, children with prolonged hypoxemia have slightly lower intelligence test scores and do not perform perceptual motor tasks as well as children with acyanotic heart disease. Newburger has found that the longer the child is hypoxemic, the greater the neurologic impairment.[23] This is supported by neuropathologic studies that demonstrate increased abnormalities of the white matter with age in children who have not undergone satisfactory palliation. This decline in neurologic function may also be attributable to increasing cumulative risk of subtle cerebrovascular accidents, stimulus deprivation resulting from diminished physical activity, or social factors. Although there are no definitive studies to differentiate between these hypotheses, Rossi et al presented provocative data supporting the role of chronic

hypoxia as an important factor producing neurologic damage.[24] They found that serum levels of brain-type creatine kinase were significantly higher in children with chronic hypoxemia than in children without hypoxemia.[24] This correlation between the degree of hypoxemia and the level of brain-type creatine kinase indicates that central nervous system damage is an ongoing process in hypoxemic children. It is noteworthy that there was no correlation between brain-type creatine kinase levels and hemoglobin levels (the degree of polycythemia).

Patients who have already undergone successful palliation of congenital cardiac defects may suffer from residual neurologic damage related to the operative procedure. Attention has generally focused on children in whom deep hypothermic circulatory arrest was employed, and controversy exists as to whether the use of this technique results in significant neurologic sequelae. Several studies have focused on comparisons between children with congenital heart disease and healthy children, including siblings.[25–28] These comparisons are confounded by many other factors, including stimulus deprivation, social conditions, and preoperative condition. Unfortunately, there is no truly objective marker for subtle neurologic injury. Blackwood et al have studied a group of children before and after deep hypothermic circulatory arrest and found no degradation of psychomotor development.[29] However, several investigators have reported various neurologic sequelae, including seizures, choreoathetosis, dyskinesias, hypotonia, pseudobulbar signs, and affective disorders. Postoperative seizures generally are not permanent[25,26,28,29]; however, it is not known if the other neurologic abnormalities also resolve with time.

Anesthetic Considerations

Preoperative evaluation should be directed toward obtaining a complete description of the anatomy and all previous surgical procedures. By its presence alone, hypoxemia indicates inadequate palliation and the existence of cardiac abnormalities. In addition to determining the degree of hypoxemia at rest, a history of hypercyanotic episodes (including precipitating factors) or recent changes in the degree of hypoxemia should be elicited. Although a decreased exercise tolerance is not specific for hypoxemia, it is an excellent indicator of overall cardiovascular function and is a part of the history that may influence anesthetic management. Hypoxemic children are generally small for age. Although distinguishing between cardiac and pulmonary causes of hypoxemia can be extremely difficult, the attempt should be made because active pulmonary infection is an indication for postponing elective surgical procedures. If there are symptoms referable to hyperviscosity or abnormal hemostasis, a hematologist should be consulted to determine the need for preoperative phlebotomy. History of previous neurologic damage resulting from surgery, embolism, or infection should be noted.

Preoperative laboratory studies should begin with a hematocrit and indices of red blood cell size. In general, the hematocrit correlates with the severity of hypoxemia. However, children or adults may suffer from iron deficiency or excessive phlebotomy, thus deceptively reducing the hematocrit. If indicated by the magnitude of the surgical procedure, adequate hemostasis should be ascertained by testing of platelet function and coagulation. A recent echocardiographic study is essential in defining the current anatomy and blood flow patterns. Transesophageal echocardiography should be considered if the precordial study is technically inadequate.

Hypoxemia alone is not an indication for invasive monitoring. The magnitude of the surgical procedure, ventricular function, anesthetic technique, and the severity of the underlying physiology are all factors that should be considered before inserting central venous or arterial catheters. Insertion of a catheter into the pulmonary artery may be technically difficult and the information obtained not easily interpreted. Obviously, a reliable oximeter signal is essential. If available, transesophageal echocardiography can provide useful data about ventricular function, end-diastolic volumes, and the magnitude of right-to-left shunting. Physiologic dead space may be increased, and end-tidal CO_2 measurements may underestimate the arterial P_{CO_2} (see subsequent section on pulmonary dysfunction).

Premedication may be especially useful if the child has a history of worsening hypoxemia when excited or agitated. Oral, rectal, or intramuscular regimens are all safe and effective.[30-32] The oral route of administration has the advantage of avoiding excitement when giving the premedication. Supplemental oxygen may be used to maintain oxygen saturation at the baseline level.

Patients who are markedly polycythemic should not be allowed to become dehydrated. The duration of the preoperative fast should be minimal for age, or an intravenous infusion should be started to prevent dehydration. Care should be taken to prevent infusion of bubbles in patients with right-to-left shunting.

The choice of anesthetic drugs is of less importance than achieving the appropriate hemodynamic goals for each cardiac defect.[33,34] Whatever the underlying cardiac defect, the primary objective is to maintain adequate tissue oxygenation. This is best accomplished by understanding the underlying cause of hypoxemia for each patient. There are two general categories of patients who suffer from hypoxemia of cardiac origin: (1) those with limited pulmonary blood flow and right-to-left shunting of blood, and (2) those with unimpeded pulmonary blood flow and significant mixing of pulmonary venous and systemic venous blood. Anesthetic management for each of these situations is quite different.

If pulmonary blood flow is limited, the source of obstruction to flow must be identified and the determinants of flow across the obstruction characterized. Figure 26–3 summarizes the principal sites where pulmonary blood flow can be obstructed and the techniques for maintaining flow. The general strategy to avoid hypoxemia during induction or maintenance of anesthesia in patients with limited pulmonary blood flow is to (1) ensure adequate hydration, (2) maintain systemic arterial blood pressure, (3) minimize additional resistance to pulmonary blood flow, and (4) avoid sudden increases in systemic oxygen demand (crying, struggling, inadequate level of anesthesia).

In those situations in which pulmonary blood flow is unimpeded but mixing of systemic venous and pulmonary venous blood occurs, arterial saturation will depend on the ratio of pulmonary to systemic blood flow (Qp/Qs ratio). In general, fully saturated arterial blood should not be expected and may not even be desirable. Excessive increases of the pulmonary to systemic flow ratio (Qp/Qs) will either increase the amount of cardiac work or result in decreased systemic perfusion if cardiovascular performance is already maximal. The primary anesthetic concerns for this category of patients include (1) maintaining ventricular performance, and (2) preventing alterations of the Qp/Qs ratio.

The pharmacokinetics of intravenously administered drugs and uptake and distribution of inhaled anesthetics in the presence of right-to-left shunting are discussed in Chapter 9. Although the effects of shunting on speed of induction should be considered, the ultimate clinical significance is minimal. Attention should focus on the important hemodynamic considerations.

Despite a reduction in the number of myocardial β receptors, newborn lambs with experimental cyanotic heart disease appear to be capable of a normal response to exogenously administered adrenergic agents.[35] An important postoperative consideration is the blunting of the chemoreceptor response to hypoxia. This situation is analogous to that of a patient after bilateral carotid endarterectomies. Profound hypoxia can occur without eliciting the normal response of increased ventilation, particularly when respiratory depressants such as narcotics have been given. Oxygen saturation should be maintained at the desired level by the use of supplemental oxygen until the child is fully awake. The mechanism of this blunted response to hypoxia is unknown, but it appears that the ventilatory response to hypoxemia returns to normal after palliative surgery to correct hypoxemia.[4] Chronic hypoxemia does not alter the ventilatory response to carbon dioxide or hydrogen ion concentration.

PULMONARY ABNORMALITIES

Cardiovascular disease imposes additional demands on the respiratory system because of its effects on gas exchange, fluid accumulation in the lung, and pulmonary mechanics. Conversely, acute pulmonary disease may

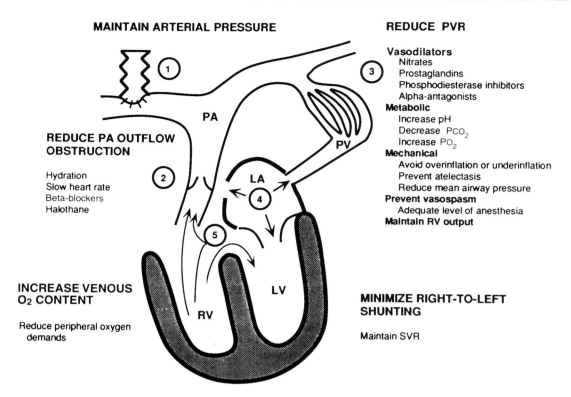

Figure 26–3. Factors that influence pulmonary blood flow in patients with reduced pulmonary blood flow. (1) Pulmonary blood flow in patients with a systemic to pulmonary artery shunt (modified Blalock-Taussig, central shunt) is dependent on the physical characteristics of the shunt (primarily length and diameter) and the pressure gradient across the shunt. Because the physical characteristics of the shunt are fixed, and the pulmonary arterial pressures are usually low relative to the systemic circulation, pulmonary blood flow is dependent primarily on systemic arterial pressure. (2) Pulmonary blood flow may be obstructed above, below, or at the level of the pulmonary valve. Infundibular stenosis (as in tetralogy of Fallot) can be thought of as a form of IHSS. Increasing right ventricular volume, slowing the heart rate, and giving β-blockers to promote relaxation of the myocardium should increase flow through the obstruction. Valvular or supravalvular obstructions may be treated surgically or by interventional catheterization. (3) At the level of the small pulmonary capillaries and vessels, pulmonary blood flow is limited by the vascular resistance and alveolar pressure. Flow can be manipulated by vasodilating drugs, metabolic factors, blunting reactive vasoconstriction, optimizing ventilatory mechanics, and maintaining right ventricular output. (4) Pulmonary blood flow can be obstructed at the junction of the pulmonary vein and left atrium, at the mitral valve, or through an atrial septal defect (if the mitral valve is restrictive or if the vein drains into the right atrium). Surgical intervention is usually required. (5) In the presence of pulmonary outflow obstruction and a ventricular septal defect (as in tetralogy of Fallot), increasing the systemic vascular resistance will "push" or prevent blood from shunting across the septal defect, thus promoting blood flow into the pulmonary artery. PA, pulmonary artery; PV, pulmonary vein; LA, left atrium; RV, right ventricle; LV, left ventricle.

stress a cardiovascular system that does not have the necessary reserves to compensate for the additional burden. In addition, patients with congenital heart defects frequently have congenital abnormalities of the airway. The anesthesiologist can classify pulmonary problems associated with congenital heart disease as those involving the head and neck that complicate laryngoscopy and intubation, those resulting in partial or complete obstruction of the large and small airways, and those associated with excessive or reduced pulmonary blood flow.

Abnormalities of the Airway

Frequently, a congenital cardiac defect is accompanied by other congenital anomalies. Abnormalities of the head and neck are of great concern to the anesthesiologist who must provide for adequate ventilation and oxygenation during anesthesia, usually by endotracheal intubation. In addition to a thorough preoperative examination of the airway, there are several syndromes or genetic disorders that are known to be present with both congenital heart defects and abnormal airway anatomy (see Appendix 26–2).

Wells[36] has recently described an association between congenital heart defects and a short trachea in neonates and infants. As a consequence of fewer cartilaginous rings, the tracheal bifurcation occurs two to three vertebral segments more cephalad than usual, thus increasing the likelihood of endobronchial intubation. This abnormality was most commonly associated with the DiGeorge anomaly (77%), skeletal dysplasia (55%), brevicollis (57%), and diaplacental rubella (40%). The majority of these dysmorphic syndromes are also associated with an increased incidence of congenital heart defects. Cardiovascular abnormalities most commonly associated with short trachea appear to be those manifested by abnormal development of the aortic valve or aortic arch, in particular, interrupted aortic arch (89%) and hypoplastic left heart syndrome (63%). Those congenital heart defects without aortic valve or arch abnormalities also have a 25% incidence of short trachea. It is not known if the trachea grows to a normal length as the infant grows.

Large and Small Airways Obstruction

In addition to the well-described obstruction of the trachea and esophagus caused by vascular rings, the trachea and large bronchi can also be compressed by an enlarged heart, pulmonary artery, aorta, or artificial conduits. Left atrial enlargement may cause an upward displacement of both major bronchi increasing the angle of the tracheal bifurcation. Pulmonary artery enlargement secondary to pulmonary hypertension can lead to compression of the superior portion of the left main bronchus, the lateral and superior portions of the right intermediate and middle bronchus, and the posterior portion of the left upper bronchus.[37] An enlarged or displaced aorta can compress the trachea on either the right or left side depending on the location of the aortic arch. Artificial conduits do not grow and require the insertion of as large a prosthesis as possible, which often leads to compression of all adjacent structures.[38]

Small airway obstruction is of great clinical significance to the infant. It is particularly common in infants with pulmonary hypertension. In addition to enlarged distal pulmonary arteries impinging on the small airways,[39] marked bronchiolar smooth muscle hyperplasia has been observed.[40] Small airway obstruction is partially reversible with bronchodilators indicating that bronchoconstriction may contribute to the clinical process. Lastly, lung parenchyma can be compressed by an enlarged heart or great vessels.

Airway obstruction produces stridor, increased work of breathing, lobar hyperinflation, atelectasis, and an increased susceptibility to infections.[41] Complete or partial obstruction of the large or small airways secondary to pulmonary hypertension is most prominent in children less than 1 year of age. In children over 1 year of age, the airways are larger, the child is better suited to compensate for the increased work of breathing, and the pulmonary blood flow may actually decrease if the pulmonary vascular resistance increases. It is not until the pulmonary vascular changes are quite advanced or ventricular failure develops that airway obstruction again becomes a significant clinical problem.

Nerve Palsy

Both phrenic and recurrent laryngeal nerve palsy have been described in children with congenital heart disease.

Compression or stretching caused by native structures, particularly the aorta, pulmonary artery, and atria, can occur in those who have not undergone palliative surgery. Surgical injury to these two nerves is secondary to retraction, thermal injury in the pericardium, internal jugular venous cannulation, or surgical transection. The left recurrent laryngeal nerve appears to be the most vulnerable because of its fixed location, which is in close proximity to the aorta, ductus, and pulmonary artery. Phrenic nerve injury rarely occurs, but when it does, it has dire consequences, particularly if the damage is bilateral.[42,43] Surgical procedures associated with nerve injury include ligation of the ductus arteriosus, repair of coarctation of the aorta, tracheostomy, and systemic to pulmonary artery shunts.

Pulmonary Abnormalities Associated with Decreased Pulmonary Blood Flow

Lees et al[44] demonstrated that children suffering from chronic hypoxemia have a slightly increased alveolar ventilation. Pulmonary venous P_{O_2} is high and pulmonary venous P_{CO_2} is lower than normal. Peripheral arterial P_{CO_2} is maintained within a narrow range. Despite the high pulmonary venous P_{O_2}, an increased alveolar to pulmonary venous gradient can be present owing to ventilation/perfusion mismatching. Because of the low pressure and blood flow in the pulmonary artery, physiologic dead space is frequently increased. The ratio of dead space to tidal volume can be as high as 0.6.[45] Factors accentuating ventilation to perfusion mismatch include decreased left atrial or pulmonary vascular pressure or increased alveolar pressure, which occur with initiation of positive-pressure ventilation, excessive continuous positive airway pressure, or severe hypovolemia.

Functional residual capacity and pulmonary compliance are generally unchanged in children with decreased pulmonary blood flow.[45–47] However, respiratory rate and tidal volume are slightly increased (Table 26–3).

Pulmonary gas exchange may be even more complicated in the presence of low pulmonary pressures and

TABLE 26–3. EFFECTS OF PULMONARY BLOOD FLOW (PBF) ON PULMONARY MECHANICS

	Increased PBF	Decreased PBF
Minute ventilation	↑	↑
Tidal volume	↓	normal
Respiratory rate	↑	normal or ↑
Functional residual capacity	normal	normal
Pulmonary compliance	↓ ↓	normal
Physiologic dead space	normal	↑ ↑
Airway resistance	↑ ↑	normal

flow in one lung and high pulmonary flow and pressures in the other, which sometimes results in unilateral pulmonary edema. This situation arises after creation of a systemic to pulmonary artery shunt[48,49] or improper pulmonary artery banding.[50] Positive-pressure ventilation worsens the ventilation to perfusion relationship because ventilation will be preferential to the more compliant (low perfusion) lung.

Pulmonary Abnormalities Associated with Increased Pulmonary Blood Flow

Manifestations of excessive pulmonary blood flow and/or pulmonary hypertension include a progressive increase in pulmonary vascular resistance, obstruction of both the large and small airways, impaired gas exchange, and alterations of pulmonary mechanics. There is great variation in both pathology and clinical presentation. Mechanisms responsible for the pathologic changes occurring in response to excessive pulmonary blood flow remain poorly understood.

Persistent elevation of pulmonary blood flow and pulmonary hypertension results in maldevelopment of the pulmonary vasculature. First, there is abnormal extension of smooth muscle along the distal vessels, followed by hypertrophy of the medial layer of the arteries. Later, there is a reduction in the number and size of the distal pulmonary arteries, a finding that indicates that the vascular changes are irreversible. The progression of histologic changes associated with increased pulmonary blood flow has been extensively reviewed, and it may be categorized by the criteria most recently refined by Rabinovitch.[39]

Although the exact mechanism producing histologic changes of the pulmonary vasculature in response to either excessive pulmonary blood flow or pulmonary hypertension is unknown, the degree to which these changes develop appears to be dependent on the nature of the cardiac defect.[39] Patients with secundum atrial septal defects seldom develop irreversible pulmonary vascular changes until adulthood. However, those with large ventricular septal defects or a large patent ductus arteriosus will generally not suffer from irreversible changes if the underlying defect is repaired before 2 years of age. A few congenital cardiac defects (including complete atrioventricular canal or truncus arteriosus) are associated with irreversible pulmonary changes before the second year of life. Abnormal pulmonary vascular development eventually leads to irreversible elevation of the pulmonary vascular resistance; a development that precludes adequate surgical palliation.

Increased pulmonary venous return to the left atrium results in enlargement of the left atrium and, occasionally, increased left atrial pressures. Elevation of the left atrial pressure can contribute to an increased lung water content[51] and increased pulmonary vascular resistance. Two other factors that have been postulated

to contribute to the development of interstitial and alveolar edema include excessive transudation of fluid secondary to mechanical damage to the endothelium and reduced pulmonary lymphatic drainage.[41]

Although children with excessive pulmonary blood flow have normal alveolar ventilation, they exhibit an increased respiratory rate and a reduced tidal volume (see Table 26–3). The functional residual capacity[47] and physiologic dead space are both normal. The two predominant alterations of pulmonary mechanics are a marked reduction of pulmonary compliance and an increased airway resistance.[46,52,53] This contributes to an increased work of breathing, which is a significant problem for the infant who is already at a mechanical disadvantage for maintaining adequate ventilation (Fig 26–4). Airway obstruction appears to resolve rapidly after surgical correction.[54]

Anesthetic Considerations

Preoperative evaluation of patients with the pulmonary sequelae of congenital heart disease should focus on three factors. First, congenital heart defects are frequently associated with abnormalities of the airways.

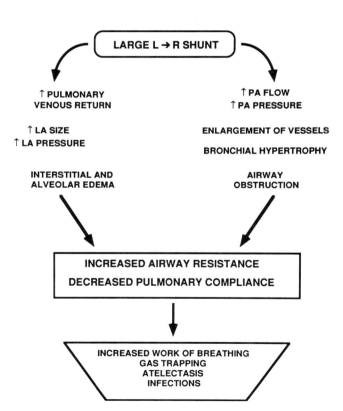

Figure 26–4. Respiratory consequences of increased pulmonary flow and pressure. Two important respiratory consequences of a large left-to-right shunt are increased airway resistance and decreased pulmonary compliance. In both infants and patients with inadequately palliated cardiac disease, these respiratory abnormalities can be the predominant clinical feature.

These abnormalities can make laryngoscopy and intubation difficult or can be a source of significant airway obstruction. Second, the amount of pulmonary blood flow (excessive or inadequate) should be determined. This is usually inferred from the anatomy, palliative surgical procedures, the presence of hypoxemia or congestive heart failure, echocardiography, or cardiac catheterization data. Lastly, intrinsic pulmonary disease (especially infectious) must be distinguished from pulmonary abnormalities secondary to cardiac disease.

Anesthetic Management of Increased Pulmonary Blood Flow.

Anesthetic considerations for patients with increased pulmonary blood flow or pulmonary hypertension vary considerably depending on the degree of pulmonary vascular pathology. Infants without increased pulmonary vascular resistance can have greatly increased pulmonary blood flow, which stresses the ability of the heart to maintain the increased volume workload. In these patients, congestive heart failure may be the primary clinical problem. Obstruction of the large and small airways results in increased resistance to airflow, which combined with relatively noncompliant lungs, increases the inspiratory pressure needed for adequate positive-pressure ventilation. In addition, the subsequent increased work of breathing may contribute to the length of time postoperative ventilation is required.

Children who have excessively developed pulmonary vascular smooth musculature are also susceptible to pulmonary vasoconstriction. Acute pulmonary vasoconstriction, occurring with inadequate anesthesia, following intense stimulation (inserting an endotracheal tube, suctioning an endotracheal tube), or associated with inadequate ventilation, can result in sudden and significant elevations of pulmonary artery pressure. Pulmonary vasoconstriction can be prevented by providing adequate anesthesia,[55] ventilation, and oxygenation. Pulmonary vasodilators are useful for severe vasoconstriction.

Chronic exposure to excessive pulmonary blood flow that ultimately produces irreversible pulmonary vasculature changes causes pulmonary vascular resistance to equal or exceed systemic vascular resistance. If there is a communication between the systemic and pulmonary circulations, a left-to-right shunt becomes a bidirectional or right-to-left shunt. The symptoms resulting from the pulmonary hypertension and right-to-left shunt are termed the Eisenmenger syndrome. These patients are usually New York Heart Association (NYHA) functional class III or IV, and anesthetic risk appears to be quite high.[56] Not only do these patients suffer from end-stage pulmonary vascular disease but also from hypoxemia, myocardial dysfunction, and dysrhythmias. The anesthetic management of these patients generally focuses on the prevention of any increase of the right-to-left shunt. However, attention should also be given to avoiding anesthetic-induced myocardial depression or triggering dysrhythmias. Hemodynamic goals are dependent on the underlying anatomy and physiology. In general, hypovolemia, increased pulmonary vascular resistance, and reductions of systemic vascular resistance should be avoided.

Anesthetic Management of Decreased Pulmonary Blood Flow

Anesthetic management of patients with decreased pulmonary blood flow is centered on the prevention of further reductions of flow (see Fig 26–3). Ventilation of these patients is generally uneventful. However, physiologic dead space increases with initiation of positive-pressure ventilation, excessive alveolar pressure, or reduction of left atrial and pulmonary artery pressures. Maintaining both intravascular volume and ventricular function are beneficial during positive-pressure ventilation. Because of the large physiologic dead space, end-tidal CO_2 measurements consistently underestimate the arterial P_{CO_2}.[45,57]

CARDIAC FAILURE

Cardiac (ventricular) failure is the condition in which the heart cannot pump enough blood to meet the metabolic demands of the body. Ventricular function refers to the interrelationship between the ability of the heart to pump blood and ventricular preload, afterload, contractility, and heart rate. Cardiac function should be distinguished from contractility, which refers only to the inotropic state of the heart. Cardiac (ventricular) reserve is the difference between resting cardiac function and maximal cardiac function. The term *limited cardiac reserve* indicates that the heart is working at or near maximum capability when the patient is at rest. The presence of acute or impending cardiac failure often necessitates major adjustments of anesthetic and monitoring techniques.

Although overt congestive heart failure is usually not difficult to detect, the seemingly normal patient who in fact has limited cardiac reserve can provide the anesthesiologist with an unpleasant surprise. Thus, an important step in the anesthetic management of patients with compromised ventricular function is determining the extent of cardiac reserve. This task is not always straightforward because several compensatory mechanisms act to maintain resting cardiac output and blood pressure despite reductions in myocardial contractility or increased cardiac workload. Clinical deterioration may not become apparent until after these compensatory mechanisms fail.

Congenital heart defects may compromise the ability of the heart to maintain adequate systemic perfusion. There are important differences in the determinants of myocardial performance, the manner in which cardiac workload is increased, and the compensatory mechanisms that occur in response to increased cardiac demand in infants and adults. These differences affect the anesthetic considerations for patients with marginal or inadequate ventricular function.

Cardiac Failure in Patients with Congenital Heart Disease

Cardiac performance is dependent on the ability of the heart to act as a muscular pump. Muscular performance is dependent on preload (end-diastolic wall tension), afterload (systolic wall tension), and contractility. The clinical equivalents of preload and afterload are end-diastolic volume and impedance to ventricular ejection, respectively. Many of the compensatory mechanisms triggered by an increased cardiac workload act to optimize preload, afterload, or contractility. Unfortunately, these compensatory mechanisms may not always be beneficial when sustained for long periods of time, or they may not increase myocardial performance enough to meet the demands placed upon the heart.

Increased Cardiac Workload. Increased cardiac workload, a common feature of congenital heart disease, can be secondary to either increased impedance to ventricular ejection (pressure overload) or increased end-diastolic and stroke volumes (volume overload). Pressure overload is associated with ventricular outflow obstruction, aortic or pulmonary artery obstruction, increased arterial vascular tone, or greatly increased blood viscosity. Volume overload occurs in association with valvular insufficiency or left-to-right shunting. In patients with congenital heart defects, it is not uncommon for the heart to be burdened by both pressure and volume overload. In addition, each ventricle may be stressed independently of the other. Ventricular pressure-volume relationships are an informative way to understand the magnitude of the increased cardiac work associated with either pressure or volume load (Fig 26–5).

Reduced Myocardial Contractility. Reduced myocardial contractility becomes a clinical feature of many patients with congenital heart disease with prolonged exposure to increased cardiac workload. Although a number of metabolic alterations have been identified in the failing heart, the fundamental defects decreasing contractility are largely unknown.[58] Proposed etiologies include an inadequate vascular supply to the heart, hyperviscosity secondary to polycythemia leading to vascular occlusions, chronic hypoxemia, and decreased perfusion secondary to elevated ventricular wall tension.[59,60] On a cellular level, abnormal mitochondrial function, alterations of the contractile proteins, and abnormalities of the sarcoplasmic reticulum have all been demonstrated. However, a single unifying biochemical defect has not been identified.[12,58,61]

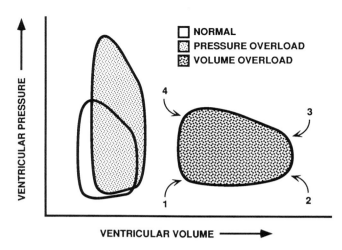

Figure 26–5. Pressure-volume relationships for normal, pressure overloaded, and volume overloaded ventricles. (1) Mitral valve opening, start of ventricular filling. (2) Mitral valve closure, beginning of isovolumic contraction. (3) Aortic valve opening, beginning of cardiac ejection. (4) Aortic valve closure (end-systolic point), beginning of isovolumic relaxation. Stroke volume is the difference in ventricular volume between points 3 and 4. Stroke work is proportional to the region inside the pressure-volume loops (hatched areas). Note that stroke work is greatly increased for both the pressure and volume overloaded ventricles.

Cardiac Dysfunction after Palliative Surgery. After cardiac surgery, cardiac dysfunction may reflect impaired myocardial contractility or increased cardiac workload secondary to residual anatomic defects. Postoperative cardiac dysfunction may be caused by several factors, including (1) cellular injury from inadequate myocardial protection, (2) inadequate coronary perfusion resulting in myocardial ischemia, (3) loss of functioning myocardium secondary to mechanical injury, (4) persistent hypoxemia, (5) persistent pressure or volume overload, (6) and persistent dysrhythmias (Table 26–4).[62] It appears that the earlier palliative surgery is undertaken to relieve hypoxemia or excessive cardiac workload, the more likely that cardiac function will be normal in the early and late postoperative periods.[62-64] Preoperative determinants of normal postoperative cardiac function after palliation of hypoxemia and/or pressure and volume overloading are currently unknown.

Assessment of Cardiac Function. A multitude of techniques are used to assess ventricular function (Table 26–5). These include measurement of the cardiac output, measurement of cardiac chamber pressures and volumes, and measures of the ability of the ventricle to relax and fill with blood (diastolic function) or contract and eject blood (systolic function). However, there are several limitations to each method. First, most techniques suffer from the inability to distinguish which determinant of ventricular function (preload, afterload, or

TABLE 26–4. CAUSES OF CARDIAC DYSFUNCTION AFTER CARDIAC SURGERY

Inadequate Myocardial Protection During the Operation
   Cardioplegia not protective
   Prolonged ischemic time
   Reperfusion injury
Inadequate Myocardial Perfusion
   Injury to coronary arteries
   Elevated oxygen demands secondary to residual pressure or volume loads
Mechanical Damage to Myocardium
   Ventriculotomy
   Retraction
Residual Hypoxemia Leading to Myocardial Ischemia
Excessive Myocardial Workload
   Residual volume load
   Residual pressure load
Dysrhythmias

contractility) is responsible for the overall inability of the heart to pump blood. Second, application of these techniques often requires both sophisticated equipment and personnel to interpret measurements. Lastly, congenital heart defects are often associated with intracardiac shunting, further complicating interpretation of these measurements. Because of these limitations, these tests seldom provide the anesthesiologist with the information desired, specifically, which determinate of cardiac performance (heart rate, preload, afterload, or contractility) can or should be optimized during the anesthetic.

TABLE 26–5. TECHNIQUES FOR ASSESSMENT OF VENTRICULAR FUNCTION

Cardiac Output
   Thermal dilution
   Dye dilution
   Fick method
   Doppler measurement of blood flow
   Echocardiographic imaging of chamber size
Pressure Measurements
   Peak rise of ventricular pressure (dp/dt)
   Ventricular end-diastolic pressure
   Atrial pressures
   Pulmonary capillary wedge pressure
Ejection Phase Indices
   Ejection fraction
   Fractional myocardial shortening (FS)
   Velocity of circumferential fiber shortening (mean and peak)
Measurements of Ventricular Volume
   Cineangiography
   Echocardiography
   Radionuclide angiography
   Gated computed tomography
   Gated magnetic resonance imaging
Pressure-Volume Relations
   Ventricular end-systolic pressure-volume relation (Emax)
   Ventricular pressure-volume loops

Compensatory Mechanisms. When an additional workload is placed on the heart, or myocardial contractility is reduced, the cardiovascular system will either compensate or fail (inadequate pumping ability to meet metabolic needs). Compensatory mechanisms that allow the heart to maintain adequate cardiac output include ventricular hypertrophy, release of myocardial and adrenal catecholamines, and retention of sodium and water by the kidney. These responses are generally adaptive and serve to maintain cardiac output. However, when sustained for long periods of time, they can become deleterious (Table 26–6).

Ventricular Hypertrophy. One of the primary adaptations to excessive volume or pressure load on the heart is an increased end-diastolic volume, which enhances the muscular function of the heart. However, acute ventricular dilation increases wall tension, which in turn reduces myocardial perfusion and increases oxygen consumption. Hypertrophy* of the ventricle returns myocardial wall tension to within normal limits, despite excessive ventricular workload, by increasing myocardial wall thickness. Interestingly, it appears that different types of cardiac stress (pressure versus volume) stimulate different hypertrophic responses.[65]

An increased pressure load results in the production of additional myofibrils parallel to existing myofibrils, thus increasing the cross-sectional area of the myocyte. The overall result is an increase in ventricular wall thickness without altering chamber size (Fig 26–6). This process allows both normal stroke volume and systolic wall tension despite an increased pressure load.[66,67]

An increased volume load stretches the ventricle, thus optimizing sarcomere length, and stimulates production of myofibrils. However, in contrast to pressure overload hypertrophy, they are also added in series (additional sarcomeres), thus increasing the length of the myocyte (see Fig 26–6). The larger chamber size with a proportional increase in wall thickness normalizes wall tension. The end-diastolic volume is greater for any end-diastolic pressure making the ventricle well suited to eject large volumes against low pressures.[66,67]

Unfortunately, with continued pressure or volume overload, myocardial exhaustion and eventual failure may occur despite ventricular hypertrophy. Myocytes become necrotic and are replaced by fibrous tissue. This places an additional burden on the remaining myocytes resulting in a vicious cycle that eventually culminates in extensive myocardial fibrosis and severely depressed contractility.[58,61]

The above discussion is predominantly based on

---

*In this context, the term *hypertrophy* refers to an increase in ventricular mass. From the cell biology standpoint, hypertrophy is an increase in the size of preexisting cells, whereas hyperplasia is an increase in the number of cells.

TABLE 26–6. SHORT-TERM AND LONG-TERM RESPONSES TO IMPAIRED CARDIAC PERFORMANCE

Response	Short-term Effects*	Long-term Effects†
Salt and water retention	Augments preload	Causes pulmonary congestion, anasarca
Vasoconstriction	Maintains blood pressure for perfusion of vital organs (brain, heart)	Exacerbates pump dysfunction (afterload mismatch); increases cardiac energy expenditure
Sympathetic stimulation	Increases heart rate and ejection	Increases energy expenditure
Sympathetic desensitization	–	Spares energy
Hypertrophy	Unloads individual muscle fibers	Leads to deterioration and death of cardiac cells; cardiomyopathy of overload
Capillary deficit	–	Leads to energy starvation
Mitochondrial density	Increase in density helps meet energy demands	Decrease in density leads to energy starvation
Appearance of slow myosin	–	Increases force, decreases shortening velocity and contractility; is energy-sparing
Prolonged action potential	–	Increases contractility and energy expenditure
Decreased density of sarcoplasmic reticulum calcium pump sites	–	Slows relaxation; may be energy-sparing
Increased collagen	May reduce dilatation	Impairs relaxation

* Short-term effects are mainly adaptive and occur after hemorrhage and in acute heart failure.
† Long-term effects are mainly deleterious and occur in chronic heart failure.
(*From Katz AM: Cardiomyopathy of overload: A major determinant of prognosis in congestive heart failure. N Engl J Med, 322:100–110, 1990, with permission.*)

observations of the adult response to increased cardiac workload. It is possible that infants with congenital heart disease may respond quite differently. The normal human heart retains its ability for hyperplasia (mitotic cell division) until approximately 3 months of age, at which time further increase in cardiac mass is accomplished by cellular hypertrophy.[68] When excessive afterload is imposed on the immature heart, hypertrophy results in "supernormal" myocardial performance that can persist into adulthood.[69,70] It has been suggested that the immature heart responds differently to an increased pressure load because the immature ventricle can undergo cellular hyperplasia in addition to cellular hypertrophy.[71]

An increase in ventricular mass is an adaptive mechanism that couples ventricular growth to ventricular workload. Regression of ventricular mass after elimination of excessive ventricular workload has been demonstrated in laboratory models, in response to deconditioning in trained athletes,[72] and following valve replacement in adults.[73] However, the consequences of removal of the excessive ventricular workload associated with congenital heart defects is largely unknown.

Adrenergic System Changes. Activation of the sympathetic nervous system occurs by stretching of atria and veins, stimulation of baroreceptors, and reduced delivery of oxygen to tissue beds. α Receptor stimulation decreases flow to the limbs, splanchnic bed, and kidneys, thereby diverting blood toward the brain and heart. β Receptor stimulation increases myocardial contractility and heart rate. Sympathetic cholinergic stimulation of the skin leads to sweating (especially in infants). It is

noteworthy that blood flow to the skin is reduced relatively early in cardiac failure.

In the adult with cardiac failure, circulating plasma norepinephrine levels are as high as two to three times normal. Circulating dopamine and epinephrine levels may also be elevated but usually to a lesser degree. The circulating norepinephrine is derived mainly from noncardiac sources and appears to correlate directly with the degree of ventricular dysfunction.[74] Severe heart failure may be precipitated in these patients by β-blockers or anesthetics that decrease sympathetic tone. Circulating catecholamines are also partly responsible for diversion of blood away from nonvital areas, thus maintaining blood pressure despite limited cardiac output. Long-term sympathetic stimulation may ultimately be detrimental because of continually elevated afterload and increased myocardial energy expenditure (see Table 26–6).

In contrast to circulating catecholamines, myocardial norepinephrine stores are depleted in patients with cardiac failure. The degree of myocardial norepinephrine depletion correlates closely with the degree of cardiac failure. Although the exact mechanism is unknown, decreased tyrosine hydroxylase activity, the enzyme that controls the rate-limiting step in the synthesis of norepinephrine, and reduced uptake of norepinephrine into nerve terminals both contribute to depletion of myocardial stores.[58] In addition, myocardial β receptor density and isoproterenol-mediated adenylate cyclase activity are both reduced with cardiac failure (Fig 26–7). This "downregulation" is probably a response to prolonged elevation of circulating norepinephrine.[14] It is not clear if

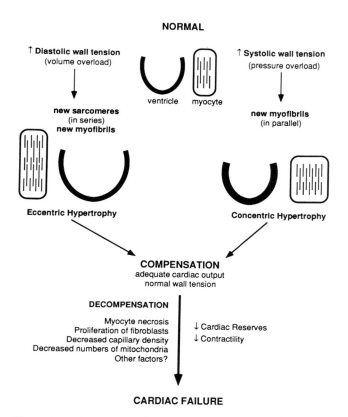

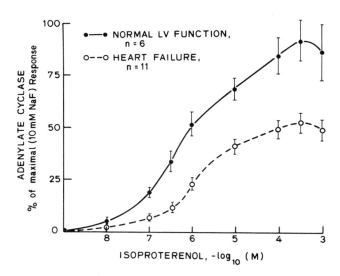

Figure 26–7. Decreased responsiveness of the failing myocardium to β agonists. Isoproterenol-stimulated adenylate cyclase activity in human left ventricles in normal human hearts (solid circles) and failing human hearts (open circles), expressed as a percentage of the response to 10 mM sodium flouride stimulation (mean ± SEM). (*From Bristow MR, Ginsburg R, Minobe W, et al: Decreased cate-cholamine sensitivity and β-adrenergic receptor density in failing human hearts. N Engl J Med 307:205–211, 1982, with permission.*)

Figure 26–6. Cardiac hypertrophy and decompensation. The normal ventricle can be subjected to pressure overload, volume overload, or both. The myocyte adapts by the addition of new myofibrils (concentric hypertrophy) and/or new sarcomeres (eccentric hypertrophy). The resulting alteration of ventricular size and thickness normalizes ventricular wall tension despite increased cardiac workload. At some point (the exact triggering mechanism is unknown), there is reduction in the number of functioning myocytes and an increase in connective tissue. Cardiac reserve is reduced until ultimately cardiac failure occurs.

this decreased response to β agonists is ultimately beneficial or deleterious in patients with cardiac failure.

Plasma norepinephrine levels in children with clinical congestive heart failure are also greatly increased.[75] The etiology of the cardiac failure does not seem to be an important factor. Plasma norepinephrine levels are increased in patients with heart failure secondary to a large left-to-right shunt and with severely decreased contractility. Circulating norepinephrine levels return to normal within months of medical management of congestive heart failure or surgical correction of the underlying cardiac defect or even cardiac transplantation.[76]

Renal System Compensation. The renal response to cardiac failure is similar to that of hypovolemia. The fall in cardiac output and diversion of blood away from the kidneys reduces renal blood flow. Retention of salt and water serves to increase venous return and end-diastolic volume, thus augmenting stroke volume by the Frank-

Starling mechanism. In addition, renin is secreted, which in turn catalyzes the conversion of angiotensin I to angiotensin II. Angiotensin II is a potent vasoconstrictor that also stimulates the release of aldosterone from the adrenal gland. Hyperaldosteronism has been documented in children with cardiac failure.

Anesthetic Considerations. The clinical presentation of heart failure often varies according to the age of the child. The major signs of cardiac failure in the infant include tachypnea, poor feeding, tachycardia, hepatomegaly, diaphoresis, diminished capillary refill, and pallor (Table 26–7). Predominant symptoms of cardiac failure in the older child with congenital heart defects include tachycardia, tachypnea, dyspnea, cool extremities, cardiac gallops, and rales. The classic radiologic findings of cardiac failure are increased cardiac size and pulmonary congestion. Although the electrocardiogram (ECG) is useful to determine the presence of a dysrhythmia that may precipitate cardiac failure, there are no ECG abnormalities specific for cardiac failure in this population. Echocardiography can be used to measure cardiac chamber sizes, circumferential fiber shortening rate, and ejection fraction. Because echocardiography is noninvasive, it is an ideal tool with which to make serial assessments of the effectiveness of therapeutic maneuvers.

Data from recent cardiac catheterization can be extremely useful in determining the cause of cardiac failure. A subjective estimate of contractility is usually

TABLE 26–7. SIGNS AND SYMPTOMS OF CARDIAC FAILURE

Decreased Systemic Perfusion
Poor feeding and failure to thrive
Tachycardia
Cardiomegaly
Gallops
Diaphoresis
Pallor or ashen color
Cold extremities
Decreased capillary refill
Decreased urine output
Pulsus paradoxus and alternans
Pulmonary Congestion
Tachypnea
Cough
Wheezing
Retractions
Rales
Hypoxemia
Dyspnea
Systemic Venous Congestion
Hepatomegaly
Jugular distension
Peripheral edema
Facial edema

provided. The presence of shunts that could contribute to volume overloading or hypoxemia can be determined. Obstruction to ventricular outflow causing increased pressure overload can also be detected. An elevated ventricular end-diastolic pressure suggests that ventricular hypertrophy has not adequately compensated for increased pressure or volume load, and preload must remain elevated to prevent cardiac failure. If cardiac catheterization data is outdated or unavailable, echocardiography provides all of this information except for the ventricular pressure measurements.

The presence or absence of cardiac failure is based primarily on the history and physical examination. If cardiac failure is evident, elective surgery should be postponed until medical or interventional therapies optimize cardiac function. If the surgery is emergent, medical therapy should be started immediately. However, most patients undergoing noncardiac surgery will not be in overt congestive heart failure at the time of surgery. Attention should then be directed toward determining the amount of cardiac reserve for each patient.

Exercise tolerance is perhaps the most informative and simplest method for estimating cardiac reserve in the patient with congenital heart disease. If the patient is sufficiently mature, formal exercise testing using graded exercise protocols, radionuclide angiography, and respiratory gas exchange measurements to assess both ventricular and pulmonary function may also be considered. Although exercise testing does not provide specific information about which determinate of ventricular function (heart rate, preload, afterload, or contractility) is

responsible for impaired cardiac function, it identifies which patients are marginally compensated. However, simply ascertaining the patient's NYHA functional class (Table 26–8) generally provides enough information for the anesthesiologist to formulate an anesthetic plan. Patients in NYHA functional classes III and IV have little cardiac reserve and are at risk for developing cardiac failure during anesthesia.

In young children and infants, evaluation of exercise tolerance is not practical. Instead, limited cardiac reserve can be assessed by evaluation of growth. Because a large proportion of metabolism is normally devoted to growth in young children and infants, those with limited cardiac reserve are generally small for age. Children who are severely growth retarded should be considered to have severely limited cardiac reserve.

The decision to use invasive monitoring should be based on the severity of the cardiac dysfunction and the magnitude of the operative procedure. A severely limited exercise tolerance (NYHA functional classes III and IV) would indicate that cardiac function is dependent on optimal preload and afterload even at rest. Arterial catheters and/or central venous catheters are extremely helpful in guiding the use of intravenous fluids or vasopressors in these patients. Pulmonary artery catheters can be difficult to insert when septal defects or abnormal anatomic relationships are present and measurements difficult to interpret in the presence of shunting. Previous surgical procedures and abnormal arterial and venous anatomy should always be considered when selecting sites for arterial or central venous catheters.

For simple surgical procedures in patients with relatively normal exercise tolerance, the choice of anesthetic is of minimal importance. If ventricular function is depressed, as evidenced by limited exercise tolerance or signs of cardiac failure, anesthetics that cause additional depression of cardiac function are best avoided. Anesthesia that is based primarily on a synthetic narcotic, such as fentanyl, appears to offer the most cardiovascular stability. Nitrous oxide or small doses of benzodiazepines

TABLE 26–8. NEW YORK HEART ASSOCIATION FUNCTIONAL CLASS

I	**No Limitation:** Ordinary physical activity does not cause undue fatigue, dyspnea, or palpitation.
II	**Slight Limitation of Physical Activity:** Such patients are comfortable at rest. Ordinary physical activity results in fatigue, palpitation, dyspnea, or angina.
III	**Marked Limitation of Physical Activity:** Although patients are comfortable at rest, less than ordinary activity will lead to symptoms.
IV	**Inability to Carry on Any Physical Activity Without Discomfort:** Symptoms of congestive heart failure are present even at rest. With any physical activity, increased discomfort is experienced.

may be used to supplement the narcotic and provide amnesia. Although ketamine is a myocardial depressant, it is frequently used because of its sympathomimetic effects. When ketamine is used in patients who are already dependent on maximal sympathetic stimulus (such as those in congestive heart failure), it may have unfavorable effects on cardiac function. Drugs that significantly slow or increase heart rate can adversely affect ventricular output and their use should be considered carefully before administration. Because circulatory time may be prolonged in patients with cardiac failure and blood flow diverted to the brain and heart, induction should proceed in a slow and controlled manner. It should be mentioned that in patients with hypertrophic subvalvular obstruction, anesthetics that depress ventricular function might actually relieve obstruction to ventricular ejection.

Cardiac failure during anesthesia is usually diagnosed by systemic hypotension, diminished heart tones, changes in oxygen saturation, decreased perfusion of the skin, decreased urine output, and the development of metabolic acidosis. As a general principle, therapy should start with optimizing the determinant of myocardial performance (cardiac rhythm, preload, contractility, or afterload) that is most impaired. If the cause of cardiac failure is not apparent from recent operative events (hypovolemia, anesthetic-induced myocardial depression) or preoperative evaluation, empiric therapy should be initiated. Sinus rhythm should be restored and bradycardia or supraventricular tachycardia treated. Despite the fact that the depressed ventricle is less responsive to increasing preload than the normal ventricle, decreased preload may have catastrophic effects in the marginally compensated circulation. Therefore, unless there is evidence of venous or pulmonary congestion, intravenous fluids should be administered. Ventricular contractility should be enhanced by avoiding myocardial depressants and administering inotropic drugs. Inotropic drugs should be titrated to effect, as chronic congestive heart failure is accompanied by a downregulation of β receptors in the heart, and greater than usual doses may be required to improve contractility (see Fig 26–7). If the systemic pressure is increased and the pathophysiology such that pulmonary blood flow would not be decreased, careful afterload reduction can reduce cardiac workload and improve cardiac output (Fig 26–8).

As a final note, congenital heart disease can sometimes result in isolated right ventricular failure. Isolated right ventricular failure can be difficult to diagnose in the operating room but should be suspected if indicated by the preoperative anatomy, physiology, or examination. The principles of management discussed above can also be applied to right ventricular failure. However, in the presence of normal pulmonary vasculature, right ventricular afterload can be significantly reduced while maintaining systemic perfusion by maintaining a high F_{IO_2},

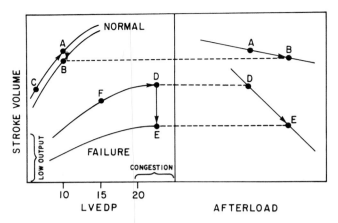

Figure 26–8. Frank-Starling relationships in the normal and failing heart. Frank-Starling curves (left panel) of a normal heart and a failing heart and the impact of increased afterload on each heart's stroke volume (right panel). An increase in afterload of the normal heart produces only a small decrement in its stroke volume (A to B). An equivalent increase in the failing heart's afterload produces a much greater decrease in its stroke volume (D to E). (*From Clark NJ, Martin RD: Anesthetic considerations for patients undergoing cardiac transplantation. J Cardiothoracic Anesth 2:519–542, 1988, with permission.*)

reduced P_{CO_2}, and an elevated pH. An attempt should be made to avoid increased airway pressures during hyperventilation as this factor may also increase pulmonary vascular resistance.

DYSRHYTHMIAS

As more children with congenital heart disease survive to adulthood, it is becoming apparent that dysrhythmias are a significant problem. Dysrhythmias can lead to hemodynamic deterioration or even sudden death. The anesthesiologist must be aware of which patients are at risk of developing dysrhythmias, what types of dysrhythmias are likely to occur, and the most effective means of therapy. Until there are clinical studies specifically addressing the anesthetic issues of children with dysrhythmias and congenital heart disease, data about the natural history of dysrhythmias in these patients must be used to guide anesthetic management.

Dysrhythmias are the result of either altered cardiac impulse generation or conduction. In patients with congenital heart disease, disorders of the conduction system, both congenital and acquired, are more common than disorders of impulse generation. There are several possible etiologies for the conduction system disturbances that produce dysrhythmias. These include (1) intrinsic anatomic or physiologic abnormalities, (2) damage resulting from chronic hypoxia or hemodynamic stress, (3) injury occurring at the time of surgery, or (4) a complex interaction of all three.

Several surgical procedures are associated with a high likelihood of postoperative dysrhythmias. These procedures include atrial correction of transposition of the great arteries (Mustard or Senning procedure), the Fontan procedure for single ventricle defects, and "repair" of tetralogy of Fallot.

Congenital Conduction System Abnormalities

Many congenital heart defects are accompanied by intrinsic ECG abnormalities (Table 26–9). The origins of these abnormalities range from simple anatomic displacement of the conduction system to severe hemodynamic or metabolic derangements causing distortion or destruction of the conduction system. There are a few congenital defects in which a conduction system abnormality is a predominant feature. These include congenital complete atrioventricular block, congenitally corrected transposition of the great arteries, the Wolff-Parkinson-White syndrome, supraventricular tachycardia, and the Ebstein anomaly.

Congenital Complete Atrioventricular Block. Congenital complete atrioventricular block (CCAVB) is the condition in which atrial impulses are not conducted to the ventricles. Although relatively rare, CCAVB is the most common intrinsic conduction defect of clinical significance that produces bradycardia. The incidence of CCAVB is 1 in 22,000 live births. The diagnosis is most often made during the newborn period. The majority of deaths secondary to complete heart block occur during infancy, and the majority of infants who die have concurrent cardiac structural defects.[77] The most common associated structural defects are congenitally corrected transposition of the great arteries (ventricular inversion) or defects of the atrial or ventricular septum. There is a strong association between maternal collagen vascular disease and CCAVB, and it has been postulated that maternal immunoglobulin (IgG) antibodies that cross the placenta damage the fetal cardiac conduction system.

Most infants with congenital heart block have a ventricular rate of less than 75 beats per minute (bpm). Rarely will the resting heart rate be greater than 100 bpm. The ability to increase heart rate in response to exercise or pharmacologic stimulation is highly variable, and some patients never increase their heart rate above 100 bpm. Children who are unable to increase their heart rate are entirely dependent on an increase of stroke volume to produce an increase in cardiac output (myocardial contractility is usually normal).

The presence of a wide QRS complex or ventricular ectopy is considered significant because it is likely that at least some of the syncopal episodes and deaths in older patients are a result of ventricular dysrhythmias rather than severe bradycardia.[78] Indications for preoperative

insertion of a permanent pacemaker are listed in (Table 26–10).

Congenitally Corrected Transposition of the Great Arteries. This cardiac defect is most commonly associated with CCAVB. Corrected transposition is characterized by an abnormal connection between the atria and the ventricles. Although there is potential for a normal circulatory pattern, other cardiac lesions are often present. Atrioventricular block can exist at birth if accessory conduction pathways are not established, or complete heart block can develop later in life. The risk of late occurrence is about 2% per year.[79] Patients who require repair of a ventricular septal defect have a 25% chance of developing complete heart block operatively, but the risk of late-onset block is not increased. If a stable escape rhythm is not present in those with complete heart block, syncope and even sudden death is possible. Anesthetic considerations are the same as those for patients with congenital complete heart block.

Supraventricular Tachycardia and Wolff-Parkinson-White Syndrome. Abnormalities of automaticity, or the presence of a reentrant phenomenon, can result in supraventricular tachycardia (SVT). Abnormal automaticity is a result of sinus node dysfunction or the presence of an ectopic atrial pacemaker. Although sinus node dysfunction is relatively common in children with congenital heart defects, it is usually characterized by a slowed firing rate. In contrast, ectopic atrial pacemakers are often present in children with chronic SVT producing heart rates between 120 and 200 bpm and sometimes resulting in myocardial dysfunction. Ectopic atrial pacemakers are a much greater problem in patients after reparative cardiac surgery.

The reentrant phenomenon is the underlying mechanism for the majority of SVTs. Reentry may occur in any cardiac tissue but is commonly associated with a well-defined pathway, as in the Wolff-Parkinson-White (WPW) syndrome, or in areas of myocardial scarring. Common causes of atrial or ventricular scar formation are surgical injury, hypertrophy associated with focal myocardial fibrosis, or myocardial ischemia.

Supraventricular tachycardia is a relatively common dysrhythmia in infants. The heart rate is usually in the 200- to 300-bpm range. As many as 25–50% of infants with SVT (and no associated cardiac defects) will have ECG evidence of the WPW syndrome when in normal sinus rhythm. SVT in the older child is even more likely to be secondary to the WPW syndrome.

The WPW syndrome is characterized by an accessory atrial connection. It is the only dysrhythmia that is unequivocally secondary to reentry phenomenon. Episodes of tachycardia are most frequent during infancy, puberty, and later adulthood. Twenty-five percent of children with WPW may have normal ECGs.

TABLE 26–9. ELECTROCARDIOGRAPHIC PATTERNS ASSOCIATED WITH CONGENITAL HEART DEFECTS

Cardiac Defect	Atrial Flutter/Fibrillation	Supraventricular Tachycardia	Ventricular Arrhythmia	Atrioventricular Block	Preexcitation Syndrome	Abnormal P Wave Orientation	Right Atrial Overload	Left Atrial Overload	Left Bundle Branch Block	Left Axis Deviation	Right Bundle Branch Block	Right Ventricular Volume Overload	Right Ventricular Pressure Overload	Left Ventricular Volume Overload	Left Ventricular Pressure Overload	Biventricular Overload	Abnormal Q Waves or Myocardial Infarction Pattern
Atrial septal defect (secundum)	++	+	0	+	0	+	++	+	+	0	+	+	+++	+	0	0	0
Prolapsed mitral valve syndrome	+	+	+	0	+	0	0	+	0	0	0	0	0	0	0	0	0
Aortic stenosis	0	0	+	+	0	0	0	++	+	+	0	0	0	0	+	0	0
Idiopathic hypertrophic subaortic stenosis	+	0	++	0	+	0	0	++	++	++	0	0	0	0	0	++	++
Pulmonary stenosis	0	0	0	0	0	0	++	+	0	0	+	+	+++	0	0	+	0
Ventricular septal defect	+	0	0	0	0	0	0	+	+	0	0	+	0	+++	0	+++	0
Patent ductus arteriosus	+	0	0	0	0	0	0	++	+	+	0	0	0	+++	0	0	0
Tetralogy of Fallot	0	0	+	0	0	0	++	0	0	0	+	0	+++	0	0	0	0
Coarctation of aorta	+	0	0	0	0	0	0	+	+	0	+	+	0	0	++	0	0
Eisenmenger syndrome	++	0	+	0	0	0	++	++	0	0	+	0	+++	0	0	++	0
Atrial septal defect (primum)	++	+	0	++	+	0	+	+	+	+	+	+++	+	+	+	0	0
Corrected transposition*	+	+++	0	+++	+	0	+++	+	+++	+	0	0	0	0	+	+	++
Ebstein anomaly	++	+++	0	+	++	0	+++	++	+	+	+++	+	0	0	0	0	0
Tricuspid atresia	+	+	+	0	0	0	+++	+	+++	+	0	0	0	+	+	+	+
Congenital anomalies of coronary arteries	+	0	++	0	0	0	0	++	+	+	+	0	0	0	+	0	+++
Transposition of great arteries (postop)	+	++	0	+	0	0	0	++	0	+	+	0	+++	0	+	0	0

Symbols: +++, almost always seen (characteristics of defect); ++, commonly seen with defect; +, sometimes seen with defect (especially with associated defects or advancing age); 0, rarely seen with defect.

* The precordial QRS progression in corrected transposition may mimic left ventricular hypertrophy, usually with ST segment abnormalities. True hypertrophy of the left-sided ventricle can occur in corrected transposition from associated left atrioventricular valvular regurgitation, ventricular septal defect, and so on.

(From Ellison RC, Sloss, LJ: Electrocardiographic features of congenital heart disease in the adult. In Roberts WC (ed): Congenital Heart Disease in Adults, Philadelphia: FA Davis, 1987, pp 168–169, with permission.)

TABLE 26–10. CRITERIA FOR PERMANENT PACEMAKER PLACEMENT FOR PATIENTS WITH CONGENITAL COMPLETE ATRIOVENTRICULAR BLOCK

Syncope
Congestive heart failure
Conduction block below the bundle of His (QRS > 0.10 s)
Presence of ventricular escape beats
Infants with a resting heart rate of <55 bpm
Older children with a heart rate of <50 bpm
Moderate or severe exercise intolerance
The presence of other debilitating cardiac defects

Ebstein Anomaly. The Ebstein anomaly is characterized by a displacement of the tricuspid valve into the body of the right ventricle. The major physiologic consequences are tricuspid insufficiency and/or stenosis, a small right ventricular chamber, massive right atrial dilation with inclusion of aneurysmal right ventricular tissue in the atrium, a right-to-left shunt through an atrial septal defect or patent foramen ovale, and dysrhythmias. Numerous ECG abnormalities are present. Atrial tachydysrhythmias are present in over 25% of these patients, many of whom exhibit a WPW pattern. The numerous accessory fibers are thought to represent persistent fetal conduction pathways. With or without surgery, a significant number of these patients are at risk for sudden death.[80,81]

If identified, accessory pathways are often destroyed during valve reconstruction procedures; however, atrial fibrillation and atrial flutter are still frequently seen in the early postoperative period and ventricular fibrillation can occur.[82] If the tricuspid valve is replaced, complete heart block may occur in 25% of patients. Late dysrhythmias are common, usually tachydysrhythmias. Atrial fibrillation or flutter will recur in over one third of patients postoperatively and the incidence of late sudden death related to dysrhythmias is as high as 7–8%. In general, if severe dysrhythmias were present preoperatively, there is a greater risk of developing dysrhythmias late after the operation.[82] Late complete heart block is uncommon.

Dysrhythmias and death during placement of intracardiac catheters have been described.[83] Stimulation of the "morphologic right ventricular" tissue situated in the right atrium resulting in ventricular fibrillation or tachycardia is thought to be the cause of these arrests. This risk should be considered carefully before proceeding with central venous catheterization. Drugs that could stimulate conduction through accessory pathways should be avoided if possible. The use of digoxin or verapamil in the treatment of supraventricular tachycardia has been associated with an increase in conduction through the accessory pathways possibly leading to ventricular tachycardia of fibrillation. Drugs slowing conduction and increasing the refractory period, such as type I antiarrhythmics, should be used instead.

Acquired Conduction System Abnormalities

Frequently, dysrhythmias do not become evident until adulthood making it difficult to determine the relative contribution of chronic hypoxia, hemodynamic stress, or other factors to their development. Nonsurgically acquired conduction defects are rare and are usually associated with infectious destruction of the conduction system, idiopathic fibrous degeneration, cardiomyopathies, tumor invasion (tuberous sclerosis), or drug overdose. During surgery, no part of the cardiac conduction system is safe from injury by cardioplegia solutions, ischemia, metabolic abnormalities, or mechanical injury (Fig 26–9).

Injury to the Sinus Node and Sinoatrial Pathways.

Injury to the sinus node can occur during any type of cardiac operation. Even cannulation of the superior vena cava or excessively tight vena caval tape can result in transient dysfunction. Permanent damage may result from incision of the sinus node or placement of sutures in its vicinity. The likelihood of permanent damage occurring is greatest for repair of sinus venosus defects, atrial septal defects, and atrial switch procedures (Mustard or Senning). In some patients with tricuspid atresia, surgical disruption of the vascular supply to the sinus node may occur during the Fontan procedure.

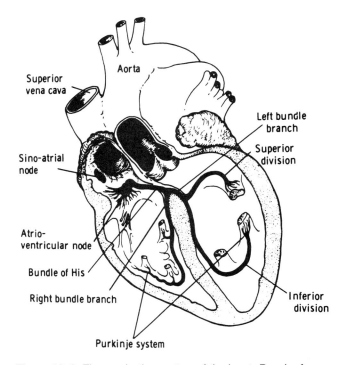

Figure 26–9. The conduction system of the heart. Repair of many cardiac defects requires work in close proximity to the atrioventricular node, bundle of His, and right bundle branch. (*From Goldman MJ: Principles of clinical electrocardiography. 7th ed. Los Altos, CA: Lange Medical Publications, 1970, p 41, with permission.*)

Clinical manifestations include sinus bradycardia, sinoatrial block, or supraventricular tachycardias. These dysrhythmias may appear immediately following surgery or years after the initial repair. Dysrhythmias appearing immediately after surgery generally resolve without specific therapy. Late-appearing dysrhythmias may be entirely asymptomatic or may provoke hemodynamic collapse and sudden death.

Injury to the Atrioventricular Node and Bundle of His.

Injury to the atrioventricular (AV) node and bundle of His may result from any surgery in close proximity to these structures (surgical closure of AV canal defects, atrial switch procedures, closure of membranous ventricular septal defects, or repair of tetralogy of Fallot). Clinical manifestations include junctional tachycardia or AV block. Junctional tachycardia is most commonly seen in the immediate postoperative period and can be extremely difficult to treat effectively. Early damage can result from interruption of the vascular supply to these structures or direct mechanical injury. Precise localization of the conduction system in many congenital heart defects has dramatically decreased the incidence of postoperative complete heart block in recent years. Late onset of AV block may occur secondary to necrosis and progressive fibrosis extending into the conduction system.

Injury to the Intraventricular Conduction System.

Intraventricular conduction defects result from injury to any of the bundle branches. Consequent electrocardiographic patterns are those of right bundle branch block (RBBB), left anterior hemiblock (LAH), or prolongation of the PR interval (trifascicular block). Surgical palliation of tetralogy of Fallot, AV canal defects, membranous ventricular septal defects, or any procedure involving right ventriculotomy may result in damage to bundle branches.

The clinical significance of bundle branch block is controversial. It has been suggested that patients with a combination of RBBB and LAH are at risk of developing complete heart block or even sudden death.[84]

Dysrhythmias Associated with Specific Surgical Procedures

Ostium Secundum Atrial Septal Defect Closure.

Preoperatively, sinus node function is abnormal in up to 80% of those patients but symptomatic bradydysrhythmias are rare.[85] The PR interval is prolonged in 20–30% of patients, which is seen more commonly in older patients.[86] Atrioventricular and infranodal conduction are usually normal.

Atrial tachydysrhythmias are uncommon in children with unrepaired atrial septal defects (ASD). However, with advancing age, atrial fibrillation and flutter become

quite prominent. As many as 50% of the patients who survive to age 60 with an ASD have tachydysrhythmias.[86] Progressive atrial fibrosis secondary to distension, hypoxemia, or surgical injury is thought to be the etiology of late-appearing tachydysrhythmias. If there is concomitant pulmonary hypertension or right heart failure, tachydysrhythmias can lead to ventricular dysrhythmias and possibly sudden death. When ventricular function is limited, loss of sinus rhythm can result in severe hemodynamic compromise.

The sinus node is particularly vulnerable during surgery, with as many as 40% of patients exhibiting bradydysrhythmias in the immediate postoperative period. However, persistent sinus node dysfunction requiring pacemaker insertion is uncommon. Late development of sinus bradycardia or atrioventricular block is also rare but has been implicated in the sudden death of a few patients.[87]

Twenty-five years after surgical repair, almost all patients with preoperative atrial fibrillation or flutter will demonstrate recurrence. In contrast, those without preoperative tachydysrhythmias have only a 5–10% chance of later development.[88] Thus, it is possible that early repair is associated with a reduced incidence of late postoperative tachydysrhythmias.

Sinus Venosus Atrial Septal Defect Closure.

Atrial ectopic foci are commonly present preoperatively. The proximity of the defect to the sinus node predisposes to injury during surgical repair, often resulting in postoperative bradydysrhythmias. Long-term considerations appear to be similar to that of secundum atrial septal defects.

Ostium Primum Atrial Septal Defect Closure.

Preoperative electrocardiograms are often abnormal, with the PR interval being prolonged in half of these patients because of displacement of the atrial conduction system and atrioventricular node. In the early postoperative period, transient complete atrioventricular block is not uncommon. Atrial fibrillation or flutter can occur late after repair in 5–10%.[89] Persistent atrioventricular block is present in approximately 5% with late occurrence in another 2%. Atrioventricular block occurs more often in ostium primum defects than ostium secundum defects, possibly because of the close proximity of the atrioventricular node and bundle of His to the repair. However, the natural course of ostium primum septal defects is otherwise similar to that of ostium secundum defects.

Ventricular Septal Defect Closure.

The preoperative electrocardiogram varies depending on the size and location of the defect. However, significant dysrhythmias are uncommon. Intraoperatively, the conduction system can be damaged with atrioventricular block, a major postoperative concern. Atrioventricular block is rare with growing knowledge of the anatomy of the conduction system. Right bundle branch block is a common postoperative finding occurring most frequently after right ventriculotomy. Ectopic atrial dysrhythmias, junctional beats, and premature ventricular contractions are seen in the immediate postoperative period but most resolve without specific therapy. Late-onset complete heart block is rare, developing in fewer than 5% of postoperative patients.[90] Patients with early postoperative atrioventricular block appear to be at increased risk. Unlike tetralogy of Fallot, late-onset ventricular dysrhythmias are rare.

Fontan Procedure for Single-Ventricle Lesions.
The ventricle in patients with univentricular heart may be of left, right, or indeterminate morphology. Those with right ventricular morphology usually have a normal PR interval and atrioventricular conduction. Those with left ventricular morphology generally have a portion of the ventricular inlet missing, thus disrupting the normal conduction system. Atrioventricular conduction time is often prolonged, and complete heart block can be present. Regardless of the type of surgical palliation, dysrhythmias leading to death may occur in as many as 30% of patients with single-ventricle lesions.[91,92] The reason for the increased incidence of morbid dysrhythmias is unclear. Excessive hemodynamic stresses (volume overload), chronic hypoxemia, and coronary insufficiency have all been implicated.

The Fontan procedure is currently being applied to the majority of patients in whom a biventricular repair is deemed impossible. Although many modifications of the original Fontan procedure are used today, all divert systemic venous blood into the pulmonary artery, thus bypassing the ventricle. As in the Mustard or Senning procedure, extensive intra-arterial surgery may be required that increases postoperative dysrhythmias, usually ectopic atrial rhythms or junctional tachycardias. Most atrial dysrhythmias resolve without specific therapy. In addition, the sinus and AV nodes are in close proximity to the operative field, and up to 10% of children may experience severe sinus bradycardia or permanent complete heart block, often requiring pacemaker placement.[93] This is more common in patients with tricuspid atresia, possibly because the vascular supply to the sinus node is transected during the repair.

Supraventricular dysrhythmias become problematic late after the repair. As many as 40% of all patients undergoing Fontan procedures may be affected, sometimes leading to hemodynamic deterioration. The prevalence of atrial dysrhythmias increases with the passage of time. Holter recordings may also show premature ventricular beats, sinus bradycardia, and transient atrioventricular blocks. The significance of these late-developing dysrhythmias is unknown, but it appears that the presence

of persistent hemodynamic abnormalities predisposes to the development of ventricular dysrhythmias.

Mustard or Senning Procedure for Transposition of the Great Arteries (TGA).
These two intra-atrial baffle procedures have been widely used for the last 25 years to "correct" most forms of TGA. Both procedures involve excision of the atrial septum and redirection of systemic venous blood into the pulmonary ventricle and return of pulmonary venous blood into the systemic ventricle. The extensive excision and suturing of the atria results in significant damage to the sinus node and conduction system. Despite surgical modifications to minimize disruption of the conduction system, the incidence of postoperative atrial dysrhythmias remains significant.[94]

In the early postoperative period, atrial dysrhythmias (tachydysrhythmias and bradydysrhythmias) are quite frequent. Most of these resolve within a few weeks, although formal electrophysiologic testing reveals a high incidence of sinus node dysfunction and atrial ectopic dysrhythmias at the time of discharge from the hospital.

As time progresses, sinus node dysfunction develops in the majority of patients,[95] and by the eighth postoperative year, only half remain in normal sinus rhythm. The types of dysrhythmias encountered include sinus bradycardia, atrioventricular block, junctional tachycardia, atrial fibrillation, and atrial flutter. A combination of one or more of the above may produce a tachycardia-bradycardia syndrome. These dysrhythmias often result in hemodynamic deterioration and should be treated promptly. Dysrhythmias have also been implicated in the 5–8% of these patients who die suddenly without anatomic cause, particularly in those experiencing supraventricular tachycardia.[95,96]

Arterial Switch Procedure for Transposition of the Great Arteries.
The arterial switch procedure does not appear to result in the long-term development of dysrhythmias. Symptomatic atrial dysrhythmias are rare and possibly related to prior atrial septostomy or septectomy. Sinus node dysfunction is uncommon. Coronary insufficiency may lead to ischemic dysrhythmias but appears to be a relatively uncommon problem.[97]

"Repair" of Tetralogy of Fallot.
Dysrhythmias are uncommon in children under 8 years of age with uncorrected tetralogy. However, 50% will have frequent (>30/h) premature ventricular contractions by the age of 15. Ventricular tachycardia resulting in syncope and even sudden death has been reported.

Electrophysiologic abnormalities are seen frequently after surgery. This is a consequence of the proximity of the operative field to the conduction system and the right ventriculotomy. In the early postoperative period, a right bundle branch block pattern is observed in over half of patients and bifascicular block (right bundle branch block and left anterior hemiblock) in up to 8% of patients. The incidence of complete heart block ranges from 0 to 22%,[64,98] but atrioventricular conduction usually returns, and fewer than 2% of patients are left with a permanent complete heart block. Patients with transient complete heart block in the immediate postoperative period appear to have a 10 times greater risk of developing delayed postoperative complete heart block.[84,98,99]

Five years postoperatively, the risk of sudden death or sustained ventricular tachycardia can be as high as 5%.[64,100–102] Although some of these deaths are related to the development of complete heart block, ventricular dysrhythmias are the major cause.[100,101] Sustained ventricular tachycardia potentially arises from the ventriculotomy site or from the ventricular septum, both regions where extensive fibrosis occurs. However, most patients who die suddenly also suffer from inadequate hemodynamic palliation manifested by right ventricular pressures greater than 60 mm Hg.[101,103] Surgical "repair" before the age of 5 appears to reduce the risk of late sudden death and significant ventricular dysrhythmias; however, the follow-up time for this group of patients has been relatively short.[64,101] These data indicate that the distension caused by sustained right ventricular pressure overload (both before and after the repair) is a contributing factor in the development of ventricular dysrhythmias. Evidence that late ventricular dysrhythmias are rare after ventriculotomy for closure of ventricular septal defect lends support to this theory.

Anesthetic Considerations

The risk of anesthesia in patients with dysrhythmias secondary to congenital heart disease has not been studied in a systematic manner. It is not known if perioperative dysrhythmias represent a significant anesthetic risk. However, their presence clearly indicates an underlying cardiac abnormality. Dysrhythmias in patients who have already had their surgical "repair" are particularly disconcerting because they may be secondary to inadequate surgical palliation resulting in progressive myocardial dysfunction or degeneration. As a general note, anesthetic management of coexistent ventricular failure or hypoxemia must be considered when planning maneuvers to avoid dysrhythmias.

Perioperative Management of Patients with Complete Heart Block (CHB). Symptoms of CHB during infancy are typically those of congestive heart failure and include tachypnea, lethargy, pallor, diaphoresis, and poor feeding. In older children with significant bradycardia, congestive heart failure is rare but syncope and reduced exercise tolerance are predominant complaints. The severity of the clinical presentation CHB is dependent on the resting heart rate and the presence of other cardiac defects.

A 24-hour Holter recording allows diagnosis of dysrhythmias in many more patients than the standard ECG, and should be considered when there are clinical symptoms attributable to dysrhythmias. Exercise testing is a more sensitive test for dysrhythmias and also can provide information about the functional status of the cardiovascular system as a whole. An occasional patient may require formal preoperative electrophysiology studies. Patients should also be thoroughly evaluated for associated congenital heart defects or inadequate surgical palliation by transthoracic or transesophageal echocardiography.

If insertion of a permanent pacemaker is not warranted, a temporary pacing device should be readily available. Transcutaneous pacing is easily and rapidly implemented, does not require central venous access, and its effectiveness has been tested in normal children weighing as little as 6 kg.[104] Transesophageal pacemakers are also easily inserted; however, in patients with AV conduction block, only ventricular capture should be expected.

It would seem prudent to avoid or minimize the use of drugs that are known to slow nodal pacemakers or myocardial conduction either directly, by decreasing sympathetic tone, or by increasing vagal tone.[105] Such drugs include halothane (although it has been used successfully in patients with CHB), most synthetic narcotics, and vecuronium when used in association with fentanyl or etomidate.[106] The use of halothane in the presence of increased serum catecholamine levels might also predispose to ventricular ectopy. Atropine and isoproterenol increase the heart rate in patients with congenital CHB by increasing the automaticity of the nodal pacemaker but neither drug significantly enhances atrioventricular conduction. Atropine also protects against vagal and drug-induced bradycardia, which is particularly important during intraoperative vagal stimulation (oculocardiac reflex). Administration of neostigmine or succinylcholine should be proceeded by atropine. In patients with poor exercise tolerance or a demonstrated inability to increase heart rate, hypovolemia must be avoided as cardiac output depends on stroke volume alone.

Anesthetic Management of Patients with Supraventricular Tachycardia (SVT). In the infant, symptoms of SVT are those of congestive heart failure. The heart rate is usually regular and in the 200- to 300-bpm range. Older children seldom present in congestive heart failure but may experience episodes of syncope, palpitations, and exhibit poor exercise tolerance. If symptoms attributable to SVT are present, a 24-hour Holter recording should be considered. History, physical examination, and echocardiography should be evaluated for evidence of associated cardiac defects.

Patients who have undergone previous surgical procedures are a unique group who warrant special preoperative evaluation. A history of preoperative or early postoperative dysrhythmias indicates a patient who could be at greater risk for late development of SVT. Because of the association of postoperative hemodynamic impairment with dysrhythmias, the adequacy of the surgical palliation should be carefully assessed. Preoperative echocardiography should specifically evaluate residual shunts, chamber enlargement, baffle obstruction, valvular insufficiency, and ventricular outflow obstruction.

Although there are no clinical studies examining which anesthetic drugs may precipitate SVT in this population of patients, a few guidelines should be considered.[107] Premedication may decrease anxiety over surgery or separation from parents, thus preventing excessive sympathetic activity during the time of induction. The use of atropine or glycopyrrolate should be avoided if possible. Volatile anesthetics, particularly halothane, may predispose to the development of supraventricular excitability in dogs. However, whether halothane enhances the development of SVT in the human has not been established. Muscle relaxants without significant vagolytic activity should be used. Central venous catheterization may precipitate SVT, especially in the patients with the Ebstein anomaly.

In the infant, vagal maneuvers are seldom effective in treating SVT. If circulatory shock is present, synchronized direct-current cardioversion is recommended. An energy setting of 0.5 J/kg is usually effective. Other therapeutic options for the infant include initiating the diving reflex, overdrive pacing, adenosine, digoxin, β-blockers, verapamil, and class I antiarrhythmics. Although digoxin may make adult patients with the WPW syndrome more susceptible to ventricular fibrillation, this rarely occurs in the pediatric population, and digoxin is commonly started after successful cardioversion. The use of verapamil for SVT has been reported to cause cardiac decompensation in infants and should be used cautiously if at all.[108] A transesophageal pacing catheter can be used for both diagnosis and overdrive pacing.[109] It is easy to insert, avoids the need for central venous cannulation, and is effective in infants and children.

In the older child, intravenous verapamil is currently the treatment of choice if vagal maneuvers fail. Adenosine is gaining popularity as a first-line therapy in the adult, and it has been reported to be successful in the young child.[110] Other therapeutic options include initiating the diving reflex, overdrive pacing, edrophonium, phenylephrine, β-blockers, and class I antiarrhythmics. Cardioversion should be used if hemodynamic instability is present.[80]

Anesthetic Management of Patients with Ventricular Dysrhythmias. Patients after ''repair'' of tetralogy of Fallot are at highest risk for malignant ventricular dys-

rhythmias. A history of syncope is suspicious of dysrhythmias, and poor exercise tolerance is suggestive of right ventricular failure. Both are strong risk factors for the eventual development of ventricular tachycardia and even sudden death.

Preoperative studies should include an ECG. The presence of a right bundle branch block is common and these patients are unlikely to degenerate into complete heart block. The prognosis of bifascicular block is not known. Patients who experienced transient complete heart block at the time of surgery appear to be at a much greater risk of recurrence. Unfortunately, this information may be difficult to obtain from perioperative records. The presence of ventricular ectopy on the standard ECG is ominous as 30% of these patients eventually die suddenly.[101] These patients should be referred for possible antiarrhythmic therapy or further palliation. Formal electrophysiologic testing of the conduction system identifies patients at the highest risk of developing complete heart block or ventricular tachycardia, but its use remains controversial. There is evidence that suppression of ventricular ectopy reduces the incidence of sudden death in patients with tetralogy of Fallot.[101]

The anesthesiologist should minimize or eliminate factors that may predispose to ventricular ectopy and be prepared to treat aggressively any ectopy that occurs. Inadequate anesthesia resulting in excessive sympathetic stimulation should be avoided. Although ketamine increases circulating catecholamines, it has been used extensively in patients with tetralogy of Fallot without report of malignant dysrhythmias. The use of large doses of epinephrine in local anesthetic solutions should be considered carefully, as should the use of halothane. Hypercarbia, acidosis, and severe hypoxemia may all lower the threshold for ventricular ectopy.

Ventricular dysrhythmias can appear when the heart is excessively burdened by increased pressure or volume load. This is particularly true in patients with tetralogy of Fallot who have persistent right ventricular outflow tract obstruction.[102] Therefore, attention should be directed toward minimizing hemodynamic stress on the right ventricle that occurs with sudden increases of the pulmonary vascular resistance, positive-pressure ventilation, positive end-expiratory pressure (PEEP), and extreme fluid overload.

PREGNANCY AND CONGENITAL HEART DISEASE

Cardiac disease, congenital and acquired, is a leading nonobstetric cause of maternal death during pregnancy. The number of women with congenital heart disease who survive to become pregnant is steadily increasing,[111,112] and the anesthesiologist must become facile in the management of these patients. Unfortunately, there are no comprehensive data with which to guide the management of these patients, and formulation of an anesthetic plan must be extrapolated from knowledge of the physiologic changes that occur during pregnancy, determination of the degree of cardiovascular impairment, anticipated effects of the anesthetics, and an understanding of the pathophysiology associated with congenital heart defects.

Normal Cardiovascular Changes During Pregnancy

The cardiovascular changes that accompany a normal pregnancy can be categorized into those that occur during gestation, labor and delivery, and the postpartum period. Major hemodynamic alterations are summarized in Table 26–11.

Beginning at 6 weeks of pregnancy, maternal blood volume steadily increases. During the second trimester, the rate of blood volume expansion accelerates reaching a plateau at 32 weeks[113] (Fig 26–10). At this time, blood volume is approximately 40% (1.5 L) greater than the pregestational state. This increase is primarily due to an expansion of plasma volume, and despite an increase in red blood cell mass, the hematocrit decreases.

Resting heart rate increases during the latter half of gestation reaching 10–15% above the pregestational rate when near term. Systemic arterial blood pressure, systemic vascular resistance, and pulmonary vascular resistance are all decreased reaching a nadir at approximately 28 weeks. Systemic vascular resistance and blood pressure both increase slightly during the latter half of the third trimester.

Stroke volume, left ventricular chamber size, and left ventricular mass progressively increase, as demonstrated by Katz and others.[114–116] The etiology of the increase in chamber size and mass is unclear. It has been

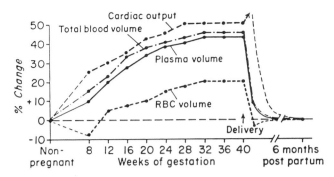

Figure 26–10. Changes in maternal blood, red cell, and plasma volume during pregnancy. The increase in plasma volume is greater than the increase in red cell volume, producing the "relative" anemia of pregnancy. Note that the cardiac output does not decline in the last few weeks of gestation. Early studies demonstrating a decline in cardiac output at the end of gestation did not account for the effects of the supine position on cardiac output. (*From Bonica JJ: Obstetric Analgesia and Anesthesia. 2nd ed. Amsterdam: World Federation Society of Anesthesiologists, 1980, p 2, with permission.*)

postulated that the left ventricle becomes more compliant during pregnancy allowing an increase in end-diastolic volume with the same distending pressure. Although stroke volume increases during this time, the ejection fraction remains constant.[116,117] There is no consensus about whether myocardial contractility changes or remains the same during pregnancy. Resolution of this problem has been difficult because only indirect measurements of contractility (systolic time intervals, velocity of circumferential shortening, ejection fraction, and shortening fraction) have been made.

At term, cardiac output is increased to nearly 40% above pregestational levels. Most of this increment is secondary to an augmentation of stroke volume, which peaks at 20–24 weeks. As pregnancy advances, the heart rate gains significance in maintaining the greater cardiac output. Estimates of changes in cardiac output during the third trimester vary widely. When it is measured with the patient in the lateral position, thereby eliminating the effects of aortocaval compression, cardiac output does not appear to decrease at term.

The cardiovascular changes that occur during labor and delivery are influenced by the frequency and force of uterine contractions, the presence or absence of pain, the type of anesthesia utilized, maternal posture, and the mode of delivery. Cardiac output increases by as much as 30–45% with each contraction, primarily because 300–500 mL of blood is expelled from the uterine circulation, thereby augmenting venous return to the heart. As labor progresses, cardiac output continues to increase with each contraction. This increase can be attenuated by a reduction of pain and anxiety.

The importance of maternal position on hemodynamics cannot be overemphasized. In the lateral recumbent position, changes in cardiac output and stroke

TABLE 26–11. EXPECTED CHANGES IN THE CARDIOVASCULAR SYSTEM DURING PREGNANCY

Variable	Average % Change
Blood volume	↑ 35
Plasma volume	↑ 45
Red blood cell volume	↑ 20
Cardiac output	↑ 40
Stroke volume	↑ 30
Heart rate	↑ 15
Total peripheral resistance	↓ 15
Mean arterial blood pressure	↓ 15
Systolic blood pressure	↓ 0–15
Diastolic blood pressure	↓ 10–20
Central venous pressure	0

(*From Cheek TG, Gutsche BB: Maternal physiologic alterations during pregnancy. In Schnider SM (ed): Anesthesia for Obstetrics. 2nd ed. Baltimore: Williams & Wilkins, 1987, p 3, with permission.*)

volume with uterine contractions are attenuated,[118] thus reducing cardiovascular demands during labor (Fig 26–11). Aortocaval compression resulting from the supine position should always be avoided in the third trimester.

The blood loss that occurs during delivery averages 500 mL for vaginal delivery and 1000 mL for cesarean section. Immediately postpartum, there is an appreciable (up to 40%) increase in cardiac output. This is thought to occur because elimination of the placental circulation and uterine contraction increase the circulating blood volume an additional 15–30%. Cardiac output then returns to prelabor levels within 1–2 hours and to pregestational levels by 2 weeks. The rapidity of restoration depends largely on the ability of the kidneys to return the plasma volume to pregestational levels.

The demands on the maternal cardiovascular system are greatest at three distinct periods: (1), at 20–24 weeks when the increase in blood volume and stroke volume is maximal, (2), during labor and delivery when significant fluctuations in the cardiac output occur, and (3) during the immediate postpartum period when the cardiac output is the greatest and maternal blood volume unpredictable. These periods represent the greatest risk

to a patient with cyanosis, impaired ventricular function, or pulmonary hypertension. In addition, patients with more common, but minor, congenital heart defects may first become symptomatic during these periods.

Anesthetic Considerations

Anesthetic management must be individualized to both the severity of the cardiovascular disease and obstetric considerations. Assessment of the severity of the cardiovascular disease consists of a complete characterization of the anatomy, including previous cardiac surgical procedures, and the degree of functional impairment. In general, maternal risk can be estimated by the NYHA functional class (Table 26–12). Specifically, the major risk factors are pulmonary vascular disease (pulmonary hypertension), ventricular failure resulting in pulmonary edema, and hypoxemia.

The history and physical examination should focus on detecting the presence of major risk factors. Unfortunately, symptoms associated with a normal pregnancy can be erroneously attributed to cardiovascular disease or, much worse, symptoms of cardiovascular impairment may be attributed to pregnancy. Dyspnea on exertion

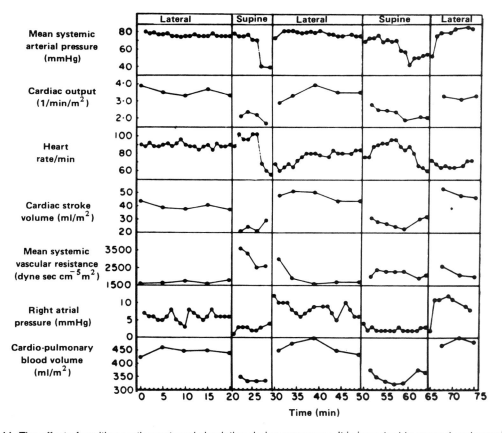

Figure 26–11. The effect of position on the maternal circulation during pregnancy. It is important to prevent aortocaval compression during pregnancy. Note that blood pressure, cardiac output, and cardiopulmonary blood volume decrease in the supine position due to decreased venous return. Lateral recumbency rapidly restores maternal cardiac output. (*From Lees, MM, et al: The circulatory effects of recumbent postural change in late pregnancy. Clin Sci 32:461, 1967, with permission.*)

and easy fatigability are present in 75% of normal pregnancies,[119] but paroxysmal nocturnal dyspnea and hemoptysis indicate underlying pathology. Peripheral edema, third heart sounds, and systolic ejection murmurs are common physical findings during normal pregnancies, but fourth heart sounds and diastolic murmurs are infrequent findings and indicate possible cardiovascular disease. Basal rales should disappear with a cough or a deep breath. A ventricular heave and prominent jugular venous pulsations are apparent in many normal patients; however, mean jugular venous pressure should not be elevated. The resting heart rate is generally less than 100 bpm.

Precordial echocardiographic examination provides almost all the information required by the anesthesiologist, including the magnitude and direction of shunts, ventricular function, and an estimation of the pulmonary artery pressure.[120] Because the information gained is so valuable, transesophageal echocardiography is indicated if the precordial examination is technically inadequate and significant cardiovascular impairment is suspected.

Numerous ECG changes occur during a normal pregnancy. These include atrial and ventricular premature complexes, minor changes in the PR and QT intervals, left or right axis deviation, Q wave in lead III or AVR, and ST segment depression or T wave inversion in the anterior precordial leads.[121] A history of exercise tolerance can provide valuable information, but formal exercise testing is usually not carried out during gestation. Cardiac catheterization provides little additional data that would impact on anesthetic management, especially in view of the possible fetal effects. Although there is currently no known risk to the fetus or mother associated with magnetic resonance imaging, the technique is not widely employed for cardiac imaging during pregnancy.

Preoperative evaluation should place a patient into one of two categories. Those with little or no functional impairment (NYHA class I or II) and those with significant functional impairment (NYHA class III or IV).[121] As cardiovascular demands increase, functional class may deteriorate one or more levels during the pregnancy.[111] For this reason, anesthesiologists should become involved early in the care of all patients with congenital heart disease and follow them throughout pregnancy.

TABLE 26–12. RELATIONSHIP BETWEEN NYHA FUNCTIONAL CLASS AND MATERNAL AND FETAL MORTALITY

Maternal Mortality	
Classes I and II	0.4%
Classes III and IV	6.8%
Fetal Mortality	
Classes I and II	None
Classes III and IV	30%

Patients with Minimal Functional Impairment. These patients are NYHA functional class I or II. The majority of patients with minimal functional impairment undergo labor and delivery in an uneventful manner and even may escape diagnosis during pregnancy. After excluding the presence of significant pulmonary hypertension, ventricular failure, dysrhythmias, and hypoxemia, anesthetic management proceeds as in the normal parturient.

Patients with Significant Functional Impairment. These patients are NYHA functional class III or IV and have a high incidence of both maternal and fetal morbidity. The presence of pulmonary vascular disease, ventricular failure, or hypoxemia can often be traced to one or more long-standing communications between the pulmonary and systemic circulations. Anesthetic management for these patients focuses on two goals. First, prevention of unfavorable changes in the direction and magnitude of existing shunts. Second, preservation of ventricular function by preventing increased ventricular workload, maintaining adequate preload, and avoiding excessive anesthetic-induced myocardial depression.

Patients with a NYHA functional class rating of I or II require only the noninvasive measurement of blood pressure, continual oximetry, and ECG. However, patients who exhibit pulmonary hypertension, ventricular failure, or hypoxemia require more extensive monitoring that should continue well into the postpartum period. Patients with pulmonary hypertension or tetralogy of Fallot are at risk for sudden death up to a week postpartum.[56] An arterial catheter provides continuous and reliable measurement of blood pressure and arterial blood gases. The site of catheter insertion should take into account previous surgical procedures. Monitoring central venous pressure allows for the detection of changes in preload that can be quite variable during labor or cesarean section. Central venous pressure measurements are especially helpful as a guide to intravenous fluid therapy during regional anesthesia. Pulmonary artery catheterization provides useful information but difficulties in placement and interpretation of measurements when intracardiac shunting is present should be considered. When central venous or pulmonary artery pressures are measured, trends rather than absolute values should guide therapy. Fetal heart rate should be monitored according to obstetric indications.

Anesthesia for Labor. Normal hemostasis should be ascertained before initiating spinal or epidural anesthesia. In addition to anticoagulant therapy, primary pulmonary hypertension and polycythemia are both associated with defective hemostasis. Epidural or intrathecal opiate administration alone may provide adequate analgesia for the first stage of labor without altering maternal hemodynamics. However, a pudendal block may be necessary during the second stage of labor.[122,123]

Regional anesthesia has been used effectively even in situations where a decrease in systemic vascular resistance would be considered detrimental.[124–126] Segmental epidural anesthesia attenuates the large increases in central venous pressure and cardiac output that occur during uterine contractions,[127] thus reducing demands on the cardiovascular system. It is preferable to insert the epidural catheter before severe pain occurs. Small incremental doses of local anesthetics should be used to achieve the desired level of analgesia in a controlled manner. If indicated by the severity of the congenital heart disease, central venous pressure measurement is useful to guide intravenous fluid therapy. Eliminating epinephrine from the test dose should be considered if there is a risk of developing dysrhythmias. Aortocaval compression must be avoided by proper maternal positioning. Most investigators advocate delivery with minimal expulsive effort in order to attenuate hemodynamic fluctuations.[121,128,129]

Anesthesia for Cesarean-Section. Vaginal delivery is considered preferable to elective cesarean section in women with congenital heart disease. However, the majority of the cases reported in the literature describe delivery by cesarean section. Continuous lumbar epidural anesthesia (CLE) has been most frequently utilized. CLE provides surgical analgesia in a controlled manner with predictable hemodynamic consequences. The onset of the sympathectomy should be slow and allow time for administration of fluids or vasopressors to compensate for decreases in preload and systemic vascular resistance. In patients with cardiomyopathy secondary to chronic pressure or volume overload, small decreases in preload can have significant effects on ventricular output. Central venous pressure monitoring is particularly helpful in these situations. Heart rate and ventricular contractility generally remain unchanged during epidural anesthesia. Epidural narcotics can be used to supplement the local anesthetics in situations in which further sympathectomy is undesirable. However, epidural narcotics alone will not provide surgical analgesia. With the extensive sympathectomy, the importance of preventing aortocaval compression cannot be overemphasized.

In the presence of right-to-left shunting, rapid decreases in systemic vascular resistance worsen hypoxemia. In addition, a decrease in preload may severely limit ventricular output in patients with ventricular hypertrophy. Prevention of major alterations in cardiac shunts and preload is preferable to treatment after cardiovascular deterioration occurs. Phenylephrine restores both preload and systemic vascular resistance. However, its use in obstetrics is controversial as it may impair uterine blood flow. Metaraminol may be preferable to

ephedrine in treating hypotension and in avoiding dysrhythmias. Nevertheless, the maternal circulation must be supported to the extent needed.

Although subarachnoid block can be utilized for cesarean section, it should be reserved for those patients with relatively minor congenital heart defects. The rapidity with which sympathectomy occurs during subarachnoid block often leads to hypotension even after prophylactic administration of ephedrine.[130]

General anesthesia has the advantage of rapid induction and maintenance of the systemic vascular resistance. However, differences in the dose response to anesthetic drugs and variations in surgical stimulation and blood loss make it difficult to predict the exact hemodynamic consequences. During induction, arterial blood may desaturate quite rapidly even after seemingly adequate preoxygenation. Induction of anesthesia with barbiturates followed by endotracheal intubation appears to maintain maternal blood pressure, possibly due to an increase in circulating catecholamines.[131,132] Ketamine usually increases both arterial blood pressure and cardiac output and does not appear to promote hypoxemia even with right-to-left intracardiac shunting.

Oxytocic drugs should be given slowly to avoid hypotension that may occur with rapid administration. Patients who have anatomy compatible with right-to-left shunting should have all intravenous lines cleared of bubbles. Antibiotics should be given just before the active phase of labor (see Appendix 26–1).

Fetal Considerations

Maternal congenital heart disease resulting in hypoxemia is associated with poor fetal growth and a high incidence of fetal complications. The risk to the fetus generally parallels the degree of hypoxemia. Neonates are smaller and perinatal mortality substantially higher.

Even though most patients with congenital heart disease have no recognizable genetic syndrome, the risk of recurrence of a congenital heart defect in the fetus may be as high as 17%.[133] Newborn children of women with congenital heart disease should be closely observed.

PROSTHETIC MATERIALS

Surgery for congenital heart defects often requires the use of prostheses for the replacement or construction of valves, conduits, and patches. The anesthesiologist should be aware of the presence of these materials. Both biologic and synthetic materials are used, each with their own advantages and disadvantages.

Biologic Materials

Biologic materials can be either endogenous or exogenous in origin. Endogenous materials include pericardium, blood vessels, and even valves. These materials are usually placed at the time of cardiac surgery. Endogenous materials have the major advantage of tissue compatibility that promotes the unimpeded regeneration of living endothelial cells. The ability of the prosthesis to resist infection is enhanced and the likelihood of thrombus formation reduced by the use of endogenous tissue. Unfortunately, the availability of endogenous materials such as pericardium is limited, and these materials may not be suitable for the fabrication of complex prostheses. In addition, the tensile strength of pericardium is not as great as that of the synthetic materials and may not be appropriate when excessive stress is expected. The use of endogenous blood vessels or valves also poses the additional risk of removing them from their natural positions.

Exogenous biologic prostheses are either homografts (from human cadavers) or xenografts (from animals). Xenografts are chemically preserved and treated to minimize antigenicity and prevent tissue deterioration. However, tissue fixing also eliminates cellular viability, which ultimately results in reduced durability. When xenografts are used in children, valve degeneration occurs more rapidly than in adults and may begin as early as 2 years after insertion.[134,135] The overall failure rate is as high as 10% per year. Xenografts do have the advantage of being widely available and relatively easy to implant. The sewing ring of xenograft valves may reduce the effective size of the valve orifice, which is problematic when a smaller valve is needed. Pressure gradients from the left ventricle to the ascending aorta can be as great as 15–20 mm Hg. Even without the use of anticoagulants, the risk of thromboembolic complications is less than 3% per year.[134]

By their nature, homograft implants are believed to have minimal antigenicity. Valve prostheses are available in continuity with the annulus and great artery, thus allowing excellent hemodynamic performance. Because of the bulk of the structures supporting the valve, it is seldom used in the mitral position. Homograft valves appear to be quite durable, commonly lasting 15–20 years, at which time about 10% per year will fail.[136] Balloon dilation may allow even longer valve life. Progressive internal obstruction secondary to pseudointimal thickening is uncommon. Thrombosis is rare making systemic anticoagulation unnecessary. These valves appear to be relatively resistant to infection. Unfortunately, homograft is not always available in sufficient quantity or appropriate size.

Synthetic Materials

Mechanical Valves. Mechanical valve prostheses include caged-ball, tilting-disk, or bi-leaflet designs (Table 26–13). Most modern valves are composed of pyrolite carbon, an extremely strong, smooth, and relatively nonthrombogenic material. The hemodynamic profile of tilting-disk valves is slightly superior to caged-ball mech-

TABLE 26–13. COMMONLY ENCOUNTERED VALVE PROSTHESES

Caged-Ball
 Starr-Edwards (Edwards CVS Division, Baxter Intl, Santa Ana, CA)
Tilting-Disc
 Bjork-Shiley (Shiley, Irvine, CA)
 Lillehei-Kastor (Medical Inc, Inver Grove Heights, MN)
 Omniscience (Medical Inc, Inver Grove Heights, MN)
 Medtronic-Hall (Hall-Kaster) (Medtronic, Inc, Eden Prairie, MN)
Bi-Leaflet
 St. Jude Medical (St. Jude Medical, St. Paul, MN)
Biologic
 Homograft
 Hancock (Medtronic, Inc, Minneapolis)
 Carpentier-Edwards (Edwards CVS Division, Baxter Intl, Santa Ana, CA)
 Ionescu-Shiley (Shiley, Irvine, CA)

anisms, but they are the most vulnerable to immobilization by thrombus or tissue. The bi-leaflet valve has the best hemodynamic characteristics of any mechanical valve, especially in the smaller sizes, and is frequently used in children.[134] All mechanical valves are exceedingly durable. With anticoagulant therapy, the risk of thromboembolism is less than 3% per year, essentially equivalent to that of xenograft valves. However, anticoagulant therapy adds the risk of hemorrhagic complications, which can be considerable for children.

Gore-Tex and Dacron. These synthetic fabrics are used as tube grafts or flat sheets. Both materials have a higher tensile strength than pericardium. Bleeding and extravasation of plasma through these materials can occur at the time of insertion, especially through needle holes; however, both fabrics soon develop a neointimal layer. If the neointimal layer is not firmly affixed to the inside of the graft, dissection and eventual obstruction to flow can occur. In addition, if high pressures exist within the graft, neointimal thickening can progress to the point of obstruction. The likelihood of obstruction is enhanced when blood flow is turbulent or there is a kink in the synthetic material. Turbulent blood flow can also result in hemolysis and thrombocytopenia. Gore-Tex (polytetrafluoroethylene; W.L. Gore Associates, Elkton, Maryland) generally forms a thinner and more stable neointimal layer than Dacron. Other late complications associated with the use of these fabrics include infection and aneurysm formation.

Umbrellas and Coils. Umbrellas are used to close atrial septal defects, muscular ventricular septal defects, and even a patent ductus. Coils are inserted into aortopulmonary collateral vessels in an effort to limit pulmonary blood flow to that supplied by the pulmonary artery (see Chapter 7). Both umbrellas and coils are designed to promote endothelial growth, and closure of the defect is often not complete until this occurs. Little is known about the long-term consequences of these devices.

MANAGEMENT OF PERIOPERATIVE ANTICOAGULATION

Perioperative management of anticoagulants (coumadin being the most commonly used today) depends predominantly on the urgency and nature of the surgical procedure. In general, the risk of allowing coagulation to normalize during the perioperative period appears to be negligible, whereas difficulties with hemostasis occur in more than 10% of patients undergoing noncardiac surgery.[137]

For elective surgery, coumadin therapy should be discontinued 1–3 days preoperatively while maintaining systemic anticoagulation with intravenous heparin. The dose of heparin should be regulated to keep the activated partial thromboplastin time one and one-half times the control value. The prothrombin time should be allowed to return to within a few seconds of normal. Intravenous heparin is then discontinued 4–6 hours before surgery and restarted within 48 hours after the operation. Coumadin therapy is resumed 1–7 days postoperatively.

Emergency noncardiac surgery necessitates the rapid reversal of hemostatic defects within a short period of time. Cessation of coumadin and administration of vitamin K will have no effect for at least 24 hours. Rapid normalization of coagulation can only be accomplished by replacement of coagulation factors, usually with fresh frozen plasma.

REFERENCES

1. Banchero N: Cardiovascular responses to chronic hypoxia. *Annu Rev Physiol* **49**:465–476, 1987
2. Heistad DD, Abboud FM: Circulatory adjustments to hypoxia. *Circulation* **61**:463–470, 1980
3. Hollenberg M, Honbo N, Samorodin AJ: Effects of hypoxia on cardiac growth in neonatal rat. *Am J Physiol* **231**:1445–1450, 1976
4. Blesa MI, Lahiri S, Rashkind WJ, Fishman AP: Normalization of the blunted ventilatory response to acute hypoxia in congenital cyanotic heart disease. *N Engl J Med* **296**:237–241, 1977
5. Teitel D, Sidi D, Bernstein D, et al: Chronic hypoxemia in the newborn lamb: Cardiovascular, hematopoietic, and growth adaptations. *Pediatr Res* **19**:1004–1010, 1985
6. Bernstein D, Teitel D, Sidi D, et al: Redistribution of regional blood flow and oxygen delivery in experimental cyanotic heart disease in newborn lambs. *Pediatr Res* **22**:389–393, 1987
7. Barragry TP, Blatchford JW, Tuna IC, et al: Left ventricular dysfunction in a canine model of chronic cyanosis. *Surgery* **102**:362–370, 1987
8. Graham TP, Erath HG, Buckspan GS, Fisher RD: Myocardial anaerobic metabolism during isoprenaline infusion in a cyanotic animal model: Possible cause of myocardial dysfunction in cyanotic congenital heart disease. *Cardiovas Res* **13**:401–406, 1979
9. Graham TP, Erath HG, Boucek RJ, Boerth RC: Left ventricular function in cyanotic congenital heart disease. *Am J Cardiol* **45**:1231–1236, 1980
10. Jarmakani JM, Graham TP, Canent RV, Jewett PH: Left heart function in children with tetralogy of Fallot before and after palliative or corrective surgery. *Circulation* **46**:478–490, 1972
11. Borow KM, Green LH, Castaneda AR, Keane JF: Left ventricular function after repair of tetralogy of Fallot and its relationship to age at surgery. *Circulation* **61**:1150–1158, 1980
12. Perloff JK: The increase in and regression of ventricular mass. In Perloff JK, Child JS (eds): *Congenital Heart Disease in Adults*. Philadelphia: WB Saunders, 1991, pp 313–322
13. Bernstein D, Voss E, Huang S, et al: Differential regulation of right and left ventricular B-adrenergic receptors in newborn lambs with experimental cyanotic heart disease. *J Clin Invest* **85**:68–74, 1990
14. Bristow MR, Ginsburg R, Minobe W, et al: Decreased catecholamine sensitivity and B-adrenergic receptor density in failing human hearts. *N Engl J Med* **307**:205–211, 1982
15. Rosove MH, Perloff JK, Hocking WG, et al: Chronic hypoxaemia and decompensated erythrocytosis in cyanotic congenital heart disease. *Lancet* **2**:313–315, 1986
16. Phornphutkul C, Rosenthal A, Nadas A, Berenburg W: Cerebrovascular accidents in infants and children with cyanotic congenital heart disease. *Am J Cardiol* **32**:329–334, 1973
17. Perloff JK, Rosove MH, Child JS, Wright GB: Adults with cyanotic congenital heart disease: Hematologic management. *Ann Intern Med* **109**:406–413, 1988
18. Gidding SS, Stockman JA: Effect of iron deficiency on tissue oxygen delivery in cyanotic congenital heart disease. *Am J Cardiol* **61**:605–607, 1988
19. Colon-Otero G, Gilchrist GS, Holcomb GR, et al: Preoperative evaluation of hemostasis in patients with congenital heart disease. *Mayo Clin Proc* **62**:379–385, 1987
20. Kontras S, Sirak H, Newton W: Hematologic abnormalities in children with congenital heart disease. *JAMA* **195**:611–615, 1976
21. Gill JC, Wilson AD, Endres-Brooks J, Montgomery RR: Loss of the largest von Willebrand factor multimers from the plasma of patients with congenital heart disease. *Blood* **67**:758–761, 1986
22. Fischbein CA, Rosenthal A, Fischer EG, et al: Risk factors for brain abscess in patients with congenital heart disease. *Am J Cardiol* **34**:97–102, 1974
23. Neuburger JW, Sibert AR, Buckley LP, Fyler DC: Cognitive function and age at repair of transposition of the great arteries in children. *N Engl J Med* **310**:1496–1499, 1984
24. Rossi RF, Ekroth R, Jansson K, Scallan M, et al: Brain type creatine kinase in relation to oxygen desaturation in the blood of children with congenital heart disease. *Scand J Thorac Cardiovasc Surg* **24**:75–77, 1990

25. Brunberg JA, Reilly EL, Doty DB: Central nervous system consequences in infants of cardiac surgery using deep hypothermia and circulatory arrests. *Circulation* 49–50(suppl II):60–68, 1974

26. Ehyai A, Fenichel GM, Bender HW: Incidence and prognosis of seizures in infants after cardiac surgery with profound hypothermia and circulatory arrest. *JAMA* 252:3165–3167, 1984

27. Wells FC, Coghill S, Caplan HL, et al: Duration of circulatory arrest does influence the psychological development of children after cardiac operation in early life. *J Thorac Cardiovasc Surg* 86:823–831, 1983

28. Wical BS, Tomasi LG: A distinctive neurologic syndrome after induced profound hypothermia. *Pediatr Neurol* 6:202–205, 1990

29. Blackwood MJA, Haka IK, Steward DJ: Developmental outcome in children undergoing surgery with profound hypothermia. *Anesthesiology* 65:437–440, 1986

30. Nicolson SC, Betts EK, Jobes DR, et al: Comparison of oral and intramuscular preanesthetic medication for pediatric inpatient surgery. *Anesthesiology* 71:8–10, 1989

31. Goldstein DMC, Davis PJ, Kretchman E, et al: Double-blind comparison of oral transmucosal fentanyl citrate with oral meperidine, diazepam, and atropine as preanesthetic medication in children with congenital heart disease. *Anesthesiology* 74:28–33, 1991

32. Stewart KG, Rowbottom SJ, Aitken AW, et al: Oral ketamine premedication for paediatric cardiac surgery—A comparison with intramuscular morphine (both after oral trimeprazine). *Anaesth Intensive Care* 18:11–14, 1990

33. Greeley WJ, Bushman GA, Davis DP, Reves JG: Comparative effects of halothane and ketamine on systemic arterial oxygen saturation in children with cyanotic heart disease. *Anesthesiology* 65:666–668, 1986

34. Laishley RS, Burrows FA, Lerman J, Roy WL: Effect of anesthetic induction regimens on oxygen saturation in cyanotic congenital heart disease. *Anesthesiology* 65:673–677, 1986

35. Bernstein D, Crane C: Comparative circulatory effects of isoproterenol and dopamine in lambs with experimental cyanotic heart disease. *Pediatr Res* 29:323–328, 1991

36. Wells AL, Wells TR, Landing BH, et al: Short trachea, a hazard in tracheal intubation of neonates and infants: Syndromal associations. *Anesthesiology* 71:367–373, 1989

37. Stanger P, Lucas RV, Edwards JE: Anatomic factors causing respiratory distress in acyanotic congenital heart disease. *Pediatrics* 43:760–769, 1969

38. Corno A, Giamberti A, Giannico S, et al: Airway obstructions associated with congenital heart disease in infancy. *J Thorac Cardiovasc Surg* 99:1091–1098, 1990

39. Rabinovitch M: Pulmonary hypertension. In Adams FH, Emmanouilides GC (eds): *Heart Disease in Infants, Children, and Adolescents.* Baltimore: Williams & Wilkins, 1983, pp 669–692

40. Motoyama EK, Tanaka T, Fricker FJ: Peripheral airway obstruction in children with congenital heart disease and pulmonary hypertension. *Am Rev Respir Dis* 133:A10, 1986

41. Lister G, Pitt BR: Cardiopulmonary interactions in the infant with congenital cardiac disease. *Clin Chest Med* 4:219–232, 1983

42. Lynn AM, Jenkens JG, Edmonds JF, Burns JE: Diaphragmatic paralysis after pediatric cardiac surgery: A retrospective analysis of 34 cases. *Crit Care Med* 11:280–282, 1983

43. Mickell JJ, Oh KS, Siewers RD, et al: Clinical implications of postoperative unilateral phrenic nerve paralysis. *J Thorac Cardiovasc Surg* 76:279–304, 1978

44. Lees MH, Burnell RH, Morgan CL, Ross BB: Ventilation-perfusion relationships in children with heart disease and diminished pulmonary blood flow. *Pediatrics* 42:778–785, 1968

45. Burrows FA: Physiologic dead space, venous admixture, and the arterial to end-tidal carbon dioxide difference in infants and children undergoing cardiac surgery. *Anesthesiology* 70:219–225, 1989

46. Bancalari E, Jesse MJ, Gelband H, Garcia O: Lung mechanics in congenital heart disease with increased and decreased pulmonary blood flow. *Pediatrics* 90:192–195, 1977

47. Thorsteinsson A, Jonmarker C, Larsson A, et al: Functional residual capacity in anesthetized children: Normal values and values in children with cardiac anomalies. *Anesthesiology* 73:876–881, 1990

48. Laver MB, Hallowell P, Goldblatt A: Pulmonary dysfunction secondary to heart disease: Aspects relevant to anesthesia and surgery. *Anesthesiology* 33:161–192, 1970

49. Albers WH, Nadas AS: Unilateral chronic pulmonary edema and pleural effusion after systemic-pulmonary artery shunts for cyanotic congenital heart disease. *Am J Cardiol* 19:861–866, 1967

50. Durmowicz AG, St Cyr JA, Clarke DR, Stenmark KR: Unilateral pulmonary hypertension as a result of chronic high flow to one lung. *Am Rev Respir Dis* 142:230–233, 1990

51. Staub NC: Pathogenesis of pulmonary edema. *Am Rev Respir Dis* 109:358–372, 1974

52. Howlett G: Lung mechanics in normal infants and infants with congenital heart disease. *Arch Dis Child* 47:707–715, 1972

53. Lister G, Talner N: Management of respiratory failure of cardiac origin. In Gregory GA (ed): *Respiratory Failure in the Child.* New York: Churchill Livingstone, 1981, pp 67–87

54. Hordof AJ, Mellins RB, Gersony WM, Steeg CN: Reversibility of chronic obstructive lung disease in infants following repair of ventricular septal defect. *Pediatrics* 90:187–191, 1977

55. Hickey PR, Hansen DD, Wessel DL, et al: Blunting of stress responses in the pulmonary circulation of infants by fentanyl. *Anesth Analg* 64:1137–1142, 1985

56. Gleicher N, Midwall J, Hochberger D, Jaffin H: Eisenmenger's syndrome and pregnancy. *Obstet Gynecol Surv* 34:721–741, 1979

57. Lindahl SG, Yates AP, Hatch DJ: Relationship between invasive and noninvasive measurements of gas exchange in anesthetized infants and children. *Anesthesiology* 66:168–175, 1987

58. Katz AM: Cardiomyopathy of overload. A major determinant of prognosis in congestive heart failure. *N Engl J Med* 322:100–110, 1990

59. Bortone AS, Hess OM, Chiddo A, et al: Functional and

structural abnormalities in patients with dilated cardiomyopathy. *J Am Coll Cardiol* **14**:613–623, 1989

60. Talner NS: Heart failure. In Adams FH, Emmanouilides GC (eds): *Heart Disease in Infants, Children, and Adolescents.* Baltimore: Williams & Wilkins, 1983, pp 708–725

61. Braunwald E: Pathophysiology of heart failure. In Braunwald E (ed): *Heart Disease: A Textbook of Cardiovascular Medicine.* Philadelphia: WB Saunders, 1988, pp 426–448

62. Moreau GA, Graham TP: Clinical assessment of ventricular function after surgical treatment of congenital heart defects. *Cardiol Clin* **7**:439–452, 1989

63. DiDonato RM, Wernovsky G, Walsh EP, et al: Results of the arterial switch operation for transposition of the great arteries with ventricular septal defect: Surgical considerations and midterm follow-up data. *Circulation* **80**:1689–1705, 1989

64. Walsh EP, Rickenmacher S, Keane JF, et al: Late results in patients with tetralogy of Fallot repaired during infancy. *Circulation* **77**:1062–1067, 1988

65. Rossi MA, Carillo SV: Cardiac hypertrophy due to pressure and volume overload: Distinctly different biological phenomena? *Int J Cardiol* **31**:133–142, 1991

66. Panidis IP, Kotler MN, Ren J, et al: Development and regression of left ventricular hypertrophy. *J Am Coll Cardiol* **3**:1309–1320, 1984

67. Grossman W: Cardiac hypertrophy: Useful adaptation of pathologic process? *Am J Med* **69**:576–584, 1980

68. Anversa P, Olivetti G, Loud AV: Morphometric study of early postnatal development in the left and right ventricular myocardium of the rat. *Circ Res* **46**:495–502, 1980

69. Donner R, Carabello BA, Black I, Spann JF: Left ventricular wall stress in compensated aortic stenosis in children. *Am J Cardiol* **51**:946–951, 1983

70. Borow KM, Colan SD, Neumann A: Altered left ventricular mechanics in patients with valvular aortic stenosis and coarctation of the aorta: Effects on systolic performance and late outcome. *Circulation* **72**:515–522, 1985

71. Assey ME, Wisenbaugh T, Spann JF, et al: Unexpected persistence into adulthood of low wall stress in patients with congenital aortic stenosis: Is there a fundamental difference in the hypertrophic response to a pressure overload present from birth? *Circulation* **75**:973–979, 1987

72. Ehsani AA, Hagberg JM, Hickson RC: Rapid changes in left ventricular dimensions and mass in response to physical conditioning and deconditioning. *Am J Cardiol* **42**:52–56, 1978

73. Monrad ES, Hess OM, Murakami T, et al: Time course of regression of left ventricular hypertrophy after aortic valve replacement. *Circulation* **77**:1345–1355, 1988

74. Thomas JA, Marks BH: Plasma norepinephrine in congestive heart failure. *Am J Cardiol* **41**:233–243, 1978

75. Ross RD, Daniels SR, Schwartz DC, et al: Plasma norepinephrine levels in infants and children with congestive heart failure. *Am J Cardiol* **59**:911–914, 1987

76. Ross RD, Daniels SR, Schwartz DC, et al: Return of plasma norepinephrine to normal after resolution of congestive heart failure in congenital heart disease. *Am J Cardiol* **60**:1411–1413, 1987

77. Michaelsson M, Engle MA: Congenital complete heart block: An international study of the natural history. In

Brest AN (ed): *Cardiovascular Clinics: Pediatric Cardiology.* Philadelphia: FA Davis, 1972, pp 85–101

78. Ross BA: Congenital complete atrioventricular block. *Pediatr Clin North Am* **37**:69–78, 1990

79. Huhta JC, Maloney JD, Ritter DG, et al: Complete atrioventricular block in patients with atrioventricular discordance. *Circulation* **67**:1374–1377, 1983

80. Gillette PC, Garson AJ, Porter CJ, McNamara DG: Dysrhythmias. In Adams FH, Emmanouilides GC (eds): *Heart Disease in Infants, Children, and Adolescents.* Baltimore: Williams & Wilkins, 1983, pp 725–741

81. Kumar AE, Fyler DC, Mietinen OS, Nadas AS: Ebstein's anomaly: Clinical profile and natural history. *Am J Cardiol* **28**:84–95, 1971

82. Oh JK, Holmers DR, Hayes DL, et al: Cardiac arrhythmias in patients with surgical repair of Ebstein's anomaly. *J Am Coll Cardiol* **6**:1351–1357, 1985

83. Watson H: Natural history of Ebstein's anomaly of tricuspid valve in childhood and adolescence. *Br Heart J* **36**:417–427, 1974

84. Wolff GS, Rowland TW, Ellison RC: Surgically induced right bundle branch block with left anterior hemiblock: An ominous sign in postoperative tetralogy of Fallot. *Circulation* **46**:587–594, 1972

85. Clark EB, Kugler JD: Preoperative secundum atrial septal defect with coexisting sinus node and atrioventricular node dysfunction. *Circulation* **65**:976–980, 1982

86. Craig RJ, Selzer A: Natural history and prognosis of atrial septal defect. *Circulation* **37**:805–815, 1968

87. Bharati S, Lev M: Conduction system in sudden unexpected death a considerable time after repair of atrial septal defect. *Chest* **94**:142–148, 1988

88. Brandenberg RO, Holmes DR, Brandenburg RO, McGoon DR: Clinical follow-up study of paroxysmal supraventricular tachyarrhythmias after repair of secundum type atrial septal defect. *Am J Cardiol* **51**:273–276, 1983

89. Vetter VL, Horowitz LN: Electrophysiologic residua and sequelae of surgery for congenital heart defects. *Am J Cardiol* **50**:588–604, 1982

90. Godman MJ, Roberts NK, Izukawa T: Late postoperative conduction disturbances after repair of ventricular septal defect and tetralogy of Fallot. *Circulation* **49**:214, 1974

91. Moodie DS, Riller DG, Tajik AJ, O'Fallon M: Long-term follow-up in the unoperated univentricular heart. *Am J Cardiol* **53**:1124–1128, 1984

92. Moodie DS, Ritter DG, Tajik AH, et al: Long-term follow-up after palliative operation for univentricular heart. *Am J Cardiol* **53**:1648–1651, 1984

93. Weber HS, Hellenbrand WE, Kleinman CS, et al: Predictors of rhythm disturbances and subsequent morbidity after the Fontan operation. *Am J Cardiol* **64**:762–767, 1989

94. Duster MC, Bink-Boelkens MT, Wampler D, et al: Long-term follow-up of dysrhythmias following the Mustard procedure. *Am Heart J* **109**:1323–1326, 1985

95. Flinn CJ, Wolff GS, Dick M, et al: Cardiac rhythm after the Mustard operation for complete transposition of the great arteries. *N Engl J Med* **310**:1635–1638, 1984

96. Southall DP, Stebbens V, Shinebourne EA: Sudden and

unexpected death between 1 and 5 years. *Arch Dis Child* **62**:700–705, 1987

97. Vetter VL, Tanner CS: Electrophysiologic consequences of the arterial switch repair of d-transposition of the great arteries. *J Am Coll Cardiol* **12**:229–237, 1988

98. Steeg CN, Krongard E, Davachi F, et al: Post-operative left anterior hemiblock and right bundle branch block following repair of tetralogy of Fallot: Clinical and etiologic considerations. *Circulation* **51**:1026–1029, 1975

99. Friedli B, Bolens M, Taktak M: Conduction disturbances after correction of tetralogy of Fallot: Are electrophysiologic studies of prognostic value? *J Am Coll Cardiol* **11**: 162–165, 1988

100. Deanfield JE, Ho SY, Anderson RH, et al: Late sudden death after repair of tetralogy of Fallot: A clinicopathologic study. *Circulation* **67**:626–631, 1983

101. Garson A, Randall DC, Gillette PC, et al: Prevention of sudden death after repair of tetralogy of Fallot: Treatment of ventricular arrhythmias. *J Am Coll Cardiol* **6**:221–227, 1985

102. Chandar JS, Wolff GS, Garson A, et al: Ventricular arrhythmias in postoperative tetralogy of Fallot. *Am J Cardiol* **65**:655–661, 1990

103. Chen D, Moller JH: Comparison of late clinical status between patients with different hemodynamic findings after repair of tetralogy of Fallot. *Am Heart J* **113**:767–772, 1987

104. Beland MJ, Hesslein PS, Finlay CD, et al: Noninvasive transcutaneous cardiac pacing in children. *Pace* **10**:1262–1270, 1987

105. Diaz J, Friesen RH: Anesthetic management of congenital complete heart block in childhood. *Anesth Analg* **58**: 334–336, 1979

106. Atlee JL, Bosnjak ZJ: Mechanisms for cardiac dysrhythmias during anesthesia. *Anesthesiology* **72**:347–374, 1990

107. Jones RM, Broadbent MP, Adams AP: Anaesthetic considerations in patients with paroxysmal supraventricular tachycardia. A review and report of cases. *Anaesthesia* **39**: 307–313, 1984

108. Kirk CR, Gibbs JL, Thomas R, et al: Cardiovascular collapse after verapamil in supraventricular tachycardia. *Arch Dis Child* **62**:1265–1266, 1987

109. Stevenson GW, Schuster J, Kross J, Hall SC: Transoesophageal pacing for perioperative control of neonatal paroxysmal supraventricular tachycardia. *Can J Anaesth* **37**: 672–674, 1990

110. Chow AE, Noble-Jamieson C: Termination of paroxysmal supraventricular tachycardia by intravenous adenosine in a child. *Anaesthesia* **44**:322–323, 1989

111. Shime J, Mocarski EJM, Hastings D, et al: Congenital heart disease in pregnancy: Short- and long-term implications. *Am J Obstet Gynecol* **156**:313–322, 1987

112. Oakley CM: Pregnancy in heart disease: Pre-existing heart disease. *Cardiovasc Clin* **19**:57–80, 1989

113. Scott DE: Anemia in pregnancy. *Obstet Gynecol Annu* **1**:219–244, 1972

114. Rubler S, Damani PM, Pinto ER: Cardiac size and performance during pregnancy estimated by echocardiography. *Am J Cardiol* **40**:534–540, 1977

115. Ueland K, Novy MJ, Peterson EN, Metcalfe J: Maternal cardiovascular dynamics IV. The influence of gestational age on the maternal cardiovascular response to posture and exercise. *Am J Obstet Gynecol* **104**:856–864, 1969

116. Katz R, Karliner JS, Resnik R: Effects of a natural volume overload state (pregnancy) on left ventricular performance in normal human subjects. *Circulation* **58**:434–441, 1978

117. Cole P, Cook F, Plappert T, et al: Longitudinal changes in left ventricular architecture and function in peripartum cardiomyopathy. *Am J Cardiol* **60**:871–876, 1987

118. Metcalfe J, Ueland K: Maternal cardiovascular adjustments to pregnancy. *Prog Cardiovasc Dis* **16**:363–374, 1974

119. Milne JA, Howie AD, Pack AI: Dyspnoea during normal pregnancy. *Br J Obstet Gynaecol* **85**:260–263, 1978

120. Stevenson JG: Comparison of several noninvasive methods for estimation of pulmonary artery pressure. *J Am Soc Echocardiogr* **2**:157–171, 1989

121. Cole PL, Sutton M: Normal cardiopulmonary adjustments to pregnancy: Cardiovascular evaluation. *Cardiovasc Clin* **19**:37–56, 1989

122. Abboud TK, Raya J, Noveihed R, Daniel J: Intrathecal morphine for relief of labor pain in a parturient with severe pulmonary hypertension. *Anesthesiology* **59**:477–479, 1983

123. Ahmad S, Hawes D, Dooley S, et al: Intrathecal morphine in a parturient with a single ventricle. *Anesthesiology* **54**:515–517, 1981

124. Baumann H, Schneider H, Drack G, et al: Pregnancy and delivery by caesarean section in a patient with transposition of the great arteries and single ventricle. *Br J Obstet Gynaecol* **94**:704–708, 1987

125. Fong J, Druzin M, Gimbel AA, Fisher J: Epidural anaesthesia for labour and caesarean section in a parturient with a single ventricle and transposition of the great arteries. *Can J Anaesth* **37**:680–684, 1990

126. Johnston TA, de Bono D: Single ventricle and pulmonary hypertension. A successful pregnancy. *Br J Obstet Gynaecol* **96**:731–734, 1989

127. Ueland K, Hansen JM: Maternal cardiovascular dynamics. III. Labor and delivery under local and caudal analgesia. *Am J Obstet Gynecol* **103**:8–18, 1969

128. Roberts SL, Chestnut DH: Anesthesia for the obstetric patient with cardiac disease. *Clin Obstet Gynecol* **30**:601–610, 1987

129. Perloff JK: Pregnancy in congenital heart disease. In Perloff JK, Child JS (eds): *Congenital Heart Disease in Adults*. Philadelphia: WB Saunders, 1991, pp 124–140

130. Gutsche BB: Prophylactic ephedrine preceding spinal analgesia for cesarean section. *Anesthesiology* **45**:462–465, 1976

131. Palahniuk RJ, Cumming M: Foetal deterioration following thiopentone-nitrous oxide anaesthesia in the pregnant ewe. *Can Anaesth Soc J* **24**:361–370, 1977

132. Shnider SM, Wright RG, Levinson G, et al: Plasma norepinephrine and uterine blood flow changes during endotracheal intubation and general anesthesia in the pregnant ewe. *Anesthesiology* **49**:A115, 1978

133. Whittemore RH, Hobbins JC, Engle MA: Pregnancy and its outcome in women with and without surgical treatment of congenital disease. *Am J Cardiol* **50**:641–651, 1982

134. Morgan RJ, David JT, Fraker T: Current status of valve prostheses. *Surg Clin North Am* **65**:699–720, 1985
135. Jamieson WR, Rosado LJ, Munro AI, et al: Carpentier-Edwards standard porcine bioprosthesis: Primary tissue failure (structural valve deterioration) by age groups. *Ann Thorac Surg* **46**:155–162, 1988
136. McGiffin DC, O'Brien MF, Stafford EG, et al: Long-

term results of the viable cryopreserved allograft aortic valve: Continuing evidence for superior valve durability. *J Cardiac Surg* **3**:289–292, 1988
137. Tinker JH, Tarhan S: Discontinuing anticoagulant therapy in surgical patients with cardiac valve prostheses. *JAMA* **239**:738–739, 1978

APPENDIX 26–1A ANTIBIOTIC PROPHYLAXIS FOR ENDOCARDITIS

Endocarditis Prophylaxis Recommended*
  By Cardiac Condition
    Prosthetic cardiac valves, including bioprosthetic and homograft valves
    Previous bacterial endocarditis, even in the absence of heart disease
    Most congenital malformations
    Rheumatic and other acquired valvular dysfunction, even after valvular surgery
    Hypertrophic cardiomyopathy
    Mitral valve prolapse with valvular regurgitation
  By Surgical Procedure
    Dental procedures known to induce gingival or mucosal bleeding, including professional cleaning
    Tonsillectomy and/or adenoidectomy
    Surgical operations that involve intestinal or respiratory mucosa
    Bronchoscopy with a rigid bronchoscope
    Sclerotherapy for esophageal varices
    Esophageal dilatation
    Gallbladder surgery
    Cystoscopy
    Urethral dilatation
    Urethral catheterization if urinary tract infection is present†
    Urinary tract surgery if urinary tract infection is present†
    Prostatic surgery
    Incision and drainage of infected tissue†
    Vaginal hysterectomy
    Vaginal delivery in the presence of infection†

Endocarditis Prophylaxis Not Recommended
  By Cardiac Condition
    Isolated secundum atrial septal defect
    Surgical repair without residua beyond 6 months of secundum atrial septal defect, ventricular septal defect, or patent ductus arteriosus
    Previous coronary artery bypass graft surgery
    Mitral valve prolapse without valvular regurgitation‡
    Physiologic, functional, or innocent heart murmurs
    Previous Kawasaki disease without valvular dysfunction
    Previous rheumatic fever without valvular dysfunction
    Cardiac pacemakers and implanted defibrillators
  By Surgical Procedure§
    Dental procedures not likely to induce gingival bleeding such as simple adjustment of orthodontic appliances or fillings above the gum line
    Injection of local intraoral anesthetic (except intraligamentary injections)
    Shedding of primary teeth
    Tympanostomy tube insertion
    Endotracheal intubation
    Bronchoscopy with a flexible bronchoscope, with or without biopsy
    Cardiac catheterization
    Endoscopy with or without gastrointestinal biopsy
    Cesarean section
    In the absence of infection for urethral catheterization, dilation and curettage, uncomplicated vaginal delivery, therapeutic abortion, sterilization procedures, or insertion or removal of intrauterine devices

* This appendix lists procedures but is not meant to be all inclusive.
† In addition to prophylactic regimen for genitourinary procedures, antibiotic therapy should be directed against the most likely pathogen.
‡ Individuals who have a mitral valve prolapse associated with thickening and/or redundancy of the valve leaflets may be at increased risk for bacterial endocarditis, particularly men who are 45 years of age or older.
§ In patients who have prosthetic heart valves, a previous history of endocarditis or surgically constructed systemic-pulmonary shunts or conduits, physicians may choose to administer prophylactic antibiotics even for low-risk procedures that involve the lower respiratory, genitourinary, or gastrointestinal tracts.
(*From Dajani AS, et al: Recommendations by the American Heart Association, Prevention of Bacterial Endocarditis. JAMA 264:2919–2922, 1990.*)

APPENDIX 26–1B. PROPHYLACTIC REGIMEN FOR DENTAL, ORAL, OR UPPER RESPIRATORY TRACT PROCEDURES IN PATIENTS WHO ARE AT RISK

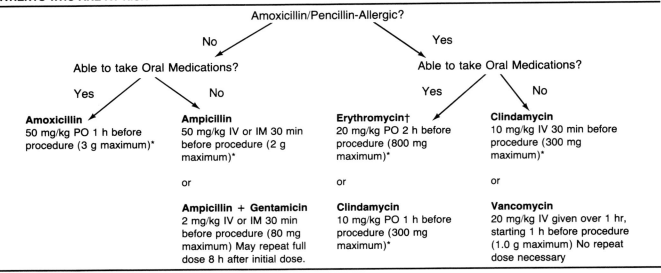

Amoxicillin
50 mg/kg PO 1 h before procedure (3 g maximum)*

or

Ampicillin
50 mg/kg IV or IM 30 min before procedure (2 g maximum)*

Ampicillin + Gentamicin
2 mg/kg IV or IM 30 min before procedure (80 mg maximum) May repeat full dose 8 h after initial dose.

Erythromycin†
20 mg/kg PO 2 h before procedure (800 mg maximum)*

or

Clindamycin
10 mg/kg PO 1 h before procedure (300 mg maximum)*

Clindamycin
10 mg/kg IV 30 min before procedure (300 mg maximum)*

or

Vancomycin
20 mg/kg IV given over 1 hr, starting 1 h before procedure (1.0 g maximum) No repeat dose necessary

* Follow-up dose: half the dose 6 h after the initial dose, may substitute oral preparation
† Erythromycin ethylsuccinate, maximum dose for erythromycin stearate is 1 g

APPENDIX 26–1C. PROPHYLACTIC REGIMENS FOR GENITOURINARY AND GASTROINTESTINAL PROCEDURES

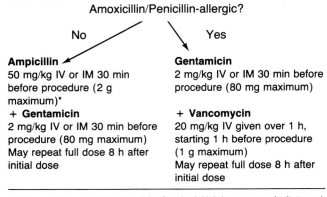

Ampicillin
50 mg/kg IV or IM 30 min before procedure (2 g maximum)*
+ Gentamicin
2 mg/kg IV or IM 30 min before procedure (80 mg maximum) May repeat full dose 8 h after initial dose

Gentamicin
2 mg/kg IV or IM 30 min before procedure (80 mg maximum)

+ Vancomycin
20 mg/kg IV given over 1 h, starting 1 h before procedure (1 g maximum) May repeat full dose 8 h after initial dose

* Follow-up dose: half the dose 6 h after the initial dose, may substitute oral preparation

APPENDIX 26–2. SYNDROMES ASSOCIATED WITH CARDIAC DEFECTS

Syndrome or Malformation	Cardiac Defect*	Frequency of Occurrence	Classification of Malformation	Other Considerations
Aase	VSD	F	Skeletal	Anemia
Alagille (arteriohepatic dysplasia)	PS, ASD, VSD, PDA, CoA	F	Miscellaneous	Biliary hypoplasia, vertebral anomalies, peculiar facies
Alcohol, fetal effects	VSD, PDA, ASD, TOF, CoA	F	Environmental	Micrognathia, cervical vertebral malformations
Antley-Bixler	ASD	O	Craniosynostosis	Midfacial hypoplasia, choanal atresia
Apert (acrocephalosyndactyly)	VSD, PA, PS	O	Craniosynostosis	Midfacial hypoplasia
Baller-Gerold	VSD	O	Craniosynostosis	
Bardet-Biedl	Miscellaneous defects	O	Miscellaneous	Obesity
Beals (contractural arachnodactyly)	Mitral valve prolapse, ASD, VSD, aortic hypoplasia	F	Connective tissue disorder	Joint contractures, micrognathia
Beckwith-Wiedemann	Miscellaneous defects	O	Miscellaneous	Macroglossia, neonatal hypoglycemia
Blepharophimosis	Miscellaneous defects	O	Facial	Hypotonia
Camptomelic dysplasia	Miscellaneous defects	O	Skeletal	Central nervous system disorganization, micrognathia, cervical vertebral anomalies, small thorax, tracheobronchiomalacia
Carpenter	VSD, PDA	O	Craniofacial	Obesity, craniosynostosis
Cat's-eye (coloboma of iris–anal atresia)	Anomalous pulmonary venous return	F	Chromosomal	Micrognathia, renal agenesis
CHARGE association	TOF, PDA, double outlet right ventricle, AV canal, VSD, ASD	F	Miscellaneous	Choanal atresia, micrognathia
Child	VSD, ASD, single coronary ostium	F	Skeletal	Unilateral hypomelia
Coffin-Lowry	Mitral insufficiency	O	Facial	Hypotonia, vertebral dysplasia
Coffin-Siris	PDA, VSD, ASD, TOF	O	Miscellaneous	Vertebral anomalies, central nervous system anomalies
Cohen	Mitral valve prolapse	O	Neuromuscular	Hypotonia, maxillary hypoplasia, mild micrognathia, seizures
Conradi-Hunermann	VSD, PDA	O	Skeletal	Tracheal calcifications and stenosis
Cornelia de Lange (Brachmann–de Lange syndrome)	VSD, TOF	O	Small stature	Micrognathia, seizures, choanal atresia, hiatal hernia
Cri-du-chat (5p-)	VSD, PDA, ASD, PS	O	Chromosomal	Hypotonia
DiGeorge sequence	Aortic arch anomalies, TOF, truncus arteriosus, VSD, PDA	F	Miscellaneous	Thymic and parathyroid hypoplasia or aplasia, short trachea
Dilantin, fetal effects	PS, AS, CoA, PDA, septal defects	O	Environmental	Short neck
Ehlers-Danlos	Mitral and tricuspid valve prolapse, aortic root dilatation, ASD	F	Connective tissue disorder	Hyperextensible joints, hyperelastic and friable skin, poor wound healing, easy bruising
Ellis–van Creveld (chondroectodermal dysplasia)	ASD	F	Skeletal	Small thorax, renal agenesis
Fabry (Anderson-Fabry, angiokeratoma corporis diffusum)	Glycolipid infiltration of the heart and valves	O	Miscellaneous	Attacks of burning pain in hands, seizures, respiratory obstruction
Fanconi pancytopenia	PDA, VSD	O	Skeletal	Pancytopenia, renal anomalies

APPENDIX 26–2. SYNDROMES ASSOCIATED WITH CARDIAC DEFECTS (continued)

Syndrome or Malformation	Cardiac Defect*	Frequency of Occurrence	Classification of Malformation	Other Considerations
FG syndrome	Miscellaneous defects	O	Facial	Hypotonia, seizures, craniosynostosis
Fraser (cryptophthalmos)	Miscellaneous defects	O	Facial	Laryngeal stenosis, renal agenesis, absence of nostril, thymic aplasia, partial absence of sternum
Geleophysic dysplasia	Progressive thickening of valves	F	Skeletal	
Goldenhar (facioauriculo-vertebral spectrum, 1st and 2nd branchial arch syndrome, hemifacial microsomia)	VSD, PDA, TOF, CoA	O	Miscellaneous	Micrognathia, maxillary hypoplasia, cervical spine anomalies
Goltz	Miscellaneous defects	O	Hamartoses	
Hay-Wells (ectodermal dysplasia, ankyloblepharon–ectodermal dysplasia–clefting syndrome)	VSD, PDA	O	Facial	Maxillary hypoplasia
Holt-Oram (cardiac-limb syndrome)	ASD, VSD, dysrhythmias, PDA, PS, miscellaneous defects	F	Skeletal	Vertebral anomalies
Homocystinuria	Aortic and pulmonary artery dilation, intravascular thrombosis	F	Connective tissue disorder	
Hurler (mucopolysaccharidosis I H)	Multivalvular and coronary disease, cardiomyopathy	F	Storage disorder	Large tongue, short neck
Hurler-Scheie compound syndrome (mucopolysaccharidosis I H/S)	Valvular anomalies	O	Storage disorder	Micrognathia
Ivemark's asplenia/polysplenia (laterality sequences)	Situs inversus, anomalous pulmonary venous return, common atrium, single ventricle, TGA, AV canal, PS, PA	F	Miscellaneous	Multiple spleens, asplenia, renal anomalies
Kartagener	Situs inversus, ASD, VSD	F	Miscellaneous	Sinusitis, bronchiectasis, thick mucus
Klippel-Feil	VSD	O	Miscellaneous	Fused cervical vertebrae, central nervous system anomalies
Larsen	Miscellaneous defects	O	Facial	Flat facies, mobile or infolding arytenoid cartilage
Marfan	Aortic dilation and possible dissection, aortic and mitral incompetence	F	Connective tissue disorder	Joint laxity, pneumothorax, respiratory infections
Maroteaux-Lamy (muco-polysaccharidosis VI)	Aortic incompetence	O	Storage disorder	Vertebral anomalies, macroglossia
Meckel-Gruber (dysen-cephalia splanchno-cystica)	septal defects, PDA, CoA, PS	O	Central nervous system	Cerebral hypoplasia, micrognathia, short neck, craniosynostosis, pulmonary hypoplasia, renal anomalies, adrenal hypoplasia
Miller (postaxial acrofacial dysostosis)	Miscellaneous defects	O	Facial	Micrognathia, malar hypoplasia
Miller-Dieker (lissencephaly syndrome)	Miscellaneous defects	F	Central nervous system	Incomplete brain development, infections

APPENDIX 26–2. SYNDROMES ASSOCIATED WITH CARDIAC DEFECTS (continued)

Syndrome or Malformation	Cardiac Defect*	Frequency of Occurrence	Classification of Malformation	Other Considerations
Morquio (mucopolysaccharidosis IV, types A and B)	Aortic incompetence	F	Storage disorder	Frequent respiratory infections, vertebral anomalies, including cervical subluxation
Mulibrey nanism (perheentupa syndrome)	Pericardial constriction	F	Small stature	Hypotonia
Multiple lentigenes (LEOPARD)	PS, hypertrophic obstructive cardiomyopathy, abnormal ECG	F	Hamartoses	
Nager (acrofacial dysostosis syndrome)	TOF	O	Facial	Micrognathia
Neurofibromatosis	PS, renal artery stenosis	O	Hamartoses	Dysplastic tumors along nerves, seizures, vertebral anomalies
Noonan (Turner-like syndrome)	Pulmonic valve dysplasia, septal defects, PDA	F	Small stature	Webbed neck, pectus excavatum
Opitz (Opitz-Frias, G syndrome)	Miscellaneous defects	O	Facial	Malformation of the larynx, short trachea, pulmonary hypoplasia
Osteogenesis imperfecta, type I	Aortic and mitral incompetence	O	Connective tissue disorder	Fragile bones, bleeding tendency
Pallister-Hall	AV canal	F	Central nervous system	Hypopituitarism, micrognathia, hypoplasia or absence of the epiglottis, dysplastic tracheal cartilage, abnormal or absent lung
Phenylketonuria, fetal effects	TOF, VSD, ASD, CoA	F	Environmental	Mandibular hypoplasia, seizures, cervical and sacral spine anomalies
Hunter (Pompe's disease, mucopolysaccharidosis II)	Congestive heart failure, coronary occlusion	O	Storage disorder	Macroglossia
Progeria (Hutchinson-Gilford)	Accelerated arteriosclerosis	F	Miscellaneous	Premature aging, skeletal hypoplasia, micrognathia
Pseudo-Hurler (polydystrophy syndrome)	Aortic valve regurgitation	F	Storage disorder	Short neck, coarse facies
Radial aplasia–thrombocytopenia (TAR syndrome)	ASD, TOF	F	Skeletal	Severe thrombocytopenia, anemia, granulocytosis, micrognathia
Retinoic acid, fetal exposure	Truncus arteriosus, TGA, TOF, double outlet right ventricle, VSD, interrupted aortic arch	F	Environmental	Micrognathia, hydrocephalus, cerebellar hypoplasia
Roberts–SC phocomelia, (pseudothalidomide)	ASD	O	Facial	Micrognathia, hypomelia, thrombocytopenia
Robinow	ASD	O	Facial	Micrognathia, macroglossia, seizures
Rubella, fetal effects	PDA, PS, ASD	F	Environmental	Thrombocytopenia or anemia, obstructive jaundice
Rubinstein-Taybi	PDA, VSD	F	Short stature	Hypoplastic maxilla
Ruvalcaba	Miscellaneous defects	O	Facial	Small mouth, vertebral anomalies, seizures
Scheie (mucopolysaccharidosis I S)	Aortic incompetence	F	Storage disorder	Short neck, macroglossia, sleep apnea
Schinzel-Giedion	ASD	O	Central nervous system	Seizures, choanal stenosis, macroglossia
Sebaceous nevus sequence	VSD, CoA	O	Hamartoses	Seizures
Short rib–polydactyly	TGA, double-outlet left and right ventricles, AV canal, tricuspid atresia	F	Skeletal	Small thorax, pulmonary hypoplasia

APPENDIX 26–2. SYNDROMES ASSOCIATED WITH CARDIAC DEFECTS (continued)

Syndrome or Malformation	Cardiac Defect*	Frequency of Occurrence	Classification of Malformation	Other Considerations
Shprintzen (velocardiofacial)	VSD, TOF, right aortic arch	F	Facial	Vertical maxillary excess, retruded mandible, hypotonia
Sly (mucopolysaccharidosis VII)	Miscellaneous valvular diseases	O	Storage disorder	Vertebral anomalies
Smith-Lemli-Opitz	VSD, PDA	O	Facial	Seizures, micrognathia
Stickler (arthro-ophthalmopathy)	Mitral valve prolapse	O	Facial	Micrognathia, hypotonia
Sturge-Weber	CoA	O	Hamartoses	Meningeal hemangiomata, seizures
Systemic lupus erythematosus, fetal effects	Complete heart block	O	Miscellaneous	
Townes	Miscellaneous defects	O	Facial	Hemifacial microsomia, renal hypoplasia
Treacher Collins (mandibulofacial dysostosis, Franceschetti-Klein	Miscellaneous defects	O	Facial	Micrognathia, pharyngeal hypoplasia, microstomia, choanal atresia
Trimethadione, fetal effects	Septal defects, TGA, TOF, hypoplastic left heart syndrome	F	Environmental	Micrognathia, midface hypoplasia
Tuberous sclerosis	Rhabdomyoma, cardiomyopathy	O	Hamartoses	Sublingual fibromatoma, seizures, cystic pulmonary changes
Valproate, fetal effects	CoA, AS, interrupted aortic arch, ASD, PA with intact septum, VSD	F	Environmental	Small mouth, meningomyelocele
VATER association	VSD	F	Miscellaneous	Vertebral anomalies, tracheoesophageal fistula, renal abnormalities
Waardenburg I and II	VSD	O	Facial	Hypoplastic alae nasi, vertebral anomalies
Warfarin, fetal effects	Miscellaneous defects	O	Environmental	Nasal hypoplasia, central nervous system anomalies
Weill-Marchesani	Miscellaneous defects	O	Skeletal	
Williams	Supravalvar aortic stenosis, PS, septal defects	F	Facial	Elfin facies, hoarse voice
XO (Turner)	CoA, bicuspid aortic valve, AS, VSD, ASD	F	Chromosomal	Webbed neck, micrognathia
XXXXX	PDA	F	Chromosomal	
XXXY and XXXXY	PDA	O	Chromosomal	Short neck
Triploidy diploid/triploid mixoploidy syndromes	Septal defects	F	Chromosomal	Dysplastic calvaria, micrognathia, hydrocephalus, adrenal hypoplasia, renal anomalies
Trisomy 4p	miscellaneous defects	O	Chromosomal	Hypertonia or hypotonia, seizures, macroglossia, micrognathia, vertebral anomalies
Trisomy 9 mosaic	Miscellaneous defects	F	Chromosomal	Micrognathia
Trisomy 9p	Miscellaneous defects	O	Chromosomal	Micrognathia
Trisomy 13	VSD, PDA, double-outlet right ventricle, ASD, anomalous venous return, PS, atretic mitral or aortic valves, CoA	F	Chromosomal	Holoprosencephaly, seizures, apnea, thrombocytopenia
Trisomy 18	VSD, PDA, polyvalvular dysplasia, ASD, CoA, numerous others	F	Chromosomal	Short sternum, small oral opening, micrognathia, hypotonia

APPENDIX 26–2. SYNDROMES ASSOCIATED WITH CARDIAC DEFECTS (continued)

Syndrome or Malformation	Cardiac Defect*	Frequency of Occurrence	Classification of Malformation	Other Considerations
Trisomy 20p	VSD, TOF	O	Chromosomal	Hypotonia, ataxia, vertebral anomalies
Trisomy 21 (Down)	AV canal, ASD, VSD, TOF, PDA	F	Chromosomal	Large tongue, hyperextensible joints, atlantoaxial dislocation
Trisomy partial 10q	Miscellaneous cardiac	F	Chromosomal	Microcephaly, renal malformations
4p-(Wolf syndrome)	VSD, PDA, ASD, PS	F	Chromosomal	Hypotonia, seizures, cranial asymmetry, micrognathia
9p-	VSD, PDA, PS	F	Chromosomal	Craniosynostosis, micrognathia, short neck
13q-	Miscellaneous defects	F	Chromosomal	Microcephaly, micrognathia
18q-	Miscellaneous defects	F	Chromosomal	Midface hypoplasia, narrow palate

* Listing is not meant to be all inclusive.

Abbreviations: VSD, ventricular septal defect; ASD, atrial septal defect; AV canal, atrioventricular canal; AS, aortic stenosis; PS, pulmonic stenosis; CoA, coarctation of the aorta, TOF, tetralogy of Fallot; PA, pulmonary atresia; TGA, transposition of the great arteries; PDA, patent ductus arteriosus.

(*Modified from Jones KL (ed): Smith's Recognizable Patterns of Human Malformation, 4th ed. Philadelphia, WB Saunders, 1988.*)

APPENDIX 26–3. CONSIDERATIONS FOR PATIENTS WHO HAVE UNDERGONE CARDIAC SURGERY

Surgical Procedure	Hypoxemia	Pulmonary Blood Flow	Ventricular Load	Dysrhythmias	Comments
Blalock-Taussig (classic, modified)	+	↑ or ↓ *	V		Subclavian artery distortion may effect blood pressure measurements; right and left PA flow may be unequal
Central shunts (Potts, Waterston, central)	+	↑ or ↓ *	V		Excessive PA flow more likely than with BT shunt
Atrial septectomy	+	↑ or ↓	V		Hypoxemia may worsen depending of direction and magnitude of flow through the defect
Glenn shunt	+	↓	V		Passive pulmonary blood flow; moderate-to-severe V/Q mismatch
Caval-pulmonary	+	↓	V		Passive pulmonary blood flow
Fontan (modified, Fontan-Kreutzer)				SB, SVT, CHB	Passive pulmonary blood flow; pericardial, pleural, abdominal effusions; cardiac output often limited by pulmonary blood flow
Atrial switch (Mustard, Sennings)			P or V	SVT	Ability of the morphologic right ventricle to function as a systemic ventricle is questionable; baffle obstruction can cause pulmonary or systemic venous congestion
Arterial switch (Jatene, anatomic)			±P		Perioperative myocardial infarction possible
Damus-Kaye-Stansel with systemic-pulmonary shunt	+	↑ or ↓ *	V		
Rastelli			P or V (right ventricular)	CHB, VENT	Sequelae of right ventriculotomy; conduit may become inadequate or obstructed; conduit may impinge on large airways
Norwood stage 1	+	↑ or ↓	V		Critical "balance" between systemic and pulmonary circulations
Tetralogy repair			P or V (right ventricular)	CHB, VENT	Sequelae of right ventriculotomy; residual shunting through ASD or PFO
Coarctation repair (subclavian flap angioplasty, tube graft, end-to-end anastomosis			P		Loss of subclavian artery may effect blood pressure measurement; restenosis can occur
AV canal repair			P or V	SVT	Pulmonary vasculature may be excessively reactive for an undetermined period of time
Atrial septal defect (suture closure, patch closure)				SVT	
Ventricular septal defect				VENT	Right ventriculotomy used for some surgical approaches

* Dependent of the amount of flow through the shunt.
P, pressure load; V, volume load; PA, pulmonary artery; BT, Blalock-Taussig; SB, sinus bradycardia; SVT, supraventricular tachycardia; CHB, complete heart block; VENT, ventricular dysrhythmias.

Index

Page numbers followed by t and f denote tables and figures, respectively.

Page numbers followed by t and f denote tables and figures, respectively.

Page numbers followed by t and f denote tables and figures, respectively.

Page numbers followed by t and f denote tables and figures, respectively.

Page numbers followed by t and f denote tables and figures, respectively.

Page numbers followed by t and f denote tables and figures, respectively.

Page numbers followed by t and f denote tables and figures, respectively.

Page numbers followed by t and f denote tables and figures, respectively.

Page numbers followed by t and f denote tables and figures, respectively.

Page numbers followed by t and f denote tables and figures, respectively.

Page numbers followed by t and f denote tables and figures, respectively.

Page numbers followed by t and f denote tables and figures, respectively.

Page numbers followed by t and f denote tables and figures, respectively.

Page numbers followed by t and f denote tables and figures, respectively.

Page numbers followed by t and f denote tables and figures, respectively.

Page numbers followed by t and f denote tables and figures, respectively.